Absolute Nephrology Review

Alluru S. Reddi

Absolute Nephrology Review

An Essential Q & A Study Guide

Second Edition

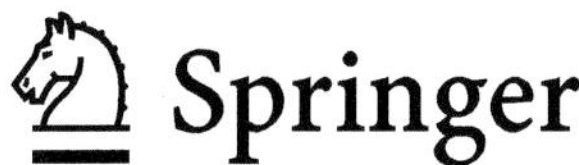

Alluru S. Reddi
Division of Nephrology and Hypertension
Rutgers New Jersey Medical School
Newark, NJ, USA

ISBN 978-3-030-85957-2 ISBN 978-3-030-85958-9 (eBook)
https://doi.org/10.1007/978-3-030-85958-9

This Springer imprint is published by the registered company Springer Nature Switzerland AG
The registered company address is: Gewerbestrasse 11, 6330 Cham, Switzerland

Rajendra Kapila MD, a friend and colleague, knew everything about the bacterium, parasite, virus, fungus, and every organ system in the body. As a great clinician and teacher, we will all miss him. It is an honor for me to dedicate this book to him.

New Nomenclature for Kidney Function and Disease[1]

In June 2019, Kidney Disease: Improving Global Outcomes (KDIGO) convened a Consensus Conference with the goal of revising and refining the nomenclature to describe kidney function and disease. For example, common terms such as renal or nephro- and end-stage renal (kidney) disease have been replaced by kidney and kidney failure, respectively. The following table summarizes some important changes proposed by KDIGO. The reader is referred to the Suggested Reading for explanation of the preferred terms.

Preferred term	Term (s) to avoid
Kidney function and disease	Renal and the prefix "nephro-" (except in the setting of specific functions, diseases, or syndromes
Kidney disease (acute kidney disease and chronic kidney disease)	Renal disease, nephropathy (except in the setting of specific diseases such as membranous nephropathy)
Kidney function	Renal function with exception of describing specific functions such as renal acidification, renal concentrating mechanism
Residual kidney function (RKF)	Residual renal function (RRF)
Kidney structure	Renal structure with the exception of describing specific structures within the kidney, such as artery, vein, capsule, parenchyma, cortex, medulla, glomeruli, tubules, interstitium, cysts, tumors
Kidney failure	Renal failure (RF); end-stage renal disease (ESRD); end-stage kidney disease (ESKD), renal disease; nephropathy; renal/kidney impairment, insufficiency, dysfunction; azotemia
Duration of kidney failure AKI stage 3 (disease duration $\leq$3 months) Kidney failure (disease duration >3 months)	 Acute renal failure; renal disease; nephropathy; renal/kidney impairment, insufficiency, dysfunction; azotemia; uremia Chronic renal failure; chronic renal disease; chronic nephropathy; chronic renal/kidney impairment, insufficiency, dysfunction; azotemia; uremia; irreversible kidney failure
Kidney replacement therapy (KRT)	Renal replacement therapy (RRT)
Dialysis AKI stage 3D CKD G5	 AKI-D, dialysis-dependent AKI ESKD, ESKF, ESRD, ESRF, dialysis-dependent CKD
Kidney transplantation	ESKD, ESKF, ESRD, ESRF
Acute kidney disease (AKD)	Acute renal failure (ARF); acute renal insufficiency (ARI)
AKI	ARF, ARI
CKD	Chronic renal failure (CRF); ESRD; renal/ kidney impairment, insufficiency, dysfunction
CKD classification [KDIGO CGA classification by cause, GFR category (G1–G5), and albuminuria category (A1–A3)]	Mild, moderate, severe, early, advanced CKD; CKD stage 1–5 (complete description preferred rather than G category alone). Patient with CKD could not be classified as "CKD G2, A1"
GFR (units must be specified as mL/min/1.73 m^2 or mL/min)	

Suggested Reading

Levey AS, Eckardt K-U, Dorman NM, et al. Nomenclature for kidney function and disease: report of a Kidney Disease: Improving Global Outcomes (KDIGO) Consensus Conference. Kidney Int 97:1117–1129, 2020.

[1] Note that old terminology was used in this book because the chapters were written prior to publication of the paper in *Kidney International.*

Preface

The purpose of the second edition of *Absolute Nephrology Review* is to have the nephrology fellows and the practicing nephrologists to learn kidney disease as a whole in the form of questions and answers. It is the intention of the author to familiarize the reader with board-like questions to provide nephrological information in thought-provoking fashion. The questions are based on a review of recent information obtained from several journals and standard textbooks and also from author's clinical experience. The questions in each chapter are geared to cover the basics of physiology, pathogenesis, and treatment strategies of a clinical problem.

Writing a pertinent question is more difficult than writing a book chapter. Each question took a lengthy time to write and even more time to provide a choice of education-enhancing answers. I strongly believe that this review book would help each graduating nephrology fellow and practicing nephrologist to learn the subject and pass their board and other examinations. The author emphasizes that this review book is not a substitute for the existing textbooks and all other available board-type question books.

This book would not have been completed without the help of many students, house staff, and colleagues, who encouraged and supported me learn kidney disease and manage patients appropriately. They have been the powerful source of my knowledge, and I am grateful to all of them. I am extremely thankful and grateful to my family, particularly to my two grandchildren, for their immense support and patience. Finally, I extend my thanks to the staff at Springer, particularly Hannah Campeanu, Associate Editor, for her constant support, help, and advice. Constructive criticism for improvement of the book is gratefully acknowledged.

Newark, NJ, USA Alluru S. Reddi

Contents

Chapter 1
Fluids, Electrolytes, and Acid–Base Disorders

Sodium and Water Abnormalities

1. A 36-year-old woman is admitted for dizziness, weakness, poor appetite, fatigue, and salt-craving for 4 weeks. She has history of asthma, and not on any medications. She has a family history of type 1 diabetes and hypothyroidism. On admission, her blood pressure (BP) is 100/60 mm Hg with a pulse rate of 100 beats/min (sitting), and 80/48 mm Hg with a pulse rate of 120 beats/min (standing). Her temperature is 99.6 °F. Laboratory values are as follows:

Na^+ = 124 mEq/L	Creatinine = 1.8 mg/dL
K^+ = 6.1 mEq/L	Glucose = 50 mg/dL
Cl^- = 114 mEq/L	Hemoglobin = 13 g/dL
HCO_3^- = 20 mEq/L	Hematocrit = 40%
BUN = 42 mg/dL	Urinary Na^+ = 60 mEq/L

Based on the above history and laboratory values, which one of the following fluids is APPROPRIATE in addition to pertinent hormone administration?

A. 5% dextrose in water (D5W)
B. 5% albumin
C. Ringer's lactate (lactated Ringer solution)
D. Normal (0.9%) saline
E. 0.45% (half-normal) saline

The answer is D

Based on the orthostatic BP and pulse changes, hyponatremia, hyperkalemia, acute kidney injury, hypoglycemia, and high urine Na^+ excretion, the most likely diagnosis is Addison's disease, which is due to glucocorticoid and mineralocorticoid deficiency. Her signs and symptoms are related to volume depletion and electrolyte abnormalities. Hypotension is related to loss of both Na^+ and water caused by deficiency of the above hormones.

In addition to administration of hydrocortisone and fludrocortisones, the patient needs normal saline administration to improve total body volume (D is correct). Both volume repletion and hormone treatment improve BP and electrolytes.

D5W may improve hyperkalemia and glucose; however, it is not adequate to improve volume as much as normal saline (A is incorrect). Five percent albumin may expand volume but is not indicated in this patient (B is incorrect). Ringer's lactate may exacerbate hyperkalemia and hypercalcemia (about 10% of patients with Addison's disease have hypercalcemia) with little effect on hyponatremia. Thus, C is incorrect. Half-normal saline is not adequate to replete the entire fluid in this patient (E is incorrect).

Suggested Reading

Griffing GT. Addison disease treatment and management. MedScape. 2018.
Sarkar SB, Sarkar S, Ghosh S, et al. Addison's disease. Contemp Clin Dent. 2012;3:484–6.
Ten S, New M, Maclaren N. Addison's disease 2001. J Clin Endocrinol Metab. 2001;86:2909–22.

A. S. Reddi, *Absolute Nephrology Review*, https://doi.org/10.1007/978-3-030-85958-9_1

2. It is always important to know how much infused crystalloid and colloid will remain in the intravascular compartment to improve volume status and hemodynamic status. **Which one of the following fluids contributes MOST to the intravascular compartment?**

   A. 5% dextrose in water (D5W)
   B. Half-normal saline
   C. Normal saline
   D. Ringer's lactate
   E. C and D

   The answer is E

   In order to answer the question, it is important to remember the percentage of total body water and its distribution in various fluid compartments. In a 70-kg man with lean body mass, the total body water accounts for 60% of body weight (42 L), and two-thirds of this water (i.e., 28 L) is in the intracellular fluid (ICF) and one-third (i.e., 14 L) is in the extracellular fluid (ECF) compartment (Fig. 1.1). Of these 14 L of ECF water, 3.5 L (25%) is present in the intravascular and 11.5 L (75%) in the interstitial compartments. Accordingly, if 1 L of D5W is infused, approximately 667 mL will move into the ICF and 333 mL will remain in the ECF compartment. Of these 336 mL, only 83 mL (25%) will remain in the intravascular compartment (Fig. 1.2).

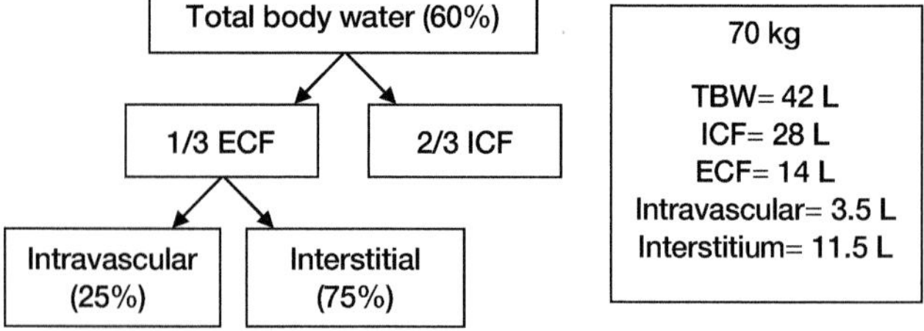

Fig. 1.1 Distribution of total body water (TBW) in a 70-kg man. ECF extracellular fluid volume, ICF intracellular fluid volume

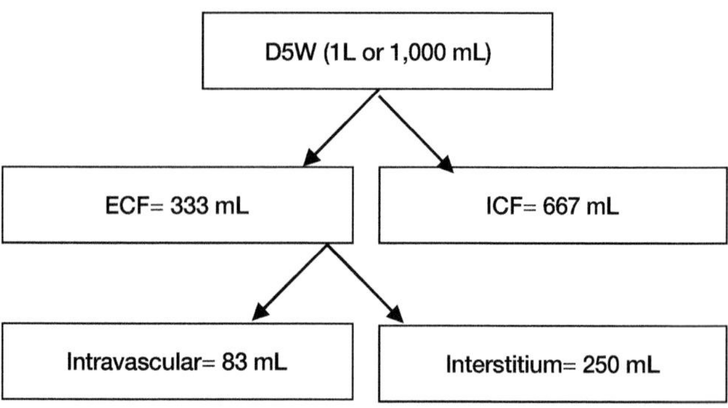

Fig. 1.2 Distribution of 5% dextrose in water (D5W) in the body. ECF extracellular fluid volume, ICF intracellular fluid volume

The retention of hypotonic solutions such as 0.45% NaCl (half-normal) is different. 0.45% NaCl is considered to be a 50:50 mixture of normal saline and free water. If 1 L of 0.45% NaCl is infused, the free water (500 mL) is distributed between ICF (333 mL) and ECF (167 mL) compartments. Of 167 mL, only 42 mL (25%) will remain in the intravascular compartment. Considering the other 500 mL, which behaves like 0.9% saline, 375 mL (75%) will move into the interstitial space and 125 mL stays in the intravascular compartment (Fig. 1.3). Thus, the total volume remaining intravascularly after 1 L of infusion would be only 167 mL (42 + 125 = 167 mL).

On the other hand, more fluid is retained in the intravascular space with isotonic fluids. If 1 L of normal saline is infused, all of the fluid will remain in the intravascular compartment, and then approximately 750 mL will move into the interstitial compartment, leaving 250 mL in the intravascular compartment (Fig. 1.4). The movement of saline into the interstitial compartment occurs approximately 30 min after infusion. During this period of intravascular stay of saline, volume status and BP improve. Urine output may or may not improve until additional volume is infused. Similar volume changes occur with Ringer's lactate. Thus, E is correct.

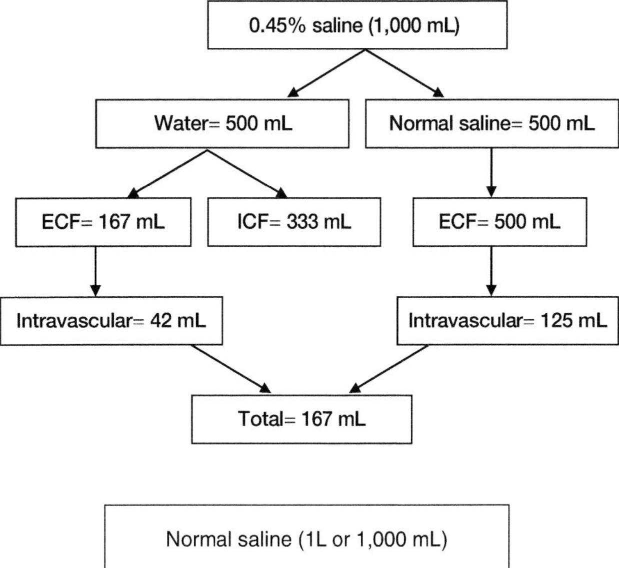

Fig. 1.3 Distribution of half-normal saline in the body. ECF extracellular fluid volume, ICF intracellular fluid volume

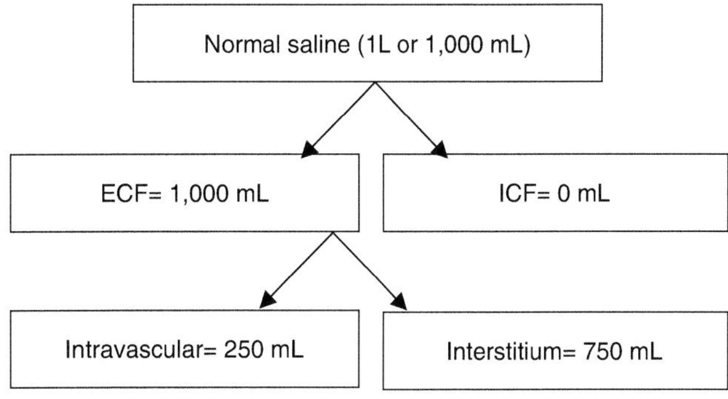

Fig. 1.4 Distribution of normal saline in the body. ECF extracellular fluid volume, ICF intracellular fluid volume

Infusion of colloids results in even much more retention of fluids in the intravascular compartment. If 1 L of 5% albumin is infused, 900 mL will stay in the intravascular compartment and 100 mL in the interstitial compartment. Albumin stays in the intravascular compartment for >16 h.

When 1 L of 25% albumin is infused, the intravascular volume will be 4 L because approximately 3 L of fluid will move from the interstitium into the intravascular compartment.

Approximate distribution of various crystalloids and colloids (albumin) in body compartments in the absence of shock or sepsis is summarized in Table 1.1.

Table 1.1 Approximate distribution of 1 L of IV fluids in body compartments

Fluid	Intracellular (mL)	Interstitial (mL)	Intravascular (mL)
D5W	664	252	83
Normal saline (0.9%)	0	752	248
Ringer's lactate	0	752	248
Albumin (5%)	0	100	900
Albumin (25%)[a]	0	−3000	4000

[a]Fluid movement from interstitial to intravascular (plasma) compartment

Suggested Reading

Nuevo FR, Vennari M, Agrò FE. How to maintain and restore fluid balance: crystalloids. In: Agrò FE, editor. Body fluid management. From physiology to therapy. Milan: Springer; 2013. p. 37–46.

Reddi AS. Intravenous fluids: composition and indications. In: Reddi AS, editor. Fluid, electrolyte and acid-base disorders. Clinical evaluation and management. 2nd ed. New York: Springer; 2018. p. 35–49.

3. A 24-year-old woman is admitted for fever with chills and weakness. She is found to be hypotensive and tachycardic. Blood cultures are positive for *Staphylococcus aureus*, and the diagnosis of septic shock is made. There is no peripheral edema. Based on the sensitivity, the patient is started on vancomycin. Pertinent labs:

Na^+ = 144 mEq/L	Glucose = 80 mg/dL
K^+ = 5.1 mEq/L	Total protein = 5.8 g/dL
Cl^- = 88 mEq/L	Albumin = 2.0 g/dL
HCO_3^- = 20 mEq/L	Hemoglobin = 10 g/dL
BUN = 30 mg/dL	Hematocrit = 30%
Creatinine = 1.7 mg/dL	Urinary Na^+ = 10 mEq/L

Which one of the following fluids is APPROPRIATE for initial resuscitation?

A. Packed red blood cells (pRBCs)
B. Half-normal saline
C. Normal saline
D. Ringer's lactate
E. Albumin

The answer is C

Relative intravascular volume depletion is usual in septic shock. This patient has evidence of intravascular volume depletion. Therefore, the choice of fluid is normal saline (C is correct). Rapid infusion of at least 1 L of saline is needed within an hour and then at least 150 to 200 mL/h until BP, tissue perfusion, and oxygen delivery are acceptable. Note that the patients with septic shock can develop pulmonary edema at pulmonary capillary wedge pressures <18 mm Hg. Raising Hb >10 g/dL is not beneficial; therefore, transfusion of pRBCs is not required (A is incorrect). However, the patient needs transfusion of pRBCs once her Hb drops below 7 g/dL.

Ringer's lactate may be considered in the absence of lactic acidosis and hyperkalemia. Because of low Cl^-, the patient is less prone to develop acute kidney injury, as compared with normal saline. However, Ringer's lactate and half-normal saline may not be appropriate (B and D are incorrect)

Albumin may help restore BP and tissue perfusion, if BP does not improve with substantial amount of normal saline and the patient has trace edema. However, peripheral edema may be present in patients with septic shock without adequate volume replacement because of extravasation of fluid into the interstitium due to increased vascular permeability. Vasopressors, in addition to albumin, may be required to improve BP, tissue perfusion, and gas exchange. However, albumin is not the initial choice of fluid resuscitation. Thus, E is incorrect.

Suggested Reading

Reddi AS. Intravenous fluids: composition and indications. In: Reddi AS, editor. Fluid, electrolyte and acid-base Disorders. Clinical evaluation and management. 2nd ed. New York: Springer; 2018. p. 35–49.
Tommasino C. Volume and electrolyte management. Best Pract Res Clin Anaesthesiol. 2007;21:497–516.

4. A 30-year-old man is admitted to the trauma service with multiple abdominal wounds that required splenectomy and repair of several organs. He has multiple surgical drainages. His blood pressure is 120/80 with a pulse rate of 80. His labs:

Na^+ = 134 mEq/L	Ca^{2+} = 7.4 mg/dL
K^+ = 3.1 mEq/L	Phosphate = 3.5 mg/dL
Cl^- = 88 mEq/L	Albumin = 4.1 d/dL
HCO_3^- = 18 mEq/L	Hemoglobin = 11 g/dL
BUN = 10 mg/dL	Hematocrit = 34%
Creatinine = 1.1 mg/dL	Urinary Na^+ = 12 mEq/L
Glucose = 80 mg/dL	Urinary K^+ = 10 mEq/L

Which one of the following fluids contributes MOST to the intravascular compartment?

A. D5W
B. Half-normal saline

C. Normal saline
D. Ringer's lactate
E. C and D

The answer is D

This patient has multiple electrolyte problems because of nonrenal losses. Therefore, the appropriate fluid for initial therapy is Ringer's lactate, which contains Na^+, Cl^-, K^+, Ca^{2+}, and lactate. This fluid should be continued until all electrolyte abnormalities are corrected (D is correct).

D5W is not an appropriate fluid for this patient, as he has hypokalemia, and dextrose would further lower serum [K^+]. This may cause weakness and arrhythmia. Also, normal saline alone is not appropriate because it may lower [K^+] even further by urinary excretion. Although normal saline with K^+ administration would minimize loss of K^+, it may not improve other electrolyte abnormalities.

Suggested Reading

Reddi AS. Intravenous fluids: composition and indications. In: Reddi AS, editor. Fluid, electrolyte and acid-base disorders. Clinical evaluation and management. 2nd ed. New York: Springer; 2018. p. 35–49.
Tommasino C. Volume and electrolyte management. Best Pract Res Clin Anaesthesiol. 2007;21:497–516.

5. A 54-year-old man with history of hypertension, type 2 diabetes, coronary artery disease with stent placement, and CHF is admitted for dyspnea at rest. He noticed swelling of his legs for 4 weeks despite salt restriction and diuretics (furosemide 40 mg BID and metolazone 2.5 mg QD). His LV ejection fraction (EF) is 40%. Physical examination shows: BP 100/60 mm Hg, pulse 102 beats/min, marked JVD, crackles, increased S_3, positive hepatojugular reflex, and pitting edema up to knees. Labs: Na^+ 134 mEq/L, K^+ 3.8 mEq/L, Cl^- 90 mEq/L, HCO_3^- 28 mEq/L, BUN 46 mg/dL, creatinine 1.8 mg/dL, eGFR <60 mL/min, and glucose 100 mg/dL. $HbA1_c$ 7%. His O_2 saturation is 87%. EKG shows tachycardia. He weighs 98 kg. **Based on the above history and lab values, which one of the following is the MOST appropriate initial management in this patient?**

A. Intravenous (IV) administration of furosemide
B. Nitroglycerine
C. Inotrope
D. All of the above
E. Increase metolazone dose

The answer is D

This patient presents with acute exacerbation of his chronic heart failure. A stepwise treatment is necessary to improve his respiratory status (hypoxemia) and hemodynamic stability. First, he needs a nonrebreather facemask with high-flow percent O_2. Oxygenation should be monitored with pulse oximetry. If respiratory distress continues, consider a noninvasive ventilation to avoid intubation. Second, improve fluid overload by IV administration of 20–40 mg of furosemide as an initial dose. However, patients with chronic heart failure should receive their regular dose of furosemide intravenously. In some patients, continuous IV furosemide (5–10 mg/h) is better than IV bolus because of established safety profile, greater urine output, and less renal impairment. Try not to exceed 160 mg/day to avoid adverse effects. Third, if diuresis is poor on furosemide, a vasodilator such as nitroglycerine at 20 μg/min should be started. Since nitroglycerine causes hypotension, monitoring of BP is extremely important, and the drug should be discontinued once systolic BP is <90 mm Hg. Finally, an inotrope should be considered if weight and edema do not improve. Increasing metolazone is inappropriate (answer E is incorrect).

Suggested Reading

Amer M, Adomaityte J, Qawum R. Continued infusion versus intermittent bolus furosemide in ADHF: an updated meta-analysis of randomized control studies. J Hosp Med. 2012;7:270–5.
Čerlinskaitė K, Javanainen T, Cinotti R, et al. On behalf of the Global Research on Acute Conditions Team (GREAT) Network. Acute heart failure management. Korean Circ J. 2018;48:463–80.
Krum H, Teerlink R. Medical therapy for heart failure. Lancet. 2011;378:713–21.
Ponikowski P, Voors AA, Anker SD, et al. 2016 ESC Guidelines for the diagnosis and treatment of acute and chronic heart failure: the Task Force for the diagnosis and treatment of acute and chronic heart failure of the European Society

of Cardiology (ESC)Developed with the special contribution of the Heart Failure Association (HFA) of the ESC. Eur Heart J. 2016;37:2129–200.

Yancy CW, Jessup M, Bozkurt B, et al. 2013 ACCF/AHA guideline for the management of heart failure: a report of the American College of Cardiology Foundation/American Heart Association Task Force on practice guidelines. Circulation. 2013;128:e240–327.

6. The above patient improved symptomatically over a 48-h period; however, his urine output and edema did not improve substantially. His weight decreased from 98 to 96 kg. Repeat labs show creatinine of 2.4 mg/dL. His BP is maintained at 100/56 mm Hg. **What would be the next appropriate step?**

   A. Increase the dose of furosemide
   B. Start nesiritide
   C. Start dobutamine
   D. Add metolazone to furosemide
   E. Observe patient for another 24 h for urine output

   The answer is C

   Inotropic agonists such as dobutamine should be considered in view of low EF. Dobutamine improves cardiac output by decreasing afterload and increasing inotropy. Renal perfusion also improves at doses of 1–2 µg/kg/min (C is correct). Other treatment options do not improve the patient's clinical status and may be harmful. The available evidence from clinical trials on nesiritide does not support its routine use in hospitalized patients with acute decompensated heart failure.

   Suggested Reading

Ponikowski P, Voors AA, Anker SD, et al. 2016 ESC Guidelines for the diagnosis and treatment of acute and chronic heart failure: the Task Force for the diagnosis and treatment of acute and chronic heart failure of the European Society of Cardiology (ESC)Developed with the special contribution of the Heart Failure Association (HFA) of the ESC. Eur Heart J. 2016;37:2129–200.

Yancy CW, Jessup M, Bozkurt B, et al. 2013 ACCF/AHA guideline for the management of heart failure: a report of the American College of Cardiology Foundation/American Heart Association Task Force on practice guidelines. Circulation. 2013;128:e240–327.

7. Despite dobutamine, the urine output did not improve significantly in 24 h. Milrinone, which is a phosphodiesterase inhibitor, was started with a bolus dose of 25 µg/kg followed by 0.1 µg/kg/min to improve inotropy. BP, urine output, and edema did not improve. BP is 90/70 mm Hg. Serum chemistry shows creatinine level of 3.2 mg/dL. **Which one of the following treatment strategies is APPROPRIATE to improve his condition?**

   A. Start peritoneal dialysis (PD)
   B. Start hemodialysis
   C. Start continuous venovenous hemodiafiltration (CVVHDF)
   D. Start tolvaptan
   E. Start aquapheresis

   The answer is C

   The patient developed type 1 cardiorenal syndrome. Diuretics, nitroglycerine, and dobutamine should be discontinued. Of all the available options, CVVHDF is the suitable option because it can improve both fluid status and creatinine (C is correct). PD is a slow process, and HD may not be helpful in view of low BP. Tolvaptan may not work that well in this patient with low EF and decreased urine output. Aquapheresis is indicated in patients with CHF, but it increases creatinine even further. Thus, starting the patient on CVVHDF is a better option than other interventions.

   Suggested Reading

Premuzic V, Basic-Jukic N, Jelakovic B, et al. Continuous veno-venous hemofiltration improves survival of patients with congestive heart failure and cardiorenal syndrome compared to slow continuous ultrafiltration. Ther Apher Dial. 2017;21:279–86.

Rangaswami J, Bhalla V, Blair JEA, et al. Cardiorenal syndrome: classification, pathophysiology, diagnosis, and treatment Strategies: a scientific statement from the American Heart Association. Circulation. 2019;139:e840–78.

8. A 50-year-old woman with alcohol abuse presents to the Emergency Department for the first time with dyspnea, worsening abdominal distention, and swollen legs for the last 4 weeks. Past medical history includes 1 pint of alcohol a day for 20 years. She is not on any medications. She eats regular diet. BP is 124/68 mm Hg with pulse rate of 80 beats/min. She has crackles, an S_3, tense ascites, and pitting edema up to the knees. Pertinent labs: serum [Na^+] 128 mEq/L; [K^+] 3.6 mEq/L; creatinine 0.8 mg/dL. Chest X-ray shows pulmonary congestion. **Which one of the following choices regarding her management is CORRECT?**

   A. Restrict fluids
   B. Furosemide 40 mg orally
   C. Furosemide 40 mg IV
   D. Furosemide and metolazone
   E. Hemodialysis

   The answer is C

   Since her major problem is Na^+ and water retention, restriction of both will help lose weight. Since the patient has crackles with pulmonary congestion, she would benefit from IV infusion of a loop diuretic such as furosemide (40 mg BID; some prefer to give 80 mg). Thus, C is correct. Once patient is stable, spironolactone at 100 mg should be started initially with up-titration every 3 days by 100 mg up to 400 mg/day. If urine output is not adequate, furosemide up to 160 mg (80 mg BID) should be tried. Bed rest is advisable to improve cardiac output and GFR. Her ascites and CHF should improve. If her ascites does not improve despite the above treatment modality, large volume paracentesis with 5% albumin (8 g/L) replacement is recommended. Daily weight, BP, and intake/output (I/O) should be recorded. Other options are not appropriate.

   Suggested Reading

   EASL Clinical Practice Guidelines for the management of patients with decompensated cirrhosis. European Association for the Study of the Liver. J Hepatol. 2018;69:406–60.

9. With the above management, she lost 14 kg in 7 days. Her serum [Na^+] is 134 mEq/L, and creatinine remains at 0.8 mg/dl. She received education about restricted Na^+ diet and obstinance from alcohol and discharged on spironolactone 400 mg QD and furosemide 80 mg BID. She is given clinic appointment in 2 weeks. In the clinic, she was found to have severe volume depletion and weight loss of another 4 kg. Her ascites did not increase during this 2-week period. **What would you do next?**

   A. Decrease spironolactone and furosemide dose and give clinic appointment in 1 week
   B. Discontinue diuretics and advise to drink water, and see her in the clinic in 1 week
   C. Admit her and hydrate her with D5W
   D. Admit her and hydrate her with 0.45% NaCl
   E. Admit her, discontinue diuretics, and start initially with 5% albumin, and if necessary normal saline

   The answer is E

   She should be hospitalized for volume replacement and stabilization. Diuretics should be stopped, and 5% albumin should be given (100 g/day). A liter of normal saline can be considered with 50 g of 5% albumin the next day. Daily weight with BP and intake/output should be followed. On discharge, furosemide dose should be decreased to 40 mg BID with reducing dose of spironolactone, as indicated. Follow-up in 1–2 weeks is needed. Choices A to D are inappropriate.

   Suggested Reading

   EASL Clinical Practice Guidelines for the management of patients with decompensated cirrhosis. European Association for the Study of the Liver. J Hepatol. 2018;69:406–60.

10. A 46-year-old man is referred to you by a primary care physician for evaluation of proteinuria and leg edema for 3 months. The patient is healthy otherwise. He is not on any medications; however, he has a long history of smoking. The patient noticed edema of lower extremities 2 months ago. He has mild shortness of breath on walking. BP is 132/80 mm Hg with a pulse rate of 74 beats/min. Physical examination is normal other than pitting edema in lower extremities. Serum chemistry and complete blood count is normal (creatinine 0.8 mg/dL). Serum albumin is 3.2 g/dL. Urinalysis reveals 4+ proteinuria and fatty casts. Urine protein to creatinine ratio is 7.2, and 24-h protein is 7.1 g. His

urinary Na^+ is 142 mEq/L. He weighs 94 kg. The patient agrees to renal biopsy, which shows membranous nephropathy. Workup for secondary causes of membranous nephropathy is negative. He has no insurance. **Which one of the following choices regarding the initial management of his edema is CORRECT?**

A. Limit fluid restriction to 750 mL/day
B. Restrict dietary Na^+ to 88 mEq (2 g) per day
C. Start furosemide 40 mg orally
D. Start an ACE-I
E. B, C, and D

The answer is E

Restriction of Na^+ (88 mEq) in the diet is the first step in the management. Furosemide 40 mg QD and lisinopril (an ACE-I) 20 mg QD should be started to improve edema and proteinuria. Limiting water at this time is not appropriate. The patient's weight, edema, BP, proteinuria, creatinine, K^+, and urinary Na^+ for compliance of diet should be followed frequently. Adding amiloride seems to lower proteinuria, if no or partial response to lisinopril is observed.

Suggested Reading

Rondon-Berrios H. New insights into the pathophysiology of oedema in nephrotic syndrome. Nefrologia. 2011;31:148–54.
Schrier RW. Renal sodium excretion, edematous disorders, and diuretic use. In: Schrier RW, editor. Renal and electrolyte disorders. 8th ed. Philadelphia: Wolters Kluwer; 2018. p. 47–85.

11. A 48-year-old woman with small cell lung cancer is brought to the Emergency Department with altered mental status of 4 days duration and questionable seizure disorder. Her husband says that the patient is sipping water frequently because of dry mouth. Her BP is 130/80 mm Hg with pulse of 74 beats/min. Following 2 L of 0.45% saline in 24 h, the following lab data are obtained:

$$\text{Serum Na}^+ = 114\,\text{mEq/L}$$
$$\text{Serum osmolality} = 238\,\text{mOsm/kg H}_2\text{O}$$
$$\text{Urine Na}^+ = 140\,\text{mEq/L}$$
$$\text{Urine K}^+ = 34\,\text{mEq/L}$$
$$\text{Urine osmolality} = 284\,\text{mOsm/Kg H}_2\text{O}$$
$$24\,\text{h urine volume} = 1\,\text{L}$$

Regarding electrolyte-free water clearance (T^e_{CH2O}), which one of the following is CORRECT?

A. –0.75 L
B. –0.52 L
C. +0.52 L
D. +0.75 L
E. −0.82 L

The answer is B

The concept of T^e_{CH2O} is used to calculate the kidneys' ability to conserve or excrete the daily intake of fluids to maintain normal serum [Na]. Whenever water balance is disturbed, either hypo- or hypernatremia develops. In such a situation, calculation of T^e_{CH2O} is helpful in evaluating serum [Na^+] by using the following formula:

$$\mathbf{T^e_{CH2O} = V\left(1-\left(U_{Na}+U_k\right)/P_{Na}\right)}$$

where V is urine volume/24 h and U_{Na}, U_K, and P_{Na} are urine Na^+, K^+, and plasma Na^+ concentrations in mEq/L. Substituting the data from the patient, we obtain

$$\mathbf{T^e_{CH2O} = 1\left(1-\left(140+34\right)/114\right) = -0.52L.}$$

Whenever the value is negative, the kidney is adding water to the body, resulting in hyponatremia. Thus, option B is correct. On the other hand, when the T^e_{CH2O} is positive, the kidney is removing water from the body with the resultant hypernatremia.

Another simple way to explain T^e_{CH2O} is to calculate the ratio of U_{Na} + U_K to P_{Na}. If the ratio is >1, the T^e_{CH2O} is negative, indicating hyponatremia. If the ratio is <1, the T^e_{CH2O} is positive, indicating hypernatremia. In this patient, the ratio is 1.5 (140 + 34/114 = 1.5).

Suggested Reading

Reddi AS. Disorders of water balance: physiology. In: Reddi AS, editor. Fluid, electrolyte and acid-base disorders. Clinical evaluation and management. 2nd ed. New York: Springer; 2018. p. 97–106.

Rose BD. New approach to disturbances in the plasma sodium concentration. 1986;81:1033–40.

Thurman JM, Berl T. Disorders of water metabolism. In: Mount DB, Sayegh MH, Singh AJ, editors. Core concepts in the disorders of fluid, electrolytes and acid-base balance. New York: Springer; 2013. p. 29–48.

12. A 72-year-old woman, who lives alone, was admitted for weakness, inability to walk, and forgetfulness over a 2-week period of time. She cooks her own meals. She is slightly lethargic. Physical examination shows BP 124/74 mm Hg, pulse 78/min, and no orthostatic hypotension. Physical examination is normal. Labs:

Serum	Urine
Na^+ = 120 mEq/L	Volume = 1 L/day
K^+ = 3.6 mEq/L	Na^+ = 20 mEq/L
Cl^- = 88 mEq/L	K^+ = 12 mEq/day
BUN = 6 mg/dL	Urea nitrogen = 246 mg
Creatinine = 0.5 mg/dL	Osmolality = 110 mOsm/kg H_2O
Glucose = 90 mg/dL	
Uric acid = 5.2 mg/dL	
Osmolality = 250 mOsm/kg H_2O	
Total protein = 6.8 g/dL	

Which one of the following is the MOST likely cause for her hyponatremia?

A. Pseudohyponatremia
B. Hypertonic hyponatremia
C. Hyponatremia due to tea and toast diet
D. Hyponatremia due to hydrochlorothiazide (HCTZ)
E. Syndrome of inappropriate antidiuresis (SIADH)

The answer is C

The patient does not have pseudohyponatremia, as serum glucose and total protein are normal. Also, she does not have hypertonic hyponatremia because her serum glucose is normal and she has no osmolal gap, suggestive of the presence of either mannitol or glycerol (answers A and B are incorrect).

Based on physical examination, the patient has euvolemic hyponatremia. Generally, the typical American diet generates a minimum of 600 mOsm per day (assuming 60 g protein intake). All of these mOsm are excreted either in 12 L of urine, if urine osmolality is 50 mOsm/kg H_2O, or 0.5 L of urine, if urine osmolality is 1200 mOsm/kg H_2O (Total mOsm/Urine osmolality or 600/50 = 12 L or 600/1200 = 0.5 L). Thus, a normal individual with intact diluting and concentrating ability can excrete urine from 0.5 L to 12 L without any change in water balance (or plasma osmolality).

The patient has urine osmolality of 110 mOsm/kg H_2O; therefore, she can excrete all her mOsm in 2.2 L of urine (110/50 = 2.2 L). However, her total mOsm were only 110, suggesting poor solute intake. If this patient drinks >2.7 L (2.2 + 0.5 L insensible loss) of fluids daily and her solute excretion is only 110 mOsm, she will be in a positive water balance with subsequent development of hyponatremia.

Lack of solute intake impairs the kidney's ability to dilute the urine to <100 mOsm/kg H_2O, as reduced solute excretion limits water excretion. Her hyponatremia will improve with diet that contains at least 60 g protein, salt (100 mEq Na^+), and 40–60 mEq K^+. Thus, the patient carries the diagnosis of hyponatremia due to tea and toast (C is correct). It should be noted that urine osmolalities <100 mOsm/kg H_2O have been reported in several cases of patients with very low solute intake.

She does not have either HCTZ-induced hyponatremia or SIADH, as other labs such as uric acid (usually low in both conditions) is normal for her age (D and E are incorrect).

Suggested Reading

Berl T. Impact of solute intake on urine flow and water excretion. J Am Soc Nephrol. 2008;19:1076–8.

Jamison RL, Oliver RE. Disorders of urinary concentration and dilution. Am J Med. 1982;72:308–22.

Reddi AS. Disorders of water balance: hyponatremia. In: Reddi AS, editor. Fluid, electrolyte and acid-base disorders. Clinical evaluation and management. 2nd ed. New York: Springer; 2018. p. 107–45.

Thaler SM, Teitelbaum I, Berl T. "Beer potomania" in non-beer drinkers: effect of low dietary solute intake. Am J Kidney Dis. 1998;31:1028–30.

13. A 44-year-old menstruating woman had abdominal surgery lasting for 4 h. Perioperatively, she received normal saline to maintain BP and urine output. Postoperatively, she received 0.45% saline at 120 mL/h, and morphine for pain. Her urine out was 110 mL/h. Twenty-four hours later, she was awake and complained of nausea and headache. The following labs were available at the time of consultation:

$$\text{Serum}\left[\text{Na}^+\right] = 130\ \text{mEq/L}$$
$$\text{Urine}\left[\text{Na}^+\right] = 100\ \text{mEq/L}$$
$$\text{Urine}\left[\text{K}^+\right] = 30\ \text{mEq/L}$$
$$\text{Urine osmolality} = 440\ \text{mOsm/kg}\,\text{H}_2\text{O}$$
$$\text{Urine output} = 110\ \text{mL/h}$$
$$\text{Pre-op serum}\left[\text{Na}^+\right] = 139\ \text{mEq/L}$$
$$\text{Weight} = 64\,\text{kg}$$

Which one of the following regarding the amount of water excess is CORRECT?

A. 4.2 L
B. 1.6 L
C. 3.2 L
D. 2.1 L
E. 3.6 L

The answer is D

The following two formulas can be used to calculate water excess:

1. Water excess = Total body water (TBW) × actual [Na⁺] = Pre-op [Na⁺] × New TBW

$$\text{Weight} = 64\,\text{kg}$$
$$\text{TBW} = 64 \times 0.5 = 32\,\text{L}$$
$$\text{Actual}\left[\text{Na}^+\right] = 130\,\text{mEq/L}$$
$$\text{Pre-op}\left[\text{Na}^+\right] = 139\,\text{mEq/L}$$
$$\text{New TBW} = 32 \times 130 / 139 = 29.92\,\text{L}$$
$$\text{Water excess} = \text{Previous TBW} - \text{New TBW or } 32 - 29.92 = 2.1\,\text{L}$$

2. Alternative calculation:

$$\text{Pre-op total body Na}^+ = \text{TBW} \times \text{serum}\left[\text{Na}^+\right] \text{or } 32 \times 139 = 4448\,\text{mEq}$$
$$\text{Positive water balance} = \text{Total body Na}^+ / \text{Actual}\left[\text{Na}^+\right] \text{or } 4448 / 130 = 34.2\,\text{L}$$
$$\text{Water excess} = 34.2 - 32 = 2.2\,\text{L}$$

Thus, choice D is correct.

Suggested Reading

Reddi AS. Disorders of water balance: hyponatremia. In: Reddi AS, editor. Fluid, electrolyte and acid-base disorders. Clinical evaluation and management. 2nd ed. New York: Springer; 2018. p. 107–45.

Thurman JM, Berl T. Disorders of water metabolism. In: Mount DB, Sayegh MH, Singh AJ, editors. Core concepts in the disorders of fluid, electrolytes and acid-base balance. New York: Springer; 2013. p. 29–48.

14. **In the above patient, which one of the following i.v. fluids is appropriate?**

A. 0.9% NaCl
B. Ringer's lactate
C. 3% NaCl
D. Furosemide and NaCl tablets
E. Restriction of fluid

The answer is C

The patient's symptoms of nausea and headache are related to acute decrease in serum [Na^+] and are probably early manifestations of impending encephalopathy in this menstruating woman. Thus, she has acute symptomatic (<48 h) hyponatremia. Therefore, 3% NaCl is appropriate. The rate of increase is 1–2 mEq/h to the maximum of 6 mEq in 3 h or until symptoms improve. Note that the rate of increase should not exceed by 6–8 mEq in a 24-h period. Thus, answer C is correct. Other answers are not appropriate for treatment of acute symptomatic hyponatremia.

Suggested Reading

Adroguè HJ, Madias NE. The challenge of hyponatremia. J Am Soc Nephrol. 2012;23:1140–8.

Arieff AI. Hyponatremia, convulsions, respiratory arrest, and permanent brain damage after elective surgery in healthy women. N Engl J Med. 1986;314:1529–35.

Sterns RH. Disorders of plasma sodium-Causes, consequences, and correction. N Engl J Med. 2015;372:55–65.

Sterns RH, Silver SM. Complications and management of hyponatremia. Curr Opin Nephrol Hypertens. 2016; 25:114–9.

15. A 27-year-old man with resection of pineal gland tumor developed persistent hyponatremia. He complains of weakness and mild dizziness. Physical exam reveals a BP of 114/70 mm Hg and a pulse rate of 100 beats/min (supine), 100/60 mm Hg and a pulse rate of 120 beats/min (standing), respiratory rate of 16/min, and a temperature of 99.1 ° F. Cardiac exam is normal. Lungs are clear to auscultation. There is no peripheral edema. He receives 2.5 L of normal saline daily.
Lab studies:

$$\begin{aligned}
&Na^+ = 122\,\text{mEq/L}\\
&K^+ = 4.2\,\text{mEq/L}\\
&Cl^- = 96\,\text{mEq/L}\\
&HCO_3^- = 27\,\text{mEq/L}\\
&\text{BUN} = 22\,\text{mg/dL}\\
&\text{Creatinine} = 1.4\,\text{mg/dL}\\
&\text{Glucose} = 80\,\text{mg/dL}\\
&\text{Total protein} = 7.69\,\text{g/dL}\\
&\text{Uric acid} = 3.5\,\text{mg/dL}\\
&\text{Urine osmolality} = 700\,\text{mOsm/kg}/H_2O\\
&\text{Urine Na} = 350\,\text{mEq/L}\\
&\text{Urine K} = 24\,\text{mEq/L}\\
&\text{Urine volume} = 4\,\text{L}/24-\text{h}
\end{aligned}$$

Which one of the following is the MOST likely cause of this patient's hyponatremia?

A. Pseudohyponatremia
B. Late vomiting
C. Adrenal insufficiency
D. Cerebral salt wasting
E. SIADH

The answer is D

Pseudohyponatremia is related to extremely high levels of proteins and triglycerides. Although triglycerides were not measured, his total protein concentration was normal. Therefore, this patient does not have pseudohyponatremia.

Vomiting is a consideration; however, serum [Cl^-] and urinary [K^+] are not consistent with vomiting. In general, patients with late vomiting conserve Na^+ and excrete low Na^+ because of volume depletion. Also, K^+ excretion is enhanced in both early and late vomiting. Therefore, option B is incorrect.

Adrenal insufficiency is also a consideration in view of normal to low BP and increased pulse rate as well as increased urinary Na^+ excretion. However, normal Cl^-, HCO_3^-, and glucose levels exclude the diagnosis of adrenal insufficiency.

Hypotonic hyponatremia, low serum uric acid level, relatively normal BP, high urine Na^+ and osmolality suggest the diagnosis of SIADH. However, high pulse rate and slightly elevated HCO_3^- and BUN levels are unusual in patients with SIADH. Patients with SIADH are euvolemic and lower their serum Na^+ levels with normal saline. The clinical presentation of this patient is suggestive of volume depletion, rather than euvolemia. Therefore, SIADH is unlikely in this patient.

Cerebral salt wasting (CSW) is the most likely cause of this patient's hyponatremia. Hypovolemia and serum as well as urine studies are consistent with CSW. Thus, option D is correct. CSW is also called cerebral/renal salt wasting by some investigators.

Suggested Reading

Maesaka JK, Imbriano LJ, Ali NM, et al. Is it cerebral or renal salt wasting. Kidney Int. 2009;76:934–8.
Oh JY, Shin JI. Syndrome of inappropriate antidiuretic hormone secretion and cerebral/renal salt wasting syndrome: similarities and differences. Front Pediatr. 2015;2 (article 146):1–5.
Reddi AS. Disorders of water balance: hyponatremia. In: Reddi AS, editor. Fluid, electrolyte and acid-base disorders. Clinical evaluation and management. 2nd ed. New York: Springer; 2018. p. 107–45.

16. A 42-year-old man was admitted for subarachnoid hemorrhage. Following clipping of the aneurysm, he develops hyponatremia (Na^+ dropped from 136 to 124 mEq/L). A tentative diagnosis of cerebral salt wasting (CSW) was made. **Which one of the following distinguishes CSW from SIADH?**

A. Ability to excrete Na^+ load
B. Low serum uric acid level
C. Normal serum K^+ level
D. Increased $FE_{uric\ acid}$ and FE_{PO4}
E. Failure to normalize $FE_{uric\ acid}$ once the underlying cause is eliminated

The answer is D

CSW occurs in patients with subarachnoid hemorrhage and other CNS disorders such as tuberculous meningitis. It is characterized by low blood and plasma volumes and negative salt balance. CSW and SIADH are characterized by hypotonic hyponatremia, ability to excrete Na^+, low serum uric acid level because of increased secretion, resulting in high $FE_{uric\ acid}$, and normal serum K^+ levels. However, $FE_{uric\ acid}$ returns to baseline once the cause of SIADH is corrected, but it will remain high in patients with CSW. Also, FE_{PO4} remains high in CSW and is normal in SIADH.

Although Na excretion is common to both, it is much higher in CSW than in SIADH. Also, the urine volume is much higher in CSW than in SIADH.

Suggested Reading

Arieff A, Gabbai R, Goldfine ID. Cerebral salt-wasting syndrome: diagnosis by urine sodium excretion. Am J Med Sci. 2017;354:350–4.

Garimella S. Cerebral salt-wasting syndrome. MedScape. 2018.

Imbriano LJ, Mattana J, Drakakis J, et al. Identifying different causes of hyponatremia with fractional excretion of uric acid. Am J Med Sci. 2016;352:385–90.

Maesaka JK, Imbriano LJ, Ali NM, et al. Is it cerebral or renal salt wasting. Kidney Int. 2009;76:934–8.

Reddi AS. Disorders of water balance: hyponatremia. In: Reddi AS, editor. Fluid, electrolyte and acid-base disorders. Clinical evaluation and management. 2nd ed. New York: Springer; 2018. p. 107–45.

17. **Which one of the following choices regarding treatment of hyponatremia is CORRECT in the above patient?**

A. Fluid restriction
B. Hypertonic saline and furosemide administration
C. Use of vasopressin antagonist
D. Salt intake and fludrocortisone
E. Use of demeclocycline and urea

The answer is D

Patients with CSW are hypovolemic with low BP and orthostatic changes because they lose salt in the urine. Therefore, the treatment to improve serum [Na$^+$] is volume expansion with NaCl and fludrocortisone. Thus, choice D is correct. Other treatment modalities do not improve serum [Na$^+$] in patients with CSW. Choices A, B, C, and E are beneficial in patients with SIADH.

Suggested Reading

Garimella S. Cerebral salt-wasting syndrome. MedScape. 2018.

Maesaka JK, Imbriano LJ, Ali NM, et al. Is it cerebral or renal salt wasting. Kidney Int. 2009;76:934–8.

Reddi AS. Disorders of water balance: hyponatremia. In: Reddi AS, editor. Fluid, electrolyte and acid-base disorders. Clinical evaluation and management. 2nd ed. New York: Springer; 2018. p. 107–45.

18. A 20-year-old woman collapses at a wild party several hours after taking ecstasy. **Which one of the following electrolyte abnormalities is MOST likely to be found in this subject?**

A. Hyperkalemia due to vigorous dancing and drug abuse
B. Hypokalemia due to excess β-adrenergic surge
C. Hypokalemic periodic paralysis precipitated by ecstasy
D. Hyponatremia due to an effect on vasopressin secretion and fluid intake
E. Hyponatremia due to vigorous dancing and fluid intake

The answer is D

Ecstasy is a popular name for a ring-substituted form of methamphetamine. It gained the popularity of a "club drug" among adolescents, young adults, and subjects attending "rave" parties. Among other side effects such as rhabdomyolysis, arrhythmias, and renal failure, ecstasy causes symptomatic hyponatremia and sudden death. Ecstasy induces vasopressin secretion and retention of water in the stomach and intestine by decreasing GI motility. Hyponatremia develops as a result of water reabsorption from the GI tract and excessive oral intake in the presence of high vasopressin levels. Thus, option D is correct. Other options have very little role in the development of hyponatremia in the presence of ecstasy.

Suggested Reading

Hall AP, Henry JA. Acute toxic effets of 'ecstasy' (MDMA) and related compounds: overview of pathophysiology and clinical management. Br J Anaestth. 2006;96:678–85.

Kalantar-Zadeh K, Nguyen MK, Chang R, et al. Fatal hyponatremia in a young woman after ecstasy ingestion. Nat Clin Pract Nephrol. 2006;2:283–8.

Reddi AS. Disorders of water balance: hyponatremia. In: Reddi AS, editor. Fluid, electrolyte and acid-base disorders. Clinical evaluation and management. 2nd ed. New York: Springer; 2018. p. 107–45.

19. A marathon runner was disoriented and delirious post-race, and was found to have a serum [Na^+] 128 mEq/L. His weight was slightly higher than pre-race weight. **Which one the following is the MOST appropriate fluid administration?**

A. 1 L of D5W
B. 1 L of 0.45% saline
C. 3% saline in small volume boluses
D. 1 L 0.9 saline
E. 0.5 L 7.5% saline

The answer is C

The recommended initial fluid management in symptomatic exercise-induced, euvolemic hyponatremic patient is 3% saline in small volume boluses. Hypotonic fluids such as 0.45% saline or isotonic D5W should be avoided because of further decrease in serum [Na^+]. Normal saline (0.9%) is the fluid of choice to replace volume, although a study reported good results with isotonic saline in athletes. Isotonic saline may not be a suitable solution to correct hyponatremia in patients with elevated or inappropriate high levels of vasopressin. Although both 3% and 7.5% saline are hypertonic, 3% saline is usually the preferred fluid for symptomatic hyponatremic patients. Thus, answer C is correct.

Suggested Reading

Reddi AS. Disorders of water balance: hyponatremia. In: Reddi AS, editor. Fluid, electrolyte and acid-base disorders. Clinical evaluation and management. 2nd ed. New York: Springer; 2018. p. 107–45.
Sterns RH. Disorders of plasma sodium. Causes, consequences, and correction. N Engl J Med. 2015;372:55–65.
Verbalis JG. Diagnosis, evaluation, and treatment of hyponatremia: expert panel recommendations. Am J Med. 2013;126(suppl 1):S1–S42.

20. A 60-year-old woman with history of lung cancer is admitted for weakness and lethargy for 4 weeks. Her serum [Na^+] is 120 mEq/L. She weighs 60 kg. Her serum osmolality is 250 mOsm/kg H_2O with urine osmolality of 616 mOsm/kg H_2O. The diagnosis of SIADH is made. **What would be her serum [Na], if she receives 1 L of isotonic saline?**

A. 122 mEq/L
B. 116 mEq/L
C. 118 mEq/L
D. 120 mEq/L
E. 124 mEq/L

The answer is C

The selection of fluids in the treatment of SIADH depends on a clear-cut understanding of the fluid, serum and urine osmolalities. In addition, the physician should evaluate the total body water (TBW) content as well as the total body Na^+ (TB_{Na}) content. I would like to use TB_{Na} content rather than total plasma osmolality, because both calculations would yield similar results. A systematic approach would yield the correct answer.

First, calculate TBW and TB_{Na} of the patient as follows:

$$\begin{aligned} \text{TBW} &= \text{Wt}(\text{kg}) \times \%\text{of water / kg} \\ &= 60 \times 0.5 = 30\,\text{L} \end{aligned}$$

$$\begin{aligned} \text{TB}_{\text{Na}} &= \text{TBW} \times \text{serum}[\text{Na}] \\ &= 30 \times 120 = 3{,}600\,\text{mEq} \end{aligned}$$

Second, calculate the amount of urine volume that is required to excrete the osmoles of a given fluid to be administered to the patient. This can be calculated by dividing urine osmolality into fluid osmolality.

In the above patient, the new serum [Na^+] can be obtained as follows:

$$\text{Osmoles}(\text{osmolality})\,\text{of } 0.9\%\text{NaCl} = 308\left(\text{Na}^+ = 154\,\text{and}\,\text{Cl}^- = 154 = 308\right)$$

$$\text{Urine osmolality} = 616\,\text{mOsm}$$

$$\text{Amount of urine required to excrete } 308 \text{ osmoles} = 308/616 = 0.5\,\text{L}$$

The patient received 1 L of 0.9% saline; however, the patient excreted all the osmoles in 0.5 L of urine. Therefore, the patient retained 0.5 L of free water, which causes the TBW to increase from 30 to 30.5 L. Assuming the TB_{Na} remains at 3600 mEq, the new serum [Na^+] would be:

$$3,600 / 30.5 = 118\,\text{mEq} / \text{L}$$

Thus, in a patient with the diagnosis of SIADH, administration of 0.9% NaCl would result in decrease rather than increase in serum [Na^+]. Thus, option C is correct.

Suggested Reading

Reddi AS. Disorders of water balance: hyponatremia. In: Reddi AS, editor. Fluid, electrolyte and acid-base disorders. Clinical evaluation and management. 2nd ed. New York: Springer; 2018. p. 107–45.

Rose BD. New approaches to disturbances in the plasma sodium concentration. Am J Med. 1986;81:1033–40.

21. An 80-year-old woman was admitted for nausea, headache, and psychosis for 2 days: Past medical history includes hypertension, and her physician increased hydrochlorothiazide (HCTZ), from 12.5 to 25 mg daily. The patient was drinking water more than usual. Her BP was 120/70 mm Hg and pulse rate of 80 beats/min. There were no orthostatic BP and pulse changes. Serum chemistry: Na^+ 112 mEq/L, K^+ 3.2 mEq/L, Cl^- 90 mEq/L, and glucose 90 mg/dL. The urine osmolality is 220 m0sm/kg H_2O. She weighs 70 kg. **Which one of the following statements regarding her hyponatremia is CORRECT?**

A. Furosemide rather than HCTZ is a frequent cause of hyponatremia
B. HCTZ impairs urine concentrating capacity
C. Electrolyte free H_2O clearance decreases with HCTZ
D. Electrolyte free H_2O clearance increases with HCTZ
E. None of the above

The answer is C

Hyponatremia is a well-documented complication of diuretic use. About 73% of cases of hyponatremia were related to thiazide diuretic use. Twenty percent of cases were attributed to a combination of thiazides and K^+-sparing diuretics, and 8% were related to furosemide use. Thus, HCTZ rather than furosemide is the most common cause of hyponatremia because thiazides impair maximum urinary dilution but not concentrating ability. Urine osmolality is usually >100 mOsm/kg H_2O among thiazide users. The expected urine osmolality for this degree of hyponatremia (118 mEq/L) with normal diluting capacity should be about 50 mOsm/kg H_2O. However, this patient is unable to lower urine osmolality <100 mOsm/kg H_2O because of the effect of HCTZ on renal water handling. HCTZ decreases free H_2O clearance (i.e., more water reabsorption) and causes inability to lower urine osmolality to <100 mOsm/kg H_2O. Thus, answer C is correct.

Furosemide impairs concentrating ability of the kidney, and free water clearance is increased rather than decreased. Therefore, furosemide alone does not cause hyponatremia, but a combination of HCTZ and furosemide can result in hyponatremia. However, some patients may develop hyponatremia with orthostatic BP and pulse changes with chronic use of furosemide due to total body Na^+ and water loss. Thus, the answers A, B, D, and E are incorrect.

Suggested Reading

Astraf N, Loursdey R, Arial AI. Thiazide-induced hyponatremia associated with death or neurologic damage in outpatients. Am J Med. 1981;70:1163–8.

Hix JK, Silver S, Sterns RH. Diuretic-associated hyponatremia. Semin Nephrol. 2011;31:553–66.

Hwang KS, Kim G-H. Thiazide-induced hyponatremia. Electrolyte Blood Press. 2010;8:51–7.

Liamis G, Filippatos TD, Elisaf MS. Thiazide-associated hyponatremia in the elderly: what the clinician needs to know. J Geriatr Cardiol. 2016;13:175–82.

Reddi AS. Disorders of water balance: hyponatremia. In: Reddi AS, editor. Fluid, electrolyte and acid-base disorders. Clinical evaluation and management. 2nd ed. New York: Springer; 2018. p. 107–45.

Spital A. Diuretic-induced hyponatremia. Am J Nephrol. 1999;191:447–52.

22. **Which one of the following strategies regarding treatment of hyponatremia is CORRECT in the above patient?**

   A. Restrict fluids to 1 L/day
   B. Discontinue HCTZ
   C. Increase serum [Na^+] from 112 to 130 mEq/L in 6 h by 3% saline
   D. Increase serum [Na^+] from 112 to 118 mEq/L in 3 h by 3% saline with a goal to 126 mEq/L in 48 h
   E. Increase serum [Na^+] from 112 to 130 mEq/L in 24 h by normal saline

   The Answer is D

   This patient has acute symptomatic hyponatremia, which requires immediate treatment. Although controversial, treatment should be prompt in view of preventing progression of cerebral edema and hypoxia, which far exceed the risk of osmotic demyelination. Initially, serum [Na^+] should be corrected by 2 mEq/L per hour from 112 to 118 mEq/L in 3–4 h until symptoms resolve. Then correction should not exceed 12–14 mEq in 48 h to 126 mEq/L with 3% or normal saline (D is correct). Administration of hypertonic saline should be adjusted to achieve the target serum [Na^+] by frequent determinations of serum [Na^+] and urine Na^+ and K^+ levels.

   Restriction of fluids and discontinuation of HCTZ are not appropriate for acute symptomatic hyponatremia, although adequate after relief of symptoms. Administration of normal saline is inadequate and inappropriate to this patient. Also, rapid connection of serum [Na^+] to 130 mEq/L in 6 hours may be a risk for osmotic demyelination. Thus, answers A, B, C, and E are incorrect.

   It has been shown that slow correction of thiazide-induced symptomatic hyponatremia in 18 to 56 h may be associated with a high rate of permanent neurologic damage. Thus, prompt correction to relieve symptoms is required.

   It should be noted that a patient with hyponatremia and hypokalemia who is admitted for weakness can be successfully treated with KCl.

   Suggested Reading

Astraf N, Loursdey R, Arial AI. Thiazide-induced hyponatremia associated with death or or neurologic damage in outpatients. Am J Med. 1981;70:1163–8.
Hix JK, Silver S, Sterns RH. Diuretic-associated hyponatremia. Semin Nephrol. 2011;31:553–66.
Hwang KS, Kim G-H. Thiazide-induced hyponatremia. Electrolyte Blood Press. 2010;8:51–7.
Liamis G, Filippatos TD, Elisaf MS. Thiazide-associated hyponatremia in the elderly: what the clinician needs to know. J Geriatr Cardiol. 2016;13:175–82.
Reddi AS. Disorders of water balance: hyponatremia. In: Reddi AS, editor. Fluid, electrolyte and acid-base disorders. Clinical evaluation and management. 2nd ed. New York: Springer; 2018. p. 107–45.
Spital A. Diuretic-induced hyponatremia. Am J Nephrol. 1999;191:447–52.

23. **Which one of the following possible mechanisms regarding thiazide-induced hyponatremia is CORRECT?**

   A. Hypovolemia-stimulated vasopressin release and increased H_2O reabsorption in the cortical collecting duct with impairment in urinary diluting mechanism
   B. Upregulation of aquaporin receptor-2 expression in the collecting duct by HCTZ
   C. Increased proximal tubule solute and water reabsorption
   D. Impaired free H_2O excretion, particularly in the elderly secondary to a relative decrease in PGE_2
   E. All of the above

   The answer is E

   Thiazides cause not only mild asymptomatic but also severe symptomatic hyponatremia, as shown in the above case. The disorder is also life-threatening in some susceptible patients. Although the mechanisms for thiazide-induced hyponatremia are not fully understood, several possible explanations have been suggested. These include: (1) volume contraction with decreased GFR; (2) decrease in urinary dilution (3) stimulated release of vasopressin and increased H_2O reabsorption; (4) upregulation of aquaporin receptor-2 expression in the collecting duct by HCTZ; (5) relative decrease in vasodilatory PG synthesis in elderly subjects with unopposed vasopressin action; and 6) increased proximal tubule solute and water reabsorption due to volume depletion. This causes less glomerular filtrate delivered to the distal tubule with resultant decrease in water excretion. Thus, options A to D are correct.

Other mechanisms include: (1) diuretic-induced hypokalemia, which may further exacerbate hyponatremia by transcellular cation exchange due to osmolality changes. During this exchange, K^+ moves out of the cell to improve hypokalemia and Na^+ moves into the cell to maintain electroneutrality and thus exacerbate hyponatremia; (2) increased water intake due to stimulated thirst mechanism; and (3) decreased solute intake causing decreased water excretion.

Suggested Reading

Astraf N, Loursdey R, Arial AI. Thiazide-induced hyponatremia associated with death or neurologic damage in outpatients. Am J Med. 1981;70:1163–8.
Hix JK, Silver S, Sterns RH. Diuretic-associated hyponatremia. Semin Nephrol. 2011;31:553–66.
Liamis G, Filippatos TD, Elisaf MS. Thiazide-associated hyponatremia in the elderly: what the clinician needs to know. J Geriatr Cardiol. 2016;13:175–82.
Palmer BF, Clegg DJ. Renal considerations in the treatment of hypertension. Am J Hypertens. 2018;31:394–401.
Reddi AS. Disorders of water balance: hyponatremia. In: Reddi AS, editor. Fluid, electrolyte and acid-base disorders. Clinical evaluation and management. 2nd ed. New York: Springer; 2018. p. 107–45.
Spital A. Diuretic-induced hyponatremia. Am J Nephrol. 1999;191:447–52.

24. **Which one of the following is a risk factor for thiazide-induced hyponatremia?**

A. Elderly subjects
B. Poor solute intake
C. Female gender
D. Low body mass
E. All of the above

The answer is E

All of the above conditions predispose to thiazide-induced hyponatremia. Other conditions that are associated with thiazide-induced hyponatremia include: (1) comorbidities such as congestive heart failure, cirrhosis, and diabetes mellitus; (2) psychogenic polydipsia; (3) concomitant use of antidepressants, NSAIDS (nonsteroidal anti-inflammatory inhibitors), and spironolactone/amiloride; and (4) increased dose of thiazides.

Suggested Reading

Hix JK, Silver S, Sterns RH. Diuretic-associated hyponatremia. Semin Nephrol. 2011;31:553–66.
Liamis G, Filippatos TD, Elisaf MS. Thiazide-associated hyponatremia in the elderly: what the clinician needs to know. J Geriatr Cardiol. 2016;13:175–82.
Palmer BF, Clegg DJ. Renal considerations in the treatment of hypertension. Am J Hypertens. 2018;31:394–401.
Spital A. Diuretic-induced hyponatremia. Am J Nephrol. 1999;191:447–52.

25. A 49-year-old male was brought to the Emergency Department for evaluation of nausea, fatigue, and weakness for 24 h. His wife says that he had been having binge drinking without any food intake. He is not taking any medications. On physical examination, he was euvolemic. His weight is 70 kg. BP is 100/60 mm Hg with a pulse rate of 82 beats/min. Serum [Na^+] is 120 mEq/L; [K^+] 3.8 mEq/L; BUN 8 mg/dL; creatinine 0.6 mg/dL; and osmolality 230 mOsm/kg H_2O. Urine studies are: osmolality 75 mOsm/kg H_2O; Na^+ 10 mEq/L; and K^+ 20 mEq/L. The diagnosis of beer potomania was made. **Assuming no urine output in 2–3 hours, which one of the following is the MOST appropriate therapy for this patient?**

A. D5W
B. 0.9% NaCl
C. 3% NaCl
D. 0.45% NaCl
E. Fluid restriction and NaCl tablets

The answer is B

Treatment of acute symptomatic hyponatremia due to binge drinking is a therapeutic challenge to physicians because of waning and waxing symptoms. A review of the literature on hyponatremia due to beer ingestion

shows administration of 0.9% NaCl, 0.45% NaCl with KCl supplementation, and 3% NaCl and fluid restriction to no treatment. Thus, treatment of hyponatremia depends on the severity and duration of onset of symptoms.

This patient has mild to moderate symptoms of hyponatremia. The appropriate treatment appears 0.9% saline rather than 3% saline (B is correct). Rapid correction of serum Na^+ from 120 to 126 mEq/L by 3% saline is not necessary in this patient. Furthermore, rapid correction of serum Na^+ to >130 mEq/L in an alcoholic may precipitate osmotic demyelination syndrome. Therefore, either infusion of 0.9% saline (1 L in 24 h) or fluid restriction to increase serum Na^+ by <10 mEq/L in 24 h or <18 mEq/L in 48 h is advisable.

D5W is not the solution of initial choice in this patient, because it is converted into free H_2O and may lower serum [Na^+] even further. D5W can be started, if caloric intake is needed after serum [Na^+] reaches approximately 128 mEq/L. Also, fluid restriction with supplementation of NaCl tablets is not the appropriate choice.

Suggested Reading

Reddi AS. Disorders of water balance: hyponatremia. In: Reddi AS, editor. Fluid, electrolyte and acid-base disorders. Clinical evaluation and management. 2nd ed. New York: Springer; 2018. p. 107–45.

Sanghavi SR, Kellerman PS, Nanovic L. Beer potomania: an unusual cause of hyponatremia at high risk of complications from rapid correction. Am J Kidney Dis. 2007;50:673–81.

26. **Which of the following risk factors may precipitate osmotic demyelination syndrome (ODS) in a patient with hyponatremia?**

    A. Hypokalemia
    B. Alcoholism
    C. Hypoxia
    D. Serum [Na^+] <105 mEq/L
    E. All of the above

    The answer is E

    All of the above conditions have been reported to precipitate ODS with overcorrection of Na^+ in a patient with chronic hyponatremia (hyponatremia present >48 h). Thus, E is correct.

Suggested Reading

Achinger S, Ayus JC. Treatment of hyponatremic encephalopathy in the critically ill. Crit Care Med. 2017;45:1762–71.

George JC, Zafar W, Bucaloiu ID, et al. Risk factors and outcomes of rapid correction of severe hyponatremia. Clin J Am Soc Nephrol. 2018;13:984–92.

27. A 28-year-old woman was admitted for nausea, vomiting, blurred vision, and questionable seizures. She was electively intubated for air-way protection. Further history was obtained from the mother, who stated that the patient had nonbloody diarrhea for 2 days and drank several liters of water. The patient is a strict vegan, and in good health, and does not take any medications. Physical examination revealed a thin female with a BP of 116/72 mm Hg with a pulse of 98 beats/min. Lung and heart examination were normal. There was no peripheral edema. Her weight was 64 kg. Six weeks ago, she delivered a healthy baby and her serum [Na^+] was 140 mEq/L. The laboratory results showed:

Serum	Urine
Na^+ = 114 mEq/L	Na^+ = <20 mEq/L
K^+ = 2.7 mEq/L	K^+ = 6 mEq/L
Cl^- = 78 mEq/L	Osmolality = 40 mOsm/kg H_2O
HCO_3^- = 17 mEq/L	
Creatinine = 0.5 mg/dL	
BUN = 4 mg/dL	
Glucose = 100 mg/dL	
Uric acid = 2.9 mg/dL	
Osmolality = 240 mOsm/kg H_2O	

Assuming her total output (diarrheal fluid, urine output, and insensible loss) is 2 L/day, how much water she may have consumed that lowered her serum [Na^+] from 140 to 114 mEq/L?

A. 8 L
B. 9 L
C. 11 L
D. 13 L
E. 15 L

The answer is C

First, calculate her total body water (TBW) and total body Na^+ prior to admission, and then calculate water excess.

$$\text{TBW} = 64 \times 0.5 = 32\,\text{L}$$

$$\text{Previous body Na}^+ = \text{TBW} \times \text{serum}\left[\text{Na}^+\right] \text{or}\, 32 \times 140 = 4480\,\text{mEq}$$

$$\text{New TBW} = 4480/114 = 39.3\,\text{L}$$

$$\text{Water excess} = 39.3 - 32 = 7.3\,\text{L}$$

Second, add total output for 2 days (4 L) to water excess of 7.3 L. Therefore, the patient may have consumed approximately 11 L of water. Thus, answer C is correct.

Suggested Reading

Reddi AS. Disorders of water balance: hyponatremia. In: Reddi AS, editor. Fluid, electrolyte and acid-base disorders. Clinical evaluation and management. 2nd ed. New York: Springer; 2018. p. 107–45.

28. In the Emergency Department, she received 100 mL of 3% NaCl, and her urine output was noted to be 200 mL/h. Repeat serum [Na^+] in 4 h was 119 mEq/L. She was extubated. The patient did not receive any IV fluids or other interventions for the next 20 h. The urine output increased to 300 mL/h. After 24 h, her serum [Na^+] was 141 mEq/L. **Which one of the following is the MOST appropriate next step in the management of her hyponatremia?**

A. D5W at 100 mL/h
B. Free water boluses at 200 mL Q6H via N/G tube
C. 0.45% saline at 100 mL/h
D. Restrict fluid to 1 L/day
E. DDAVP 1–2 μg i.v. or 4 μg subcutaneously with free water boluses or D5W (10 mL/kg)

The answer is E

Although serum [Na^+] can be corrected rapidly in polydipsic patients, the increase of 27 mEq in 24 h is too rapid because of increased urine output. Serum [Na^+] may further increase, if urine output does not decrease. Therefore, the appropriate management at this time is to prevent further increase in serum [Na^+], decrease urine output, and prevent demyelination. These changes can be reversed by administration of DDAVP and hypotonic fluids. Studies in animals and humans suggest that this type of management is appropriate to prevent further increase in serum [Na^+]. DDAVP 1–2 μg i.v. should be started with free water boluses or D5W. Thus, option E is correct. Infusion of hypotonic solutions alone is not sufficient to reverse demyelination. Also, restriction of fluid will take long time to lower serum [Na^+]. It should be noted that administration of DDAVP alone is not appropriate because it would prevent further increase but does not decrease serum [Na^+].

Suggested Reading

Achinger SG, Ayus JC. Use of desmopressin in hyponatremia: foe or friend. Kidney Med. 2019;1:65–70.
Reddi AS. Disorders of water balance: hyponatremia. In: Reddi AS, editor. Fluid, electrolyte and acid-base disorders. Clinical evaluation and management. 2nd ed. New York: Springer; 2018. p. 107–47.
Sterns RH. Disorders of plasma sodium. Causes, consequences, and correction. N Engl J Med. 2015;372:55–65.
Sterns RH, Hix JK, Silver S. Treating profound hyponatremia: a strategy for controlled correction. Am J Kidney Dis. 2010;56:774–9.

29. A 32-year-old woman with AIDS was referred to the renal clinic for evaluation of persistent hyponatremia. There was no history of recent infections but admits to daily intake of beer and at times depression. The patient is thin but not cachectic. BP is 120/80 mm Hg with a pulse of 78 beats/min. There are no orthostatic changes. Examination of the lung and heart is normal. No peripheral edema is appreciated. Serum and urine chemistries:

Serum	Urine
Na^+ = 126 mEq/L K^+ = 4.2 mEq/L Cl^- = 94 mEq/L HCO_3^- = 23 mEq/L BUN = 12 mg/dL Creatinine = 0.5 mg/dL Glucose = 104 mg/dL Albumin = 3.4 g/dL Normal liver function tests and cortisol Osmolality = 264 mOsm/kg H_2O	Osmolality = 578 mOsm/kg H_2O Na^+ = 80 mEq/L K^+ = 40 mEq/L

Which one of the following treatments is INAPPROPRIATE in this patient?

A. Water restriction
B. Lithium
C. Demeclocycline
D. Selective serotonin reuptake inhibitor (SSRI)
E. Dilantin

The answer is D

Except for SSRI, other treatment modalities have been tried to improve chronic asymptomatic hyponatremia in patients with ectopic production or stimulation of ADH. SSRIs such as setraline, paroxetine, and duloxetine inhibit the reuptake of serotonin, thus causing hyponatremia. SSRIs induce SIDAH by several mechanisms that include: (1) stimulation of ADH secretion; (2) augmentation of ADH action in the renal medulla; (3) resetting the osmostat that lowers the threshold for ADH secretion; and (4) interaction of SSRIs with other medications via p450 enzymes, resulting in enhanced action of ADH. Thus, D is correct. Dilantin inhibits ADH secretion, so that it will improve hyponatremia.

Suggested Reading

Jacob S, Spinler SA. Hyponatremia associated with selective serotonin-reuptake inhibitors in older adults. Ann Pharmacother. 2006;40:1618–22.
Lien Y-HH, Commentary. Antidepressants and hyponatremia. Am J Med. 2018;131:7–8.
Mort JR, Aparasu RR, Baer RK. Interaction between selective serotonin reuptake inhibitors and nonsteroidal anti-inflammatory drugs: Review of the literature. Pharmacotherapy. 2006;26:1307–13.
Sahoo S, Grover S. Hyponatremia and psychotropics. J Geriatr Mental Health. 2016;3:108–22.

30. A 65-year-old man with small cell cancer of left lung is found to have hyponatremia due to SIADH. He is seen by a nephrologist, who started him on a fluid restriction of 1 L/day. Patient refused to take demeclocycline because of his alcohol use and urea for gastrointestinal upset. For a while, his serum [Na^+] was maintained between 130 and 135 mEq/L. The patient was given a follow-up visit in 3 months, at which time he presented with weakness, fatigue, and inability to concentrate during conversation. He also complained that he had a sense of falling. He checked his BP which was 140/78 mm Hg. He admitted to drinking >1 L of fluids/day because of increased thirst. His serum [Na^+] is 124 mEq/L, and euvolemic. His urine osmolality is 550 mOsm/kg H_2O and 24-h urine volume 1.2 L. Urine Na^+ and K^+ are 80 and 54 mEq/L, respectively. Other laboratory results are consistent with SIADH. **What is the appropriate step in the management of his hyponatremia?**

A. Fluid restriction under supervision
B. Normal saline
C. Tolvaptan

D. 3% saline
E. Salt tablets

The answer is C

The patient is symptomatic from his chronic hyponatremia. Impairment in cognitive function and falls with fractures are not uncommon in patients with chronic hyponatremia. The patient should be admitted to the hospital for two reasons: (1) to improve symptoms with an increase in serum [Na^+] to 128–130 mEq/L in a 24-h period. Starting 3% saline is appropriate; and (2) consideration for an oral vaptan, as the patient is noncompliant to fluid restriction. Tolvaptan is the oral form that is available as 15, 30, and 60 mg tablets.

Tolvaptan should be started in a hospital setting for monitoring of serum [Na^+] during the dosage-titration phase. The drug is started at 15 mg once daily and titrated up to 60 mg daily without fluid restriction. Once this patient's symptoms improve, he can be discharged 2–3 days on a fixed dose of tolvaptan.

Tolvaptan is indicated in euvolemic and hypervolemic hyponatremic patients. It should not be used in patients with hypovolemic hyponatremia. Clinical studies have shown beneficial effects of tolvaptan.

The SALT trials, which included patients with SIADH, CHF, and cirrhosis, showed that tolvaptan increased serum [Na^+] by 4.5 mEq/L on day 4, and 7.4 mEq/L over a 30-day period compared with fluid restriction alone. The patients were also followed-up for a mean of 701 days. Mean serum [Na^+] increased from 131 to >135 mEq/L.

This patient will benefit from tolvaptan use to increase his serum [Na^+] and prevent falls and fractures. Thus, C is correct. Other options do not help long-term hyponatremia.

Suggested Reading

Fiordoliva M, Meletani T, Baleani MG, et al. Managing hyponatremia in lung cancer: latest evidence and clinical implications. Ther Adv Med Oncol. 2017;9:711–9.

Reddi AS. Disorders of water balance: hyponatremia. In: Reddi AS, editor. Fluid, electrolyte and acid-base disorders. Clinical evaluation and management. 2nd ed. New York: Springer; 2018. p. 107–45.

Rondon-Barrios H, Berl T. Vasopressin receptor antagonists in hyponatremia: uses and misuses. Front Med. 2017;Article 141:1–8.

Thurman JM, Berl T. Disorders of water metabolism. In: Mount DB, Sayegh MH, Singh AJ, editors. Core concepts in the disorders of fluid, electrolytes and acid-base balance. New York: Springer; 2013. p. 29–48.

Zhang X, Zhao M, Du W, et al. Efficacy and safety of vasopressin receptor antagonists for euvolemic or hypervolemic hyponatremia: a meta-analysis. Medicine. 2016;95(15):e3310.

31. **What are the possible explanations for the failure of water restriction to improve serum [Na^+] in the above patient?**

A. Urine osmolality >500 mOsm/kg H_2O
B. Urine volume <1500 mL/day
C. The ratio of urine Na^+ plus K^+ to serum Na^+ >1
D. All of the above
E. A and C only

The answer is D

Fluid restriction is the initial treatment of choice for asymptomatic patients with SIADH. In real world, fluid restriction does not always work because of weather conditions and changes in thirst (to name a few). When urine osmolality is >500 mOsm/kg H_2O, the electrolyte free water excretion is decreased, suggesting that the patient is retaining water due to excess ADH secretion. Thus, urine osmolality >500 mOsm/kg H_2O is a risk factor for failure of fluid restriction. Also, urine volume <1500 mL/day suggests water retention due to high circulating ADH levels, causing failure of water restriction to improve serum [Na^+].

Determination of urine Na^+ and K^+ is useful in calculating electrolyte free water excretion, which is calculated as the sum of the concentrations of urine Na^+ and K^+ divided by serum Na^+. If the ratio is >1, it indicates negative electrolyte free water clearance and hyponatremia, and the ratio <1 suggests positive free water clearance and, therefore, hypernatremia.

In this patient, the ratio is >1 (urine Na^+ 80 mEq/L and K^+ 54 mEq/L = 134 mEq/L divided by serum Na^+ 124 mEq/L gives a ratio of 1.08). Decreased electrolyte free water excretion is another explanation for failure of water restriction to increase serum [Na^+] in this patient. Thus, answer D is correct.

A prospective study of fluid restriction in SIADH patients showed that high urinary Na^+ levels (≥130 mEq/L) and high urine osmolality (≥500 mOsm/kg H_2O) were significantly associated with nonresponse to fluid restriction. Also, lower levels of serum mid-regional pro-atrial natriuretic peptide and high serum urea nitrogen were associated with nonresponse to fluid restriction.

Suggesting Reading

Furst H, Hallows KR, Post J, et al. The urine/plasma electrolyte ratio: a predictive guide to water restriction. Am J Med Sci. 2000;319:240–4.

Verbalis JG. Diagnosis, evaluation, and treatment of hyponatremia: expert panel recommendations. Am J Med. 2013;126(suppl 1):S1–S42.

Winzeler B, Lengsfeld S, Nigro N, et al. Predictors of nonresponse to fluid restriction in hypernatremia due to the syndrome of inappropriate antidiuresis. J Intern Med. 2016;280:609–17.

32. After 3 months use of tolvaptan, the above patient was found to have high levels of aminotransferases on routine serum chemistry. The patient admits to daily drinking of beer. After extensive discussion, the patient decides to discontinue tolvaptan and wants to go on fluid restriction. He prefers regular diet with Na^+ intake of 102 mEq (6 g of salt). Physical examination and blood pressure are normal. Labs:

Serum	Urine
Na^+ = 134 mEq/L K^+ = 4.0 mEq/L Cl^- = 95 mEq/L HCO_3^- = 23 mEq/L BUN = 12 mg/dL Creatinine = 0.5 mg/dL Glucose = 90 mg/dL Abnormal liver function tests Osmolality = 272 mOsm/kg H_2O	Volume = 1.5 L Osmolality = 500 mOsm/kg H_2O Na^+ = 60 mEq/L K^+ = 30 mEq/L

Assuming daily insensible loss of 700 mL, which one of the following approximate amounts of daily water intake you recommend for this patient that wound increase his serum [Na^+] to 135 mEq/L?

A. 1.00 L
B. 1.20 L
C. 1.40 L
D. 1.60 L
E. 1.60 L

The answer is B

The major objective in the management of this patient is to maintain serum [Na^+] around 134 mEq/L in the absence of tolvaptan. As the patient agrees to fluid restriction, the best way to restrict is to calculate electrolyte free water clearance (see question 11), which approximates the amount of water that will not change his serum [Na^+]. Electrolyte free water clearance ($T^e{}_{CH2O}$) can be calculated by the following formula:

$$\mathbf{T^{e}{}_{CH2O} = V\left(1-\left(U_{Na}+U_{k}\right)/P_{Na}\right)}$$

where V is urine volume, U_{Na} and U_K are urine Na^+ and urine K^+, respectively, and P_{Na} is plasma Na^+. Substituting the data from the patient, we obtain:

$$\mathbf{T^{e}{}_{CH2O} = 1.5\left(1-\left(60+30/134\right)\right) = 0.49\,L}$$

Adding daily 700 mL as insensible loss to 0.49 L of electrolyte free water clearance, daily intake of 1.19 L will increase serum [Na^+] to 135 mEq/L. On the other hand, if fluid is restricted to 1 L, serum [Na^+] increases to 136 mEq/L. Thus, answer B is correct.

Suggested Reading

Ellison DH, Berl T. The syndrome of inappropriate antidiuresis. N Engl J Med. 2007;356:1064–72.
Rose BD. New approach to disturbances in the plasma sodium concentration. 1986;81:1033–40.
Verbalis JG, Greenberg A, Burst V, et al. Diagnosing and treating the syndrome of inappropriate antidiuretic hormone secretion. Am J Med. 2016;129(537):29–537.e23.

33. **Which one of the following conditions is contraindicated for the use of vaptans?**

A. Hypovolemia
B. Symptomatic hyponatremia
C. Impaired thirst mechanism
D. Concomitant use of drugs that increase vaptan levels
E. All of the above

The answer is E

Vaptans are contraindicated in hypovolemic hyponatremia because of their exacerbation of hypotension. Also, they are not useful in the treatment of symptomatic hyponatremia, which requires immediate increase in serum [Na^+] to improve symptoms. Vaptans increase electrolyte free water excretion, and the patients need to drink water to replenish water loss and maintain euvolemia. Otherwise the patients become volume depleted, if they do not drink water because of impaired thirst mechanism with resultant hypernatremia. Vaptans are metabolized by CYP3A4 cytochrome system, and inhibitors of this system such as ketoconazole or other drugs elevate vaptan levels when used concomitantly. Vaptan dose needs to be adjusted whenever both drugs are used concomitantly. Thus, answer E is correct. Interestingly, conivaptan inhibits CYP3A4; therefore, it is limited to 4 days of i.v. use only.

Suggested Reading

Rondon-Barrios H, Berl T. Vasopressin receptor antagonists in hyponatremia: uses and misuses. Front Med. 2017;Article 141:1–8.
Zhang X, Zhao M, Du W, et al. Efficacy and safety of vasopressin receptor antagonists for euvolemic or hypervolemic hyponatremia: a meta-analysis. Medicine. 2016;95(15):e3310.

34. A 3-month-old male infant is admitted for irritability. Physical examination is unremarkable other than a BP of 128/92 mm Hg. Serum [Na] is 123 mEq/L, creatinine <0.3 mg/dL; BUN 5 mg/dL, vasopressin <1 pg/ml (normal 1–13.3), urine osmolality 284, and urine Na^+ 35; other chemistries are normal. **Which one of the following is the MOST likely diagnosis in this infant?**

A. Classical syndrome of inappropriate antidiuretic hormone secretion (SIADH)
B. Nephrogenic SIADH (NSIADH)
C. Congestive heart failure (CHF)
D. Dehydration
E. Drug-induced hyponatremia

The answer is B

NSIADH is similar to SIADH, but rare. It was first described in 2005 in infants with hyponatremia and high urine osmolality. Unlike SIADH, patients with NSIADH have undetectable or extremely low ADH levels. NSIADH is a gain of function mutation in vasopressin V2 receptor (B is correct). Treatment is fluid restriction, urea, and a combination of low dose furosemide and NaCl tablets. Other drugs such as lithium, demeclocycline, or vaptans are generally not recommended. NSIADH was also described in adult patients. This genetic disease was described in a large five-generation family. Other options are incorrect because these conditions are associated with high ADH levels. It should be noted that in drug-induced hyponatremia, the ADH levels may be normal or high.

Suggested Reading

Decaux G, Vandergheynst F, Bouko Y, et al. Nephrogenic syndrome of inappropriate antidiuresis in adults: High phenotypic variability in men and women from a large pedigree. J Am Soc Nephrol. 2007;18:606–12.

Feldman BJ, Rosenthal SM, Vargas GA, et al. Nephrogenic syndrome of inappropriate antidiuresis. N Engl J Med. 2005;352:1884–90.
Reddi AS. Disorders of water balance: hyponatremia. In: Reddi AS, editor. Fluid, electrolyte and acid-base Disorders. clinical evaluation and management. 2nd ed. New York: Springer; 2018. p. 107–45.
Thurman JM, Berl T. Disorders of water metabolism. In: Mount DB, Sayegh MH, Singh AJ, editors. Core concepts in the disorders of fluid, electrolytes and acid-base balance. New York: Springer; 2013. p. 29–48.

35. **Which one of the following is the LEAST likely cause of isotonic hyponatremia?**

A. Granulated sugar (sucrose)
B. Hyperproteinemia
C. Hypercholesterolemia
D. Hypertriglyceridemia
E. Methanol

The answer is E

In a case report, topical application of granulated sugar to an infected wound resulted in hypertonic hyponatremia. Unlike oral sucrose, directly absorbed sucrose from a wound into circulation does not metabolize into glucose and fructose. This results in hypertonic hyponatremia. Elevated proteins as in multiple myeloma, a different form of cholesterol found in lipoprotein X (2) or triglycerides cause isotonic hyponatremia. Lipoprotein X has been described in patients with cholestatic liver disease such as primary biliary cirrhosis. Patients with severe triglyceridemia will have a lactescent serum. However, methanol causes osmolal gap but not nonhypotonic hyponatremia.

Suggested Reading

Rao N, Jain A, Goyale A, et al. Lipoprotein X in autoimmune liver disease causing interference in routine and specialist biochemical investigations. Clin Lipidol. 2017;12:8–13.
Reuters R, Boer W, Simmermacher R, et al. A bag full of sugar makes your sodium go down. Nephrol Dial Transplant. 2005;20:2543–4.
Turchin A, Seifter JL, Seely EW. Mind the gap. N Engl J Med. 2003;349:1465–8.

36. A 52-year-old woman was admitted with weakness and confusion for 2 days. She admits to drinking alcohol for the last 6 days. She has the history of central diabetes insipidus and was on desmopressin. One week prior to admission, she was euvolemic and her serum chemistry was normal. She weighs 70 kg. Admitting labs:

Serum	Urine
Na^+ = 114 mEq/L	Na^+ = <20 mEq/L
K^+ = 2.2 mEq/L	K^+ = 30 mEq/L
Cl^- = 92 mEq/L	Osmolality = 100 mOsm/kg H_2O
HCO_3^- = 22 mEq/L	Ethanol = 0 mg/dL
Creatinine = 0.5 mg/dL	
BUN = 6 mg/dL	
Glucose = 90 mg/dL	
Osmolality = 238 mOsm/kg H_2O	

Which one of the following is an APPROPRIATE initial fluid management in this patient?

A. D5W
B. Normal saline
C. 3% saline
D. KCl
E. KCl and D5W

The answer is D

This patient has profound hypokalemia. D5W and normal saline would lower K^+ even further; therefore, these are not appropriate fluids for this patient. Three percent saline increases serum [Na^+] but does not improve serum [K^+]. Therefore, 3% saline is not an appropriate choice of fluid. KCl and D5W is not an appropriate fluid for this patient, as this fluid may not normalize serum [K^+]. The appropriate fluid is administration of KCl, which improves both K^+ and Na^+ levels, as described below:

$$\textbf{Serum}\left[\textbf{Na}^+\right] = \textbf{Total body Na}^+ + \textbf{Total body K}^+ / \textbf{Total body water}$$

Thus, potassium supplementation as KCl will improve [Na^+]. Therefore, answer D is correct.

Suggested Reading

Reddi AS. Disorders of water balance: hyponatremia. In: Reddi AS, editor. Fluid, electrolyte and acid-base disorders. Clinical evaluation and management. 2nd ed. New York: Springer; 2018. p. 107–45.

37. A 32-year-old man was referred to the renal clinic for evaluation of persistent hyponatremia (130 mEq/L) despite fluid restriction. The patient has been paraplegic for 4 years following a gunshot wound. He is alert, oriented, and not in any distress. He is on regular diet with 1.5 L fluid restriction. He is on 10 mg of oxycodone, as needed. His only complaint is occasional weakness, which he attributes to immobility. His labs: Na^+ 130 mEq/L, K^+ 4.5 mEq/L, Cl^- 96 mEq/L, HCO_3^- 23 mEq/L, BUN 14 mg/dl, creatinine 0.8 mg/dL, and glucose 90 mg/dL. Total protein and lipids are normal. Liver, thyroid, and adrenal function tests are normal. Urine osmolality is 580 mOsm/kg H_2O, and Na^+ is 80 mEq/L. Following 1 L of normal saline, his serum Na^+ remains at 129 mEq/L. In order to understand the etiology of his hyponatremia, a water loading test is performed by giving 1 L of water orally. The results of the test are shown in the following table.

Time (min)	Serum Na^+ (mEq/L)	Urine Na^+ (mEq/L)	Urine osmolality (mOsm/kg H_2O)	Urine volume (mL)
0	130	80	580	0
30	129	58	480	100
90	130	30	240	350
120	129	20	90	450

Based on the above data, which one of the following is the MOST likely diagnosis in this patient?

A. Pseudohyponatremia
B. Poor oral intake
C. Syndrome of inappropriate antidiuretic hormone secretion (SIADH)
D. Nephrogenic syndrome of inappropriate antidiuresis (NSIAD)
E. Reset osmostat

The answer is E

Pseudohyponatremia is unlikely, because glucose, total protein, and lipids are normal. Thus, answer A is incorrect. Patients with poor oral intake are unable to concentrate their urine to 580 mOsm/kg H_2O, although they can dilute to 100 mOsm/kg H_2O. Also, high urine Na^+ excretion rules out poor solute intake. Patients with SIADH and NSIAD are unable to dilute their urine osmolality to <100 mOsm/kg H_2O. Also, these patients cannot excrete the water load in a short period of time because of ADH activity. Thus, answers B–D are incorrect. This patient has the diagnosis of reset osmostat, as he can concentrate or dilute his urine appropriately. Because of this ability, patients with reset osmostat can excrete most of the water load in <4 h and maintain their serum [Na^+] at their preset level despite changes in water intake. Thus, answer E is correct.

Suggested Reading

Reddi AS. Disorders of water balance: hyponatremia. In: Reddi AS, editor. Fluid, electrolyte and acid-base disorders. Clinical evaluation and management. 2nd ed. New York: Springer; 2018. p. 107–45.

Robertson GL. Regulation of arginine vasopressin in the syndrome of inappropriate antidiuresis. Am J Med. 2006;119:S36–42.

38. A 65-year-old man with long history of smoking was admitted initially for treatment of non-small cell lung cancer and chemotherapy. His chemotherapy regimen includes cisplatin, gemcitabin, paclitaxel, and bevacizumab. He started having polyuria and weakness with orthostatic blood pressure and pulse changes. His labs:

Serum	Urine
Na^+ = 124 mEq/L	Na^+ = 90 mEq/L
K^+ = 2.8 mEq/L	K^+ = 60 mEq/L
Cl^- = 112 mEq/L	Osmolality = 500 mOsm/kg H_2O
HCO_3^- = 22 mEq/L	
Creatinine = 1.5 mg/dL	
BUN = 36 mg/dL	
Glucose = 90 mg/dL	

Which one of the following is the MOST likely cause of his hyponatremia?

A. Syndrome of inappropriate antidiuretic hormone secretion (SIADH)
B. Nephrogenic syndrome of inappropriate antidiuresis (NSIAD)
C. Reset osmostat
D. Cisplatin-induced hyponatremia
E. Cerebral salt wasting (CSW)

The answer is D

This patient developed cisplatin-induced nephrotoxicity. Polyuria develops 24–48 h after cisplatin dose, which is related to defective concentrating ability of the kidneys. Cisplatin also induces proximal tubular injury and Fanconi syndrome. As a result, Na^+ is lost in the urine with other ions, and the patient develops volume depletion and hyponatremia. Thus, answer D is correct. Increase in creatinine is related to both volume depletion and cisplatin-induced proximal tubular injury. SIADH, NSIAD, and reset osmostat can be excluded based on orthostatic changes, as these conditions are associated with euvolemia. Thus, answers A–C are incorrect. CSW causes volume depletion, orthostatic changes, hyponatremia, elevation in creatinine, and urinary Na^+ loss, but not hypokalemia and kaliuresis. Thus, answer E is incorrect.

Suggested Reading

Hamdi T, Latta S, Jallad B, et al. Cisplatin-induced renal salt wasting syndrome. South Med J. 2010;103:793–9.
Pham P-C, Reddy P, Qaqish S, et al. Cisplatin-Induced renal salt wasting requiring over 12 Liters of 3% saline replacement. Case Rep Nephrol. 2017;Article ID 8137078, 4 pages.

39. A 50-year-old hypertensive man is admitted for headache and altered mental status. A CT scan of the head shows subarachnoid hemorrhage. He is receiving hyperalimentation, and his urine output is 4 L/day. Also, the nurse notices diarrhea of 1-day duration. His serum Na^+ is 149 mEq/L, K^+ 3.3 mEq/L, HCO_3^- 26 mEq/L, BUN 44 mg/dL, creatinine 1.6 mg/dL, and glucose 200 mg/dL. His urine Na^+ is 70 mEq/L, and urine osmolality 380 mOsm/kg H_2O. His volume status is adequate. **Which one of the following is the MOST likely cause of his hypernatremia?**

A. Nephrogenic diabetes insipidus
B. Partial central diabetes insipidus
C. Osmotic diarrhea
D. Osmotic diuresis
E. 7.5% NaCl administration to improve brain edema

The answer is D

Patients with either nephrogenic diabetes insipidus or partial central diabetes insipidus have mostly water diuresis rather than high solute diuresis. The osmolal excretion is normal in diabetes insipidus. Patients with diabetes insipidus have low urine osmolality despite a high serum osmolality or hypernatremia. The patient is excreting a total of 1520 mOsm/day (380 × 4 = 1520). Therefore, the patient has solute diuresis. Thus, options A and B are unlikely in this patient. Option C is also unlikely because the urinary Na^+ level is low rather than high in diarrhea

because the kidney conserves Na^+. Option E is also unlikely because the patient does not have any volume expansion due to hypertonic saline infusion, and the patient should have a sodium diuresis. The patient has osmotic diuresis, which is the cause of his hypernatremia (D is correct). In general, the urine osmolality in osmotic diuresis is relatively higher than serum osmolality. The following flow diagram shows the differential diagnosis of polyuria.

Suggested Reading

Oster JR, Singer I, Thatte L, et al. The polyuria of solute diuresis. Arch Intern Med. 1997;157:721–9.

Reddi AS. Disorders of water balance: hypernatremia. In: Reddi AS, editor. Fluid, electrolyte and acid-base disorders. Clinical evaluation and management. 2nd ed. New York: Springer; 2018. p. 147–64.

Thurman JM, Berl T. Disorders of water metabolism. In: Mount DB, Sayegh MH, Singh AJ, editors. Core concepts in the disorders of fluid, electrolytes and acid-base balance. New York: Springer; 2013. p. 29–48.

40. A 74-year-old man is admitted from the nursing home for lethargy, disorientation, and confusion. The nurse's record shows that the patient had cerebrovascular accident 5 years ago. The patient did not have any fever, diarrhea, or fluid loss. Urine output is recorded as 700 mL/day.

On admission, the BP is 100/70 mm Hg with a pulse rate of 100 beats/min (supine) and 80/60 mm Hg with a pulse rate of 110 beats/min (sitting). Physical examination is normal except for dry mucous membranes. He weighs 70 kg. Laboratory values are:

Serum	Urine
Na^+ = 168 mEq/L	Na^+ = 12 mEq/L
K^+ = 4.6 mEq/L	Osmolality = 600 mOsm/kg H_2O
Cl^- = 114 mEq/L	
HCO_3^- = 26 mEq/L	
Creatinine = 1.9 mg/dL	
BUN = 64 mg/dL	
Glucose 110 mg/dL	

What would his water deficit be when calculated for desired serum [Na^+] of 140 mEq/L?

A. 3–4 L
B. 4.1–5 L
C. 5.1–6 L
D. 6.1–7 L
E. >8 L

The answer is E

Any one of the following formulas can be used to calculate water deficit:

Formula 1

$$\text{Water deficit} = \text{Previous total body water}(\text{TBW}) \times \text{actual}\left[\text{Na}^+\right] = \text{Desired}\left[\text{Na}^+\right] \times \text{New TBW}$$

$$\text{New TBW} = \frac{\text{Previous TBW} \times \left[\text{Actual Na}^+\right]}{\text{Desired}\left[\text{Na}^+\right]}$$

$$\text{Example : Weight} = 70\,\text{kg}$$

$$\text{Previous TBW} = 70 \times 0.6 = 42\,\text{L}$$

$$\text{Actual}\left[\text{Na}^+\right] = 168\,\text{mEq / L}$$

$$\text{Desired}\left[\text{Na}^+\right] = 140\,\text{mEq / L}$$

$$\text{New TBW} = 42 \times 168 / 140 = 50.4\,\text{L}$$

$$\text{Water deficit} = \text{New TBW} - \text{Previous TBW or } 50.4 - 42 = 8.4\,\text{L}$$

Formula 2

$$\text{Water deficit} = \frac{\text{Previous TBW} \times \left([\text{Actual}\left[\text{Na}^+\right] - 1\right)}{\text{Desired}\left[\text{Na}^+\right]}$$

By using the above example, we obtain:

$$\frac{42 \times (168 - 1)}{140} = 8.4\,\text{L}$$

Formula 3 (a rough estimate)

An editorial by Stern and Silver (QJM 96:549–552, 2003) suggests that administration of 3–4 mL/kg of electrolyte-free water can lower serum [Na$^+$] by 1 mEq/L in a lean individual. Total water deficit can be calculated as weight in kg × mL to be administered (3 or 4 mL) × the difference between the actual and desired [Na$^+$].

If we apply 4 mL/kg to a 70 kg individual to reduce serum [Na$^+$] from 168 to 140 mEq/L, the water deficit would be: 70 × 4 × 28 or 280 × 28 = 7.84 L.

All formulas resulted in >7 L of water loss. Thus, choice E is correct.

Suggested Reading

Reddi AS. Disorders of water balance: hypernatremia. In: Reddi AS, editor. Fluid, electrolyte and acid-base disorders. Clinical evaluation and management. 2nd ed. New York: Springer; 2018. p. 147–64.

Thurman JM, Berl T. Disorders of water metabolism. In: Mount DB, Sayegh MH, Singh AJ, editors. Core concepts in the disorders of fluid, electrolytes and acid-base balance. New York: Springer; 2013. p. 29–48.

41. **Assuming the patient had no oral intake and daily urine output of 700 mL, approximately how many days it would have taken to develop serum [Na$^+$] from 140 to 168 mEq/L?**

 A. 2 days
 B. 3 days
 C. 5 days
 D. 7 days
 E. 9 days

The answer is C

To answer this question, one needs to calculate the total daily fluid loss. This can be calculated from daily urine output and insensible loss (approximately 700 mL/day). Thus, the patient's daily fluid loss is: 700 mL + 900 mL = 1600 mL (1.6 L).

The patient's total water deficit is 8.4 L; dividing 8.4 by 1.6 gives 5.25. Thus, it would have taken approximately 5 days for this patient to increase serum [Na] from 140 mEq/L to 168 mEq/L. Thus, answer C is correct.

Suggested Reading

Reddi AS. Disorders of water balance: hypernatremia. In: Reddi AS, editor. Fluid, electrolyte and acid-base disorders. Clinical evaluation and management. 2nd ed. New York: Springer; 2018. p. 147–64.

42. A patient received 2 L of normal saline, and his BP improved. His mental status improved, and he says he is hungry and thirsty. His serum [Na$^+$] remains at 167 mEq/L and glucose 198 mg/dL. His 24 h urine output is 1.2 L. **What is your further management of this patient to improve hypernatremia?**

 A. Continue normal saline
 B. Ringer's lactate
 C. Free water by mouth
 D. Half-normal saline
 E. Half-normal saline and D5W

The answer is C

The patient requires free-water repletion. In a mentally alert patient, oral ingestion of water is strongly advised. In other patients, IV administration of D5W is preferred. In a diabetic patient, 0.45% (half-normal saline) is

preferable. The rate of correction (decrease) should not exceed 10–12 mEq/L/24 h. However, a maximum safe rate of correction for chronic hypernatremia has not been established in adult patients. However, a retrospective study of 250 patients with chronic hypernatremia suggested that a 30-day mortality was similar in those who had rapid correction of Na^+ >12 mEq/L in 24 h compared to those who had <12 mEq/L of correction in 24 h. It seems that chronic hypernatremic patients behave differently than those of hyponatremic patients in terms of Na^+ correction in a 24-h period.

Suggested Reading

Chauhan K, Pattharanitima P, Patel N, et al. Rate of correction of hypernatremia and health outcomes in critically ill patients. Clin J Am Soc Nephrol. 2019;14:656–63.

Reddi AS. Disorders of water balance: hypernatremia. In: Reddi AS, editor. Fluid, electrolyte and acid-base disorders. Clinical evaluation and management. 2nd ed. New York: Springer; 2018. p. 147–64.

Thurman JM, Berl T. Disorders of water metabolism. In: Mount DB, Sayegh MH, Singh AJ, editors. Core concepts in the disorders of fluid, electrolytes and acid-base balance. New York: Springer; 2013. p. 29–48.

43. Following water intake, the urine output improved to 1.4 L/day. His weight remains at 70 kg. Labs show:

$$\begin{aligned}
&Na^+ = 166\,mEq/L\\
&K^+ = 3.9\,mEq/L\\
&Cl^- = 115\,mEq/L\\
&HCO_3^- = 26\,mEq/L\\
&\text{Creatinine} = 1.5\,mg/dL\\
&\text{BUN} = 40\,mg/dl\\
&\text{Glucose} = 100\,mg/dL\\
&\text{Serum osmolality} = 351\,mOsm/kg\,H_2O\\
&\text{Urine osmolality} = 331\,mOsm/kg\,H_2O\\
&\text{Urine } Na^+ = 50\,mEq/L\\
&\text{Urine } K^+ = 32\,mEq/L\\
&\text{Urine volume/day} = 1.4\,L
\end{aligned}$$

Assuming daily insensible loss of 900 mL, which one of the following amounts of fluid that is required to lower serum [Na^+] from 166 mEq/L to 154 mEq/L in a 24-h period?

A. 3.0 L
B. 4.0 L
C. 5.0 L
D. 6.0 L
E. 7.0 L

The answer is C

In order to lower serum [Na^+] from 166 to 154 mEq/L (a 12 mEq/L drop), you need to include three components of fluid:

1. **Total fluid deficit**
2. **Electrolyte free water clearance**
3. **Insensible loss**

Total fluid deficit can be easily calculated at bed side from the rough estimate of Sterns and Silver (QJM 96:549–552, 2003), using 4 mL/kg × 12 mEq/L. This gives a fluid deficit of 3.36 L (70 × 4 × 12 = 3.36 L).

Electrolyte free water clearance (T^e_{CH2O}) can be calculated by the following formula:

$$\mathbf{T^e{}_{CH2O} = V\left(1 - \left(U_{Na} + U_K\right)/P_{Na}\right)}$$

where V is urine volume/day, U_{Na}, U_K, and P_{Na} are urine Na^+, K^+, and plasma Na^+ concentrations in mEq/L. Substituting the data from the patient, we obtain:

$$T^e_{CH2O} = 1.4\left(1-\left(50+32\right)/166\right) = 0.71\,L$$

$$\text{Insensible loss} = 0.9\,L\left(900\,mL/day\right)$$

Total amount of fluid needed to lower serum [Na^+] from 166 to 154 mEq/L is:

$$3.36 + 0.71 + 0.9 = 4.97\,L.\text{Thus, answer C is correct.}$$

Suggested Reading

Popli S, Tzamaloukas AH, Ing TS. Osmotic diuresis-induced hypernatremia: better explained by solute-free water clearance or electrolyte-free water clearance? Int Urol Nephrol. 2014;46:207–10.

Rose BD. New approaches to disturbances in the plasma sodium concentration. Am J Med. 1986;81:1033–40.

44. A 1-week-old boy was brought to the Emergency Department for irritability, polyuria, vomiting milk soon after ingestion, dehydration, hypernatremia, and hyperthermia. The patient responds adequately to volume replacement. **Which one of the following statements regarding this infant is FALSE?**

    A. The clinical presentation is consistent with the diagnosis of X-linked nephrogenic diabetes insipidus (NDI)
    B. X-linked NDI is due to loss-of-function mutation in vasopressin V2 receptor (AVPR2)
    C. Dehydration in infants with X-linked NDI can be so severe that can lead to low BP and impairment in oxygenation to the kidneys, brain, and other organs
    D. The clinical presentation is consistent with NDI due to mutations in the aquaporin 2 (AQP2) gene
    E. Combination of a thiazide diuretic and indomethacin is the most effective therapy to improve polyuria

The answer is D

All options other than D are consistent with the diagnosis of X-linked NDI. The other form of congenital NDI has either autosomal dominant or recessive mode of inheritance (10% of cases) and is caused by loss-of-function mutation of AQP gene. Polyuria, dehydration, and hypernatremia are also common in this form of congenital DI.

Suggested Reading

Christ-Crain M, Bichet DG, Fenske WK. Diabetes insipidus. Nat Rev Dis Premere. 2019;5:54 (1–20).

Reddi AS. Disorders of water balance: hypernatremia. In: Reddi AS, editor. Fluid, electrolyte and acid-base disorders. Clinical evaluation and management. 2nd ed. New York: Springer; 2018. p. 147–64.

Sands JM, Bichet DG. Nephrogenic diabetes insipidus. Ann Intern Med. 2006;144:186–94.

45. A 36-year-old man is admitted for nausea, vomiting, confusion, and gait disturbances. He is on lithium for bipolar disorder and Lisinopril 40 mg for hypertension. His sister says that he has frequent urination. He is hypotensive and serum Na^+ concentration is 152 mEq/L with creatinine of 2.4 mg/dL. Serum lithium (Li) level is 3.8 mEq/L (therapeutic level 0.8–1.2 mEq/L). Urine osmolality is 350 mOsm/kg H_2O. **Which one of the following is APPROPRIATE in the management of Li toxicity?**

    A. Hydration with normal saline
    B. Discontinue lisinopril
    C. Start hemodialysis (HD) following adequate hydration and stabilization of patient
    D. Discontinue HD once serum Li <1 mEq/L
    E. All of the above

The answer is E

Li is frequently used for the treatment of bipolar disorder. However, the therapeutic and toxic range is very narrow. Li is handled by the kidney similar to that of Na^+. Any condition that reduces glomerular filtration rate (GFR) increases serum Li levels.

In this patient, treatment of hypertension by lisinopril may have reduced his GFR. His frequent urination and urine osmolality suggest that he developed Li-induced nephrogenic diabetes insipidus. The management includes

volume replacement with 0.9% saline, which improves blood pressure and urinary excretion of Li. Lisinopril should be discontinued. After stabilizing the patient, commencing HD is appropriate. HD is effective as Li is easily dializable because it is water soluble and minimally protein-bound and has low apparent volume of distribution. HD should be discontinued once Li levels are <1 mEq/L. Rebound of Li is rather common; therefore, frequent determination of Li levels is necessary. Thus, all answers are correct.

Suggested Reading

Haussmann R, Bauer M, von Bonin, et al. Treatment of lithium intoxication: facing the need for evidence. Int J Bipolar Disord. 2015;5(23):1–5.
Timmer RT, Sands JM. Lithium intoxication. J Am Soc Nephrol. 1999;10:666–74.

46. **Which one of the following drugs is useful in the management of lithium (Li)-induced nephrogenic diabetes insipidus (NDI)?**

   A. Hydrochlorothiazide (HCTZ)
   B. Lisinopril
   C. Nonsteroidal anti-inflammatory drugs (NSAIDs)
   D. Amiloride
   E. None of the above

The answer is D

Li causes polyuria, polydipsia, and inability to concentrate the urine. Thus, patients become volume depleted. Therefore, patients must consume water to prevent volume depletion. HCTZ causes volume depletion by promoting excretion of solute and water. As a result, Li is absorbed in the proximal tubule causing high serum levels of Li. HCTZ also causes hypokalemia, which can perpetuate NDI. ACE-Is such as lisinopril may lower GFR and can impair Li excretion. Similar to ACE-Is, NSAIDs also decrease GFR with resultant decrease in excretion of Li. Thus, answers A to C are incorrect.

Amiloride is the drug of choice for LI-induced NDI. It reduces the uptake of Li since it blocks sodium epithelial channel (ENaC), thereby reducing the incidence of Li overdose unless the patient develops acute or chronic kidney injury. Amiloride also reduces urine volume with chronic Li use. Thus, answer D is correct.

Suggested Reading

Haussmann R, Bauer M, von Bonin, et al. Treatment of lithium intoxication: facing the need for evidence. Int J Bipolar Disord. 2015;5(23):1–5.
Timmer RT, Sands JM. Lithium intoxication. J Am Soc Nephrol. 1999;10:666–74.

47. A 76-year-old man is admitted from a nursing home for evaluation of persistent hypernatremia and mild confusion. He was admitted previously with similar presentation. He has a history of stroke with full recovery. An MRI done during previous admission showed no hypothalamic or pituitary lesions. On the transfer note, the nurse mentioned that he never asks for water, and water in the pitcher is always full. On physical examination, he is found to be slightly confused but oriented to place. Except for orthostatic blood pressure and pulse changes, the rest of the examination is normal. Serum [Na^+] before stroke was normal. Pertinent labs:

$$\text{Serum Na}^+ = 154\,\text{mEq/L}$$
$$\text{Serum osmolality} = 346\,\text{mOsm/kg H}_2\text{O}$$
$$\text{Urine osmolality} = 606\,\text{mOsm/kg H}_2\text{O}$$

He received 2 L of normal saline with improvement in blood pressure and pulse. He subsequently drank another 2 L of water. His repeat labs:

$$\text{Serum Na}^+ = 146\,\text{mEq/L}$$
$$\text{Serum osmolality} = 302\,\text{mOsm/kg H}_2\text{O}$$
$$\text{Urine osmolality} = 308\,\text{mOsm/kg H}_2\text{O}$$

Based on the above labs before and after hydration, the diagnosis of hypodipsic hypernatremia was made. **Which one of the following daily prescriptions is the MOST appropriate for this patient?**

A. Normal saline
B. D5W (5% dextrose in water)
C. 0.45% saline
D. Encourage water intake
E. Mandatory pharmacologic order of water intake

The answer is E

This patient carries the diagnosis of hypodipsic (adipsic) hypernatremia, which is characterized by absent or inadequate sensation of thirst with decreased water intake despite water availability. It arises as a result of complete or partial destruction of osmoreceptors for thirst. ADH release to osmotic stimuli may be normal or blunted, but response to nonosmotic stimuli (hypovolemia, hypotension, nausea) is preserved. These hypodipsic patients develop not only hypernatremia, hyperosmolality but also a decrease in blood volume and elevated blood urea nitrogen. Patients with mild hypernatremia can present with confusion and drowsiness, whereas those with severe hypernatremia can develop seizures, rhabdomyolysis, and coma. Hypodipsic patients have been shown to have pathologic lesions in the brain such as neoplastic, nonneoplastic, granulomatous, vascular, or other lesions.

This patient's serum [Na^+] was normal before he had stroke, but his thirst mechanism has been lost after stroke. However, he was able to suppress his ADH and capable of diluting urine following hydration.

The appropriate management of his serum Na^+ level is not simply encouraging water intake but writing a mandatory pharmacologic order of a specific amount of water after documenting urine output and insensible loss. Thus, answer E is correct. Other answers are not appropriate for this patient.

Suggested Reading

Miller PD, Krebs RA, Neal BJ, et al. Hypodipsia in geriatric patients. Am J Med. 1982;73:354–6.
Phiilips PA, Rolls BJ, Ledingham JGG, et al. Reduced thirst after water deprivation in healthy elderly men. N Engl J Med. 1984;311:753–9.
Reddi AS. Disorders of water balance: hypernatremia. In: Reddi AS, editor. Fluid, electrolyte and acid-base disorders. Clinical evaluation and management. 2nd ed. New York: Springer; 2018. p. 147–64.

48. A 46-year-old woman is admitted for polyuria, polydipsia, and nocturia. She fulfills her thirst mostly with ice water. Her serum [Na^+] is 158 mEq/L with urine osmolality of 98 mOsm/kg H_2O. **Which one of the following urine osmolalities (mOsm/kg H_2O) is consistent with her diagnosis?**

	Osmolality (mOsm) before dehydration	**Osmolality (mOsm) after 12-h dehydration**	**Osmolality (mOsm) after vasopressin**
A	600	1100	1080
B	100	120	360
C	180	350	500
D	300	310	314
E	120	500	520

The answer is B

Based on the history and urine osmolality, the patient has central diabetes insipidus (CDI). Option B is consistent with CDI. Options A, C, D, and E are consistent with normal subject, partial CDI, nephrogenic DI, and psychogenic polydipsia, respectively.

Suggested Reading

Oster JR, Singer I, Thatte L, et al. The polyuria of solute diuresis. Arch Intern Med. 1997;157:721–9.
Reddi AS. Disorders of water balance: hypernatremia. In: Reddi AS, editor. Fluid, electrolyte and acid-base disorders. Clinical evaluation and management. 2nd ed. New York: Springer; 2018. p. 147–64.

49. A 24-year-old pregnant woman in her third trimester was admitted for polyuria (urine volume 4.2 L/day). Her serum [Na^+] is 146 mEq/L with urine osmolality of 114 mOsm/kg H_2O. Polyuria improves only transiently despite administration of vasopressin. **Which one of the following treatments is APPROPRIATE to improve both polyuria and hypernatremia?**

    A. Increase vasopressin dose to 50 U twice daily
    B. Limit fluid intake to improve polyuria
    C. Match intake and output to maintain fluid status
    D. Administer dDAVP to improve polyuria
    E. Do nothing until delivery

    The answer is D

    Infrequently, pregnant women in their late gestation develop polyuria, thirst, and polydipsia. The urine is dilute, and vasopressin administration transiently increases the osmolality; however, vasopressin levels decrease within 30 min due to degradation by the enzyme, vasopressinase. This enzyme is produced by the placenta, and women with polyuria have high circulating levels of vasopressinase. Polyuria, which is called transient diabetes insipidus of pregnancy, disappears after delivery. Vasopressinase degrades vasopressin, but not its synthetic analogue dDAVP (desmopressin). Therefore, women with transient diabetes insipidus of pregnancy respond to treatment with dDAVP. Thus, option D is correct. Other options are inappropriate for this woman.

    Suggested Reading

Ananthakrishnan S. Diabetes insipidus during pregnancy. Best Pract Res Clin Endocrinol Metab. 2016;30:305–15.
Durr A, Hoggard JG, Hunt JM, Schrier RW. Diabetes insipidus in pregnancy associated with abnormally high circulating vasopressinase activity. N Engl J Med. 1987;316:1070–4.

50. A 54-year-old man with subarachnoid hematoma was seen in neurosurgery unit for hypernatremia and polyuria. He was on several i.v. drips for control of hypertension and high protein supplementation. He weighs 80 kg. Pertinent labs: Na^+ 158 mEq/L, K^+ 3.6 mEq/L, Cl^- 112 mEq/L, HCO_3^- 24 mEq/L, creatinine 1.4 mg/dL, BUN 24 mg/dL, and glucose 98 mg/dL. Urine studies: volume 5 L/day, osmolality 420 mOsm/kg H_2O, Na^+ 100 mEq/L, K^+ 40 mEq/L, and urea nitrogen 350 mg/dL. **Which one of the following choices is appropriate to decrease urine output?**

    A. Desmopressin 1 μg subcutaneously Q12-h
    B. Desmopressin 1 μg i.v. Q12-h
    C. Hydrochlorothiazide (HCTZ) 25 mg daily
    D. Decrease solute load
    E. Restrict fluid intake

    The answer is D

    Based on urine osmolality, the patient has solute diuresis (see Fig. 1.5). Polyuria is related to very large administration of solute in the form of saline and protein. This is clearly evident from urine osmolality of 420 mOsm/kg H_2O. When this osmolality is multiplied by urine output of 5 L, the patient is excreting 2100 (420 × 5 = 2100)

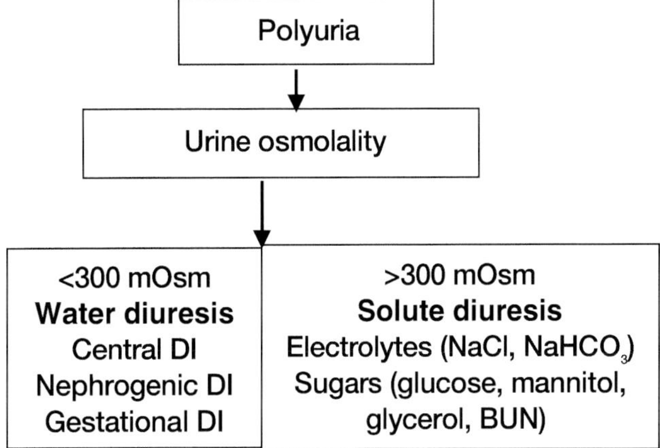

Fig. 1.5 Diagnostic approach to the patient with polyuria

mOsm/day. This is a large solute load, which obligates a high urine output. Therefore, reducing solute load is important in decreasing urine output. Desmopressin may transiently decrease urine output, but this is not a correct way of managing this condition. Fluid restriction may lower urine output, but worsens hypernatremia. HCTZ may be helpful transiently, but not as effective as reducing solute load. Thus, answer D is correct.

The millimoles that are excreted can also be calculated from urine chemistry, as follows:

$$\begin{aligned}
&\textbf{Urine volume} = 5\,\text{L}\\
&\textbf{Urine Na}^{+} = 100\,\text{mEq / L or } 500\,\text{mEq / total volume}\\
&\textbf{Urine K}^{+} = 40\,\text{mEq / L or } 200\,\text{mEq / total volume}\\
&\textbf{Urine urea nitrogen} = 350\,\text{mg / dL or } 3{,}500\,\text{mg / L or } 17{,}500\,(17.5\,\text{g}) / \text{total volume}\\
&\textbf{Milliosmoles generated from urea nitrogen} = 17.5\,\text{g} / 28 / \text{mol} = 0.625\,\text{mol or } 625\,\text{mmol / day},\\
&\quad \text{where } 28 \text{ is molecular weight of urea nitrogen}\\
&\textbf{Total osmolar excretion} = (\text{total urine Na}^{+} + \text{total urine K}^{+})\,2 + \text{mosmol from urea nitrogen}\\
&\qquad = (500 + 200)\,2 = 1{,}400 + 625 = 2{,}025, \text{ where 2 used for total anions excreted with cations}
\end{aligned}$$

The total osmolar excretion can be calculated easily by multiplying urine osmolality by total urine volume, as shown above. Both calculations yield approximately similar values.

Total protein administration can be calculated as follows:

$$\begin{aligned}
&\textbf{Total protein intake} = \text{Urinary urea nitrogen} + \text{Nonurea nitrogen excretion}\,(0.031\,\text{g / kg})\\
&\textbf{This patient's urea nitrogen excretion} = 17.5\,\text{g}\\
&\textbf{Patient's weight} = 80\,\text{kg}\\
&\textbf{Nonurea nitrogen excretion} = 0.031 \times 80 = 2.48\,\text{g}\\
&\textbf{Total nitrogen excretion} = 17.5 + 2.48 = 19.98\\
&\textbf{1 g urea nitrogen} = 6.25\,\text{g protein (or protein content is } 16\%\text{ of urea nitrogen)}
\end{aligned}$$

Therefore, total administration of protein in this patient = 19.98 × 6.25 = 124.9 g/day

Suggested Reading

Berl T. The impact of solute intake on urine flow and water excretion. J Am Soc Nephrol. 2008;19:1076–8.

Bhasin B, Velez JCQ. Evaluation of polyuria: the roles of solute loading and water diuresis. Am J Kidney Dis. 2016;67:507–11.

Potassium and Acid-Base Disorders

1. A 42-year-old woman was seen by her primary care physician (PCP) for routine physical check-up in the middle of July. Two days later, she was called by her PCP and informed that her serum [K^+] is low (3.2 mEq/L), and a repeat test is necessary. She told her PCP that she eats a regular diet with lot of fruits and she does not have any vomiting or diarrhea. **What would be the reason for her relative hypokalemia?**

   A. Laboratory error
   B. Seasonal pseudohypokalemia
   C. False history of eating regular diet and fruits
   D. Increased red blood cell (RBC) count
   E. A and D

   The answer is B

   Pseudohypokalemia is rather rare. However, it has been described at least in two conditions: (1) in patients with high white blood cell (WBC) count; and (2) in summer months with high ambient temperature. Both conditions seem to increase K^+ uptake and also stimulate glucose metabolism. Pseudohypokalemia has been reported in patients with myeloproliferative disorders. Delayed analysis of the blood sample (prolonged time between

collection of blood and the time of determination) seems to be the reason for hypokalemia. Increased RBCs may release K^+ by hemolysis, causing hyperkalemia. Spurious hypokalemia does not have any clinical consequences. Thus, answer B is correct.

Suggesting Reading

Maters PW, Lawson N, Marenah CB, et al. High ambient temperature: a spurious cause of hypokalemia. BMJ. 1996;312:1653–9.

Naparstek Y, Gutman A. Case report: spurious hypokalemia in myeloproliferative disorders. Am J Med Sci. 1984;288:175–7.

Sodi R, Davison AS, Holmes E, et al. The phenomenon of seasonal pseudohypokalemia: effects of ambient temperature, plasma glucose and role for sodium–potassium-exchanging-ATPase. Clin Chem. 2009;42:813–8.

2. A 24-year-old Asian woman is admitted for weakness and inability to get up from bed in the morning. These symptoms started following a birthday party last night. She has no significant medical history and does not take any medication. Serum chemistry is normal except for [K^+] of 2.4 mEq/L. Her sister had a similar episode 2 months ago, and the symptoms resolved spontaneously. The diagnosis of familial hypokalemic periodic paralysis (HypoPP) is considered in this patient. **Which one of the following statements is FALSE regarding familial HypoPP?**

   A. The most common familial form (60–70%), an autosomal dominant disorder, is due to mutations in the muscle Ca^{2+} channel α1 subunit gene
   B. A smaller number (10–20%) of the familial form of the disorder is due to mutations in the skeletal muscle Na^+ channel
   C. Carbonic anhydrase inhibitor frequently reduces the number of paralysis attacks in patients with familial hypoPP
   D. High carbohydrate intake precipitates paralytic attacks in many Asian population
   E. Paralytic attacks are best treated with IV infusion of KCl at the rate of 30 mEq/h

   The answer is E

   All of the above statements other than E are correct for familial hypoPP. It is prudent to infuse KCl at a rate of 10 mEq/h in order to avoid rebound hyperkalemia.

   Suggested Reading

Fialho D, Griggs RC, Matthews E. Handb Clin Neurol. 2018;148:505–20.

Fontaine B. Periodic paralysis. Adv Genet. 2008;63:3–23.

3. An 18-year-old male comes to the Emergency Department with a complaint of severe muscle weakness and dizziness. His systolic BP is 94 mm Hg with orthostatic change. He says that he craves for Chinese food with added salt. He is not on any medications, and he does not use any illicit drugs. He complains of arthritic-like knee pain. X-rays of the knees shows Ca^{2+} deposition. Pertinent laboratory results:

Serum	Urine (24 h)
Na^+ = 137 mEq/L	Na^+ = 120 mEq/L
K^+ = 2.9 mEq/L	K^+ = 80 mEq/L
Cl^- = 84 mEq/L	Ca^{2+} = 50 mg/dL
HCO_3^- = 30 mEq/L	pH = 6.2
Ca^{2+} = 8.5 mg/dL	Osmolality = 300 mOs/kg H_2O
Mg^{2+} = 0.8 mg/dL	Diuretic screening = negative
Blood pH = 7.48	

   Which one of the following disorders is the MOST likely diagnosis in this patient?

   A. Bartter syndrome with mutation in ROMK channel (type 2)
   B. Liddle syndrome
   C. Gitelman syndrome
   D. Hereditary mineralocorticoid excess syndrome
   E. Acquired mineralocorticoid excess syndrome

   The answer is C

Based on the blood pressure, options B, D, and E can be excluded, as these disorders are characterized by hypertension. Type 2 Bartter syndrome and Gitelman syndrome are characterized by hypokalemia, metabolic alkalosis, and hypo- or normal blood pressure. Type 2 Bartter syndrome is usually present in neonates, whereas Gitelman syndrome occurs in adolescents. Thus, the patient described above has Gitelman syndrome, as his urine Ca^{2+} excretion is low. In Bartter syndrome, Ca^{2+} excretion is normal to high. Patients with Gitelman syndrome have hypomagnesemia due to increased loss of Mg^{2+} in the urine. The patient's dizziness is related to volume depletion caused by Na^{+} diuresis.

Suggested Reading

Al Shibli A, Narchi H. Bartter and Gitelman syndromes: spectrum of clinical manifestations caused by different mutations. World J Methodol. 2015;5:55–61.

Bonnardeaux A, Bichet DG. Inherited disorders of the renal tubule. In: Yu ASL, Chertow GM, Luyckx VA, et al., editors. Brenner & Rector's the kidney. 11th ed. Philadelphia: Elsevier Saunders; 2020. p. 1450–89.

Kleta R, Bockenhaur D. Salt-losing nephropathies in children: what's new, what's controversial? J Am Soc Nephrol. 2018;29:727–39.

Seyberth HW. Pathophysiology and clinical presentations of salt-losing tubulopathies. Pediatr Nephrol. 2016;31:407–18.

4. **Which one of the following strategies in the management of the above patient is CORRECT?**

   A. High salt intake
   B. KCl
   C. Mg sulfate
   D. Eplerenone
   E. All of the above

   The answer is E

   This patient needs lifelong supplementation of high salt intake, KCl, and $MgCl_2$ (magnesium sulfate or magnesium oxide, which causes more diarrhea than magnesium chloride). Eplerenone (spironolactone-receptor blocker) seems better than either spironolactone or amiloride to maintain serum normal [K^{+}].

   Suggested Reading

Al Shibli A, Narchi H. Bartter and Gitelman syndromes: spectrum of clinical manifestations caused by different mutations. World J Methodol. 2015;5:55–61.

Bonnardeaux A, Bichet DG. Inherited disorders of the renal tubule. In: Yu ASL, Chertow GM, Luyckx VA, et al., editors. Brenner & Rector's the kidney. 11th ed. Philadelphia: Elsevier Saunders; 2020. p. 1450–89.

Kleta R, Bockenhaur D. Salt-losing nephropathies in children: what's new, what's controversial? J Am Soc Nephrol. 2018;29:727–39.

Koulouridis E, Koulouridis I. Molecular pathophysiology of Bartter's and Gitelman's syndromes. World J Pediatr. 2015;11:113–25.

Seyberth HW. Pathophysiology and clinical presentations of salt-losing tubulopathies. Pediatr Nephrol. 2016;31:407–18.

5. A 1-month-old child is admitted for severe volume depletion. History of the child includes polyhydramnios, premature birth, episodes of salt and water loss in the neonatal period, hypokalemic metabolic alkalosis, hypercalciuria, and early onset nephrocalcinosis. **Which one of the following transporter mutations characterizes the above clinical manifestations of the child?**

   A. Na/Cl cotransporter in distal convoluted tubule (DCT)
   B. Na/K/2Cl cotransporter in thick ascending limb of Henle's loop (TALH)
   C. Basolateral Cl channel (ClC-kb) of TALH
   D. Renal outer medullary K channel (ROMK) of TALH
   E. Basolateral calcium-sensing receptor (CaSR) of TALH

   The answer is B

   The history and clinical presentation suggests the diagnosis of type 1 Bartter syndrome (BS), which is due to mutation in Na/K/2Cl cotransporter located in TALH. Thus, answer B is correct. Mutation in Na/Cl cotransporter causes Gitelman syndrome. Other types of BS are shown in Table 1.2. Other answers are, therefore, incorrect.

Table 1.2 Types of Bartter syndrome

Type of transporter	Disease	Some clinical features	Inheritance
Apical Na/K/2Cl cotransporter	Neonatal Bartter syndrome type 1	Hypokalemia, metabolic alkalosis, hypercalciuria, hypotension	AR
Apical K channel (ROMK)	Neonatal Bartter syndrome type 2	Hypokalemia, metabolic alkalosis, hypotension	AR
Basolateral Cl channel (ClC-kb)	Classic Bartter syndrome type 3 (infantile)	Hypokalemia, metabolic alkalosis, hypotension, or normal BP	AR
Basolateral Cl channel (ClC-kb/barttin)	Bartter syndrome type 4	Hypokalemia, metabolic alkalosis, hypotension, sensorineural deafness	AR
Activation of basolateral Ca^{2+}-sensing receptor	Bartter syndrome type 5	Salt wasting, hypokalemia, metabolic alkalosis, hypercalciuria	AD

AR autosomal recessive, *AD* autosomal dominant

Suggested Reading

Al Shibli A, Narchi H. Bartter and Gitelman syndromes: spectrum of clinical manifestations caused by different mutations. World J Methodol. 2015;5:55–61.

Bonnardeaux A, Bichet DG. Inherited disorders of the renal tubule. In: Yu ASL, Chertow GM, Luyckx VA, et al., editors. Brenner & Rector's the kidney. 11th ed. Philadelphia: Elsevier Saunders; 2020. p. 1450–89.

Kleta R, Bockenhaur D. Salt-losing nephropathies in children: what's new, what's controversial? J Am Soc Nephrol. 2018;29:727–39.

Koulouridis E, Koulouridis I. Molecular pathophysiology of Bartter's and Gitelman's syndromes. World J Pediatr. 2015;11:113–25.

Seyberth HW. Pathophysiology and clinical presentations of salt-losing tubulopathies. Pediatr Nephrol. 2016;31:407–18.

6. A 30-year-old man visits the Emergency Department with acute exacerbation of asthma. **Which one of the following drugs does NOT cause hypokalemia?**

   A. Insulin
   B. β_2-agonists
   C. Clenbuterol
   D. Propranolol
   E. Gentamicin

   The answer is D

   Insulin, β_2-agonists, and clenbuterol promote K^+ from extracellular to intracellular compartment, whereas gentamicin binds to Ca^{2+}-sensing receptor located at the basolateral membrane of the thick ascending limb of Henle's loop, causing inhibition of ROMK channel. This results in urinary K^+ loss and hypokalemia. Propranolol is a nonspecific β-adrenergic antagonist, causing elevation in serum [K^+]. Thus, choice D is correct.

Suggested Reading

Reddi AS. Disorders of potassium: hypokalemia. In: Reddi AS, editor. Fluid, electrolyte, and acid-base disorders. Clinical evaluation and management. 2nd ed. New York: Springer; 2018. p. 175–91.

7. A 26-year-old man is seen in the Emergency Department for anxiety, palpitations, tachypnea following heroin intake with his friends. He is alert, oriented, afebrile without any respiratory distress. His pupils are normal. Blood pressure and pulse rate are 110/70 and 114 per min, respectively. Labs: Na^+ 140 mEq/L, K^+ 2.6 mEq/L, Cl^- 106 mEq/L, HCO_3^- 24 mEq/L, creatinine 0.9 mg/dl, BUN 16 mg/dl, and glucose 164 mg/dl. EKG shows prolonged QT interval and Q waves without ST segment changes. Troponin levels are normal. Urine drug screen is positive only for opiates. He refuses naloxone, as he says that his symptoms are not related to heroin alone. **Which one the following is the MOST likely cause of his hypokalemia?**

   A. Caffeine
   B. Theophylline
   C. Clenbuterol-tainted heroin
   D. Cocaine and heroin
   E. None of the above

The answer is C

The patient does not demonstrate classic symptoms of heroin abuse, such as CNS and respiratory depression, miosis, or bradycardia. Although caffeine and theophylline can cause hypokalemia by cellular shift, urine toxicology was negative for these substances. Clenbuterol is a β_2-agonist that is approved to treat bronchospasm in the horse. In addition, clenbuterol has been shown to increase muscle mass while simultaneously decreasing fat mass in lambs, horses, broiler chickens, and steers. Clenbuterol is similar to salbutamol, and it has been used as a bronchodilator in humans in Europe. Because of its anabolic and lipolytic effects, clenbuterol has been used by body builders illicitly to gain muscle mass. In the United States, foods-containing clenbuterol have been banned.

In 2005, the CDC reported 26 suspected or confirmed cases of clenbuterol-tainted heroin in New Jersey, New York, Connecticut, and North and South Carolina. Because of its β_2-adrenergic effects, clenbuterol causes profound hypokalemia by shifting K^+ into the cell. It is not known whether heroin is sold in the street as heroin tainted with clenbuterol or clenbuterol sold as heroin. Thus, choice C is correct.

The combination of cocaine and heroin rarely causes hypokalemia unless a β_2-adrenergic drug is contaminated. Thus, answers D and E are incorrect.

Suggested Reading

Kearns CF, McKeever KH. Clenbuterol and the horse revisited. Vet J. 2009;182:384–9.

Koopman R, Ryall JG, Church JE, et al. The role of beta-adrenoceptor signaling in skeletal muscle: therapeutic implications for muscle wasting disorders. Curr Opin Nutr Metab Care. 2009;12:601–6.

Reddi AS. Disorders of potassium: hypokalemia. In: Reddi AS, editor. Fluid, electrolyte, and acid-base disorders. Clinical evaluation and management. 2nd ed. New York: Springer; 2018. p. 175–91.

8. **Which one of the following electrolyte abnormalities may precipitate hepatic encephalopathy?**

   A. Hypercalcemia
   B. Hypocalcemia
   C. Hypomagnesemia
   D. Hyperkalemia
   E. Hypokalemia

The answer is E

Patients with hepatic encephalopathy have increased circulating levels of NH_3. During the conversion of glutamine to glutamate, NH_3 is formed. This reaction is catalyzed by the enzyme phosphate-dependent glutaminase (PDG). Hypokalemia stimulates the activity of this enzyme, resulting in high levels of NH_3 with resultant precipitation of hepatic encephalopathy. Thus, answer E is correct. On the other hand, hyperkalemia inhibits PDG. As a result, NH_3 production is decreased. The other electrolyte abnormalities have little or no significant effect on NH_3 production.

Suggested Reading

Abu Hossain S, Chaudhry FA, Zahedi K, et al. Cellular and molecular basis of increased ammoniagenesis in potassium deprivation. Am J Physiol Renal Physiol. 2011;301:F969–76.

Fraley DS, Adler S, Rankin B, et al. Relationship of phosphate-dependent glutaminase activity to ammonia excretion in potassium deficiency and acidosis. Miner Electrolyte Metab. 1985;11:140–9.

Gaduputi V, Chandrala C, Abbas N, et al. Prognostic significance of hypokalemia in hepatic encephalopathy. Hepatogastroenterology. 2014;61:1170–4.

9. A 27-year-old man is admitted for headache, shortness of breath, and chest pain for 4 days. He has a family history of hypertension (HTN). His blood pressure (BP) is 180/100 mm Hg, pulse rate of 64 beats/min. He is on three antihypertensive medications, including a thiazide diuretic. He has no orthostatic changes. Pertinent labs:

$$Na^+ = 148\,mEq/L$$
$$K^+ = 2.8\,mEq/L$$
$$Cl^- = 90\,mEq/L$$
$$HCO_3^- = 32\,mEq/L$$
$$BUN = 22\,mg/dL$$
$$Creatinine = 1.8\,mg/dL$$
$$Glucose = 80\,mg/dL$$
$$Venous\ blood\ pH = 7.47$$
$$Plasma\ renin\ activity = <1\,ng/mL/h\,(normal\ 0.2-1.6\,ng/mL/h)$$
$$Plasma\ aldosterone\ activity = 150\,ng/dL\,(normal\ 3-16\,ng/dL)$$

Which one of the following diagnoses is MOST likely in this patient?

A. Type 1 Bartter syndrome
B. Gitelman syndrome
C. Liddle syndrome
D. Renal artery stenosis
E. Primary aldosteronism

The answer is E

BP and plasma renin and aldosterone levels are extremely important in making the diagnosis in this patient. Bartter and Gitelman syndromes are associated with low to normal BP. Therefore, answers A and B are incorrect. Liddle syndrome needs to be considered, but both plasma renin and aldosterone are low in this condition. Renal artery stenosis is also likely, but it is associated with high plasma renin and aldosterone levels. Thus, answers C and D are incorrect.

Primary aldosteronism is the most likely diagnosis in this patient, which presents with HTN, low renin and high aldosterone levels. Aldosterone to renin ratio is very high. High levels of aldosterone are due to increased secretion of this hormone by either adrenal cortical adenoma or bilateral hyperplasia of the gland. Aldosterone promotes Na^+ reabsorption and K^+ secretion in the distal nephron. As a result, plasma volume is increased with an increase in serum [Na^+] and volume-dependent HTN. Hypernatremia may also be caused by relative suppression of ADH due to volume expansion. Plasma renin level is low because of volume expansion; however, aldosterone levels are high due to autonomous secretion of this hormone by the adenoma or bilateral hyperplasia of the adrenal gland. Primary aldosteronism is commonly seen in young patients with refractory hypertension (HTN), hypokalemia, hypernatremia, and saline-resistant metabolic alkalosis. Spironolactone or amiloride is the drug of choice for HTN management. Thus, answer E is correct.

BP and pertinent serum values are summarized in Table 1.3 for the patients described above.

Table 1.3 BP and pertinent serum values of patients discussed in question 10

Disease	BP	Na^+	K^+	HCO_3^-	Renin	Aldosterone
Type 1 Bartter syndrome	↓/N	↓/N	↓	↑	↑	↑
Gitelman syndrome	↓/N	↓/N	↓	↑	↑	↑
Liddle syndrome	↑	N/↑	↓	↑	↓	↓
Renal artery stenosis	↑	↓	↓	↑	↑	↑
Primary aldosteronism	↑	↑	↓	↑	↓	↑

↑ increase, ↓ decrease, *BP* blood pressure, *N* normal

Suggested Reading

Byrd JB, Turcu AF, Auchus RJ. Primary aldosteronism. Practical approach to diagnosis and management. Circulation. 2018;138:823–35.

Funder JW, Carey RM, Mantero F, et al. The management of primary aldosteronism: case detection, diagnosis, and treatment: An Endocrine Society clinical practice guideline. J Clin Endocrinol Metab. 2016;101:1889–916.

Kumar B, Swee M. Aldosterone-renin ratio in the assessment of primary aldosteronism. JAMA. 2014;312:184–5.

Maiolini G, Rossitto G, Bisogni V, et al. Quantitative value of Aldosterone-Renin ratio for detection of Aldosterone-Producing Adenoma: The Aldosterone-Renin Ratio for Primary Aldosteronism (AQUARR) Study. J Am Heart Assoc. 2017;6:e005574. https://doi.org/10.1161/JAHA.117.005574.

Reddi AS. Disorders of potassium: hypokalemia. In: Reddi AS, editor. Fluid, electrolyte, and acid-base disorders. Clinical evaluation and management. 2nd ed. New York: Springer; 2018. p. 175–91.

10. **Match the following clinical histories of patients with the molecular defects:**

A. An 18-year-old man with low renin and aldosterone levels, hypokalemia, and severe hypertension, who responds to amiloride but unresponsive to spironolactone	1. Mutations in the cytoplasmic COOH-terminus of the β- and γ-subunits of the epithelial sodium channel (ENaC)126
B. A child with low renin-aldosterone levels, hypokalemia, severe hypertension, poor growth, short stature, and nephrocalcinosis	2. Loss-of-function mutations in 11β-hydroxysteroid dehydrogenase type 2 (11β-HSD2) enzyme
C. A 16-year-old man with mild hypertension, mild hypokalemia (3.4 mEq/L), and HCO_3^- concentration of 29 mEq/L. His hypertension is unresponsive to angiotensin converting enzyme-inhibitors (ACE-Is) and β-blockers, but responsive to glucocorticoids	3. A chimeric gene duplication from unequal crossover between 11β-hydroxylase and aldosterone synthase genes
D. A 20-year-old pregnant woman develops severe hypertension without proteinuria during her third trimester. Her 17-year-old brother is also hypertensive whose blood pressure rises on spironolactone	4. A missense mutation in mineralocorticoid receptor

Answers: A = 1; B = 2; C = 3; D = 4. The patient described in choice A has Liddle syndrome, which is an autosomal dominant disorder. It is caused by mutations in the cytoplasmic COOH-terminus of the β-and γ- subunits of the ENaC. Activation of this channel results in increased Na reabsorption with blunted Na excretion, hypokalemia, and low-renin-aldosterone hypertension. Hypertension (HTN) responds to triamterene or amiloride, but not to spironolactone. Affected patients are at increased risk for cerebrovascular and cardiovascular disease.

The child described in choice B carries the diagnosis of the syndrome of apparent mineralocorticoid excess (AME), which is a rare autosomal recessive disorder. It is due to a loss-of-function mutation in the gene encoding the enzyme 11β-hydroxysteroid dehydrogenase type 2 (11βHSD2). This enzyme converts cortisol to the inactive cortisone. As a consequence of the mutation, the 11β-HSD2 enzyme activity is decreased with resultant accumulation of cortisol. Cortisol acts like a mineralocorticoid by occupying its receptor, causing Na^+ reabsorption, hypokalemic metabolic alkalosis, and low-renin-aldosterone HTN. Suppression of renin and aldosterone is due to volume excess caused by Na^+ and water retention. Children with AME demonstrate low birth weight and nephrocalcinosis, the latter is due to hypokalemic nephropathy. HTN responds to salt restriction, amiloride, or triamterene but not to regular doses of spironolactone. Licorice ingestion induces a similar syndrome. Complications include cardiac events, including stroke and renal failure.

The clinical history described in choice C is consistent with the diagnosis of glucocorticoid-remediable hyperaldosteronism (GRA). This disorder, also called familial hyperaldosteronism type 1, is caused by a chimeric gene duplication from unequal crossover between aldosterone synthase and 11β-hydroxylase. Some patients with GRA may have severe HTN, hypokalemia, and metabolic alkalosis. Some other patients may have mild HTN, normal to low serum K^+, and mild increase in serum HCO_3^- concentrations. Plasma renin is suppressed, but aldosterone levels are increased. Aldosterone secretion is stimulated by ACTH and not by angiotensin II. Therefore, administration of glucocorticoid suppresses excessive aldosterone secretion and improves HTN.

The possible diagnosis of the patient presented in choice D is a case of early-onset HTN with severe exacerbation during pregnancy. This disorder is caused by an activating heterozygous missense mutation in the mineralocorticoid receptor (MR) gene called S810L mutation. Clinically the patient presents with HTN before age 20 years with low plasma K^+, renin and aldosterone levels. Pregnancy exacerbates HTN without proteinuria, edema, or neurologic changes. Aldosterone levels, which are elevated during pregnancy, are extremely low in MR gene mutation. MR antagonists such as spironolactone become agonists and increase blood pressure in patients with mutation in MR gene. Therefore, spironolactone is contraindicated in these patients. Progesterone also increases

blood pressure in patients with MR gene mutation, since this hormone levels are extremely high in these patients. It should be remembered that heterozygous loss-of-function mutations in the MR gene (locus symbol NR3C2) results in pseudohypoaldosteronism type I (PHA I), an autosomal disorder, that causes salt wasting and hypotension. This disease remits with age.

Suggesting Reading

Ehret GB. Genetics of hypertension. In: Bakris GL, Sorrentino MJ, editors. Hypertension. A companion to Braunwald's heart disease. 3rd ed. Philadelphia: Elsevier; 2018. p. 52–9.
Sarkar T, Singh NP. Epidemiology and genetics of hypertension. J Assoc Physicians India. 2015;63:61–8.

11. A 70-year-old woman with chronic kidney disease (CKD) stage 4 fell and sustained hip fracture. Following hip surgery, she developed watery diarrhea, which did not respond to fasting for 24 h. She complained of abdominal pain. An abdominal X-ray shows dilatation of the colon, and acute pseudo-obstruction (Ogilvie syndrome) was diagnosed. Her stool volume was 876 mL/day. Over a period of 4 days, her serum [K^+] fell from 4.2 to 2.2 mEq/L. **Which one of the following is MOST likely overexpressed transporter in the colon causing hypokalemia?**

A. Na/K/2 Cl cotransporter
B. Na/Cl cotransporter
C. Big K (BK) channel
D. Epithelial Na Channel (ENaC)
E. None of the above

The answer is C

The patient has secretory diarrhea, as it did not respond to fasting (osmotic diarrhea responds to fasting). Several case reports suggest that secretory diarrhea develops following the onset of pseudo-obstruction and loss of K^+ in the stool in the order of 130–170 mEq/L. This extensive loss of K^+ is attributed to overexpression of BK channels in the colon. Thus, option C is correct.

Suggested Reading

Reddi AS. Disorders of potassium: hypokalemia. In: Reddi AS, editor. Fluid, electrolyte, and acid-base disorders. Clinical evaluation and management. 2nd ed. New York: Springer; 2018. p. 175–91.
Sandle GI, Hunter M. Apical potassium (BK) channels and enhanced potassium secretion in human colon. Q J Med. 2010;103:85–9.

12. A 32-year-old man is referred to you for evaluation of persistent hyperkalemia (5.9 mEq/L) and HTN. Two members in his family have similar clinical presentation. Other labs are as follows: Na^+ 140 mEq/L, Cl^- 114 mEq/L, HCO_3^- 16 mEq/L, creatinine 0.8 mg/dL, and glucose 90 mg/dL. Minor work up reveals low renin and aldosterone levels. Urinary Na^+ levels were 30 mEq/L. An ABG shows hyperchloremic metabolic acidosis. He is not on any medications. **Which one of the following therapeutic regimens is APPROPRIATE for this patient?**

A. Furosemide (Lasix)
B. Hydrochlorothiazide (HCTZ)
C. Spironolactone
D. Acetazolamide (Diamox)
E. Salt substitute

The answer is B

In any young male, the presence of hyperkalemia, hypertension, hyperchloremic metabolic acidosis, low renin, low or normal aldosterone, and normal kidney function should suggest pseudohypoaldosteronism type II (PHA II) (Gordon syndrome) as the most likely diagnosis. PHA II is considered a "mirror image" of Gitelman syndrome. Overexpression and activity of Na/Cl cotransporter in the distal tubule results in PHA II, which is an autosomal dominant disease. It is caused by mutations in genes that encode WNK kinases. Only mutations in WNK1 and WNK4 cause PHAII.

Under normal conditions, WNK4 inhibits the activities of Na/Cl cotransporter and ROMK but enhances the paracellular Cl transport. The activity of WNK4 is suppressed by WNK1. When mutations in WNK1 occur, there is an abundance of WNK1 which then removes the inhibitory effect of WNK4 on Na/Cl cotransporter activity.

This results in excessive reabsorption of NaCl and thus volume-dependent hypertension. Mutations in WNK4 also result in similar enhancement of NaCl reabsorption.

As mentioned earlier, WNK4 inhibits ROMK by endocytosis of the channel. Mutations in WNK4 enhance the inhibitory effect of ROMK and thus hyperkalemia. Also, L-WNK1 suppresses ROMK and thus contributing to hyperkalemia. Hyperkalemia is, therefore, related to the combined effect of both WNK4 and WNK1.

WNK4 has also been shown to phosphorylate claudins, which are tight junction proteins involved in paracellular Cl^- transport. Thus, mutations in WNK4 cause enhanced transcellular NaCl and paracellular Cl^- transport with inhibition of K^+ secretion, resulting in volume expansion, hyperkalemia, and hypertension as seen in PHA II. Volume expansion leads to suppression of renin and at times aldosterone levels. Urine Na^+ concentration decreases because of its enhanced reabsorption in the distal tubule.

PHA II responds to thiazide diuretics such as HCTZ, as overactivity of Na/Cl cotransporter is suppressed. Therefore, option B is correct. Furosemide is a loop diuretic, and it does not act on Na/Cl cotransporter that is localized in the distal tubule. Spironolactone is K^+-sparing diuretic, which increases serum K^+ levels even further. Diamox is a carbonic anhydrase inhibitor, which prevents HCO_3^- regeneration in the proximal tubule. Hyperchloremic metabolic acidosis is further exacerbated by diamox. Generally, salt substitutes contain K^+ and are not indicated in this subject. Therefore, options A, C, D, and E are incorrect.

Suggested Reading

Furgeson SB, Linas S. Mechanisms of type I and type II Pseudohypoaldosteronism. J Am Soc Nephrol. 2010;21: 1842–5.
Hadchouel J, Delaloy C, Faure S, et al. Familial hyperkalemic hypertension. J Am Soc Nephrol. 2006;17:208–17.
Reddi AS. Disorders of potassium: hyperkalemia. In: Reddi AS, editor. Fluid, electrolyte, and acid-base disorders. Clinical evaluation and management. 2nd ed. New York: Springer; 2018. p. 193–210.
Shekarabi M, Zhang J, Khanna AR, et al. WNK kinase signaling in ion homeostasis and human disease. Cell Metab. 2017;25:285–99.

13. **Which one of the following is NOT associated with hyperkalemic periodic paralysis (HperPP) compared to hypokalemic periodic paralysis (HypoPP)?**

    A. Familial form of HyperPP is due to mutations in skeletal muscle Na channel. The secondary form of HyperPP can mimic Guillain-Barré syndrome with respiratory failure and diaphragmatic paralysis.
    B. The familial form of HyperPP predominantly presents with myopathic weakness during high K^+ intake or rest after exercise compared to the secondary form of HyperPP.
    C. Younger age (<10 year or infancy to childhood) of onset, greater frequency of attacks with faster recovery, and frequent attacks during fasting distinguish familial form of HyperPP from that of HypoPP.
    D. High carbohydrate intake, insulin stimulation, and epinephrine release are frequently the causes of attacks in HyperPP.

    The answer is E

    Except for option E, all other options characterize HperPP, which is precipitated by exposure to cold, rest after exercise and high K^+ diet. Answer E is the cause that precipitates hypokalemic periodic paralysis.

Suggested Reading

Patangi SO, Garner M, Powell H. Management of a patient with hyperkalemic periodic paralysis requiring coronary artery bypass grafts. Ann Card Anaesth. 2012;15:302–4.
Reddi AS. Disorders of potassium: hyperkalemia. In: Reddi AS, editor. Fluid, electrolyte, and acid-base disorders. Clinical evaluation and management. 2nd ed. New York: Springer; 2018. p. 193–210.

14. **Which one of the following statements about pseudohyperkalemia is CORRECT?**

    A. Erythrocytosis, leukocytosis, and thrombocytosis cause pseudohyperkalemia by releasing K^+ from cells
    B. Clenching of fist or tourniquet use results in K^+ leak from muscle cells and cause pseudohyperkalemia
    C. Reverse pseudohyperkalemia is a phenomenon in which plasma K^+ levels are higher than serum K^+ levels because of heparin-induced cell membrane damage

D. Familial forms of pseudohyperkalemia have been reported due to increased permeability of K^+ from erythrocytes
E. All of the above

The answer is E

Pseudohyperkalemia needs to be ruled out before the treatment of true hyperkalemia is considered. All of the above statements are true. Thus, answer E is correct.

Suggested Reading

Meng QH, Wagar EA. Pseudohyperkalemia: a new twist on an old phenomenon. Crit Rev Clin Lab Sci. 2015;52:45–55.
Mount DB. Disorders of potassium balance. In: Yu ASL, Chertow GM, Luyckx VA, et al., editors. Brenner & Rector's the kidney. 11th ed. Philadelphia: Elsevier; 2020. p. 537–79.
Reddi AS. Disorders of potassium: hyperkalemia. In: Reddi AS, editor. Fluid, electrolyte and acid-base disorders. Clinical evaluation and management. 2nd ed. New York: Springer; 2018. p. 193–210.

15. A 50-year-old man is brought to the Emergency Department by the family for weakness and fatigue. He missed two hemodialysis treatments. His serum [K^+] is 7.6 mEq/L. EKG shows widened peaked T waves. **Which one of the following is NOT indicated in the management of his hyperkalemia with EKG changes?**

A. Calcium gluconate
B. Hypertonic (3%) saline
C. Albuterol
D. Hemodialysis
E. Peritoneal dialysis

The answer is E

Calcium antagonizes the membrane effects of hyperkalemia without lowering serum [K^+] by reducing the threshold potential of cardiac myocytes. Calcium gluconate (10%) is preferred to calcium chloride because the latter causes necrosis if it extravasates into the tissue. Calcium salts can be given over a 10–15 min period in an individual not on digitalis. However, in a patient on digitalis and hyperkalemic EKG changes, calcium can be given slowly over a period of 30 minutes. It is of interest to note that a patient with unrecognized digitalis toxicity and hyperkalemia was successfully treated with calcium chloride.

Hypertonic (3%) saline has been shown to reverse the EKG changes due to hyperkalemia in a patient with hyponatremia. It is given as a bolus of 50 mL. Whether or not this treatment is effective in normonatremic individual is unknown. The effect is due to changes in the electrical properties of cardiac myocytes rather than a change in serum [K^+].

Albuterol (10 mg) by nebulization has been shown to lower plasma [K^+] by 0.6 mEq/L in patients with normal or decreased renal function. An additive effect of insulin/glucose has been reported with albuterol. Plasma K^+-lowering effect of albuterol is due to its transport into the cell.

Hemodialysis is the most effective way of removing K^+ from the body. Rapid removal of K^+ may precipitate ventricular arrhythmias in some patients; therefore, continuous EKG monitoring is recommended.

Peritoneal dialysis (PD) also removes K^+ in maintenance of PD patients with modest hyperkalemia; however, it is not the choice of treatment for severe hyperkalemia with EKG changes. It should be noted that glucose in the peritoneal fluid can transport K^+ into the cell without affecting total body K^+ stores. Thus, option E is incorrect.

Suggested Reading

Dépret F, Peacock WF, Liu KD, et al. Management of hyperkalemia in the acutely ill patient. Ann Intensive Care. 2019;9:32. https://doi.org/10.1186/s13613-019-0509.
Mount DB. Disorders of potassium balance. In: Yu ASL, Chertow GM, Luyckx VA, et al., editors. Brenner & Rector's the kidney. 11th ed. Philadelphia: Elsevier; 2020. p. 537–79.
Ng KE, Lee C-S. Updated treatment options in the management of hyperkalemia. US Pharm. 2017;42:HS15–8.
Shingarev R, Allon M. A physiologic-based approach to the treatment of acute hyperkalemia. Am J Kidney Dis. 2010;56:578–84.

16. A 22-year-old female student presents to her student health clinic for fatigue and weakness of her lower extremities following her routine jogging. Her complaints started 6 weeks ago when her physician started a new oral contraceptive (OC). She has no significant medical history, and not on any medication other than OC. Serum chemistry other than K^+ (5.9 mEq/L) is normal. **Which one of the following oral contraceptives predisposes to hyperkalemia?**

    A. Ethinyl estradiol and norethindrine
    B. Ethinyl estradiol and norgestrel
    C. Ethinyl estradiol and desogestrel
    D. Ethinyl estradiol and drospirenone
    E. None of the above

    The answer is D

    Millions of women worldwide use combined OCs (COCs). COCs contain both estrogen and a progestin. Ethinyl estradiol is the estrogen component of the COCs; however, the progestin component varies and may include a first-generation progestin (option A), a second-generation progestin (option B), a third-generation progestin (option C), or a newly added progestin (option D), which is a spironolactone derivative. Review of her COC confirmed drospirenone, which was discontinued with return of her serum [K^+] to normal.

    Suggested Reading

Bird ST, Pepe SR, Etminan M, et al. The association between drospirenone and hyperkalemia: a comparative-safety study. BMC Clin Pharmacol. 2011;11:23. http://www.biomedcentral.com/1472-6904/11/23

Reddi AS. Disorders of potassium: hyperkalemia. In: Reddi AS, editor. Fluid, electrolyte, and acid-base disorders. Clinical evaluation and management. 2nd ed. New York: Springer; 2018. p. 193–210.

17. A typical North American diet generates 1 mmol/kg/day of endogenous nonvolatile acid. **Which one of the following sources contributes to the acid production?**

    A. Carbohydrates (glucose)
    B. Triglycerides
    C. Phosphoproteins
    D. Anionic amino acids (glutamate, aspartate)
    E. A, B, and C

    The answer is E

    Diet generates both acids and bases. Generally, meat generates acid (H^+) and vegetables produce base (HCO^-). Table 1.4 summarizes the dietary sources of acid and base.

Table 1.4 Sources of dietary acid and base production

Source	Acid produced	Base produced
Sulfur-containing amino acids (cysteine, cystine, methionine)	Sulfuric acid	
Phosphoproteins, phospholipids	Phosphoric acid	
Glucose	Lactic acid, pyruvic acid	
Triglycerides	Acetoacetic acid, β-hydroxybutyric acid	
Nucleoproteins	Uric acid	
Organic cations	HCl	
Diet with anionic amino acids (glutamate, aspartate)		HCO_3^-
Citrate, lactate		HCO_3^-

Suggested Reading

Gennari FJ. Regulation of acid-base balance: overview. In: Gennari FJ, Adrogué HJ, Galla JH, Madias NE, editors. Acid–base disorders and their treatment. Boca Raton: Taylor & Francis; 2005. p. 177–208.

Hamm LL, DuBose TD Jr. Disorders of acid-base balance. In: Yu ASL, Chertow GM, Luyckx VA, et al., editors. Brenner & Rector's the kidney. 11th ed. Philadelphia: Elsevier; 2020. p. 496–536.

Reddi AS. Acid-base disorders. Clinical evaluation and management. New York: Springer; 2020.
Scialla JJ, Anderson CAM. Dietary acid load: a novel nutritional target in chronic kidney disease? Adv Chronic Kidney Dis. 2013;20:141–9.

18. Net acid excretion (NAE) responds appropriately to changes in acid–base balance. **Which one of the following conditions *increases* NAE?**

A. Metabolic alkalosis
B. Metabolic acidosis
C. Hypokalemia
D. Increased NH_3 synthesis
E. B, C, and D

The answer is E

As stated previously, the H ions that are generated as fixed (nonvolatile) acids must be excreted daily in the urine to maintain normal acid–base balance. These H^+ are not excreted as free ions. Instead, they are excreted in the form of titratable acidity (TA), which is phosphate in the form of $HPO_4^{2-}/H_2PO_4^-$ and NH_4^+. Only a small amount of H^+ is excreted as free ions. Each liter of urine contains approximately 0.04 mmol of free H^+. Because of this negligible amount of free H^+, the urine pH is maintained between 4.5 and 6.0. Another reason for the maintenance of acid urine pH is the relatively low concentration of HCO_3^- (<3 mEq/L of urine). Urinary loss of HCO_3^- greater than 5 mEq would generally raise the pH above 6.0 and make the urine alkaline. HCO_3^- loss in the urine is generally equated as a gain of H^+ to the body.

The excretion of H^+ as TA and NH_4^+ is quantified as NAE. NAE is defined as the sum of TA and NH_4^+ minus any urinary HCO_3^- concentration. Therefore, NAE is calculated as follows:

$$NAE = TA + NH_4^+ - HCO_3^-.$$

Metabolic acidosis, hypokalemia, and increased NH_3 synthesis increase whereas as metabolic alkalosis decreases NAE. Thus, answer E is correct.

Suggested Reading

Hamm LL, DuBose TD Jr. Disorders of acid-base balance. In: Yu ASL, Chertow GM, Luyckx VA, et al., editors. Brenner & Rector's the kidney. 11th ed. Philadelphia: Elsevier; 2020. p. 496–536.
Hamm LL, Nakhoul N, Hering-Smith KS. Acid-base homeostasis. Clin J Am Soc Nephrol. 2015;10:2232–42.
Reddi AS. Acid-base disorders. Clinical evaluation and management. New York: Springer; 2020.

19. A 50-year-old man is admitted to the intensive care unit with anterior wall myocardial infarction. Six hours later, he develops shortness of breath. Physical exam and chest X-ray are consistent with pulmonary edema. Electrolytes and ABG values:

Na^+ = 140 mEq/L	pH = 7.36
K^+ = 5.2 mEq/L	pCO_2 = 34 mm Hg
Cl^- = 94 mEq/L	pO_2 = 80 mm Hg
HCO_3^- = 16 mEq/L	HCO_3^- = 22 mEq/L
BUN = 30 mg/dL	
Creatinine = 1.4 mg/dL	
Glucose = 200 mg/dL	

Which one of the following BEST characterizes the acid–base disturbance?

A. Metabolic acidosis and respiratory alkalosis
B. Metabolic alkalosis and metabolic acidosis
C. Respiratory acidosis and metabolic acidosis
D. Respiratory alkalosis and metabolic alkalosis
E. None of the above

The answer is E

The acid–base disorder should be analyzed systematically. Once the laboratory values are available, the next step is to check whether the pH is correct or not. One must use the Henderson equation to obtain the [H⁺] and then the pH. The Henderson equation is:

$$\left[H^{+}\right] = 24 \times \frac{PCO_2}{\left[HCO_3^{-}\right]}$$

Substituting the values, we obtain:

$$\left[H^{+}\right] = 24 \times \frac{34}{16} = 51$$

Remember the following approximate [H⁺] to clinically relevant pH values:

$$\begin{aligned} &\text{pH}\,7.50 = 30 \\ &\text{pH}\,7.40 = 40 \\ &\text{pH}\,7.30 = 50 \\ &\text{pH}\,7.20 = 60 \\ &\text{pH}\,7.10 = 80 \\ &\text{pH}\,7.10 = 100 \end{aligned}$$

The [H⁺] of 51 corresponds to a pH of 7.30. Therefore, the pH reported from the laboratory is incorrect. Also, there is a large difference between the measured and calculated HCO_3^-. In view of this, it is difficult to interpret the ABG (E is correct). Both electrolytes and ABG should be repeated within few minutes apart. This case emphasizes the need for checking the accuracy or internal consistency of the pH value.

Suggested Reading

Hamm LL, DuBose TD Jr. Disorders of acid-base balance. In: Yu ASL, Chertow GM, Luyckx VA, et al., editors. Brenner & Rector's the kidney. 11th ed. Philadelphia: Elsevier; 2020. p. 496–536.

Reddi AS. Acid-base disorders. Clinical evaluation and management. New York: Springer; 2020.

20. A 72-year-old woman with a history of type 2 diabetes mellitus, congestive heart failure (CHF), and renal failure is admitted for nausea, vomiting, and shortness of breath. Her medications include insulin and furosemide. Her weight is 60 kg. Admission laboratory values:

Na^+ = 140 mEq/L	pH = 7.40
K^+ = 4.1 mEq/L	pCO_2 = 40 mm Hg
Cl^- = 95 mEq/L	pO_2 = 90 mm Hg
HCO_3^- = 24 mEq/L	HCO_3^- = 24 mEq/L
Creatinine = 4.1 mg/dL	
BUN = 52 mg/dL	
Glucose = 145 mg/dL	
Albumin = 4.1 g/dL	

Which one of the following acid–base disturbance is CORRECT?

A. Metabolic acidosis and respiratory alkalosis
B. Metabolic acidosis and metabolic alkalosis
C. Respiratory acidosis and metabolic acidosis
D. Respiratory alkalosis and metabolic alkalosis
E. Metabolic acidosis, metabolic alkalosis, and respiratory alkalosis

The answer is B

Although the ABG values look normal, in fact, they are abnormal once the anion gap (AG) is calculated. The patient has an AG of 21. If this were a pure metabolic acidosis, the pH, serum [HCO_3^-], and pCO_2 levels would be lower than normal. Since the patient has vomiting and she is also taking furosemide for her CHF, she developed metabolic alkalosis. The coexistence of metabolic acidosis and metabolic alkalosis normalizes ABG values and gives the impression of no underlying disturbance (B is correct). The clue for the diagnosis of this mixed metabolic acidosis and metabolic alkalosis is the presence of a high AG. Thus, this case emphasizes the importance of calculating AG in the analysis of any acid–base disturbance.

Suggested Reading

Kurtz I. Acid-base case studies. 2nd ed. Victoria: Trafford Publishing; 2006.
Hamm LL, DuBose TD Jr. Disorders of acid-base balance. In: Yu ASL, Chertow GM, Luyckx VA, et al., editors. Brenner & Rector's the kidney. 11th ed. Philadelphia: Elsevier; 2020. p. 496–536.
Reddi AS. Acid-base disorders. Clinical evaluation and management. New York: Springer; 2020.

21. A 51-year-old man is admitted for painless growth in right temporal area for a 3-week period. The only complaint he had was poor appetite with 4 lb weight loss. He has no history of any other chronic disease and is not on any medications. He has not seen a physician in 10 years. Admitting laboratory values:

Na^+ = 124 mEq/L	pH = 7.39
K^+ = 3.9 mEq/L	pCO_2 = 39 mm Hg
Cl^- = 100 mEq/L	pO_2 = 94 mm Hg
HCO_3^- = 23 mEq/L	HCO_3^- = 22 mEq/L
Creatinine = 1.0 mg/dL	
BUN = 16 mg/dL	
Glucose = 102 mg/dL	
Serum osmolality = 284 mOsm/kg H_2O	

What is the MOST clinically evident abnormality in the assessment of acid–base disturbance in this patient?

A. Anion gap (AG)
B. Albumin
C. Total protein
D. All of the above
E. None of the above

The answer is D

From the above electrolytes, it is obvious that the AG is only 1. This is abnormal that warrants further evaluation. Hypoalbuminemia is the most common cause of low AG in hospitalized, and also in ambulatory patients. Serum albumin level came back as 4.5 g/dl. Therefore, hypoalbuminemia is not the cause for his low AG.

In view of hyponatremia and normal serum osmolality, ordering serum total protein is very important at this time. His total protein is 14.2 g/dL, which is causing hyponatremia. The increase in total protein warrants serum and urine protein immunoelectrophoresis, which showed very high IgG levels. Along with pathology report, the diagnosis of IgG multiple myeloma was made.

IgG molecules carry a positive charge at pH of 7.4, and thus an increase in unmeasured cations, and this increase in unmeasured cations causes low AG. Although low AG is the most evident abnormality in this patient, measurement of albumin is important to evaluate the AG, and total protein is also important to evaluate isotonic hyponatremia (D is correct).

Suggested Reading

Emmett M. Approach to the patient with a negative anion gap. Am J Kidney Dis. 2016;67:143–50.
Emmett M, Narins RG. Clinical use of the anion gap. Medicine. 56:38–54.

22. A 54-year-old woman was admitted to the Emergency Department (ED) for shortness of breath, "unwell" feeling, and weakness of few days duration. Her BP was 114/51 mm Hg with a pulse rate of 69 beats per minute. She was afebrile.

Her medical history is significant for cervical and lumbosacral disc disease, hypertension, depression, anxiety, ataxia, and chronic pulmonary obstructive disease. She had carpal tunnel and cervical disc surgery, cholecystectomy, and hysterectomy. Her medications included combivent (ipratropium bromide 18 μg and albuterol 90 μg) 1 puff every 8 h, metoprolol 12.5 mg twice daily, klonopin (clonazepam) 0.5 mg every 8 h, as needed, and vicodin ES (hydrocodone bitartrate 7.5 mg and acetaminophen 750 mg) every 8 h, as needed. The patient was previously admitted with similar complaints and found to have a high AG metabolic acidosis and acute kidney injury, requiring short-term hemodialysis.

Labs are shown in the following table. Hemoglobin was 13.4 g% and a platelet count of 430,000. Serum glucose was 80 mg/dl. ABG: pH of 7.20, pCO_2 15 mm Hg, pO_2 91 mm Hg, and calculated HCO_3^- of 6 mEq/L. The AG was 16. Other pertinent labs are normal. Serum osmolality was 293 mOsm/L. Serum ketones and lactate were negative, and urinalysis was normal.

Hospital day	Na^+ (mEq/L)	K^+ (mEq/L)	Cl^- (mEq/L)	HCO_3^{--} (mEq/L)	Creatinine (mg/dL)	BUN (mg/dL)	AG (mEq/L)	Albumin (g/dL)	pH
Admission	138	4.6	114	8	0.87	10	16	4.4	7.20
Day 2	143	4.8	119	11	0.59	11	13	3.9	7.31
Day 3	141	3.6	109	18	0.55	9	14	3.4	
Day 4	142	3.2	107	25	0.48	8	10	3.3	
Day 5	140	4.1	100	33	0.55	8	7	3.6	

Which one of the following acid–base disturbances is CORRECT?

A. Metabolic acidosis and respiratory alkalosis
B. Metabolic acidosis and metabolic alkalosis
C. Respiratory acidosis and metabolic acidosis
D. Respiratory alkalosis and metabolic alkalosis
E. Metabolic acidosis, metabolic alkalosis, and respiratory alkalosis

The answer is A

Based on pH and pCO_2 and serum $[HCO_3^-]$, the acid–base disorder is a high AG metabolic acidosis and respiratory alkalosis (A is correct).

23. **Which one of the following tests you order at this time?**

A. Serum osmolal gap
B. Serum aspirin levels
C. Urinary pyroglutamic acid
D. Serum D-lactate levels
E. Serum L-lactate levels

The answer is C

In this patient, the osmolal gap is 6 mOsm/L, which is normal. This normal osmolal gap excludes acidosis due to methanol, ethylene glycol, ketones, and possibly lactic acid. Lactate levels were normal, and ketones were negative.

The initial acid–base disorder in aspirin overdose is respiratory alkalosis followed by the development of high AG metabolic acidosis. In this patient, serum salicylate levels were normal, excluding the diagnosis of aspirin overdose (B is incorrect).

Patients with D-lactic acidosis usually present with neurologic signs and symptoms, and this patient has symptoms related to acid–base disturbance and acute kidney injury (D is incorrect).

This patient is on high doses of acetaminophen (750 mg Q8 h); and urinary pyroglutamic acid levels were ordered. Her urinary pyroglutamic acid levels came back at >11,500 mmol/mol creatinine (reference range 0–100 mmol/mole creatinine). Also, acetaminophen and its metabolites were present. Therefore, the diagnosis was pyroglutamic acidosis due to daily high doses of acetaminophen (Tylenol) use (C is correct). Tylenol depletes GSH, which promotes pyroglutamic acid production. She was started on Fentanyl patch, and her serum $[HCO_3^-]$ for the last 3 years has been normal.

Suggested Reading

Fenves AZ, Kirkpatrick HM III, Patel VV, et al. Increased anion gap metabolic acidosis as a result of 5-oxoproline (pyroglutamic acid): a role for acetaminophen. Clin J Am Soc Nephrol. 2006;1:441–7.

Reddi AS, Kunadi AR. Recurrent anion gap metabolic acidosis in a woman with vertebral disease. Am J Emerg Med. 2011;29:962–3.

24. A 40-year-old woman with history of short-bowl surgery is seen for slurred speech, confusion, weakness, impaired motor coordination, and irritability. She likes ice cream and develops mild neurologic problems following large quantities of ice cream. She is not on any medications or special diets. ABG: pH 7.27, pCO_2 24 mm Hg, and calculated HCO_3^- 16. Urine ketones are negative. Serum lactate levels are 1.5 mmol/L. Serum creatinine is normal. The anion gap is 20, but osmolal gap is normal. **Which one of the following is the MOST likely cause of this acid–base disturbance in this patient?**

    A. L-Lactic acid
    B. Pyroglutamic acid
    C. D-Lactic acid
    D. Methanol
    E. Topiramate

    The answer is C

    Except for topiramate, all other causes generate high AG metabolic acidosis. Topiramate causes non-AG metabolic acidosis due to inhibition of carbonic anhydrase. Serum lactate is normal; therefore, lactic acidosis is excluded. Also, methanol intoxication is excluded based on normal osmolal gap. There is no history of medication (Tylenol or Tylenol-containing narcotics) or antibiotic use. Therefore, pyroglutamic acidosis is ruled out. Based on the surgical history, high carbohydrate intake, and neurologic manifestations, the most likely diagnosis is D-lactic acidosis. Thus, option C is correct.

Suggested Reading

Gurukripa Kowlgi N, Chhabra L. D-lactic acidosis: an underrecognized complication of short bowl syndrome. Gastroenterol Res Pract. 2015; Article ID 476215, 8 pages

Kang KP, Lee S, Kang SK. D-Lactic acidosis in humans: review of update. Electrolyte Blood Press. 2006;4:53–6.

25. The above patient (case 23) is admitted for management of neurologic manifestations and high AG metabolic acidosis. **Which one of the following medications improves her clinical status?**

    A. Oral vancomycin
    B. Metronidazole
    C. Ciprofloxacin
    D. Rifamixin
    E. All of the above

    The answer is E

    All of the above medications are indicated in the treatment of D-lactic acidosis. Duration of antibiotic therapy has not been established, but 7–14 days therapy is recommended until symptoms improve. Appropriate antibiotics are oral vancomycin (125–500 mg 1–4 times/day), metronidazole (500 mg 3 times/day), ciprofloxacin (500 mg 2 times/day), and rifamixin (550 mg 2–3 times/day). Thus, answer E is correct.

    Neomycin and trimethoprim-sulfamethoxazole should be avoided, as they may be associated with episodes of D-lactate encephalopathy.

Suggested Reading

Gurukripa Kowlgi N, Chhabra L. D-lactic acidosis: an underrecognized complication of short bowl syndrome. Gastroenterol Res Pract. 2015; Article ID 476215, 8 pages

Kang KP, Lee S, Kang SK. D-Lactic acidosis in humans: review of update. Electrolyte Blood Press. 2006;4:53–6.

Reddi AS. Acid-base disorders. Clinical evaluation and management. New York: Springer; 2020.

26. A 17-year-old female student is admitted for confusion and acute kidney injury. She is able to give some history that she had a fight with her boyfriend 2 days ago, and she drank some liquid that was in their garage. She has no other significant medical or illicit drug history. In the Emergency Department, her vital signs are stable. Other than altered mental status and confusion, her physical exam is normal. She weighs 60 kg. Laboratory values:

Serum	Urine
Na^+ = 141 mEq/L K^+ = 4.2 mEq/L Cl^- = 110 mEq/L HCO_3^- = 7 mEq/L BUN = 28 mg/dL Creatinine = 1.8 mg/dL Glucose = 72 mg/dL Serum osmolality = 312 mOsm/kg H_2O ABG = pH = 7.21, pCO_2 = 17 mm Hg, pO_2 = 94 mm Hg, HCO_3^- = 6 mEq/L	Osmolality = 320 mOsm/kg H_2O pH = 5.2 Protein = trace Blood = negative Urine sediment = envelope-like crystals (see figure below)

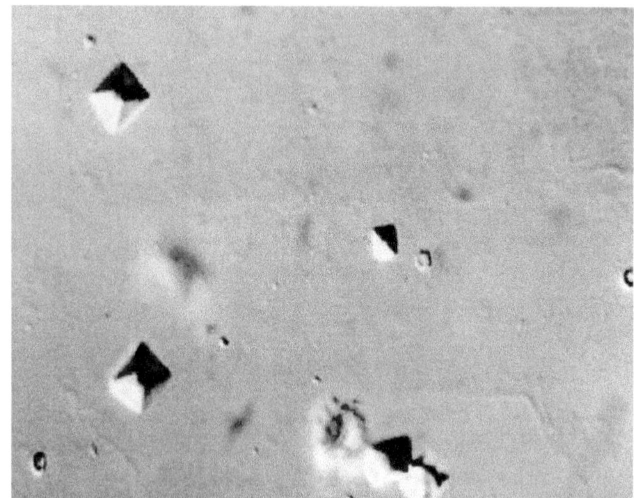

Which one of the following alcohol ingestions is the MOST likely cause of her symptoms?

A. Ethanol
B. Ethylene glycol
C. Methanol
D. Toluene
E. Isopropyl alcohol

The answer is B

This patient has a high AG metabolic acidosis with respiratory alkalosis. She has also an osmolal gap of 16, which is elevated. The presence of calcium oxalate crystals (envelope-like) in the urine sediment is the clue for her acid–base disturbance, which is ethylene glycol ingestion (B is correct). One of the final products of ethylene glycol is oxalic acid, which is excreted as oxalate.

Antidote for ethylene glycol is fomepizole. The initial dose is 15 mg/kg followed by 10 mg/kg every 12 h for four doses. Continue fomepizole, if ethylene glycol levels are not below 20 mg/dL. At the same time, hydration with D5W and 3 ampules (150 mEq) of $NaHCO_3$ to run at 120 mL/h to improve volume status should be started. Hemodialysis is indicated, if no improvement in kidney function and metabolic acidosis following adequate hydration and $NaHCO_3$ administration is observed.

Suggested Reading

Barceloux DG, Krenzelok EP, Olson K, et al. American academy of clinical toxicology practice guidelines on the treatment of ethylene glycol poisoning. J Toxicol Clin Toxicol. 1999;37:537–60.

Brent J. Fomepizole for ethylene glycol and methanol poisoning. N Engl J Med. 2009;360:2216–23.

Kraut JA, Xing SX. Approach to the evaluation of a patient with an increased serum osmolal gap and high-anion gap metabolic acidosis. Am J Kidney Dis. 2011;58:480–4.
Reddi AS. Acid-base disorders. Clinical evaluation and management. New York: Springer; 2020.

27. A 55-year-old man with chronic alcoholism presents to the Emergency Department with agitation, blurred vision, and eye pain. Blood pressure and pulse rate are normal. He is afebrile. He has a high AG metabolic acidosis with an osmolal gap of 26 mOsm/L. **Which one of the following toxic alcohol ingestions is the MOST likely cause of his symptoms?**

   A. Ethanol
   B. Ethylene glycol
   C. Methanol
   D. Toluene
   E. Isopropyl alcohol

   The answer is C

   Of all of the above alcohols, only methanol can cause the patient's symptoms because formic acid that is formed from methanol is toxic to the optic nerve, causing visual impairment, blurred vision, eye pain, and blindness. Therefore, early institution of fomepizole is recommended to inhibit alcohol dehydrogenase and conversion of methanol to formaldehyde and formic acid (C is correct).

   Suggested Reading

Brent J. Fomepizole for ethylene glycol and methanol poisoning. N Engl J Med. 2009;360:2216–23.
Kraut JA, Xing SX. Approach to the evaluation of a patient with an increased serum osmolal gap and high-anion gap metabolic acidosis. Am J Kidney Dis. 2011;58:480–4.
Reddi AS. Acid-base disorders. Clinical evaluation and management. New York: Springer; 2020.

28. A 50-year-old man was admitted with severe abdominal pain and vomiting. CT of abdomen was normal. The patient has no complaints of eye problems. Labs indicate an increase in serum creatinine, osmolality, and osmolal gap. Arterial blood gas shows a high AG metabolic acidosis. He became oliguric and hyperkalemic, requiring hemodialysis. Two days later, he developed bilateral facial palsy. Urinalysis is normal. **Which of the following alcohols is MOST likely responsible for his clinical status?**

   A. Ethanol
   B. Ethylene glycol
   C. Methanol
   D. Diethylene glycol
   E. Isopropyl alcohol

   The answer is D

   The clinical manifestations, particularly, bilateral facial palsy (seventh nerve palsy) is rather common in patients with diethylene glycol intoxication. Thus, answer D is correct.

   Ethanol and methanol rarely cause neurologic complications. Although ethylene glycol may present with neurologic complications, the urinalysis is normal (without oxalate crystals). Therefore, ethylene glycol poisoning is unlikely. Thus, answers A, B, C, and E are incorrect.

   Suggested Reading

Kraut JA, Xing SX. Approach to the evaluation of a patient with an increased serum osmolal gap and high-anion gap metabolic acidosis. Am J Kidney Dis. 2011;58:480–4.
Reddi AS. Acid-base disorders. Clinical evaluation and management. New York: Springer; 2020.
Schep LJ, Slaughiter RJ, Temple WA, et al. Diethylene glycol poisoning. Clin Toxicol. 2009;47:525–35.

29. **Which one of the following agents initially causes respiratory alkalosis and then high AG metabolic acidosis in an adult subject?**

   A. Toluene
   B. Tenofovir
   C. Acetylsalicylic acid (ASA)

D. Flucloxacillin
E. None of the above

The answer is C

ASA causes initially respiratory alkalosis due to stimulation of medullary respiratory center and hyperventilation. Subsequently, metabolic acidosis develops due to lactic acid and ketoacid production. Respiratory alkalosis seems to be the main reason for lactic acid production. Thus, answer C is correct. In children, metabolic acidosis is the initial presentation of ASA ingestion

Toluene causes hippuric acid and tenofovir causes lactic acid, whereas flucloxacillin causes pyroglutamic acid.

Suggested Reading

O'Malley GF. Emergency department management of the salicylate-poisoned patient. Emerg Med Clin N Am. 2007;25:333–46.
Reddi AS. Acid-base disorders. Clinical evaluation and management. New York: Springer; 2020.

30. A 45-year-old man was brought by his wife to the Emergency Department for confusion and acetone breath. As per his wife, he drinks alcohol every day. Pertinent labs reveal a high serum osmolality with large osmolal gap and normal acid–base values. **Based on the above information, which one of the following alcohol he consumed?**

A. Ethanol
B. Methanol
C. Ethylene glycol
D. Isopropyl alcohol
E. Diethylene glycol

The answer is D

Isopropyl alcohol is usually called rubbing alcohol, and alcoholics occasionally drink it when ethanol is not available. It is metabolized to acetone, and urine is positive for ketones. One needs to rule out diabetic ketoacidosis because of acetone breath by determining serum glucose levels, which are normal in individuals with isopropyl alcohol ingestion. There are no acid–base disorders other than high serum osmolality and large osmolal gap because of isopropyl alcohol. Thus, answer D is correct. Treatment is supportive, as the intoxication is self-limited. However, hemodialysis is indicated in individuals with serum levels of isopropyl alcohol >200 mg/dL and hypotension.

Other answers are incorrect because they cause acid–base disorders as well as electrolyte abnormalities.

Suggested Reading

Reddi AS. Acid-base disorders. Clinical evaluation and management. New York: Springer; 2020.
Slaughter RJ, Mason RW, Beasley DM, et al. Isopropanol poisoning. Clin Toxicol. 2014;52:470–8.

31. Two type 1 diabetic patients are admitted to the intensive care unit for management of severe diabetic ketoacidosis (DKA). One patient has acute kidney injury (AKI), glucosuria, and ketonuria. The other patient is on hemodialysis (HD) with no urine output. Their DKA was precipitated by pneumonia. Serum [HCO_3^-] is 8 mEq/L in both patients. You decide to treat both patients with normal saline and bicarbonate ($NaHCO_3$). **Which one of the following patients requires more fluid and bicarbonate to improve volume status and acidosis?**

A. Both require equal quantity of saline and bicarbonate
B. HD patient requires both more than the AKI patient
C. AKI patient requires both more than the HD patient
D. HD patient requires more bicarbonate than saline
E. AKI patient requires only saline

The answer is C

Volume status is different in both patients. The patient with AKI loses more water and electrolytes than HD patient with no urine formation. This is evident from glucosuria and ketonuria, which obligate water and salt loss. Therefore, volume depletion is rather severe in the patient with urine output due to osmotic diuresis and requires more fluid than the HD patient. Because ketones are lost in the urine and infusion of saline further lowers

bicarbonate, recovery of serum [HCO_3^-] from these ketone bodies is slow once insulin is started. Therefore, the patient with AKI requires substantial repletion of volume and bicarbonate. Thus, answer C is correct.

Because of no urine output, the HD patient does not lose any ketones, and therefore, these ketones are retained in the body. Also, there is no osmotic diuresis and consequently no water loss. Following insulin administration, these ketones are converted into bicarbonate and serum [HCO_3^-] improves much faster than that of the patient with AKI. Therefore, the patient requires less volume and little or no bicarbonate. Thus, other answers are incorrect.

Suggested Reading

Adrogué HJ, Madias NE. Diabetic and other forms of ketoacidosis. In: Gennari FJ, Adrogué HJ, Galla JH, Madias NE, editors. Acid-base disorders and their treatment. Boca Raton: Taylor & Francis; 2005. p. 313–50.

Dhatariya KK, Velllanki P. Treatment of diabetic ketoacidosis (DKA)/hyperglycemic hyperosmolar state (HHS): Novel advances in the management of hyperglycemic crises (UK versus USA). Curr Diab Rep. 2017;17:33.

Fayfman M, Pasquel FJ, Umpierrez GE. Management of hyperglycemic crises. Diabetic ketoacidosis and hyperglycemic hyperosmolar state. Med Clin N Am. 2017;101:587–606.

32. A type 2 diabetic man is on sodium-glucose cotransporter-2 (SGLT-2) inhibitor for 1 year. He presents to his primary care physician with complaints of nausea, vomiting, weakness, and abdominal pain for 4 days. He has some burning on urination. His blood pressure and pulse are normal. Serum glucose is 148 mg/dL, and he has acetone breath. **Which one the following is the MOST likely diagnosis in this patient?**

A. Alcohol ketoacidosis
B. Starvation ketoacidosis
C. Euglycemic diabetic ketoacidosis (DKA)
D. Lactic acidosis
E. Ingestion of isopropyl alcohol

The answer is C

Many case reports of euglycemic DKA have been reported since the introduction of SGLT-2 inhibitors in both type 1 and type 2 diabetic patients with normal or slightly elevated glucose levels. Relative lack of insulin and infection seem to precipitate DKA in these patients who are on SGLT-2 inhibitors. These patients have high glucagon levels, which may promote ketogenesis. Discontinuation of SGLT-2 inhibitor and institution of insulin improve ketoacidosis. Thus, answer C is correct.

Alcohol and starvation ketoacidosis are unlikely in view of slightly elevated glucose levels, as these two conditions are usually associated with low glucose levels. Lactic acid is also unlikely in view of normal blood pressure. Isopropyl alcohol is metabolized to acetone, but metabolic acidosis is unlikely in view of normal blood pressure. Thus, answers A, B, D, and E are incorrect.

Suggested Reading

Goldenberg RM, Berard LD, Cheng AYY, et al. SGLT2 inhibitor-associated diabetic ketoacidosis: clinical review and recommendations for prevention and diagnosis. Clin Therapuet. 2016;38:2654–64.

Rosenstock J, Ferrannini E. Euglycemic diabetic ketoacidosis: a predictable, detectable, and preventable safety concern with SGLT2 inhibitors. Diabetes Care. 2015;38:1638–42.

33. **Match the drug effects of lactic and pyroglutamic acids shown in Column A with the mechanisms of action shown in Column B.**

Column A	Column B
A. Metformin	1. Inhibition of mitochondrial protein synthesis
B. Tenofovir	2. Uncoupling of oxidative phosphorylation
C. Linezolid	3. Inhibition of pyruvate dehydrogenase complex
D. Propofol	4. Inhibition of alcohol dehydrogenase
E. Fomepizole	5. Inhibition of 5-oxoprolinase
F. Flucloxacillin	6. Increase in NADH/NAD$^+$ ratio, inhibition of gluconeogenesis from lactate, inhibition of mitochondrial respiration
G. Thiamine deficiency	

Answers: A = 6; B = 1; C = 1; D = 2; E = 4; F = 5; G = 3

Suggested Reading

Reddi AS. Acid-base disorders. Clinical evaluation and management. New York: Springer; 2020.

34. **Match the following causes with their renal tubular acidosis (RTAs).**

Cause	RTA
A. Obstructive uropathy	1. Classic distal RTA
B. Spironolactone	2. Hyperkalemic distal RTA with alkaline urine
C. Valproic acid	3. Type 4 RTA with acid urine
D. Ifosfamide	4. Proximal RTA
E. Amiloride	
F. Cyclosporine	
G. NSAIDs	
H. Medullary sponge kidney	

Answers: A = 2; B = 3; C = 4; D = 4; E = 2; F = 1; G = 3; H = 1

Suggested Reading

Alexander RT, Bitzan M. Renal tubular acidosis. Pediatr Clin North Am. 2019;66:135–57.
Batlle D, Arruda J. Hyperkalemic forms of renal tubular acidosis: clinical and pathophysiological aspects. Adv Chronic Kidney Dis. 2018;25:321–33.
Hall AM, Bass P, Unwin RJ. Drug-induced renal Fanconi syndrome. QJ Med. 2014;107:261–9.
Reddi AS. Acid-base disorders. Clinical evaluation and management. New York: Springer; 2020

35. An 18-year-old woman is admitted to the hospital for worsening weakness and problems with breathing for the last 2 weeks. She loves ice cream since childhood. She states that she had 4–6 urinary tract infections (UTIs) in recent years, which were treated. She is not on any medications. Admitting laboratory values are:

Serum	Urine
Na^+ = 138 mEq/L	pH = 6.6
K^+ = 1.2 mEq/L	Glucose = negative
Cl^- = 118 mEq/L	Blood = positive (had recent menstruation)
HCO_3^- = 12 mEq/L	Ketones = negative
Creatinine = 0.6 mg/dL	Protein = 3+
BUN = 22 mg/dL	Na^+ = 60 mEq/L
Glucose =90 mg/dL	K^+ = 100 mEq/L
ANA = positive	Cl^- = 110 mEq/L
Complement = low	
ABG: pH 7.2, pCO_2 26 mm Hg, HCO_3^- 11 mEq/L	

Which one of the following is the MOST likely cause of her symptoms?

A. Exacerbation of systemic lupus erythematosus (SLE)
B. Proximal RTA
C. Distal RTA
D. Type 4 RTA
E. Hypokalemic periodic paralysis

The answer is C

The patient's weakness and respiratory distress are related to hypokalemia rather than exacerbation of SLE. Although glomerular disease is common in SLE, tubular dysfunction is uncommon in the presence of normal renal function. However, hypokalemia-related clinical manifestations have been described prior to the diagnosis of SLE. The serum and urine findings in this patient are suggestive of distal RTA (hyperchloremic metabolic acidosis and alkaline urine pH despite acidosis). A few cases of distal RTA have been reported in the literature. The pathophysiology of distal RTA in lupus patients is unclear; however, destruction of distal nephron by immunoglobulins has been suggested. Proximal RTA in this patient is unlikely as she has no manifestations of Fanconi

syndrome. Also, patients with proximal RTA can acidify their urine at a serum [HCO_3^-] of 12 mEq/L. Although type 4 RTA has been described in lupus patients, hypokalemia rules out this diagnosis in this patient. Hypokalemic periodic paralysis is also unlikely because of positive ANA, lupus nephritis, and urine [K^+] of 100 mEq/L. In hypokalemic periodic paralysis, urine K^+ is low because of transcellular distribution.

Suggested Reading

Batlle D, Haque SK. Genetic causes and mechanisms of distal renal tubular acidosis. Nephrol Dial Transplant. 2012;27:3691–704.

Reddi AS. Acid-base disorders. Clinical evaluation and management. New York: Springer; 2020.

Trepiccione F, Prosperi F, Rosenburch de la Motte L, et al. New findings on the pathogenesis of distal renal tubular acidosis. Kidney Dis. 2017;3:98–105.

Vallės PG, Batlle D. Hypokalemic distal renal tubular acidosis. Adv Chronic Kidney Dis. 2018;25:303–20.

36. A 19-year-old thin female student is brought to the Emergency Department by her friends for altered mental status, euphoria, dizziness, and dizziness after a rave party. She has no history of drug abuse, and not on any medications. Physical exam is normal except for a blood pressure of 90/60 mm Hg with pulse rate of 102 beats/min. Labs on admission and 18 h later are:

On admission	18 h later
Na^+ = 142 mEq/L	Na^+ = 138 mEq/L
K^+ = 3.5 mEq/L	K^+ = 2.2 mEq/L
Cl^- = 100 mEq/L	Cl^- = 118 mEq/L
HCO_3^- = 12 mEq/L	HCO_3^- = 14 mEq/L
Creatinine = 1.8 mg/dL	Creatinine = 0.9 mg/dL
BUN = 22 mg/dL	BUN = 12 mg/dL
Glucose =96 mg/dL	Glucose =100 mg/dL
ABG: pH 7.24, pCO_2 28 mm Hg, HCO_3^- 11 mEq/L	ABG: pH 3.2, pCO_2 29, HCO_3^+ 13
Urine pH =5.2	Urine pH =6.5

It is evident that the patient has a high AG metabolic acidosis with appropriate respiratory compensation on admission, and 18 h later, the acid–base disorder is hypokalemic hyperchloremic metabolic acidosis, and respiratory compensation is appropriate. **Which one of the following agents causes these types of acid–base disorders?**

A. Topiramate
B. Ifosfamide
C. Toluene
D. Cisplatin
E. Tenofovir

The answer is C

Toluene is initially metabolized to hippurate, which causes a high AG metabolic acidosis. Subsequently, hippurate is rapidly excreted in the urine with volume expansion, and the AG disappears. The typical acid–base disorder is hyperchloremic metabolic acidosis with severe hypokalemia. Hypokalemia is related to more distal delivery of Na^+ with hippurate, leaving Cl^- behind. Some of the patients are unable to acidify their urine due to impaired H^+ secretion. All other drugs cause proximal RTA with adequate urinary acidification once serum [HCO_3^-] is below18 mEq/L.

Suggested Reading

Batlle D, Haque SK. Genetic causes and mechanisms of distal renal tubular acidosis. Nephrol Dial Transplant. 2012;27:3691–704.

Reddi AS. Acid-base disorders. Clinical evaluation and management. New York: Springer; 2020.

Trepiccione F, Prosperi F, Rosenburch de la Motte L, et al. New findings on the pathogenesis of distal renal tubular acidosis. Kidney Dis. 2017;3:98–105.

Vallės PG, Batlle D. Hypokalemic distal renal tubular acidosis. Adv Chronic Kidney Dis. 2018;25:303–20.

37. A 34-year-old man, brought to the Emergency Department by his friend, complains of weakness, fatigue, poor appetite, and dizziness for 2 weeks. He has not seen any physician for 5 years. Other than daily cocaine use, he has no significant medical history. He is not on any prescription medications. Physical examination reveals orthostatic blood pressure and pulse changes. Except for anal condyloma acuminata, the remaining exam is unremarkable. Rapid HIV test is positive. Laboratory values on admission:

Serum	Urine
Na^+ = 126 mEq/L	pH = 5.2
K^+ = 6.5 mEq/L	Glucose = negative
Cl^- = 110 mEq/L	Blood = negative
HCO_3^- = 13 mEq/L	Protein = negative
Creatinine = 2.1 mg/dl	Na^+ = 101 mEq/L
BUN = 42 mg/dl	K^+ = 30 mEq/L
Glucose =60 mg/dl	Cl^- = 40 mEq/L
ABG: pH 7.29, pCO_2 28 mm Hg, HCO_3^- 12 mEq/L	

Which one of the following acid–base disorder is CORRECT?

A. Proximal RTA (type II)
B. Distal RTA (type I)
C. Incomplete RTA (type III)
D. Type 4 RTA with hypoaldosteronism
E. Hyperkalemic RTA with a defect in voltage gradient

The answer is D

This patient has hyperkalemic hyperchloremic (non-AG) metabolic acidosis with appropriate respiratory compensation. Serum and urine chemistry and orthostatic changes suggest Addison disease, which causes type 4 RTA. Hypoaldosteronism due to adrenal gland destruction by viruses (HIV, CMV), and bacteria (mycobacterium tuberculosis), or fungal agents has been described. Patients with type 4 RTA due to aldosterone deficiency can acidify their urine.

Proximal RTA is unlikely because of hyponatremia and hyperkalemia. Note that patients with proximal RTA can acidify their urine at this level of serum [HCO_3^-], as all of this HCO_3^- can be reabsorbed and generate an acid urine.

Patients with incomplete RTA cannot acidy their urine even after an acid load. Also, hyperkalemic distal RTA patients with a defect in voltage gradient cannot acidify their urine. Therefore, options A, B, C, and E are incorrect.

Suggested Reading

Batlle D, Arruda J. Hyperkalemic forms of renal tubular acidosis: clinical and pathophysiological aspects. Adv Chronic Kidney Dis. 2018;25:321–33.

Karet FE. Mechanisms in hyperkalemic renal tubular acidosis. J Am Soc Nephrol. 2009;20:251–4.

Reddi AS. Acid-base disorders. Clinical evaluation and management. New York: Springer; 2020.

38. A 42-year-old man presents to his primary care physician for left flank pain and hematuria. Urinalysis reveals a pH of 6.9 and hematuria only. There is no evidence of UTI. Renal ultrasound shows the presence of kidney stones. He has no deafness. Serum chemistry and ABG show mild hypokalemic hyperchloremic metabolic acidosis. Serum creatinine is normal. He has a family history of kidney stones, and several members have mild hypokalemic hyperchloremic metabolic acidosis. **Which one of the following renal tubular acidosis (RTAs) is the MOST likely diagnosis in this patient?**

A. Proximal RTA
B. Distal RTA
C. Type IV RTA with aldosterone deficiency
D. Incomplete RTA
E. Hyperkalemic RTA with inability to acidic urine

The answer is B

This patient has hereditary form of distal RTA with autosomal dominant inheritance. It occurs in adults. Autosomal recessive forms are diagnosed in infancy and childhood with or without deafness. Hyperkalemic RTA with a defect in voltage gradient is seen in patients with mild to moderate renal dysfunction. Type 4 RTA patients

with aldosterone deficiency have mild renal impairment and can acidify their urine. Patients with incomplete RTA may have a combination of both proximal and distal RTA. They may present with acid urine, but the diagnosis is established only after an acid load. Proximal RTA patients present with severe hypokalemia, but nephrolithiasis is uncommon. Thus, options A, C, D, and E are incorrect.

Suggested Reading

Batlle D, Haque SK. Genetic causes and mechanisms of distal renal tubular acidosis. Nephrol Dial Transplant. 2012;27:3691–704.

Reddi AS. Acid-base disorders. Clinical evaluation and management. New York: Springer; 2020.

39. **What is the genetic defect in the above patient?**

A. Mutations in the gene encoding Cl/HCO_3 exchanger (Anion Exchange 1, AE1)
B. Mutations in the gene encoding B1 subunit of H-ATPase
C. Mutations in the gene encoding a4 subunit of H-ATPase
D. Mutations in the gene encoding carbonic anhydrase II (CA II) enzyme
E. Deficiency of Na/H exchanger (NHE3)

The answer is A

Autosomal dominant distal RTA is caused by mutations in the gene encoding the basolateral Cl/HCO_3 exchanger. They are unable to acidify their urine. They have mild hypokalemia and mild hyperchloremic acidosis. They have hypercalciuria with hypocitraturia with development of nephrocalcinosis/lithiasis later in life.

Gene mutations stated in options B and D cause autosomal recessive distal RTA with or without deafness, respectively. Deficiency of CA II enzyme causes distal RTA with osteopetrosis and cerebral calcifications. It occurs mostly in Arab populations of the Middle East. At times patients present with clinical manifestations of both proximal and distal RTA. Deficiency of Na/H exchanger causes possibly autosomal dominant form of proximal RTA, and so far no gene mutations have been reported. Thus, options B, C, D, and E are incorrect.

Suggested Reading

Batlle D, Haque SK. Genetic causes and mechanisms of distal renal tubular acidosis. Nephrol Dial Transplant. 2012;27:3691–704.

Reddi AS. Acid-base disorders. Clinical evaluation and management. New York: Springer; 2020.

40. A 44-year-old woman with Sjögren's syndrome with hypergammaglobulinemia and tubulointerstitial disease is referred to renal clinic for evaluation of documented hypokalemic hyperchloremic metabolic acidosis. She was treated with corticosteroids for tubulointerstitial disease. Her serum [HCO_3^-] is 16 mEq/L and eGFR is 56 ml/min. Serum phosphate, uric acid, and glucose levels are normal. **What other pertinent laboratory test you order at this time?**

A. Arterial blood gas
B. Kidney biopsy to know the extent of interstitial disease
C. Urinalysis
D. Serum renin and aldosterone levels
E. None

The answer is C

It is important to know whether the patient is able to acidify or alkalinize her urine. Patients with Sjögren's syndrome can develop type I or type II RTA. At times, they can present with both type I and type II RTAs. Urine pH is an important determinant in the diagnosis of the type of RTA. All other tests are not important at this time.

Suggested Reading

Gil-Peña H, Mejia M, Santos F. Renal tubular acidosis. J Pediatr. 2014;164:691–8.

Reddi AS. Acid-base disorders. Clinical evaluation and management. New York: Springer; 2020.

Golembiewska E, Ciechanowski K. Renal tubular acidosis-underrated problem? Acta Biochim Pol. 2012;59:213–7.

Niewold TB, Short DK, Albright RC. 27-Year-old woman with numbness and weakness of the extremities. Mayo Clin Proc. 2003;78:95–8.

41. **Which one of the following statements is TRUE regarding distal RTA?**

   A. Inability to acidify urine
   B. Prone to develop calcium phosphate stones
   C. Urinary citrate excretion is low
   D. Urinary NH_4^+ excretion is low
   E. All of the above

The answer is E

All of the above statements are correct. Thus, answer E is correct. Of particular importance is the development of calcium phosphate stones because calcium phosphate is soluble in alkaline pH and can precipitate in renal tubules. On the other hand, calcium oxalate stones are formed in acidic pH.

Suggested Reading

Reddi AS. Acid-base disorders. Clinical evaluation and management. New York: Springer; 2020.
Vallės PG, Batlle D. Hypokalemic distal renal tubular acidosis. Adv Chronic Kidney Dis. 2018;25:303–20.

42. An 18-year-old female student is admitted for weakness, tiredness, and loose stools for 1 week. She denies diarrhea or any type of medications but admits to frequent urination. Physical exam reveals a thin female with no apparent distress. Blood pressure is 100/60 mm Hg with a pulse rate of 94 beats per minutes with orthostatic changes. She is afebrile. Lungs and heart are normal. Abdomen is soft with no tenderness. There is no peripheral edema. Laboratory values:

Serum	Urine
Na^+ = 132 mEq/L	pH = 6.4
K^+ = 2.8 mEq/L	Osmolality = 800 mOsm/kg H_2O
Cl^- = 115 mEq/L	Na^+ = 20 mEq/L
HCO_3^- = 15 mEq/L	K^+ = 15 mEq/L
Creatinine = 1.5 mg/dl	Cl^- = 55 mEq/L
BUN = 30 mg/dl	
Glucose = 90 mg/dl	
Albumin = 4.2 g/dl	
ABG: pH = 7.32; PCO_2 = 30; PO_2 = 98; HCO_3 = 14	

Which one of the following best describes the observed abnormalities in serum chemistry?

   A. Distal RTA
   B. Diuretic abuse
   C. Laxative abuse
   D. Proximal RTA
   E. Surreptitious vomiting

The answer is C

This patient has hyperchloremic metabolic acidosis (HCMA) with appropriate respiratory compensation. Based on the urine pH and HCMA, distal RTA can be considered; however, urine electrolytes do not support this diagnosis. Diuretic abuse may cause volume depletion and orthostatic changes, but urine pH, osmolality, and electrolyte pattern do not support diuretic abuse. Also, diuretics such as furosemide and hydrochlorothiazide cause metabolic alkalosis rather than metabolic acidosis. Carbonic anhydrase inhibitors such as acetazolamide cause HCMA with alkaline urine pH and proximal RTA; however, urine lytes do not support acetazolamide abuse. Proximal RTA is also unlikely because the urine pH is usually <5.5 with serum [HCO_3^-] of 15 mEq/L. Urine pH and electrolytes do not suggest late vomiting, as early and late vomiting cause low Cl^- and high K^+ excretion. During early vomiting, the urine pH is alkaline because of HCO_3^- excretion, and acid pH during late vomiting because of H^+ secretion. Thus, options A, B, D, and E are incorrect.

The patient agreed to laxative abuse, which was confirmed by stool testing with NaOH. Laxative abusers will have diarrhea-induced volume depletion, and the electrolyte abnormalities, as described above.

In this patient, the U_{AG} is negative ($U_{Na} + U_K - U_{Cl}$ or 20 + 15 – 55 = –20), suggesting high NH_4^- excretion. This test also rules out both proximal and distal RTAs as well.

Suggested Reading

Gennari FJ, Weise WJ. Acid-base disturbances in gastrointestinal disease. Clin J Am Soc Nephrol. 2008;3:1861–8.
Reddi AS. Acid-base disorders. Clinical evaluation and management. New York: Springer; 2020.

43. **Match the following electrolyte and ABG values with the case histories.**

A. Patient with simple diarrhea
B. Patient with diarrhea and vomiting
C. Patient with diarrhea and lactic acidosis
D. Patient with diarrhea and respiratory alkalosis due to pneumonia

Option	Na^+ (mEq/L)	K^+ (mEq/L)	Cl^-(mEq/L)	HCO_3^- (mEq/L)	pH	pCO_2 (mm Hg)
1	138	2.4	120	9	7.32	18
2	140	3.2	116	5	7.13	14
3	134	2.8	104	23	7.40	38
4	136	3.1	114	12	7.28	26

Answers: A = 4; B = 3; C = 2; D = 1

Calculation of serum AG is helpful because lactic acidosis is associated with elevated AG. The serum AG in option 2 is 19, and therefore, associated with case C. All other cases have normal serum AG.

Patient with diarrhea and vomiting should have near normal serum [HCO_3^-] compared to other cases, because vomiting is associated with low serum [Cl^-]. Serum pH should be normal. (Diarrhea causes low pH and vomiting raises pH. When both coexist, the pH becomes normal.) Thus, option 3 corresponds to case B.

Patient with diarrhea and respiratory alkalosis should have relatively low HCO_3^-, high Cl^-, and near normal pH. Electrolytes and ABG described in option 1 are consistent with case D.

Uncomplicated diarrhea is associated with moderate acidemia, and electrolyte and ABG pattern is consistent with option 4.

Suggested Reading

Gennari FJ, Weise WJ. Acid-base disturbances in gastrointestinal disease. Clin J Am Soc Nephrol. 2008;3:1861–8.
Reddi AS. Acid-base disorders. Clinical evaluation and management. New York: Springer; 2020.

44. The patient is a 65-year-old man who was brought to the Emergency Department (ED) after being found on the floor at home due to a fall. He was awake and alert but oriented to place and time only. He was then noted to have a draining wound of his left foot that was wrapped in plastic. The patient complained of generalized weakness with muscle cramps and poor appetite for a few days. He also admitted to difficulty in walking from his foot ulcer. While in the ED, the patient became agitated, requiring intubation for airway protection. Past medical history includes only foot ulcers for 2 years. He was hospitalized 2 weeks prior to this admission at another hospital. He was treated with intravenous antibiotics for 1 week and discharged. He was not on any medications.

On admission, his BP was 131/77 mm Hg with a regular pulse rate of 82/ min. He was afebrile. His body mass index was 18.2. He was well developed but poorly nourished. Except for a well demarcated left lower foot ulcer with unclean margins extending from distally one-third of foot to toes, the rest of the physical exam was unremarkable. The ulcers were foul-smelling with serous but not purulent discharge and wrapped with white powder in plastic.

Chest X-ray was unremarkable. The EKG showed normal sinus rhythm with pulse rate of 80 beats/min, normal axis, first degree AV block, QT prolongation (536 ms), 1 VPC, ST depression in V3–V6 and inferior leads. Because of agitation, a CT scan of head was done, which was negative. Initial and subsequent lab data are shown below:

Lab value	Day 1	Day 2	Day 3	Day 4	Day 5
Na^+ (mEq/L)	148	142	140	137	138
K^+ (mEq/L)	1.8	2.9	2.9	2.5	3.6
Cl^- (mEq/L)	73	92	92	96	100
HCO_3^- (mEq/L)	54	45	40	38	32
Creatinine (mg/dL)	3.4	2.7	2.4	1.6	1.2
Albumin (g/dL)	2.7	–	–	–	–
Lactate (mmol/L)	2.2	–	–	–	–
Urine (U) pH	6.0	6.0	–	8.0	–
U_{Na} (mEq/L)	21	27	43	74	–
U_K (mEq/L)	58	90	59	4	–
U_{Cl} (mEq/L)	<10	<10	26	37	–
Ketones	Negative	–	–	–	–
ABG					

Lab value	Day 1	Day 2	Day 3	Day 4	Day 5
pH	7.69	7.55	7.48	7.48	7.46
pCO_2	45	56	59	51	34
pO_2	48	218	134	101	94
CK (U)	5604	1846	1335	771	–
Troponin	28.32	5.16	–	–	–

What is the acid–base disturbance in this patient?

A. Metabolic alkalosis
B. Metabolic acidosis and respiratory alkalosis
C. Metabolic alkalosis, respiratory alkalosis, and metabolic acidosis
D. Metabolic acidosis, metabolic alkalosis, and respiratory acidosis
E. Metabolic alkalosis, respiratory alkalosis, and respiratory acidosis

The answer is C

Based on elevated pH and HCO_3^-, the primary acid–base disorder is metabolic alkalosis. However, calculation of respiratory compensation and AG would help to characterize the acid–base disturbance in this patient. The expected pCO_2 should be 61; however, the reported pCO_2 is 45. This indicates that the patient is hyperventilating, and therefore, respiratory alkalosis is also present.

The AG is 21, which is not due to entirely metabolic alkalosis. Despite volume depletion, his albumin is only 2.7 g/dL, which could not account for elevated AG. Also, ketoacidosis or lactic acidosis is not the cause. We believe that either renal insufficiency or other organic acid may have caused elevated AG.

Thus, the acid–base disorder is a primary metabolic alkalosis with superimposed respiratory alkalosis and a high AG metabolic acidosis (C is correct).

In a 24-h period, the patient received a total of 7 L of 0.9% saline, 2 L of 0.45% saline, 360 mEq of KCl, and 8 mEq of $MgSO_4$. The blood pressure improved. The patient received only one dose of acetazolamide 250 mg, after adequate hydration. In a 4-day period, the patient received a total of 7 L of 0.9% saline, 19 L of 0.45% saline, and 960 mEq of KCl. The EKG abnormalities had resolved, and an ECHO showed no wall motion or valvular abnormalities.

After extubation, the patient admitted to eating baking soda (a palm full with water) and covering the foot ulcer with adequate amount of baking soda ($NaHCO_3$) for a year and half.

Suggested Reading

John RS, Simoes S, Reddi AS. A patient with foot ulcer and severe metabolic alkalosis. Am J Emerg Med. 2012;260: e5–8.

Marston N, Kehl D, Copp J, et al. Alkalotics anonymous: severe metabolic alkalosis. Am J Med. 2014;127:25–7.

45. A 17-year-old Caucasian medical student is seen in the ED for persistent headache for a 2-week duration. She has no history of HTN, migraine, or diabetes. She has been healthy and not on any medication. There is no family history of hypertension other than obesity. Physical exam shows a blood pressure of 200/142 mm Hg and pulse rate of 94 beats per minute. Her blood pressure was normal 6 months ago. Funduscopic examination reveals hypertensive retinopathy without papilledema. There are no crackles, S_4 or S_3, abdominal bruits, or edema. Neurologic exam is normal. Laboratory values:

Serum	Urine
Na^+ = 136 mEq/L	pH = 6.2
K^+ = 2.8 mEq/L	Osmolality = 1000 mOsm/kg H_2O
Cl^- = 84 mEq/L	Na^+ = 80 mEq/L
HCO_3^- = 35 mEq/L	K^+ = 55 mEq/L
Creatinine = 1.5 mg/dL	Cl^- = 75 mEq/L
BUN = 32 mg/dL	
Glucose = 92 mg/dL	
Albumin = 4.2 g/dL	
ABG: pH = 7.48; PCO_2 = 47 mm Hg; HCO_3 = 34 mEq/L	

What is the acid–base disturbance?

A. Respiratory alkalosis
B. Respiratory alkalosis and respiratory acidosis
C. Metabolic alkalosis with appropriate respiratory compensation
D. Metabolic alkalosis and respiratory alkalosis
E. None of the above

The answer is C

Both blood pH and serum [HCO_3^-] are increased; therefore, the primary acid–base disturbance is metabolic alkalosis with appropriate respiratory response (C is correct).

Suggested Reading

Reddi AS. Acid-base disorders. Clinical evaluation and management. New York: Springer; 2020.
Soleimani M. Potassium-depletion metabolic alkalosis. In: Gennari FJ, Adrogué HJ, Galla JH, Madias NE, editors. Acid-base disorders and their treatment. Boca Raton: Taylor & Francis; 2005. p. 553–84.

46. This student has significant metabolic alkalosis, and urine Cl^- determination is very important to distinguish Cl^--responsive from Cl^--resistant metabolic alkalosis. This patient has Cl^--resistant metabolic alkalosis. **Which one of the following diagnoses you need to consider in her?**

A. Primary aldosteronism
B. Cushing syndrome
C. Malignant hypertension (HTN)
D. Renal artery stenosis
E. All of the above

The answer is E

All of the above diagnoses are correct (E). In order to distinguish one from the other, plasma renin and aldosterone levels should be obtained. Both of them were elevated. This rules out primary aldosteronism because renin is suppressed in this form of HTN (A is incorrect). She has no features of Cushing syndrome (B is incorrect).

Malignant HTN is also unlikely in view of normal BP 6 months ago. Although retinopathy supports the diagnosis of long-standing HTN, the absence of papilledema does not support the diagnosis of malignant HTN (C is incorrect).

Renin secreting tumor is a possibility; however, patients with this tumor have resistant HTN prior to diagnosis of this tumor. Although the occurrence of this tumor in many case reports is in young patients (18–24 years), they all had prior HTN. Also, retinopathy has not been described (to my knowledge). After exclusion of the above conditions, possible renal artery stenosis was entertained.

After volume expansion and controlling BP, an MR angiography was done because of its 100% sensitivity and 94% specificity for detecting renal artery stenosis. This patient was found to have unilateral renal artery stenosis due to fibromuscular dysplasia (D is correct).

Suggested Reading

Reddi AS. Acid-base disorders. Clinical evaluation and management. New York: Springer; 2020.
Soleimani M. Potassium-depletion metabolic alkalosis. In: Gennari FJ, Adrogué HJ, Galla JH, Madias NE, editors. Acid-base disorders and their treatment. Boca Raton: Taylor & Francis; 2005. p. 553–84.

47. A 24-year-old man was referred to the renal clinic for evaluation of recent onset hypertension (HTN) noted on a routine physical checkup. He has a strong family history of HTN at an early age. He is not on any medications. BP is 190/104 mm Hg with a pulse rate of 74 beats/min. There are no orthostatic changes. His laboratory values are consistent with hypokalemic metabolic alkalosis. He has high urine Cl^- relative to Na^+ and K^+, which are also high. His plasma renin and aldosterone levels are extremely low. **Which one of the following is the MOST likely diagnosis in this patient?**

A. Primary aldosteronism
B. Renal artery stenosis
C. Liddle syndrome

D. Gitelman syndrome
E. Bartter syndrome

The answer is C

Primary aldosteronism and renal artery stenosis are associated with hypertension and high aldosterone levels. Patients with Gitelman and Bartter syndromes present with normal to low blood pressure. Renin and aldosterone levels are high rather than low in these syndromes. Therefore, the patient has Liddle syndrome, which is a genetic disorder due to mutations in ENaC. Renin and aldosterone levels are usually low, but normal values have also been reported. These low levels have been attributed to volume expansion and/or sclerosis of renin-producing cells in the juxtaglomerular apparatus.

Suggested Reading

Reddi AS. Metabolic alkalosis. In: Reddi AS, editor. Fluid, electrolyte, and acid-base disorders. Clinical evaluation and management. 2nd ed. New York: Springer; 2018. p. 403–27.
Reddi AS. Acid-base disorders. Clinical evaluation and management. New York: Springer; 2020.

48. **Which one of the following drugs is APPROPRIATE for this patient?**

A. Spironolactone
B. Eplerenone
C. Hydrochlorothiazide
D. Metolazone
E. Amiloride

The answer is E

Patients with Liddle syndrome respond only to amiloride or triamterene and not to the other drugs mentioned above (E is correct). In contrast, patients with primary aldosteronism respond to either spironolactone or amiloride. Thus, control of HTN with spironolactone or eplerenone suggests the diagnosis of primary aldosteronism, whereas failure to control BP suggests either Liddle syndrome or essential hypertension. BP improves with amiloride in Liddle syndrome, whereas it may not improve in essential hypertension. The latter requires probably more than one drug.

Suggested Reading

Reddi AS. Metabolic alkalosis. In: Reddi AS, editor. Fluid, electrolyte, and acid-base disorders. Clinical evaluation and management. 2nd ed. New York: Springer; 2018. p. 403–27.
Reddi AS. Acid-base disorders. Clinical evaluation and management. New York: Springer; 2020.

49. **Match the serum and urinary electrolyte pattern with patient history.**

	Serum $[Na^+]$[a]	Serum $[K^+]$	Serum $[Cl^-]$	Serum $[HCO_3^-]$	Blood pH	Urine $[Na^+]$	Urine $[K^+]$	Urine $[Cl^-]$	Urine $[Ca^{2+}]$	Urine pH
A	136	3.0	89	28	7.48	100	40	15	200	7.2
B	135	2.8	86	32	7.50	40	30	15	150	5.8
C	136	3.0	86	32	7.51	80	44	60	250	6.1
D	137	2.9	84	30	7.48	120	80	60	50	6.2

[a]mEq/L

1. An 18-year-old man with craving for salty food and a mutation in Na/Cl cotransporter
2. A 12-year-old boy with a documented mutation in Na/K/2Cl cotransporter
3. A 27-year-old woman with vomiting for <2 days
4. A 40-year-old man with protracted vomiting for >7 days

Answers: 1 = D; 2 = C; 3 = A; 4 = B

The 18-year-old man carries the diagnosis of Gitelman syndrome, whereas the 12-year-old boy has Bartter syndrome. Clinically, both syndromes behave similarly. Urinary excretion of Ca^{2+} levels is the most important determinant of these syndromes. Hypocalciuria characterizes the Gitelman syndrome, whereas Ca^{2+} excretion is

normal in Bartter syndrome. Labs shown in D and C are consistent with Gitelman and Bartter syndromes, respectively.

From the above table, it is evident that early and late vomiting can be diagnosed based only on the urine electrolytes and urine pH. In early vomiting, the kidneys try to get rid of excess Na^+ and HCO_3^- in the urine to maintain near normal serum levels of these electrolytes. The urine pH is alkaline because of the presence of HCO_3^-. If this vomiting continues, the intravascular volume is depleted, and metabolic alkalosis is sustained. This causes Na^+ and HCO_3^- reabsorption, resulting in low levels of these electrolytes and acidification of urine pH. During the correction phase of metabolic alkalosis, urine pH becomes alkaline because of HCO_3^- excretion. Thus, labs shown in A and B correspond to early and late vomiting, respectively.

Suggested Reading

Reddi AS. Metabolic alkalosis. In: Reddi AS, editor. Fluid, electrolyte, and acid-base disorders. Clinical evaluation and management. 2nd ed. New York: Springer; 2018. p. 403–27.

Reddi AS. Acid-base disorders. Clinical evaluation and management. New York: Springer; 2020.

50. A 36-year-old woman was admitted for weakness, dizziness, and inability to walk for 2 weeks. She has a childhood history of hypothyroidism and sensorineural deafness. She denied vomiting. Her medications include synthroid for hypothyroidism and hydrochlorothiazide (HCTZ) for endolymph excess in the ear. Except for palpable goiter and low blood pressure, her physical examination is otherwise normal. Two months ago, her labs were normal. Current labs:

Serum	Urine
Na^+ = 134 mEq/L	pH = 6.0
K^+ = 2.6 mEq/L	Osmolality = 400 mOsm/kg H_2O
Cl^- = 84 mEq/L	Na^+ = 40 mEq/L
HCO_3^- = 36 mEq/L	K^+ = 50 mEq/L
Creatinine = 1.1 mg/dL	Cl^- = 20 mEq/L
BUN = 10 mg/dL	
Glucose = 90 mg/dL	
Albumin = 4.0 g/dL	
ABG: pH = 7.48, pCO_2 = 47 mm Hg HCO_3^- = 35 mEq/L	

Which one of the following transport mechanisms is IMPLICATED for her childhood disease and metabolic alkalosis?

A. Na/H-ATPase
B. Na/K/2Cl cotransporter
C. Na/Cl cotransporter
D. Epithelial Na^+ channel (ENaC)
E. Cl/HCO_3 exchanger

The answer is E

This patient carries the diagnosis of Pendred syndrome, which is an autosomal recessive disorder. This disorder is characterized by sensorineural deafness and goiter due to defect in iodide organification. Pendred syndrome is caused by biallelic mutations in the solute carrier family 26A4 gene, which encodes pendrin. In the kidney, pendrin functions as a Cl/HCO_3 exchanger in the β-intercalated cell where Cl^- is reabsorbed and HCO_3^- is excreted into the lumen (Chap. 2). This suggests that pendrin may protect against development of either salt loss or metabolic alkalosis under basal conditions because excess generation of HCO_3^- from any source is transported into the lumen and Cl^- is reabsorbed.

Under basal conditions, patients with Pendred syndrome do not develop any electrolyte or acid–base abnormalities. This suggests that there is a compensatory mechanism that prevents these abnormalities. Studies have shown that thiazide-sensitive Na/Cl cotransporter in the distal tubule takes over the function of pendrin as a Cl^-transporter. Conversely, when Na/Cl cotransporter is inhibited by a thiazide, pendrin expression and activity are increased. When both transporters are inhibited, volume depletion and metabolic alkalosis develop due to loss of NaCl in the urine. This happens when a Pendred syndrome patient is treated with a thiazide diuretic for

endolymph accumulation in the ear. The mechanism by which this crosstalk between Na/Cl cotransporter and Cl/HCO_3 exchanger occurs is not completely understood.

Our patient with Pendred syndrome developed hypokalemia, hypochloremia, metabolic alkalosis, and volume depletion (low blood pressure) because of mutation in pendrin and inhibition of Na/Cl cotransporter by HCTZ. Discontinuation of HCTZ and hydration with normal saline and KCl would improve her electrolyte abnormalities and metabolic alkalosis. Thus, choice E is correct. Although pendrin interacts with other transporters, their deficiency or activation does not cause Pendred syndrome. Thus, choices A–D are incorrect.

Suggested Reading

Kandasamy N, Fugazola L, Evans M, et al. Life-threatening metabolic alkalosis in pendred syndrome. Eur J Endocrinol. 2011;165:167–70.
Soleimani M. The multiple roles of pendrin in the kidney. Nephrol Dial Transplant. 2015;30:1257–66.
Wall SM, Laza-Fernandez Y. The role of pendrin in renal physiology. Annu Rev Physiol. 2015;77:363–78.

51. **Which one of the following conditions of metabolic alkalosis does NOT respond to infusion of normal saline?**

A. Vomiting
B. Nasogastric suction
C. Bartter syndrome
D. Gitelman syndrome
E. C and D

The answer is E

Both vomiting and nasogastric suction cause saline-responsive metabolic alkalosis, whereas Bartter syndrome and Gitelman syndrome are saline-resistant conditions of metabolic alkalosis. Thus, answer E is correct.

Suggested Reading

Reddi AS. Metabolic alkalosis. In: Reddi AS, editor. Fluid, electrolyte, and acid-base disorders. Clinical evaluation and management. 2nd ed. New York: Springer; 2018. p. 403–27.
Reddi AS. Acid-base disorders. Clinical evaluation and management. New York: Springer; 2020.

52. A 64-year-old woman with COPD develops diarrhea of 1 week duration. She says that she took enough fluids "to keep up with diarrhea," but abdominal cramps and slight dizziness brought her to the ED. She is alert and oriented. Her BP is 120/60 mm Hg with a hear rate of 96 beats/min. Respiratory rate is 19/min. She has orthostatic BP and pulse changes. Laboratory values:

Serum	ABG
Na^+ = 136 mEq/L	pH = 7.27
K^+ = 3.2 mEq/L	pCO_2 = 62 mm Hg
Cl^- = 100 mEq/L	pO_2 = 88 mm Hg
HCO_3^- = 28 mEq/L	HCO_3^- = 27 mEq/L
Creatinine = 1.0 mg/dL	
BUN = 24 mg/dL	
Glucose = 92 mg/dL	

What is the acid–base disturbance?

A. Metabolic acidosis and respiratory alkalosis
B. Metabolic acidosis and metabolic alkalosis
C. Respiratory acidosis and metabolic acidosis
D. Respiratory acidosis and metabolic alkalosis
E. Respiratory acidosis, metabolic acidosis, and metabolic alkalosis

The answer is C

Low pH and high pCO_2 and HCO_3^- indicate that the primary acid–base disorder is chronic respiratory acidosis. If she had acute respiratory acidosis, her serum HCO_3^- would have been 26 (24 + 2) rather than 28 mEq/L.

The pH and serum [HCO_3^-] are low for chronic respiratory acidosis. Since she has diarrhea, she developed non-AG metabolic acidosis, which lowered HCO_3^- and pH. Note that pCO_2 may have been slightly lowered because of mild increase in respiratory rate. Thus, the patient has chronic respiratory acidosis and metabolic acidosis.

Suggested Reading

Reddi AS. Metabolic alkalosis. In: Reddi AS, editor. Fluid, electrolyte, and acid-base disorders. Clinical evaluation and management. 2nd ed. New York: Springer; 2018. p. 403–27.

Reddi AS. Acid-base disorders. Clinical evaluation and management. New York: Springer; 2020.

53. A 56-year-old man with history of COPD and essential hypertension is admitted for recently exacerbated shortness of breath and easy fatiguability. He is on bronchodilators and hydrochlorothiazide (HCTZ). Laboratory values:

Serum	ABG
Na^+ = 134 mEq/L	pH = 7.42
K^+ = 3.6 mEq/L	pCO_2 = 59 mm Hg
Cl^- = 91 mEq/L	pO_2 = 62 mm Hg
HCO_3^- = 37 mEq/L	HCO_3^- = 36 mEq/L
Creatinine = 0.9 mg/dL	
BUN = 14 mg/dL	
Glucose = 90 mg/dL	
Albumin = 4.5 g/dL	

What is the acid–base disturbance?

A. Metabolic acidosis and respiratory alkalosis
B. Metabolic acidosis and metabolic alkalosis
C. Respiratory acidosis and metabolic acidosis
D. Respiratory acidosis and metabolic alkalosis
E. Respiratory acidosis, metabolic acidosis, and metabolic alkalosis

The answer is D

The increases in HCO_3^- and pCO_2 with slightly elevated pH indicate that the acid–base disorder is metabolic alkalosis. Based on the respiratory response for metabolic alkalosis, the expected pCO_2 should be (ΔHCO_3^- = 13 (37 − 24) × 0.7 = 13) 53 (40 + 13) mm Hg. However, the reported pCO_2 is 59 mm Hg. Therefore, the acid–base is metabolic alkalosis superimposed on chronic respiratory acidosis. The coexistence of metabolic alkalosis is due to HCTZ.

Suggested Reading

Reddi AS. Metabolic alkalosis. In: Reddi AS, editor. Fluid, electrolyte, and acid-base disorders. Clinical evaluation and management. 2nd ed. New York: Springer; 2018. p. 403–27.

Reddi AS. Acid-base disorders. Clinical evaluation and management. New York: Springer; 2020.

54. A 24-year-old woman with asthma is seen in the Emergency Department for acute exacerbation due to upper respiratory tract infection. Prior to bronchodilator and corticosteroid therapy, laboratory values were drawn, which show:

Serum	ABG
Na^+ = 139 mEq/L	pH = 7.55
K^+ = 3.4 mEq/L	pCO_2 = 22 mm Hg
Cl^- = 96 mEq/L	pO_2 = 88 mm Hg
HCO_3^- = 21 mEq/L	HCO_3^- = 20 mEq/L
Creatinine = 0.6 mg/dL	
BUN = 18 mg/dL	
Glucose = 92 mg/dL	

What is the acid–base disturbance?

A. Metabolic acidosis
B. Metabolic alkalosis
C. Acute respiratory alkalosis
D. Chronic respiratory alkalosis
E. Respiratory alkalosis and metabolic acidosis

The answer is C

Based on alkaline pH, low HCO_3^-, and low pCO_2, the acid–base disturbance is respiratory alkalosis. It is acute respiratory alkalosis, as the decrease in serum [HCO_3^-] from 24 to 21 mEq/L (for each mm Hg decrease in pCO_2, HCO_3^- decreases by 0.2 mEq/L) is consistent with uncomplicated acute respiratory alkalosis. Hypocapnia due to hyperventilation is common during exacerbation of asthma.

Suggested Reading

Reddi AS. Metabolic alkalosis. In: Reddi AS, editor. Fluid, electrolyte, and acid-base disorders. Clinical evaluation and management. 2nd ed. New York: Springer; 2018. p. 403–27.
Reddi AS. Acid-base disorders. Clinical evaluation and management. New York: Springer; 2020.

55. A 66-year-old man with COPD is admitted for increasing shortness of breath, and swollen legs for 10 days. He is on bronchodilators and furosemide. Physical examination reveals crackles and an S_3, and 2+ pitting edema in lower extremities. The patient receives IV furosemide 60 mg Q12H for 3 days, and his shortness of breath and edema improved. EKG is normal. Laboratory values:

Serum electrolytes and ABG On admission	Serum electrolytes and ABG on fourth day
Na^+ = 136 mEq/L	Na^+ = 134 mEq/L
K^+ = 3.3 mEq/L	K^+ = 3.2 mEq/L
Cl^- = 104 mEq/L	Cl^- = 96 mEq/L
HCO_3^- = 18 mEq/L	HCO_3^- = 21 mEq/L
Creatinine = 1.1 mg/dL	Creatinine = 1.2 mg/dL
BUN = 28 mg/dL	BUN = 38 mg/dL
Glucose = 102 mg/dL	Glucose = 112 mg/dL
ABG	ABG
pH = 7.45	pH = 7.48
pCO_2 = 26 mm Hg	pCO_2 = 28 mm Hg
pO_2 = 90 mm Hg	pO_2 = 92 mm Hg
HCO_3^- = 17 mEq/L	HCO_3^- = 20 mEq/L

What is the acid–base disturbance on admission?

A. Metabolic acidosis
B. Metabolic alkalosis
C. Acute respiratory alkalosis
D. Chronic respiratory alkalosis
E. Respiratory alkalosis and metabolic acidosis

The answer is D

Based on alkaline pH, low serum [HCO_3^-] and pCO_2, the acid–base disturbance is respiratory alkalosis. The expected serum [HCO_3^-] from secondary response for acute respiratory alkalosis is 21 mEq/L (24 – 3 = 21 mEq/L). For chronic respiratory alkalosis, the expected serum [HCO_3^-] from secondary response is 18 (24 – 6 = 18 mEq/L). Therefore, the patient has uncomplicated chronic respiratory alkalosis.

56. **What is the acid–base disorder on the fourth day?**

A. Metabolic acidosis
B. Metabolic alkalosis
C. Acute respiratory alkalosis
D. Chronic respiratory alkalosis
E. Chronic respiratory alkalosis and metabolic alkalosis

The answer is E

Although the patient had chronic respiratory alkalosis on admission, the pH, serum [HCO_3^-], and pCO_2 are elevated following treatment, suggesting superimposed metabolic alkalosis caused by administration of furosemide. The induction of metabolic alkalosis due to loop diuretics is not uncommon in patients with CHF and edema.

Suggested Reading

Reddi AS. Metabolic alkalosis. In: Reddi AS, editor. Fluid, electrolyte, and acid-base disorders. Clinical evaluation and management. 2nd ed. New York: Springer; 2018. p. 403–27.
Reddi AS. Acid-base disorders. Clinical evaluation and management. New York: Springer; 2020.

57. **For each set of laboratory data, select the appropriate acid–base disturbance.**

Option	Na^+ (mEq/L)	Cl^- (mEq/L)	HCO_3^- (mEq/L)	pH	pCO_2 (mm Hg)	HCO_3^- [a] (mEq/L)
A	130	95	10	7.34	19	9
B	136	94	24	7.39	39	23
C	130	85	29	7.50	36	28
D	140	100	20	7.27	44	19
E	142	100	32	7.41	52	31

[a]Calculated HCO_3^-

1. Metabolic alkalosis and respiratory acidosis
2. Metabolic acidosis and respiratory alkalosis
3. Metabolic acidosis and respiratory acidosis
4. Metabolic acidosis and metabolic alkalosis
5. Metabolic alkalosis and respiratory alkalosis

Answers: A = 2; B = 4; C = 3; D = 5; E = 1 or (1 = E; 2 = A; 3 = D; 4 = B; 5 = C)

To answer these questions, it is important to calculate the AG. The AG and an understanding of the pathogenesis of the above mixed acid–base disorders provide important clues for their identification. The AG for the values shown in options A to E is 25, 18, 16, 20, and 10 mEq/L, respectively. Regarding the pathogenesis of the acid–base disorder in answer 1, either vomiting or diuretic (thiazide or loop diuretic) use generally causes metabolic alkalosis and emphysema or any disorder causing retention of CO_2 results in respiratory acidosis. Lab data shown in option E are consistent with metabolic alkalosis and respiratory acidosis. Both disorders cause a normal to high pH and elevated HCO_3^- and pCO_2. The AG is usually normal or slightly elevated, if metabolic alkalosis predominates.

The acid–base disturbance given in answer 2 may be caused by diseases such as renal failure, lactic acidosis, ketoacidosis, or ingestion of toxins such as methanol or ethylene glycol, which lower serum [HCO_3^-] and elevate AG. The appropriate response for metabolic acidosis is hyperventilation. This results in low pCO_2. Data shown in option A are consistent with metabolic acidosis and respiratory alkalosis. Metabolic acidosis may exist alone (pure) or may exist with another primary disorder (mixed). In order to distinguish between the two disorders, the expected PCO_2 should be calculated, as shown under the discussion of mixed metabolic acidosis and respiratory alkalosis. If the ABG shown in option A were a pure metabolic acidosis, the pCO_2 would have been between 21 and 25 mm Hg. Instead, the pCO_2 is 19 mm Hg. Therefore, respiratory alkalosis is superimposed on metabolic acidosis.

The acid–base disturbance given in answer 3 is generally caused by a condition that generates lactic acid acutely such as sudden cardiac arrest or severe hypotension superimposed on a patient with underlying emphysema with CO_2 retention. The combination of metabolic acidosis and respiratory acidosis lowers pH below 7.40 and [HCO_3^-] below 24 mEq/L with normal to slightly elevated pCO_2. The AG is usually elevated because of accumulation of lactic acid or a similar anion. Lab data shown in option D are consistent with both metabolic and respiratory acidosis.

The acid–base disorder given in answer 4 occurs in a patient with renal failure who develops vomiting or on a thiazide or loop diuretic. Renal failure causes high AG metabolic acidosis with low pH, low [HCO_3^-], and low pCO_2. On the other hand, metabolic alkalosis results in a high pH, elevated [HCO_3^-], and a high pCO_2 due to hypoventilation. When both disorders coexist, the pH, [HCO_3^-], and pCO_2 are normalized. The only clue to this acid–base disorder is elevated AG, because both metabolic acidosis and metabolic alkalosis cause elevated

AG. However, metabolic acidosis due to diarrhea or renal tubular acidosis does not elevate AG. The combination of normal AG metabolic acidosis and metabolic alkalosis generally causes slight elevation in AG because of the latter acid–base disorder. Lab data shown in option B are consistent with metabolic acidosis and metabolic alkalosis.

The acid–base disturbance given in answer 5 is seen in a patient who has liver failure with hyperventilation. This causes respiratory alkalosis. If this patient is also being treated with a diuretic, such as furosemide, or experienced vomiting, the patient develops metabolic alkalosis. In such a patient, the pH is usually >7.40, the [HCO_3^-] is normal to high, and pCO_2 is normal to slightly low. Lab data shown in option C are consistent with respiratory and metabolic alkalosis. A similar acid–base disorder can be seen in a normal pregnant woman with severe vomiting.

Suggested Reading

Reddi AS. Metabolic alkalosis. In: Reddi AS, editor. Fluid, electrolyte, and acid-base disorders. Clinical evaluation and management. 2nd ed. New York: Springer; 2018. p. 403–27.

Reddi AS. Acid-base disorders. Clinical evaluation and management. New York: Springer; 2020.

58. A 38-year-old man with history of type 1 diabetes and pancreatitis is admitted for nausea, vomiting, and severe abdominal pain for the last 4 days. He did not take insulin because of poor oral intake. Laboratory results:

Serum	ABG
Na^+ = 120 mEq/L	pH = 7.47
K^+ = 3.9 mEq/L	pCO_2 = 23 mm Hg
Cl^- = 60 mEq/L	pO_2 = 109 mm Hg
HCO_3^- = 17 mEq/L	HCO_3^- = 16 mEq/L
Creatinine = 3.1 mg/dL	
BUN = 88 mg/dL	
Glucose = 776 mg/dL	
Ketones = positive	

Which one of the following describes the BEST of his acid–base status?

A. Metabolic acidosis and metabolic alkalosis
B. Metabolic alkalosis and respiratory alkalosis
C. Metabolic acidosis and respiratory acidosis
D. Respiratory alkalosis, metabolic acidosis, and metabolic alkalosis
E. Metabolic acidosis, respiratory acidosis, and metabolic alkalosis

The answer is D

Using the Henderson equation, the [H^+] is 32, which corresponds to a pH of 7.48 and close to the patient's pH. From the ABG values, the initial disturbance is respiratory alkalosis, and calculation of secondary response suggests that it is chronic rather than acute respiratory alkalosis. Hyperventilation due to abdominal pain accounts for this acid–base disturbance.

The calculated AG is 43, which is not due to alkalosis, but entirely to the presence of metabolic acidosis. Insulin withdrawal and subsequent generation of ketoacids (ketone positive) account for this high AG metabolic acidosis.

Assuming the normal AG of 10, this patient has an excess of 33 (43 − 10 = 33; ΔAG = 33) anions. If 1 H^+ is buffered by 1 HCO_3^-, the patient should not have any measurable HCO_3^- in the serum. However, his measured HCO_3^- is 17 mEq/L, suggesting that he had a high level of serum HCO_3^- before the development of metabolic acidosis. Thus, he had metabolic alkalosis prior to the development of metabolic acidosis. This was confirmed by the patient that his vomiting started before he withdrew insulin injections. Thus, the patient has a triple acid–base disorder of chronic respiratory alkalosis and high AG metabolic acidosis and metabolic alkalosis.

The $\Delta AG/\Delta HCO_3^-$ ratio can be helpful in this patient, as the ratio >2 is indicative of metabolic alkalosis. In this patient, the $\Delta AG/\Delta HCO_3^-$ ratio is 4.71 (ΔAG = 33; ΔHCO_3^- = 7 (24 − 17); ratio = 33/7 = 4.71). However, it is not necessary to depend on $\Delta AG/\Delta HCO_3^-$ ratio all the time. For example, this patient's serum [HCO_3^-] is disproportionately high compared to the increase in AG, suggesting an underlying metabolic alkalosis.

Suggested Reading

Reddi AS. Metabolic alkalosis. In: Reddi AS, editor. Fluid, electrolyte, and acid-base disorders. Clinical evaluation and management. 2nd ed. New York: Springer; 2018. p. 403–27.

Reddi AS. Acid-base disorders. Clinical evaluation and management. New York: Springer; 2020.

59. A 31-year-old woman with alcohol abuse and pancreatitis is admitted for shortness of breath, confusion, profuse vomiting, and abdominal pain. She is electively intubated and sedated. The following laboratory values are obtained:

Serum	ABG
Na^+ = 136 mEq/L	pH = 7.01
K^+ = 4.9 mEq/L	pCO_2 = 26 mm Hg
Cl^- = 87 mEq/L	pO_2 = 67 mm Hg
HCO_3^- = 7 mEq/L	HCO_3^- = 6 mEq/L
Creatinine = 4.1 mg/dL	
BUN = 7 mg/dL	
Glucose = 72 mg/dL	
Ketones = Positive	

What is the acid–base disturbance?

A. Metabolic acidosis and metabolic alkalosis
B. Metabolic alkalosis and respiratory alkalosis
C. Metabolic acidosis and respiratory acidosis
D. Respiratory alkalosis, metabolic acidosis, and metabolic alkalosis
E. Metabolic acidosis, respiratory acidosis, and metabolic alkalosis

The answer is E

Based on low pH and serum [HCO_3^-], and the AG of 42, the patient has a high AG metabolic acidosis due to alcoholic ketoacidosis.

Since the expected pCO_2 for this degree of acidemia is 18.5 mm Hg (range 16.5–20.5), the patient has respiratory acidosis (hypercapnia), which is due to the sedative.

As in case 86, there is a disproportionate relationship between the increase in AG and decrease in HCO_3^-, suggesting an underlying metabolic alkalosis. This is evident from low serum [Cl^-], which is due to vomiting. The $\Delta AG/\Delta HCO_3^-$ ratio is 1.9 ($\Delta AG = 42 - 10 = 32$; $\Delta HCO_3^- = 24 - 7 = 17$; ratio 32/17 = 1.9; close to 2), which also supports the underlying metabolic alkalosis.

Thus, the acid–base disorder is a high AG metabolic acidosis, respiratory acidosis, and metabolic alkalosis.

Suggested Reading

Reddi AS. Metabolic alkalosis. In: Reddi AS, editor. Fluid, electrolyte, and acid-base disorders. Clinical evaluation and management. 2nd ed. New York: Springer; 2018. p. 403–27.

Reddi AS. Acid-base disorders. Clinical evaluation and management. New York: Springer; 2020.

60. A 60-year-old woman with HIV/AIDS is admitted for diarrhea and polysubstance abuse. She is hypotensive (systolic blood pressure of 90 mm Hg) with heart rate of 112 beats/min. Laboratory values:

Serum	ABG
Na^+ = 130 mEq/L	pH = 7.06
K^+ = 5.5 mEq/L	pCO_2 = 28 mm Hg
Cl^- = 112 mEq/L	pO_2 = 84 mm Hg
HCO_3^- = 9 mEq/L	HCO_3^- = 8 mEq/L
Creatinine = 1.5 mg/dL	
BUN = 38 mg/dL	
Glucose = 80 mg/dL	
Albumin = 2.3 g/dL	
Urine toxicology: positive for cocaine and heroin	

Which one of the following describes the BEST of her acid–base status?

A. Metabolic acidosis and metabolic alkalosis
B. Metabolic alkalosis and respiratory alkalosis
C. Metabolic acidosis and respiratory acidosis
D. Respiratory acidosis, metabolic alkalosis, and metabolic acidosis
E. Metabolic acidosis, respiratory alkalosis, and metabolic alkalosis

The answer is C

The patient has a high AG metabolic acidosis and respiratory acidosis. Her AG is 14 when corrected for normal albumin level of 4.3 g/dL. Note that the AG decreases by 2.5 for each gram decrease in serum albumin from normal values of 4–4.5 g/dL. The superimposed respiratory acidosis is caused by her illicit drug use, which inhibits the medullary respiratory center. The high anion gap seems to be due to lactic acid production (hypotension) and acute kidney injury.

In this patient, the $\Delta AG/\Delta HCO_3^-$ ratio is 0.5 ($\Delta AG = 14 - 10 = 4$; $\Delta HCO_3^- = 24 - 9 = 15$; ratio 4/15 = 0.3). The $\Delta AG/\Delta HCO_3^-$ ratio <1 is suggestive of diarrhea as a cause of abnormal ABG in a patient who does not give adequate history of diarrhea.

Suggested Reading

Reddi AS. Metabolic alkalosis. In: Reddi AS, editor. Fluid, electrolyte, and acid-base disorders. Clinical evaluation and management. 2nd ed. New York: Springer; 2018. p. 403–27.
Reddi AS. Acid-base disorders. Clinical evaluation and management. New York: Springer; 2020.

61. A 48-year-old woman is admitted for weakness, myelopathy, and fatigue for few weeks. Her past medical history includes type 2 diabetes and is on metformin. Physical exam reveals a thin female and appears chronically ill. Examination of other systems is unremarkable except for a BP of 190/98 mm Hg and a pulse rate of 84 beats/min. Her BP improved with spironolactone. Labs:

Serum	Urine
Na^+ = 130 mEq/L	pH = 5.8
K^+ = 2.5 mEq/L	Osmolality = 480 mOsm/kg H_2O
Cl^- = 84 mEq/L	Na^+ = 60 mEq/L
HCO_3^- = 39 mEq/L	K^+ = 20 mEq/L
Creatinine = 1.5 mg/dL	Cl^- = 50 mEq/L
BUN = 38 mg/dL	Creatinine = 100 mg/dL
Glucose =280 mg/dL	
Albumin = 2.3 g/dL	
Plasma renin activity = <0.1 ng/mL/h (normal 0.2–1.6 ng/mL/h)	
Plasma aldosterone concentration = 1.5 ng/dL (normal 3–16 ng/dL)	
ABG: pH = 7.49, pCO_2 = 48, pO_2 = 90 mm Hg, HCO_3^- = 38 mEq/L	

Which of the following diagnoses is MOST likely in this patient?

A. Primary aldosteronism
B. Renal artery stenosis
C. Gitelman syndrome
D. Liddle syndrome
E. Endogenous Cushing syndrome

The answer is E

Based on plasma renin activity (PRA) and plasma aldosterone concentration (PAC), primary aldosteronism (low PRA and high PAC) and renal artery stenosis (both PRA and PAC high) are excluded. Gitelman syndrome has high PRA and PAC, but BP is normal to low. Thus, answers A, B, and C are incorrect. Patients with Liddle syndrome have low PRA and PAC and their BP does not improve with spironolactone (answer D is incorrect).

Based on the symptoms of the patient and diabetes, plasma cortisol was ordered, which was very high. Biochemical and imaging studies suggested ectopic production of adreno- corticotrophic hormone (ACTH) causing Cushing syndrome. A small mass in the right lung lower lobe producing ACTH was identified. Resection of the mass and medical therapy with mifepristone blocks the action of cortisol by antagonizing the cortisol receptors.

Cortisol is severalfold more potent and has more affinity for mineralocorticoid receptor than aldosterone. For this reason, cortisol is converted into inactive cortisone by the enzyme 11β-hydroxysteroid dehydrogenase type 2 present in the kidney. Deficiency or inactivation of this enzyme causes excessive circulating levels of cortisol, which functions like a mineralocorticoid. As a result, Na^+ is retained and K^+ is secreted with resultant volume expansion, HTN, and hypokalemia. Volume expansion causes lower concentrations of both PRA and PAC. Hypokalemia maintains metabolic alkalosis. Studies have shown that ectopic ACTH inhibits 11β-hydroxysteroid dehydrogenase type 2 activity and thus elevated cortisol levels. Thus, Cushing syndrome causes hypokalemia, metabolic alkalosis, and HTN (answer E is correct).

Suggested Reading

Seow CJ, Young WF Jr. An overlooked cause of hypokalemia. Am J Med. 2017;130:e433–5.

Torpy DJ, Mullen N, Ilias J, et al. Association of hypertension and hypokalemia with Cushing's syndrome caused by ectopic ACTH secretion. A series of 58 cases. Ann N Y Acad Sci. 2002;970:134–44.

Walker BR, Campbell JC, Fraser R, et al. Mineralocorticoid excess and inhibition of 11β-hydroxysteroid dehydrogenase in patients with ectopic ACTH syndrome. Clin Endocrinol (Oxf). 1992;37:483–92.

62. **Which one the following primary acid–base disorder is Most commonly seen in intensive care unit (ICU)?**

A. Respiratory alkalosis
B. Respiratory acidosis
C. High AG metabolic acidosis
D. Metabolic alkalosis
E. Respiratory acidosis and metabolic alkalosis

The answer is C

Although any one of the above the above acid–base disturbance can occur in ICUs, the most likely disturbance is high AG metabolic acidosis due to sepsis, ketoacidosis, and ingestion of toxins. Thus, answer C is correct. Mixed acid–base disorders are also rather common; however, metabolic alkalosis superimposed on respiratory acidosis is usually induced during the management of the patient. In contrast, mixed metabolic acidosis and respiratory alkalosis is rather common.

Suggested Reading

Al-Jaghbeer M, Kellum JA. Acid-base disturbances in intensive care patients: etiology, pathophysiology and treatment. Nephrol Dial Transplant. 2015;30:1104–11.

Fencl V, Rossing TH. Acid-base disorders in critical care medicine. Annu Rev Med. 1989;40:17–29.

Reddi AS. Acid-base disorders. Clinical evaluation and management. New York: Springer; 2020.

63. **Which one of the following nutrients is implicated in weaning of the patient with impaired lung function MOST difficult?**

A. Glutamate
B. Aspartate
C. Essential fatty acids
D. Glucose
E. None of the above

The answer is D

Studies have shown that excess use of glucose-containing solutions or high carbohydrate feeds generate CO_2, which makes weaning of the patient difficult. Thus, answer D is correct. Other nutrients are not involved in generating excess CO_2.

Suggested Reading

Al-Jaghbeer M, Kellum JA. Acid-base disturbances in intensive care patients: etiology, pathophysiology and treatment. Nephrol Dial Transplant. 2015;30:1104–11.
Fencl V, Rossing TH. Acid-base disorders in critical care medicine. Annu Rev Med. 1989;40:17–29.
Reddi AS. Acid-base disorders. Clinical evaluation and management. New York: Springer; 2020.

64. A 36-year-old man with cirrhosis is admitted for management of hepatic encephalopathy. Arterial blood gas (ABG) shows the following values:

$$pH = 7.45$$
$$pO_2 = 90 \text{ mm Hg}$$
$$pCO_2 = 26 \text{ mm Hg}$$
$$\text{Serum } HCO_3^- = 18 \text{ mEq / L}$$

What is the acid–base disorder in this patient?

A. Metabolic acidosis and metabolic alkalosis
B. Respiratory acidosis and metabolic acidosis
C. Metabolic alkalosis and respiratory alkalosis
D. Respiratory alkalosis with appropriate respiratory compensation
E. Respiratory alkalosis and metabolic acidosis

The answer is D

The ABG values suggest only chronic respiratory alkalosis with appropriate secondary physiologic response (compensation). Metabolic alkalosis is unlikely because of low HCO_3^- concentration. Both pH and HCO_3^- level do not suggest respiratory acidosis. This is not a mixed acid–base disturbance because of appropriate renal compensation. Thus, answer D is correct.

Suggested Reading

Ahya SN, Soler MJ, Levitsky J, Battle D. Acid-base and potassium disorders in liver disease. Semin Nephrol. 2006;26:466–70.
Bernardi M, Predieri S. Editorial. Disturbance of acid-base balance in cirrhosis: a neglected issue warranting further insights. Liver Int. 2005;25:463–6.
Scheiner B, Lindner G, Reiberger T, et al. Acid-base disorders in liver disease. J Hepatol. 2017;67:1062–73.

65. A 40-year-old woman with cirrhosis is admitted for management of ascites. She is on 200 mg of spironolactone daily. **Which one of the following acid–base disturbance is MOST likely in this patient?**

A. Respiratory alkalosis and high anion gap (AG) acidosis
B. Respiratory alkalosis and normal AG acidosis
C. Respiratory alkalosis and metabolic alkalosis
D. Respiratory alkalosis only
E. Metabolic alkalosis only

The answer is B

A patient with cirrhosis and ascites usually has respiratory alkalosis because of hyperventilation. Spironolactone causes hyperchloremic (non-AG) metabolic acidosis. Unless the patient has sepsis or hypoxia or other conditions that cause acid production, metabolic acidosis is uncommon in cirrhotic patients. Patients on loop diuretics for management of ascites usually develop metabolic alkalosis superimposed on respiratory alkalosis. Single acid–base disturbance is present only in uncomplicated cirrhotic patient. Thus, answer B is correct.

Suggested Reading

Ahya SN, Soler MJ, Levitsky J, Battle D. Acid-base and potassium disorders in liver disease. Semin Nephrol. 2006;26:466–70.

Bernardi M, Predieri S. Editorial. Disturbance of acid-base balance in cirrhosis: a neglected issue warranting further insights. Liver Int. 2005;25:463–6.
Scheiner B, Lindner G, Reiberger T, et al. Acid-base disorders in liver disease. J Hepatol. 2017;67:1062–73.

66. A 46-year-old malnourished woman with cirrhosis and ascites undergoes large volume paracentesis as an outpatient. Four days later she comes to the Emergency Department (ED) with complaints of nausea, vomiting, abdominal pain, and dizziness. In ED, she is found to have hypotension with orthostatic blood pressure and pulse changes. Labs and ABG show:

Serum chemistry	ABG
Na^+ = 140 mEq/L	pH = 7.36
K^+ = 5.4 mEq/L	pO_2 = 84 mm Hg
Cl^- = 102 mEq/L	pCO_2 = 25 mm Hg
HCO_3^- = 14 mEq/L	HCO_3^- = 13 mEq/L
Creatinine 4.4 mg/dL	
Albumin = 3.2 g/dL	

Which one of the following BEST characterizes the acid–base disturbance in this patient?

A. High anion gap (AG) acidosis and respiratory alkalosis
B. Respiratory alkalosis and normal AG acidosis
C. Respiratory alkalosis and metabolic alkalosis
D. Respiratory alkalosis only
E. Metabolic acidosis only

The answer is A

The patient has a high AG metabolic acidosis due to acute kidney injury (AKI) precipitated by large volume paracentesis without albumin infusion. Albumin corrected AG is 26.5, which is high for renal failure alone. The secondary response (compensation) for metabolic acidosis is respiratory with low pCO_2. The expected pCO_2 is 29 mm Hg (27–31 mm Hg). However, the patient's pCO_2 is 25, suggesting that respiratory alkalosis is superimposed on metabolic acidosis. Thus, answer A is correct.

As noted above, AKI alone will not give an AG of 26.5. Usually AKI will give an AG of 18, and the difference between 26.5 and 18 is 8.5. This difference in AG may be due to other anions such as lactic acid, ketoacids, or other anions. Based on hypotension and relative hypoxemia on ABG, lactic acidosis and uremic acidosis seem responsible for this high AG. Indeed, serum lactate levels were 9 mmol/L. Other answers are incorrect.

Suggested Reading

Ahya SN, Soler MJ, Levitsky J, Battle D. Acid-base and potassium disorders in liver disease. Semin Nephrol. 2006;26:466–70.
Bernardi M, Predieri S. Editorial. Disturbance of acid-base balance in cirrhosis: a neglected issue warranting further insights. Liver Int. 2005;25:463–6.
Scheiner B, Lindner G, Reiberger T, et al. Acid-base disorders in liver disease. J Hepatol. 2017;67:1062–73.

67. A 52-year-old man underwent abdominal surgery for intestinal perforation complicated by sepsis, requiring intubation. Two weeks later, he was started on TPN with 10% glucose. **Which one of the following complications develops following glucose TPN?**

A. Hypercapnia
B. Increased O_2 consumption
C. Increased tidal volume
D. Increased respiratory rate
E. All of the above

The answer is E

TPN-induced hypercapnia has been known for a long time. In addition, infusion of large quantities of glucose was found to increase O_2 consumption, energy expenditure, tidal volume, and respiratory rate. Thus, answer E is correct.

Suggested Reading

Dark DS, Pingleton SK, Kerby GR. Hypercapnia during weaning. A complication of nutritional support. Chest. 1986;88:141–3.

Dounousi E, Zikou X, Koulouras V, et al. Metabolic acidosis during parenteral nutrition: pathophysiological mechanisms. Indian J Crit Care Med. 2015;19:270–4.

Kushner RF. Total parenteral nutrition-associated metabolic acidosis. J Parenter Enteral Nutr. 1986;10:306–10.

68. Current TPN solutions contain several classes of amino acids. **Which amino acids generate H^+ following their metabolism during TPN administration?**

A. Aspartate and glutamate
B. Methionine, cysteine, and cystine
C. Lysine, arginine, and histidine
D. B and C
E. All of the above

The answer is D

Newer TPN solutions contain cationic (lysine, arginine, and histidine), anionic (aspartate and glutamate), and sulfur-containing amino acids (methionine, cysteine, and cystine). When cationic amino acids are metabolized, H^+ is generated at the rate of 1 mol per 1 mol of amino acid. Metabolism of sulfur-containing amino acids yields 2 mol of H^+ per 1 mol of amino acid. On the other hand, metabolism of anionic amino acids consumes H^+ with generation of HCO_3^-. Thus, oxidation of aspartate and glutamate, which are anionic amino acids, reduces acid load to the body. Thus, answer D is correct.

Suggested Reading

Dark DS, Pingleton SK, Kerby GR. Hypercapnia during weaning. A complication of nutritional support. Chest. 1986;88:141–3.

Dounousi E, Zikou X, Koulouras V, et al. Metabolic acidosis during parenteral nutrition: pathophysiological mechanisms. Indian J Crit Care Med. 2015;19:270–4.

Kushner RF. Total parenteral nutrition-associated metabolic acidosis. J Parenter Enteral Nutr. 1986;10:306–10.

69. **Which one of the following is an important cause of metabolic alkalosis in patients on TPN?**

A. Vomiting and gastric suction
B. Lysine acetate
C. Volume depletion due to osmotic diuresis
D. All of the above
E. A only

The answer is D

Metabolic alkalosis is not uncommon in patients on TPN. Both the underlying disease processes requiring nasogastric suction, duodenal obstruction causing vomiting, and excess acetate infusions can increase serum HCO_3^- level with resultant metabolic alkalosis. Also, osmotic diuresis-induced volume depletion can raise serum HCO_3^- level and causes metabolic alkalosis. Thus, answer D is correct.

Suggested Reading

Dark DS, Pingleton SK, Kerby GR. Hypercapnia during weaning. A complication of nutritional support. Chest. 1986;88:141–3.

Dounousi E, Zikou X, Koulouras V, et al. Metabolic acidosis during parenteral nutrition: Pathophysiological mechanisms. Indian J Crit Care Med. 2015;19:270–4.

Kushner RF. Total parenteral nutrition-associated metabolic acidosis. J Parenter Enteral Nutr. 1986;10:306–10.

Reddi AS. Acid-base disorders. Clinical evaluation and management. New York: Springer; 2020.

70. **Which one of the following acid–base disorders is MOST likely during pregnancy?**

A. High anion gap (AG) metabolic acidosis
B. Metabolic alkalosis

C. Respiratory alkalosis
D. Respiratory acidosis
E. Metabolic acidosis and metabolic alkalosis

The answer is C

Respiratory alkalosis is the most common acid–base disorder in pregnancy because of increased progesterone levels, which stimulate medullary respiratory center. Also, increased minute ventilation decreases pCO_2 levels. Thus, answer C is correct.

Metabolic acidosis is not that common unless the patient develops diabetic or starvation ketosis. Metabolic alkalosis is also uncommon unless the patient has vomiting or hyperemesis gravidarum. Metabolic alkalosis is usually superimposed on respiratory alkalosis. Respiratory acidosis is extremely rare.

Suggested Reading

Alkhasoneh M, Jacobs J, Kaur G. A case of severe metabolic acidosis during pregnancy. Clin Case Rep. 2019;7:550–2.
Frise C, Noori M, Williamson C. Severe metabolic alkalosis in pregnancy. Obstret Med. 2013;6:138–40.
Hankins GDV, Clark SL, Harvey CJ, et al. Third trimester arterial blood gas and acid-base values in normal pregnancy at moderate altitude. Obstet Gynecol. 1996;88:347–50.
McAulifffe F, Kametas N, Krampl E, et al. Blood gases in pregnancy at sea level and at high altitude. BJOG. 2001;108:980–5.
Omo-Aghoja L. Maternal and fetal acid-base chemistry: a major determinant of perinatal outcome. Ann Med Health Sci Res. 2014;4:8–17.

71. **Which one of the following strategies for managing respiratory alkalosis is APPROPRIATE in pregnancy?**

A. Opiates to suppress respiratory rate
B. A rebreather (Ambu bag)
C. $NaHCO_3$
D. No treatment
E. Delivery

The answer is D

Respiratory alkalosis is self-limited in uncomplicated pregnancy, which improves following delivery at the end of gestation. Therefore, no treatment is needed. Other treatment modalities are not necessary. Thus, answer D is correct.

Suggested Reading

Hankins GDV, Clark SL, Harvey CJ, et al. Third trimester arterial blood gas and acid-base values in normal pregnancy at moderate altitude. Obstet Gynecol. 1996;88:347–50.
McAulifffe F, Kametas N, Krampl E, et al. Blood gases in pregnancy at sea level and at high altitude. BJOG. 2001;108:980–5.
Omo-Aghoja L. Maternal and fetal acid-base chemistry: a major determinant of perinatal outcome. Ann Med Health Sci Res. 2014;4:8–17.
Reddi AS. Acid-base disorders. Clinical evaluation and management. New York: Springer; 2020.

72. A 50-year-old woman had abdominal surgery for intestinal perforation. Postoperatively, she received opiates for abdominal pain. **Which one of the following primary acid–base disturbances is MOST likely to be present in the patient?**

A. Metabolic acidosis
B. Metabolic alkalosis
C. Respiratory acidosis
D. Respiratory alkalosis
E. Respiratory acidosis and respiratory alkalosis

The answer is C

Opiates inhibit medullary respiratory center. As a result, hypercapnia develops, leading to respiratory acidosis. Thus, answer C is correct.

Suggested Reading

Clark J, Walker WF. Acid-base problems in surgery. World J Surg. 1983;7:590–8.

Lawton TO, Quinn A, Fletcher SJ. Perioperative metabolic acidosis: the Bradford Anaesthetic Department Acidosis Study. J Intensive Care Soc. 2019;20:11–7.

Mostert M, Bonavia A. Starvation ketoacidosis as a cause of unexplained metabolic acidosis in the perioperative period. Am J Case Rep. 2016;17:755–8.

Reddi AS. Acid-base disorders. Clinical evaluation and management. New York: Springer; 2020.

Waters JH, Miller LR, Clack S, et al. Cause of metabolic acidosis in prolonged surgery. Crit Care Med. 1996;27:2142–6.

73. An 18-year-old man is admitted for observation following motor vehicle accident. He is kept NPO (nothing per mouth) for series of imaging studies and is receiving half-normal saline. He gave the history of driving whole night without food intake other than black coffee. Following 16 h waiting for the tests, serum chemistry shows bicarbonate of 18 mEq/L. Venous pH is 7.39. Respiratory rate is 12 per min. **Which one of the following primary acid–base disturbances is MOST likely in this patient?**

A. Respiratory alkalosis
B. Metabolic acidosis
C. Metabolic alkalosis
D. Respiratory acidosis
E. Metabolic acidosis and metabolic alkalosis

The answer is B

The reason for low bicarbonate is probably starvation ketosis because the patient has net been eating for more than 24 h. The simple and best test is urinalysis, which may show the presence of ketones. It is not unusual to see an elderly developing starvation ketosis awaiting surgery or imaging studies in a busy hospital with trauma center.

Chronic respiratory alkalosis also lowers serum HCO_3^- level to this level, but time to develop chronicity is >2–3 days. Also, this patient's respiratory rate is normal. Therefore, respiratory alkalosis is unlikely. Serum HCO_3^- concentration is >24 mEq/L in both metabolic alkalosis and respiratory acidosis. In metabolic acidosis and metabolic alkalosis, serum HCO_3^- concentration is usually within normal limits. Thus, all the other answers are incorrect.

Suggested Reading

Clark J, Walker WF. Acid-base problems in surgery. World J Surg. 1983;7:590–8.

Lawton TO, Quinn A, Fletcher SJ. Perioperative metabolic acidosis: the Bradford Anaestetic Department Acidosis Study. J Intensive Care Soc. 2019;20:11–7.

Mostert M, Bonavia A. Starvation ketoacidosis as a cause of unexplained metabolic acidosis in the perioperative period. Am J Case Rep. 2016;17:755–8.

Reddi AS. Acid-base disorders. Clinical evaluation and management. New York: Springer; 2020.

Waters JH, Miller LR, Clack S, et al. Cause of metabolic acidosis in prolonged surgery. Crit Care Med. 1996;27:2142–6.

74. **Which one of the following acids causes metabolic acidosis during intraoperative surgery?**

A. Acetoacetic acid
B. β-Hydroxybutyric acid
C. Hippuric acid
D. Lactic acid
E. None of the above

The answer is D

Lactic acidosis is the most likely acid generated during intraoperative period because of hypotension, hemorrhage, hypoxia, etc. Thus, answer D is correct. Other acid production is unlikely.

Suggested Reading

Clark J, Walker WF. Acid-base problems in surgery. World J Surg. 1983;7:590–8.

Lawton TO, Quinn A, Fletcher SJ. Perioperative metabolic acidosis: the Bradford Anaestetic Department Acidosis Study. J Intensive Care Soc. 2019;20:11–7.

Reddi AS. Acid-base disorders. Clinical evaluation and management. New York: Springer; 2020.

Waters JH, Miller LR, Clack S, et al. Cause of metabolic acidosis in prolonged surgery. Crit Care Med. 1996;27:2142–6.

Chapter 2
Glomerular, Tubulointerstitial, and Vascular Diseases

1. A 20-year-old athletic man with no significant past medical history is found to have isolated asymptomatic microscopic hematuria on routine physical examination (phys exam). He is not on any medications and does not use illicit drugs. **Which one of the following observations is suggestive of glomerular hematuria?**

   A. Presence of many isomorphic red blood cells (RBCs) in urine sediment
   B. Presence of many isomorphic RBCs and white blood cells (WBCs) in urine sediment
   C. Presence of many dysmorphic RBCs or acanthocytes in urine sediment
   D. Presence of many "decoy cells" in urine sediment
   E. All of the above

   The answer is C

   Urinary RBCs or erythrocytes are of two types: isomorphic and dysmorphic. Isomorphic RBCs have regular shapes and contours. These RBCs generally originate from lower urinary tract. Dysmorphic RBCs have irregular shapes and contours and originate from renal parenchyma (glomeruli). Thus, hematuria is considered either glomerular or nonglomerular in origin. Hematuria is also seen in several nonrenal conditions such as exercise, fever, and/or menstruation.

   Glomerular hematuria is considered when ≥40% dysmorphic RBCs or 5% acanthocytes or RBC casts are present. Dysmorphic RBCs are best visualized by phase contrast microscopy.

   RBCs acquire dysmorphism while they are passing through gaps of the glomerular basement membrane. Also, physicochemical insults occur when RBCs pass through the renal tubules. It has been shown that the number of dysmorphic RBCs is higher in proliferative glomerulonephritis than in nonproliferative glomerulonephritis.

   The presence of "decoy cells," in the urine is from a virus called BK polyomavirus. It is a double-stranded DNA virus that affects about 90% of the general population. Interestingly, a number of kidney transplant patients develop renal as well as graft failure due to infection of this virus. The "decoy cells" bear viral inclusion bodies, and their presence in the urine indicates the infection with BK virus. Decoy cells show glossy appearing intranuclear viral inclusion bodies mostly coming from the uroepithelium.

   In this individual, there is no evidence of infection or renal disease. His hematuria can be attributed to exercise. Thus, options A, B, D, and E are incorrect.

   Suggested Reading

   Fogazzi GB, Garigali G. Urinalysis. In: Feehally J, Floege J, Tonelli M, et al., editors. Comprehensive clinical nephrology. 6th ed. Philadelphia: Elsevier; 2019. p. 39–52.

   Fogazzi GB, Edfonti A, Garigali G, et al. Urinary erythrocyte morphology in patients with microscopic hematuria caused by a glomerulopathy. Pediatr Nephrol. 2008;23:1093–110.

2. An 18-year-old adult is found to have persistent asymptomatic isolated microscopic hematuria (PAIMH) >5 RBCs/hpf during phys exam for military service. There is no significant personal or family history of renal or urologic disease. He is not on any medications. Phys exam, blood pressure, and serum chemistry are normal. There is no proteinuria on urine dipstick. **In view of the available evidence, which one of the following statements is CORRECT?**

A. S. Reddi, *Absolute Nephrology Review*, https://doi.org/10.1007/978-3-030-85958-9_2

A. He is at risk for progressive kidney disease
B. He warrants testing for genetic disease
C. He is not at risk for any kidney disease
D. He is at low risk for future kidney disease and needs follow-up
E. He does not need any follow-up and ignore hematuria

The answer is D

PAIMH, once thought to be a benign disease, seems to carry a low risk for future development of either hereditary nephritis, thin basement membrane disease, IgA nephropathy, or other diseases with progression to end-stage kidney disease (ESKD). In a retrospective study, Vivante et al. from Israel reported that 0.3% (3690 out of 1,203,626 subjects) of young adults aged 16–25 years had PAIMH. At a follow-up of 22 years, 26 of 3690 (0.7%) participants with PAIMH developed treated ESKD, compared to only 0.045% of participants without hematuria. A multivariate analysis showed that the hazard ratio for treated ESKD with hematuria versus non-hematuria was 18.5%. However, the absolute risk of progression is low (3 ESKD/1000). Thus, PAIMH carries a low absolute risk for ESKD in Israeli young adults. Whether or not PAIMH carries such a risk for ESKD in other populations remains to be seen. Thus, option D is correct.

Suggested Reading

Kovacević Z, Jovanović D, Rabrenović V, et al. Asymptomatic microscopic hematuria in young males. Int J Clin Pract. 2008;62:406–12.
Vivante A, Afek A, Frenkel-Nir Y, et al. Persistent asymptomatic isolated microscopic hematuria in Israeli adolescents and young adults and risk for end-stage renal disease. JAMA. 2011;306:729–36.

3. A 16-year-old adolescent is found to have orthostatic proteinuria (1.2 g/day). **Which one of the following do you suggest regarding his risk for future development of kidney disease?**

A. High risk and treatment required
B. Low risk and no treatment required
C. No risk and no treatment required
D. Kidney biopsy is required to assess risk
E. Repeat proteinuria is required in 2 weeks to assess risk

The answer is C

Orthostatic proteinuria is common in children and adolescents. It is uncommon in individuals older than 30 years of age. Orthostatic proteinuria is defined as the presence of proteinuria (up to 2 g) in upright position and very little proteinuria (<50 mg) in supine position. The pathogenesis of proteinuria is unclear; however, renal hemodynamic changes and entrapment (kinking) of left renal vein between aorta and superior mesenteric artery have been implicated. Long-term (20-year) follow-up of subjects with orthostatic proteinuria showed no progression of renal disease. Proteinuria resolves in 50% of subjects after 10 years and 87% after 20 years. Therefore, orthostatic proteinuria is a benign condition, and no treatment or kidney biopsy is required. Thus, option C is correct.

Suggested Reading

Devarajan P. Mechanisms of orthostatic proteinuria: lessons from a transplant donor. J Am Soc Nephrol. 1993;4:36–9.
Shintaku N, Takahashi Y, Akaishi K, et al. Entrapment of left renal vein in children with orthostatic proteinuria. Pediatr Nephrol. 1990;4:324–7.
Springberg PD, Garrett Jr LE, Thompson Jr AL, et al. Fixed and reproducible orthostatic proteinuria: results of a 20-year follow-up study. Ann Intern Med. 1982;97:516–9.

4. A 30-year-old Caucasian man is referred to you by a primary care physician for evaluation of 2+ (100 mg/dL) proteinuria confirmed on three different visits on a routine urinalysis. There is no hematuria. The personal and family history is unremarkable. He is not on any medications. A 24-h proteinuria is 1.2 g. Blood pressure is normal. Serum creatinine is 0.8 mg/dL with an estimated glomerular filtration rate (eGFR) >60 mL/min/1.73 m^2. **Regarding the status of his kidney function in the next 7–10 years, which one of the following statements is CORRECT?**

A. Difficult to predict at this time
B. Kidney biopsy is required to evaluate kidney function
C. No relationship exists between isolated proteinuria and kidney function

D. Annual estimation of eGFR is required to evaluate kidney function status
E. There is a possibility that his eGFR may decline >5%/year from baseline in the next 7 years

The answer is E

Persistent isolated proteinuria has been found to be strongly associated with progression of kidney disease, and cardiovascular as well as all-cause mortality. In population studies, dipstick proteinuria was identified as an important predictor of ESKD. Also, routine testing for proteinuria using dipstick can predict future kidney function decline.

Clark et al. evaluated the predictive value of dipstick proteinuria of different levels for rapid kidney function decline (RKFD) in 2574 Canadian participants (18–92 years of age) over a median of 7 years follow-up. RKFD was defined as a >5% annual eGFR change from baseline. Overall, 2.5% (*N* = 63) had ≥100 mg/dL (≥1 g/L) or ≥2+ proteinuria. Of these, 8.5% experienced RKFD during a 7-year follow-up. One in 2.6 patients with proteinuria >100 mg/dl experienced RKFD. Participants >60 years of age and eGFR <60 mL/min were at higher risk for RKFD. Dipstick proteinuria >100 mg/dL correctly identified RKFD in 91%, incorrectly in 1.7% and missed RKFD in 7.7% of participants.

In this study, proteinuria was found to be a strong predictor for RKFD than albuminuria. After adjusting for age, hypertension, diabetes, cardiovascular disease, obesity, and family history of diabetes were all significantly associated with increased risk for RKFD. The detection of trace protein or greater had more than twofold increase in the risk of RKFD. Thus, inexpensive dipstick screening for proteinuria can detect those individuals at risk for RKFD. Of all the options, option E is, therefore, correct.

Suggested Reading

Clark WF, Macnab JJ, Sontrop JM, et al. Dipstic proteinuria as a screening strategy to identify rapid renal decline. J Am Soc Nephrol. 2011;22:1729–36.
Iseki K, Iseki C, Ikemiya Y, et al. Risk of developing end-stage renal disease in a cohort of mass screening. Kidney Int. 1996;49:800–5.
Ishani A, Grandits GA, Grim RH, et al. Association of single measurements of dipstic proteinuria, estimated glomerular filtration rate, and hematocrit with 25-year incidence of end-stage renal disease in the multiple risk factor intervention trial. J Am Soc Nephrol. 2006;17:1444–52.

5. A 35-year-old woman was found to have asymptomatic hematuria with albumin:creatinine ratio <0.02 mg/mg. **Which one of the following diagnoses is MOST likely on a kidney biopsy?**

A. IgA nephropathy
B. X-linked Alport syndrome
C. Autosomal dominant Alport syndrome (previously called thin basement membrane disease, TBD)
D. MPGN (type I)
E. Lupus nephritis (Class I)

The answer is C

In a study by Hall et al., patients with asymptomatic microscopic hematuria and normal albumin excretion rate (<20 mg/day or albumin:creatinine ratio (ACR) <0.02 mg/mg or <30 mg/day) were found to have mostly autosomal dominant Alport syndrome (43.1%). About 20.1% had IgA nephropathy, 20.1% had nondiagnostic abnormalities, and 18.1% had normal findings.

Other studies have shown that 50–90% of patients with albuminuria (ACR >0.02 mg/mg or >30 mg/day) and microscopic hematuria were found to have IgA nephropathy. On the other hand, patients with hematuria with normal albumin excretion rate were found to have mostly autosomal Alport syndrome. Shen et al. reported in Chinese that adult subjects with isolated microscopic hematuria and elevated serum IgA/C3 ratio (~4.5) and an ACR of 96 mg/g are more common in IgA nephropathy than subjects with autosomal Alport syndrome. Thus, the degree of albuminuria in a patient with microscopic hematuria can predict the type of kidney disease on a kidney biopsy.

Suggested Reading

Assadi FK. Value of urinary excretion of microalbuminuria in predicting glomerular lesions in children with isolated microscopic hematuria. Pediatr Nephrol. 2005;20:1131–5.
Eardley KS, Ferreira MA, Howie AJ, et al. Urinary albumin excretion: A predictor of glomerular findings in adults with microscopic hematuria. QJM. 2004;97:297–301.

Hall CL, Bradley R, Kerr A, et al. Clinical value of renal biopsy in patients with asymptomatic microscopic hematuria with and without low-grade proteinuria. Clin Nephrol. 2004;62:267–72.

Kashtan CE, Ding J, Garosi G, et al. Alport syndrome: a unified classification of genetic disorders of collagen IV α345: a position paper of the Alport syndrome Classification Working Group. Kidney Int. 2018;93:1045–51.

Shen P, He L, Jiang Y, et al. Useful indicators for performing renal biopsy in adult patients with isolated microscopic hematuria. Int J Clin Pract. 2007;61:789–94.

6. A 50-year-old housewife visits her physician for extreme wrist and knee pain. She has been taking ibuprofen for a number of years with partial relief of her pain. She denies fatigue, weakness, and lower extremity edema. Blood pressure is elevated. Urinalysis shows >300 mg proteinuria with a protein to creatinine ratio of 4.5 (mg/mg). There is no hematuria. **Which one of the following glomerular diseases is MOST likely found on a kidney biopsy?**

   A. Focal segmental glomerulosclerosis (FSGS)
   B. Minimal change disease
   C. Membranoproliferative glomerulonephritis (MPGN)
   D. Amyloidosis
   E. Chronic GN (glomerulonephritis)

   The answer is B

   The patient has been taking ibuprofen for many years. The ingestion of nonsteroidal anti-inflammatory drugs (NSAIDs) such as ibuprofen can cause proteinuria from nonnephrotic range to nephrotic range. Generally, nephrotic syndrome is due to a glomerular lesion, most commonly minimal change disease. Few reports have also described nephrotic syndrome due to membranous nephropathy in NSAID users. FSGS and MPGN have also been described.

   Bakhriansyah et al. conducted a matched case-control study of 2620 patients with a diagnosis of nephrotic syndrome and 10,454 matched controls. Of these 2620 patients, kidney biopsy findings were available in 288 patients. MN was the diagnosis in 30%, FSGS in 20%, minimal change disease in 9%, and diffuse mesangial proliferative glomerulonephritis in 6%. Among NSAIDs, indomethacin, diclofenac, ketorolac (acetic acid derivatives) and ibuprofen, naproxen, and ketoprofen (propionic acid derivatives) were associated with a higher risk of nephrotic syndrome. This analytical study requires validation. Until then minimal change, disease seems to be the most common glomerular disease associated with NSAIDs.

   Amyloidosis with nephrotic syndrome can be seen in patients with rheumatoid arthritis, but the patient does not have any other manifestations of amyloidosis. Chronic GN is a possibility, but the absence of hematuria rules out this disease. Also, nephrotic syndrome is less likely in chronic GN. Thus, option B is correct.

   Suggested Reading

Bakhriansyah M, Souverein PC, van den HoogenMWF, et al. Risk of nephrotic syndrome for non-steroidal antiinflammatory drug users: A case-control study. Clin J Am Soc Nephrol. 2019;14:1355–62.

Mérida E, Manuel Praga M. NSAIDs and nephrotic syndrome. Clin J Am Soc Nephrol. 2019;14:1280–2.

Palmer BF. Nephrotoxicity of nonsteroidal anti-inflammatory agents, analgesics, and inhibitors of the renin-angiotensin system. In: Coffman TM, Falk RJ, Molitoris BA, et al., editors. Schrier's diseases of the kidney. 9th ed. Philadelphia: Wolters Kluwer/Lippincott Williams & Wilkins; 2013. p. 943–58.

7. A 12-year-old female student with nephrotic syndrome (10 g/day) is seen in renal clinic for management of her proteinuria. She is started on oral prednisone with good response (proteinuria 250 mg/day) in 9 weeks. Prednisone was slowly tapered to 5 mg every other day. She is not hypertensive; however, she is just started on 2.5 mg of enalapril. After 2 years of remission, she presents to the clinic with peripheral edema, and urinary protein excretion increased to 6.5 g/day. Her kidney function is normal. **Which one of the following urinary findings is suggestive of relapse her nephrotic syndrome?**

   A. Urinary albumin:protein ratio
   B. Urinary neutrophil gelatinase-associated lipocalin (NGAL)
   C. Monocyte chemoattractant protein-1 (MCP-1)
   D. Urinary CTLA-4
   E. Urinary CD80

The answer is E

Garin et al. reported a urine marker for relapse of idiopathic minimal change disease mostly in children. It is named CD80 (also known as B7.1), which is expressed on podocytes in various animal models of nephrotic syndrome. CD80 is a transmembrane protein that provides a co-stimulatory signal for T cell activation. Its expression is always activation-induced. It is reported that induction of CD80 by podocytes causes proteinuria and fusion of foot processes in mice. Garin et al. have shown that urinary CD80 levels are increased during relapse and normalization during remission in children with minimal change disease. Elevation in urinary CD80 was not observed in other glomerular diseases.

T regulatory cells also secrete soluble CTLA-4, which binds to CD80 and can block its co-stimulatory activation of T cells. Unlike CD80, the urinary levels of soluble CTLA-4 are not elevated during relapse of minimal change disease. However, the ratio of CD80/CTLA-4 is elevated. Thus, option D is incorrect.

MCP-1 levels are increased in the urine during lupus flare and not in minimal change disease. Urinary NGAL is elevated in AKI prior to an increase in serum creatinine levels. Increased urinary albumin:protein ratio differentiates glomerular from nonglomerular causes of hematuria. Thus, options A to D are incorrect.

Suggested Reading

Garin EH, Diaz LN, Mu W, et al. Urinary CD80 excretion increases in idiopathic minimal-chamge disease. J Am Soc Nephrol. 2009;20:260–6.

Ohisa N, Yoshida K, Matsuki R, et al. A comparison of urinary albumin-total protein ratio to phase-contrast microscopic examination of urine sediment for differentiating glomerular and nonglomerular bleeding. Am J Kidney Dis. 2008;52:235–41.

8. The above patient has relapse of her nephrotic syndrome and insists on renal biopsy findings to know why she relapsed. The family supported her request. The renal biopsy findings are consistent with minimal change disease (normal appearing glomerulus on light microscopy and foot processes effacement on electron microscopy). **Which one of the following therapies do you start on her?**

   A. Calcineurin inhibitors (cyclosporine, tacrolimus)
   B. Corticosteroids (prednisone, prednisolone)
   C. Cyclophosphamide
   D. Mycophenolate mofetil (MMF)
   E. Rituximab

The answer is B

Corticosteroids are the first-line therapy for minimal change disease (MCD) in children and adults. The corticosteroids commonly used include prednisone or prednisolone. The above patient has steroid-sensitive nephrotic syndrome.

The most common cause of idiopathic nephrotic syndrome in children is MCD, which responds, as mentioned above, to corticosteroids. Patients are treated initially with prednisone without a renal biopsy. The protocols that include optimal dose, duration of treatment, and the route of administration are variable. However, one approach is to start prednisone at 60 mg/m^2/day (maximum 80 mg/day) for 4 weeks and follow the proteinuric response. If there is a response, the dose should be reduced to 35–40 mg/m^2/day on alternate days for 4–8 weeks, and then taper off over 4–6 weeks. If there is a relapse, prednisone should be started again as above (answer B is correct). If there are frequent relapses, a renal biopsy is required (in this case biopsy was done at the patient's request). If the biopsy confirms minimal change disease, either cyclosporine (4–6 mg/kg/day) for 1 year or cyclophosphamide (2 mg/kg/day) for 8–12 weeks should be considered.

Webb et al. studied 237 children aged 1–14 years and treated steroid-sensitive nephrotic syndrome with prednisolone either 16 weeks or 8 weeks to observe the pattern of disease relapse. They found no significant difference in time to first relapse or in the incidence of frequently relapsing nephrotic syndrome between the two treatment groups. However, 16-week treatment was associated with a short-term health economic benefit through reduced resource use and increased quality of life. Thus, extended steroid therapy beyond 8 weeks may seem to improve quality of life in children; however, the adverse effects of extended use of steroids were not documented.

There is no indication of steroid resistance in this patient. Although calcineurin inhibitors, cyclophosphamide, MMF, and rituximab have shown remission of nephrotic syndrome in patients with MCD, they are recommended for patients with steroid resistance or to decrease exposure to steroids or patients who develop complications from steroids.

Suggested Reading

Vivarelli M, Massella L, Ruggiero B, et al. Minimal change disease. Clin J Am Soc Nephrol. 2017;12:332–45.

Webb NJA, Woolley RL, Lambe T, et al. PREDNOS Collaborative Group. Long term tapering versus standard prednisolone treatment for first episode of childhood nephrotic syndrome: Phase III randomised controlled trial and economic evaluation. BMJ. 2019;365:l1800. https://doi.org/10.1136/bmj.l1800.

9. **Which one of the following statements regarding management of nephrotic syndrome in patients with minimal change disease (MCD) is CORRECT?**

A. In adult patients, daily or alternate-day corticosteroid therapy shows no differences in remissions, time to remission, relapse rate, or time to relapse
B. Remission and relapse rates are similar in patients treated with tacrolimus monotherapy after short-term IV methylprednisolone and conventional glucocorticoid treatment for adult-onset MCD with nephrotic syndrome
C. In adult patients, treatment with low-dose prednisone plus enteric-coated mycophenolate sodium was not superior to a standard high-dose prednisone (1 mg/kg/day) regimen in inducing complete remission of nephrotic syndrome
D. Rituximab is more effective than tacrolimus in maintaining disease remission and minimizing corticosteroid exposure in children with steroid-dependent nephrotic syndrome
E. All of the above

The answer is E

All of the above statements are correct (E is correct). Waldman et al. treated 65 adult patients with daily steroids and 23 received alternate-day steroids initially. There were no differences in remissions, time to remission, relapse rate, or time to relapse between daily- and alternate-day-treated patients (A is correct).

CNIs (cyclosporine and tacrolimus) were used as first-line therapy for MCD. Use of CNIs reduced the exposure to steroids. Li and colleagues randomized 119 patients with adult-onset MCD to receive either steroid or tacrolimus therapy after IV methylprednisolone for 10 days. The treatment was continued for 16–20 weeks with gradual tapering over 18 weeks. Mean time to remission and to relapse of nephrotic syndrome were similar, suggesting that tacrolimus monotherapy is noninferior to steroid monotherapy (B is correct).

Rémy et al. randomized 116 adults to receive either low-dose prednisone (0.5 mg/kg/day, maximum 40 mg/day) plus enteric-coated mycophenolate sodium 720 mg twice daily (test group; $N = 58$) or high-dose prednisone (1 mg/kg/day, maximum 80 mg/day) (control group; $N = 58$) for 24 weeks. The primary endpoint was complete remission after 4 weeks of treatment, and 109 of 116 participants achieved the primary endpoint with no significant difference between the test and control groups. Secondary endpoint was remission after 8 and 24 weeks of treatment, which was similar between the two groups. Median time to relapse was similar in both groups. Thus, the study showed that treatment with low-dose prednisone plus enteric-coated mycophenolate sodium was not superior to a standard high-dose prednisone regimen to induce complete remission in adults with minimal change nephrotic syndrome (C is correct).

Rituximab has been shown to be effective for the treatment of patients with steroid-dependent nephrotic syndrome or frequently relapsing nephrotic syndrome in children. Basu et al. compared the efficacy of rituximab and tacrolimus in maintaining relapse-free survival among children with steroid-dependent nephrotic syndrome. In their study, 120 children aged 3–16 years were randomized to receive either tacrolimus (along with tapering alternate-day prednisolone) for 12 months or a single course of rituximab (two infusions of 375 mg/m^2). All but three completed 1 year of follow-up. Relapse-free survival rate was higher in the rituximab than in the tacrolimus group. Also, the median time to first relapse was 40 weeks in the rituximab group compared to 29 weeks in the tacrolimus group. Frequency of relapse rate was lower (>1 relapse in 2 patients) in the rituximab group than in the tacrolimus group (>1 relapse in 10 patients). The cumulative corticosteroid dose during the 12-month study period was lower with rituximab compared with tacrolimus. Thus, rituximab is more effective than tacrolimus in prolonging remission of nephrotic children (D is correct).

Suggested Reading

Basu B, Sander A, Roy B, et al. Efficacy of rituximab vs tacrolimus in pediatric corticosteroid-dependent nephrotic syndrome: a randomized clinical trial. JAMA Pediatr. 2018;172:757–64.

Li X, Liu Z, Wang L, et al. Tacrolimus monotherapy after intravenous methylprednisolone in adults with minimal change nephrotic syndrome. J Am Soc Nephrol. 2017;28:1286–95.

Rémy P, Audard V, Natella PA, et al. MSN Trial Investigators. An open-label randomized controlled trial of low-dose corticosteroid plus enteric-coated mycophenolate sodium versus standard corticosteroid treatment for minimal change nephrotic syndrome in adults (MSN Study). Kidney Int. 2018;94:1217–26.
Waldman M, Crew RJ, Valeri A, et al. Adult minimal-change disease: clinical characteristics, treatment, and outcomes. Clin J Am Soc Nephrol. 2007;2:445–53.

10. **Match the following therapies with adult minimal change disease nephrotic syndrome (See Table 2.1).**

Table 2.1 Therapy for adult minimal change nephrotic syndrome (adapted from Vivarelli et al.)

A. Initial detection of nephrotic syndrome	1. Prednisone or prednisolone 1 mg/kg/day or 2 mg/kg every other day (maximum 80 mg/day or 120 mg every other day for 4–16 weeks with gradual tapering over a period of 6 months after remission)
B. Infrequent relapses	2. Prednisone or prednisolone 1 mg/kg/day or 2 mg/kg every other day (maximum 80 mg/day or 120 mg every other day for 4–16 weeks with gradual tapering over a period of 6 months after remission)
C. Frequent relapses and steroid dependency	3. Cyclophosphamide (CPA) 2–2.5 mg/kg/day for 8 weeks (single course) If relapse occurs despite CPA or to preserve fertility: cyclosporine 3–5 mg/kg/day in two divided doses for 1–2 years or tacrolimus 0.05–0.1 mg/kg/day in two divided doses until 3 months after remission, then taper to the minimum effective dose for 1–2 years If intolerant to prednisone, CPA, cyclosporine, or tacrolimus: Mycophenolate mofetil 500–1000 mg 2 times daily for 1–2 years

Answers: A = 1; B = 2; C = 3

Suggested Reading

Vivarelli M, Massella L, Ruggiero, B, et al. Minimal change disease. Clin J Am Soc Nephrol. 2017;12:332–45.

11. A 60-year-old man is admitted for nephrotic syndrome and a serum creatinine concentration of 2.6 mg/dL. A kidney biopsy shows minimal change disease (MCD). **Which one of the following statements is LEAST likely in this patient when compared to a similar-aged male with MCD and normal renal function (creatinine 1.10 mg/dL)?**

A. Increased systolic blood pressure (SBP)
B. Renal failure due to renal ischemia
C. Proteinuria much higher despite similar glomerular disease
D. Evidence of AKI and atherosclerosis in addition to minimal change disease
E. Irreversible acute kidney disease (AKI)

The answer is E

A reversible moderate reduction in GFR was observed in approximately 30% of children and adults with nephrotic syndrome and MCD. The association of minimal change disease with AKI has been described much more commonly in adults than in children. Studies have shown that patients with this association were older, had a higher SBP and proteinuria, and their renal biopsies showed evidence of atherosclerosis, renal ischemic changes as well as acute tubular injury. Follow-up studies of a small number of patients showed that the AKI reversed spontaneously or in some patients after dialytic therapy. Thus, AKI is reversible.

Suggested Reading

Meyrier A, Niaudet P. Acute kidney injury complicating nephrotic syndrome of minimal change disease. Kidney Int. 2018;94:861–9.
Smith JD, Heyslett JP. Reversible renal failure in the nephrotic syndrome. Am J Kidney Dis. 1992;19:201–13.

12. An 18-year-old African American man is found to have hematuria and 3+ proteinuria on urinalysis during a routine phys exam. He is referred to a nephrologist for further evaluation. A 24-h urine collection shows 5.2 g of proteinuria. His BP is 148/86 mm Hg and has a pulse rate of 76 beats/min. Except for trace edema, his phys exam is otherwise normal. Serum chemistry and CBC are normal. Serum complement and ASO titers are normal. ANA and anti-DNA antibodies are negative. A renal biopsy shows the following:

- Light microscopy (LM): normal glomerular appearance
- Electron microscopy (EM): mesangial immune complex dense deposits
- Immunofluorescence (IF) microscopy: 2+ IgG, 2+ IgM, 2+ C3, and 4+ C1q and absent κ and λ chains in glomerular mesangium

Which one of the following choices is the MOST likely diagnosis in this patient?

A. Minimal change disease
B. Focal segmental glomerulosclerosis (FSGS)
C. Lupus nephritis (Class I)
D. C1q nephropathy
E. Orthostatic proteinuria

The answer is D

The diagnosis in this young patient is C1q nephropathy, which is a rare renal disease that resembles histologically lupus nephritis. C1q nephropathy is seen predominantly in young (15–30 years of age) subjects with male dominance. African Americans and Hispanics may have a higher incidence. The clinical manifestations include proteinuria in the nephrotic range or nephrotic syndrome with normal to decreased GFR. Hematuria, edema, and hypertension are present in substantial number of patients. Interestingly, C1q nephropathy is usually diagnosed during a routine phys exam. In these patients, LM findings vary from normal appearing glomeruli (mimicking minimal change disease) to FSGS. IF and EM show the presence of dominant or co-dominant deposits of C1q with less staining for immunoglobulins and C3 and electron-dense deposits in the mesangial region. The staining for κ and λ chains is absent. Serum complement levels are normal. Renal survival at 3 years of follow-up is 84%, and proteinuria does not always respond to corticosteroids.

Based on the IF microscopy findings, C1q nephropathy may be confused with class 1 or class 2 lupus nephritis. However, absence of lupus serology and normal serum complement levels, absence of tubuloreticular inclusion bodies, lack of staining for κ and λ chains, and absence of anti-C1q antibodies exclude the diagnosis of lupus nephritis.

The presence of immune deposits excludes the diagnosis of both minimal change disease and FSGS. Orthostatic proteinuria, which is defined as the presence of proteinuria in the upright position and the absence of proteinuria in the supine position, should be considered in any young individual with proteinuria around 1–2 g/day. In these subjects, the renal biopsy is normal, and the course of proteinuria is benign. Follow-up in 6–12 months is needed to ascertain that the degree or pattern of proteinuria has not changed, and corticosteroid treatment is not indicated.

Suggested Reading

Devasahayam J, Erode-Singaravelu G, Bhat Z, et al. C1q nephropathy: the unique underrecognized pathological entity. Analyt Cell Pathol. 2015;2015:490413, 5 pages.

Fogo AB, Lusco MA, Najafian B, et al. AJKD Atlas of Renal Pathology: C1q Nephropathy. Am J Kidney Dis. 2015;66(3):e13–4.

Sharman A, Furness P, Feehally J. Distinguishing C1q nephropathy from lupus nephritis. Nephrol Dial Transplant. 2004;19:1420–6.

Vizjak A, Ferluga D, Rozic M, et al. Pathology, clinical preserntations, and outcomes of C1q nephropathy. J Am Soc Nephrol. 2008;19:2237–44.

13. **Match the following glomerular lesions (variants) of primary (idiopathic) focal segmental glomerulosclerosis (FSGS) with the renal outcomes, as described from 1 to 4.**

A. Figure 2.1a
B. Figure 2.1b
C. Figure 2.1c
D. Figure 2.1d

1. Patients with severe nephrotic syndrome and deteriorating renal function with time
2. Patients with severe nephrotic syndrome and least impaired renal function with time
3. Patients with lowest frequency of nephrotic syndrome and highest frequency of hypertension
4. Similar to perihilar variant with less severe glomerular sclerosis and tubulointerstitial injury

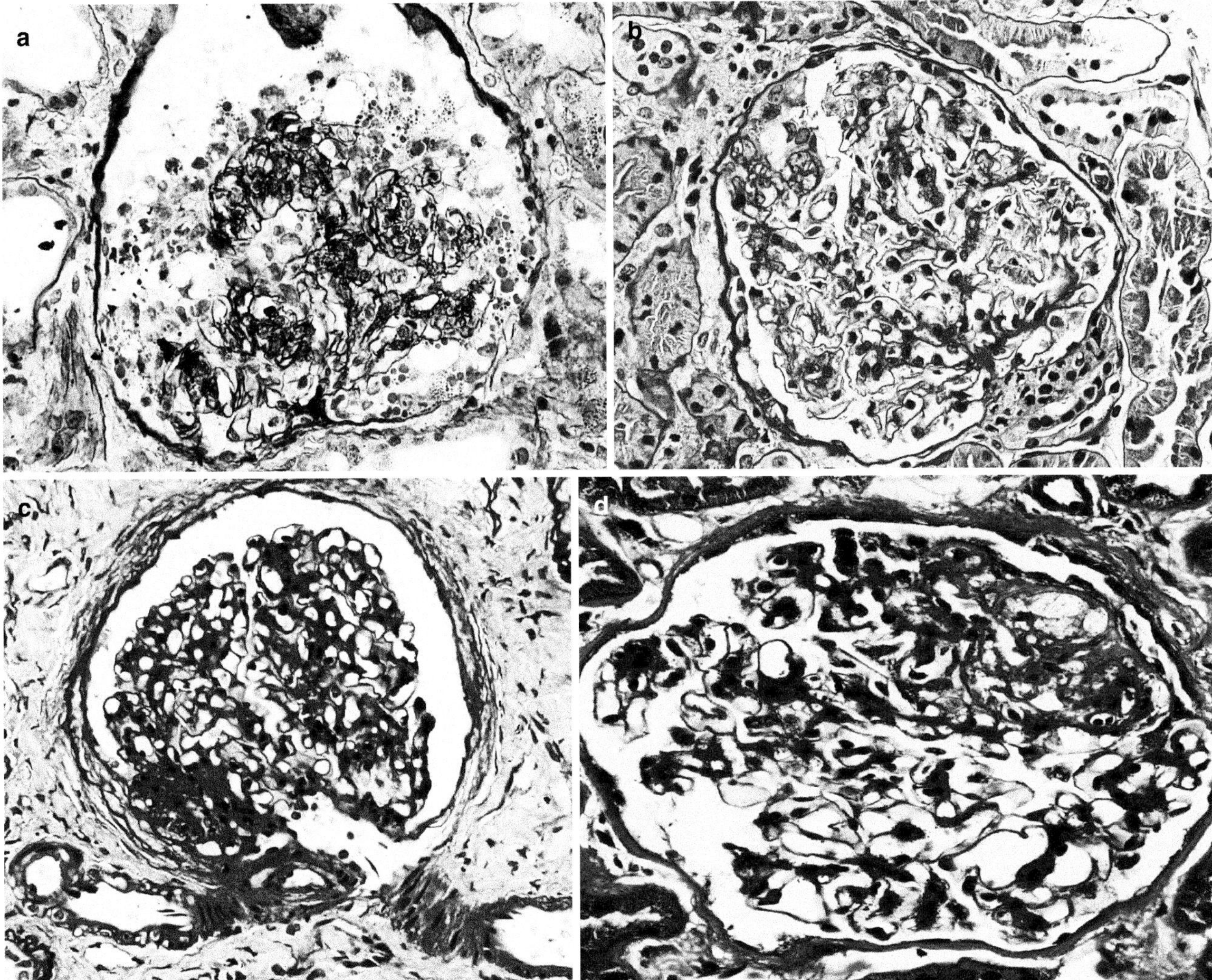

Fig. 2.1 Variants of idiopathic focal segmental glomerulosclerosis

Answers: A = 1; B = 2; C = 3; D = 4

Primary focal segmental glomerulosclerosis (FSGS) has been classified into five variants based on histologic features and renal outcomes. They are (1) collapsing FSGS, (2) tip lesion FSGS, (3) cellular FSGS, (4) perihilar FSGS, and (5) FSGS not otherwise specified (FSGS NOS). Thomas et al. reviewed the biopsy specimens of 282 patients with 20 years of follow-up and compared the clinical outcomes and response to treatment among these 5 variants. Collapsing variant had a striking predilection for African Americans, and patients with this form had severe nephrotic syndrome, substantial renal insufficiency, and poor renal survival. Only 14% of patients were in complete remission at the end of follow-up. Therefore, Fig. 2.1a is consistent with option 1 (collapsing FSGS).

Tip lesion FSGS was present in low percentage of patients; however, they have severe nephrotic syndrome, but the initial and final serum creatinine levels were least affected. Of all FSGS variants, patients with tip lesion variant had the highest rate of complete remission as well as the highest rate of renal survival. Thus, Fig. 2.1b is compatible with option 2 (tip lesion FSGS).

Patients with perihilar FSGS had the lowest frequency of nephrotic syndrome and the highest frequency of hypertension. Although these patients had good renal survival, their complete and partial remission was poor. This lesion did not have a predilection for African Americans. Thus, Fig. 2.1c is consistent with option 3 (perihilar FSGS).

The clinical features of patients with FSGS NOS are similar to those of the perihilar FSGS. Hypertension and nephrotic syndrome were common, and complete remission was low. Glomerulosclerosis and chronic tubulointerstitial injury were not severe. Therefore, Fig. 2.1d is consistent with option 4 (FSGS NOS).

The frequency of cellular FSGS was only 3%. Therefore, no conclusions regarding clinical features or renal outcomes could be reached with this lesion (Figure not shown).

In summary, the clinical features and complete remission were worst in patients with collapsing FSGS and more favorable in patients with tip lesion FSGS.

Suggested Reading

D'Agati V. The spectrum of focal segmental glomerulosclerosis: new insights. Curr Opin Nephrol Hypertens. 2008;17:271–81.

D'Agati VD, Fogo AB, Bruijn JA, et al. Pathologic classification of focal segmental glomerulosclerosis: a working proposal. Am J Kidney Dis. 2004;43:368–82.

Fogo AB, Kashgarian M. Diagnostic atlas of renal pathology. 3rd ed. Philadelphia: Elsevier, Inc.; 2017. p. 20–49.

Thomas DB, Franceschini N, Hogan SL, et al. Clinical and pathologic characteristics of focal segmental glomerulosclerosis pathologic variants. Kidney Int. 2006;69:920–6.

14. **Which one of the following mechanisms involved in the pathogenesis of primary focal segmental glomerulosclerosis (FSGS) is CORRECT?**

A. Podocyte injury, apoptosis, detachment, and loss of podocytes
B. Soluble urokinase plasminogen activator receptor (suPAR)
C. Circulating cardiotrophin-like cytokine factor 1 (CLCF1)
D. Circulating anti-CD40 IgG
E. All of the above

The answer is E

There is substantial evidence to show that podocyte injury is at the center of the development of FSGS. It is the earliest morphologic feature of FSGS, which is observed in recurrent FSGS in the allograft kidney by electron microscopy prior to the development of overt sclerosis. Both animal and human studies have shown apoptosis, detachment, and loss of podocytes. Loss of podocytes leaves the glomerular basement membrane (GBM) nude, thus allowing the remaining podocytes to hypertrophy to cover the denuded GBM. Proteins pass through the denuded GBM, causing proteinuria. However, hypertrophied podocytes may not be sufficient to cover the denuded GBM. Consequently, parietal epithelial cells differentiate into podocytes and contribute to functional recovery partially. Proteinuria decreases but does not reduce completely. However, hypertrophied podocytes cause mechanical stress and hyperfiltration, which triggers further podocyte detachment and causes decreased ability of differentiation of parietal epithelial cells into podocytes. This leads to proteinuria and progressive scar formation with progression to FSGS (A is correct).

Studies from animals and humans have implicated the presence of certain circulating permeability factors in the pathogenesis of FSGS. These factors include suPAR, CLCF1, anti CD40 IgG, and apA1b (an isoform of ApoA1). Serum suPAR levels were found to be elevated in children and adults with FSGS. Also, an inverse relationship was reported between suPAR and eGFR levels (B, C, and D are correct).

Suggested Reading

Ahn W, Bomback AS. Approach to diagnosis and management of primary glomerular diseases due to podocytopathies in adults: core curriculum 2020. Am J Kidney Dis. 2020;75:955–64.

Shabaka A, Ribera AT, Fernández-Juárez G. Focal segmental glomerulosclerosis: state-of-the-art and clinical perspective. Nephron. 2020;144:413–27.

Wada T, Nangaku M. A circulating permeability factor in focal segmental glomerulosclerosis: the hunt continues. Clin Kidney J. 2015;8:708–15.

15. **Regarding the treatment of nephrotic syndrome due to primary focal segmental glomerulosclerosis (FSGS), which one of the following statements is CORRECT?**

A. Corticosteroids have been the first-line therapy at 1 mg/kg/day for ≥16 weeks
B. Calcineurin inhibitors (CNIs) are generally used as second-line agents

C. Rituximab can enhance remission, if used with immunosuppressive drugs
D. Mycophenolate mofetil (MMF) is likely inferior to CNIs
E. All of the above

The answer is E

The treatment of primary FSGS should be individualized on the basis of histologic variants of FSGS and also factors such as age and comorbidities. Immunosuppressive drugs need to be used in patients with nephrotic syndrome, as renin-angiotensin inhibitors are not adequate to lower massive proteinuria.

In general, the degree of proteinuria determines the prognosis of kidney survival in patients with idiopathic FSGS. It has been shown that about 50% of patients with proteinuria <10 g/day progress to ESKD in 5–10 years; however, patients with proteinuria >10 g/day may progress to ESKD within 5 years. Thus, patients with primary FSGS may benefit from reduction in proteinuria. One approach is to start prednisone at 1 mg/kg/day (maximum 80 mg/day) or 2 mg/kg on alternate days for ≥16 weeks in patients with nephrotic syndrome and serum creatinine level <2–3 mg/dL. If there is a response, prednisone should be tapered over a period of 3–6 months. Steroids should be tried again for a relapse after prolonged remission. If there is no response after 4 weeks or intolerant to prednisone, cyclosporine at 2–4 mg/kg/day (~100 mg twice daily) should be tried for at least 6 months with concurrent use of prednisone (15 mg/day). Note that continuation of low-dose steroid (15 mg/day) may potentiate the response to cyclosporine (answers A and B are correct). It should be noted that long-term use of cyclosporine causes nephrotoxicity, particularly in those with reduced kidney function (eGFR <30 mL/min). Cyclosporine can be used as the first-line therapy in patients who relapse frequently or resistant to steroids or develop complications to steroids.

Tacrolimus has been used in patients with cyclosporine resistant or dependent FSGS. However, the remission rates are only 15%, but the relapse rates remained at 72% after tacrolimus discontinuation.

Rituximab has been shown to improve proteinuria in both children and adults with FSGS who are steroid dependent or who relapse frequently. In combination with other immunosuppressive drugs, rituximab causes increased rates of remission, decreased rates of relapses, and reduced doses of other immunosuppressive drugs (C is correct).

Kidney survival to corticosteroid treatment depends on the proteinuria response. If remission of proteinuria is complete or partial (40–80%) after 12–16 weeks, the patient has a better kidney survival compared to a patient with little or no reduction in proteinuria. This patient is considered to have steroid-resistant proteinuria with poor kidney survival. If the patient relapses during the period of tapering steroid dose, the patient is considered to be steroid dependent, and the kidney survival is intermediate.

The study of Gipson et al. compared the efficacy of a 12-month course of cyclosporine to a combination of oral pulse dexamethasone and MMF in children and adults with steroid-resistant primary FSGS. Their study did not find a difference in rates of proteinuria remission in a 12-month period between cyclosporine and the combination of MMF and steroids, suggesting treatment superiority of cyclosporine over MMF (D is correct).

The Nephrotic Syndrome Study Network (NEPTUNE) assessed the efficacy of immunosuppressive therapy on complete remission of proteinuria in a cohort of 441 patients with primary diagnosis of MCD, FSGS, and membranous nephropathy (MN). The study findings were that 46% of the cohort achieved a complete remission. The complete remission was 75% in MCD, 34% in FSGS, and 31% in MN patients. Previous studies reported frequencies of complete remission ranging from 70% to 87% in MCD, 20–34% in FSGS, and 60% in MN. Thus, complete remission in proteinuria with immunosuppressive therapy and renin-angiotensin inhibitors can be achieved in some patients. However, complete remission of proteinuria is dependent on the degree of proteinuria and kidney pathology at baseline.

ACTH seems to improve proteinuria in some patients with steroid-dependent or steroid-resistant FSGS. In a study of 24 patients, treatment with subcutaneous ACTH gel (80 units twice weekly) showed complete or partial remission of proteinuria in 7 patients after a mean follow-up of 16 months but 2 of them relapsed. Thus, ACTH may be used in difficult patients, but its cost limits its use for many such patients.

Suggested Reading

Ahn W, Bomback AS. Approach to diagnosis and management of primary glomerular diseases due to podocytopathies in adults: core curriculum 2020. Am J Kidney Dis. 2020;75:955–64.

Gipson DS, Trachtman H, Kaskel FJ, et al. Clinical trial of focal segmental glomerulo-sclerosis in children and young adults. Kidney Int. 2011;80:868–78.

Gipson DS, Troost JP, Lafayette RA, et al. Complete remission in the Nephrotic Syndrome Study Network (NEPTUNE). Clin J Am Soc Nephrol. 2016;11:81–9.
Rosenberg AZ, Kopp JB. Focal segmental glomerulosclerosis. Clin J Am Soc Nephrol. 2017;12:502–17.
Shabaka A, Ribera AT, Fernández-Juárez G. Focal segmental glomerulosclerosis: state-of-the-art and clinical perspective. Nephron. 2020;144:413–27.

16. **Which one of the following conditions is NOT associated with FSGS?**

A. Morbid obesity
B. Hepatitis C infection
C. Sickle cell disease
D. HIV infection
E. Low nephron number

The answer is B

FSGS is a disease of podocyte injury. Generally, FSGS is classified into primary, genetic, and secondary forms. Since FSGS is a podocytopathy, a new classification was introduced for all cytopathies based on their pathogenesis into (1) permeability factor-induced, (2) toxic, (3) genetic, and (4) hyperfiltration-mediated categories. For simplicity, we follow secondary causes of FSGS to answer the question.

Except for hepatitis C infection which causes mostly MPGN type I, all other conditions are associated with FSGS and nephrotic syndrome. FSGS in obesity and decreased number of nephrons may result from intraglomerular hypertension (hyperfiltration), whereas that in sickle cell anemia it may be due to hypoxemia. How HIV infection causes FSGS is not clearly understood; however, the involvement of NEF gene has been implicated.

Suggested Reading

Ahn W, Bomback AS. Approach to diagnosis and management of primary glomerular diseases due to podocytopathies in adults: core curriculum 2020. Am J Kidney Dis. 2020;75:955–64.
Appel GB, D'Agati VD. Primary and secondary (non-genetic) causes of focal and segmental glomerulosclerosis. In: Feehally J, Floege J, Tonelli M, et al., editors. Comprehensive clinical nephrology. 6th ed. Philadelphia: Elsevier; 2019. p. 219–31.
De Vriese AS, Sethi S, Nath KA, et al. Differentiating primary, genetic, and secondary FSGS in adults: a clinicopathologic approach. J Am Soc Nephrol. 2018;29:759–74.
Kopp JB, Anders H-J, Susztak K, et al. Podocytopathies. Nat Rev Primer. 2020;6:68.

17. **Which one of the following factors at diagnosis in predicting the long-term kidney survival in patients with FSGS is FALSE?**

A. Nephrotic-range proteinuria (≥3.5 g/day) and absence of remission
B. eGFR <60 mL/min
C. Hypoalbuminemia
D. Interstitial fibrosis and tubular atrophy
E. Black race

The answer is E

Several factors that predict the long-term kidney survival in patients with FSGS have been identified. Forster et al. evaluated demographics, clinical characteristics, histopathology, and immunosuppressive therapy on long-term kidney survival in ethnically diverse, adult cohort of 338 patients with biopsy-proven FSGS who had long-term treatment with renin-angiotensin inhibitors using data from the US Department of Defense healthcare network. Median follow-up after biopsy diagnosis was 9.5 years. Multivariate analysis showed that nephrotic-range protein, eGFR <60 mL/min, hypoalbuminemia, interstitial fibrosis and tubular atrophy, and interstitial inflammation at diagnosis and the absence of remission were all associated with worse long-term kidney survival (A-D correct). Black race with hazard ratio of 0.9 (CI 0.5–1.8; $p = 0.77$) was not found to be a risk factor (E is false).

Immunosuppressive therapy and absence of remission were not associated with improved kidney survival in the whole cohort, or in a subgroup with nephrotic-range proteinuria. However, immunosuppressive therapy was associated with better renal survival in a subgroup of patients with FSGS with both nephrotic-range proteinuria and hypoalbuminemia or hypoalbuminemia alone. Table 2.2 shows hazard ratios (CI not included for simplicity) for several factors.

Table 2.2 Multivariate analysis of various variables and hazard ratios

Variable	Hazard ratio	Significance
Age	1.07	Yes
Black race	0.7	No
Proteinuria >3.5 g/day	5.7	Yes
Complete remission	0.04	Yes
Partial remission	0.12	Yes
Albumin ≤3.0 g/dL	2.0	No
eGFR >60 mL/min	0.17	No
Interstitial fibrosis and tubular atrophy >15%	2.6	Yes
Immunosuppressive therapy	0.55	No

Adapted from Forster et al.

Suggested Reading

Forster BM, Nee R, Little DJ, et al. Focal segmental glomerulosclerosis, risk factors for end stage kidney disease, and response to immunosuppression. Kidney. 2021;360(2):105–13.

18. **Which one of the following statements regarding the circulating permeability factor to increased albumin permeability in patients with glomerular disease is FALSE?**

A. A high circulating permeability factor is responsible for recurrence of FSGS and proteinuria in a kidney transplant patient
B. Patients with steroid-responsive nephrotic syndrome or with membranous nephropathy after kidney transplant have low circulating levels of permeability factor
C. Plasmapheresis treatment has no effect either on permeability factor level or proteinuria in patients with recurrent FSGS
D. Patients with FSGS but without kidney transplants have very high circulating levels of permeability factor
E. Patients with ESKD due to hypertension or polycystic kidney disease have normal circulating levels of permeability factor

The answer is C

Savin et al. identified in plasma from patients with FSGS a factor that increases glomerular permeability to albumin and named it a permeability factor. Subsequently, this factor was found to be increased and responsible for recurrence of the disease and proteinuria after a kidney transplant in patients with primary FSGS. Following plasmapheresis in six patients with recurrences, both the permeability factor and proteinuria were significantly reduced. Therefore, option C is false. The permeability factor levels were low in other patients with steroid-sensitive nephrotic syndrome, or in patients with membranous nephropathy after kidney transplantation, or in patients with ESKD due to hypertension or polycystic kidney disease. This permeability factor was subsequently identified as cardiotrophin-like cytokine factor 1 (CLCF1).

CLCF1 belongs to the IL-6 family of B-cell-stimulating cytokine, and its levels were 100 times higher in patients with recurrent FSGS than in controls, CLCF1 likely causes FSGS due to destabilization of the actin cytoskeleton of podocytes. In one study, it was found that CLCF-1 decreased nephrin expression in isolated rat glomeruli and cultured murine podocytes.

Not only plasmapheresis but also plasma immunoadsorption by protein A column reduced permeability factor and proteinuria in patients with FSGS. Pharmacologic agents including indomethacin and cyclosporine can block in vitro activity of permeability factor.

Suggested Reading

Moriconi L, Lenti C, Puccini R, et al. Proteinuria in focal segmental glomerulosclerosis: role of circulating factors and therapeutic approach. Ren Fail. 2001;23:533–41.
Savin VJ, Sharma R, Sharma M, et al. Circulating factor associated with increased glomerular permeability to albumin in recurrent focal segmental glomerulosclerosis. N Engl J Med. 1996;334:878–83.
Savin VJ, McCarthy ET, Sharma M. Permeability factors in focal segmental glomerulosclerosis. Sem Nephrol. 2003;23:147–60.

Shojia J, Mii A, Terasaki M, et al. Update on recurrent focal segmental glomerulosclerosis in kidney transplantation. Nephron. 2020;144(suppl 1):65–70.

Wada T, Nangaku M. A circulating permeability factor in focal segmental glomerulosclerosis: the hunt continues. Clin Kidney J. 2015;8:708–15.

19. **Which one of the following findings distinguishes primary from secondary forms of focal segmental glomerulosclerosis (FSGS)?**

A. Increase in mesangial matrix
B. Focal sclerosis only in some parts of the glomerulus in primary FSGS
C. Serum albumin and width of foot processes (effacement of foot processes)
D. Tram-tract appearance of the basement membrane
E. None of the above

The answer is C

The causes of FSGS may be primary or secondary. The secondary forms are generally characterized by glomerular hyperfiltration and glomerular hypertrophy. It was suggested that serum albumin and the degree of foot processes effacement can distinguish primary from secondary forms of FSGS. Praga et al. reported that serum albumin levels are <3 g/dL in those with biopsy-proven primary FSGS, compared to >3.5 g/dL in those patients with secondary FSGS. A histopathologic study by Deegens et al. showed that the width of foot processes is significantly higher (3200 nm) in primary FSGS, as compared with 1098 nm in secondary FSGS (normal 562 nm). Overall, foot process width over 1500 nm differentiated idiopathic from secondary FSGS with high sensitivity and specificity. This signifies that patients with primary FSGS have complete effacement of foot processes compared to patchy effacement in secondary FSGS. Thus, option C is correct. Other options are incorrect.

It should be noted from the study of Deegens et al. and others that effacement of foot processes depends on the type of glomerular disease rather than the degree of proteinuria.

Suggested Reading

Deegens JKJ, Dijkman HBPM, Borm GF, et al. Podocyte foot process effacement as a diagnostic tool in focal segmental glomerulosclerosis. Kidney Int. 2008;74:1568–78.

Praga M, Morales E, Herrero J, et al. Absence of hypoalbuminemia despite massive proteinuria in focal segmenal glomerulosclerosis secondary to hyperfiltration. Am J Kidney Dis. 1999;33:52–8.

20. Primary (idiopathic) membranous nephropathy is now considered an antibody (Ab)-mediated autoimmune glomerular disease with complement activation. **Which one of the following antigens seems to play a pathogenic role in the development of membranous nephropathy?**

A. Phospholipase A_2 receptor
B. Thrombospondin type-1 domain-containing 7A (THSD7A)
C. Neural epidermal growth factor-like 1 (NELL-1)
D. Semaphorin3B (Sema3B)
E. All of the above

The answer is E

Membranous nephropathy (MN) is traditionally divided into primary MN when it has no association with any disease and secondary MN when it has a disease association such as autoimmune disease, malignancy, infection, or drugs. There is sufficient evidence to suggest that primary MN is an autoimmune disease. The search for target antigens is currently underway.

In 2009, Beck et al. identified a target antigen called M-type phospholipase A_2 receptor (PLA$_2$R), which is expressed on podocytes. In their study, circulating autoantibodies to PLA$_2$R were identified in 26 of 37 (70%) patients with primary MN. Both PLA$_2$R and its autoantibody were isolated from immune complexes of patients with MN. The autoantibodies, which belong to the IgG4 subclass of the immunoglobulins, are specific to primary MN, as these antibodies were detected in 70% of patients with primary MN and were absent in patients with secondary MN. Six cohort studies from Europe and China have identified anti-PLA2R antibodies in 57, 74, 75, 78, 80, and 82% of patients with primary MN. Thus, option A is correct.

THSD7A was the second antigen that was identified in 2014. Like PLA2R, THSD7A a transmembrane protein expressed on podocytes. THSD7A antigen is responsible for approximately 3% of patients with primary MN and 10% of primary MN patients who are negative for anti-PLA2R. This antigen may also be involved in the pathogenesis of some cases of malignancy-associated MN. In some cases of primary MN, both THSD7A and PLA2R have been reported.

With the use of laser microdissection and tandem mass spectrometry, additional antigens were identified. Two of them, NELL-1 and sema3B, were identified in primary MN. NELL-1 antigen seems responsible in approximately 16% of cases of PLA2R-negative primary MN. Antibodies to this antigen were found in PLA$_2$R-negative primary MN patients but not in patients with secondary MN, minimal change disease, or IgA nephropathy. The predominant IgG subclass in this disease is IgG1 rather than IgG4. Although NELL-1 antigen is predominantly found in primary MN cases, it may be present in malignancy-associated MN.

Sema3B was identified as the target antigen in a unique form of PLA2R-negative primary MN mostly children (73% of cases) and young adults (27%). The mean age of children was 6.9 years and 36.3 years in young adults. Sema3B antigen is present in 1–3% of all primary MN, and IgG subtyping reveals predominantly IgG1.

Among the four antigens that were identified by the laser microdissection and mass spectrometry, two of them were described above. The remaining two are exotosin 1 and 2 and PCDH7. These are associated with secondary MN. Exotosin 1/2 are present in secondary (autoimmune) MN. PCDH7 antigen is not associated with either autoimmune disease or infection but found in a patient with MN associated with prostate carcinoma.

Suggested Reading

Beck LH, Bongio RGB, Lambeau G, et al. M-type phospholipase A$_2$ receptor as target antigen in idiopathic membranous nephropathy. N Engl J Med. 2009;361:11–21.

Couser WG. Primary membranous nephropathy. Clin J Am Soc Nephrol. 2017;12:983–97.

Sethi S. New 'antigens' in membranous nephropathy. J Am Soc Nephrol. 2021;32:268–78.

21. **Which one of the following statements regarding anti-PLA$_2$R antibodies and membranous nephropathy (MN) is CORRECT?**

A. Anti-PLA2R antibody titers correlate with disease activity, provide prognostic information about severity of disease, and can serve as a useful biomarker for assessing treatment efficacy
B. Occurrence of spontaneous remission is more common in patients with low antibody titers than those with high antibody titers
C. High antibody titers are associated with lower response to immunosuppressive therapy and longer time to remission
D. Anti-PLA2R titers may also predict progression from nonnephrotic proteinuria to nephrotic-range proteinuria
E. All of the above

The answer is E

All of the above statements are correct. In addition, high antibody titers are associated with high risk of progressive kidney failure. Although antibody titers are important, glomerular staining for PLA$_2$R is more sensitive than circulating anti-PLA$_2$R antibodies in diagnosing PLA$_2$R-associated MN. Patients have a higher rate of spontaneous remission when their IgG4 antibody is directed only at the cysteine-rich epitope of PLA$_2$R. Of note that >50% of pediatric cases are PLA$_2$R-positive, and steroid treatment is ineffective in children <2 years of age if antibody titers are not measured.

Suggested Reading

Bech AP, Hofstra JM, Brenchley PE, et al. Association of anti-PLA(2)R antibodies with outcomes after immunosuppressive therapy in idiopathic membranous nephropathy. Clin J Am Soc Nephrol. 2014;9:1386–92.

Couser WG. Primary membranous nephropathy. Clin J Am Soc Nephrol. 2017;12:983–97.

Glassock RJ. Antiphospholipase A2 receptor autoantibody guided diagnosis and treatment of membranous nephropathy: a new personalized medical approach. Clin J Am Soc Nephrol. 2014;9:1341–3.

Hofstra JM, Beck LH Jr, Beck DM, et al. Anti-phospholipase A(2) receptor antibodies correlate with clinical status in idiopathic membranous nephropathy. Clin J Am Soc Nephrol. 2011;6:1286–91.

Hoxha E, Harendza S, Pinnschmidt H, et al. PLA2R antibody levels and clinical outcome in patients with membranous nephropathy and non-nephrotic-range proteinuria under treatment with inhibitors of the renin-angiotensin system. PLoS One. 2014;9:e11068.

22. A 55-year-old Caucasian man presents with periorbital and lower extremity edema. He does not take any medication and has no other significant past medical history. After appropriate lab tests, a kidney biopsy was done which is consistent with primary membranous nephropathy (Stage II). Serum creatinine is 1.2 mg/dL, and 24-h urine protein is 5.4 g. **Which one of the following statements is the LEAST likely predictor of progressive kidney disease in this patient?**

    A. Female sex and Stage I or II glomerulopathy on kidney biopsy
    B. Persistent proteinuria of 8 g/day or more for 6 months or longer
    C. Male sex, age >50 years and uncontrolled hypertension
    D. Interstitial fibrosis and tubular atrophy at the time of kidney biopsy
    E. Urinary excretion of β_2-microglobulin >54 µg/mmol creatinine, IgG >250 mg/day C5b-9 >7 mg/mg creatinine

    The answer is A

    The natural course of primary membranous nephropathy (MN) is that about 25–33% of patients will have spontaneous remission in 3–4 years. Despite spontaneous remission, several studies have estimated the prognosis of kidney survival in patients with MN. Male sex, age >50 years, persistent proteinuria >8 g/day for 6 months or longer, decreased kidney function, uncontrolled hypertension, interstitial fibrosis, and tubular atrophy were shown to be predictors of progressive kidney disease in patients with primary MN. Also, advanced glomerulopathy (Stages III or IV) or the presence of crescents on renal biopsy may portend a poor prognosis.

    Some studies have shown that urinary excretion of β_2-microglobulin, IgG, and C5b-9 may have a prognostic value for assessing renal survival. If β_2-microglobulin excretion is >54 µg/mmol creatinine, IgG excretion >250 mg/day, and C5b-9 >7 mg/mg creatinine, the progression of kidney disease is much greater in patients with MN than in those who have lower excretions of these proteins.

    Female sex and less severe glomerulopathy (Stages I or II) seem to have a low predictive value as indicators of kidney disease progression. Thus, choice A is incorrect.

    Suggested Reading

Cattran DC, Pei Y, Greenwood CM, et al. Validation of a predictive model of idiopathic membranous nephropathy: its clinical and research implications. Kidney Int. 1997;51:901–7.

Salant DJ, Cattran DC. Membranous nephropathy. In: Feehally J, Floege J, Tonelli M, et al., editors. Comprehensive clinical nephrology. 6th ed. Philadelphia: Elsevier; 2019. p. 240–53.

23. Patients with primary membranous nephropathy (MN) and nephrotic syndrome are at increased risk for venous thromboembolic events (VTEs). **Which one of the following statements is a risk factor for VTE?**

    A. Serum albumin concentration of 3.8 g/dL
    B. Serum albumin concentration of 3.5 g/dL
    C. Serum albumin concentration of 3.2 g/dL
    D. Serum albumin concentration of 3.0 g/dL
    E. Serum albumin concentration of 2.2 g/dL

    The answer is E

    One of the complications of nephrotic syndrome is VTEs, which include renal vein thrombosis, deep venous thrombosis, and pulmonary embolism. Of the primary glomerular diseases, MN is the most common disorder that predisposes patients to VTEs. In patients with MN, the single most important risk factor was found to be hypoalbuminemia. The risk for VTEs increased with serum albumin levels <2.8 g/dL. Patients with FSGS and IgA nephropathy were recently found to be at risk for VTEs but not to the extent of patients with MN. In 1313 patients with nephrotic syndrome, the adjusted hazard ratio for VTE was 10.8 for MN and 5.9 for FSGS compared with IgA nephropathy.

    In MN, a serum albumin level of <2.8 g/dL was associated with a 2.5-fold increased risk of VTE compared to patients with a serum albumin of ≥2.8 g/dL. Each 1.0 g/dL decrease in serum albumin from 2.8 g/dL resulted in a 2.13-fold increased risk of VTE. The VTE risk was 5.8-fold when serum albumin level was <2.2 g/dL.

    The benefit-to-risk ratio for patients at low risk for bleeding was calculated to be 4.5:1 and 13.1:1 for serum albumin levels of <3 and <2 g/dL, respectively, which indicated there is benefit for anticoagulation at any serum albumin level <3 g/dL.

The duration of anticoagulation in patients with nephrotic syndrome is not clear at this time. It is, however, recommended that anticoagulation should be continued, while the patient remains nephrotic (serum albumin <3.0 g/dL).

It was suggested that proteinuria of any degree was not found to be an independent risk factor for VTEs; however, massive proteinuria has been suggested to be a strong predictor of VTE.

Suggested Reading

Barbour SJ, Greenwald A, Djurdjev O, et al. Disease-specific risk of venous thromboembolic events is increased in idiopathic glomerulonephritis. Kidney Int. 2012;81:190–5.

Glassock RJ. Prophylactic anticoagulation in nephrotic syndrome: a clinical conundrum. J Am Soc Nephrol. 2007;18:2221–5.

Gordon-Cappitelli JJ, Choi MJ. Prophylactic anticoagulation in adult patients with nephrotic syndrome. Clin J Am Soc Nephrol. 2020;15:123–5.

Lin R, McDonald G, Jolly T, et al. A systematic review of prophylactic anticoagulation in nephrotic syndrome. Kidney Int Rep. 2020;5:435–47.

Lionaki S, Derebail VK, Hogan SL, et al. Venous thromboembolism in patients with membranous nephropathy. Clin J Am Soc Nephrol. 2012;7:43–51.

24. **Which one of the following strategies regarding the treatment of primary membranous nephropathy (MN) is CORRECT?**

A. Conservative management controlling fluids and blood pressure (BP) as initial treatment
B. Cyclophosphamide or chlorambucil with steroids
C. Calcineurin inhibitors (cyclosporine or tacrolimus)
D. Rituximab
E. All of the above

The answer is E

Conservative management is extremely important in patients at any level of proteinuria. One needs to manage fluid overload in the form of edema, high BP, thromboembolic state, and control other risk factors such as hyperlipidemia to prevent cardiovascular disease. Edema treatment requires fluid and sodium restriction, judicious use of thiazide diuretics, and, if necessary, amiloride to block epithelial Na^+ channel. Renin-angiotensin-aldosterone inhibitors control not only BP but also reduce proteinuria. Thus, answer A is correct.

In many patients, conservative management is not sufficient to reduce proteinuria. In such cases, immunosuppressive therapy is indicated. Unlike FSGS, patients with MN do not usually respond to steroids alone. A meta-analysis reported that corticosteroids conferred no benefit in reducing proteinuria or preserving renal function. On the other hand, a beneficial effect of alkylating agents was found with cyclophosphamide giving fewer adverse reactions than chlorambucil. The recommended regimen is oral prednisone (0.5 mg/kg/day) or methylprednisolone I g IV for 3 days only on months 1, 3, and 5 and oral cyclophosphamide (2–2.5 mg/day) on months 2, 4, and 6 (Ponticelli regimen). Thus, answer B is correct. However, this regimen has several adverse effects, including opportunistic infections and malignancy. Therefore, care must be taken to apply this regimen.

Initial study by Cattran et al. showed that cyclosporine was effective in reducing proteinuria and slowing the rate of kidney function decline in patients with progressive loss of kidney function. Cyclosporine should be started at 3–5 mg/kg/day in two divided doses for at least 6 months. Cyclosporine levels should be monitored and maintained its trough levels between 120 and 200 μg/L. Concomitant use of prednisone at 10 mg every other day is found to be useful along with cyclosporine. Tacrolimus was also found to reduce proteinuria, but the relapse rate is high after discontinuation of the drug (C is correct). It should be remembered that calcineurin inhibitors can reduce proteinuria, but long-term use of them may cause nephrotoxicity. Thus, the benefit/risk ratio should be evaluated in the use of these drugs. Also, a UK study showed that cyclosporine treatment is no better than conservative management.

Rituximab (RTX) is a monoclonal antibody directed against CD20 that depletes B cells. Initial reports from Italy demonstrated that administration of RTX (375 mg/m^2) weekly for 4 weeks reduced proteinuria in primary MN with treatment-refractory nephrotic syndrome. A number of studies followed this report and showed long-term partial (>50%) or complete remission of proteinuria with low adverse effect compared to alkylating agents/corticosteroids. A recent study reported that RTX was noninferior to cyclosporine in inducing complete or partial

remission of proteinuria at 12 months and was superior in maintaining proteinuria remission up to 24 months in MN. Because of its efficacy in reducing proteinuria and lowering circulating anti-PLA$_2$R antibody titers with low adverse effects, RTX is recommended as first-line therapy in patients with MN (D is correct). For a detailed description of various studies on RTX in MN, the reader is referred to the Suggested Reading.

Suggested Reading

Bomback AS, Fervenza FC. Membranous nephropathy: approaches to treatment. Am J Nephrol. 2018;47(suppl 1):30–42.

Cattran DC, Appel GB, Hebert LA, et al. Cyclosporine in patients with steroid-resistant membranous nephropathy: a randomized trial. Kidney Int. 2001;59:1484–90.

Fervenza FC, Appel GB, Barbour SJ, et al. Rituximab or cyclosporine in the treatment of membranous nephropathy. N Engl J Med. 2019;381:36–46.

Howman A, Chapman TL, Langdon MM, et al. Immunosuppression for progressive membranous nephropathy: a UK randomised controlled trial. Lancet. 2013;381:744–51.

Loulwa Alsharhan L, Beck Jr LH. Membranous nephropathy: core curriculum 2021. Am J Kidney Dis. 2021;77:440–53.

Ponticelli C, Altieri P, Scolari F, et al. A randomized study comparing methylprednisolone plus chlorambucil versus methylprednisolone plus cyclophosphamide in idiopathic membranous nephropathy. J Am Soc Nephrol. 1998;9:444–50.

van de Logt A-E, Wetzels JF. Rituximab is preferable to cyclophosphamide for treatment of membranous nephropathy: CON. Kidney. 2021;360.

van den Brand JA, van Dijk PR, Hofstra JM, et al. Long-term outcomes in idiopathic membranous nephropathy using a restrictive treatment strategy. J Am Soc Nephrol. 2014;25:150–8.

25. **According to the Oxford classification of IgA nephropathy, which one of the following pathologic features is LEAST predictive of the rate of eGFR decline and ESKD?**

A. Mesangial hypercellularity score
B. Endocapillary hypercellularity
C. Segmental sclerosis or adhesion/ interstitial fibrosis/tubular atrophy
D. Cellular and fibrocellular crescents
E. All of the above

The answer is E

Although IgA nephropathy is the most common primary glomerular disease worldwide, there is now an international consensus for its pathologic or clinical classification. This classification, called the Oxford classification of IgA nephropathy, was introduced in 2009 to identify specific pathologic features that would predict the risk for progression of the disease and treatment response to ACE-Is and/or ARBs as well as immunosuppressive agents. This new Oxford classification of IgA nephropathy is based on 265 kidney biopsy findings with clinical data that were collected internationally from Asia, Europe, North America, and South America. The following histopathological features were identified for reproducibility:

1. **Mesangial cell hypercellularity (>4 mesangial cells)**
2. **Segmental sclerosis or adhesion**
3. **Global glomerulosclerosis**
4. **Endocapillary hypercellularity (hypercellularity due to increased number of cells within glomerular capillary lumina, causing narrowing of the lumina)**
5. **Cellular or fibrocellular crescents**
6. **Interstitial fibrosis/tubular atrophy**
7. **Arteriosclerosis**

However, only four independent histopathological features with reproducibility and predictive power were selected in the first classification:

1. **Mesangial hypercellularity (M)**
2. **Endocapillary hypercellularity (E)**
3. **Segmental sclerosis or adhesion (S)**
4. **Interstitial fibrosis/tubular atrophy (T)**

The association between the above histopathological features and kidney prognosis was retrospectively assessed during 69 months of median follow-up period. The clinical endpoints were a 50% decline in eGFR and the development of ESKD. During the 69 months follow-up period, 22% of them developed a 50% reduction in eGFR and 13% reached ESKD. By multivariate linear regression model, only segmental sclerosis or adhesion and interstitial fibrosis/tubular atrophy but not mesangial cell hypercellularity were strongly associated with decline in eGFR after adjustment for baseline or follow-up mean arterial pressure, proteinuria, and eGFR. By Cox proportional hazard models, mesangial hypercellularity and interstitial fibrosis/tubular atrophy but not segmental sclerosis or adhesion were associated with a decline in eGFR and ESKD. Considering both models, only mesangial cell hypercellularity, segmental sclerosis, or adhesion and interstitial nephritis/tubular atrophy have significant predictive power of renal prognosis.

A large study showed that E lesions are predictive of outcome in children and adults, but only in those without immunosuppression. However, fibrocellular crescents were found to have no prognostic importance in the original study. Subsequently, crescents or fibrocellular crescents were also found to be predictive of poor renal outcomes in patients with an estimated GFR <30 mL/min, and they were included in the MEST score to be reported as MEST-C score (answer E is correct).

Based on the above results, the Oxford classification recommends reporting mesangial cell hypercellularity, endocapillary proliferation, segmental sclerosis or adhesion, interstitial fibrosis/tubular atrophy, and crescents (MEST-C) score as histopathological prognostic features in a biopsy specimen of a patient with IgA nephropathy.

Suggested Reading

Cattran DC, Coppo R, Cook HT, et al. The Oxford classification of IgA nephropathy: rationale, clinicopathological correlations, and classification. Kidney Int. 2009;76:534–45.

Roberts ISD, Cook HT, Troyanov S, et al. The Oxford classification of IgA nephropathy: pathology, definitions, correlations, and reproducibility. Kidney Int. 2009;76:546–56.

Trimarchi H, Barratt J, Cattran DC, et al. on behalf of the IgAN Classification Working Group of the International IgA Nephropathy Network and the Renal Pathology Society. Oxford classification of IgA nephropathy 2016: an update from the IgA Nephropathy Classification Working Group. Kidney Int. 2017;91:1014–21.

26. A 28-year-old Filipino man is referred to a nephrologist for further evaluation of microscopic hematuria. His younger sister and brother, who live in the Philippines, are also found to have macroscopic hematuria following an upper respiratory infection. His BP is 146/84 mm Hg and has a pulse rate of 72 beats/min. The rest of the phys exam is unremarkable. Urinalysis shows 2+ blood and trace protein. Urine sediment reveals 30–40 dysmorphic RBCs without RBC casts. A 24-h urine collection has 300 mg of protein. His serum creatinine is 0.7 mg/dL. Serum complement level is normal and ANA is negative. **Which one of the following statements explains the BEST regarding the pathogenesis of his hematuria?**

A. Mutations involving the COL4A5 gene (α-5 chain of type IV collagen)
B. Mutations involving the COL4A3 or COL4A4 gene
C. Immune complex deposition in the subendothelial and mesangial region
D. Glomerular basement membrane thickness <200 nm in diameter
E. A defect in galactosylation of serum IgA1 hinge glycopeptides

The answer is E

This patient carries the diagnosis of IgA nephropathy (IgAN), which is the most common form of idiopathic GN in the world. IgAN is typically diagnosed in young adults (second and third decades of life), and the disease is more common in males than females. About 40–50% of patients present with microscopic hematuria at the time of their presentation. Episodes of macroscopic hematuria occur 1–2 days following upper respiratory infection. About 30–40% present with asymptomatic microscopic hematuria. The pathogenesis of hematuria in IgAN is incompletely understood. However, recent studies have shown that there is under galactosylation of the IgA1 hinge glycopeptides. IgA occurs in two isoforms: IgA_1 and IgA_2. It is the IgA_1 that is mostly deposited in IgAN. The human IgA_1 molecule is a glycoprotein that is formed by the attachment of a protein with an O-linked oligosaccharide in the hinge region. This oligosaccharide consists of N-acetylgalactosamine, which is usually substituted

with terminal galactose. In IgAN, the IgA_1 molecule contains less terminal galactose compared to IgA_1 in healthy controls. This under galactosylation may promote self-aggregation of IgA_1 with less clearance from circulation and thus deposition in the kidney.

Mutations in genes encoding the α3, α4, and α5 chains of type IV collagen (COL4A3, COL4A4, and COL4A5, respectively) result in Alport syndrome. Microscopic hematuria is a common abnormality in patients with Alport syndrome. Three genetic forms of Alport syndrome are described. About 80% of patients have X-linked form of the disease because of mutations in COL45 gene encoding the α5 chain of type IV collagen. About 15% of patients have autosomal recessive form of Alport syndrome, which is due to mutations in the COL4A3 or COL4A4 gene encoding α3 or α4 chains. About 5% of patients develop autosomal dominant form of Alport syndrome because of heterozygous mutations in COL4A3 or COL4A4 genes. Therefore, options A and B are incorrect.

Option D refers to thin basement membrane disease (autosomal dominant Alport syndrome). Normal basement membrane thickness in adults varies from 326 nm in females to 373 nm in males. Adult patients with thin basement membrane disease have typically <200 nm in thickness, which may be due to mutations in COL4A3 or COL4A4 genes. Hematuria in these patients, therefore, is not due to immune complexes.

Deposition of immune complex deposits predominantly in the subendothelial region and also in the mesangium is seen in patients with type I MPGN, who also present with hematuria. Although immune deposits are present in IgAN, they are exclusively or predominantly deposited in the mesangium. Another characteristic feature of IgAN is more intensive staining for λ light chains than for k light chains.

Suggested Reading

Nachman PH, Jennette JC, Falk RJ. Primary glomerular disease. In: Brenner BM, editor. Brenner & Rector's the kidney. 8th ed. Philadelphia: Saunders; 2008. p. 987–1066.

Suzuki H, Kiryluk K, Novak J, et al. The pathophysiology of IgA nephropathy. J Am Soc Nephrol. 2011;22:1795–1803.

van der Boog PJM, van Kooten C, de Jizter JW, et al. Role of macromolecular IgA in IgA nephropathy. Kidney Int. 2005;67:813–21.

27. The patient described above (question 26) asks you whether or not he requires treatment of his hematuria and hypertension (HTN). **Which of the following do you suggest at this time?**

A. No need for treatment and observation only
B. Fish oil daily
C. Low maintenance dose of corticosteroids
D. Treatment with ACE-I or ARB
E. Tonsillectomy

The answer is D

This patient has not only hematuria but HTN as well. Treatment of HTN is indicated. Several studies have shown that either an ACE-I or an ARB is the drug of choice in hypertensive IgAN patients with normal renal function and mild proteinuria (<500 mg/day). The suggested target BP is 125/75 mm Hg, particularly in those with proteinuria >1.0 g/day. Therefore, option D is correct. It is generally accepted that no specific treatment is required for microscopic hematuria in a patient with normal renal function. Similarly, macroscopic hematuria with normal renal function may not require a specific treatment.

One study showed that consumption of fish oil containing β-3 fatty acids (12 g/day) was beneficial in reducing proteinuria and preserving renal function. Other studies failed to confirm the results of this study. Thus, strong evidence in support of the use of expensive fish oil as a treatment for IgAN is lacking at the present time, although individualized treatment may be recommended.

Strong supportive care at least for 6 months is recommended before immunosuppressive therapy is started. Corticosteroids, either daily or on alternate-day basis, have been used extensively in the treatment of IgAN. An Italian study demonstrated long-time (10 years after treatment) renal survival was much better in steroid-treated than nonsteroid-treated patients with serum creatinine level of 1.0–1.1 mg/dL and proteinuria between 1.8 and 2.0 g/day. The 2012 KDIGO guideline also suggests that corticosteroids should be initiated in high-risk patients only if proteinuria is >1 g/day after supportive care has been optimized for 3–6 months and only if GFR remains above 50 mL/ min.

However, the benefit of corticosteroids has been challenged by two recent studies. The German STOP-IgAN trial did not show any additional benefit of corticosteroid addition in reducing proteinuria or decline in eGFR compared to supportive care involving renin-angiotensin. The Chinese TESTING trial had to be terminated early because the patients on corticosteroids experienced severe and at times fatal infections. Both these studies recommend strong supportive care and suggest that immunosuppressive therapy wound not add any benefit in the management of IgA nephropathy.

In our patient with normal renal function and proteinuria of 300 mg/day, however, corticosteroid therapy is not indicated. If proteinuria progresses to >1 g/day despite HTN control (BP <125/75 mm Hg) with maximum renin-angiotensin blockade, corticosteroids should be considered.

Tonsillitis and upper respiratory infections precede recurrent macroscopic hematuria in IgAN. Therefore, tonsillectomy has been proposed as a means of preventing recurrent bouts of macroscopic hematuria as well as progression of the disease. Although some studies have proven tonsillectomy to be effective, other studies suggest no benefit. Thus, tonsillectomy is not indicated in our patient.

Suggested Reading

Floege J, Feehally J. The therapy of IgA nephropathy. Nat Rev Nephrol. 2013;9:320–7.

Lv J, Xu D, Perkovic V, et al. Corticosteroid therapy in IgA nephropathy. J Am Soc Nephrol. 2012;23:1108–16.

Lv J, Zhang H, Wong MG, et al. TESTING Study Group. Effect of oral methylprednisolone on clinical outcomes in patients with IgA nephropathy: the TESTING randomized clinical trial. JAMA. 2017;318:432–42.

Rauen T, Eitner F, Fitzner C, et al. Intensive supportive care plus immunosuppression in IgA nephropathy. N Engl J Med. 2015;373:2225–36.

Tesar V, Troyanov S, Bellur S, et al. Corticosteroids in IgA nephropathy: a retrospective analysis from the VALIGA Study. J Am Soc Nephrol. 2015;26:2248–58.

28. During the follow-up of the above patient, you have done a kidney biopsy which showed normal looking glomeruli with few mesangial deposits that stained 2+ for IgA. The patient asks you about his kidney prognosis. **Which one of the following prognostic factors regarding kidney survival is FALSE?**

A. Sustained HTN
B. Persistent proteinuria >1 g/day or nephrotic syndrome
C. Acute kidney injury associated with macroscopic hematuria
D. Tubulointerstitial disease
E. Male sex and older age at the onset of disease

The answer is C

Except for acute kidney injury associated with macroscopic hematuria (option C), all other features presented were found to predict poor prognosis. A kidney biopsy is indicated if kidney function does not improve within 3–4 days of supportive treatment in a patient with macroscopic hematuria and acute kidney injury. The biopsy should distinguish ATN which is self-limiting from crescentic IgA nephropathy (IgAN) which requires intensive immunosuppression. Similarly, macroscopic hematuria, due to inflammation, may also be self-limiting. Acute kidney injury due to ATN has been reported with recurrent bouts of macroscopic hematuria. Thus, option C is false. In contrast to macroscopic hematuria, persistent microscopic hematuria is associated with a poor prognosis.

The amount of proteinuria 1 year after diagnosis was found to predict kidney survival. Patients with <500 mg/day had no kidney failure within a 7-year follow-up, whereas those with >3 g/day had approximately a 60% chance of reaching ESKD.

Magistroni et al. developed a clinical prognostic index (CPI) using clinical and pathologic data from 310 patients with biopsy-proven IgAN. They assigned two points for serum creatinine level >1.4 mg/dL, one point for proteinuria >1 g/day, one point for HTN, and one point for age >30 years at biopsy. Patients with a CPI score of 0–2 (low CPI score) had a 10-year kidney survival rate of 91.7% compared with 35% for patients with a CPI score of 3–5 (high CPI score). Barbour et al. combined MEST score with cross-sectional clinical data at biopsy and suggested that combined data can provide earlier risk prediction in IgAN than other methods that use 2 years of follow-up data.

Suggested Reading

Barbour SJ, Espino-Hernandez G, Reich HN, et al. The MEST score provides earlier risk prediction in IgA nephropathy. Kidney Int. 2016;89:167–75.

Floege J, Feehally J. The therapy of IgA nephropathy. Nat Rev Nephrol. 2013;9:320–7.

Magistroni R, Furci L, Leonelli M, et al. A validated model of disease progression in IgA nephropathy. J Nephrol. 2006;19:32–40.

29. **Rituximab, a monoclonal antibody directed against CD20, has been found to be LEAST likely useful in the treatment of which one of the following kidney diseases?**

A. Idiopathic membranous nephropathy
B. Minimal change disease
C. Class IV lupus nephritis
D. ANCA-positive renal disease
E. Diabetic nephropathy

The answer is E

Rituximab, a monoclonal antibody directed against CD20 antigen, has been successfully used as a therapeutic agent in a variety of renal diseases, including idiopathic membranous nephropathy, cryoglobulinemia-associated MPGN, class IV lupus nephritis, and ANCA-positive renal diseases. The CD20 antigen is found on immature and mature B cells, as well as on malignant B cells, and rituximab treatment has been shown to prevent B cells from proliferation because of apoptosis and lysis through complement-dependent and complement-independent mechanisms. Rituximab might also inhibit T cell activation. Thus, rituximab affects production of antibodies as well as regulation of immunoglobulin maturation by B cells. Improvement in proteinuria, and vasculitis, as well as disappearance of HCV has been observed with rituximab therapy. Rituximab has also been used in kidney transplant patients to lower alloreactive antibodies, and to treat rejection associated with B cells and antibodies. Steroid-dependent nephrotic syndrome due to minimal change disease is found to respond to rituximab. However, rituximab has not been used in patients with diabetic nephropathy. Thus, choice E is incorrect. It should be noted that rituximab can cause fatal pulmonary fibrosis.

Suggested Reading

Ahmed MS, Wong CF. Rituximab and nephrotic syndrome: a new therapeutic hope? Nephrol Dial Transplant. 2008;23:11–7.

Francois H, Daugas E, Bensman A, et al. Unexpected efficacy of rituximab in multirelapsing minimal change nephrotic syndrome in the adult: first case report and pathophysiological considerations. Am J Kid Dis. 2007;49:158–61.

Gilbert RD, Hulse E, Rigden S. Rituximab therapy for steroid-dependent minimal change nephrotic syndrome. Pediatr Nephrol. 2006;21:1698–700.

Jones RB, Tervaert JWC, Hauser T, et al. Rituximab versus cyclophosphamide in ANCA-associated renal vasculitis. N Engl J Med. 2010;363:211–20.

Salama AD, Pusey CD. Drug insight: rituximab in renal disease and transplantation. Nat Clin Pract Nephrol. 2006;2:221–30

30. A 64-year-old Caucasian woman presents to her primary care physician for severe headache. Her BP is found to be 180/100 mm Hg. Physical exam is normal except for trace edema. A urinalysis reveals hematuria, 3+ proteinuria, and RBC casts. Serum creatinine is 2.8 mg/dL and BUN 60 mg/dL. She is referred to a nephrologist. Kidney biopsy (Fig. 2.2) shows:

- LM (Left): mesangial cell proliferation with lobular pattern. Congo red stain negative
- EM (Right): randomly arranged fibrils ranging from 15 to 30 nm in diameter distributed throughout the glomerulus
- IF: prominent, but sludgy IgG and C3, k and l light chains in mesangial areas

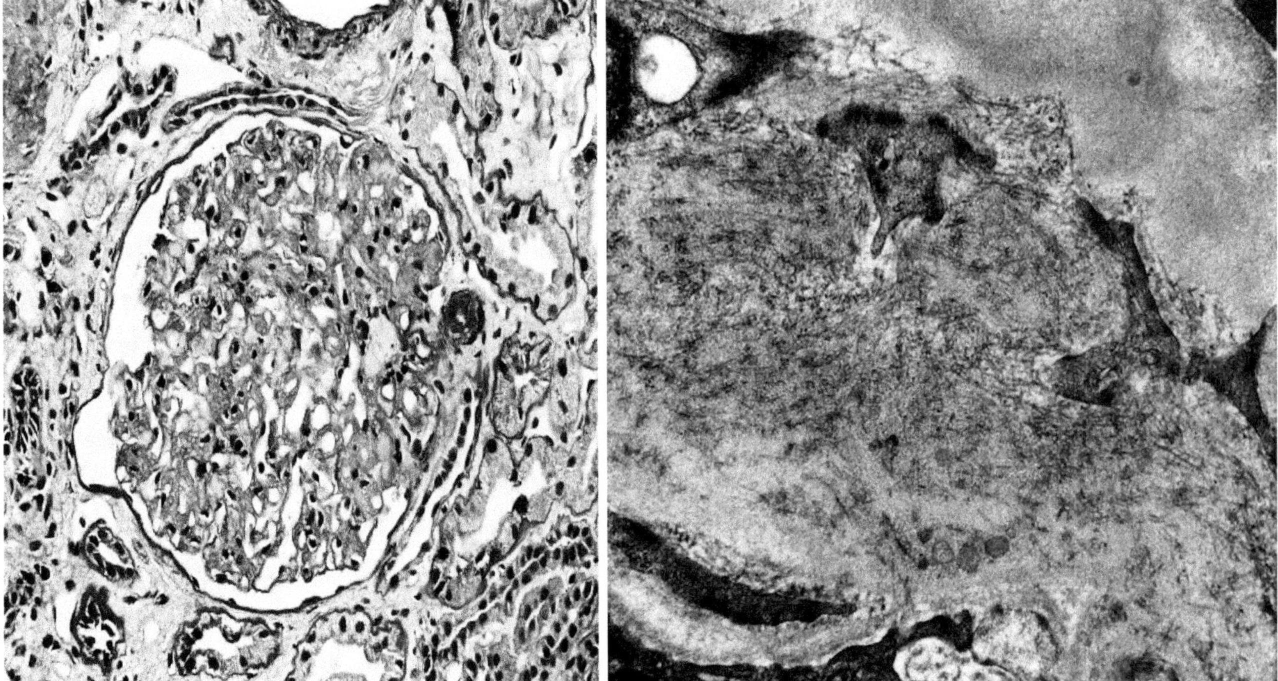

Fig. 2.2 Light (left) and electron (right) photomicrographs of the patient described above

Based on the above information, which one of the following is the MOST likely diagnosis?

A. Membranoproliferative glomerulonephritis (MPGN)- type I
B. Lupus nephritis (Class III)
C. Monoclonal immunoglobulin deposit disease
D. Immunotactoid glomerulopathy
E. Fibrillary glomerulonephritis (GN)

The answer is E

Based upon the size of the fibrils, the patient has fibrillary GN rather than immunotactoid glomerulopathy. Light microscopic findings may not distinguish fibrillary GN from other glomerular diseases, as mentioned in options from A to D, because fibrillary GN is pleomorphic and presents as lobular glomerulopathy as type 1 MPGN, membranous or crescentic GN. The definitive diagnosis of fibrillary GN is usually made by electron microscopy, which shows nonbranching fibrils ranging from 15 to 25 nm in diameter, as opposed to immunotactoid glomerulopathy that demonstrates fibrils with >30 nm in diameter. Furthermore, immunotactoid glomerulopathy is found in association with lymphoproliferative diseases. There is no known effective therapy for fibrillary GN, although steroids alone or in combination with cyclophosphamide or rituximab have been used with variable success. Kidney transplantation is a viable option, but recurrence of the disease is common. Lupus nephritis and monoclonal immunoglobulin deposit disease do not demonstrate fibrils on EM.

Suggested Reading

Andeen NK, Troxell Ml, Riazy M, et al. Fibrillary glomerulonephritis. Clinicopathologic features and atypical cases from a multi-institutional cohort. Clin J Am Soc Nephrol. 2019;14:1741–50.
Nasr SH, Fogo AB. New developments in the diagnosis of fibrillary glomerulonephritis. Kidney Int. 2019;96:581–92.
Rosenstock JL, Markowitz GS. Fibrillary glomerulonephritis: an update. Kidney Int Rep. 2019;4:917–22.

31. A 15-year-old female was brought to the physician by her parents for loss of fat in the upper part of the body, rapid growth (5′ 11″ tall), muscular hypertrophy, subcutaneous nodules, and macroglossia. Urinalysis showed proteinuria and hematuria. A spot urine protein to creatinine ratio was 3.2. C4 was normal, but C3 was very low. Serum creatinine was 1.4 mg/dL. A kidney biopsy showed the following:

    - LM (Fig. 2.3a): endocapillary proliferation with thickened glomerular basement membranes (GBM). The involved portions of the GBM resemble a "string of sausages"
    - EM (Fig. 2.3b): dense deposits in the basement membrane, Bowman capsule, and tubules
    - IF (Fig. 2.3c): Strong irregular C3 staining along the capillary wall. Immunoglobulins absent

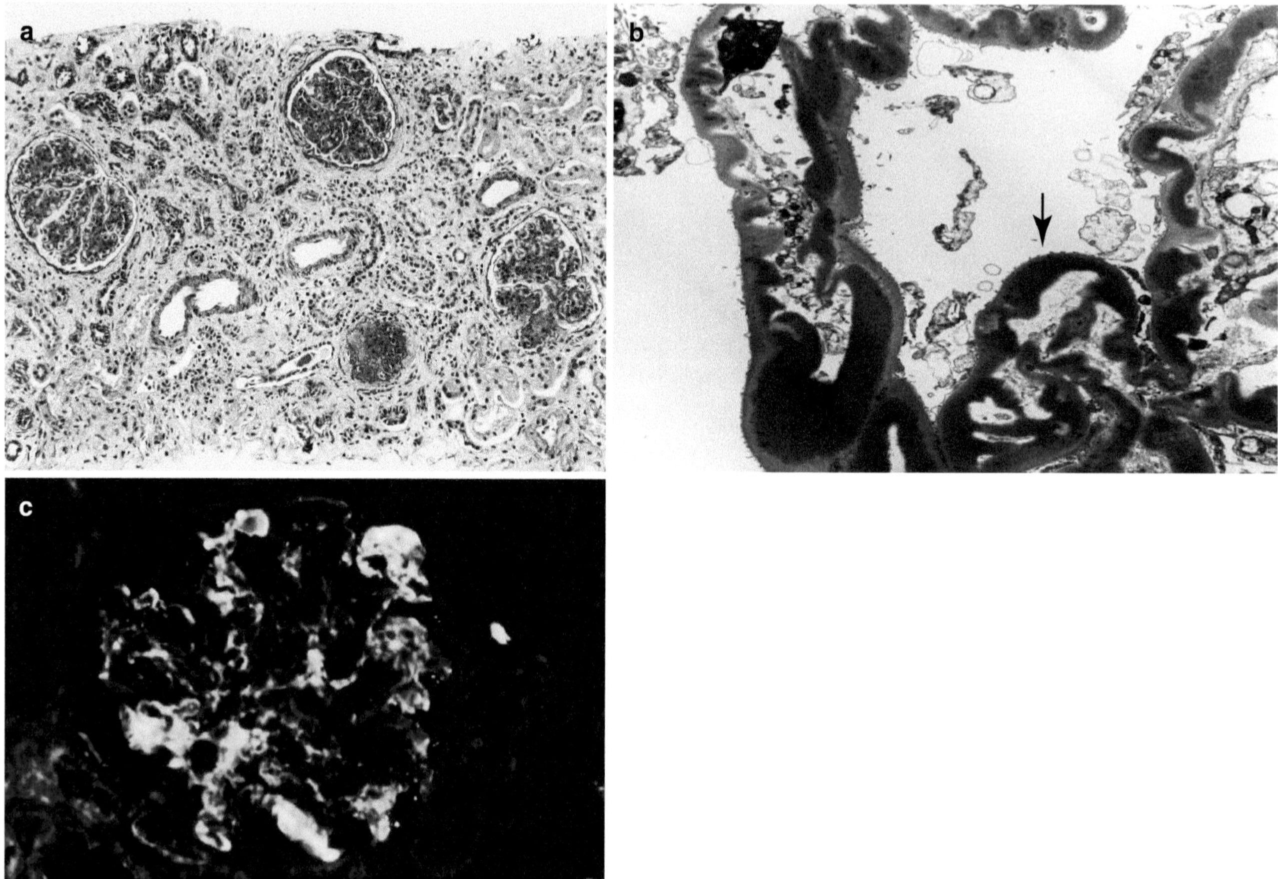

Fig. 2.3 (**a**) Pattern of glomerular injury observed by light microscopy. (**b**) Electron micrograph (EM) showing dense appearance of the GBM (arrow). (**c**) Immunofluorescence (IF) staining pattern (irregular) of C3

The clinical presentation and kidney pathology findings are MOST consistent with which one of the following diagnoses?

A. Lupus nephritis (Class IV)
B. C3 glomerulonephritis
C. Dense deposit disease
D. Amyloidosis
E. C1q nephropathy

The answer is C

C3 glomerulopathy is a term that comprises two diseases: (1) C3 glomerulonephritis (C3 GN) and (2) dense deposit disease (DDD). C3 GN was formerly called membranoproliferative GN I and III (MPGN 1 and III), and DDD was called MPGN II. The term C3 glomerulopathy was introduced in 2012 based on the pathogenic mechanism that involves dysregulation of alternative pathway of complement with excessive deposition of C3 without immune complexes in the glomerular basement membrane and mesangium.

The patient described in the question has partial lipodystrophy (PLD), which is most commonly seen in girls between 5 and 15 years of age. The most common kidney disease that is associated with PLD is dense deposit disease (DDD). Therefore, option C is correct. Renal disease occurs in 20–50% of patients with PLD, and PLD occurs in 10% of patients with DDD. Apart from kidney disease, patients with PLD, similar to total lipodystrophy patients, may have several metabolic and systemic abnormalities, including tall stature, muscular hypertrophy, subcutaneous nodules, macroglossia, hyperinsulinemia, insulin resistance, and diabetes.

The kidney biopsy findings with low C3 and normal C4 are consistent with DDD. Patients are noted to have asymptomatic proteinuria and microhematuria, but nephrotic syndrome is occasionally present. The pathogenesis of the acquired form of PLD is believed to be an autoimmune disorder. It has been reported that DDD or PLD or both are associated with dysfunction of the complement system. Subsequently, an IgG autoantibody was detected called the C3 nephritic factor (C3NeF). The target of this autoantibody is the alternative pathway C3 convertase C3bBb. Thus, diminished complement C3 levels in association with the C3NeF are the most prominent serologic abnormality in patients with DDD and PLD. The glomerular disease progresses rapidly to ESKD. Plasmapheresis has been shown to be beneficial in patients with C3NeF.

In C3 glomerulonephritis and lupus nephritis, both C4 and C3 are generally depressed, but the complement levels are normal in patients with amyloidosis and C1q nephropathy (D and E are incorrect).

Suggested Reading

Appel GB. C3 glomerulopathy: a new disease comes of age. Mayo Clin Proc. 2018;93:968–9.

Pickering MC, D'Agati VD, Nester CM, et al. C3 glomerulopathy: consensus report. Kidney Int. 2013;84:1079–89.

Schena FP, Esposito P, Rossini M. A narrative review on C3 glomerulopathy: a rare renal disease. Int J Mol Sci. 2020;21:525.

Sethi S, Fervenza FC. Membranoproliferative glomerulonephritis-a new look at an old entity. N Engl J Med. 2012;366:1119–31.

Smith RJ, Appel GB, Blom AM, et al. C3 glomerulopathy- understanding a rare complement-driven renal disease. Nat Rev Nephrol. 2019;15:129–43.

32. **Match the following disease states with the electron microscopy findings of the glomeruli.**

   1. Amyloidosis
   2. Immunotactoid glomerulopathy
   3. Fibrillary glomerulonephritis (GN)

      A. Microtubular structure with 30–50 nm in diameter (Fig. 2.4a)
      B. Randomly arranged fibrils with 15–30 nm in diameter (Fig.2.4b)
      C. Randomly arranged fibrils with 8–12 nm in diameter (Fig.2.4c)

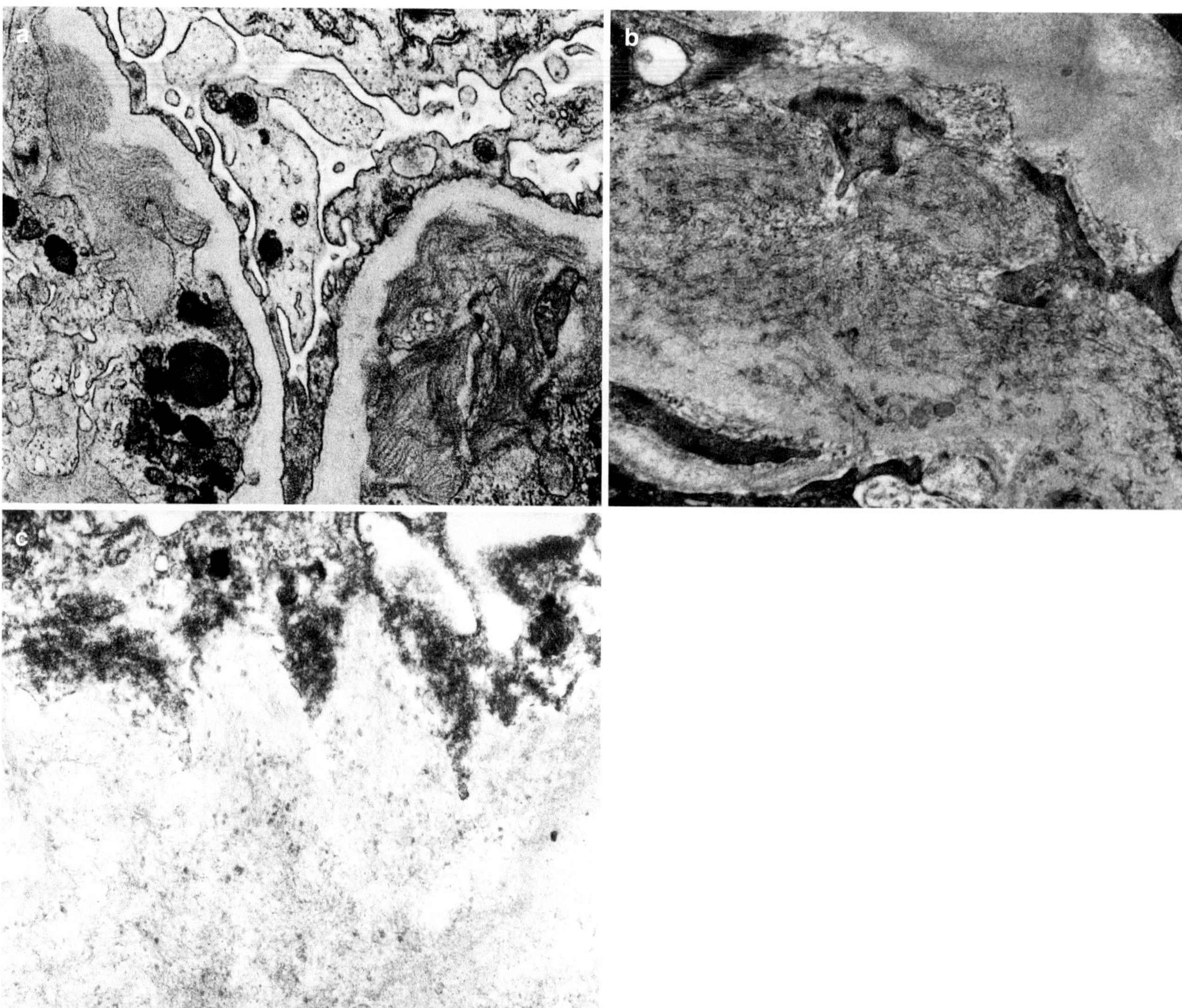

Fig. 2.4 EM micrographs showing fibrils with different widths

Answers: 1 = Fig. 2.4b; 2 = Fig. 2.4c; 3 = Fig. 2.4a

Light microscopy does not distinguish amyloidosis from either fibrillary or immunotactoid GN. All three diseases will give the appearance of nodules or lobules resembling diabetic glomerulosclerosis or membranoproliferative GN. However, these diseases can be distinguished by the size of the fibrils seen on electron microscopy. The fibrils in amyloidosis are randomly arranged and range from 8 to 12 nm in diameter (Fig. 2.4c), whereas in fibrillary or immunotactoid GN the diameters of the fibrils range from 15 to 30 nm (Fig. 2.4b) and 30 to 50 nm (Fig. 2.4a), respectively. In fibrillary GN, the fibrils are also randomly arranged as in amyloidosis, but they are larger. In immunotactoid GN, the fibrils appear as large microtubular deposits and are arranged in parallel arrays giving the appearance of a "stacked wood" arrangement (Fig. 2.4a).

Suggested Reading

Bonsib SM, editor. Atlas of medical renal pathology. New York: Springer; 2013. p. 1–266.
Fogo AB, Kashgarian M. Diagnostic atlas of renal pathology. 3rd ed. Philadelphia: Elsevier, Inc.; 2017. p. 1–546.

33. **Match the following LM pictures with the clinical presentations.**

A. A 56-year-old Caucasian man with isolated nephrotic syndrome
B. A 10-year-old boy with nephrotic syndrome

C. An 18-year-old woman with hematuria and proteinuria and low C3
D. A 19-year-old African American man with nephrotic syndrome

Answers: A = Fig. 2.5d, e; B = Fig. 2.5a; C = Fig. 2.5c; D = Fig. 2.5b

The frequent cause of isolated nephrotic syndrome in a 56-year-old Caucasian man is membranous nephropathy. The "spike and dome" appearances of the GBM shown in Fig. 2.5d, e are consistent with the presentation of the patient.

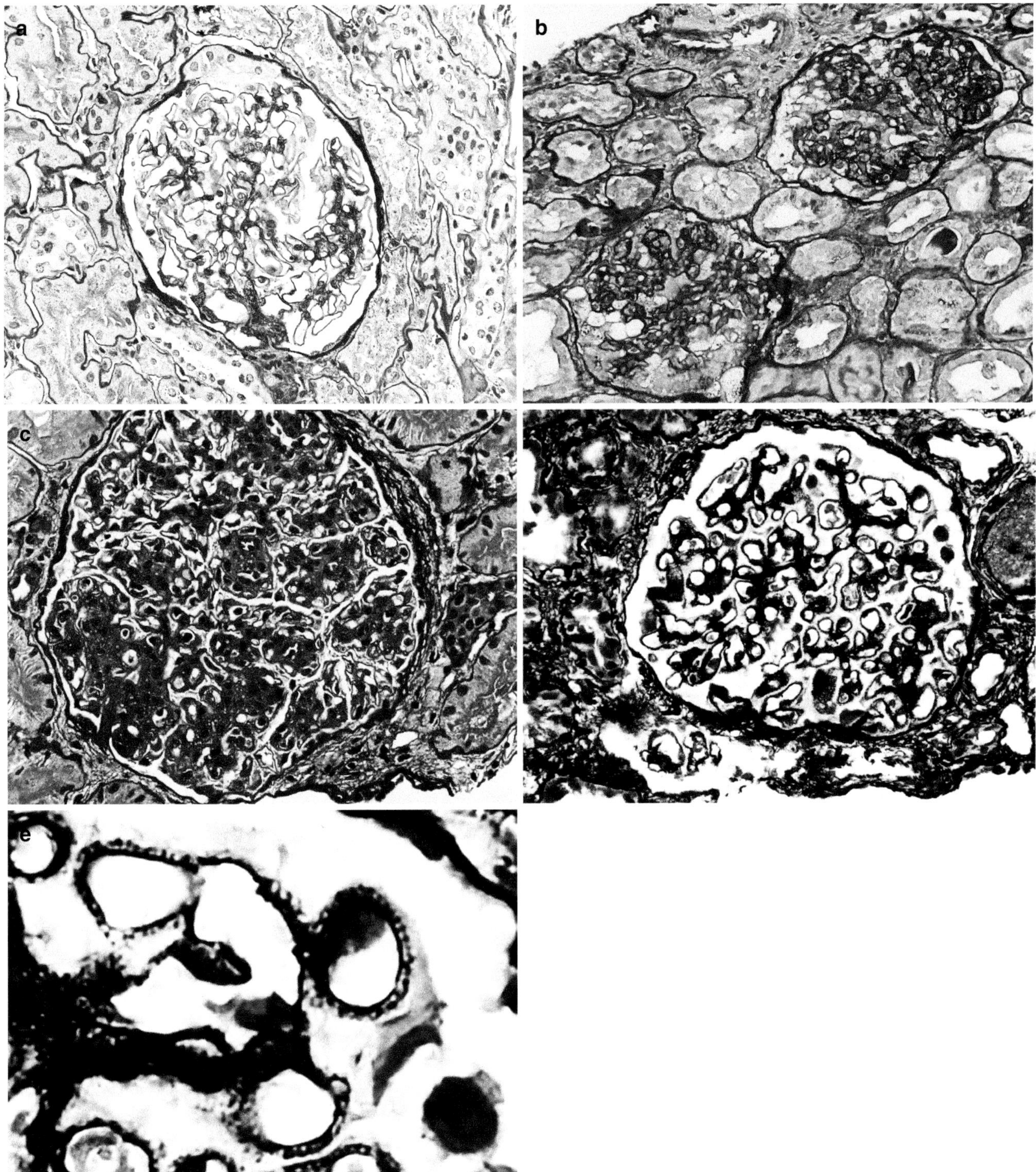

Fig. 2.5 Pattern of glomerular injury observed by light microscopy

The most common cause of nephrotic syndrome in children is minimal change disease, and the glomerulus appears normal on light microscopy. Figure 2.5a shows normal glomerular appearance, which is consistent with the description of the patient in choice B.

Figure 2.5c shows hypercellularity, mostly mesangial cells and infiltrating leukocytes and lobular appearance, consistent with C3 glomerulonephritis. Patients often have low C3 and total hemolytic complement (CH50). Thus, the description of Fig. 2.5c is consistent with the presentation of the patient given in choice C.

The most likely glomerular disease in the 19-year-old African American male with nephrotic syndrome is collapsing variant of FSGS, and Fig. 2.5b is consistent with this diagnosis.

Suggested Reading

Bonsib SM, editor. Atlas of medical renal pathology. New York: Springer; 2013. p. 1–266.
Fogo AB, Kashgarian M. Diagnostic atlas of renal pathology. 3rd ed. Philadelphia: Elsevier, Inc.; 2017. p. 1–546.

34. A 22-year-old African American woman with HIV disease presents to the Emergency Department with nausea, vomiting, hematuria, proteinuria, and swollen legs. She used heroin and cocaine 7 years ago. She got HIV transmission from a sexual contact. Pertinent labs include a creatinine level of 3.4 mg/dL and albumin concentration of 2.4 g/dL. ANA was weakly positive (titer <1:80). Antidouble-stranded DNA is negative. Serum complements are normal. A 24-h urine protein reveals 6.5 g. The kidneys are large on ultrasound. Kidney biopsy findings are

- LM: diffuse glomerulonephritis with endocapillary cell proliferation (Class IV)
- EM: mesangial and subendothelial electron-dense deposits with tubuloreticular inclusion bodies in endothelial cells
- IF: granular glomerular staining (>1+) for IgG, IgM, IgA, C3, C1q, κ and λ chains

The biopsy results suggest which one of the following glomerular findings?

A. Focal segmental glomerulosclerosis (FSGS) of collapsing variant
B. IgA nephropathy
C. Lupus-like glomerulonephritis (GN)
D. Immune complex GN other than lupus-like GN
E. Minimal change disease

The answer is C

HIV-associated glomerular diseases can be classified into podocytopathies and immune complex-mediated categories. Podocytopathies include classic HIV-associated nephropathy (HIVAN), FSGS not otherwise specified, and infrequently minimal change disease and diffuse mesangial hypercellularity. Classically, FSGS of collapsing variant is the most common glomerular lesion found in HIV patients. IF staining is usually absent. This classic lesion is generally referred to HIVAN.

The HIV-associated immune complex kidney disease once referred to as HIVICK may occur in various forms: (1) diffuse proliferative GN (postinfectious GN) or lupus-like disease, (2) IgA nephropathy, (3) membranous nephropathy, and (4) cryoglobulinemic GN. The common histologic features of these four glomerular diseases are the presence of mesangial and glomerular basement membrane immune complexes associated with HIV antigens. Instead of HIVICK, the 2018 KDIGO guideline recommends specific description of the immune complex disease in the context of HIV disease because other causes of these immune complex diseases should be ruled out with appropriate tests.

The findings described in the patient are consistent with lupus-like GN rather than other glomerular diseases. Haas et al. reported 14 HIV patients with lupus-like GN (Class IV), characterized by a "full house" pattern of immunoglobulin and complement deposition in glomeruli. However, these patients had no strong serology for lupus. However, some patients had weakly positive (titer <1:80) ANA titers, but no antidouble-stranded DNA. Thus, lupus-like GN with immunohistologic features without serologic markers of lupus is another glomerular disease associated with HIV/AIDS patients.

Most of these patients have long-standing (>10 years) HIV viremia. Clinical features include hematuria, proteinuria, hypertension, and decreased renal function. Renal outcome is poor in these patients.

Suggested Reading

Booth JW, Hamzah L, Jose S, et al. Clinical characteristics and outcomes of HIV-associated immune complex kidney disease. Nephrol Dial Transplant. 2016;31:2099–107.

Cohen AH, Nast CC. Renal injury associated with human immunodeficiency virus infection. In: Jennette JC, Olson JL, Schwartz MM, Silva FG, editors. Heptinstall's pathology of the kidney. 6th ed. Philadelphia: Lippincott Williams & Wilkins; 2006. p. 397–422.
Haas M, Kaul S, Eustace JA. HIV-associated immune complex glomerulonephritis with "lupus-like" features. A clinicopathologic study of 14 cases. Kidney Int. 2005;67:1381–90.
Swanepoel CR, Atta MG, D'Agati VD, et al. Kidney disease in the setting of HIV infection: conclusions from a Kidney Disease: Improving Global Outcomes (KDIGO) Controversies Conference. Kidney Int. 2018;93:545–59.

35. **Regarding the treatment of HIV-associated nephropathy (HIVAN), which one of the following statements is INCORRECT?**

A. Antiretroviral therapy is effective in improving kidney function and proteinuria
B. Antiretroviral therapy reduces the rate of progression of kidney disease to ESKD by a significant percentage
C. Improvement in kidney function with antiretroviral therapy correlates with the reversal of histologic changes of HIVAN
D. Antiretroviral therapy continues to have beneficial effects on kidney function even after its discontinuation
E. ACE-Is and ARBs reduce proteinuria and improve kidney survival

The answer is D

The treatment and prevention of HIVAN are based on the premise that the glomerular lesions are caused by active viral infection of the kidney. Therefore, antiretroviral therapy is considered the major therapeutic modality for HIVAN. It was shown that treatment with antiretroviral agents immediately after diagnosis of HIVAN is effective in improving kidney function and proteinuria and reducing the progression of kidney disease to ESKD by 38%. It has also been shown that the observed improvement in GFR by antiretroviral agents correlates with an improvement in histologic changes of the kidney. Loss of podocyte markers such as synaptopodin was reacquired the following antiretroviral therapy. Conservative management of proteinuria with inhibition of renin-angiotensin system has been found to be effective in reducing proteinuria and prolonging kidney survival in patients with HIVAN. Thus, ACE-Is and ARBs are found to be add-on drugs for treatment of HIVAN.

Once antiretroviral therapy is discontinued, kidney lesions progress at an accelerated rate. Therefore, continuation of antiretroviral therapy is indicated to improve both kidney function and proteinuria in HIVAN. Thus, option D is incorrect.

Studies have shown that atazanavir and lopinavir/ritonavir are associated with rapid decline in eGFR in incident CKD patients. Switching from ritonavir-boosted atazanavir or lopinavir to boosted darunavir has been associated with improved kidney function.

Suggested Reading

Hughes K, Jerry Chang J, Stadtler H, et al. HIV-1 infection of the kidney: mechanisms and implications. AIDS. 2021;35:359–67.
Kalayjian RC. The treatment of HIV-associated nephropathy. Adv Chronic Kidney Dis. 2010;17:59–71.
Swanepoel CR, Atta MG, D'Agati VD, et al. Kidney disease in the setting of HIV infection: conclusions from a Kidney Disease: Improving Global Outcomes (KDIGO) Controversies Conference. Kidney Int. 2018;93:545–59.

36. Nephrotoxicity is one of the serious side effects of antiretroviral therapy. **Which one of the following statements regarding the mechanisms of renal injury is FALSE?**

A. Increase in intracellular concentration of antiretroviral drugs through human organic anion transporter1-controlled mechanisms in the tubule
B. Apoptosis (programmed cell death) via the mitogen-activated protein kinase (MAPK) pathway
C. Mitochondrial damage disrupting fatty acid oxidation and energy production
D. Crystal deposition and vascular injury
E. Decreased renal blood flow and glomerular hypertension

The answer is E

Antiviral drug-induced nephrotoxicity is a major problem in HIV/AIDS patients. The mechanisms by which these drugs cause nephrotoxicity are (1) transport defects, (2) apoptosis, (3) mitochondrial injury, and (4) crystal deposition and vascular injury.

Basically, human organic anion transporter1 (hOAT1), human organic cation transporter1 (hOCT1), and multidrug resistance-associated protein type 2 (MRP2) controlled mechanisms mediate renal tubular uptake and excretion of antiviral drugs. When these mechanisms are defective, the intracellular concentration of some antiviral drugs increases, causing tubular dysfunction. Acyclic nucleotide phosphonates (cidofovir and adefovir) toxicity is due to transport defects.

Apoptosis (programmed cell death) can occur in concert with immune-mediated injury via activation of the MAPK pathway, resulting in barrier dysfunction in renal epithelial cells. Interferon causes renal dysfunction through this pathway.

Drugs such as nucleoside reverse transcriptase inhibitors (zidovudine, didanosine, stavudine) enter mitochondria by cellular diffusion and/or transport mechanisms and disturb respiratory-chain enzymes or mitochondrial DNA. This results in oxidative stress with ensuing anaerobic metabolism, lactic acidosis, decreased energy production, and triglyceride accumulation (microvascular fat within cells). Drugs such as acyclovir or indinavir can form crystals in renal tubules and cause AKI by intratubular obstruction. Interferon and valacyclovir have been shown to cause thrombotic microangiopathies. Changes in renal hemodynamics such as decreased renal blood flow and glomerular hypertension have not been studied in patients on antiviral drugs. Therefore, option E is incorrect.

Suggested Reading

Berns JS, Kasbekar N. Highly active antiretroviral therapy and the kidney: an update on antiretroviral medications for nephrologists. Clin J Am Soc Nephrol. 2006;1:117–29.

Daugas E, Rougier J-P, Hill G. HAART-related nephropathies in HIV-infected patients. Kidney Int. 2005;67:393–403.

Izzedine H, Launay-Vacher V, Deray D. Antiviral drug-induced nephrotoxicity. Am J Kidney Dis. 2005;45:804–17.

Jao J, Wyatt CM. Antiretroviral medications: adverse effects. Adv Chronic Kidney Dis. 2010;17:72–82.

37. A 30-year-old man with HIV-associated nephropathy (HIVAN) is on maintenance hemodialysis. **Which one of the following drugs needs dose reduction in the patient?**

   A. Norvir (Ritonavir, a protease inhibitor)
   B. Viread (Tenofovir, a nucleotide reverse transcriptase inhibitor)
   C. Sustiva (Efavirenz, a non-nucleotide reverse transcriptase inhibitor)
   D. Fugeon (Enfuvirtide, an entry fusion inhibitor)
   E. None of the above

The answer is B

Except for viread (tenofovir), the other drugs do not require any dose adjustments in patients with CKD or on dialysis. Nucleoside/nucleotide, reverse transcriptase inhibitors primarily undergo kidney elimination, and the other categories of drugs are metabolized in the liver. Detailed pharmacokinetic studies, however, for fugeon have not been done in patients with low GFR, but dose adjustment is not necessary.

Suggested Reading

Berns JS, Kasbekar N. Highly active antiretroviral therapy and the kidney: an update on Semustine antiretroviral medications for nephrologists. Clin J Am Soc Nephrol. 2006;1:117–29.

Daugas E, Rougier J-P, Hill G. HAART-related nephropathies in HIV-infected patients. Kidney Int. 2005;67:393–403.

Izzedine H, Launay-Vacher V, Deray D. Antiviral drug-induced nephrotoxicity. Am J Kidney Dis. 2005;45:804–17.

38. **Match the following chemotherapeutic drugs with the reported kidney toxicity.**

   A. Semustine
   B. Cisplatin
   C. Mitomycin C
   D. Cyclophosphamide
   E. Interleukin-2
   F. Adriamycin

      1. Acute kidney injury (AKI) and tubulointerstitial (TID) disease
      2. Hemolytic uremic syndrome (HUS)
      3. Chronic kidney disease 3 years after therapy

4. AKI with high dose
5. Hyponatremia and hemorrhagic cystitis
6. Collapsing glomerulopathy

Answers: A = 3; B = 1; C = 2; D = 5; E = 4; F = 6

Semustine is a nitrosourea compound that crosses the blood-brain barrier easily and is therefore used in malignant brain tumors. High-dose (1500 mg/m²) therapy in children has been shown to cause CKD 3–5 years after completion of the treatment.

Cisplatin is an effective chemotherapeutic agent that has been used to treat many tumors, including bladder cancer. Nephrotoxicity is a troublesome complication of cisplatin, which is dose dependent. TID with heavy proteinuria is commonly observed with hyaline droplets in the proximal tubular cells, tubular necrosis, and degeneration of tubular BM. Tubular defect results in magnesium and phosphate wasting and AKI. Concomitant use of other nephrotoxins can potentiate cisplatin nephrotoxicity. Hydration with brisk diuresis and administration of sodium thiosulfate have been shown to reduce cisplatin-induced nephrotoxicity.

Mitomycin C is used in combination with 5-fluorouracil in treatment of gastrointestinal carcinoma. High doses of mitomycin C (>60 mg/m²) have been shown to cause HUS.

Cyclophosphamide is active against lymphomas and hematologic malignancies. It causes hyponatremia due to its antidiuretic effect in the distal nephron without causing an increase in ADH levels. Also, cyclophosphamide causes hemorrhagic cystitis.

Interleukin-2, which has a killer cell function, causes AKI in high doses. It reduces GFR by renal vasoconstriction. Adriamycin use is associated with the development of proteinuria and also collapsing glomerulopathy.

Suggested Reading

Palmer BF, Henrich WL. Toxic nephropathy. In: Brenner BM, editor. Brenner & Rector's the kidney. 7th ed. Philadelphia: Saunders; 2004. p. 1625–58.

Safirstein RL. Renal diseases induced by antineoplastic agents. In: Schrier, editor. Diseases of the kidney & urinary tract. 8th ed. Philadelphia: Lippincott Williams & Wilkins; 2007. p. 1068–81.

39. **Match the following drugs with the reported nephrotoxicity.**

A. Acyclovir
B. Foscarnet
C. Indinavir
D. Adefovir
E. Pentamidine

1. Hypocalcemia, hypomagnesemia, and hyperkalemia with prolonged therapy
2. Hypocalcemia, hyperphosphatemia, and increased serum PTH levels
3. AKI due to intratubular precipitation of needle-shaped crystals
4. Crystalluria and nephrolithiasis
5. Proximal tubular injury, low-grade proteinuria, and an increase in serum creatinine level

Answers: A = 3; B = 2; C = 4; D = 5; E = 1

Acyclovir is an antiviral agent, which is excreted by the kidney. It causes AKI by intratubular precipitation of acyclovir crystals. Urinalysis shows needle-shaped crystals under polarizing light. Volume depletion precipitates ARF.

Foscarnet is used to treat CMV infection in transplant patients and is excreted by the kidney. It causes AKI, hypocalcemia, hyperphosphatemia, and elevated PTH levels. Hydration with normal saline reduces nephrotoxicity.

Indinavir is a protease inhibitor that causes crystalluria and nephrolithiasis due to precipitation of the drugs in renal tubules. Long-term use of the drug includes interstitial inflammation, granuloma formation, interstitial fibrosis, and finally renal failure.

Adefovir is a nucleoside inhibitor that causes proximal tubular injury, resulting in phosphaturia, proteinuria, and AKI due to mitochondrial toxicity. It is excreted by the kidney.

Pentamidine is clinically used to treat pneumocystis carinii pneumonia. Frequent doses accumulate in the kidney and cause tubular injury. Hypocalcemia, hypomagnesemia, and hyperkalemia have been reported with prolonged therapy.

Suggested Reading

Izzedine H, Launay-Vacher V, Deray D. Antiviral drug-induced nephrotoxicity. Am J Kidney Dis. 2005;45:804–17.
Palmer BF, Henrich WL. Toxic nephropathy. In: Brenner BM, editor. Brenner & Rector's the kidney. 7th ed. Philadelphia: Saunders; 2004. p. 1625–58.

40. **Match the following clinical histories with the LM figures of the kidney.**

A. A 65-year-old man with nephrotic syndrome, hematuria, and hypertension. Glomerulus with multiple nodules and these nodules are PAS-positive, but silver stain-negative. Hypocomplementemic and hepatitis C-positive
B. A 70-year-old man with hematologic malignancy and deposits with microtubular fibrils >30 nm in diameter on EM
C. A 22-year-old woman with hematuria, hypertension, and low complement levels 2 weeks following an upper respiratory tract infection
D. A 20-year-old woman with hematuria, proteinuria, and normal complement levels 2 days following an upper respiratory infection

Answers: A = Fig. 2.6c; B = Fig. 2.6b; C = Fig. 2.6d; D = Fig. 2.6a

The diagnosis in the 65-year-old man (choice A) with nephrotic syndrome, hematuria, hypertension, hypocomplementemia, and hepatitis C with glomerular nodules on kidney biopsy seems to have monoclonal immunoglobulin deposition disease, which comprises light, heavy, and light-and-heavy chains. Although the clinical and pathologic characteristics are similar in all three diseases, hypocomplementemia and false-positive hepatitis C antibody are characteristics of heavy-chain deposition disease (HCDD). Thus, Fig. 2.6c is consistent with HCDD.

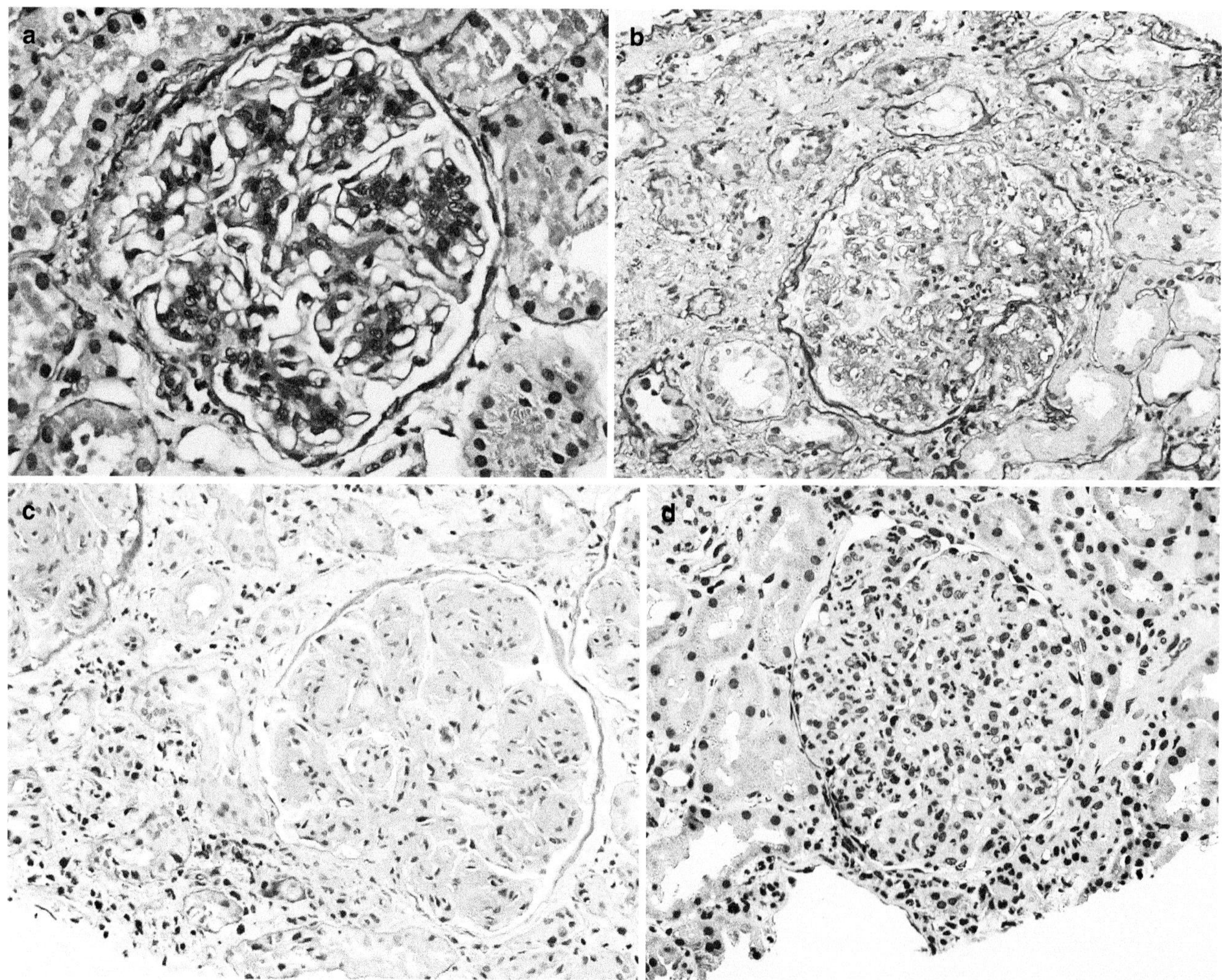

Fig. 2.6 Pattern of glomerular injury observed by light microscopy

The patient described in choice B seems to have immunotactoid glomerulopathy. Kidney biopsy in patients with immunotactoid glomerulopathy shows either membranous nephropathy or MPGN type 1. Thus, light microscopy of the glomerulus shows lobular pattern with nodule-like appearance in some patients. Generally, the nodules are silver stain negative. Figure 2.6b is consistent with immunotactoid glomerulopathy.

The clinical features of the patient in choice C are consistent with acute poststreptococcal glomerulonephritis, and the glomerular findings shown in Fig. 2.6d are consistent with this diagnosis. The glomerular lesions are characterized by diffuse endocapillary (mesangial and endothelial) hypercellularity and infiltration of leukocytes. IF microscopy shows the deposition of C3, IgG, IgM, and properdin in glomerular capillary loops and mesangium.

Figure 2.6a, by process of elimination, is compatible with the description of the patient given in choice D. This patient carries the diagnosis of IgA nephropathy. The earliest light microscopy expression of IgA nephropathy is either focal or diffuse mesangial hypercellularity and in some cases endothelial hypercellularity. Figure 2.6a shows segmental mesangial cell hypercellularity with deposition of mesangial matrix. Influx of leukocytes is also seen in some patients. The glomerular lesions are similar to those seen in class II lupus nephritis.

Suggested Reading

Bonsib SM, editor. Atlas of medical renal pathology. New York: Springer; 2013. p. 1–266.
Fogo AB, Kashgarian M. Diagnostic atlas of renal pathology. 3rd ed. Philadelphia: Elsevier, Inc.; 2017. p. 1–546.

41. An 82-year-old obese Caucasian woman with history of hypertension and proteinuria of 1.5 g/day. She is on ACE-I and a β-blocker. Her glycated HbA1c is 6%, and not on any oral hypoglycemic medications. You are asked to see the patient for an increase in proteinuria to 4.6 g/day. Urinalysis is positive for albumin without RBCs or WBCs. **Which one of the following diagnoses is LEAST likely on a kidney biopsy?**

A. Membranous nephropathy
B. Amyloidosis
C. Minimal change disease
D. Focal segmental glomerulosclerosis (FSGS)
E. Fibrillary glomerulonephritis (GN)

The answer is E

Studies on kidney biopsy in the very elderly (≥80 years) are sparse. Kidney abnormalities in the elderly have been attributed to aging, hypertension, and other conditions. Nair et al. identified, in a retrospective analysis, 100 patients aged 80 years or older with kidney biopsies for various reasons. Crescentic GN was the most common glomerular lesion, and membranous nephropathy accounted for only 15%. Of the 100 biopsies, 40 of them showed a kidney condition that would benefit from therapeutic intervention, and the remaining biopsies provided useful information that can prevent harmful intervention. Thus, a kidney biopsy in the very elderly is needed for the diagnostic, prognostic, and therapeutic purposes.

Moutzouris et al. performed an analysis of another retrospective kidney biopsy study in 235 elderly (≥80 years) patients, and the results were compared to a control group of 264 patients aged between 60 and 61 years. The indications for biopsy were AKI, chronic progressive kidney disease, nephrotic syndrome, nephrotic syndrome with AKI, and isolated proteinuria. The most common diagnoses are shown in Table 2.3.

Table 2.3 Kidney biopsy findings in the very elderly with various indications for biopsy

Disease	Percent
Pauci-immune GN	19
Hypertensive nephrosclerosis	7.1
FSGS secondary to hypertension and aging	7.6
IgA nephropathy	7.1
Membranous nephropathy	7.1
Amyloidosis	5
Minimal change disease	5
Myeloma cast nephropathy	5

Interestingly, kidney biopsies done in patients with nephrotic syndrome alone had different diagnoses (Table 2.4).

Table 2.4 Kidney biopsy findings in the very elderly with nephrotic syndrome

Disease	Percent
Membranous nephropathy	22
Amyloidosis	18
Minimal change disease	16
IgA nephropathy	6
Pauci-immune GN	4
Membranoproliferative GN	4
Diabetic glomerulosclerosis	4
FSGS (primary)	4

Overall, the kidney biopsy study in the very elderly provided diagnostic information that modified the treatment in 67% of those patients with AKI and nephrotic syndrome. Thus, kidney biopsy should be done in the very elderly, if indicated.

In the study of Uezono et al., the elderly (65 years and older) had FSGS (23%), minimal change disease (19%), and membranous nephropathy (15%) as the primary diagnosis for their nephrotic syndrome. Also, 71% of the elderly who presented with AKI had MPO-ANCA-positive crescentic GN on kidney biopsy.

Fibrillary GN in the very elderly is unlikely because the median age is around 50 years. Thus, option is incorrect.

Suggested Reading

Moutzouris D-A, Herlitz L, Appel GB, et al. Renal biopsy in the very elderly. Clin J Am Soc Nephrol. 2009;4:1073–82.
Nair R, Bell JM, Walker PD. Renal biopsy in patients aged 80 years and older. Am J Kidney Dis. 2004;44:618–26.
Uezono S, Hara S, Sato Y, et al. Renal biopsy in elderly patients: a clinicopathological analysis. Ren Fail. 2006;28:549–55.

42. A 56-year-old Caucasian man with type 2 diabetes, proteinuria (2 g/day), eGFR of 54 mL/min, and blood pressure (BP) of 136/84 mm Hg sees you in your office for evaluation of his medications and advice for management of his kidney disease. His medications include hydrochlorothiazide (HCTZ) (12.5 mg), diltiazem CD (240 mg), losartan (100 mg), and atorvastatin (40 mg). **Keeping evidence-based practice in mind, which one of the following changes you would make to reduce proteinuria in this patient?**

A. Discontinue diltiazem CD and start Nifedipine XL 60 mg to improve BP
B. Continue the current antihypertensives and advice the patient to consume 8 g of NaCl in the diet
C. Continue HCTZ and diltiazem CD but switch from losartan to telmisartan (80 mg/day)
D. Substitute chlorthalidone for HCTZ and continue other medications
E. Re-evaluate medications in 1 year

The answer is C

Several studies have shown beneficial effects of ACE-Is or angiotensin-receptor blockers (ARBs) in reducing proteinuria in both type 1 and type 2 diabetic patients. Also, thiazide diuretics (HCTZ or chlorthalidone) and nondihydropyridine calcium blockers (long-acting diltiazem or verapamil) were found to be beneficial in type 2 diabetic patients with proteinuria.

A multicenter trial evaluated the superiority of telmisartan, an ARB, over another ARB, losartan in type 2 diabetic patients with a mean albumin:creatinine ratio of approximately 1400 mg/g, eGFR of 50 mL/min, and blood pressure >130/80 mm Hg. The primary endpoint was the difference in the urinary albumin to creatinine ratio between the groups at 52 weeks. Although the reduction in blood pressure was similar in both groups, the mean reduction in albuminuria was greater in the telmisartan than in the losartan group. Thus, this study found superiority over losartan in reducing albuminuria in type 2 diabetic patients with hypertension and CKD. Thus, evidence-based medicine suggests switching losartan to telmisartan.

Suggested Reading

Bakris G, Burgess E, Weir M, et al. on behalf of the AMADEO Study Investigators. Telmisartan is more effective than losartan in reducing proteinuria in patients with diabetic nephropathy. Kidney Int. 2008;74:364–9.

43. You are asked by a primary care physician to see a type 1 diabetic patient with albuminuria of 10 mg/day. He has been on enalapril 20 mg/day. His BP is 122/72 mm Hg. His glycated HbA1c is 7.5%. The primary care physician seeks your advice for change of enalapril to losartan 50 or 100 mg/day in view of clinical trials that showed a kidney benefit in type 2 diabetic patients. **In view of an important study, which one of the following suggestions do you recommend to the primary care physician?**

A. Switch enalapril to losartan
B. Continue enalapril
C. Add losartan to enalapril
D. Change enalapril to another ACE-I
E. Discontinue enalapril as BP is good

The answer is B

Several studies have shown that inhibition of renin-angiotensin-aldosterone system in type 1 and type 2 diabetic subjects by ACE-Is or ARBs is kidney-protective. Most of these studies have been done in patients with micro- (category A1 albuminuria; <30 mg/day) or moderate to severe albuminuria (categories A2-A3 albuminuria) with or without hypertension. However, studies in patients with normoalbuminuria (<30 mg/day) and normotension have been sparse. The study of Mauer et al. reported such a study in type 1 diabetic subjects. They conducted a multicenter, controlled trial of 285 normotensive and normoalbuminuric type 1 diabetic subjects. They were divided into three groups: One group received enalapril (20 mg daily), an ACE-I; the second group losartan (100 mg daily), an ARB; and the third group did not receive any medication and served as placebo. Both groups were followed for 5 years. The primary end point was a change in the fractional mesangial volume per glomerulus over a 5-year period in kidney biopsy specimens done before and after the study. Also, progression of retinopathy was evaluated. The results showed that the mesangial fractional volume per glomerulus did not differ significantly between the placebo and treated groups. However, albuminuria increased in the losartan group but not in the enalapril group as compared with the placebo group. However, the progression of retinopathy was reduced in the treated groups as compared with the placebo group. Thus, early blockade of the renin-angiotensin-aldosterone system in type 1 diabetic subjects did not slow nephropathy progression but slowed the progression of retinopathy.

From the above discussion, it appears that continuation of enalapril is appropriate in the patient (option B is correct), and other options are incorrect. The combination of ACE-I and ARB is not suggested at this time in view of a large trial, using a combination of ramipril and telmisartan (the ONTARGET study).

Suggested Reading

Mann JFE, Schmieder RE, McQueen M, et al. Renal outcomes with telmisartan, ramipril, or both, in people at high vascular risk (the ONTARGET study): a multicentre, randomized, double-blind, controlled trial. Lancet. 2008;372:547–53.

Mauer M, Zinman B, Gardiner R, et al. Renal and retinal effects of enalapril and losartan in type 1 diabetes. N Engl J Med. 2009;361:40–51.

44. A 48-year-old man with recently diagnosed type 2 diabetes sees his primary care physician for new-onset lower extremity edema. His medications include glipizide 5 mg, lisinopril 20 mg, and HCTZ 12.5 mg. He has no retinopathy. Lungs are clear. There is no S_3. Lower extremities show 3+ edema. HbA1c is 7%. He is referred to you for a kidney biopsy. **Which one of the following is NOT an indication for kidney biopsy in a diabetic patient?**

A. Proteinuria or nephrotic syndrome of sudden onset, appearing less than 5–10 years of type I diabetes
B. Proteinuria and/or impaired renal function in the presence of retinopathy mostly in type 1 diabetes
C. Proteinuria associated with a nephritic syndrome characterized by micro- or macrohematuria, renal insufficiency with RBC casts in types 1 and 2 diabetes
D. Unexplained kidney failure with or without proteinuria
E. Presence of a systemic disease with abnormal serologic findings and clinical renal disease

The answer is B

Occasionally, patients with established diabetes present with dipstick positive or heavy proteinuria that is not expected for the duration or control of hyperglycemia. Also, unexpected deterioration in kidney function is seen. Such atypical presentation is more common in type 2 diabetic than type 1 diabetic patients. These patients require a thorough clinical workup of proteinuria. Such patients usually undergo a kidney biopsy to establish diabetic kidney disease (DKD) and its various stages, but also to document existence of a nondiabetic kidney disease alone or superimposed on DKD. In addition to a definitive diagnosis, the histopathologic findings provide pertinent prognostic information as well as a direction for appropriate therapy and management. The indications for kidney biopsy are shown in Table 2.5.

Table 2.5 Indications for kidney biopsy in diabetic patients with kidney disease

1. Proteinuria or nephrotic syndrome of sudden onset, appearing less than 5–10 years of type I diabetes
2. Proteinuria and/or impaired kidney function in the absence of retinopathy in type 1 diabetes[a]
3. Proteinuria associated with a nephritic syndrome characterized by micro- or macrohematuria, renal insufficiency with RBC casts in types 1 and 2 diabetes
4. Unexplained kidney failure with or without proteinuria
5. Presence of a systemic disease with abnormal serologic findings and clinical kidney disease
6. Abnormal imaging studies such as ultrasonography and Doppler studies, after excluding reno-vascular disease
7. Absence of urologic disease or infection

[a]The prevalence of retinopathy is less predictable for diabetic kidney in type 2 diabetes

When kidney biopsies were performed in patients with atypical presentation, as shown in the table, a variety of nondiabetic kidney diseases were observed. Such kidney lesions were present either alone or superimposed on DKD, making management more difficult. The following glomerular lesions have been documented.

- Minimal change nephrotic syndrome/focal segmental glomerulosclerosis
- Membranous glomerulopathy
- Crescentic glomerulonephritis (GN)
- Postinfectious GN
- IgA nephropathy-primary/secondary
- Lupus nephritis
- HCV-associated GN
- Fibrillary GN
- Monoclonal immunoglobulin-mediated diseases
- Collapsing glomerulopathy

It is, therefore, suggested that the nephrologist should include nondiabetic kidney lesions in the differential diagnosis of abnormal proteinuria. It is believed that type 1 diabetic patients with retinopathy will have kidney disease, and kidney biopsy is usually not indicated. Thus, option B is correct.

Suggested Reading

Reddi AS. Pathology of the kidney in type 1 diabetes. In: Diabetic nephropathy: theory & practice. East Hanover: College Book Publishers, LLC; 2004. p. 109–29.

Seshan SV, Reddi AS. Albuminuria-proteinuria in diabetes mellitus. In: Lerma EV, Batuman V, editors. The kidney in diabetes. New York: Springer; 2014. p. 107–17.

45. **Which one of the following agents is MOST likely to cause the progression of kidney disease?**

A. Pirfenidone
B. Hepatocyte growth factor
C. Transforming growth factor-β1
D. ACE inhibitors
E. Relaxin

The answer is C

Several antifibrotic agents have been tried to prevent fibrosis in the kidney and thus progression of the kidney disease in both diabetic and nondiabetic individuals. These agents include pirfenidone, hepatocyte growth factor,

ACE inhibitors, and relaxin. Transforming growth factor-β1 (TGF-β1) is a cytokine that has been shown to cause fibrosis in the kidney, and anti-TGF-β1 treatment ameliorates kidney disease in animal models of diabetes.

Suggested Reading

Coppo R, Amore A. New perspectives in treatment of glomerulonephritis. Pediatr Nephrol. 2004;19:256–65.
Kania DS, Smith CT, Nash CL, et al. Potential new treatments for diabetic kidney disease. Med Clin N Am. 2013;97:115–34.
Klinkhammer BM, Goldschmeding R, Floege J, et al. Treatment of renal fibrosis—turning challenges into opportunities. Adv Chronic Kidney Dis. 2017;24:117–29.
Mathew A, Cunard R, Sharma K. Antifibrotic treatment and other new strategies for improving renal outcomes. Contrib Nephrol. 2011;170: 217–27.
Negri AL. Prevention of progressive fibrosis in chronic renal diseases: antifibrotic agents. J Nephrol. 2004;17:496–503.
Samuel CS, Hewitson TD. Relaxin in cardiovascular and renal disease. Kidney Int. 2006;69:1498–502.
Shihab FS. Do we have a pill for renal fibrosis? Clin J Amer Soc Nephrol. 2007;2:876–8.

46. A 48-year-old woman with long-standing type 2 diabetes is referred to a nephrologist for evaluation of CKD (eGFR 58 mL/min), hematuria, and chronic flank pain. On history, she had frequent UTIs with E. coli infection and an episode of decreased urine output secondary to urinary tract obstruction. The patient is not ill and has no dysuria. A kidney biopsy shows macrophages with abundant, foamy, and multinucleated giant cells with owl eye appearance and positive PAS staining. **The history and kidney biopsy findings are MOST consistent with which of the following diagnoses?**

A. Acute pyelonephritis
B. Xanthogranulomatous pyelonephritis
C. Malakoplakia
D. Active renal tuberculosis (TB)
E. Diabetic nephropathy

The answer is C

Acute pyelonephritis presents with nausea, vomiting, fever, flank or colicky pain, dysuria, and frequent urination. Generally, patients are volume depleted with low BP and always ill-looking. The patient presented in the case is not ill and did not present with any one of the above clinical manifestations. Therefore, option A is incorrect.

The diagnosis of xanthogranulomatous pyelonephritis is a good possibility; however, the kidney biopsy findings are not consistent with this disease. Also, the renal pathology is not consistent with diabetic nephropathy.

Renal TB is the most common extrapulmonary TB, which remains clinically silent for many years with irreversible renal damage. Acutely, urogenital TB may present with dysuria, hematuria, flank pain, and pyuria. Unexplained sterile pyuria and hematuria in a clinically silent patient should prompt the clinician to consider renal TB in the differential diagnosis. Pathologic changes in the kidney include granulomatous inflammation with papillary necrosis. The patient presented in the case does not seem to carry the diagnosis of renal TB.

Based upon the history and kidney pathology, the patient carries the diagnosis of malakoplakia, which is a rare granulomatous disease with many clinical similarities to xanthogranulomatous pyelonephritis. Malakoplakia is common in middle-aged women with chronic UTI. It is caused by enteric bacteria and affects many organs but frequently the urinary tract. The gross lesion appears as a soft yellow-brown plaque of variable size. Histologically, the plaques show large macrophages with foamy cytoplasm. The cytoplasm contains PAS-positive granules and crystals called Michaelis-Gutmann bodies. These bodies contain calcium and iron. Malakoplakia seems to be due to a defect in macrophage function that blocks the lysosomal enzymatic degradation of engulfed bacteria and accumulates in the cytoplasm as bacterial debris. E. coli is the most common organism cultured in the urine. Malakoplakia is commonly seen in immunosuppressive patients. Treatment with antimicrobial agents for UTI and cholinergic agonist, bethanechol, has been proven beneficial in some patients.

Suggested Reading

Diwakar R, Else J, Wong W, et al. Enlarged kidneys and acute renal failure-why is renal biopsy necessary for diagnosis and treatment. Nephrol Dial Transplant. 2008;23:401–3.
Kobayashi A, Utsunimiya Y, Kono M, et al. Malakoplakia of the kidney. Am J Kidney Dis. 2008;51:326–30.

47. A 36-year-old woman with rheumatoid arthritis for several years is admitted for hematuria, proteinuria, and worsening kidney function. Her medications include prednisone, methotrexate, and an ACE inhibitor. Her arthritis was controlled for 8 years, but joint pain became worse 6 months ago. At that time, she was started on etanercept (TNFα-antagonist) and her symptoms improved. Her serum creatinine was 0.8 mg/dL. She had no either hematuria or proteinuria at the start of etanercept. On admission, her serum creatinine is 6.2 mg/dL. ANA and antidouble-stranded DNA are positive. Urinalysis reveals 2+ blood, 4+ proteinuria, RBCs, and RBC casts. Spot urine protein to creatinine ratio is 8. **Which one of the following is the MOST likely diagnosis in this patient?**

A. ACE inhibitor-induced acute kidney injury (AKI)
B. Amyloidosis
C. Glomerulonephritis induced by etanercept
D. Glomerulonephritis due to long-term rheumatoid arthritis
E. Methotrexate-induced chronic tubulointerstitial disease (TID)

The answer is C

The presence of RBCs, RBC casts, and AKI are consistent with glomerulonephritis with endocapillary (endothelial and mesangial cells) proliferation. ACE inhibitors may cause AKI in patients with bilateral renal artery stenosis or in those with decreased effective arterial blood volume. In addition, they may rarely cause membranous nephropathy. However, the clinical picture of the patient is not consistent with ACE inhibitor use. Amyloidosis with nephrotic syndrome develops in patients with rheumatoid arthritis. However, the findings on urinalysis are not consistent with amyloidosis. Similarly, glomerulonephritis (GN) can occur in rheumatoid arthritis, but the kidney course is atypical. Also, the occurrence of nephrotic syndrome in chronic TID due to methotrexate is unusual. Thus, options A, B, D, and E are incorrect.

It has been shown that TNFα-antagonists (etanercept, adalimumab, and infliximab) lead to formation of antibodies, including ANA, antidouble-stranded DNA, and anticardiolipin antibodies in some patients with rheumatoid arthritis, resulting in reversible lupus-like syndrome. Stokes and colleagues reported their data on five patients with long-standing rheumatoid arthritis who developed new-onset glomerular disease, proteinuria >1 g/day, and AKI. Kidney biopsies showed lupus nephritis (classes III and IV) in two patients, pauci-immune necrotizing crescentic GN in one patient, pauci-immune necrotizing crescentic GN and amyloidosis in one patient, and membranous nephropathy and renal vasculitis in another patient. Median duration of therapy was 6 months (3–30 months). Similarly, Chin et al. described a psoriatic patient who developed nephrotic syndrome due to membranous nephropathy following infliximab administration. In both studies, discontinuation of TNFα-antagonists improved proteinuria and kidney function. Thus, use of TNFα-antagonists may induce kidney disease in some patients. Since our patient developed kidney disease and lupus serology in 6 months following therapy with etanercept, option C is the correct answer.

Suggested Reading

Chin G, Luxton G, Harvey JM. Infliximab and nephrotic syndrome. Nephrol Dial Tansplant. 2005;20:2824–26.
De Bandt. Lessons for lupus from tumour necrosis factor blockade. Lupus. 2006;15:762–7.
Stokes MB, Foster K, Markowitz GS, et al. Development of glomerulonephritis during anti-TNF-α therapy for rheumatoid arthritis. Nephrol Dial Tansplant. 2005;20:1400–6.

48. **Match the following light microscopic (LM) findings of the glomerulus with the associated kidney diseases.**

A. Normal glomerular appearance
B. Spike-like appearance of capillary loops
C. Lobular with tram-track appearance of capillary loops
D. Wire loop appearance of capillary loops
E. Nodular appearance of mesangial matrix
F. Collapsing form of FSGS with severe microcystic tubular injury and tubulointerstitial inflammation

1. Minimal change disease
2. Systemic lupus erythematosus (SLE)
3. Amyloidosis

4. Membranous nephropathy (Stage II)
5. MPGN type I
6. HIVAN

Answers: A = 1; B = 4; C = 5; D = 2; E = 3; F = 6

Certain LM findings are characteristic of some common glomerular diseases. Patients with minimal change disease have normal appearing glomeruli, and diagnosis of the disease is made by electron microscopy which demonstrates effacement or fusion of foot processes.

Patients with active lupus nephritis demonstrate the presence of wire loops, a descriptive term for thickened glomerular capillary walls due to the presence of large subendothelial deposits. The capillary walls have a thick and rigid appearance (wire loop-like) that can be detected by light microscopy. This lesion is seen in class III and IV lupus nephritis.

The presence of nodules or nodular appearance of mesangial matrix is not only characteristic of diabetic nephropathy but also seen in other glomerular diseases such as amyloidosis, MPGN (type 1), and monoclonal immunoglobulin deposition disease, and fibrillary GN.

Spike-like appearance of the glomerular capillary is seen with Jones silver methenamine stain in membranous nephropathy (stage II), which is due to the growth of the GBM as projections between subepithelial immune deposits. Spikes are also seen in amyloidosis. In this disease, amyloid deposits in the peripheral GBM form spicular hair-like projections that resemble the spikes of membranous nephropathy.

Lobulations of glomerular capillary walls are seen in MPGN (mostly type 1). This disorder is characterized by global capillary wall thickening and endocapillary (endothelial and mesangial cell) hypercellularity. Mesangial hypercellularity is accompanied by excessive mesangial matrix expansion, which gives the appearance of nodules as well as lobulation. On Jones silver methenamine stain, the GBM appears duplicated because of the production of BM material between the original BM and endothelium with resultant formation of a new BM. This doubling or duplicated BM appears like tram-tracking on LM.

Patients with HIVAN have FSGS of collapsing variant. Associated morphologic changes include severe tubulointerstitial lesions with cystic dilation of tubules and tubular degeneration. With advanced disease, interstitial fibrosis and tubular atrophy occur.

Suggested Reading

Bonsib SM, editor. Atlas of medical renal pathology. New York: Springer; 2013. p. 1–266.

Fogo AB, Kashgarian M. Diagnostic atlas of renal pathology. 3rd ed. Philadelphia: Elsevier, Inc.; 2017. p. 1–546.

49. **Match the following electron microscopic (EM) findings of the glomerulus with appropriate kidney disease.**

A. Effacement of foot processes only
B. Tubuloreticular inclusion bodies
C. Diffuse global subepithelial deposits with surrounding basement membrane (BM) material
D. Hump-shaped subepithelial deposits without surrounding BM material
E. Predominantly subendothelial deposits with endocapillary proliferation and few mesangial deposits
F. Ribbon-like BM appearance with dense deposits in the glomerular and tubular BM

1. HIVAN
2. Minimal change disease (MCD)
3. Acute and chronic postinfectious GN
4. Membranous nephropathy (Stages II and III)
5. Dense deposit disease (C3 glomerulopathy)
6. MPGN type 1

Answers: A = 2; B = 1; C = 4; D = 3; E = 6; F = 5

Effacement or fusion of foot processes on EM is the only finding in patients with MCD, as glomeruli on LM appear normal. IF microscopy in MCD shows no immunoglobulin or complement deposition. Effacement of foot processes is a common observation in proteinuric conditions in association with other morphologic changes (see Fig. 2.7 with foot process effacement).

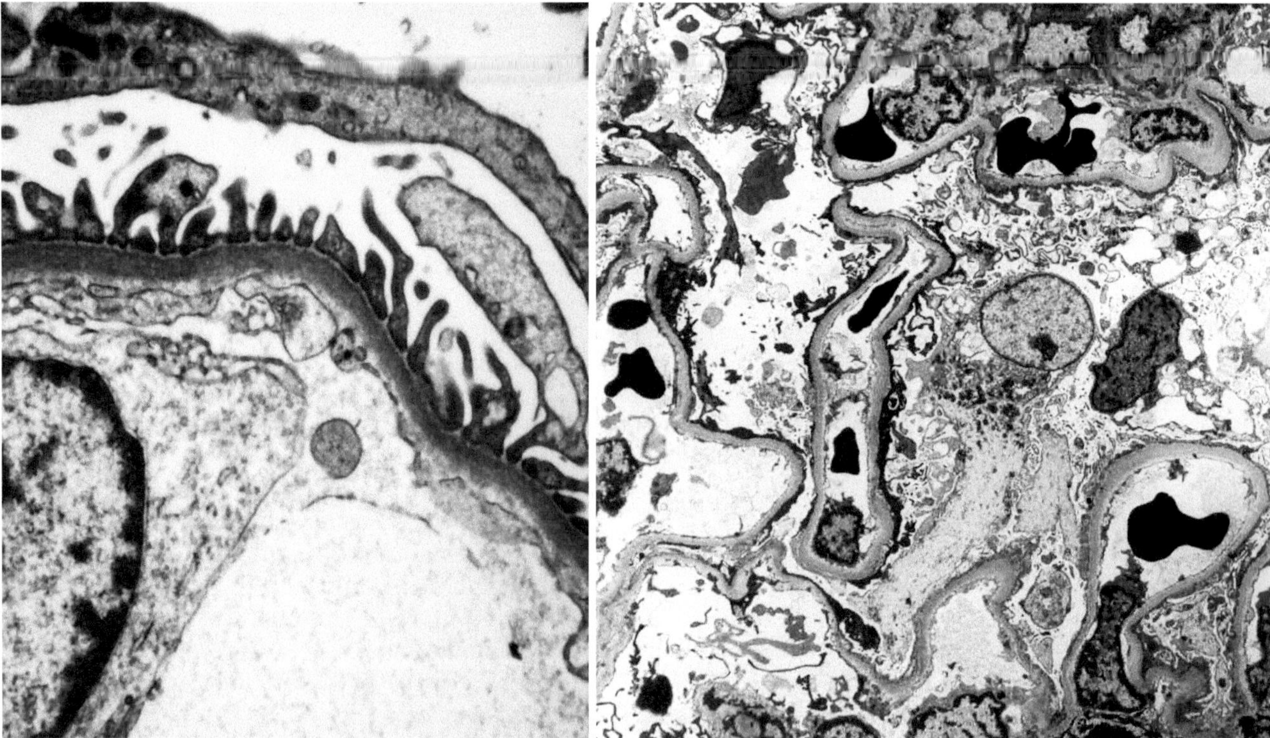

Fig. 2.7 EM micrograph showing foot processes effacement (compare with normal basement membrane with foot processes on left)

Tubuloreticular inclusion bodies (TRIs), approximately 24 nm in diameter, are found in the endoplasmic reticulum of glomerular and vascular endothelial cells of the HIV patients (Fig. 2.8). The presence of these TRIs is suggestive of HIV infection in otherwise asymptomatic individuals. Such TRIs, resembling myxoviruses, are also present in patients with SLE. The significance of TRIs is unclear; however, they are inducible by interferon-α.

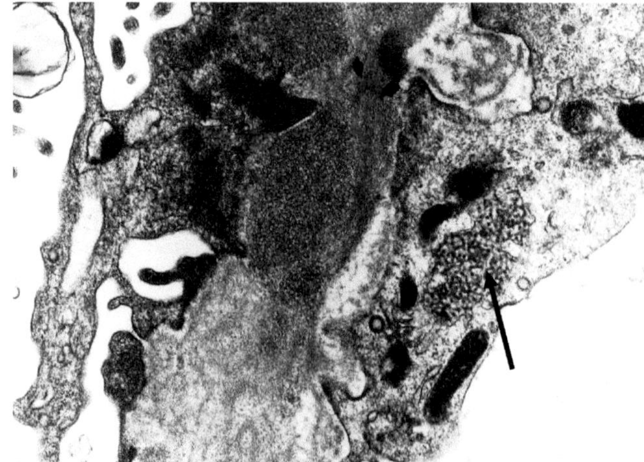

Fig. 2.8 EM micrograph showing tubuloreticular inclusion bodies in the endothelial cell (arrow) of the glomerulus

The characteristic EM finding in membranous nephropathy is the presence of immune complex deposits between the epithelial cells and basement membrane (BM) starting with stage I membranous nephropathy. In stage II membranous nephropathy, the BM matrix forms spike-like projections around the deposits, which then encircles the deposits to form stage IV membranous nephropathy. In stage IV, the deposits are resorbed with resultant lucent areas in irregularly thickened BMs (Fig. 2.9).

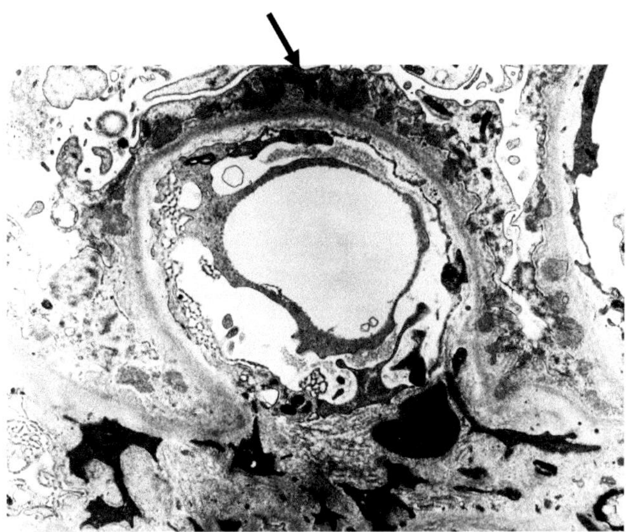

Fig. 2.9 EM micrograph showing subepithelial deposits (arrow) between epithelial cells and basement membrane in membranous nephropathy

The presence of numerous subepithelial hump-shaped immune deposits without surrounding BM matrix is characteristic of acute poststreptococcal GN (Fig. 2.10). Occasional subendothelial and mesangial deposits are also present. In the chronic phase of the disease, the subepithelial humps disappear and mesangial deposits predominate with a few subendothelial deposits.

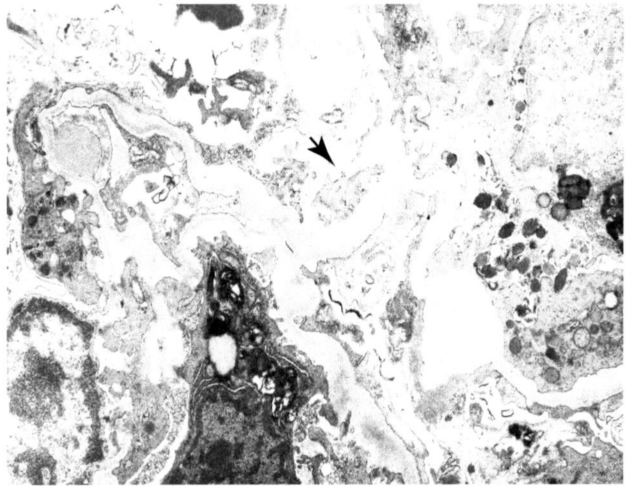

Fig. 2.10 EM micrograph showing hump-shaped subepithelial deposits (arrow) in acute postinfectious glomerulonephritis

In patients with MPGN type 1, the ultrastructural changes of the kidney are characterized by endocapillary proliferation and numerous immune deposits in the subendothelial portions of the capillary walls and mesangial regions (Fig. 2.11). In addition, a separation of the endothelium from the BM is seen with new BM matrix synthesis under the endothelial cells that have become detached from the original BM. Between the new and old layers of BMs interposed mesangial, endothelial, and mononuclear cells are found, giving the duplicated appearance of the BM by the LM. In contrast, the dense deposit disease is characterized by the presence of the electron-dense band of homogenous material in some parts of the BM. This homogenous material represents small immune deposits, which are also found in the mesangial region.

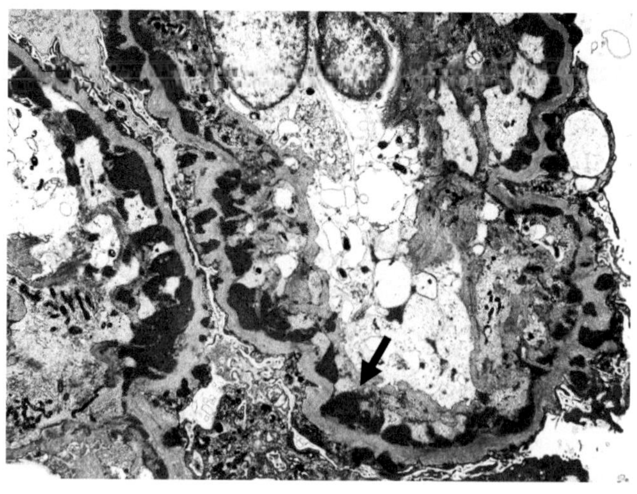

Fig. 2.11 EM micrograph showing subendothelial deposits (arrow) in MPGN type 1

Suggested Reading

Bonsib SM, editor. Atlas of medical renal pathology. New York: Springer; 2013. p. 1–266.
Fogo AB, Kashgarian M. Diagnostic atlas of renal pathology. 3rd ed. Philadelphia: Elsevier, Inc.; 2017. p. 1–546.

50. **Select the predominant immunoglobulin pattern with the appropriate mesangial proliferative GN:**

A. Mesangial IgG deposits (±IgM, IgA +C3)
B. Mesangial IgA deposits (±IgM +C3)
C. Mesangial C3 deposits
D. Mesangial Clq deposits (±IgG, IgM +C3)
E. Mesangial IgM deposits (±C3)

1. SLE
2. Clq nephropathy
3. IgA nephropathy
4. Resolving poststreptococcal GN
5. IgM nephropathy

Answers: A = 1; B = 3; C = 4; D = 2; E = 5

IF pattern of mesangial deposits is characteristic of certain glomerular diseases. In SLE, the predominant immunoglobulin that is deposited is IgG (Fig. 2.12) followed by IgM and IgA. Both C3 and Clq with intense staining for the latter are also commonly identified.

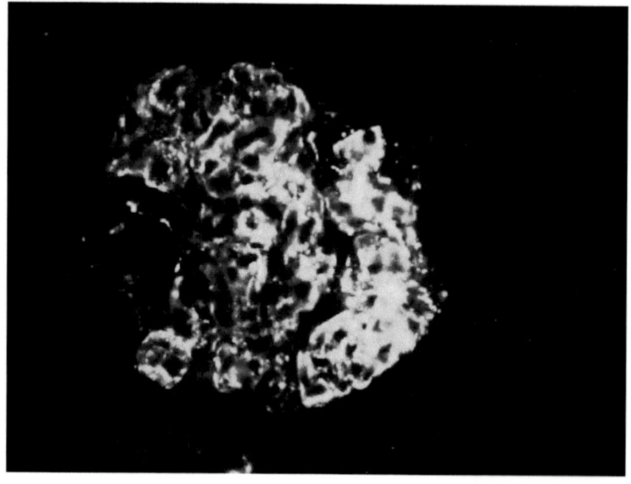

Fig. 2.12 Granular pattern of IgG in a patient with lupus nephritis

Although IgG is the predominant immunoglobulin found in the subepithelial deposits of the BM in patients with membranous nephropathy (Fig. 2.13), the presence of mesangial deposits is extremely rare in primary membranous nephropathy.

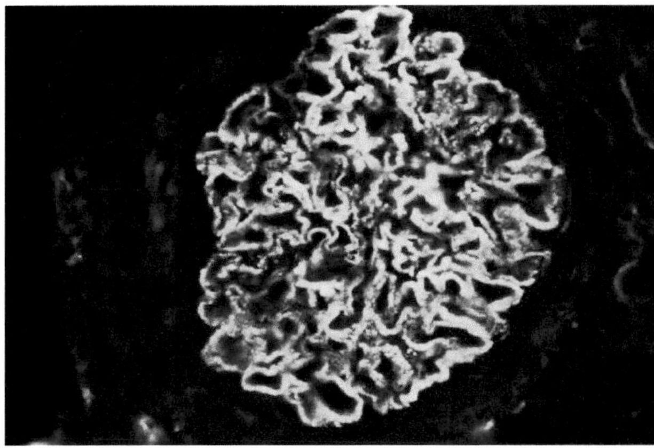

Fig. 2.13 IF pattern in membranous nephropathy with evenly granular capillary loop and subepithelial deposit distribution of IgG

In IgA nephropathy, the mesangial deposit staining for IgA is much stronger than for IgG or IgM. Substantial mesangial staining for C3 as well as absent or weak staining for Clq has been demonstrated in IgA nephropathy specimens. If the specimen demonstrates intense staining for IgA and IgG, the possibility of lupus nephritis rather than IgA nephropathy should be considered.

Clq nephropathy is diagnosed by conspicuous and the dominant mesangial staining for Clq. This predominant staining for Clq is accompanied by staining for IgG, IgM, and C3.

In poststreptococcal GN, the immune deposits in the GBM and mesangium stain with IgG and C3 with predominance of the latter. IgG and IgA staining are minimal or absent. Although garland, starry sky, and mesangial patterns of immune staining have been described, the mesangial pattern with predominantly C3 staining corresponds to the resolving phase of poststreptococcal GN.

IgM nephropathy is predominantly characterized by glomerular deposits of IgM and C3. The disease presents with nephrotic syndrome at least in 50% of patients and hematuria with a poor response to glucocorticoids.

In contrast to the granular pattern, linear pattern of immunoglobulin and complement deposition is seen in many conditions, including anti-GBM disease, diabetic kidney disease, and anti-GBM disease (see Fig. 2.14).

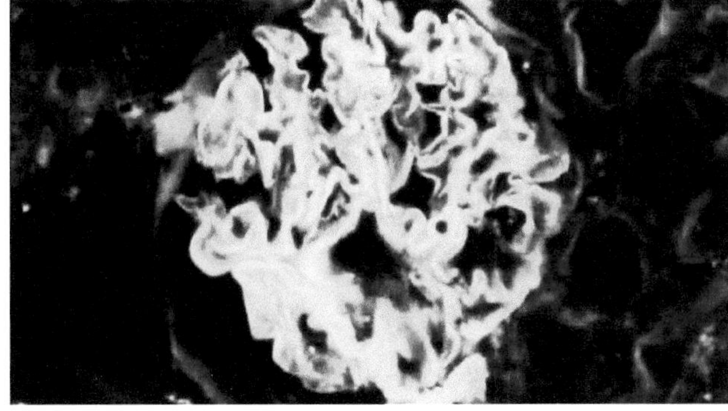

Fig. 2.14 Linear pattern of IgG in a patient with anti-GBM disease

Suggested Reading

Bonsib SM, editor. Atlas of medical renal pathology. New York: Springer; 2013. p. 1–266.
Fogo AB, Kashgarian M. Diagnostic atlas of renal pathology. 3rd ed. Philadelphia: Elsevier, Inc.; 2017. p. 1–546.

51. **Match the following drugs with the commonly described glomerular diseases.**

A. Gold
B. Penicillamine
C. Pamidronate
D. NSAIDs
E. Lithium
F. Interferon-α
G. Hydrocarbons
H. Mitomycin, quinine, ticlopidine, clopidogrel, oral contraceptives
I. Antivascular endothelial growth factor antibody (Anti-VEGF Ab)

1. Membranous nephropathy and minimal change disease (MCD)
2. Membranous nephropathy (MN)
3. MCD and MN
4. FSGS (collapsing variant)
5. MCD and FSGS
6. MCD, FSGS, and crescentic GN
7. Anti-GBM Ab disease
8. Thrombotic thrombocytopenic purpura (TTP)
9. Thrombotic microangiopathy with proteinuria

Answers: A = 1; B = 2; C = 4; D = 3; E = 5; F = 6; G = 7; H = 8; I = 9

A number of drugs have been found to cause a variety of glomerular and vascular changes. Treatment of patients with gold was found to develop proteinuria and nephrotic syndrome due to MN and MCD. Similarly, penicillamine was found to cause MN. Treatment of pamidronate may induce predominantly collapsing variant of FSGS. NSAIDs were found to induce MCD and MN. Lithium treatment causes MCD and FSGS. Interferon-α was found associated with MCD, FSGS, crescentic GN, and thrombotic microangiopathy. Exposure to hydrocarbons is a risk factor for the development of anti-GBM-Ab disease. Drugs such as mitomycin, quinine, ticlopidine, clopidogrel, and estrogen-containing oral contraceptives were found associated with TTP. Bevacizumab (anti-VEGF Ab) and related drugs have been shown to cause glomerular thrombotic microangiopathy with proteinuria in the nephrotic range. Thus, a careful history of drug ingestion should be taken in patients with proteinuria and vascular changes of the kidney.

Suggested Reading

Awdishu L, Mehta RL. The 6R's of drug induced nephrotoxicity. BMC Nephrol. 2017;18:124.
Palmer BF, Henrich WL. Toxic nephropathy. In: Brenner BM, editor. Brenner & Rector's the kidney. 7th ed. Philadelphia: Saunders; 2004. p. 1625–58.
Perazella MA, Shirali AC. Nephrotoxicity of cancer immunotherapies: past, present and future. J Am Soc Nephrol. 2018;29:2039–52.

52. **Match the following infectious agents with the commonly described glomerular diseases.**

A. Parvovirus 19
B. Hepatitis B
C. Hepatitis C
D. HIV
E. Plasmodium malaria
F. Schistosomiasis
G. Syphilis
H. E. coli O157:H7

1. Membranous nephropathy (MN)
2. FSGS (collapsing variant)

eculizumab may be one of the beneficial monoclonal antibodies for the treatment of dense deposit disease. Thus, option D is correct. Thalidomide is used in patients with multiple myeloma, and its efficacy has not been tested in dense deposit disease.

Suggested Reading

McCaughan JA, O'Rourke DM, Courtney AE. Recurrent dense deposit disease after renal transplantation: an emerging role for complementary therapies. Am J Transplant. 2012;12:1046–51.
Nester CM, Smith RJ. Treatment options for C3 glomerulopathy. Curr Opin Nephrol Hypertens. 2013;22:231–7.
Ricklin D, Lambris JD. Complement targeted therapeutics. Nat Biotechnol. 2007;25:1265–75.
Schena FP, Esposito P, Rossini M. A narrative review on C3 glomerulopathy: a rare renal disease. Int J Mol Sci. 2020;21:525.
Smith RJ, Appel GB, Blom AM, et al. C3 glomerulopathy- understanding a rare complement-driven renal disease. Nat Rev Nephrol. 2019;15:129–43.

56. A 30-year-old Caucasian man is admitted for painless palpable purpura, arthralgias (knee and ankle), and abdominal pain with bloody diarrhea for 7 days. The rash is predominantly located on the extensor surfaces of lower extremities with spread to buttocks. Blood pressure and kidney function are normal. Urinalysis shows microscopic hematuria. A tentative diagnosis of Henoch-Schönlein purpura (HSP) is entertained. **Which one of the following statements regarding HSP is FALSE?**

A. HSP is more prevalent in children, although it may occur at any age
B. Renal involvement in subjects with HSP is associated with extensive deposition of IgA in the mesangium
C. In contrast to IgA nephropathy (IgAN), HSP nephropathy has been described in association with hypersensitivity reactions
D. In HSP, the circulating immune complexes are larger and IgE levels are higher than in IgAN
E. Prospective, randomized studies of IgAN and HSP nephropathy without crescents yielded similar beneficial effects of a combination of cyclophosphamide and rituximab

The answer is E

HSP is predominantly a disease of childhood, although it may occur at any age. In both children and adults, males are affected more often than females. HSP is more common in Caucasians than in African Americans. HSP may be considered a systemic counterpart of IgAN. LM studies vary from normal looking glomeruli to glomeruli demonstrating diffuse proliferative lesions with or without crescents. IF studies show predominant IgA1 deposits in the mesangium and peripheral capillary loops. One feature that distinguishes HSP nephropathy from other forms of IgA nephropathy is the frequent presence of IgG and occasionally IgM.

In contrast to IgAN, HSP nephropathy has been found to be associated with hypersensitivity. Several drugs such as ACE-Is, cocaine, ciprofloxacin, and vancomycin have been found to induce HSP. HSP nephropathy is characterized by plasma levels of larger IgA1 immune complexes and elevated levels of IgE compared to IgAN.

The clinical outcome of HSP nephropathy is different between children and adults. A large retrospective study in adults with a follow-up of 14.8 years showed clinical remission (absence of hematuria, proteinuria, and normal renal function) in only 20%.

There are no prospective, randomized clinical studies in IgAN and HSP nephropathy patients, using a combination of cyclophosphamide and rituximab. Rituximab alone has been shown to improve kidney function in some patients. Cyclophosphamide has not been found to be effective in noncrescentic HSP nephropathy. Also, glucocorticoids do not improve HSP nephropathy, although they may improve abdominal pain. Thus, option E is false.

Suggested Reading

Davin J-C, tenBerge IJ, Weening JJ. What is the difference between IgA nephropathy and Henoch-Schönlein purpura nephritis? Kidney Int. 2001;59:823–34.
Haas M. IgA nephropathy and Henoch-Schönlein purpura nephritis. In: Jennette JC, Olson JL, Schwartz MM, Silva FG, editors. Heptinstall's pathology of the kidney. 6th ed. Philadelphia: Lippincott Williams & Wilkins; 2006. p. 423–86.
Phillebout E, Thervet E, Hill G, et al. Henoch-Schönlein purpura in adults: outcome and prognostic factors. J Am Soc Nephrol. 2002;13:1271–78.

57. A 28-year-old African American man was admitted for nausea, vomiting, weakness, cough, progressive dyspnea, and occasional hemoptysis of 2-week duration. He was treated with antibiotics with temporary improvement in his respiratory symptoms. However, dyspnea and hemoptysis continued, requiring hospitalization. He smokes two packs of cigarettes per day. Physical exam and pertinent labs:

- BP: 120/80 mm Hg, pulse 80 (supine)
- BP: 100/60 mm Hg, pulse 100 (standing)
- Conjunctiva: pale, no icterus
- Lungs: crackles
- Heart: S_1 S_2 normal; 2/6 SEM left sternal border; no S_3 or rub
- Abd: benign
- Ext: trace edema
- Hgb: 9 g/dL
- Platelets: 340,000
- Na^+ = 136 mEq/L
- K^+ = 5.6 mEq/L
- Cl^- = 102 mEq/L
- HCO_3^-:= 14 mEq/L
- BUN = 100 mg/dL
- Creatinine = 7.1 mg/dL
- Serum complement = Normal
- pANCA = Positive
- Urinalysis = 2+ blood, 1+ protein, 20–30 RBCs and erythrocyte casts
- Chest X-ray = Fluffy infiltrates
- Kidney biopsy = Crescentic glomerulonephritis (GN) with fibrinoid necrosis and strong linear IgG deposition of the glomerular basement membrane (GBM)

Which one of the following is the MOST likely diagnosis?

A. Granulomatosis with polyangiitis (Wegener's granulomatosis)
B. Microscopic polyangiitis
C. Anti-GBM disease
D. Systemic lupus erythematosus (SLE)
E. Classic polyarteritis nodosa

The answer is C

The immunofluorescence findings on kidney biopsy rule out granulomatosis with polyangiitis and microscopic polyangiitis, as both are considered pauci-immune vasculitides, although crescentic GN, pulmonary hemorrhage, and ANCAs are present. Thus, options A and B are incorrect.

In active lupus nephritis, pANCA is positive, and complements are generally low. In classic polyarteritis nodosa, a disease of medium-sized arteries, ANCAs are absent. Also, crescentic GN is not a typical presentation of classic polyarteritis nodosa. Thus, options D and E are also incorrect.

The kidney biopsy findings are suggestive of anti-GBM disease, which consists of GN, lung hemorrhage, and anti-GBM-antibodies (answer C is correct). Generally, anti-GBM disease and Goodpasture syndrome are used together because Goodpasture described the first case of kidney failure and lung hemorrhage in a young man due to influenza in 1919. Many specialists in the field are comfortable to use the term anti-GBM disease because it is an autoimmune disease, causing vasculitis of small vessels affecting the capillary beds of the kidneys and lungs.

Most of the patients with anti-GBM disease have crescentic GN and kidney dysfunction at the time of clinical presentation. Glomeruli with crescents may have fibrinoid necrosis in adjacent arteries and arterioles. Linear staining of immunoglobulins, particularly IgG, is seen in all GBMs.

Suggested Reading

Gulati K, McAdoo SP. Anti-glomerular basement membrane disease. Rheum Dis Clin N Am. 2018;44:651–73.
McAdoo SP, Pusey CD. Anti-glomerular basement membrane disease. Clin J Am Soc Nephrol. 2017;12:162–72.

58. **Which one of the following factors is associated with anti-GBM disease?**

A. Exposure to hydrocarbons
B. Cigarette smoking
C. Influenza A and Covid-19 infection
D. Use of alemtuzumab
E. All of the above

The answer is E

Environmental factors play an important role in anti-GBM disease. Among them exposure or inhalation of hydrocarbons may initiate the onset of the disease. It is suggested that local inflammation caused by inhaled toxins may cause increased capillary permeability by disturbing alveolar basement membranes. This may provide access to pathogenic autoantibodies into the lung, causing lung hemorrhage (A is correct). Cigarette smoking is an added insult to lung hemorrhage (B is correct).

Seasonal clustering of anti-GBM disease has been reported. Influenza A is a seasonal infectious disease; the case reported by Goodpasture had exposure to influenza. Recently, case series described a cluster of cases occurring in association with the outbreak of the novel coronavirus, SARS-CoV-2. This association is logical, and answer C is probably correct.

Alemtuzumab (Campath-1H) is a humanized anti-CD52 monoclonal antibody, and its administration causes profound B- and T-lymphocyte depletion. It is an induction agent in kidney transplantation. Also, it is used in multiple sclerosis and chronic lymphocytic leukemia. Clatworthy, Wallin, and Jayne used alemtuzumab in two patients with multiple sclerosis and nonrenal ANCA-associated vasculitis and found that both patients developed acute kidney injury due to anti-GBM disease 9–10 months later. Thus, the nephrologists should be aware of this complication of alemtuzumab (answer D is correct).

Suggested Reading

Bombassei GJ, Kaplan AA. The association between hydrocarbon exposure and anti-glomerular basement membrane antibody-mediated disease (Goodpasture's syndrome). Am J Ind Med. 1992;21:141–53.
Clatworthy MR, Wallin EF, Jayne DR. Anti-glomerular basement membrane disease after alemtuzumab. N Engl J Med. 2008;359:768–9.
Prendecki M, Clarke C, Cairns T, et al. Anti-glomerular basement membrane disease during the COVID-19 pandemic. Kidney Int. 2020;98:780–1.
Wilson CB, Smith RC. Goodpasture's syndrome associated with influenza A2 virus infection. Ann Intern Med. 1972;76:91–4.

59. **Which one of the following treatment plans for the patient with anti-GBM disease is CORRECT?**

A. Corticosteroids alone
B. Corticosteroids and azathioprine
C. Plasma exchange, corticosteroids, cyclophosphamide, and hemodialysis
D. Corticosteroids, cyclophosphamide, and anticoagulants
E. Hemodialysis only because of high serum creatinine, and immunosuppression may not have any further benefit

The answer is C

The major principles of anti-GBM disease therapy are (1) removal of circulating anti-GBM-antibodies, (2) stop antibody production, and (3) correct underlying cause of the disease. Prior to immunosuppressive therapy,

patients with anti-GBM disease (Goodpasture syndrome or disease) died shortly after pulmonary hemorrhage or kidney failure. The introduction of immunosuppressive therapy and plasma exchange has dramatically improved the prognosis of this disease.

For an active disease, daily plasma exchange (plasmapheresis) should be started immediately with removal of 2–4 L of plasma with 5% albumin replacement. Patients with lung hemorrhage may benefit from fresh frozen plasma replacement to replete clotting factors. Plasma exchange should be continued at least for 14 days and until the disappearance of circulating anti-GBM-antibodies. We prefer to follow the antibody titers every month because rebound may be seen.

Next, oral corticosteroids should be started at a dose of 1 mg/kg/day (60 mg daily) for 1 week, then reduce dose weekly to 20 mg by 6 weeks, and then gradually taper until complete discontinuation at 6–9 months. Some nephrologists prefer IV methylprednisolone at the dose of 1 g/day for three doses and then oral prednisone 60 mg/day. Note that methylprednisolone may increase the risk of infection.

Simultaneously with the above treatments, oral cyclophosphamide at a dose of 2–3 mg/kg/day should be started and continued for 3 months. Others prefer to continue for 6–12 months. For IV administration, the starting dose should be 0.5 mg/m^2 body surface area. Adjustment of cyclophosphamide dosage is required based upon kidney function and white cell count. Also, patients >55 years of age require a reduced dose.

Hemodialysis rather than other forms of renal replacement therapies is required to improve uremic signs and symptoms.

The combination of plasma exchange, corticosteroids, and cyclophosphamide has improved both patient and kidney survival dramatically.

Historical evidence suggests that treatment with corticosteroids alone or corticosteroids plus azathioprine is less effective. Therefore, options A and B are incorrect.

The major prognostic factor for disease progression to ESKD is the serum creatinine level at the time of presentation. Aggressive immunosuppression is unlikely to recover renal function without dialysis in patients with serum creatinine level >6.6 mg/dL and oliguric. However, active (not completely fibrotic) crescents and lung hemorrhage warrants plasma exchange and immunosuppression. On the other hand, immunosuppression may be withheld in those without lung hemorrhage, nonoliguric but creatinine levels >6.6 mg/dL, ANCA negative, and irreversible kidney damage on biopsy. Therefore, option D is incorrect.

Some investigators used anticoagulants in addition to corticosteroids and cyclophosphamide because of the presence of fibrin in glomerular lesions. Currently, no proven benefit has been documented with this regimen. Interestingly, anticoagulants have been shown to increase pulmonary hemorrhage. Option E, therefore, is incorrect.

Prophylaxis for oropharyngeal fungal infection, peptic ulcer, and PCP while receiving high dose is usually recommended.

Suggested Reading

Gulati K, McAdoo SP. Anti-glomerular basement membrane disease. Rheum Dis Clin N Am. 2018;44:651–73.
McAdoo SP, Pusey CD. Anti-glomerular basement membrane disease. Clin J Am Soc Nephrol. 2017;12:162–72.

60. A 60-year-old Caucasian man with history of hypertension, hepatitis C, and chronic lower extremity ulcers (see Fig. 2.15) is admitted for shortness of breath of 1-week duration and painful ulcer. He is not on any medications. Blood pressure is 152/94 mm Hg with pulse of 102 beats per minute. Lungs show crackles, heart exam reveals an S_3, skin shows 2 cm circular ulcer over left pre-tibia, 3 necrotic ulcers on right pre-tibia with necrotic tissue and pain. Lower extremities show 2+ pitting edema. Pertinent labs:

- Na^+ = 144 mEq/L
- K^+ = 4.4 mEq/L
- Cl^- = 112 mEq/L
- HCO_3^- = 19 mEq/L
- Creatinine = 2.4 mg/dL
- BUN = 66 mg/dL
- Glucose = 120 mg/dL
- Hgb = 9.6 g/dL
- Urinalysis: SG 1.011, pH 5.5, protein 100 mg/dL, blood positive, RBCs 80, WBCs 16
- Cryoglobulins 5%

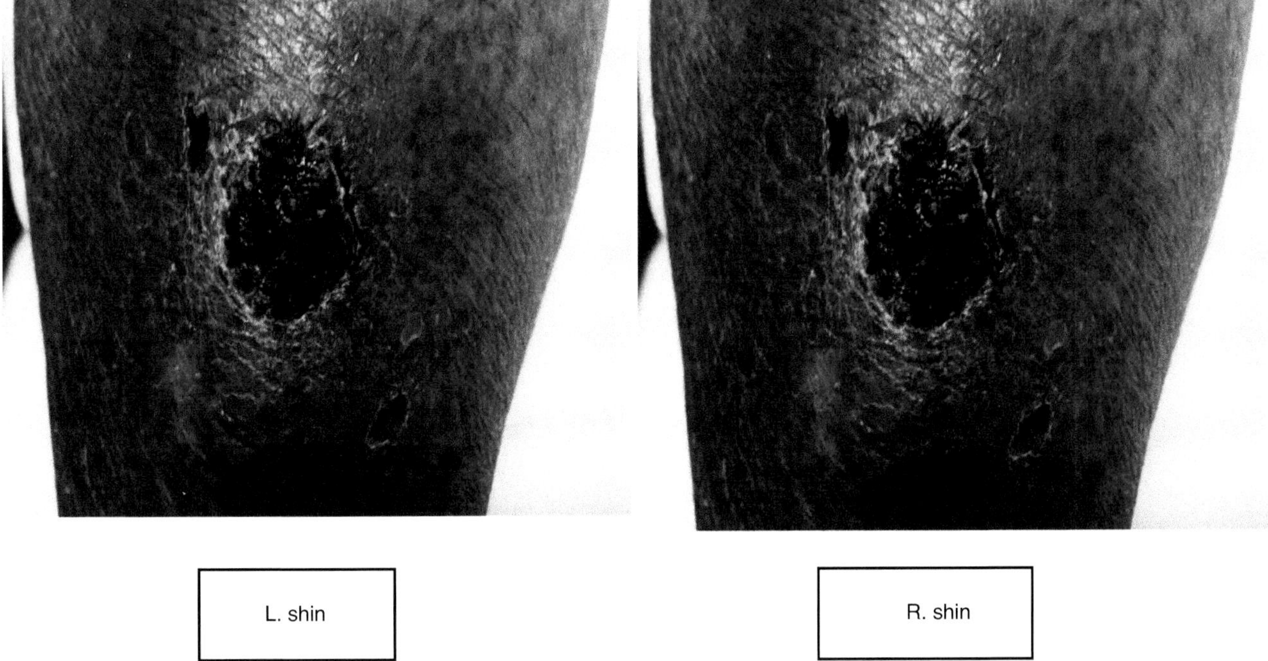

Fig. 2.15 Left and right shins of the above patient

The patient receives IV furosemide and his shortness of breath improves. Following stabilization, a kidney biopsy was done, which showed MPGN type 1. **Based on his findings, which one of the following treatments is APPROPRIATE at this time?**

A. Plasmapheresis
B. Zepatier
C. Ribavirin
D. Interferon-α and ribavirin
E. Hemodialysis

The answer is A

This patient's skin lesions did not improve with antibiotics. Since the patient has the history of hepatitis C infection for many years, cryoglobulinemia-induced vasculitis has been considered. Plasmapheresis is an effective way of removing the immune complexes and improves vasculitic lesions. Thus, option A is the appropriate choice of treatment for this patient. Generally, hepatitis C virus-associated cryoglobulinemia responds to antiviral therapy, and direct antiviral therapy with zepatier can be started following plasmapheresis. Hemodialysis is not indicated at this time. Some studies have shown that rituximab is effective in improving vasculitis and kidney function. It also inhibits the production of cryoglobulins. However, the treatment is expensive.

Suggested Reading

Ostojic P, Jeremic IR. Managing refractory cryoglobulinemic vasculitis: challenges and solutions. J Inflam Res. 2017;10:49–54.

Terrier B, Cacoub P. Cryoglobulinemia vasculitis: an update. Curr Opin Rheumatol. 2013;25:10–8.

61. A 55-year-old Caucasian man is admitted for fever, cough, weight loss, and pain in knees. Past medical history includes recurrent nasal discharge mixed with blood, frequent rhinitis, headaches, and ear pain. CT of the sinus showed pansinusitis. He takes a 2-week course of antibiotics. BP is 150/90 mm Hg with a pulse of 82 and afebrile. Positive findings on

phys exam include clotted blood in both nares, mild discharge in the left ear, and crackles in both lung fields. Serum creatinine is 4.5 mg/dL (1.1 mg/dL 1 month ago). cANCA is positive, but ANA negative. Urinalysis shows 1+ proteinuria, 3+ blood, 20–30 RBCs, and RBC casts. CXR shows bilateral infiltrates. **Based on the above information, which one of the following findings is LEAST likely in this patient?**

A. Detection of cANCA by both indirect immunofluorescence and antigen-specific assays
B. Presence of focal segmental necrotizing and crescentic GN by light microscopy
C. Frequent absence of glomerular staining for immunoglobulins by immunofluorescence microscopy
D. Glomeruli with necrotizing lesions show areas of capillary wall disruption, focal gaps in Bowman capsule, capillary thrombi, endothelial swelling and denudation and subendothelial accumulation of fibrin, platelets, and amorphous electron-dense material of nonimmune type
E. The degree of kidney failure always correlates well with the percentage of glomerular necrotizing lesions and the number of crescents

The answer is E

The triad of upper respiratory tract infection, lung, and kidney abnormalities are highly suggestive of granulomatosis with polyangiitis (Wegner's granulomatosis), and cANCA with anti-proteinase 3 is highly positive in such a patient. The patient has active kidney disease. Kidney biopsy findings suggested in options B, C, and D are seen in patients with granulomatosis with polyangiitis. Thus, options A to D are correct.

Patients with more severe form of the kidney disease have decreased GFR. However, the degree of kidney failure does not always correlate well with the percentage of glomerular necrotizing lesions, the number of active glomerular crescents, or the presence of interstitial granulomas or vasculitis. Therefore, option E is incorrect.

Suggested Reading

Hunter RW, Welsh N, Farrah TE, et al. ANCA asosiated vasculitis. BMJ. 2020;369:m1070.
Kitching AR, AndersH-J, Basu N, et al. ANCA-associated vasculitis. Nat Rev Dis Primers. 2020;6:71.
Yates M, Watts R. ANCA-associated vasculitis. Clin Med. 2017;1:60–4.

62. **Which one of the following therapies is indicated in the above patient?**

A. Corticosteroids alone
B. Trimethoprim-sulfamethoxazole and low-dose corticosteroids
C. Combined corticosteroids with either rituximab or cyclophosphamide
D. Intravenous immunoglobulins and tumor necrosis factor inhibitor-α (TNF-α)
E. Corticosteroids, methotrexate, and plasma exchange

The answer is C

The treatment of granulomatosis with polyangiitis or small-vessel vasculitis, in general, includes three phases: (1) induction of remission phase, (2) maintenance of remission phase, and (3) treatment of relapse. Induction of remission is defined as improvement in kidney function and resolution of hematuria and vasculitis in other organs.

This patient has severe renal disease. Current guidelines for such a patient recommend oral prednisone with either rituximab or cyclophosphamide. However, the use of the latter two drugs depends on the availability and cost of these drugs. When available and feasible, corticosteroids and rituximab are preferred by many nephrologists. Two randomized studies showed noninferiority of rituximab to cyclophosphamide. Also, rituximab is preferred for young patients or when patients are intolerant or resistant to cyclophosphamide. Some nephrologists prefer IV methylprednisolone (1 g/day) for 3 days, followed by oral prednisone (60 mg/day), although both pulse and oral therapy have equivalent potency (C is correct).

A combination of corticosteroids with rituximab and IV low-dose cyclophosphamide achieved remission in 6 months in 94% of patients with kidney ANCA vasculitis. This combination also caused lower death and relapse rates with decreased exposure to corticosteroids.

In two studies, mycophenolate mofetil (MMF) was compared with IV cyclophosphamide for induction of remission followed by azathioprine for maintenance of remission in patients with active disease. These studies showed that MMF was noninferior to cyclophosphamide in inducing remission (67% vs. 61%), but more relapses were observed in the MMF group (33% vs. 19%) with similar serious infectious risk. Thus, MMF can also be used in patients with pANCA vasculitis.

A variety of medications such as rituximab, azathioprine, methotrexate, MMF, and corticosteroids have been used for maintenance remission in ANCA vasculitis. Although the results are variable, the use of low-dose rituximab (500 mg on days 0 and 14, then months 6, 12, and 18) showed long-term maintenance remission compared to azathioprine in patients with ANCA vasculitis.

Corticosteroids alone are associated with lower rate of kidney and patient survival. Therefore, option A is incorrect.

Trimethoprim-sulfamethoxazole (T/S) has been used prophylactically to improve respiratory infections because airway stimulation has been postulated for disease expression and relapse. On the contrary, a controlled trial showed T/S to increase the chance of relapse and therefore, T/S alone or in combination with prednisone is not indicated for either active disease or maintenance of remission in patients with granulomatosis with polyangiitis. Therefore, option B is incorrect.

IV immunoglobulins (IgG) and TNF-α receptor antagonist (infliximab) have been tried, but this kind of therapy may be reserved for patients who failed the standard treatment; however, a recent study with TNF-α receptor antagonist failed to show a benefit of kidney survival. Option D is, therefore, incorrect.

Studies on methotrexate in combination with corticosteroids yielded variable results. Currently, methotrexate is not recommended for patients with serum creatinine level >2 mg/dL.

Similarly, studies on plasma exchange yielded no benefit over immunosuppressive therapy in patients who do not require dialysis. However, there are two indications for plasma exchange: (1) pulmonary hemorrhage and (2) serum creatinine levels >500 μmol (>5.7 mg/dL). Many nephrologists prefer to add plasma exchange (7–10 treatments in a 2-week period) in addition to standard immunosuppressive therapy in patients with pulmonary hemorrhage or AKI or both. Option E, therefore, is incorrect.

In summary, treatment of ANCA-positive small-vessel vasculitis (granulomatosis with polyangiitis or microscopic polyangiitis) should be based on disease severity. The reader is referred to voluminous literature for a detailed review of the subject.

Suggested Reading

Charles P, Perrodeau E, Samson M, et al. Long-term rituximab use to maintain remission of antineutrophil cytoplasmic antibody-associated vasculitis: a randomized trial. Ann Intern Med. 2020;173:179–87.

Jain K, Jawa P, Derebail VK, et al. Treatment updates in antineutrophil cytoplasmic autoantibodies (ANCA) vasculitis. Kidney. 2021;360. https://doi.org/10.34067/KID.0007142020.

Jones RB, Tervaert JW, Hauser T, et al. for the RAVE-ITN Research Group Rituximab versus cyclophosphamide in ANCA-associated renal vasculitis. N Engl J Med. 2010;363:211–20.

Jones RB, Hiemstra TF, Ballarin J, et al. European Vasculitis Study Group (EUVAS): mycophenolate mofetil versus cyclophosphamide for remission induction in ANCA-associated vasculitis: a randomised, non-inferiority trial. Ann Rheum Dis. 2019;78:399–405.

Kidney Disease: Improving Global Outcomes (KDIGO) Glomerulonephritis Work Group. KDIGO clinical practice guideline for glomerulonephritis. June 2020.

McAdoo SP, Medjeral-Thomas N, Gopaluni S, et al. Long-term follow-up of a combined rituximab and cyclophosphamide regimen in renal anti-neutrophil cytoplasm antibody-associated vasculitis. Nephrol Dial Transplant. 2019;34:63–73.

Stone JH, Merkel PA, Spiera R, et al. for the RAVE-ITN Research Group. Rituximab versus cyclophosphamide for ANCA-associated vasculitis. N Engl J Med. 2010;363:221–32.

Wallace ZS, Miloslavsky EM. Management of ANCA associated vasculitis. BMJ. 2020;368:m421.

Walsh M, Merkel PA, Peh CA, et al. for the PEXIVAS Investigators. Plasma exchange and glucocorticoids in severe ANCA-associated vasculitis. N Engl J Med. 2020;382:622–31.

63. **Regarding the assay of ANCA, which one of the following statements is FALSE?**

A. Indirect immunofluorescence assay (IFA) alone should not be used for detection of ANCA
B. Clinicians ordering ANCA should ensure that ANCA by IFA testing is confirmed by antigen-specific testing (immunoassays) for both proteinase 3 (PR3) and myeloperoxidase (MPO), and combining both assays may yield high specificity for both PR3-ANCA and MPO-ANCA
C. The new 2017 international consensus statement proposes that high-quality immunoassays can be used as the primary screening method for patients suspected of having the ANCA-associated vasculitides without the categorical need for IFA

D. Patients with connective disorders (rheumatoid arthritis or lupus) are positive for ANCA, with an antigenic target for MPO or PR3
E. Drugs such as hydralazine, propylthiouracil, or minocycline may be associated with high-titer MPO-ANCA reactivity with or without an associated vasculitis

The answer is D

ANCAs were originally defined by IFA and divided into cytoplasmic (cANCA) and perinuclear (pANCA) categories. The antigens responsible for these patterns have also been identified: PR3 and MPO, respectively. Occasionally, other antigens such as bactericidal permeability-inducing protein may produce cANCA reactivity. However, PR3 is responsible for >90% of cANCA positivity.

Unlike cANCA, pANCA reactivity is induced by several other antigens, including elastase, cathepsin G, lysozyme, lactoferrin, and azurocidin. Antinuclear antibodies may also yield a pANCA pattern. Therefore, pANCA positivity is not specific to microscopic polyangiitis only.

In order to associate cANCA with granulomatosis with polyangiitis and pANCA with microscopic pANCA, antigen-specific (PR3 or MPO) immunoassays should be performed in addition to IFA. Both assays provide >90% specificity for these diseases.

The immunoassays have undergone several modifications over the years with the intention to avoid IFA. As a result, the revised 2017 international consensus statement proposes that high-quality antigen-specific assays for proteinase 3 cANCAs and myeloperoxidase pANCAs should be used as the primary screening method for ANCA without the categorical need for IFA. However, IFA can be used in cases of negative cANCA or pANCA and clinical suspicion is strong for small-vessel vasculitis to increase the specificity for the disease.

Patients with connective tissue disorders and inflammatory bowel disease may have ANCA positivity. However, this positivity is largely due to non-MPO-ANCA or non-PR3-ANCA types. Therefore, answer D is incorrect.

Drugs such as hydralazine, propylthiouracil, D-penicillamine, and minocycline give false-positive ANCA reactions, which are associated with high-titer MPO-ANCA with or without an associated vasculitic syndrome.

A large multicenter cooperative European trial reported that a significant number of patients with idiopathic small-vessel vasculitis are ANCA negative, and a negative ANCA test in no way eliminates the diagnosis of such a patient with high probability of the disease. Clinical as well as other laboratory tests will indicate the appropriate treatment of the disease. Except for option C, other options are correct regarding the assays for ANCA.

Suggested Reading

Bossuyt X, Cohen Tervaert JW, Arimura Y, et al. Position paper: revised 2017 international consensus on testing of ANCAs in granulomatosis with polyangiitis and microscopic polyangiitis. Nat Rev Rheumatol. 2017;13:683–92.

64. A 52-year-old man presents to the Emergency Department with headache, nausea, vomiting, and shortness of breath. He says that he has been using cocaine and heroin for 20 years. Past medical history includes hypertension, for which he does not take any medications. His blood pressure is 200/112 mm Hg with a pulse rate of 100 beats per minute. Pertinent labs: creatinine 10.4 mg/dL, BUN 102 mg/dL, pANCA positive, proteinuria 600 mg/dL, 100 RBCs in urine sediment, and 2 RBC casts. After controlling blood pressure with antihypertensives and hemodialysis, a kidney biopsy was performed (see Fig. 2.16).

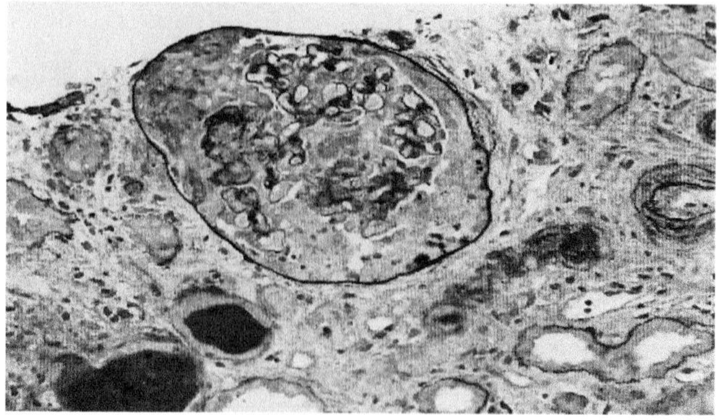

Fig. 2.16 Glomerulus showing crescents

Which one of the following agents is the MOST likely cause of this glomerular lesion?

A. Cocaine without contaminants
B. Heroin without contaminants
C. Cocaine with levamisole as a contaminant
D. Marijuana
E. Phencyclidine

The answer is C

It is known that cocaine causes vasculitis and ANCA formation. Also, cocaine induces several other autoantibodies, including ANA. In a retrospective study, McGrath et al. reported 30 cases of cocaine-induced ANCA and associated kidney disease. All cases had pANCA positivity. cANCA was positive in 50%. Abnormal urinary findings, including proteinuria, hematuria, and RBC casts, were present in eight patients. Two patients developed acute kidney injury. Kidney biopsy in one patient showed pauci-immune focal necrotizing crescentic glomerulonephritis. All these findings were attributed to contaminated cocaine with levamisole. Thus, option C is correct.

Approximately, 70% of illicit use of cocaine in the United States is contaminated with levamisole, which is an immunomodulating agent. Levamisole use has been shown to cause systemic and cutaneous vasculitis. Although levamisole induces several autoantibodies, the mechanism by which it causes the production of ANCA is not known. The other unadulterated drugs mentioned in the question have not been implicated in the generation of ANCA-induced vasculitis.

Suggested Reading

McGrath MM, Isakova T, Rennke HG, et al. Contaminated cocaine and antineutrophil cytoplasmic antibody-associated disease. Clin J Am Soc Nephrol. 2011;6:2799–805.

Nyenaber S, Mistry-Burchardi N, Rust C, et al. PR3-ANCA-positive multi-organ vasculitis following cocaine abuse. Acta Derm Venereol. 2008;88:594–6.

65. A 56-year-old Caucasian man is admitted for evaluation of weight loss (40 lbs in 4 months), fatigue, weakness, and abdominal pain. He has a history of new-onset asthma and receives oral prednisone and montelukast (10 mg daily). His BP is 135/70 mm Hg and has a pulse rate of 80 beats/min. On admission, pertinent laboratory values are

- WBCs = 31,000 (neutrophils 46%; lymphocytes 5.3%; monocytes 4.4%, eosinophils 43.6%)
- Serum creatinine = 0.8 mg/dL
- Urinalysis: pH = 5.5; SG = 1.25; 1+ proteinuria; 2+ blood; sediment: RBCs 5–10; WBCs 15–20; WBC casts and no RBC casts
- ANCA = negative
- Complements = normal
- Kidney biopsy = cellular crescents in 25% glomeruli

Based on the above information, the diagnosis of eosinophilic granulomatosis with polyangiitis (Churg-Strauss) (EGPA) is made. **Which of the following statements regarding EGPA is CORRECT?**

A. pANCA is always positive
B. Kidney disease is present in 100% of patients at time of diagnosis
C. Leukotriene receptor antagonists (montelukast)-induced EGPA is always associated with pANCA
D. Patients without kidney disease require glucocorticoids and cyclophosphamide
E. ANCA-positive patients with necrotizing and crescentic glomerulonephritis require the treatment as other patients with ANCA-positive small-vessel vasculitis

The answer is E

EGPA is characterized by asthma, peripheral and tissue eosinophilia, and vasculitis of the small-to-medium-sized vessels. It is grouped with granulomatosis with polyangiitis and microscopic polyangiitis, or kidney-limited vasculitis under ANCA-associated small-vessel vasculitis. EGPA is associated with pANCA. Generally, ANCA is positive in only 39–75% of patients with EGPA. In one study of 112 patients, pANCA was positive in 38% of the patients. When ANCA was positive, it was associated with kidney involvement, peripheral neuropathy, and biopsy-proven vasculitis. ANCA-negative patients had mostly heart disease and fever. In another study of 116

patients, ANCA was positive in 75% of patients with nephropathy, as compared with 26% of patients without nephropathy. Overall, kidney abnormalities were present only in 31 of 116 (27%) of the patients. Of these 31 patients, rapidly progressive kidney insufficiency was documented in 16 (13.8%) patients, urinary abnormalities in 14 (12.1%), and chronic kidney injury in 1 patient. Kidney biopsies were done in 16 patients: 11 had necrotizing crescentic GN, and the remaining 5 had eosinophilic interstitial nephritis, mesangial GN, and focal sclerosis. Of importance is the observation that all patients with necrotizing crescentic GN were ANCA-positive. Thus, the kidney disease is confined to mostly those with ANCA positivity. Options A and B are, therefore, incorrect.

Leukotriene receptor antagonists (zafirlukast, montelukast, and pranlukast) have been associated with the exacerbation or new onset of EGPA. However, pANCA is not elicited by these leukotriene receptor antagonists, and ANCA is negative. Thus, option C is incorrect.

Patients without kidney involvement may do well with glucocorticoid therapy alone, whereas patients with ANCA positivity and necrotizing crescentic GN require not only glucocorticoids but also cyclophosphamide or rituximab and other appropriate cytotoxic therapeutic agents. Thus, option E is correct.

Suggested Reading

Della Rossa A, Baldini C, Tavoni, A, et al. Churg-Strauss syndrome: clinical and serological features of 19 patients from a single Italian centre. Rheumatology. 2002;41:1286–94.

Hagen EC, Daha MR, Hermans J, et al. Diagnostic value of standardized assays for anti-neutrophil cytoplasmic antibodies in idiopathic systemic vasculitis. EC/BCR project for ANCA Assay Standardization. Kidney Int. 1998;53:743–53.

Hogan SL, Falk RJ, Chin H, et al. Predictors of relapse and treatment resistance in antineutrophil cytoplasmic antibody-associated small-vessel vasculitis. Ann Intern Med. 2005;143:621–31.

Kidney Disease: Improving Global Outcomes (KDIGO) Glomerulonephritis Work Group. KDIGO clinical practice guideline for glomerulonephritis. June 2020.

McGregor JG, Nachman PH, Jennette JC, et al. Vasculitic diseases of the kidney. In: Coffman TM, Falk RJ, Molitoris BA, et al., editors. Schrier's diseases of the kidney. 9th ed. Philadelphia: Wolters Kluwer/Lippincott Williams & Wilkins; 2013. p. 1325–63.

Reid AJ, Harrison BD, Watts RA, et al. Churg-Strauss syndrome in district hospital. QJM. 1998;91:219–29.

66. **Which one of the following risk factors is NOT associated with the relapse of ANCA-associated small-vessel vasculitis?**

 A. Persistence of anti-PR3 positivity
 B. Lung disease
 C. Upper respiratory tract involvement
 D. Upper airway colonization with Staph. aureus
 E. African American race

The answer is E

About 85% of patients with ANCA-associated small-vessel vasculitis (granulomatosis with polyangiitis, microscopic polyangiitis, eosinophilic granulomatosis with polyangiitis, and kidney-limited vasculitis) respond to corticosteroids and cyclophosphamide. However, 11–57% of them have a relapse. Little is known about the predictors of relapse. Hogan et al. followed a cohort of 350 patients with ANCA-associated vasculitis for a median of 49 months. Of these, 334 patients were treated, and 16 patients were not treated. Among the treated group, remission occurred in 258 (77%) patients, and the remaining 76 (23%) patients were treatment resistance. Of these 76 treatment-resistant patients, 60 developed ESKD in a median of 2 months, 12 died of disease- or therapy-related complications, and 4 had continued disease symptoms.

Of the 258 patients who attained a remission, 109 (42%) relapsed over a median of 44 months. The predictors of relapse were persistence of anti-PR3 positivity and diseases of the lung or upper respiratory tract. The increased risk for relapse was independent of age, sex, ethnicity, ANCA-specificity, and kidney function at time of biopsy. Although upper airway colonization with Staph aureus was not evaluated in the study of Hogan et al., it was found that colonization with this organism was associated with a higher relapse rate in patients with granulomatosis.

As stated above, the study of Hogan et al. did not find African American race as a predictor of relapse; however, they reported that female, African American patients, or patients with severe kidney disease may be resistant to initial treatment more often than other patients with ANCA-associated vasculitis.

Suggested Reading

Hogan SL, Falk RJ, Chin H, et al. Predictors of relapse and treatment resistance in antineutrophil cytoplasmic antibody-associated small-vessel vasculitis. Ann Intern Med. 2005;143:621–31.

Saha MK, Pendergraft III WF, Jennette JC. Primary glomerular diseases. In: Yu ASL, Chertow GM, Luyckx VA, et al., editors. Brenner & Rector's the kidney. 11th ed. Philadelphia: Elsevier Saunders; 2020. p. 1007–91.

Stegeman CA, Tervaert JW, Sluiter WJ, et al. Association of chronic nasal carriage of Staphylococcus aureus and higher relapse rate in Wegener granulomatosis. Ann Intern Med. 1994;120:12–7.

67. **Regarding patients with pauci-immune vasculitis, which one of the following statements is CORRECT?**

A. Only those patients with seropositive cANCA demonstrate severe glomerular pathology
B. Only those patients with seropositive pANCA demonstrate severe glomerular pathology
C. Only those patients with both cANCA and pANCA demonstrate severe glomerular pathology
D. Patients with negative ANCA (either cANCA or pANCA) demonstrate as severe kidney disease as those with positive ANCA
E. Patients with negative ANCA demonstrate no kidney disease

The answer is D

Pauci-immune vasculitis with fibrinoid necrosis and active cellular crescents is usually associated with the presence of either cANCA or pANCA. However, ANCAs are absent in 5–30% of patients with pauci-immune vasculitis. These ANCA-negative patients may have severe kidney disease as ANCA-positive patients. Eisenberger et al. studied 20 such patients (17 with microscopic polyangiitis, 2 with granulomatosis with polyangiitis, and 1 with renal-limited vasculitis) whose ANCA could not be detected with indirect immunofluorescence. Kidney biopsy findings included active crescents, glomerular necrosis as well as sclerosis and diffuse interstitial nephritis that were similar to ANCA-associated disease. Thus, a negative ANCA test does not rule out an active kidney disease, and the prognosis of ANCA-negative patients is similar to that of ANCA-positive patients. If clinical findings are suggestive of pauci-immune vasculitis, a kidney biopsy is indicated, and the treatment should be the same as ANCA-positive patients.

Suggested Reading

Eisenberger U, Fakhouri F, Vanhille P, et al. ANCA-negative pauci-immune renal vasculitis: histology and outcome. Nephrol Dial Transplant. 2005;20:1392–99.

Saha MK, Pendergraft III WF, Jennette JC. Primary glomerular diseases. In: Yu ASL, Chertow GM, Luyckx VA, et al., editors. Brenner & Rector's the kidney. 11th ed. Philadelphia: Elsevier Saunders; 2020. p. 1007–91.

68. A 19-year-old African American woman was admitted for hematuria, proteinuria, and bilateral flank pain of 4-week duration. Patient was diagnosed with SLE 4 years ago, and she is on prednisone (10 mg/day) which she takes irregularly. She does not keep up with her physicians' appointments. Her 36-year-old mother is also a lupus patient, and she is on maintenance doses of prednisone.

On phys exam, the patient did not appear ill. BP was 130/80 mm Hg. Except for mild CVA tenderness and 4+ pitting edema in lower extremities, the rest of the exam was unremarkable. Pertinent labs:

Hemoglobin:	10.1 g
Platelets:	100,000
Creatinine:	1.4 mg/dL
Albumin:	1.6 g/dL
ANA:	Positive
Complements (C3 + C4):	Normal
Urinalysis:	4+ protein; blood 2+; 30–40 RBCs, 10 WBCs, no RBC casts
24-h protein:	18 g
Duplex Doppler study of renal vein:	thrombosis bilaterally

Based on the physical examination and laboratory tests, which one of the following tests do you order next?

A. CT of the abdomen with contrast
B. Anti-sm-antibody
C. Double-stranded DNA antibody
D. Antiphospholipid antibody
E. ANCA

The answer is D

This patient has bilateral renal vein thrombosis due to hypercoagulable state, a complication of nephrotic syndrome. The appropriate test to be ordered is antiphospholipid antibody, which includes lupus anticoagulant antibody, anticardiolipin antibody, and anti-β_2 glycoprotein 1 antibody. Therefore, choice D is correct.

Antiphospholipid (APL) antibody syndrome can be either primary or secondary. This patient seems to have secondary APL antibody syndrome secondary to SLE. The APL antibody syndrome is one of several prothrombotic conditions in which thrombosis occurs in both the arterial and venous beds. A substantial number of lupus patients demonstrate lupus anticoagulant and anticardiolipin antibodies. Interestingly, lupus patients with high titers of IgG anticardiolipin antibodies may have greater incidence of thrombosis and thrombocytopenia. Lupus patients with APL antibody are at risk for the development of irreversible chronic kidney disease compared to those without APL antibody.

Patients with APL antibody syndrome without thrombosis may benefit from daily aspirin therapy. However, our patient needs full anticoagulation. Studies have shown that maintenance of INR (International Normalized Ratio) >3 is more effective than maintenance of INR between 2 and 2.9 with warfarin to prevent recurrent thrombosis. An INR value <1.9 does not confer significant protection.

Choices A, B, C, and E would not provide any useful clinical information in this patient.

Suggested Reading

Bienaimé F, Legendre C, Terzi F, et al. Antiphospholipid syndrome and kidney disease. Kidney Int. 2017;91:34–44.
Tektonidou MG. Antiphospholipid syndrome nephropathy: from pathogenesis to treatment. Front Immunol. 2018;9:1181.
Turrent-Carriles A, Herrera-Felix JP, Amigo MC. Renal involvement in antiphospholipid syndrome. Font Immunol. 2018;9:1008.

69. Following stabilization of the above patient (question 68), a kidney biopsy was performed after normalization of INR for a day. The biopsy showed pure membranous lupus nephritis (Class V) without any hypercellularity. **Which one of the following therapies do you recommend to the patient?**

A. Corticosteroids only
B. Mycophenolate mofetil (MMF) and corticosteroids
C. Corticosteroids and plasma exchange
D. Corticosteroids, cyclosporine, and cyclophosphamide
E. No treatment

The answer is B

Pure membranous lupus nephritis (MLN) is categorized as Class V lupus nephritis. At times, it may be associated with Class III (focal) or Class IV (diffuse) lupus nephritis. Pure MLN usually presents with nephrotic syndrome which is not a benign disease. Since patients with MLN are at substantial risk for complications of the nephrotic syndrome and also for ESKD, nephrologists may prefer to use immunosuppressive therapy. In support of this view are the encouraging results of MoK et al. who treated 38 patients with a combination of prednisone (5–10 mg/day) and azathioprine (1–2 mg/kg/day as tolerated). At 12 months of follow-up, 67% of patients ($N = 24$) achieved complete remission in serum creatinine and proteinuria, 22% ($N = 8$) achieved partial remission, and 11% ($N = 4$) were resistant to treatment. Further follow-up showed that the cumulative risk of renal relapse was 12% at 36 months and 16% at 60 months. Thus, the combination of prednisone and azathioprine seems to be efficacious in lupus patients with Class V nephritis.

Another clinical study from the NIH investigators compared prednisone alone (1 mg/kg/day on alternate days for 8 weeks with gradual tapering) with oral cyclosporine (5 mg/kg/day every 12 h) or intermittent pulse

cyclophosphamide (0.5–1.0 g/m² body surface area every other month for a total of 6 doses) in 42 patients with MLN to characterize the potential risks and benefits of these regimens. At 1 year, patients randomized to cyclosporine or pulse cyclophosphamide were found more likely to achieve complete or partial remission than patients randomized to prednisone alone. However, relapse of proteinuria occurred more frequently after discontinuation of cyclosporine than cyclophosphamide. Thus, cyclosporine and pulse cyclophosphamide alone are more effective than prednisone alone in inducing remission of proteinuria in patients with MLN.

Mycophenolate mofetil (MMF) seems to be equally effective in inducing remission of MLN, particularly in African Americans, as compared with IV cyclophosphamide. Thus, option B is correct. If the patient is intolerant or contraindicated to MMF, IV cyclophosphamide and corticosteroids can be used. Cyclosporine can be used instead of cyclophosphamide because of fertility issues and prone to leukopenia. Rituximab alone or with MMF have been tried. All patients with nephrotic syndrome should be on renin-angiotensin inhibitors, other medications for BP control, statins for hyperlipidemia, and anticoagulants for serum albumin levels <2.2 g/dL.

Studies have shown that addition of plasma exchange to immunosuppression does not have any benefit in inducing remission. No controlled studies have been available with the combination of corticosteroids, cyclosporine, and cyclophosphamide. Therefore, choices A, C, D, and E are incorrect. Figure 2.17 shows a logical approach to the management of MLN.

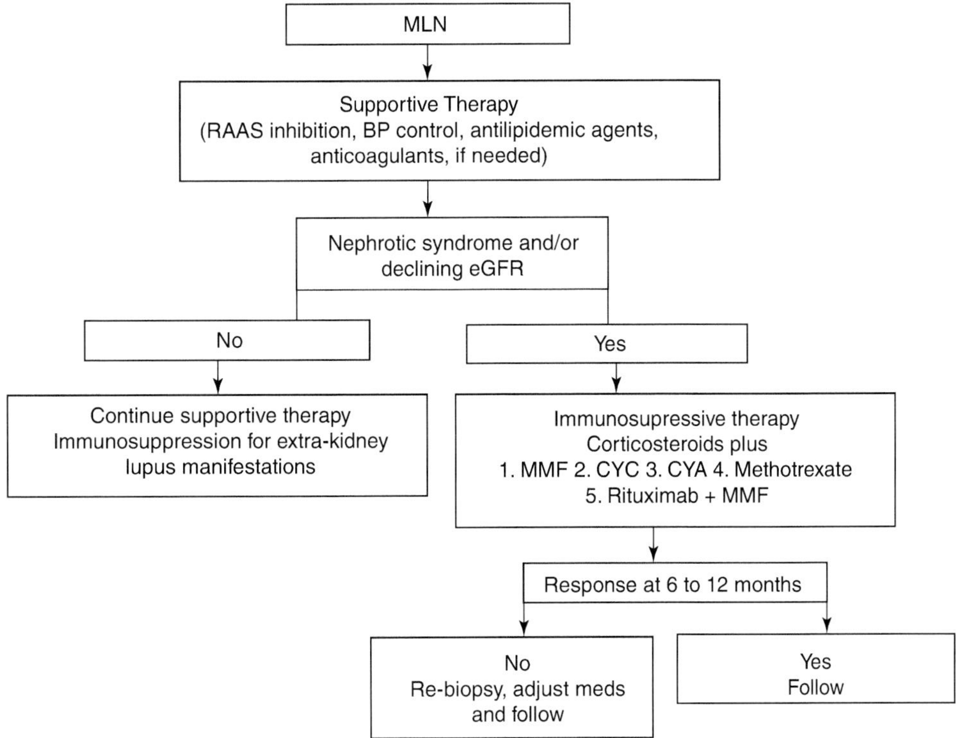

Fig. 2.17 An approach to the management of membranous lupus nephropathy (MLN) with nephrotic syndrome. Numbers 1–5 refer to the order of preference

Suggested Reading

Almaani S, Parikh S. Membranous lupus nephritis: a clinical review. Adv Chronic Kidney Dis. 2019;26:393–403.

Austin III HA, Illei GG, Braun MJ, Balow JE. Randomized, controlled trial of prednisone, cyclophosphamide, and cyclosporine in lupus membranous nephropathy. J Am Soc Nephrol. 2009;20:901–11.

Ginzler EM, Dooley MA, Aranow C, et al. Mycophenolate mofetil or intravenous cyclophosphamide for lupus nephritis. N Engl J Med. 2005;353:2219–28.

Kidney Disease: Improving Global Outcomes (KDIGO) Glomerulonephritis Work Group. KDIGO clinical practice guideline for glomerulonephritis. June 2020.

Mok CC, Ying KY, Lau CS, et al. Treatment of pure membranous lupus with prednisone and azathioprine. Am J Kidney Dis. 2004;43:269–76.

Radhakrishnan J, Moutzouris DA, Ginzler EM, et al. Mycophenolate mefetil and intravenous cyclophosphamide are similar as induction therapy for class V lupus nephritis. Kidney Int. 2010;77:152–60.

70. A 24-year-old African American woman is referred to a nephrologist for proteinuria, hematuria, and rising serum creatinine level for the last 2 weeks. She is on prednisone, 10 mg/day. Her serum creatinine is 2.1 mg/dL; anti-DNA antibody titer is markedly increased, and serum complement levels are low. Urinalysis reveals 4+ proteinuria, 3+ blood, 40 RBCs, and a few RBC casts. Kidney biopsy shows diffuse proliferative lupus nephritis (Class IV). **As per the current management, which one of the following is a better alternative to a combination of steroids and cyclophosphamide for the induction therapy of class IV lupus nephritis?**

A. Prednisone 60 mg/day orally
B. Methylprednisolone 1 g/day intravenously for 3 days followed by oral prednisone 60 mg/day
C. Oral prednisone 60 mg/day and plasma exchange
D. Oral prednisone 1 mg/kg/day with 10–20% tapering at 1-week or 2-week intervals and mycophenolate mofetil (MMF) at 500 mg twice daily to a maximum dose of 1 gram 3 times a day is as effective as IV cyclophosphamide
E. Oral prednisone 1 mg/kg/day with 10–20% tapering at 1-week or 2-week intervals and monthly intravenous cyclophosphamide (0.5 g–1 g/m^2) is superior to prednisone and MMF

The answer is D

A meta-analysis identified 25 randomized controlled trials that evaluated the benefits and risks of immunosuppressive therapies for Class IV lupus nephritis. Most of the studies compared cyclophosphamide or azathioprine plus steroids or steroids alone. Cyclophosphamide plus steroids reduced the risk for doubling of serum creatinine level as compared with steroids alone without any effect on overall mortality. Similarly, azathioprine plus steroids reduced all-cause mortality, as compared with steroids alone without any effect on kidney outcome.

The addition of plasma exchange to the above treatments did not have any further benefit. Thus, choices A, B, and C are incorrect.

Ginzler et al. conducted a 24-week trial comparing oral MMF with monthly intravenous (IV) cyclophosphamide as induction therapy for active lupus nephritis (about 55% of patients had Class IV lupus nephritis). Complete remission in 22.5% and partial remission in 29.6% occurred in patients who received MMF, as compared with 5.8% and 24.6%, respectively, in those who received cyclophosphamide. Serious infections were fewer in MMF than cyclophosphamide group. Other studies such as the Aspreva Lupus Management Study (ALMS) have shown that MMF is equally effective as IV cyclophosphamide for induction therapy of active lupus nephritis with different side effects. Currently, MMF with steroids is the preferred protocol for treatment of diffuse lupus nephritis (Class IV).

Suggested Reading

Appel GB, Contreras G, Dooley MA, et al. Aspreva Lupus Management Study Group (ALMS). Mycophenolate mofetil versus cyclophosphamide for induction treatment of lupus nephritis. J Am Soc Nephrol. 2009;20:1103–12.

Ginzler EM, Dooley MA, Aranow C, et al. Mycophenolate mofetil or intravenous cyclophosphamide for lupus nephritis. N Engl J Med. 2005;353:2219–28.

Kidney Disease: Improving Global Outcomes (KDIGO) Glomerulonephritis Work Group. KDIGO clinical practice guideline for glomerulonephritis. June 2020.

Rovin BH, Birmingham DJ, Nadasdy T. Renal involvement in systemic lupus erythmatosis. In: Coffman TM, Falk RJ, Molitoris BA, et al., editors. Schrier's diseases of the kidney. 9th ed. Philadelphia: Wolters Kluwer/Lippincott Williams & Wilkins; 2013. p. 1522–56.

71. **Which one of the following statements regarding the predictors of poor kidney survival in lupus patients is FALSE?**

A. Black race
B. Poor socioeconomic status

C. Anemia
D. High activity and chronicity index on a biopsy
E. Abnormal serology (low complement levels, high titers of anti-dsDNA)

The answer is E

The kidney survival in lupus patients depends on the severity of kidney disease, response to therapy, flare-ups of the disease, and complications of immunosuppressive therapy. Patients whose kidney disease is confined to the mesangium only have an excellent prognosis, whereas those with focal proliferative disease have variable course.

In patients with diffuse proliferative lupus nephritis, kidney survival has improved with intensive regimens. One study reported kidney survival of 89% at 1 year and 71% at 5 years. Patients with pure membranous lupus nephritis seem to have a 10-year kidney survival rate of 75% in the United States compared to 93% in Italy.

In most of these studies, black race, poor economic status, low hematocrit levels, and high activity and chronicity index on kidney biopsy portend poor kidney survival. Thus, choices A to D are correct.

Serologic abnormalities such as low complement levels or high titers of anti-DNA antibodies were not found to correlate with long-term kidney prognosis, as these abnormalities revert to normal following immunosuppressive therapy.

Suggested Reading

Contreras G, Lenz O, Pardo V, et al. Outcomes in African Americans and Hispanics with lupus nephritis. Kidney Int. 2006;69:1846–51.

Radhakrishnan J, Appel GB, D'Agati VD. Secondary glomerular disease. In: Yu ASL, Chertow GM, Luyckx VA, et al., editors. Brenner & Rector's the kidney. 11th ed. Philadelphia: Elsevier Saunders; 2020. p. 1092–164.

Rovin BH, Birmingham DJ, Nadasdy T. Renal involvement in systemic lupus erythmatosis. In: Coffman TM, Falk RJ, Molitoris BA, et al., editors. Schrier's diseases of the kidney. 9th ed. Philadelphia: Wolters Kluwer/Lippincott Williams & Wilkins; 2013. p. 1522–56.

72. An 81-year-old man with history of hypertension and on a calcium-blocker is admitted to the hospital for shortness of breath, 2–3 pillow orthopnea, and recent-onset lower extremity edema for 2 weeks. There is no history of diabetes but admits to smoking for over 45 years. Based upon jugular vein distention, crackles, and an S_3, the diagnosis of heart failure was made. An ECHO shows restrictive cardiomyopathy. Urinalysis is remarkable for 2+ proteinuria with a protein to creatinine ratio of 8 (mg/mg). Pertinent labs:

- Na^+ = 136 mEq/L
- K^+ = 3.9 mEq/L
- Cl^- = 100 mEq/L
- HCO_3^- = 22 mEq/L
- Creatinine = 1.8 mg/dL
- Glucose = 90 mg/dL
- Albumin = 2.6 g/dL
- C3 and C4 = within normal limits
- ANA = negative
- ANCA = negative
- Hepatitis B and C = negative
- Serum protein electrophoresis = no monoclonal spike

Kidney biopsy:

- LM = nodular glomerulosclerosis (Fig. 2.18a)
- IF = positive for λ (lambda) and absent for κ (kappa) chains (Fig. 2.18b)
- EM = fibrils (8–12 nm in diameter)

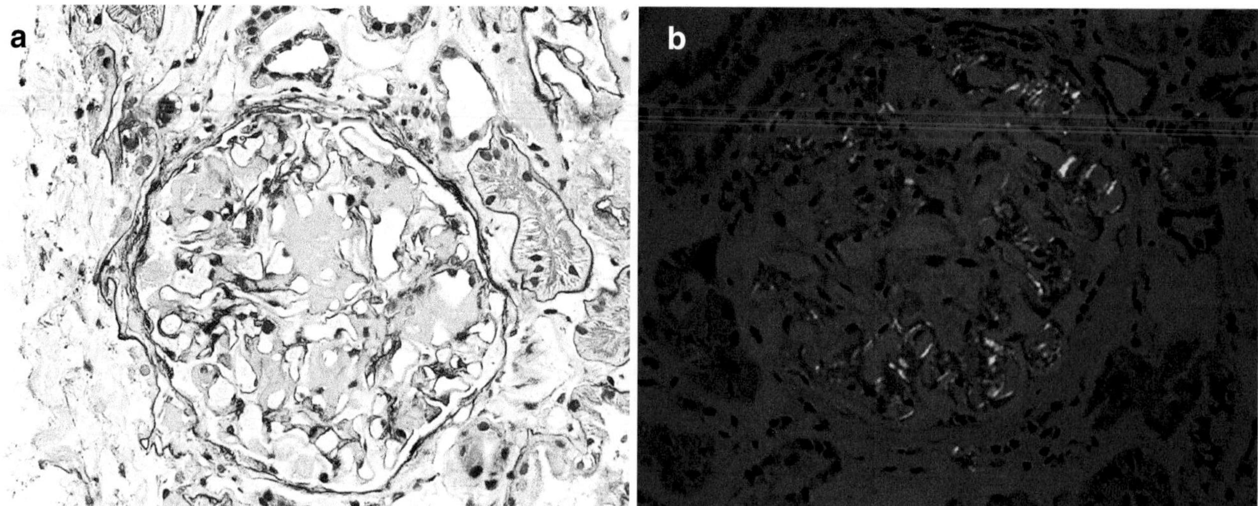

Fig. 2.18 LM (top) and IF (bottom) pattern of glomerulus in the above patient

Based on the above history, laboratory values, and kidney biopsy, which one of the following diagnoses is MOST likely in this patient?

A. Membranous nephropathy
B. Light-chain deposition disease (LCDD)
C. Amyloidosis
D. Multiple myeloma
E. Smoking-related glomerulosclerosis

The answer is C

The history, ECHO findings, urinalysis with less dipstick proteinuria and 8 g of proteinuria, and the appearance of nodules on LM as well as the presence of λ chains on IF suggest amyloidosis. The presence of nodules excludes membranous nephropathy. However, nodular glomerulosclerosis is often present in LCDD, multiple myeloma with light-chain deposition, smoking, and diabetes. In these conditions, the Congo red stain is absent. Except in multiple myeloma (not always), the urinalysis shows >2+ for proteinuria.

In LCDD, the IF shows the presence of κ chains only, and λ chains are absent. The absence of monoclonal spike on serum electrophoresis rules out the possibility of multiple myeloma. Subjects with long history of smoking do develop nephrotic syndrome, and kidney biopsy shows Congo red negative glomerular nodules. On IF microscopy, staining for both κ and λ chains is absent. Thus, options A, B, D, and E are incorrect.

Suggested Reading

Bonsib SM, editor. Atlas of medical renal pathology. New York: Springer; 2013. p. 1–266.
Fogo AB, Kashgarian M. Diagnostic atlas of renal pathology. 3rd ed. Philadelphia: Elsevier, Inc.; 2017. p. 1–546.

73. **Which one of the following pathologic findings distinguishes primary (AL) from secondary (AA) amyloidosis?**

A. Nodular appearance and positive Congo red stain of affected glomeruli by LM
B. Randomly distributed fibrils 8–12 nm in diameter by EM
C. Negative staining for immunoglobulin light chains and complements in secondary amyloidosis by IF
D. Positive staining for immunoglobulin light chains and complements in primary amyloidosis by IF
E. None of the above

The answer is C

Besides history and clinical findings, pathologic findings of the kidney also distinguish primary from secondary amyloidosis. Amyloid deposition in the mesangium and basement membrane stains positive with Congo red in

both types of amyloidosis. Also, the amyloid appears as nodules by LM. EM demonstrates nonbranching 8–12-nm-wide fibrils that are randomly distributed in the mesangium and basement membranes in both forms of amyloidosis. It is only the staining of immunoglobulin light chains and complement components that distinguishes primary from secondary amyloidosis. In primary amyloidosis, IF gives predominant staining for λ light chain than for κ light chain, and this staining is negative in secondary amyloidosis. Furthermore, staining for SAA protein is negative in primary and strongly positive in secondary amyloidosis. Thus, choice C is correct.

Suggested Reading

Radhakrishnan J, Appel GB, D'Agati VD. Secondary glomerular disease. In: Yu ASL, Chertow GM, Luyckx VA, et al., editors. Brenner & Rector's the kidney. 11th ed. Philadelphia: Elsevier Saunders; 2020. p. 1092–164.

74. A 56-year-old woman is admitted for nausea, vomiting, and weight loss. BP is 150/90 mm Hg. Except for pitting edema in lower extremities, phys exam is otherwise unremarkable. Serum creatinine is 8.4 mg/dL, BUN 100 mg/dL, albumin 2.1 g/dL, glucose 80 mg/dL, C3 and C4 normal, and ANA negative. Urinalysis reveals 4+ protein, 1+ blood, and 24-h proteinuria is 8.1 g. Urine immunoelectrophoresis demonstrates a monoclonal spike. Following stabilization on hemodialysis, a kidney biopsy shows nodular glomerulosclerosis by LM and strong staining for κ light chains. Congo red staining is negative (see Fig. 2.19).

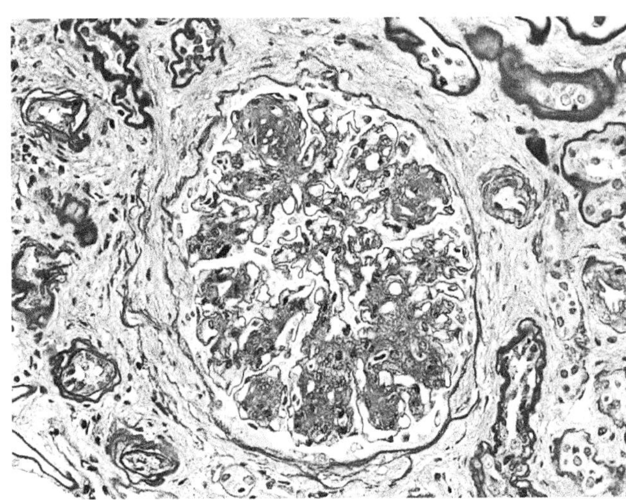

Fig. 2.19 Glomerular appearance by LM in the above patient

Which one of the following is the MOST possible diagnosis in this patient?

A. Primary (AL) amyloidosis
B. Diabetic glomerulosclerosis (GS)
C. MPGN (type I)
D. Light-chain deposition disease (LCDD)
E. Heavy-chain deposition disease (HCDD)

The answer is D

All of the diseases stated above demonstrate nodular GS. However, light (LM) immunofluorescence (IF) and electron microscopy (EM) distinguish among all types of glomerular lesions (see Table 2.6). Congo red staining is positive in patients with amyloidosis and absent in other forms of glomerular diseases. κ light-chain staining is strongest in LCDD, whereas λ light-chain staining is predominant in primary amyloidosis. Staining of both light chains is absent in HCDD. Double contour (tram-track) of glomerular basement membrane and subendothelial deposits are diagnostic of type I MPGN. Fibrils are absent in MPGN, LCDD, and HCDD.

Table 2.6 Predominant pathologic findings in some glomerular diseases with nodular appearance

Disease	LM	IF	EM
Amyloidosis	Nodules are Congo red positive	Predominantly λ chain staining	Fibrils 8–12 nm in diameter
Diabetic GS	Nodules are Congo red negative	Infrequently IgG, κ, and λ chain staining. Congo red negative	Thickening of GBM, and fibrils with variable size
MPGN type I	Lobules with double BMs (tram-track appearance). Congo red negative	IgG, IgM, and C3 staining	Subendothelial deposits. No fibrils
LCDD	Nodules are Congo red negative	Predominantly κ chain staining	No fibrils
HCDD	Nodules are Congo red negative	Predominantly heavy-chain (γ) staining. No κ or λ chain staining	No fibrils
Fibrillary GN	Nodules are Congo red negative	IgG and to a lesser extent C3 staining in mesangium and GBM. IgG4 is the dominant subclass	Fibrils 12–20 nm in diameter
Immunotactoid glomerulopathy	Nodules are Congo red negative	Predominant for IgG with lesser staining for IgA, IgM, C3, and C1q in capillary loops than in the mesangium	Microtubular structures >30 nm in diameter
Smoking	Nodules are Congo red negative	Less strong linear staining for IgG and albumin along GBM and TBM. Absent IgM, IgA, C3, C1q, κ, and λ staining	Diffuse thickening of GBM and increase in mesangial matrix

The predominant staining for κ light chains by IF and clinical features support the diagnosis of LCDD, which is one of the subtypes and most common form of monoclonal immunoglobulin deposition disease. Nephrotic syndrome and dialysis dependency are present in about 25% of patients at time of presentation. Most patients with LCDD are also hypertensive, and hematuria is present in a substantial number of patients. Thus, option D is correct.

The presence of nodules is also seen in other glomerular diseases such as fibrillary glomerulonephritis, immunotactoid glomerulopathy, thrombotic microangiopathy, fibronectin glomerulopathy, collagen III glomerulopathy, and in subjects with smoking history. The term "idiopathic nodular GS" is used to describe a glomerular lesion that has been demonstrated in nondiabetic subjects with history of smoking and chronic hypertension.

Table 2.6 shows some pathologic findings that distinguish some glomerular diseases that demonstrate nodules on LM.

Suggested Reading

Bonsib SM, editor. Atlas of medical renal pathology. New York: Springer; 2013. p. 1–266.

Fogo AB, Kashgarian M. Diagnostic atlas of renal pathology. 3rd ed. Philadelphia: Elsevier, Inc.; 2017. p. 1–546.

Nasr SH, D'Agati VD. Nodular glomerulosclerosis in the nondiabetic smoker. J Am Soc Nephrol. 2007;18:2032–6.

Surya Venkataseshan V, Churg J. Diabetes and other metabolic diseases. In: Silva FG, D'Agati VD, Nadasdy T, editors. Renal biopsy interpretation. New York: Churchill Livingstone; 1996. p. 221–57.

75. **Which one of the following kidney manifestations in patients with multiple myeloma is FALSE?**

A. Acute tubular necrosis
B. Cast nephropathy
C. AL amyloid as well as light-chain deposition disease (LCDD)
D. Interstitial fibrosis and tubular atrophy
E. Focal segmental glomerulosclerosis (FSGS)

The answer is E

The kidney is affected in several ways in multiple myeloma. Acute kidney injury (AKI) due to tubular necrosis is at times an early presentation in patients with multiple myeloma. AKI is usually precipitated by volume depletion, hypercalcemia, or nephrotoxins. Some light chains may be toxic to proximal tubule cells, resulting in acute tubular necrosis.

Myeloma cast nephropathy (previously called myeloma kidney) refers to the presence of large and numerous casts in the distal tubule, the collecting duct, and also the proximal tubule. The casts are composed mainly of light

chains, either λ or κ light chains. When an increased load of light chains is delivered to the tubule, they aggregate with Tamm-Horsfall protein and co-precipitate as casts. Colchicine prevents the aggregation and separates light chains from Tamm-Horsfall protein.

Patients with cast nephropathy present with AKI alone or AKI superimposed on chronic kidney disease due to obstruction by casts in the tubular segments as well as injury to the proximal tubule cells.

Deposition of AL amyloid in glomeruli, tubules, and blood vessels leads to the presence of amyloidosis. A distinction between myeloma-associated AL amyloidosis and primary amyloidosis is difficult to make clinically because they represent two ends of the same entity. However, the prognosis in primary amyloidosis is dependent on the pathogenic role of light chains than the underlying hematologic disease in multiple myeloma. Also, light-chain deposition is seen in some patients. About 20–40% of LCDD patients have the evidence of multiple myeloma. Like AL amyloidosis, LCDD is often the presenting disease that leads to the diagnosis of multiple myeloma at an early stage.

The presence of casts leads not only to obstruction but also tubulointerstitial disease. In addition to proximal tubular necrosis, interstitial fibrosis and tubular atrophy have been documented. When such chronic changes are seen, chances of recovery in renal function are extremely rare. Glomeruli generally show mild mesangial changes unless amyloidosis or LCDD is present. FSGS has not been demonstrated as a part of multiple myeloma. Thus, choice D is false.

Suggested Reading

Bonsib SM, editor. Atlas of medical renal pathology. New York: Springer; 2013. p. 1–266.

Fogo AB, Kashgarian M. Diagnostic atlas of renal pathology. 3rd ed. Philadelphia: Elsevier, Inc.; 2017. p. 1–546.

Korbet SM, Schwartz MM. Multiple myeloma. J Am Soc Nephrol. 2006;17:2533–45.

Saha MK, Pendergraft III WF, Jennette JC. Primary glomerular diseases. In: Yu ASL, Chertow GM, Luyckx VA, et al., editors. Brenner & Rector's the kidney. 11th ed. Philadelphia: Elsevier Saunders; 2020. p. 1007–91.

76. A 50-year-old African American woman with hepatitis C virus (HCV) is admitted for maculopapular rash in lower extremities and joint pains. There are no skin ulcers. She is not on any medications. Her BP is 140/80 mm Hg. Serum creatinine is 2.8 mg/dL and stable (serum creatinine was 1.1 mg/dL 1 month ago) with an eGFR of 49 mL/min. ANA is negative with normal C3 but depressed C4 level. Cryoglobulins are strongly positive. Urinalysis shows 4+ protein, 1+ blood with 4–6 RBCs. There are no RBC casts. A 24-h proteinuria is 5.4 g. A kidney biopsy reveals membranoproliferative glomerulonephritis (MPGN) type I without crescents.

Which one of the following therapies is APPROPRIATE for this patient?

A. Corticosteroids only
B. Corticosteroids and plasma exchange for 2 weeks
C. Pegylated (peg) interferon-α and ribavirin
D. Corticosteroids and rituximab followed by direct-acting antiviral agents (DAAs)
E. Corticosteroids, interferon-α, and ribavirin

The answer is D

Cryoglobulins are circulating immunoglobulins that precipitate at cold temperature and dissolve at warm temperature. This patient has mixed cryoglobulinemia and MPGN due to HCV infection. The goals of treatment for this patient are to improve her symptoms and eliminate HCV infection.

Previous studies have shown steroids, and cytotoxic drugs were used to suppress cryoglobulins produced; however, in selected patients, addition of plasma exchange was beneficial. Therefore, choices A and B do not entirely apply to the patient because antiviral therapy is not included.

Earlier studies reported that interferon-α improved kidney function, proteinuria, and viremia in HCV-induced kidney disease. Addition of ribavirin has shown better response, but the drug may not be well tolerated in severe kidney failure. Combination of steroids with interferon-α and ribavirin may not have adequate response in this patient. Thus, choices C and E are incorrect.

The introduction of DAAs made the use of interferon and/or ribavirin therapy obsolete. DAA not only abolishes viral RNA titers but also improves kidney lesions caused by cryoglobulins. Initially, corticosteroids (1 mg/kg/day or 60 mg/day) should be started to suppress inflammation and improve the patient's symptoms. Simultaneously, rituximab (375 mg/m^2 weekly for 4 weeks) should be started or rituximab monotherapy, as

suggested by a few randomized control trials. DAAs need to be started to completely abolish viral RNA levels. Thus, answer D is correct.

With this treatment, viral RNA titers and cryoglobulins were undetectable and her symptoms improved with reduction in creatinine and urine protein levels.

Suggested Reading

Kidney Disease: Improving Global Outcomes (KDIGO) Hepatitis C Work Group. KDIGO 2018 clinical practice guideline for the prevention, diagnosis, evaluation, and treatment of hepatitis C in chronic kidney disease. Kidney Int Suppl. 2018;8:91–165.

77. An 80-year-old Caucasian man is admitted for nausea, vomiting, weakness, and poor appetite. BP is 170/90 mm Hg. Serum creatinine is 10 mg/dL. Urinalysis shows hematuria, pyuria, proteinuria, and few RBC casts. His serum creatinine level was 1.8 mg/dL 6 weeks ago. He has no history of upper respiratory tract infection. **Which one of the following glomerular lesions would MOST likely be found in this patient?**

A. Membranous nephropathy (MN)
B. Fibrillary glomerulonephritis (GN)
C. Amyloidosis
D. Pauci-immune crescentic GN
E. Acute poststreptococcal GN (APSGN)

The answer is D

The findings on urinalysis are suggestive of acute nephritis. Acute GN in the elderly develops most commonly due to rapidly progressive GN. Amyloidosis and MN do not usually cause acute nephritic syndrome unless superimposed by crescentic GN. There is no history of sore throat or pharyngitis to suggest APSGN, although about 23% incidence of APSGN has been reported in patients older than 55 years of age.

Fibrillary GN is a good possibility; however, the mean age of patients presenting with fibrillary GN is 49 years (range from 21 to 75 years). Kidney dysfunction, hematuria, hypertension, and proteinuria in the nephrotic range are clinical features at time of presentation in these patients.

The most likely possibility in the patient presented with acute nephritic syndrome is pauci-immune crescentic GN, which is the commonly found kidney disease in elderly patients >80 years of age. In one study, pauci-immune crescentic GN was the diagnosis for AKI in 79 (31.2%) of 259 biopsies in adults aged 60 years or older. Another study reported pauci-immune GN, the most frequently observed disease on biopsy, in 19.2% of patients older than 80 years of age. Thus, choice D appears to be the correct answer for this patient.

Suggested Reading

Choudhury D, Raj DSC, Levi M. Effect of aging on renal function and disease. In: Brenner BM, editor. Brenner & Rector's the kidney. 7th ed. Philadelphia: Saunders; 2004. p. 2305–41.

Haas M, Spargo BH, Wit EJ, et al. Etiologies and outcome of acute renal insufficiency in older adults: a renal biopsy study of 259 cases. Am J Kidney Dis. 2000;35:433–47.

Moutzouris D-A, Herlitz L, Appel GB, et al. Renal biopsy in the very elderly. Clin J Am Soc Nephrol. 2009;4:1072–82.

78. A 64-year-old obese woman is being treated with vancomycin and cefepime for 10 days and you are consulted for rising serum creatinine from 0.6 mg/dL to 2.4 mg/dL. Her random vancomycin levels are 40 ng/mL. Her serum K^+ is 5.9 mEq/L, Cl^- 114 mEq/L, and HCO_3^- 16 mEq/L. A urinalysis reveals trace blood, 1+ protein, 6–10 RBCs, 30–40 WBCs, and occasional WBC casts. You make the diagnosis of acute tubulointerstitial disease (TID). **Which one of the following choices regarding acute TID is FALSE?**

A. The triad of fever, rash, and eosinophilia occurs only in one-third of patients
B. Acute TID usually presents clinically with sudden decrement in kidney function, most commonly in an asymptomatic patient who was treated with a new medication, or experienced an intervening illness
C. On kidney biopsy, the glomeruli and blood vessels are usually spared. The interstitium contains a few neutrophils, but mostly T cells ($CD4^+$ and $CD8^+$), macrophages, and eosinophils
D. Gallium (^{67}Ga) scan definitely distinguishes acute TID from acute tubular necrosis (ATN)
E. Kidney failure is usually oliguric with FE_{Na} >2% and hyperkalemia disproportionate to the degree of kidney failure

The answer is D

Drug-induced acute TID, particularly penicillin, has been shown to clinically present with skin rash in <50%, fever in 75%, and eosinophilia in 80% of patients. However, most studies reported that the triad is present in approximately 33% of the patients. Eosinophiluria has a poor positive predictive value (38%) for acute TID. Furthermore, eosinophiluria is documented in individuals with cystitis, prostatitis, and pyelonephritis

The typical presentation in patient with acute TID is a sudden decrease in kidney function with oliguria and a defect in K^+ secretion, resulting in hyperkalemia that is disproportionate to the degree of kidney dysfunction. Also, the tubular reabsorption of sodium is decreased, resulting in FE_{Na} >2%. Oliguric kidney failure is more frequent than nonoliguric kidney failure. Oliguria may be related to severe interstitial inflammation and edema causing tubular obstruction and decreased urine flow.

In certain cases, acute TID is not clear. The only way to establish the diagnosis is performing a kidney biopsy, which shows cellular infiltration, tubulitis, breaks in tubular basement membrane, atrophy, and loss of tubules (see Fig. 2.20). Fibrosis may be seen as early as 10 days after the onset of illness. Extensive fibrosis carries a poor kidney prognosis. Although neutrophils are common, mononuclear cells, including T lymphocytes and macrophages, remain the predominant cell types. Overall $CD4^+$ T cells predominate relative to $CD8^+$ T cells.

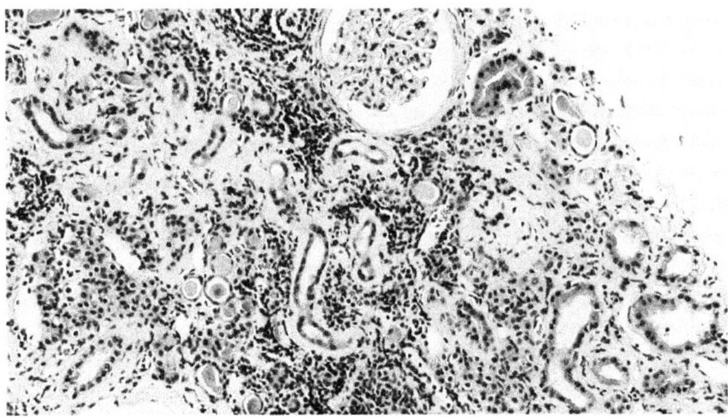

Fig. 2.20 LM photograph of acute tubulointerstitial nephritis showing interstitial edema, infiltrates of lymphocytes, monocytes, and plasma cells. The glomerulus (top) is normal

In acute TID, the glomeruli are normal looking and arterial or arteriolar changes are usually absent. When present, they may represent age-related changes.

In early 1980s, it was reported that drug-induced acute TID had increased renal uptake of ^{67}Ga in contrast to patients with ATN in whom ^{67}Ga uptake was minimal. It was subsequently shown that ^{67}Ga uptake was positive only in 58% of patients with acute TID. Also, ^{67}Ga is positive in minimal change disease and cortical necrosis. Thus, ^{67}Ga test has low predictive value for acute TID, and the choice D, therefore, is false.

Suggested Reading

Graham F, Lord M, Froment D, et al. The use of gallium-67 scintigraphy in the diagnosis of acute interstitial nephritis. Clin Kidney J. 2016;9:76–81.

Linton AL, Richmond JM, Clark WF, et al. Gallium67 scintigraphy in the diagnosis of acute renal disease. Clin Nephrol. 1985;24:84–7.

Perazella MA, Rosner MH. Tubulointerstitial *d*iseases. In: Yu ASL, Chertow GM, Luyckx VA, et al., editors. Brenner & Rector's the kidney. 11th ed. Philadelphia: Elsevier Saunders; 2020. p. 1196–222.

Rossert JA, Fischer EA. Acute interstitial nephritis. In: Feehally J, Floege J, Tonelli M, et al., editors. Comprehensive clinical nephrology. 6th ed. Philadelphia: Elsevier; 2019. p. 729–37.

Wood BC, Sharma JN, Germann DR, et al. Gallium citrate Ga 67 imaging in noninfectious interstitial nephritis. Arch Intern Med. 1978;138:1665–6.

79. **Regarding treatment of acute tubulointerstitial disease (TID), which one of the following therapeutic interventions is FALSE?**

   A. Withholding the offending agent or drug
   B. Institution of corticosteroids within 2 weeks of acute TID is superior to institution of corticosteroids 3 weeks after acute TID in maintaining serum creatinine ~1 mg/dL in those who do not improve kidney function in <2 weeks and without infection
   C. Consider combination therapy with cyclophosphamide in patients with severe acute TID who do not respond to corticosteroids within 2–3 weeks
   D. Consider corticosteroids, cyclophosphamide, and plasma exchange in patients with antitubular basement membrane antibodies
   E. Corticosteroids alone or in combination with cyclophosphamide is the preferred form of therapy for severe interstitial fibrosis to prevent progression of the disease

   The answer is E

   Removal or withholding the drug with supportive care improves kidney function in many patients. However, continued exposure to the drug may cause irreversible kidney damage, requiring renal replacement therapy. It is of interest to note that acute TID accounts for 18.6% of cases of acute kidney injury in patients older than 60 years of age. Also, of interest to note that discontinuation of the drug does not guarantee complete recovery of kidney function. Therefore, immunosuppressive therapy is indicated in some patients; however, the therapy is controversial.

   Corticosteroids at 1 mg/kg/day orally or an equivalent dose intravenously have been used successfully. If patients show improvement in kidney function within 7–10 days, the drug should be continued for 4–6 weeks and then tapered over the next several weeks. If no improvement in 2–3 weeks, therapy can either be discontinued or addition of cyclophosphamide (2 mg/kg/day) may be considered and continued for 5–6 weeks. If no response, the drug should be discontinued. In responders, cyclophosphamide should be continued for 1 year. Steroids should be tapered and discontinued. The dose of cyclophosphamide is adjusted based upon the WBC count, kidney function, and age. The time of initiation of therapy is important in preserving the kidney function. When therapy was initiated within 2 weeks, the serum creatinine remained ~1 mg/dL, whereas serum creatinine stabilized at 3 mg/dL 3 weeks after initiation of therapy. Mycophenolate mofetil has been tried in those who are intolerant to steroids or steroid resistance. These patients include diabetics, obese, or other patients in whom steroids are not an ideal agent.

   Corticosteroids (1 mg/kg/day), cyclophosphamide (2 mg/kg/day), and plasma exchange (10 treatments in a 2-week period) may be considered in patients with documented acute TID due to antitubular basement membrane antibodies.

   The presence of significant fibrosis may not warrant immunosuppressive therapy because toxicity may outweigh the benefit of the therapy. Thus, choice E is false.

   Suggested Reading

Lerma EV. Acute tubulointerstitial nephritis. In: Lerma EV, Berns JS, Nissenson AR, editors. Current diagnosis & treatment: nephrology & hypertension. New York: McGraw Hill; 2009. p. 313–9.
Neilson EG. Pathogenesis and therapy of interstitial nephritis. Kidney Int. 1989;35:1257–70.
Smith JP, Neilson EG. Treatment of acute interstitial nephritis. In: Wilcox CS, editor. Therapy in nephrology and hypertension. Philadelphia: Saunders/Elsevier; 2008. p. 313–9.

80. A 56-year-old housewife, recently migrated from Belgium, is referred to you for bilateral flank pain, chronic headache, nausea, vomiting, and poor appetite. BP is 160/90 mm Hg with a pulse rate of 74 beats/min. Her serum creatinine is 5.2 mg/dL, BUN 100 mg/dL, and uric of 4.1 mg/dL. A urinalysis reveals 1+ blood, 3+ protein, many WBCs (30–40), 10–12 RBCs, and no RBC casts. A tentative diagnosis of analgesic nephropathy is made. **Which one of the following choices regarding analgesic nephropathy is FALSE?**

   A. Analgesic nephropathy accounts for 10–20% of patients with ESKD in Belgium, Scotland, and Australia
   B. On presentation, patients frequently have nocturia, sterile pyuria, hypertension, and evidence of papillary necrosis
   C. Analgesic nephropathy develops only in those who take combination of analgesics including aspirin, acetaminophen, phenacetin, caffeine, or codeine, but not in those who ingest acetaminophen only
   D. Light microscopy of the kidney shows tubular atrophy, fibrosis of the interstitium, predominance of lymphocytes, and thickened tubular basement membranes
   E. Papillary calcification, reduced kidney volume, and bumpy kidney contour on noncontrast CT of kidneys

   The answer is C

Epidemiologic studies have shown an association between long-term ingestion of analgesics and chronic tubulointerstitial disease (TID) and papillary necrosis, which varies among different countries. Analgesic nephropathy is a common cause of CKD in Belgium, Scotland, and Australia, and accounts for 10–20% of patients with ESKD.

Analgesic nephropathy is 5–7 times more frequent in women than men. One needs to ingest at least 6 tablets daily for >3 years (or 2–3 g of the index drug) to develop CKD. Because of long-term ingestion, patients, particularly women, do not seek medical attention until CKD is far advanced. On presentation, patients complain of nocturia due to decreased concentrating ability, hypertension, and symptoms of CKD. Sterile pyuria is very common. In some patients, concomitant glomerular disease is also present because of nephrotic-range proteinuria as well as papillary necrosis.

Anemia is extremely common, which is due to both kidney disease and blood loss from peptic ulcer disease. Hypouricemia is also common secondary to decreased absorption by the damaged tubules.

Kidney biopsy findings are consistent with chronic TID, including tubular atrophy, severe interstitial fibrosis, dilatation of tubules with flattened epithelial cells, and thickened tubular basement membranes. Cellular infiltrates in the interstitium and between tubules and a few neutrophils, plasma cells, or eosinophils are frequently seen. As chronic TID progresses, glomerular abnormalities are also seen, including periglomerular fibrosis, segmental sclerosis, and ultimate global sclerosis (see Fig. 2.21)

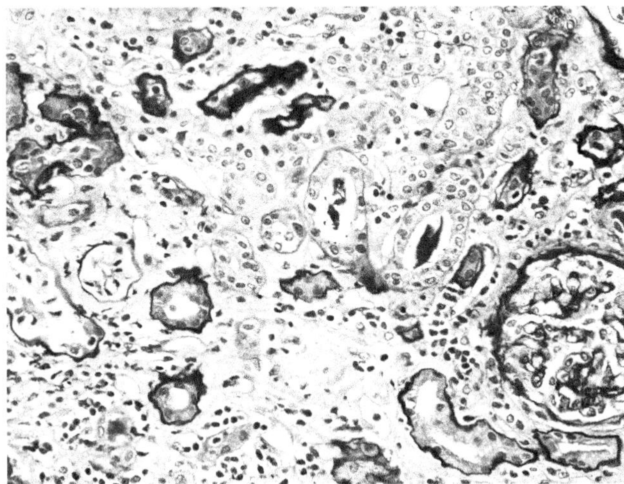

Fig. 2.21 Chronic tubulointerstitial nephritis showing tubular atrophy, tubular basement membrane thickening, tubular fibrosis, lymphocytic infiltration, periglomerular thickening, and an increase in mesangial matrix

Recent studies have shown that noncontrast CT may reveal some kidney abnormalities that are suggestive of analgesic nephropathy. These abnormalities include papillary calcification, reduced kidney volume, and bumpy kidney contours. Of these, papillary calcification has a high sensitivity and specificity for analgesic nephropathy.

In the United States, the incidence of analgesic nephropathy varies among different geographical areas. Of interest is the observation that analgesic use in North Carolina is associated with increased risk for kidney disease in those patients with excessive ingestion of only acetaminophen. Thus, not only the combination drugs, but acetaminophen ingestion alone can cause kidney disease. Therefore, choice C is false.

Suggested Reading

Perazella MA, Rosner MH. Tubulointerstitial diseases. In: Yu ASL, Chertow GM, Luyckx VA, et al., editors. Brenner & Rector's the kidney. 11th ed. Philadelphia: Elsevier Saunders; 2020. p. 1196–222.

Rossert JA, Fischer EA. Acute interstitial nephritis. In: Feehally J, Floege J, Tonelli M, et al., editors. Comprehensive clinical nephrology. 6th ed. Philadelphia: Elsevier; 2019. p. 729–37.

81. A 50-year-old man presents with toe pain on and off for over 6 months. Significant past medical history includes alcohol abuse and questionable exposure of kidneys to radiation 20 years earlier because of motor vehicle accident. He has been diagnosed with hypertension 1 year ago, and is being treated with losartan, an angiotensin-receptor blocker (ARB) 100 mg daily. He admits to occasional moonshine ingestion. Serum creatinine is 0.9 mg/dL, and uric acid is 7.8 mg/dL. Hemoglobin is 13.2 g. **Based on the above history, his toe pain and hypertension may be related to which one of the following conditions?**

A. Analgesic nephropathy
B. Cadmium nephropathy

C. Lead nephropathy
D. Balkan nephropathy
E. Radiation nephritis

The answer is C

The most likely diagnosis in this patient is lead nephropathy which causes chronic tubulointerstitial disease (TID) with interstitial fibrosis, tubular atrophy, and nephrosclerosis. History of moonshine ingestion is an important historical clue to the ingestion of lead and its clinical sequelae, including hyperuricemia, hypertension, and recurrent gouty attacks (saturnine gout). Lead is preferentially deposited in S3 portion of the proximal tubule, and nuclear inclusions in cells of this tubule are characteristic of lead nephropathy.

Excretion of lead >0.6 mg (or >600 μg) in a 24-h urine sample after two 1 g doses of CaNA2 EDTA confirms the diagnosis of lead nephropathy. EDTA has been advocated not only as a diagnostic tool but also as a therapeutic modality to prevent or reverse progression of renal disease. Analgesic ingestion is possible because of motor vehicle accident. However, analgesic nephropathy frequently presents with nocturia, hypertension, and sterile pyuria. Serum uric acid level is low to normal because of decreased absorption due to tubular dysfunction despite an increase in serum creatinine level. Thus, choice A is incorrect.

Cadmium nephropathy is common in subjects with chronic low-dose exposure. This metal-containing compound is widely used in plastic, metal, alloys, and electrical equipment manufacturing industries. Cadmium is mostly stored in the kidneys and to some extent, in the liver. Proximal tubular dysfunction is rather common. Also, distal renal tubular acidosis with osteomalacia and nephrolithiasis (due to hypercalciuria) has been described in cadmium nephropathy. Clinically, patients present with hypertension, bone pain, and CKD. Chronic TID is a common pathologic finding on a renal biopsy. A major outbreak of cadmium toxicity occurred in the 1950s, which was characterized by severe bone pain with bone fractures in older women. This disease was named "itai-itai or ouch-ouch" disease. There is no effective treatment for cadmium nephropathy. The patient presented in the question does not have any industrial exposure to cadmium. Therefore, choice B is incorrect.

Balkan nephropathy is a form of chronic TID with slow progression to ESKD, which is exclusively confined to areas in former Yugoslavia, Bulgaria, and Romania. Hypertension occurs in the late stages of the disease. Therefore, choice D is incorrect.

Radiation nephritis is a consideration in this patient. In the acute form of radiation nephritis, which occurs within 1 year of radiation, hypertension is rather common. However, anemia and edema are also present. The chronic form of radiation nephritis is characterized by hypertension, proteinuria, and progressive kidney disease with eventual development of ESKD. The histologic features of the kidney include chronic TID as well as arteriolar thrombotic changes, leading to glomerular sclerosis. The patient presented in the question does not have either anemia or CKD. Therefore, choice E is incorrect.

Suggested Reading

Perazella MA, Rosner MH. Tubulointerstitial diseases. In: Yu ASL, Chertow GM, Luyckx VA, et al., editors. Brenner & Rector's the kidney. 11th ed. Philadelphia: Elsevier Saunders; 2020. p. 1196–222.

Rossert JA, Fischer EA. Acute interstitial nephritis. In: Feehally J, Floege J, Tonelli M, et al., editors. Comprehensive clinical nephrology. 6th ed. Philadelphia: Elsevier; 2019. p. 729–37.

82. A 25-year-old Filipino man is seen in the outpatient clinic for dysuria and occasional flank pain for 6 months. He is not on any medications. A urinalysis reveals blood, proteinuria, 20–30 RBCs, and 30–40 WBCs. There are no RBC or WBC casts. Leukocyte esterase is negative. Gram stain and cultures are negative. Patient was sent home on doxycycline 100 mg twice daily.

Ten days later, he comes back with similar complaints. Repeat urinalysis shows similar findings. Serum creatinine is 1.8 mg/dL. A KUB shows nephrocalcinosis. An ultrasound of the kidneys reveals normal size kidneys with 1 cm stones. A CXR is normal. **Based upon the above history and clinical findings, which one of the following is the MOST likely diagnosis?**

A. IgA nephropathy
B. Acute uncomplicated cystitis
C. Nephrolithiasis
D. Recurrent cystitis
E. Tuberculosis (TB) of the kidney

The answer is E

The most likely diagnosis in this patient is TB of the kidney because of dysuria, hematuria, and sterile pyuria. Renal calcification further supports the diagnosis of TB of the kidney. In one study, dysuria, hematuria, pyuria, and flank pain were the most frequent symptoms of active urinary TB. Gram stain shows no bacteria, but acid-fast stain demonstrates mycobacterium tuberculosis in 90% of patients with active disease, and routine urine cultures are negative.

Sterile pyuria is seen in patients with analgesic or NSAID-induced tubulointerstitial disease, or in some patients with xanthogranulomatous pyelonephritis, and in patients with chlamydial infections.

Although KUB demonstrates renal calcification, either CT or IVP shows strictures of the ureters, cavities, or renal calcifications alone or in combination in patients with TB of the kidney.

TB of the kidney results from pulmonary TB. However, the clinical presentation of kidney TB may not be apparent for many years even after pulmonary TB had subsided. In fact, the patient presented here was inadequately treated for active pulmonary TB 5 years ago in the Philippines prior to his emigration to the United States. This is the reason why his CXR is normal despite active TB of the kidney.

IgA nephropathy is considered because of his geographic location and hematuria. However, IgA nephropathy does not usually present with dysuria or flank pain.

Bacteriuria is common in patients with either acute uncomplicated or recurrent cystitis, although dysuria and hematuria are present in these patients. Antibiotic treatment improves these symptoms.

Nephrolithiasis may present with flank pain and hematuria. However, dysuria may implicate lower urinary tract infection in patients with nephrolithiasis, which responds to antibiotics. Thus, choices A to D are incorrect.

Suggested Reading

Merchant S, Bharati A, Merchant N. Tuberculosis of the genitourinary system-urinary tract tuberculosis-Part 1. Indian J Radiol Imaging. 2013;23:46–63.

Visweswaran RK, Jayakumar KP. Tuberculosis of the urinary tract. In: Feehally J, Floege J, Tonelli M, et al., editors. Comprehensive clinical nephrology. 6th ed. Philadelphia: Elsevier; 2019. p. 639–49.

83. A 40-year-old woman presents to the Emergency Department with weakness of lower extremities and difficulty in ambulation. She started having these symptoms gradually over a 4-week period. She denies taking any medications other than some herbal medications for "slimming" her body. Her BP is 150/88 mm Hg with a heart rate of 90 bpm. Serum chemistry is as follows: Sodium 136 mEq/L, potassium 2.2 mEq/L, chloride 110 mEq/L, bicarbonate 16 mEq/L, creatinine 3.6 mg/dL, and BUN 80 mg/dL. Based on the history and serum chemistry, you make the diagnosis of aristolochic acid nephropathy (previously known as Chinese herb nephropathy). **Which one of the following statements regarding aristolochic acid nephropathy is FALSE?**

A. Aristolochic acid nephropathy is similar to Balkan endemic nephropathy with similar clinical course
B. Most patients with aristolochic acid nephropathy have rapid progression of kidney disease to ESKD within months
C. Initially presentation may be hypokalemia with renal K wasting, hyperchloremic metabolic acidosis, hypouricemia, hypophosphatemia, and glucosuria
D. Kidney biopsy shows extensive interstitial fibrosis with tubular atrophy, intimal thickening of interlobular arteries, and global sclerosis of glomeruli
E. Transitional cell carcinoma is a frequent occurrence in patients with aristolochic acid nephropathy

The answer is A

In early 1990s, an outbreak of rapidly progressive kidney failure to ESKD occurred in association with ingestion of Chinese herbs as a weight-reduction regimen in Belgium. Kidney failure did not improve after discontinuation of herbal medication. This syndrome was incorrectly named Chinese herb nephropathy. Similar outbreaks occurred in Taiwan and Japan following the consumption of a similar herbal medication and named herbal nephropathy. Chemical analysis of this herbal medication revealed aristolochic acid, as one of the constituents. The nephrotoxicity of aristolochic acid was proven in experimental animals. Thus, the disease is renamed aristolochic acid nephropathy.

In many ways, aristolochic acid nephropathy resembles Balkan nephropathy except for its clinical course which is rapid and ESKD occurs in months in the former disease rather than years (>20 years) as in Balkan nephropathy. There is some evidence that the pathogenesis in Balkan nephropathy involves ingestion of aristolochic acid from wheat contaminated with seeds of Aristolochia clematitis. Thus, choice A is false.

Clinically, patients with aristolochic acid nephropathy present with Fanconi syndrome and kidney failure. Hypokalemia due to increased K wasting is commonly seen with weakness and symmetric paralysis of lower extremities, as in the case. A kidney biopsy shows advanced interstitial fibrosis with tubular atrophy and loss of cortex. Interlobular arteries demonstrate fibromucoid intimal thickening, and glomeruli show global sclerosis. Although these changes are irreversible, corticosteroid treatment prevented the need for kidney replacement therapy in some patients as compared with the control subjects.

In a substantial number of patients with aristolochic acid nephropathy, urothelial carcinoma (mostly in the ureter) was rather common accounting for 46% in prevalence, and bilateral nephrectomy with removal of ureters was suggested as a preventive measure of the carcinoma.

Suggested Reading

Cosyns JP. Aristolochic acid and 'Chinese herbs nephropathy': a review of the evidence to date. Drug Saf. 2003;26:33–42.

Debelle FD, Vanher weghem J-L, Nortier JL. Aristolochic acid nephropathy: a worldwide problem. Kidney Int. 2008;74:158–69.

Gökman MR, Cosyns J-P, Arlt VM, et al. The epidemiology, diagnosis, and management of aristolochic acid nephropathy. A narrative review. Ann Intern Med. 2013;158:469–77.

Jadot I, Declèves A-E, Nortier J, et al. An Integrated view of aristolochic acid nephropathy: Update of the literature. Int J Mol Sci. 2017;18(2):297.

Nortier JL, Martinez MC, Schmeiser HH, et al. Urothelial carcinoma associated with the use of a Chinese herb (Aristolochia fangchi). N Engl J Med. 2000;342:1686–92.

84. A 62-year-old man presents to the Emergency Department with complaints of vague but constant abdominal pain and jaundice. His past medical history is significant for hypertension which is diet controlled. He denies diabetes or alcoholism. He urinates normally. Pertinent laboratory values: serum creatinine 1.9 mg/dL (eGFR 44 mL/min), BUN 18 mg/dL, total bilirubin 3.2 mg/dL with direct bilirubin 2.1 mg/dL, total protein 8.4 g/dL with albumin 3.8 g/dL, and normal liver function tests. Lipase and amylase levels are slightly elevated. Urinalysis shows 30 mg/dL protein (total protein 0.5 g/day) without blood. ANA is positive at 1:600, but antibodies to double-stranded DNA are absent. Serum C4 levels are low. CT of abdomen shows enlarged pancreas and kidneys. **Which one of the following tests is MOST likely to explain this patient's elevated creatinine?**

A. Kidney scan
B. ANCA
C. Rheumatoid factor
D. Serum IgG and IgG4
E. Renal ultrasound for size of the kidney

The answer is D

The patient seems to have no urinary tract obstruction, as his urination is normal. Therefore, kidney scan does not add any additional diagnostic information other than actual GFR. In the absence of hematuria or other clinical manifestations of glomerular disease, determination of ANCA may not yield additional information on kidney disease. Similarly, determination of rheumatoid factor may not be that helpful. CT of abdomen revealed large kidneys, and kidney ultrasound may show increased echogenicity or edema, which does not explain the cause for increased creatinine. Thus, options A, B, C, and E are incorrect.

The clue to the diagnosis is CT of the abdomen of possible pancreatitis or pancreatic cancer, and elevated globulin levels. Therefore, determination of serum IgG and IgG4 levels seems appropriate to make the diagnosis of IgG4-related kidney disease. Thus, option D is correct.

Suggested Reading

Culver EL, Bateman AC. General principles of IgG4-related disease. Diag Histopathol. 2013;10:111–8.

Guma M, Firestein GS. IgG4-related diseases. Best Pract Res Clin Rheumatol. 2012;26:425–38.

Stone JH. IgG4-related disease: nomenclature, clinical features, and treatment. Sem Diag Pathol. 2012;29:177–90.

85. **Which one of the following histopathologic features of the kidney is MOST likely in the above patient?**

A. Minimal change disease
B. Lupus membranous nephropathy
C. Chronic tubulointerstitial disease (TID)
D. Mesangioproliferative immune complex glomerulonephritis (GN)
E. Membranoproliferative glomerulonephritis (MPGN)

The answer is C.

The list of IgG4-related diseases is rapidly growing. Originally described as autoimmune pancreatitis, the IgG4 disease has been described in every organ of the body, including the kidney. The most common manifestation in the kidney is TID. Histologic features of TID include plasma cell-rich infiltrate, eosinophils in some cases, and immune complex deposits along the tubular basement membrane. Interstitial fibrosis is common. Immunostaining shows the presence of IgG4 in granular pattern.

Although IgG4-related kidney disease is mostly TID (C is the most reasonable answer), glomeruli are also affected in some cases. The common glomerular lesions are membranous nephropathy, MPGN, IgA nephropathy, and mesangioproliferative immune complex GN. IgG4-related plasma cell arteritis has also been described in the kidney. It can also present as acute kidney injury or CKD. Imaging studies of the kidney may show enlargement as well as masses mimicking kidney carcinoma.

In patients with IgG4-related kidney or systemic disease, serum levels of IgG and IgG4 are elevated. ANA is usually positive, but antibodies to double-stranded DNA are absent, thus excluding the diagnosis of lupus nephritis. Other glomerular diseases mentioned in options A, D, and E usually present with hematuria and proteinuria, and thus are excluded in this patient. This patient has IgG4-related disease in the pancreas and biliary duct as well.

Suggested Reading

Cornell LD. IgG4-related tubulointerstitial nephritis. Kidney Int. 2010;78:951–3.
Cornell LD. IgG4-related kidney disease. Curr Opin Nephrol Hypertens. 2011;21:279–88.
Cornell LD. IgG4-related kidney disease. Sem Diag Pathol. 2012;29:245–50.
Mbengue M, Goumri N, Niang A. IgG4-related kidney disease: pathogenesis, diagnosis, and treatment. Clin Nephrol. 2021. https://doi.org/10.5414/CN110492.
Raissian Y, Nasr SH, Larsen CP, et al. Diagnosis of IgG4-related tubulointerstitial nephritis. J Am Soc Nephrol. 2011;22:1343–52.
Saeki T, Kawano M. IgG4-related kidney disease. Kidney Int. 2014;85:251–7.
Saeki T, Nishi S, Imai N, et al. Clinicopathological characteristics of patients with IgG4-related tubulointerstitial nephritis. Kidney Int. 2010;78:1016–23.
Salvadori M, Tsalouchos A. Immunoglobulin G4-related kidney diseases: an updated review. World J Nephrol. 2018;7:29–40.

86. **Which one of the following treatments for IgG4-related (kidney) diseases is FALSE?**

A. Corticosteroids
B. Mycophenolate mofetil (MMF)
C. Cyclophosphamide
D. Rituximab
E. Plasmapheresis

The answer is E

The treatment choice is corticosteroids. Two treatment regimens have been tried. The Japanese experience suggests prednisone 0.6 mg/kg for 2–4 weeks followed by tapering to 5 mg/day for 3–6 months. The maintenance dose is 2.5–5 mg/day for 3 years. Another treatment regimen is that of Mayo clinic experience. Prednisone is started at 40 mg/day for 4 weeks and then tapering to nothing over a period of 12 weeks.

Corticosteroid-sparing therapy during remission period has been suggested using drugs such as methotrexate, azathioprine, MMF, cyclophosphamide, and rituximab. Bortezomib, a proteasome inhibitor, has also been tried. However, plasmapheresis has not been tried yet. Thus, option E is false.

Suggested Reading

Alamino RP, Espinoza LR, Zea AH. The great mimicker: IgG4-related disease. Clin Rheumatol. 2013;32:1267–73.

Alexander M, Larsen CP, Gibson IW, et al. Membranous glomerulonephritis is a manifestation of IgG4-related disease. Kidney Int. 2013;83:455–62.

Fervenza FC, Downer G, Beck LH Jr. IgG4-related tubulointerstitial nephritis with membranous nephropathy. Am J Kidney Dis. 2011;58:320324.

Saeki T, Kawano M, Mizushima I, et al. The clinical course of patients with IgG4-related kidney disease. Kidney Int. 2013;84:826–33.

Stone JH. IgG4-related disease: nomenclature, clinical features, and treatment. Sem Diag Pathol. 2012;29:177–190.

Salvadori M, Tsalouchos A. Immunoglobulin G4-related kidney diseases: an updated review. World J Nephrol. 2018;7:29–40.

87. **Which one of the following tubular functions is LEAST likely in patients with acute tubulointerstitial nephritis (TID)?**

A. Decreased absorption of Na^+, HCO_3^-, urate, and PO_4^- reabsorption by the proximal tubule
B. Decreased secretion of K^+ and H^+ by the distal tubule
C. Decreased response to ADH by the collecting duct
D. Increased secretion of K^+ and H^+ by the distal tubule
E. Increased excretion of glucose and amino acids

The answer is D

In acute TID, variable degrees of tubular injury are present, but tubular atrophy is absent. As a result, both cortical and medullary tubular functions are disturbed. Reabsorption of Na^+, HCO_3^-, urate, PO_4^-, glucose, and amino acids is decreased in the proximal tubule, resulting in Fanconi syndrome and proximal RTA. Similarly, the secretion of K^+ and H^+ by the distal tubule is decreased resulting in hyperkalemia and distal RTA. Hyperkalemia is disproportionate to the degree of renal dysfunction. Thus, option D is incorrect. The urine pH is generally alkaline in nature. Since Na^+ and K^+ are lost in the urine due to dysfunction of loop of Henle and distal nephron, the medullary hyperosmolality is decreased. This results in less responsiveness to ADH.

Suggested Reading

Perazella MA, Rosner MH. Tubulointerstitial diseases. In: Yu ASL, Chertow GM, Luyckx VA, et al., editors. Brenner & Rector's the kidney. 11th ed. Philadelphia: Elsevier Saunders; 2020. p. 1196–222.

Rossert JA, Fischer EA. Acute interstitial nephritis. In: Feehally J, Floege J, Tonelli M, et al., editors. Comprehensive clinical nephrology. 6th ed. Philadelphia: Elsevier; 2019. p. 729–37.

88. **Which one of the following drugs is LEAST likely to cause acute tubulointerstitial disease (TID)?**

A. Omeprazole (Proton pump inhibitor)
B. Sunitinib (Tyrosine kinase inhibitor)
C. Trimethoprim/sulfamethoxazole (Sulfonamides)
D. Amlodipine, diltiazem (Calcium-channel blockers)
E. Adriamycin (Antineoplastic agent)

The answer is E

Except for adriamycin, which induces proteinuria and nephrotic syndrome, all other drugs have been shown to cause acute TID. However, the onset of acute TID varies from drug to drug. Proton pump inhibitors may take 1–12 weeks, whereas tyrosine kinase inhibitors may take 3 weeks, and other drugs may take weeks to months to cause acute TID. Thus, option E is incorrect.

Suggested Reading

Brewster UC, Perazella MA. Acute kidney injury following proton pump inhibitor therapy. Kidney Int. 2007;71:589–93.

Perazella MA, Rosner MH. Tubulointerstitial diseases. In: Yu ASL, Chertow GM, Luyckx VA, et al., editors. Brenner & Rector's the kidney. 11th ed. Philadelphia: Elsevier Saunders; 2020. p. 1196–222.

Rossert JA, Fischer EA. Acute interstitial nephritis. In: Feehally J, Floege J, Tonelli M, et al., editors. Comprehensive clinical nephrology. 6th ed. Philadelphia: Elsevier; 2019. p. 729–37.

Winn SK, Ellis S, Savage P, et al. Biopsy-proven acute interstitial nephritis associated with the tyrosine kinase inhibitor sunitinib: a class effect? Nephrol Dial Transplant. 2009;24:673–5.

89. A 62-year-old Caucasian woman with long-standing history of cigarette smoking is admitted for exacerbation of asthma. Past medical history is significant for hypertension (HTN) and CKD stage 2. Her primary care physician started hydrochlorothiazide (HCTZ) for her HTN. BP is 150/84 mm Hg. Except for expiratory wheezing, the remainder of the phys exam is within normal limits. Serum creatinine is 1.8 mg/dL, and uric acid is 6.4 mg/dL. A recently performed glycated HbA1c is 6.1%. Urinalysis reveals 3+ proteinuria and a few RBCs. A 24-h proteinuria is 2.6 g. All serologies are normal. Renal ultrasound reveals normal size kidneys. **Which one of the following lesions is MOST likely to be found on a kidney biopsy?**

A. Membranous nephropathy
B. FSGS (NOS)
C. Dense deposit disease
D. Pauci-immune crescentic glomerulonephritis (GN)
E. Nodular glomerulosclerosis (GS)

The answer is E

Long history of smoking and HTN in nondiabetic subjects has been linked to the development of diffuse and nodular mesangial sclerosis with thickening of glomerular and tubular basement membranes as well as arteriolosclerosis. Deposition of immunoglobulins or albumin is minimal. These glomerular changes resemble diabetic nephropathy and other diseases with glomerular nodules or nodule-like appearance (see Fig. 2.22).

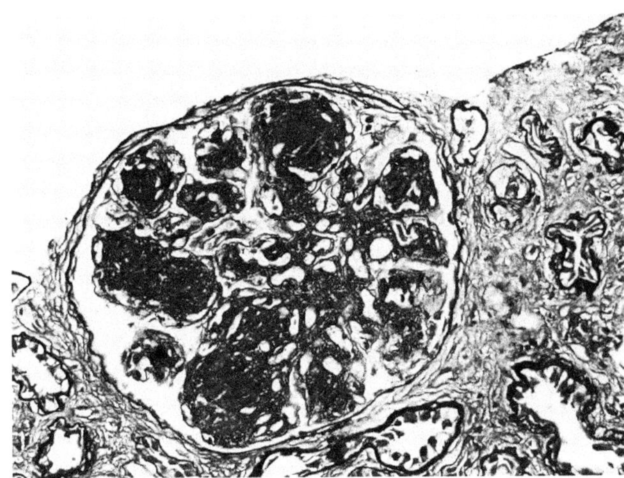

Fig. 2.22 Glomerulus from a smoker showing nodules, resembling diabetic nodular glomerulosclerosis

The pathogenesis of smoking-associated nodular GS may be related to several mechanisms, including oxidative stress, advanced glycation end products, and fibrosis-induced cytokines.

Suggested Reading

Andronesi AG, Ismail G, Fetecău A-C, et al. Smoking-associated nodular glomerulosclerosis, a rare renal pathology resembling diabetic nephropathy: case report. Rom J Morphol Embryol. 2016;57:1125–29.

Kuppachi S, Idris N, Chander PN, et al. Idiopathic nodular glomerulosclerosis in a non-diabetic hypertensive smoker: Case report and review of literature. Nephrol Dial Transplant. 2006;21:3571–5.

Nasr SH, D'Agati VD. Nodular glomerulosclerosis in the nondiabetic smoker. J Am Soc Nephrol. 2007;18:2032–6.

90. A 64-year-old man is admitted for constitutional symptoms, hematuria, proteinuria (2+ on dipstick), and rapidly increasing serum creatinine levels. There is no history of cough or hemoptysis. A kidney biopsy shows pauci-immune necrotizing crescentic GN. His serum creatinine stabilized at 6.4 mg/dL. **Which one of the following treatment modalities is APPROPRIATE in order to maintain dialysis independence at 3 months and kidney and patient survival at 1 year?**

A. Hemodialysis, plasma exchange, oral steroids, and oral cyclophosphamide
B. Pulse steroids, hemodialysis, oral steroids, and oral cyclophosphamide
C. Plasma exchange, oral steroids, and oral cyclophosphamide
D. Pulse steroids followed by oral steroids and monthly IV cyclophosphamide
E. Hemodialysis and rituximab

The answer is A

A report by European Vasculitis Study group evaluated the beneficial effect of two treatment regimens in newly diagnosed ANCA-associated systemic vasculitis patients with advanced renal insufficiency (serum creatinine >5.8 mg/dL). A total of 137 patients were followed and divided into two groups. One group (*N* = 67) was treated with IV methylprednisolone (a total of 3 g), and the second group (*N* = 70) received a total of seven plasma exchanges in a 2-week period. Both groups received oral cyclophosphamide and oral prednisolone. Oral cyclophosphamide was started at 2.5 mg/kg/day (2 mg/kg/day for age >60 years), reduced to 1.5 mg/day at 3 months, and stopped at 6 months. Thereafter, azathioprine 2 mg/kg/day was started as maintenance therapy. Oral prednisolone was tapered from 1 mg/kg/day at entry to 0.25 mg/kg/day by 10 weeks, 15 mg/day at 3 months, and 10 mg/day from 5 to 12 months. About 69% of patients required hemodialysis. The primary endpoint was dialysis independence at 3 months. Secondary endpoints were kidney and patient survival at 1 year and severe adverse event rates. At 3 months, 49% (*N* = 33) of patients on methylprednisolone and 69% (*N* = 48) patients on plasma exchange were alive and independent of dialysis. As compared with IV methylprednisolone, plasma exchange was associated with a 24% reduction in risk for progression to ESKD at 1 year. Patient survival and adverse event rates were similar between the groups; however, plasma exchange was associated with increased kidney recovery when compared with methylprednisolone. Thus, choice A is correct.

Suggested Reading

Jayne DRW, Gaskin G, Rasmussen N, et al. On behalf of the European Vasculitis Study Group. Randomized trial of plasma exchange or high-dose methylprednisolone as adjunctive therapy for severe renal vasculitis. J Am Soc Nephrol. 2007;18:2180–8.

Nachman PH, Denu-Ciocca CJ. Vasculitidies. In: Lerma EV, Berns JS, Nissenson AR, editors. Current diagnosis & treatment: nephrology & hypertension. New York: McGraw Hill; 2009. p. 265–75.

91. **Match the following therapeutic modalities with the various forms of amyloidosis.**

A. High-dose melphalan (200 mg/m^2), steroid, and autologous stem cell transplantation
B. Kidney and liver transplantation
C. Control of infection or inflammation and glycosaminoglycan (GAG) mimetics
D. Colchicine and kidney transplantation
E. Kidney transplantation

1. AA amyloidosis other than familial Mediterranean fever (FMF)
2. FMF with CKD (stages 3–4)
3. AL amyloidosis
4. Transthyretin amyloidosis and ESKD
5. Dialysis-related amyloidosis

Answers: A = 3; B = 4; C = 1; D = 2; E = 5

AA amyloidosis, also called secondary amyloidosis, occurs in patients with chronic inflammatory conditions. Some of the causes in developed countries include rheumatoid arthritis, inflammatory bowel disease, and FMF. Osteomyelitis and TB also cause AA amyloidosis in some parts of the world.

Kidneys are affected more than other organs in AA amyloidosis. Control of infection improves AA amyloidosis. Pharmacologic reduction in circulating levels of serum-associated A (SAA) protein to <10 mg/L by anti-inflammatory or immunosuppressive agents improves clinical outcome in AA amyloidosis.

Amyloid deposits consist mainly of amyloid fibrils. In addition, they also contain nonfibrillary components such as heparan and dermatan sulfate GAGs which contribute to amyloidogenesis. GAG mimetic agents such as Fibrillex can inhibit the binding of GAGs with amyloid fibrils in AA patients and animals.

Chemotherapy and autologous stem cell transplantation to suppress production of monoclonal immunoglobulin light chains have been successful in some patients. However, high-dose melphalan and autologous stem cell

therapy did not prove to be universally superior to the standard therapy that includes melphalan plus prednisone for patients with AL amyloidosis.

Other treatment modalities for AL amyloidosis include lenalidomide in combination with melphalan and dexamethasone and anti-CD38-directed monoclonal antibody daratumumab. This monoclonal antibody has improved hematologic response rates in both multiple myeloma and amyloidosis.

Orthotopic liver transplantation is considered the definitive treatment for patients with transthyretin amyloidosis. Colchicine and kidney transplantation are advocated for amyloidosis associated with FMF and CKD. Dialysis-associated amyloidosis may respond to kidney transplantation with the resultant decrease in circulating levels of β_2-microglobulins.

Suggested Reading

Dember LM. Amyloidosis-associated kidney disease. J Am Soc Nephrol. 2006;17:3458–71.

Gillmore JD, Hawkins PN. Drug insight: emerging therapies for amyloidosis. Nat Clin Pract Nephrol. 2006;2:263–70.

Hegenbart U, Bochtler T, Benner A, et al. Lenalidomide/melphalan/dexamethasone in newly diagnosed patients with immunoglobulin light chain amyloidosis: results of a prospective phase 2 study with long-term follow up. Haematologica. 2017;102(8):1424–31.

Kaufman GP, Schrier SL, Lafayette RA, et al. Daratumumab yields rapid and deep hematologic responses in patients with heavily pretreated AL amyloidosis. Blood. 2017;130:900–2.

Palladini G, Milani P, Foli A, et al. Melphalan and dexamethasone with or without bortezomib in newly diagnosed AL amyloidosis: a matched case-control study on 174 patients. Leukemia. 2014;28:2311–6.

92. A 30-year-old Caucasian woman is referred to a nephrologist for evaluation of nephrotic syndrome. Past medical history includes recurrent UTIs, requiring antibiotic use. She also uses Ibuprofen 600 mg a day for >2 years. BP and serum chemistry are normal. VDRL is nonreactive. ANA is negative, and complements are normal. HIV, hep B, and C are negative. Urinalysis reveals >10 WBCs, 2–4 RBCs, 3+ proteinuria, 1–3 hyaline casts, and a few eosinophils. A 24-h urine reveals 4.6 g of proteinuria. **In view of changing pattern of primary glomerular diseases in the United States, which one of the following diagnoses seems MOST likely in this patient?**

A. Minimal change disease (MCD)
B. Focal segmental GS (FSGS)
C. Membranous nephropathy (MN)
D. Membranoproliferative GN-type 1 (MPGN)
E. IgA nephropathy

The answer is B

Several kidney biopsy series have reported that a primary glomerular disease is present in approximately 50% of all native kidney biopsies. However, the pattern of glomerular disease varies depending on the geographic location and country. For example, increasing incidence of FSGS as the primary glomerular disease has been reported in the United States, Brazil, and India. Although a higher incidence of FSGS is reported in African Americans, some studies observed a significant increase in FSGS in Caucasians and Hispanic population.

In European countries, IgA nephropathy is the most common histologically diagnosed primary glomerular disease with the exception of the Republic of Macedonia where MN and MPGN in Romania are the primary diseases. A study in Northern Ireland reported primarily IgA nephropathy accounting for almost 39% and FSGS for 5.7% of all the biopsies done over a 30-year period. Thus, IgA nephropathy seems to be the primary glomerular disease in the United Kingdom.

In the patient described above, the glomerular lesion can be either MCD or MN due to NSAID use or FSGS due to increasing incidence in Caucasians, as observed in the Olmsted County in Minnesota.

IgA nephropathy or MPGN is possible in this patient. However, isolated nephrotic syndrome without much hematuria and normal BP and serum chemistry makes these diagnoses less likely. Indeed, the patient had a kidney biopsy, which showed primary FSGS.

Suggested Reading

Hanko JB, Mullan RN, O'Rourke DM, et al. The changing pattern of adult primary glomerular disease. Nephrol Dial Transplant. 2009;24:3050–4.

Swaminathan S, Leung N, Lager DJ, et al. Changing incidence of glomerular disease in Omsted County, Minnesota: a 30-year renal biopsy study. Clin J Am Soc Nephrol. 2006;1:483–7.

93. A 68-year-old African American woman is admitted for nausea, vomiting, constipation, abdominal pain, fatigue, weakness, loss of 10 lbs in 4 weeks, and frequent urination, particularly at nighttime. She has long-standing history of hypertension, for which she is on hydrochlorothiazide (HCTZ) 25 mg/day. She just noticed a growing and painless "bump" on left temporal area for the last 2 weeks. Phys exam is normal except for a nonmobile, nontender, and nonerythematous mass (2–3 cm) on left temporal area. Pertinent laboratory values:

- Na^+ = 132 mEq/L
- K^+ = 4.2 mEq/L
- Cl^- = 101 mEq/L
- HCO_3^- = 14 mEq/L
- Creatinine = 10.2 mg/dL
- BUN = 102 mg/dL
- Glucose = 88 mg/dL
- Total protein 10.1 g/dL
- Albumin = 3.2 g/dL
- Ca^{2+} = 10.8 mg/dL
- Phosphate = 6.1 mg/dL
- Uric acid = 9.2 mg/dL
- Hgb = 8.6 g/dL
- Urinalysis = 2+ protein with protein:creatinine ratio of 8.2
- Renal ultrasound = normal size kidneys with increased echogenicity

The creatinine did not improve despite adequate hydration, requiring hemodialysis. After stabilization, a kidney biopsy was performed (see Fig. 2.23).

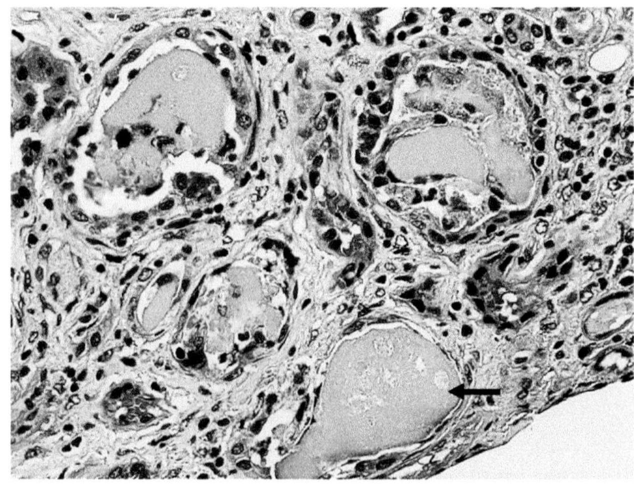

Fig. 2.23 Tubulopathy (cast in the tubule; arrow)

Which one of the following is the MOST likely diagnosis?

A. Amyloidosis
B. Acute tubulointerstitial disease (TID)
C. Myeloma cast nephropathy
D. Monoclonal gammopathy of unknown significance (MGUS)
E. Prerenal azotemia

The answer is C

The LM findings of kidney biopsy show tubules containing pale staining casts (arrow) surrounded by a multinucleated giant cell. These findings are consistent with light-chain (Bence Jones) cast nephropathy or myeloma cast nephropathy.

The kidney biopsy findings and hyponatremia, hypercalcemia, hyperuricemia, with 2+ proteinuria on urine dipstick are consistent with multiple myeloma and myeloma cast nephropathy. The casts do not usually stain with PAS. Protein electrophoresis showed an M spike, and free light chains were increased in serum. These light chains

were of λ type. Constipation and frequent urination due to nephrogenic diabetes insipidus are related to hypercalcemia. The mass on left temporal area is an extramedullary plasmacytoma, and on biopsy 90% of plasma cells were found. Thus, option C is correct.

The International Myeloma Working Group established the diagnostic criteria for multiple myeloma, as follows:

A. Presence of serum or urinary monoclonal protein without any cutoff value
B. Presence of clonal plasma cells in the bone marrow or a plasmacytoma
C. Presence of end organ damage (1 or more)

- [C] Elevated calcium >11 mg/dL
- [R] Renal insufficiency, creatinine >2 mg/dL or <40 mL/min
- [A] Anemia, Hgb <10 g/dL
- [B] Lytic bone lesions

Based on urinalysis, amyloidosis should also be considered. However, Congo red staining was negative, and no fibrils were observed on electron microscopy. Acute TID due to HCTZ is a possibility, but lab data and proteinuria of 8.2 g are not consistent with acute TID. MGUS is defined as the presence of serum monoclonal (M) protein <3 g/dL, bone marrow plasma cells <10%, and the absence of end organ damage. Failure to improve serum creatinine on adequate hydration rules out the possibility of prerenal azotemia. Thus, options A, B, D, and E are incorrect.

Suggested Reading

Dimopoulos MA, Sonneveld P, Leung N, et al. International Myeloma Working Group recommendations for the diagnosis and management of myeloma-related renal impairment. J Clin Oncol. 2016;34:1544–57.

Irish AB. Myeloma and the kidney. In: Feehally J, Floege J, Tonelli M, et al., editors. Comprehensive clinical nephrology. 6th ed. Philadelphia: Elsevier; 2019. p. 767–75.

Korbet SM, Schwartz MM. Multiple myeloma. J Am Soc Nephrol. 2006;17:2533–45.

Rajkumar SV, Dimopoulos MA, Palumbo A, et al. International Myeloma Working Group updated criteria for the diagnosis of multiple myeloma. Lancet Oncol. 2014;15:e538–48.

94. **Match the following urinary sediment (microscopic) findings with the clinical history of the patients.**

A. A 40-year-old man with alcohol abuse with severe high anion gap metabolic acidosis and high osmolal gap. He forms calcium dehydrate crystals
B. A 38-year-old woman with recurrent urinary tract infections (UTI) with klebsiella
C. An 18-year-old woman with cystinuria and nephrolithiasis
D. A 24-year-old man with HIV develops calcium oxalate monohydrate crystals
E. A 35-year-old HIV man with pulmonary TB on ethambutol with AKI receives CT of abdomen with contrast.
F. A kidney transplant patient on immunosuppressive therapy with AKI and the presence of decoy cells on urinalysis.

Answers: A = 4; B = 1; C = 2; D = 5; E = 3; F = 6

The patient described in A seems to have ingested antifreeze, which contains ethylene glycol. The end product of ethylene glycol is oxalic acid and oxalate crystals. Calcium oxalate dihydrate crystals give "envelope-like" appearance on examination of the urinary sediment. Figure 2.24.4 has "envelope-like" crystals, which have the following appearance under the microscope.

The patient described in B has UTIs with precipitation of ammonium magnesium phosphate crystals, which have "coffin-lid" appearance, as shown in Fig. 2.24.1.

The patient described in C has cystinuria and the cystine crystals take the form of a benzene ring (hexagonal), as shown in Fig. 2.24.2.

Calcium oxalate monohydrate crystals may have spindle, oval, or dumb-bell shape, as shown in Fig. 2.24.5. These crystals are also seen in excess oxalate intake, or in ethylene glycol ingestion.

Contrast promotes urate and oxalate excretion. The patient described in E is on ethambutol, which increases serum uric acid levels. When such a patient receives contrast, AKI results from intratubular obstruction of urate crystals which have no definite shape. At times, the appearance of urate crystals in the urinary sediment may take rhomboid to barrel or football shape, as shown in Fig. 2.24.3.

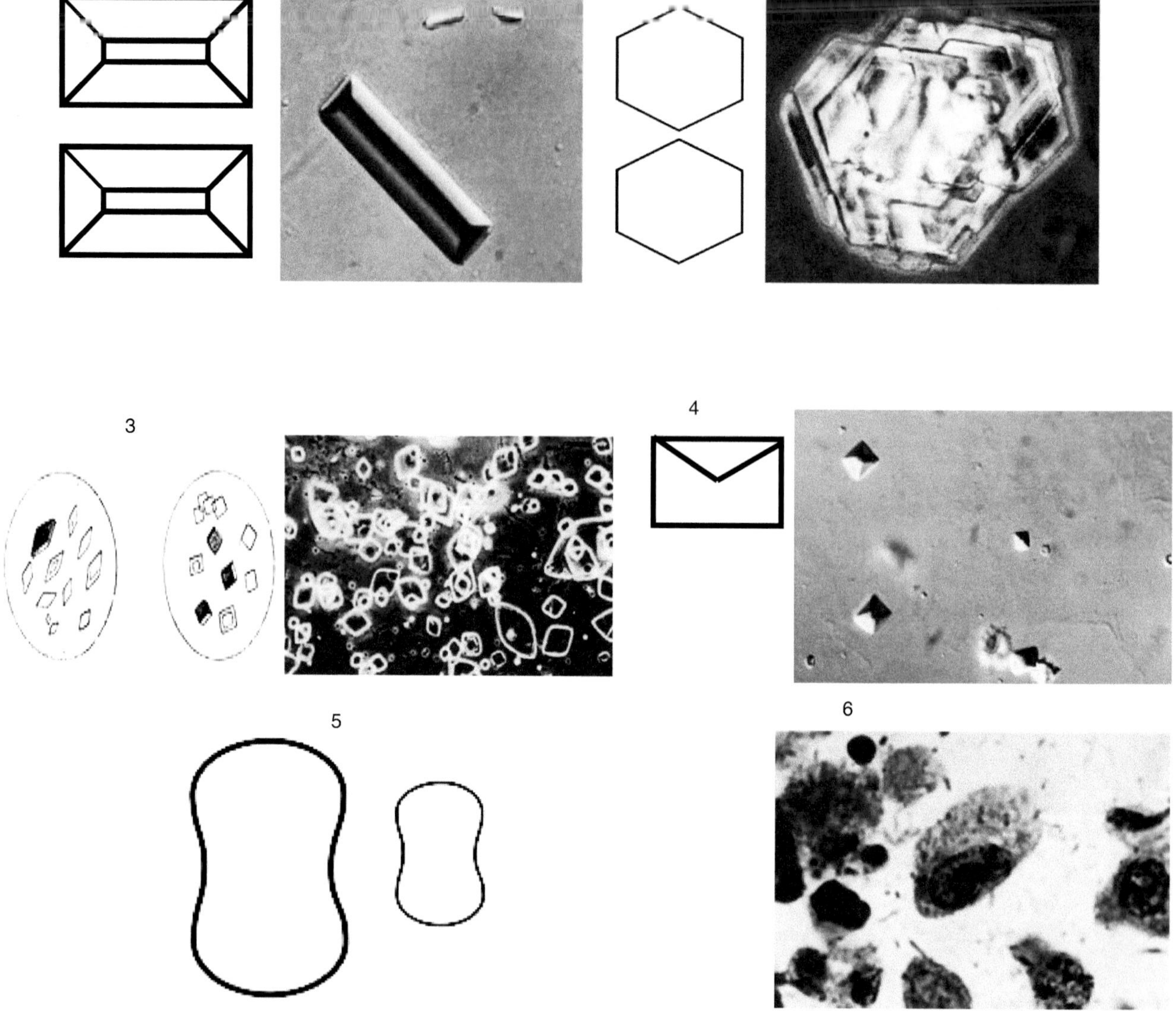

Fig. 2.24 Specific findings of the urinary sediment

Figure 2.24.6 describes the presence of a decoy cell with inclusion body within nucleus of BK virus in a kidney transplant patient on immunosuppressive therapy.

Suggested Reading

Fogazzi GB. Urinalysis. In: Floege J, Johnson RJ, Feehally J, editors. Comprehensive clinical nephrology. 4th ed. Philadelphia: Saunders/Elsevier; 2010. p. 39–55.

Fogazzi GB, Garigali G. The clinical art and science of urine microscopy. Curr Opin Nephrol Hypertens. 2003;16:625–32.

95. **Match the following drug-induced urinary crystals with the patient history.**

A. A patient on sulfadiazine
B. A patient with urinary tract infection and on ciprofloxacin
C. An HIV patient on indinavir
D. A patient treated with acyclovir
E. A patient treated with amoxicillin
F. A patient with calcium phosphate crystals

Answers: A = 5; B = 2; C = 1; D = 4; E = 3; F = 6

Drug-induced crystalluria is rather common, and in several instances the presence of these crystals is not pathologic. In some situations, however, these crystals may confirm the diagnosis of acute kidney injury. Examples include acyclovir, sulfadiazine, and indinavir. Acyclovir crystals are birefringent needle-shaped crystals (Fig. 2.25.4). Sulfadiazine crystals are also birefringent and appear as "shocks of wheat" or shells with striations (Fig. 2.25.5). Indinavir crystals are strongly birefringent and have various appearances such as fan-shaped or starburst form (Fig. 2.25.1). Ciprofloxacin crystals have star-like appearance (Fig. 2.25.2). Amoxicillin crystals appear like a branch of a broom bush (Fig. 2.25.3), whereas calcium phosphate crystals resemble a star (Fig. 2.25.6).

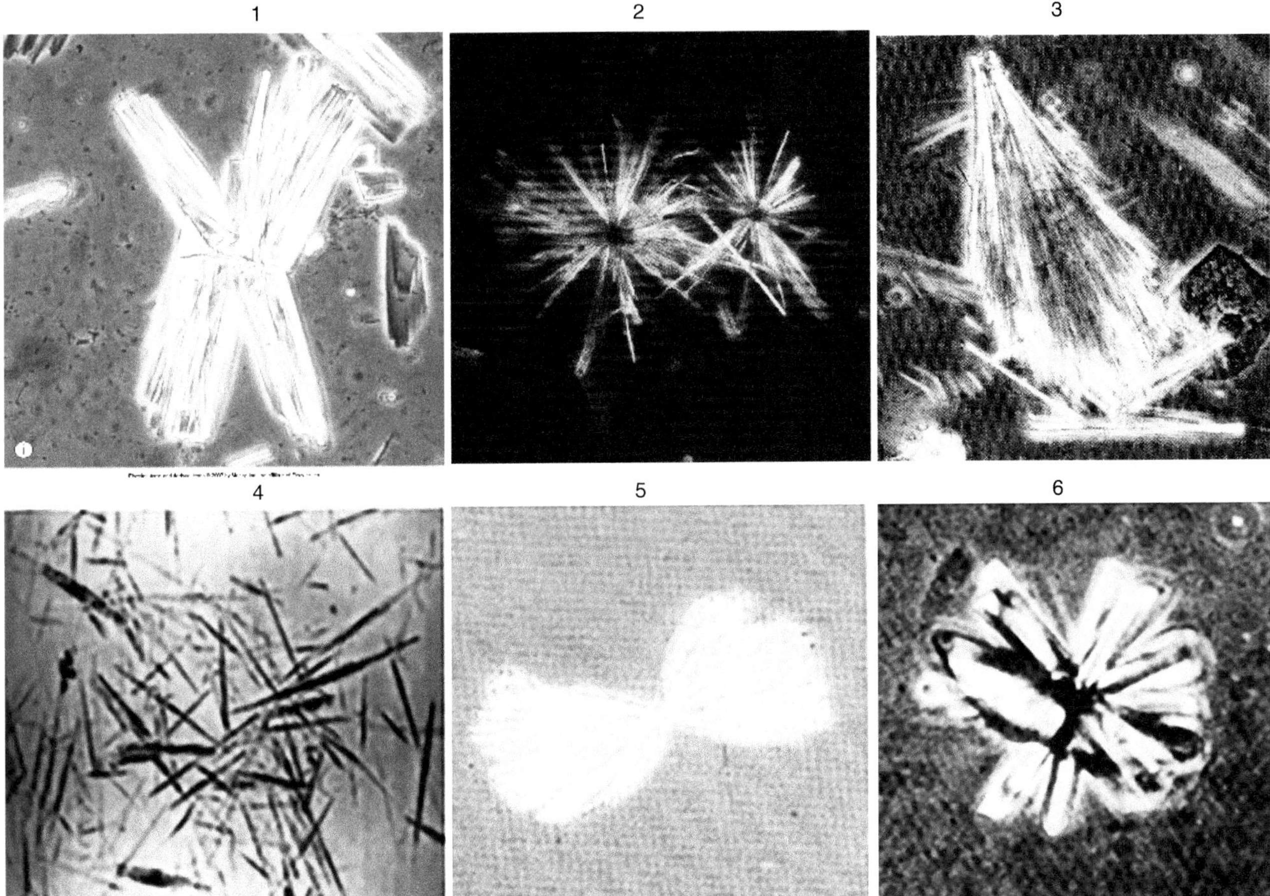

Fig. 2.25 Drug-induced urinary crystals

Suggested Reading

Fogazzi GB. Urinalysis. In: Floege J, Johnson RJ, Feehally J, editors. Comprehensive clinical nephrology. 4th ed. Philadelphia: Saunders/Elsevier; 2010. p. 39–55.

Mason WJ, Nicols HH. Crystalluria from acyclovir use. N Engl J Med. 2008;358:i3.

Perazella MA. Drug-induced acute renal failure: update on new medications and unique mechanisms of nephrotoxicity. Am J Med Sci. 2003;325:349–62.

96. **In a patient with sickle cell disease, which one of the following combinations is LEAST likely?**

A. Hematuria and renal infarction
B. Hyperkalemia and inability to concentrate urine
C. Glomerulomegaly and glomerular hypertension
D. Renal cortical carcinoma and papillary necrosis
E. MPGN and FSGS

The answer is D

Patients with sickle cell disease demonstrate hematuria due to renal infarction and extravasation of blood in the renal medulla. Hematuria is usually unilateral and originates from the left kidney in about 80% of patients. The

left-sided origin is related to "Nutcracker" phenomenon which is caused by compression of the left renal vein between the superior mesenteric artery and aorta. As a result of this compression, pressure in the renal vein increases causing anoxia and sickling of red cells in the left kidney.

Although the exact mechanism is unknown, patients with sickle cell disease have inability to secrete K causing hyperkalemia. This is independent of aldosterone. Also, patients with sickle cell disease have a defect in concentrating their urine due to loss of the countercurrent mechanism in the renal medulla. However, the diluting capacity is maintained.

Another defect is the inability to lower urine pH below 5.0. Thus, the patients develop an incomplete form of distal RTA.

Glomerular hypertrophy and glomerular hypertension have been described in young subjects with sickle cell disease. Also, these subjects demonstrate increased RPF and GFR.

Although the most common glomerular disease is FSGS, MPGN type 1 has also been described in some patients. MPGN may be related to hepatitis C from multiple blood transfusions.

Papillary necrosis occurs in more than 23% of patients. It results from obliteration of the vasa recta with medullary necrosis and fibrosis. Papillary necrosis causes painless hematuria.

Kidney medullary rather than cortical carcinoma has been described. Thus, choice D is incorrect.

Suggested Reading

Hassell KL, Statius van Eps LW, deJong PE. Sickle cell disease. In: Schrier, editor. Diseases of the kidney & urinary tract. 8th ed. Philadelphia: Lippincott Williams & Wilkins; 2007. p. 1997–2012.

Sharpe CC, Arogundade FA. Sickle cell diseases and the kidney. In: Feehally J, Floege J, Tonelli M, et al., editors. Comprehensive clinical nephrology. 6th ed. Philadelphia: Elsevier; 2019. p. 597–605.

97. An 18-year-old woman is referred to the Emergency Department by the primary care physician (PMD) for evaluation of elevated serum creatinine, altered mental status, and questionable seizure noticed by her mother. The patient had bloody diarrhea for 6 days after eating a large hamburger. The PMD gave an antibiotic, but diarrhea continued. Initial labs: Na^+ 132 mEq/L, K^+ 3.2 mEq/L, Cl^- 110 mEq/L, HCO_3^- 14 mEq/L, creatinine 3.6 mg/dL, BUN 81 mg/dL, and glucose 90 mg/dL. Complete blood count: WBC 14,000, Hgb 7.4 g/dL, platelets 64,000/μL. She has urine output of 400 mL in 16 hours. **Which one of the following is the MOST likely diagnosis in this patient?**

A. Atypical hemolytic uremic syndrome (aHUS)
B. Thrombotic thrombocytopenic purpura (TTP)
C. Shiga toxin-producing E. coli-associated hemolytic uremic syndrome (STEC-HUS)
D. Acute bilateral renal cortical necrosis
E. Ischemic acute tubular necrosis (ATN)

The answer is C

The thrombotic microangiopathies (TMAs) are a group of disorders characterized by a triad of microangiopathic hemolytic anemia, thrombocytopenia, and varying degrees of kidney failure. Of all TMAs, HUS and TTP are commonly encountered clinical conditions in a hospital setting. HUS is of two types: STEC-HUS and atypical HUS (aHUS). STEC-HUS is typically associated with bacterial infections, most commonly with E. coli 0157:H7. Shiga-like toxins are produced by these bacteria, which are responsible for diarrhea and HUS. However, HUS produced by streptococcus pneumoniae is not associated with Shiga-like toxins. The vast majority of patients with STEC-HUS are children who experience a prodromal, bloody diarrhea 1 week prior to developing HUS. Major outbreaks of STEC-HUS have been reported from consuming contaminated and uncooked hamburgers, commercial salami, alfalfa, and radish sprouts. Thus, the patient carries the diagnosis of STEC-HUS. Altered mental status and seizures have also been reported as extrarenal manifestations of STEC-HUS, which may be confused with TTP.

About 10% of patients with HUS present with aHUS. aHUS is a disease that is not associated with any infections, and occurs in 2 per million in the United States. The prognosis of patients with aHUS is poor than those with STEC-HUS, and many progresses to ESKD. aHUS is classified as sporadic or familial. Familial aHUS is defined as the presence of HUS in at least two members of the same family with clinical manifestations 6 months apart. Sporadic form develops in patients who do not have any family history of HUS. Sporadic forms can be either idiopathic or secondary due to systemic illness (infection, cancer, drugs, or pregnancy). Both sporadic and familial forms are characterized by uncontrolled activation of the complement system. Genetic and acquired

abnormalities of the alternative complement system have been described. Thus, the patient described above does not have aHUS.

TTP is a consideration because of her mental status changes as 20% of STEC-HUS patients have neurologic abnormalities at time of presentation. However, this patient has clinical manifestations of STEC-HUS, thus excluding the diagnosis of TTP.

Acute cortical necrosis can occur due to infections and many other causes. It usually presents with anuria and rising creatinine. Since this patient has nonoliguric acute kidney injury, acute cortical necrosis can be ruled out.

Ischemic ATN is a consideration, but thrombocytopenia, severe anemia, and neurologic manifestations are uncommon in ATN. Thus, option E is incorrect.

Suggested Reading

Brocklebank V, Wood KM, Kavanagh D. Thrombotic microangiopathy and the kidney. Clin J Am Soc Nephrol. 2018;13:300–17.

Fakhouri F, Scully M, Provôt F, et al. and the International Working Group on Pregnancy-Related Thrombotic Microangiopathies. Management of thrombotic microangiopathy in pregnancy and postpartum: report from an international working group. Blood. 2020;136:2103–17.

Kavanagh D, Sheerin N. Thrombotic microangiopathies. In: Yu ASL, Chertow GM, Luyckx VA, et al., editors. Brenner & Rector's the kidney. 11th ed. Philadelphia: Elsevier Saunders; 2020. p. 1178–95.

Noris M, Remuzzi G. Atypical hemolytic-uremic syndrome. N Engl J Med. 2009;36:1676–87.

Noris M, Ruggenenti PL, Remuzzi G. Thrombotic microangiopathies, including hemolytic uremic syndrome. In: Feehally J, Floege J, Tonelli M, et al., editors. Comprehensive clinical nephrology. 6th ed. Philadelphia: Elsevier; 2019. p. 343–56.

98. The above patient received appropriate fluids and electrolyte replacement. Although diarrhea improved, her serum creatinine increased to 5.6 mg/dL, and platelets decreased to 36,000/μL. Her mentation appears to be deteriorating. **Which one of the following therapies is APPROPRIATE at this time?**

A. Steroids alone
B. Platelet infusion
C. Intravenous antibiotics
D. Hemodialysis
E. Plasma exchange with fresh frozen plasma (FFP)

The answer is E

Steroids alone are ineffective in severe cases of HUS. Platelet infusion should be avoided as further organ damage can occur. However, platelet infusion is recommended when the patient is bleeding and in preparation for a surgical procedure. Antibiotics and antimotility agents should also be avoided. Studies have shown that antibiotics may enhance the release of Shiga-like toxins. Hemodialysis may improve serum creatinine levels, but it fails to correct ongoing thrombocytopenia. Thus, options A–D are incorrect.

Plasma exchange with FFP is the appropriate treatment for this severely ill patient because of deteriorating kidney function and mental status. Although supportive therapy is important in this patient, it does not alone improve the ongoing thrombocytopenia.

The patient received plasma exchange only twice and her platelets and creatinine improved without hemodialysis. She recovered her kidney function and platelets with continuing supportive therapy.

Suggested Reading

Brocklebank V, Wood KM, Kavanagh D. Thrombotic microangiopathy and the kidney. Clin J Am Soc Nephrol. 2018;13:300–17.

Kavanagh D, Sheerin N. Thrombotic microangiopathies. In: Yu ASL, Chertow GM, Luyckx VA, et al., editors. Brenner & Rector's the kidney. 11th ed. Philadelphia: Elsevier Saunders; 2020. p. 1178–95.

Noris M, Ruggenenti PL, Remuzzi G. Thrombotic microangiopathies, including hemolytic uremic syndrome. In: Feehally J, Floege J, Tonelli M, et al., editors. Comprehensive clinical nephrology. 6th ed. Philadelphia: Elsevier; 2019. p. 343–56.

99. A 17-year-old sexually active female student is admitted for evaluation of fatigue, weakness, and headache. There is no history of diarrhea. Family history for hemolytic uremic syndrome (HUS) is negative. She is not on any medications. Phys exam is normal except for blood pressure of 142/84 mm Hg. Laboratory values: WBC 12,000, Hgb 8.1 g/dL, platelets 90,000/μL, creatinine 2.4 mg/dL, BUN 63 mg/dL, C4 normal, and C3 low. Coomb's test is negative. Peripheral blood smear shows many schistocytes. **Based on the above history and laboratory values, which one of the following is the MOST likely diagnosis?**

A. Diarrhea-associated HUS (STEC-HUS)
B. Thrombotic thrombocytopenic purpura (TTP)
C. Familial atypical HUS (aHUS)
D. Sporadic aHUS
E. Ischemic acute tubular necrosis (ATN)

The answer is D

The patient has no diarrhea, which was confirmed by negative stool cultures. Therefore, STEC-HUS is unlikely. There is no family history of aHUS; therefore, familial aHUS is also unlikely. Less than 20% of cases are familial. The labs other than decreased kidney function are not consistent with ischemic ATN. Thus, options A, C, and E are incorrect.

Although TTP is a strong consideration, low C3 levels favor the diagnosis of sporadic aHUP. Thus, option D is correct.

Suggested Reading

Brocklebank V, Wood KM, Kavanagh D. Thrombotic microangiopathy and the kidney. Clin J Am Soc Nephrol. 2018;13:300–17.

Kavanagh D, Sheerin N. Thrombotic microangiopathies. In: Yu ASL, Chertow GM, Luyckx VA, et al., editors. Brenner & Rector's the kidney. 11th ed. Philadelphia: Elsevier Saunders; 2020. p. 1178–95.

Noris M, Remuzzi G. Atypical hemolytic-uremic syndrome. N Engl J Med. 2009;36:1676–87.

Noris M, Ruggenenti PL, Remuzzi G. Thrombotic microangiopathies, including hemolytic uremic syndrome. In: Feehally J, Floege J, Tonelli M, et al., editors. Comprehensive clinical nephrology. 6th ed. Philadelphia: Elsevier; 2019. p. 343–56.

100. **Which one of the following laboratory tests confirms your diagnosis in the above patient?**

A. Antiphospholipid antibody
B. Complement factor H (CFH)
C. Complement factor I (CFI)
D. Membrane cofactor protein (MCP)
E. B, C, and D

The answer is E

The patient has sporadic form of aHUS, which is due to activation of alternative complement system with low C3 and normal C4. C4 is low when classic pathway is activated. CFH regulates the alternative pathway in three ways: (1) competing with complement factor B for C3b recognition, (2) acting as a cofactor for CFI, and (3) dissociating C3 convertase. CFI is a serine protease that cleaves C3b and C4b in the presence of other cofactors, thus participating in all three complement pathways. MCP blocks C3 activation on glomerular endothelium. Genetic mutations in either CFH, CFI, or MCP cause both familial and sporadic aHUS. Therefore, screening for all three mutations is a reasonable diagnostic approach in this patient.

Sporadic aHUS can be triggered by HIV infection, anticancer drugs, immunotherapeutic agents, antiplatelet agents, malignancies, transplantation, and pregnancy. Table 2.7 summarizes the genetic abnormality and frequency of aHUS.

Table 2.7 Genetic abnormality and frequency of aHUS

Form	Gene mutation	Frequency (%)
Familial	CFH	25–30
	CFI	5–10
	MCP	7–15
	C3	2–8
	CFB	1–2
	CD46	10
	THBD[a]	9
Sporadic		
Idiopathic	CFH	15–20
	CFI	3–6
	MCP	6–10
	C3	4–6
	CFB	<1
	THBD	2
Pregnancy	CFH	20
	CFI	15
Drugs	Unknown	
HIV	Unknown	
Organ transplantation (de novo)	CFH CFI	15 16
Cancer	Unknown	

[a]Thrombomodulin

Determination of antiphospholipid antibody is helpful, but it is not an etiologic test for aHUS. Since the patient is sexually active, pregnancy and HIV test are indicated. Thus, option E is correct.

Suggested Reading

Brocklebank V, Wood KM, Kavanagh D. Thrombotic microangiopathy and the kidney. Clin J Am Soc Nephrol. 2018;13:300–17.

Kavanagh D, Sheerin N. Thrombotic microangiopathies. In: Yu ASL, Chertow GM, Luyckx VA, et al., editors. Brenner & Rector's the kidney. 11th ed. Philadelphia: Elsevier Saunders; 2020. p. 1178–95.

Noris M, Remuzzi G. Atypical hemolytic-uremic syndrome. N Engl J Med. 2009;36:1676–87.

Noris M, Ruggenenti PL, Remuzzi G. Thrombotic microangiopathies, including hemolytic uremic syndrome. In: Feehally J, Floege J, Tonelli M, et al., editors. Comprehensive clinical nephrology. 6th ed. Philadelphia: Elsevier; 2019. p. 343–56.

101. **Which one of the following therapeutic modalities is APPROPRIATE for this patient?**

A. Fresh frozen plasma (FFP)
B. Steroids only
C. Plasma exchange with FFP
D. Eculizumab
E. Platelet infusion

The answer is D

FFP restores CFH, CFI, CFB, and C3, but does not improve the levels of mutated genes. Steroids alone are not adequate to stabilize the patient. Platelet infusion is generally contraindicated because of worsening thrombotic microangiopathy. Platelet infusion is considered when a surgical procedure is anticipated and the patient is bleeding with <30,000/μl platelets. Thus, options A, B, and E are incorrect.

Eculizumab is a recombinant, humanized monoclonal IgG antibody which targets C5 and blocks its cleavage to C5b, thus preventing the generation of C5b and the cytotoxic membrane attack complex C5b-9. It may be appropriate for this patient (D is correct).

Studies have shown that eculizumab improves platelet count, glomerular filtration rate, and health-related quality of life in patients with aHUS. Also, dialysis may not be necessary for some patients with deteriorating kidney function. However, eculizumab is expensive, but its use may be cost-effective in some patients with frequent relapses of the disease. One should also note that some patients may relapse frequently and resistant to eculizumab. In such cases, genetic testing for complement variants and antibodies is warranted.

In case eculizumab is not available or otherwise, daily plasma exchange with FFP can be started. At least 6–8 treatments are required, or until symptoms and platelet count are improved.

Suggested Reading

Brocklebank V, Wood KM, Kavanagh D. Thrombotic microangiopathy and the kidney. Clin J Am Soc Nephrol. 2018;13:300–17.

Kavanagh D, Sheerin N. Thrombotic microangiopathies. In: Yu ASL, Chertow GM, Luyckx VA, et al., editors. Brenner & Rector's the kidney. 11th ed. Philadelphia: Elsevier Saunders; 2020. p. 1178–95.

Legendre CM, Licht C, Muus P, et al. Terminal complement inhibitor eculizumab in atypical hemolytic-uremic syndrome. N Engl J Med. 2013;368:2169–81.

Loirat C, Frèmeaux-Bacchi V. Atypical hemolytic uremic syndrome. Orphn J Rare Dis. 2011;6:60.

NesterCM, Brophy PD. Eculizumab in the treatment of atypical haemolytic uraemic syndrome and other complement-mediated renal diseases. Curr Opin Pediatr. 2013;25:225–31.

Noris M, Ruggenenti PL, Remuzzi G. Thrombotic microangiopathies, including hemolytic uremic syndrome. In: Feehally J, Floege J, Tonelli M, et al., editors. Comprehensive clinical nephrology. 6th ed. Philadelphia: Elsevier; 2019. p. 343–56.

Wada T, Nangaku M. Novel roles of complement in renal diseases and their therapeutic consequences. Kidney Int. 2013;84:441–50.

102. A 30-year-old woman with no significant past family and medical history is admitted for fever, nausea, vomiting, weakness, altered mental status, and petechial rash in lower extremities for 1-week duration. She has no diarrhea and is not on any medications. Her WBC count is normal, but her Hgb is 9.1 g/dL with a platelet count of 15,000/μL. Her serum creatinine is 2.4 mg/dL. Both PT/PTT are normal. Lactate dehydrogenase is elevated. Peripheral blood smear shows many schistocytes. **What are the possible diagnoses in this patient?**

A. Atypical hemolytic uremic syndrome (aHUS)
B. Disseminated intravascular coagulation (DIC)
C. Thrombotic thrombocytopenic purpura (TTP)
D. Atheroembolic disease
E. A and C

The answer is E

DIC is unlikely in view of normal PT/PTT. Also, atheroembolic disease is unlikely because of lack of risk factors or any interventional studies. Clinically, it is difficult to distinguish between aHUS and TTP, although severe neurologic changes and less kidney impairment are suggestive of TTP. Thus, diagnosis of aHUS/TTP seems appropriate in this patient.

Suggested Reading

Clark WF, Hildebrand A. Attending rounds: microangiopathic hemolytic anemia with renal insufficiency. Clin J Am Soc Nephrol. 2012;7:342–7.

George JN. Thrombotic thrombocytopenic purpura. N Engl J Med. 2006;354:1927–35.

Tsai H-M. Current concepts in thrombotic thrombocytopenic purpura. Annu Rev Med. 2006;57:419–36.

103. **Which one of the following tests distinguishes TTP from aHUS?**

A. Antiphospholipid antibody
B. Complementary factor H

C. Serum C3 and C4
D. ADAMTS 13 (a distintegrin and metalloprotease with thrombospondin-1-like domains)
E. Blood smear for schistocytes

The answer is D

Patients with TTP have a genetic defect that is characterized by the inability to cleave ultralarge vWF (von Willebrand factor). Generally, monomers of vWF are synthesized by the endothelium and are linked together by disulfide bonds to form ultralarge multimers. These ultralarge multimers of vWF promote thrombus formation. This thrombus formation is prevented by a metalloprotease that cleaves these ultralarge multimers into monomers, thereby preventing formation of microthrombi. This cleaving metalloprotease is called ADAMTS 13. Usually, 5% of its activity is enough to cleave the multimers. Patients with familial TTP have absent or <5% of normal ADAMTS 13 activity in their plasma. The absence of this enzyme activity is due to either homozygous or double heterozygous mutations in each of the two genes that encode ADAMTS 13. As a consequence of the deficiency of ADAMTS 13, patients with familial TTP have ultralarge multimers of vWF in their plasma. Acquired deficiency of ADAMTS 13 due to the formation of anti-ADAMTS 13 autoantibodies has also been described in some patients. Thus, genetic (familial) and acquired forms of TTP have been reported.

In the above patient, ADAMTS 13 is the only test that distinguishes TTP from aHUS. The other tests do not distinguish between these two clinically similar but genetically different disorders.

Suggested Reading

Brocklebank V, Wood KM, Kavanagh D. Thrombotic microangiopathy and the kidney. Clin J Am Soc Nephrol. 2018;13:300–17.
Clark WF, Hildebrand A. Attending rounds: microangiopathic hemolytic anemia with renal insufficiency. Clin J Am Soc Nephrol. 2012;7:342–7.
George JN. Thrombotic thrombocytopenic purpura. N Engl J Med. 2006;354:1927–35.
Kavanagh D, Sheerin N. Thrombotic microangiopathies. In: Yu ASL, Chertow GM, Luyckx VA, et al., editors. Brenner & Rector's the kidney. 11th ed. Philadelphia: Elsevier Saunders; 2020. p. 1178–95.
Noris M, Ruggenenti PL, Remuzzi G. Thrombotic microangiopathies, including hemolytic uremic syndrome. In: Feehally J, Floege J, Tonelli M, et al., editors. Comprehensive clinical nephrology. 6th ed. Philadelphia: Elsevier; 2019. p. 343–56.
Tsai H-M. Current concepts in thrombotic thrombocytopenic purpura. Annu Rev Med. 2006;57:419–36.

104. **Which one of the following therapeutic modalities for TTP is FALSE?**

A. Plasma exchange with FFP replacement (40 mL/kg) is the treatment of choice
B. Plasma exchange in combination with steroids may decrease relapse rates in some patients
C. Patients with cancer or chemotherapy-induced HUS/TTP benefit from extracorporeal immunoadsorption with protein A columns
D. Platelet transfusion at time of diagnosis induces an immediate and sustained response
E. Patients refractory to plasma exchange therapy may benefit from either vincristine or rituximab treatment

The answer is D

HUS/TTP does not appear to be a single entity because of different but overlapping pathogenic mechanisms. A variety of therapeutic modalities have been adapted, including steroids and plasma infusion alone or together. However, plasma exchange with fresh frozen plasma replacement has proven to be the treatment of choice in patients with TTP.

In some patients, plasma exchange in combination with steroids has been shown to delay the relapse rates of TTP. Cancer and/or chemotherapy-induced HUS/TTP can respond to extracorporeal immunoadsorption with protein A columns, which remove circulating immune complexes and improve survival of the patients. It has been shown that adult patients with TTP can benefit from either rituximab or vincristine therapy, if long-term plasma exchange has failed to improve the disease.

Platelet transfusion, once used, should be avoided to prevent microthrombi and further organ damage. Thus, statements A, B, C, and E are correct, and statement D is incorrect.

Suggested Reading

Brocklebank V, Wood KM, Kavanagh D. Thrombotic microangiopathy and the kidney. Clin J Am Soc Nephrol. 2018;13:300–17.

Clark WF, Hildebrand A. Attending rounds: microangiopathic hemolytic anemia with renal insufficiency. Clin J Am Soc Nephrol. 2012;7:342–7.

George JN. Thrombotic thrombocytopenic purpura. N Engl J Med. 2006;354:1927–35.

Kavanagh D, Sheerin N. Thrombotic microangiopathies. In: Yu ASL, Chertow GM, Luyckx VA, et al., editors. Brenner & Rector's the kidney. 11th ed. Philadelphia: Elsevier Saunders; 2020. p. 1178–95.

Moake JL. Thrombotic microangiopathies. N Engl J Med. 2002;347:589–600.

Noris M, Ruggenenti PL, Remuzzi G. Thrombotic microangiopathies, including hemolytic uremic syndrome. In: Feehally J, Floege J, Tonelli M, et al., editors. Comprehensive clinical nephrology. 6th ed. Philadelphia: Elsevier; 2019. p. 343–56.

Tsai H-M. Current concepts in thrombotic thrombocytopenic purpura. Annu Rev Med. 2006;57:419–36.

105. In the above 30-year-old (question 102), a tentative diagnosis of TTP was made, and she received plasma exchange with FFP replacement. She feels better after four plasma exchanges. Additional laboratory studies show undetectable ADAMTS 13 levels, but positive ADAMTS 13 inhibitor (anti-ADAMTS 13 IgG) titers. After seven plasma exchanges, she completely recovered and was discharged. She asks the physician about prognosis and relapse of her disease. **Which one of the following prognostic factors PREDICTS the risk for relapse?**

A. Age >30 years
B. Female sex
C. ADAMTS 13 levels >5% during remission
D. ADAMTS 13 levels <5% at time of initial presentation
E. Presence of ADAMTS 13 inhibitor at time of initial presentation

The answer is E

Relapse of TTP occurs in 20–60% of patients, with most relapses occurring during the first month after the acute episode and infrequently thereafter. Many conditions may precipitate relapses, including pregnancy, infectious diarrhea, surgery, or systemic infections. At times the etiologic or triggering agent is unclear. Age >30 years and female sex may have little or no role in precipitating relapse. Also, ADAMTS 13 activity >5% is sufficient to suppress relapse unless the patient has antibodies to ADAMTS 13 enzyme activity. Ferrari et al. followed a cohort of 35 patients with TTP who were treated with steroids and plasma exchange and then followed for a period of 18 months. Remission was achieved in 32 patients, and 3 patients died after treatment. Six patients relapsed once or twice during the follow-up. In their study, patients with or without the presence of ADAMTS 13 activity had relapses. However, it was the presence of ADAMTS 13 inhibitor (anti-ADAMTS 13 IgG) at the time of presentation that was predictive of relapse within 18 months. Thus, choice E is correct.

Suggested Reading

Ferrari S, Scheiflinger F, Reiger M, et al. for the French Clinical and Biological Network on Adult Thrombotic Microangiopathies. Prognostic value of anti-ADAMTS 13 antibody features (Ig isotype, titer, and inhibitory effect) in a cohort of 35 adult French patients undergoing a first episode of thrombotic microangiopathy with undetectable ADAMTS 13 activity. Blood. 2007;109:2815–22.

Tsai H-M. Current concepts in thrombotic thrombocytopenic purpura. Annu Rev Med. 2006;57:419–36.

106. **Regarding familial TTP, which one of the following statements is FALSE?**

A. Patients with familial TTP have large multimers of vWF in their plasma
B. In most patients with this disorder, plasma levels of ADAMTS 13 are zero or <5% of normal
C. Familial TTP is a recessive disorder caused by homozygous or double heterozygous mutations in genes that encode ADAMTS 13
D. Episodes of TTP begin in infancy or childhood or may not occur in some until precipitated by pregnancy
E. Infusion of FFP that contains ADAMTS 13 or cryosupernatant that does not contain vWF every 12 months is sufficient to prevent episodes of TTP. Frequent plasma exchange is necessary

The answer is E

Familial TTP is a rare recessive disorder. It may start in infancy or childhood and recur at regular intervals of about 3 weeks. In some patients, the disease may not be clinically apparent for years until a precipitating event such as pregnancy occurs.

Microvascular thrombi occur in most organs in patients with TTP. These thrombi contain vWF antigen but not fibrin. Patients with familial TTP have absent or <5% of normal ADAMTS 13 activity in their plasma. This absence of the enzyme activity is due to either homozygous or double heterozygous mutations in each of the two genes that encode ADAMTS 13. As a consequence of the deficiency of ADAMTS 13, patients with familial TTP have ultralarge multimers of vWF in their plasma.

Since recurrent episodes of TTP occur every 3 weeks, infusion of platelet-poor FFP or cryosupernatant, which contains the enzyme, is required only about every 3 weeks to prevent these episodes. Plasma exchange is not necessary. Therefore, statement E is false.

Suggested Reading

George JN. Thrombotic thrombocytopenic purpura. N Engl J Med. 2006;354:1927–35.

Karnib HH, Badr KF. Microvascular diseases of the kidney. In: Brenner BM, editor. Brenner & Rector's the kidney. 7th ed. Philadelphia: Saunders; 2004. p. 1601–23.

Matock CC, Marsden PA. Molecular insights into the thrombotic microangiopathies. In: Mount DB, Pollack MR, editors. Molecular and genetic basis of renal disease. A companion to Brenner & Rector's the kidney. Philadelphia: Saunders; 2008. p. 453–80.

Moake JL. Thrombotic microangiopathies. N Engl J Med. 2002;347:589–600.

107. **Regarding familial (atypical) HUS (aHUS), which one of the following statements is FALSE?**

A. The mortality rate in patients with aHUS is similar to that of diarrhea-associated HUS (D+HUS)
B. About one-third of patients with aHUS require maintenance dialysis, and the disease recurs in renal allografts
C. Mutations in genes for complement factor H (CFH), factor I (CFI), and membrane cofactor protein (MCP, also known as CD46) occur in patients with aHUS
D. Autosomal recessive form due to CFH mutations is associated with 10–50% normal levels of CFH and low serum C3 with the development of HUS at a young age
E. Autosomal dominant form due to CFH mutations is associated with functionally abnormal CFH protein and normal serum C3 levels with delayed onset of HUS which may be precipitated by pregnancy or infection

The answer is A

Familial or aHUS is a genetic disorder of alternative complement system. It is caused by mutations in the genes for CFH, CFI, and MCP. aHUS occurs in 5–10% of all cases of the disorder. The mortality rate is approximately 54% in patients with aHUS compared to 3–5% in D+HUS. Therefore, statement A is false. Supportive care is enough in most of the patients with D+HUS, and dialysis is required for those who do not respond to supportive care alone. On the other hand, plasma exchange with FFP replacement is required for patients with aHUS. However, plasma exchange does not always prevent relapse or progression of the renal disease. Kidney transplantation is complicated by the recurrence of the disease in the allograft in approximately 50% of patients. The recurrence rate is much higher in patients with CFH mutations than in those without CFH mutations. Surprisingly, a small study showed no recurrence in the renal allografts of patients with an MCP mutation.

Both recessive and autosomal forms of inheritance due to mutations in CFH have been described. Autosomal recessive form results from aberrant protein folding and decreased secretion, whereas the dominant form is due to functionally abnormal CFH.

Suggested Reading

George JN. Thrombotic thrombocytopenic purpura. N Engl J Med. 2006;354:1927–35.

Karnib HH, Badr KF. Microvascular diseases of the kidney. In Brenner BM, editor. Brenner & Rector's the kidney. 7th ed. Philadelphia: Saunders; 2004. p. 1601–23.

Matock CC, Marsden PA. Molecular insights into the thrombotic microangiopathies. In: Mount DB, Pollack MR, editors. Molecular and genetic basis of renal disease. A companion to Brenner & Rector's the kidney. Philadelphia: Saunders; 2008. p. 453–80.

Moake JL. Thrombotic microangiopathies. N Engl J Med. 2002;347:589–600.

108. A 68-year-old man develops fever, headache, myalgias, weight loss, and oliguric kidney failure 10 days following an angiographic procedure. Physical exam reveals "purple" toes and toe gangrene. **Which one of the following labs and histologic findings is FALSE?**
   A. Nephrotic-range proteinuria with FSGS or global sclerosis on renal biopsy
   B. Eosinophilia and eosinophiluria
   C. Hypocomplementemia and thrombocytopenia
   D. Normal ESR, leukopenia, and normal hemoglobin levels
   E. Occlusion of interlobular artery with cholesterol crystals

   The answer is D

   This is the typical presentation of atheroembolic disease, induced by dislodgement of atherosclerotic plague by catheter insertion in an elderly subject. Typically, clinical manifestations occur 1–14 days after the angiographic procedure, and characterized by fever, myalgias, headache, and weight loss. Cutaneous manifestations include livedo reticularis, purple toes, and toe gangrene due to cholesterol embolization. Lab findings include elevated ESR, leukocytosis, anemia, elevated creatinine, and BUN. Hypocomplementemia and thrombocytopenia have been described. In some patients, nephrotic-range proteinuria, microscopic hematuria, and FE_{Na} >1% have been demonstrated. On kidney biopsy, FSGS as well as global sclerosis with cholesterol crystals in small arteries and arterioles have been documented. Acute kidney injury leading to ESKD, requiring dialysis is observed in some patients. Cholesterol embolic diseases have been reported in renal allografts. Except for statement D, other statements are correct.

   Suggested Reading

   Meyrier A. Cholesterol crystal embolism: diagnosis and treatment. Kidney Int. 2006;69:1308–12.
   Scolari F, Ravani P. Atheroembolic renal disease. Lancet. 2010;375:1650–60.

109. **Which one of the following therapeutic modalities is found to have a favorable clinical outcome in patients with atheroembolic kidney disease?**
   A. Anticoagulants
   B. Vasodilators
   C. Surgical excision of atheromatous plagues in the suprarenal region of the aorta
   D. Dialysis only
   E. Discontinuation of anticoagulants, control of BP <140/80 and CHF, dialysis and nutritional support, and use of statins

   The answer is E

   There is no effective treatment for atheroembolic diseases, which is associated with about 64% mortality due to kidney failure. Various therapeutic modalities have been tried, including corticosteroids, vasodilators, surgical removal of atherosclerotic plaques, and hemodialysis. Anticoagulants should be avoided because of the risk for increased embolization. Belenfant et al. reported a 1-year survival of 87% in patients with acute kidney injury who were maintained on a strict regimen of anticoagulant discontinuation, postponement of surgical procedure, control of BP <140/80 mm Hg as well as CHF and continuation of dialysis therapy with adequate nutritional support. A prospective study showed that statins may have favorable kidney and patient outcome in patients with cholesterol crystal embolism. Therefore, option E is correct.

   Suggested Reading

   Belenfant X, Meyrier A, Jacquot C. Supportive treatment improves survival in multivisceral cholesterol crystal embolism. Am J Kid Dis. 1999;33:840–50.
   Scolari F, Ravani P. Atheroembolic renal disease. Lancet. 2010;375:1650–60.
   Scolari F, Ravani P, Pola P, et al. Predictors of renal and patient outcomes in atheroembolic renal disease: a prospective study. J Am Soc Nephrol. 2003;14:1584–90.

110. A 28-year-old woman is admitted for gross hematuria with left flank pain radiating to groin and thigh for 2 days. She denies dysuria or burning on urination. She had a similar episode 2 months ago, and her pain improved with codeine. Her past medical history includes depression, which she attributes to her marital problems. Her BP and serum chemis-

try and complement levels are normal. She is euvolemic. Urinalysis reveals numerous RBCs, 2–4 WBCs without any casts or proteinuria. Her medications include codeine as needed and estrogen-containing oral contraceptive pill. She denies any family history of kidney disease. **Which one of the following findings is MOST likely to be found in this patient?**

A. Kidney stones on spiral CT of abdomen
B. Subendothelial and mesangial deposits on EM
C. Intrarenal hemorrhages and thrombosis on renal angiogram
D. Presence of E. coli on urine culture
E. Lobular appearance of glomeruli and double-contour basement membranes

The answer is C

This patient with hematuria and flank pain with radiation to groin and thigh with normal kidney function and complement may have renal colic or upper urinary tract infection (UTI). Both of these conditions usually present with dehydration and at times prerenal azotemia. An unenhanced spiral CT of abdomen is helpful to rule out renal colic. If spiral CT is normal, the diagnosis of renal colic can be excluded. Urine culture is also important to consider the diagnosis of upper UTI. If no growth, UTI can be excluded. The presence of subendothelial and mesangial deposits on LM may suggest lupus nephritis, but the patient has no proteinuria or hypertension. Furthermore, complements are normal. Thus, lupus nephritis can be excluded. The findings in option E are suggestive of MPGN (type I); however, MPGN, type 1, presents with proteinuria, and at times with hypertension. Thus, MPGN, type 1, is unlikely. The most likely diagnosis seems to be the loin pain hematuria syndrome (LPHS), and the findings described in option C are consistent with this diagnosis.

LPHS is a condition of recurrent flank pain with radiation to groin and thigh and either microscopic or macroscopic hematuria. It has been described predominantly in women, and clinical manifestation may usually occur in the third decade of life, although LPHS may manifest from the first to the sixth decade of life. Pain may be unilateral or bilateral, and hematuria may be absent during pain-free period.

Acute episodes of LPHS may be associated with fever and flank pain, resembling that of acute pyelonephritis and renal colic, but appropriate tests may exclude these diagnoses. Patients with LPHS may have a history of estrogen-containing oral contraceptives and psychiatric disorders such as depression and narcotic-seeking habit. Hypertension and proteinuria are typically absent, thus excluding proteinuric conditions.

The pathogenesis of LPHS is uncertain. Renal angiographic studies have shown small-vessel narrowing, thrombi, infarction of the kidney, and spasm of small intrarenal vessels. Renal parenchymal edema with stretching of the renal capsule seems to cause pain. Also, pain may be due to intratubular obstruction of RBCs and microcrystals consisting of calcium and urate.

It is currently believed that hematuria in LPHS is of glomerular origin. Kidney biopsy in 34 patients with primary LPHS showed thin basement membrane disease (Autosomal Alport syndrome) in 26.5% and unusually thick basement membrane in 32.4%. It should be noted that LPHS may resemble IgA nephropathy in clinical presentation.

Treatment of LPHS includes nonsurgical and surgical interventions. Nonsurgical management includes analgesics, and surgical management involves nephrectomy, renal denervation, sympathectomy, and kidney autotransplantation, which includes placement of the native kidney in a different location. All of these procedures have met with some success. Spontaneous resolution of pain has occurred in 25% of these patients after conservative management with pain medications.

Suggested Reading

Dube GK, Hamilton SE, Ratner LE, et al. Loin pain hematuria syndrome. Kidney Int. 2006;70:2152–55.
Spetie DN, Nasady T, Nasady G, et al. Proposed pathogenesis of idiopathic loin pain-hematuria syndrome. Am J Kidney Dis. 2006;47:419–27.

111. A 58-year-old man is admitted for gross hematuria with left flank pain for 7 days. He denies dysuria or burning on urination. He had a similar episode 4 months ago, and his pain improved with codeine, but continues to have blood in urine. His past medical history includes hypertension and atrial fibrillation. He had been adequately anticoagulated, and his blood pressure is controlled. He is euvolemic. Phys exam is normal. Serum chemistry is normal except for creatinine of 1.8 mg/dL and lactate dehydrogenase of 1200 IU/L. Urinalysis reveals numerous RBCs, WBCs without casts or proteinuria. **Which one of the following is the MOST likely diagnosis in this patient?**

A. Nephrolithiasis
B. Urinary tract infection (UTI)
C. Renal infarction
D. Renal atheroembolic disease
E. Renal vein thrombosis

The answer is C

In this patient, UTI is less likely because of lack of symptoms. Also, the patient had persistent hematuria for the last 4 months. Renal vein thrombosis is less likely in the absence of proteinuria unless the patient has predisposing nonrenal causes. Nephrolithiasis is a possibility, but euvolemia and other symptoms make this diagnosis less likely. The patient is adequately anticoagulated, and therefore, atheroembolic disease is also unlikely. In atheroembolic disease, the deterioration in kidney function is fast. Thus, options A, B, D, and E are less likely diagnoses.

Patients with atrial fibrillation are at risk for renal infarction, which is frequently unrecognized. CT of abdomen shows a wedge-shaped hypodensity in renal parenchyma in over 90% of patients. Splenic infarction is also seen in about 30% of patients. Thus, atrial fibrillation is the most common cause of renal infarction in several of the published reports.

Suggested Reading

Autopolsky M, Simanovsky N, Staminkowicz R, et al. Renal infarction in the ED: 10-year experience and review of the literature. Am J Emerg Med. 2012;30:1055–60.
Korzets Z, Plotkin E, Bernheim J, et al. The clinical spectrum of acute renal infarction. Ise Med Assoc J. 2002;4:781–4.
Taourel P, Thuret R, Houquet MD, et al. Computed tomography in the nontraumatic renal cause of acute flank pain. Sem Ultrasound CT MR. 2008;29:241–52.

112. Infection, mostly bacteria-related glomerulonephritis (IRGN), is rather common in the elderly and immunocompromised individuals. In these individuals, the improvement in kidney function does not occur compared to IRGN in children. **On kidney biopsy, which one of the following pathologic features is COMMON in adult IRGN?**

A. Diffuse endocapillary proliferative and exudative GN with numerous intercapillary neutrophils on light microscopy (LM)
B. C3-dominant or co-dominant glomerular staining on immunofluorescence microscopy (IM)
C. In some cases of staphylococcal infection-related GN, predominantly IgA deposition rather than C3 deposition can be seen by IM
D. Subepithelial hump-shaped electron-dense deposits on electron microscopy (EM)
E. All of the above

The answer is E

IRGN in adults, particularly in diabetics and elderly, has poor kidney prognosis. Clinical manifestations include acute nephritic syndrome, HTN, mild to moderate proteinuria, edema, and reduced kidney function. Unlike children, adults require a kidney biopsy to exclude crescentic GN and other forms of GN that require immediate immunosuppressive therapy, or plasma exchange.

Histologically, all of the described LM, IM, and EM features have been described by D'Agati and her colleagues. These investigators described a separate immunopathologic IRGN which they called "IgA-dominant acute postinfectious glomerulonephritis." This form of IRGN is caused by staphylococcus sp. Unlike children, the source of infection in adults is heterogeneous (upper respiratory tract, skin, bone, lung, heart (endocarditis), urinary tract abscesses). Thus, IRGN is a serious complication in adults with poor kidney prognosis.

Suggested Reading

Nasr SH, Markowitz GS, Whelan JD, et al. IgA-dominant acute poststphylococcal glomerulonephritis complicating diabetic nephropathy. Hum Pathol. 2003;34:1235–41.
Nasr SH, Radhakrishnan J, D'Agati VD. Bacterial infection-related glomerulonephritis in adults. Kidney Int. 2013;83:792–803.

113. A 65-year-old type 2 diabetic patient is admitted for right flank pain, fever, and leukocytosis. Urinalysis shows numerous red blood cells, white cells, and proteinuria. His serum creatinine is 2.4 mg/dL, which increased from 1.8 mg/dL in 1 week. A kidney biopsy shows superimposed infection-related GN (IRGN) on diabetic kidney disease. **Which one of the following is an independent risk factor for progression of kidney failure in this patient?**

A. Older age
B. Serum creatinine level at the time of kidney biopsy
C. Degree of tubulointerstitial disease
D. Diabetes
E. All of the above

The answer is E

D'Agati and her group studied 86 patients and found that older age, high serum creatinine at the time of biopsy, more interstitial fibrosis, and comorbid conditions such as diabetes are independent renal risk factors in adults with IRGN (E is correct). Outcome studies were done in 52 patients, and 11 patients had IRGN superimposed on diabetic kidney disease. Of these 11 patients, 9 (82$) progressed to ESKD in ≥3 months. Thus, underlying diabetic kidney disease is a strong risk factor for progression to ESKD. How IRGN causes rapid progression is unclear.

Suggested Reading

Nasr SH, Markowitz GS, Stokes MB, et al. Acute postinfectious glomerulonephritis in the modern era: experience with 86 adults and review of the literature. Medicine (Baltimore). 2008;87:21–32.

Nasr SH, Radhakrishnan J, D'Agati VD. Bacterial infection-related glomerulonephritis in adults. Kidney Int. 2013;83:792–803.

Chapter 3
Calcium, Phosphorus, and Magnesium Disorders and Kidney Stones

1. You are asked to see a 70-year-old woman, a nursing home resident, for a serum Ca^{2+} level of 7.2 mg/dL and phosphate level of 1.9 mg/dL. Serum albumin and Mg^{2+} levels are normal. Renal and liver functions, except for alkaline phosphatase, are normal. She has a history of type 2 diabetes, and her diabetes is controlled with diet. Other than bone pain, she does not have any complaints.

   On physical examination, she appears tired. BP is 146/84 mm Hg with a pulse rate of 82 beats/min. Trousseau's and Chvostek's signs are negative, but calf and thigh muscle tenderness is significant. The following laboratory values are available:

Test	Value	Range
Ionized Ca^{2+}	3.5 mg/dL	4.5–5.0 mg/dL
PTH	74 pg/mL	10–65 pg/mL
$25(OH)D_3$	10 ng/mL	>30 ng/mL
$1,25(OH)_2D_3$	80 pg/mL	20–75 pg/mL
Alkaline phosphatase	300 U/L	30–120 U/L

   Which one of the following is the most LIKELY diagnosis?

   A. Hyperparathyroidism
   B. Pseudohypothyroidism
   C. Vitamin D deficiency
   D. Low Ca^{2+} intake
   E. Type 2 diabetes

   The answer is C

   Elevated PTH, $1,25(OH)_2D_3$, and alkaline phosphatase levels are observed in hyperparathyroidism; however, hypercalcemia is frequently associated with this disease. Pseudohypoparathyroidism is characterized by elevated phosphate and PTH levels, normal $25(OH)D_3$, and reduced $1,25(OH)_2D_3$ levels. Low Ca^{2+} intake does not cause hypocalcemia, as Ca^{2+} levels are maintained by bone resorption. Type 2 diabetes is associated with vitamin D deficiency, but other biochemical abnormalities observed in this patient are very unlikely caused by diabetes. Thus, options A, B, D, and E are incorrect.

   Vitamin D deficiency is the most likely diagnosis in this patient because of low $25(OH)D_3$. Active vitamin D_3 ($1,25(OH)_2D_3$) levels may be normal, slightly elevated, or reduced. Normal levels may be seen when all $25(OH)D_3$ is metabolized to $1,25(OH)_2D_3$, low levels are seen in the elderly as 1,α-hydroxylase enzyme activity is reduced. High levels are seen in some patients secondary to hypophosphatemia-enhanced 1,α-hydroxylase enzyme activity.

   In this patient, vitamin D deficiency is due to decreased sun exposure, age, and lack of sufficient intake of milk and milk products. Vitamin D deficiency has been reported in 50% of nursing home residents. Lack of vitamin D leads to decreased gut absorption of Ca^{2+} and phosphate. The resultant hypocalcemia stimulates PTH secretion, which, in turn, promotes phosphate excretion and hypophosphatemia. Elevated PTH also increases bone turnover, resulting in high alkaline phosphatase activity and bone pain.

A. S. Reddi, *Absolute Nephrology Review*, https://doi.org/10.1007/978-3-030-85958-9_3

Suggested Reading

Chonchol M, Smogorzewski MJ, Stubs JR, et al. Disorders of calcium, magnesium, and phosphate balance. In: Yu ASL, Chertow GM, Luyckx VA, et al., editors. Brenner & Rector's the kidney. 11th ed. Philadelphia: Elsevier Saunders; 2020. p. 580–613.

Holick MF, Binkley NC, Bischoff-Ferrari HA, et al. Evaluation, treatment, and prevention of vitamin D deficiency: an Endocrine Society clinical practice guideline. J Clin Endocrinol Metab. 2011;96:1911–30.

Lips P. Vitamin D physiology. Prog Biophys Mol Biol. 2006;92:4–8.

Naeem Z, Vitamin D deficiency-an ignored epidemic. Int J Health Sci (Qassim). 2010;4:V–VI.

2. A 70-year-old man was admitted for a suspicious lung mass. His BP, physical examination, and laboratory data are normal except for a creatinine of 1.2 mg/dL (eGFR 60 mL/min). An EKG is also normal. He had an MRI of his chest, which showed a well-demarcated mass. The next morning you are called by the lab for serum Ca level of 6.5 mg with normal PO_4 and albumin. The patient is asymptomatic. **Which one of the following choices is CORRECT regarding the evaluation of his hypocalcemia?**

   A. Obtain an EKG
   B. Call either an endocrinologist or nephrologist for evaluation of Ca_{2+}
   C. Order ionized Ca^{2+}
   D. Repeat Ca^{2+} immediately
   E. None of the above

   The answer is C

   This is pseudohypocalcemia secondary to MRI contrast agents. Serum Ca^{2+} is usually measured by the colorimetric assay, which uses a color-producing agent. This agent binds to Ca^{2+} and changes color in relation to the Ca^{2+} concentration. Of the four MRI contrast agents, gadodiamide (Omniscan) and gadoversetamide (OtiMARK) compete with Ca^{2+} for the colorimetric reagent and chelate Ca^{2+}, leading to falsely low Ca^{2+} concentration. Hypocalcemia persists as long as the contrast agent is in the blood. This pseudohypocalcemia does not occur with the remaining contrast agents, namely gadopentetate dimeglumine (Magnevist) or gadoteridol (Prohance). Once pseudohypocalcemia is recognized, an EKG and a consult to either an endocrinologist or nephrologist are not necessary. To clarify pseudohypocalcemia, one can order ionized Ca^{2+}, which is usually measured by ion-specific electrode method. Thus, option C is correct.

Suggested Reading

Choyke PL, Knopp MV. Pseudohypocalcemia with MR imaging contrast agents: a cautionary tale [editorial]. Radiology. 2003;227:627–8.

Williams SF, Meek SE, Moraghan TJ. Spurious hypocalcemia after gadodiamide administration. Case report. Mayo Clin Proc. 2005;80:1655–7.

3. A 71-year-old alcoholic man is admitted for profuse lower GI bleed, requiring 12 units of packed RBCs in 6 h. Hemoglobin improved, but BP was slightly low. Although he is alert and oriented, he complains of oral tingling. His serum Ca^{2+} dropped from 9.2 mg/dL to 6.0 mg/dL with normal Mg^{2+} level. His ionized Ca^{2+} is at the lower limit of normal. His liver function tests are slightly elevated. **Which one of the following is the MOST possible cause for his hypocalcemia?**

   A. Hypokalemia-induced hypocalcemia due to blood transfusion
   B. Hypocalcemia due to liver disease
   C. Hypocalcemia due to blood transfusion
   D. Hypocalcemia due to transfusion-related coagulopathy
   E. None of the above

   The answer is C

   Except for C, other answers are incorrect. Stored blood is usually anticoagulated with citrate (3 g of citrate per each unit). Although the healthy liver metabolizes 3 g of citrate every 5 min, he has a heavy load of citrate from packed RBCs. He has a mild liver disease, which may impair citrate metabolism and result in citrate toxicity. Although total Ca^{2+} determination may not be that helpful because of hemodilution related to massive transfusion, ionized Ca^{2+} is helpful.

Citrate toxicity causes tetany, prolonged QT interval, hypotension due to decreased peripheral vascular resistance, decreased myocardial contractility, and muscle tremors. IV Ca^{2+} is the appropriate treatment of transfusion-induced hypocalcemia.

Generally, hyperkalemia is the common abnormality with blood transfusion; however, hypokalemia is infrequently observed once metabolic alkalosis ensues due to conversion of citrate into HCO_3^-. Mild liver disease may not cause symptomatic hypocalcemia. Coagulopathy is also a complication of massive blood transfusion, but no relationship to hypocalcemia.

Suggested Reading

DiFrancesco NR, Gaffney TP, Lashley JL, et al. Hypocalcemia and massive blood transfusions: a pilot study in a level I trauma center. J Trauma Nurs. 2019;26:186–92.

Shiler KC, Napolitano LM. Complications of massive transfusion. Chest. 2010;137:209–20.

4. A 50-year-old man is admitted for impending alcohol withdrawal. He complains are of tingling around his lips and generalized weakness. His BP is 150/88 mm Hg with a pulse rate of 96 beats/min. Abnormal laboratory values include: K^+ 2.8 mEq/L; Ca^{2+} 6.8 mg/dL; Mg^{2+} 1.4 mg/dL; PO_4 2.1 mg/dL; and albumin 3.2 g/dL. EKG shows prolonged QT interval. **Which one of the following treatments will relieve his oral tingling?**

   A. Administration of KCl
   B. Administration of Ca gluconate
   C. Administration of $MgSO_4$
   D. Administration of D5W with KCl
   E. Administration of KCl, Ca gluconate, and $MgSO_4$

The answer is C

Hypokalemia, hypocalcemia, hypomagnesemia, and hypophosphatemia are typical electrolyte abnormalities in a patient with either acute or chronic alcoholism. There are several mechanisms for hypomagnesemia in an alcoholic patient, which in turn can cause hypokalemia and hypocalcemia.

Hypokalemia in an alcoholic patient may be due to poor dietary intake, respiratory alkalosis, diarrhea, β-adrenergic stimulation during alcohol withdrawal, and Mg^{2+} deficiency.

Hypocalcemia is caused by hypomagnesemia by two mechanisms. First, hypomagnesemia impairs PTH secretion; and second, hypomagnesemia causes skeletal resistance to PTH action. Both mechanisms result in low PTH and Ca^{2+} levels. Also, levels of $1,25(OH)_2D_3$ were found to be low in hypomagnesemia because of decreased conversion from 25-hydroxyvitamin D_3.

Alcoholism causes hypophosphatemia by poor dietary intake, transcellular distribution due to respiratory alkalosis and glucose intake, and hypomagnesemia. Since hypomagnesemia is responsible for other electrolyte abnormalities, it is the Mg^{2+} administration that corrects hypokalemia, hypocalcemia, and hypophosphatemia. Thus, option C is correct.

Unlike hypocalcemia induced by Mg^{2+} deficiency, hypocalcemia that is associated with gentamicin-induced hypomagnesemia may not improve with Mg^{2+} alone.

Suggested Reading

Agus ZS. Hypomagnesemia. J Am Soc Nephrol. 1999;10:1616–22.

Chonchol M, Smogorzewski MJ, Stubs JR, et al. Disorders of calcium, magnesium, and phosphate balance. In: Yu ASL, Chertow GM, Luyckx VA, et al., editors. Brenner & Rector's the kidney. 11th ed. Philadelphia: Elsevier Saunders; 2020. p. 580–613.

5. A 65-year-old man was admitted with acute kidney injury. His medical history is significant for diet-controlled hypertension. On serum chemistry, he was found to have Ca^{2+} levels of 19.4 mg/dL with total protein of 12.2 g/dL and albumin of 3.7 g/dL. Hypercalcemia was confirmed on repeat labs. Ionized Ca^{2+} was normal. He was asymptomatic from hypercalcemia. Serum protein electrophoresis and immunofixation showed very high levels of immunoglobulins of IgG type. **Based on the above information, which one of the following is the cause for his hypercalcemia?**

   A. Multiple myeloma
   B. Primary hyperparathyroidism
   C. Pseudohypercalcemia
   D. Diet
   E. None of the above

The answer is C

Pseudohypercalcemia is defined as elevated total serum Ca^{2+} level in the presence of normal ionized Ca^{2+} concentration. In this patient, total serum Ca^{2+} level is high, but the ionized serum Ca^{2+} level is normal. Thus, the patient has pseudohypercalcemia, which is not uncommon in a patient with IgG myeloma. No treatment for pseudohypercalcemia is required. Thus, answer C is correct.

Generally, Ca^{2+} binds to albumin; however, its binding to globulins is extremely small. When globulin levels are high (>8.0 g/dL), the binding of Ca^{2+} to globulins is increased. In particular, the IgG myeloma proteins have a much higher binding capacity with Ca^{2+}. Because of this globulin-Ca^{2+} binding, measurement of total Ca^{2+} level is high with normal ionized Ca^{2+} concentration.

Hypercalcemia is seen in about 30% of myeloma patients because of increased bone resorption. In this condition, both total and ionized Ca^{2+} levels are elevated. Also, the patient does not have any symptoms of hypercalcemia due to myeloma or primary hyperparathyroidism. The patient is not on any medications for hypercalcemia. Thus, answers A, B, and D are incorrect.

Suggested Reading

Ashrafi F, Iraj B, Nematollahi P, et al. Pseudohypercalcemia in multiple myeloma: a case report. Int J Hematol Oncol Stem Cell Res. 2017;11:246–9.

Liamis G, Liberopoulous E, Barkas E, et al. Spurious electrolyte disorders: A diagnostic challenge for clinicians. Am J Nephrol. 2013;38:50–7.

6. A 47-year-old man from New Guinea is admitted for complaints of productive cough with blood-tinged sputum, dyspnea for 1 week, and abdominal pain for 4 months. He also complained of nausea, vomiting, and dizziness for 1 week. The family noticed gradual weight loss and change in mental status. No history of kidney stones; however, he was diagnosed with tuberculosis at the age of 14 and was treated adequately. He is not on any prescription medications. He drinks milk and takes antacid for "heart burn." Chest X-ray shows bilateral infiltrates. EKG shows left bundle branch block. His BP is 130/62 mm Hg with a pulse rate of 84 beats/min (sitting); and 100/50 mm Hg with a pulse rate of 102 beats/min (standing). There is no evidence of vascular calcifications. Laboratory values are as follows:

$$Na^+ = 140\,mEq/L$$
$$K^+ = 4.1\,mEq/L$$
$$Cl^- = 96\,mEq/L$$
$$HCO_3^- = 28\,mEq/L$$
$$\text{Creatinine} = 2.7\,mg/dL$$
$$\text{BUN} = 52\,mg/dL$$
$$\text{Glucose} = 82\,mg/dL$$
$$Ca^{2+} = 21.6\,mg/dL$$
$$\text{Phosphate} = 5.3\,mg/dL$$
$$Mg^{2+} = 2.2\,mg/dL$$
$$\text{Total protein} = 7.2\,g/dL$$
$$\text{Albumin} = 4.0\,g/dL$$
$$\text{Alkaline phosphatase} = 105\,IU/L$$
$$\text{WBC} = 15{,}000$$
$$\text{Hemoglobin} = 13.8\%$$
$$\text{Platelets} = 327{,}000$$
$$\text{Active vitamin } D_3\left(1{,}25(OH)_2 D_3\right) = \text{low}$$

Based on the above data, which one of the following is the MOST likely diagnosis in this patient?

A. Primary hyperparathyroidism (PHPT)
B. Granulomatous disease (reactivation of TB)
C. Malignancy
D. Vitamin D excess
E. Familial hypocalciuric hypercalcemia (FHH)

The answer is C

Normal Cl^-, slightly elevated HCO_3^-, normal phosphate, normal alkaline phosphatase, and low $1,25(OH)_2D_3$ levels exclude the diagnosis of PHPT (A is incorrect). Reactivation of TB is possible, but the extent of Ca^{2+} and low $1,25(OH)_2D_3$ levels make this diagnosis unlikely (B is incorrect). Also, vitamin D and FHH are unlikely because of the extent of Ca^{2+} (D and E are incorrect). This patient seems to have an underlying malignancy that is causing very high levels of Ca^{2+} (C is correct). About 30% of patients with malignancy have hypercalcemia.

Suggested Reading

Goldner W. Cancer-related hypercalcemia. J Oncol Pract. 2016;12:426–32.
Reddi AS. Disorders of calcium: Hypercalcemia. In: Reddi AS, editor. Fluid, electrolyte and acid-base disorders. Clinical evaluation and management. 2nd ed. New York: Springer; 2018. p. 233–50.

7. **Which one of the following tests is APPROPRIATE to make the diagnosis of humoral hypercalcemia of malignancy in addition to serum and urine protein electrophoresis?**

A. PTH-related protein (PTH_rP)
B. PTH
C. Kidney biopsy with HIV testing and serum and renal tissue HTLV-1
D. CT of chest, abdomen, and brain
E. All of the above

The answer is E

All of the above tests are pertinent in this patient. The test results were available in 2 days later, which showed: PTH <10 pg/mL (low), PTH_rP 20 pmol/L (reference <2 pmol/L), normal $25(OH)D_3$, and normal serum and urine protein electrophoresis. CT of abdomen showed enlarged lymph nodes in his abdomen. HIV test was negative. Renal biopsy was done because of increasing creatinine despite adequate hydration, which showed acute tubular necrosis. However, serum HTLV-1 titers were positive. Testing of renal tissue was also positive for HTLV-1 virus, and the final diagnosis of hypercalcemia secondary to HTLV-1-induced adult T-cell lymphoma/leukemia was made.

HTLV-1 infection is endemic in Caribbean islands, parts of Africa, South and Central America, Japan, and southern USA, and hypercalcemia is the significant abnormality in individuals coming from these endemic areas.

Suggested Reading

Lyell V, Khatamzas E, Allain T. Severe hypercalcemia and lymphoma in an HTLV-1 positive Jamaican woman: a case report. J Med Case Rep. 2007;1:56.
Mirrakhimov AE. Hypercalcemia of malignancy: an update on pathogenesis and management. N Am J Med Sci. 2015;7:483–93.
Reddi AS. Disorders of calcium: hypercalcemia. In Reddi AS, editor. Fluid, electrolyte and acid-base disorders. Clinical evaluation and management. 2nd ed. New York: Springer. 2018. p. 233–50.

8. A 62-year-old man is brought to the Emergency Department with altered mental status. Physical examination shows a confused well-developed male with labored breathing. He required intubation to protect the airways. His BP is 132/78 mm Hg with a pulse rate of 100 beats/min. Except for lower extremity ulcer, which was rapped with a bandage containing white powder, the rest of the examination is otherwise normal. His laboratory values:

$Na^+ = 148\,mEq/L$

$K^+ = 1.8\,mEq/L$

$Cl^- = 73\,mEq/L$

$HCO_3^- = 54\,mEq/L$

$Creatinine = 3.4\,mg/L$

$BUN = 22\,mg/dL$

$Glucose = 110\,mg/dL$

$Ca^{2+} = 9.2\,mg/dL$

$Phosphate = 5.6\,mg/dL$

$Total\ protein = 7.1\,g/dL$

$Albumin = 2.7\,g/dL$

EKG : Normal sinus rhythm with prolonged QT interval

ABG : $pH = 7.69, PO_2 = 45, PCO_2 = 48$, and $HCO_3 = 53$

Urine : pH 5.8, Na^+ 81 mEq/L, K^+ 58 mEq/L, $Cl^- < 10$ mEq/L, and Ca^{2+} 150 mg/L

Urine toxicology : negative

Chest x ray : normal

After vigorous hydration with normal saline and K^+ supplementation, electrolytes, creatinine, and pH improved. BP rose to 160/90 mm Hg. The patient was successfully extubated. His iPTH and $1,25(OH)_2D_3$ were low normal.

Which one of the following is the MOST likely diagnosis of his hypercalcemia?

A. Sarcoidosis
B. Hypercalcemia related to calcium-containing medications (milk-alkali syndrome)
C. Familial hypocalciuric hypercalcemia (FHH)
D. Occult malignancy
E. Thiazide treatment

The answer is B

Sarcoidosis is excluded based on normal $1,25(OH)_2D_3$ level, although normal values in some cases were observed. Also, FHH is unlikely because of normal Ca^{2+} excretion. Hypercalcemia is almost asymptomatic in FHH. Also, Ca^{2+} excretion is low in FHH. Occult malignancy is possible; however, the patient does not have any evidence of malignancy. His chest x-ray and total protein concentration are normal. Further testing is necessary to completely rule out occult malignancy. Urine Cl^- <10 and urine Ca^{2+} 150 mg exclude the diagnosis of thiazide use. Based on the white powder that was covering the leg ulcer, the patient may be using a substance that contains Ca^{2+}. Indeed, the patient admitted to using baking soda ($CaHCO_3$) for the last 6 months as a remedy for leg ulcers. Thus, option B is correct.

Baking soda has been used as a home remedy for a number of conditions, including peptic ulcer disease and wound healing. Excessive ingestion or skin application of baking soda causes metabolic alkalosis, hypokalemia, hypercalcemia, volume contraction, and acute kidney injury. Hypercalcemia impairs HCO_3^- excretion, leading to metabolic alkalosis, volume contraction, and renal insufficiency, resulting in milk (calcium)-alkali syndrome.

Calcium-alkali (milk-alkali) syndrome can also develop without renal insufficiency. PTH and $1,25(OH)_2D_3$ are usually suppressed but normal values also have been reported. Hydration and electrolyte replacements, as required, are generally sufficient to treat calcium-alkali syndrome. At times, renal insufficiency and hypercalcemia may slowly resolve. The definitive long-term treatment is withdrawal of the offending agent.

Suggested Reading

Fitzibbons LJ, Snoey ER. Severe metabolic alkalosis due to baking soda ingestion: Case reports of two patients with unsuspected antacid overdose. J Emerg Med. 1999;17:57–61.

Medarov BI. Milk-alkali syndrome. Mayo Clin Proc. 2009;84:261–7.

Patel, AM, Goldfarb S. Got calcium? Welcome to the calcium-alkali syndrome. J Am Soc Nephrol. 2010;21:1440–3.

9. A 20-year-old man is found to have a serum Ca^{2+} level of 10.9 mg/dL , which was confirmed by determining ionized Ca^{2+} on a routine physical exam. His Mg^{2+} is also slightly elevated and phosphate is low. His intact PTH level is 70 pg/mL, and vitamin D levels are normal. All other labs are normal. He is not on any medications. Physical examination is normal. He also had elevated serum Ca^{2+} 10 years ago when he was admitted to hospital for cough and sputum production. **Which one of the following is the MOST likely diagnosis in this subject?**

   A. Primary hyperparathyroidism (PHPT)
   B. Secondary hyperparathyroidism
   C. Familial hypocalciuric hypercalcemia (FHH)
   D. Milk (calcium)-alkali syndrome
   E. Subclinical granulomatous disease

   The answer is C

   The laboratory findings are consistent with asymptomatic PHPT and FHH. The distinction between PHPT and FHH in adults can be difficult. Parathyroidectomy is the cure for PHPT, whereas all the above biochemical abnormalities persist even after parathyroidectomy in patients with FHH. One way to distinguish between PHPT and FHH is to calculate the Ca^{2+}-to-creatinine clearance ratio, which is <0.01% in FHH and >0.01% in PHPT. Renal function is normal; therefore, secondary hyperparathyroidism is unlikely. Also, normal vitamin D and elevated PTH levels exclude the diagnoses of milk (calcium)-alkali syndrome and granulomatous diseases.

   A 24-h urinary excretion of Ca^{2+} and creatinine was done, and Ca^{2+} excretion was 54 mg with a Ca^{2+} and creatinine clearance ratio <0.01%. This adult subject carries the diagnosis of FHH. Thus, option C is correct.

   Suggested Reading

Christensen SE, Nissen PH, Vestergaard P, et al. Familial hypocalciuric hypercalcaemia: a review. Curr Opin Endocrinol Diabetes Obes. 2011;18:359–70.

Shinall MC Jr, Dahir KM, Broome JT. Differentiating familial hypocalciuric hypercalcemia from primary hyperparathyroidism. Endocr Pract. 2013;19:697–702.

10. Excess PTH in patients with CKD has deleterious effects on various organ systems, including the cardiovascular system (CVS). **Of the following, which is NOT the effect of PTH on CVS?**

   A. Impaired myocardial contractility
   B. Increased myocardial interstitial fibrosis
   C. Vascular and valvular calcification
   D. Arterial vasodilation
   E. Left ventricular hypertrophy (LVH) and arrhythmias

   The answer is D

   For years, PTH has been considered a potent toxin with several adverse effects such as anemia, bone disease, neuromuscular myopathy, insulin resistance, and dyslipidemia. In addition, PTH has several deleterious effects on CVS. These include impaired myocardial contractility, leading to both systolic and diastolic dysfunction, myocardial and interstitial fibrosis, LVH, valvular calcifications, and arrythmias. All of these change lead to impaired myocardial contractility. There are certain blood pressure-independent effects of PTH, including thickening of intramyocardial arterioles and impaired endothelial vasodilatory functions, and the latter may lead to arterial vasoconstriction and hypertension. Thus, option D is incorrect.

   Suggested Reading

Amann K, Ritz E. Cardiac disease in chronic uremia: pathophysiology. Adv Ren Replace Ther. 1997;4:212–24.

Brown SJ, Ruppe MD, Tabatabai LS. The parathyroid gland and heart disease. Methodist Debakey Cardiovasc J. 2017;13:49–54.

Pascale AV, Finelli R, Giannotti R, et al. Vitamin D, parathyroid hormone and cardiovascular risk: the good, the bad and the ugly. J cardiovas Med. 2018;19:62–6.

Rostand SG, Drucke TB. Parathyroid hormone, vitamin D, and cardiovascular disease in chronic renal failure. Kidney Int. 1999;56:383–92.

11. **High PO_4 stimulates PTH through which one of the following mechanisms?**

A. Inhibits Ca-sensing receptor (CaSR) expression in the parathyroid gland
B. Inhibits PTH degradation
C. Increases FGF-23
D. Increases parathyroid cell proliferation and growth
E. All of the above

The answer is E

High PO_4 intake or high phosphate circulating levels stimulate PTH synthesis and secretion by all of the above mechanisms. Thus, control of PO_4 maintains near-normal levels of PTH in CKD patients.

Suggested Reading

Christov M, Sprague SM. Chronic kidney disease-mineral bone disorder. In: Yu ASL, Chertow GM, Luyckx VA, et al., editors. Brenner & Rector's the kidney. 11th ed. Philadelphia: Elsevier; 2020. p. 1805–37.
Silver J, Naveh-Many T. Phosphate and the parathyroid. Kidney Int. 2009;75:898–905.

12. **Which one of the following drugs is NOT associated with hypercalcemia?**

A. Vitamin A
B. Omeprazole
C. Silicone
D. Lithium
E. Chloroquine

The answer is E

Except for ketoconazole, all other medications have been shown to cause hypercalcemia. Vitamin A intoxication causes bone resorption and elevates serum [Ca]. Also, vitamin A analogs, used in dermatologic and malignant conditions, cause hypercalcemia.

Omeprazole, a proton pump inhibitor (PPI), has been shown to cause acute tubulointerstitial granulomatous disease and hypercalcemia with normal PTH levels. PPIs may also cause hypocalcemia.

The use of liquid silicone for soft tissue augmentation (breast and hip) has been shown to induce granulomas and hypercalcemia. Renal stones and renal failure due to obstruction and hypercalcemia do occur in some patients. Hypercalcemia improves with steroids. TNF-α inhibitors have also been used to prevent granuloma formation as TNF-α induces granuloma formation.

Lithium has been known for years to cause hypercalcemia by stimulating PTH secretion. This effect occurs probably through interaction with Ca-sensing receptor to alter the set point for PTH secretion in relation to plasma [Ca^{2+}].

Chloroquine causes hypocalcemia by decreasing the production of 1,25-dihydroxycholecalciferol. Thus, option E is correct.

Suggested Reading

Jacobs TP, Bilezikian JP. Rare causes of hypercalcemia. J Clin Endocrinol Metab. 2005;90:6316–22.
Khan O, Sim JJ. Silicone-induced granulomas and renal failure. Dial Transpl. 2010;39:254–60.
Wall CAM, Gaffney EF, Mellotte GJ. Hypercalcemia and acute interstitial nephritis associated with omeprazole therapy. Nephrol Dial Transpl. 2000;15:1450–2.

13. A 70-year-old woman is on hydrochlorothiazide (HCTZ) for hypertension for 7 years. Her BP and pulse are normal. Except for a recent increase in Ca^{2+} of 10.8 mg/dL, all her serum chemistry is normal. Her physician discontinued HCTZ and started her on an ACE-I. Follow-up of the patient showed hypercalcemia despite discontinuation of thiazide. **Which one of the following statements is FALSE regarding HCTZ and Ca^{2+}?**

A. HCTZ and other thiazides cause hypocalciuria
B. Volume contraction after chronic thiazide treatment increases Ca^{2+} reabsorption in the proximal tubule
C. Chronic thiazide treatment causes an increase both in TRPV5 channel and Ca^{2+} reabsorption in the distal tubule
D. The patient may have underlying primary hyperparathyroidism
E. Thiazides inhibit Na/Cl cotransporter in the distal tubule, causing loss of NaCl and volume depletion

The answer is C

Thiazide diuretics reduce calcium excretion. Two mechanisms have been postulated for this hypocalciuria: (1) the tubule Na^+ concentration is reduced by inhibiting Na/Cl cotransporter, which increases Na/Ca exchange and Ca^{2+} reabsorption, and (2) by inhibiting NaCl reabsorption in the distal tubule, thiazides promote NaCl loss and induce volume contraction. This volume contraction promotes passive paracellular Ca^{2+} transport in the proximal tubule. Studies with TRPV5 knockout mice have shown that thiazides promote Ca^{2+} reabsorption as wild-type mice, indicating that TRPV5 is not involved in thiazide-induced hypocalciuria. Thus, option C is false.

Wermers et al. determined the incidence of thiazide-associated hypercalcemia in 72 patients residing in Olmsted County, Minnesota, and found that 33 patients (64%) had persistent hypercalcemia after discontinuation of thiazide diuretic. Of these 33 patients, 20 had underlying primary hyperparathyroidism. The authors suggested that underlying primary hyperparathyroidism is common in patients who develop severe hypercalcemia while taking thiazide diuretics.

Suggested Reading

Griebeler ML, Kearns AE, Ryu E, et al. Thiazide-associated hypercalcemia: Incidence and association with primary hyperparathyroidism over two decades. J Clin Endocrinol Metab. 2016;101:1166–73.

Mensenkamp AR, Hoenderop JGJ, Bindels RJM. Recent advances in renal tubular calcium reabsorption. Curr Opin Nephrol Hypertens. 2004;15:524–9.

Wermers RA, Kearns AK, Jenkins GD, et al. Incidence and clinical spectrum of thiazide-associated hypercalcemia. Am J Med. 2007;120:911.e9–15.

14. **Regarding the PTH assay, which one of the following statements is FALSE?**

A. The first-generation radioimmunoassay (RIA) measures either C-terminal (53–84) or midregion (48–68) PTH molecule
B. The second-generation immunoradiometric assays (IRMA) measure intact (1-84) and other degradation fragments (7–84)
C. The actions of intact PTH (1–84) are different than that of 7–84 fragment
D. The ratio of 1–84 to 7–84 discriminates low-turnover from high-turnover bone disease in dialysis patients
E. The third-generation IRMA measures the biointact (1–84) and not 7–84 fragment of PTH

The answer is D

The intact PTH is a single-chain 84 amino acid peptide hormone. The Kidney Disease Outcomes Quality Initiative (K/DOQI) guidelines recommend that serum PTH levels of patients with CKD should be measured regularly and maintained within target ranges. For this reason, the methodology for PTH should be accurate because treatment decisions are made on the levels of PTH.

The first-generation RIA was described in 1963. It used polyclonal antibodies directed toward C-terminal or midregion PTH molecule. In addition, PTH fragments were also measured. Therefore, the PTH levels were greatly elevated. Thus, the first-generation assays became obsolete.

The second-generation PTH assays were introduced in mid-1980s as first- and second-generation assays. The first second-generation IRMA used two different antibodies; one directed toward the 39–84 portion and the second toward the 15–20 portion of the PTH molecule. These second-generation assays were called "INTACT PTH" assays as they were thought to measure only the full-length 1–84 PTH. Soon it was realized that these assays had certain limitations, in particular, their values were high and overestimated (in the range of 400–500 pg/mL) because of recognition of another fragment with amino acids from 7–84 of the PTH molecule. The high-intact PTH values in dialysis patients made the physician to take steps for suppression by either medical or surgical interventions, leading to low-turnover bone disease.

Further studies have shown that the newly measured 7–84 fragment has effects that are opposite to the intact 1–84 PTH, such as a decrease in serum Ca and urine PO_4 excretion and inhibition of bone resorption. These inhibitory effects of the 7–84 fragment seem to be mediated through a receptor called PTHR1, which is different from PTH/PTHrp receptor.

The third-generation PTH assay was first developed in 1999. It also used two antibodies; one directed toward C-terminal amino acids, and the second toward the first amino acids (1–4). Thus, the third-generation IRMA does not recognize the 7–84 fragment, and therefore, measures the biointact PTH (1–84).

Subsequently, some authors suggested that the ratio 1–84 PTH to 7–84 PTH (measured by the third- and second-generation assays, respectively) can discriminate between low- and high-turnover bone disease better than either one of the assays. However, it was later proven that the ratio has little discriminatory effect on bone disease. Thus, option D is false.

Table 3.1 summarizes the merits and pitfalls of the above described assays of PTH in dialysis patients.

Table 3.1 Merits and pitfalls of PTH assays

Assay/Yr	Method	Merits	Pitfalls
First-generation/1963	RIA	First method of PTH assay	Poor affinity and specificity Currently not used
Second-generation/1987 (intact PTH)	IRMA	Most widely used and follows current guideline recommendations Less expensive compared to third-generation assay	High intermethod variability Measures 7-84 PTH fragment
Third-generation/1999 (biointact PTH)	IRMA	Measures biologically active PTH Does not measure 7-84 PTH fragment May have better correlation with mortality	Expensive Less widely used Not adopted by current guidelines

RIA radioimmunoassay, *IRMA* immunoradiometric assays

Suggested Reading

Christov M, Sprague SM. Chronic kidney disease-mineral bone disorder. In: Yu ASL, Chertow GM, Luyckx VA, et al., editors. Brenner & Rector's the kidney. 11th ed. Philadelphia: Elsevier; 2020. p. 1805–37.

Friedman PA, Goodman WA. PTH (1-84)/PTH (7-84): a balance of power. Am J Physiol Renal Physiol. 2006; 290:F975–84.

Komaba H, Goto S, Fukagawa M. Critical issues of PTH assays. Bone. 2009;44:666–70.

Soliman M, Hassan W, Yaseen M, et al. PTH assays in dialysis patients: practical considerations. Sem Dial. 2019;32:9–14.

Souberbielle J-CP, Roth H, Fouque DP. Parathyroid hormone measurement in CKD. Kidney Int. 2010;77:93–100.

15. Measurements of PTH levels by the second- and third-generation assays were used to assess bone disease and mortality in ESKD patients. **Which one of the following statements is INCORRECT regarding PTH assays?**

    A. In choices for healthy outcomes in caring for end-stage renal disease (CHOICE) study, elevations of PTH values as measured by the third-generation assay rather than the second-generation assay were significantly associated with an increased risk of mortality
    B. Treatment of hemodialysis (HD) patients with maxacalcitol had lower ratios of third- to second-generation (1–84/7–84) PTH values
    C. Treatment of HD patients with cinacalcet lowered PTH levels determined by both third- and second-generation assays, but the ratio of third- to second-generation PTH values did not change
    D. PTH values are similar with both third- and second-generation assays
    E. In patients with parathyroid carcinoma and severe primary as well as secondary hyperparathyroidism, the third-generation assay measures a new molecular form of PTH with an intact N-terminus

The answer is D

The third-generation assay measures only biointact or whole PTH (1–84 amino acids) molecule, whereas the second-generation assays detect not only intact (1–84 amino acids) but also another fragment containing 7–84 amino acid molecule. Therefore, the PTH values determined by the second-generation assays are much higher than those values measured by the third-generation assay. Thus, option D is incorrect.

The CHOICE study showed that elevated levels of PTH as measured by the third-generation assay were strongly associated with increased risk of mortality in incident HD patients than those values measured by the second-generation assays

A study using maxacalcitol (22-oxa-calcitriol), a vitamin D analogue, found a decreased ratio of calculated biointact (equivalent to third-generation assay)-to-measured intact (second-generation) PTH ratio throughout the 24-week study period in HD patients without any change in serum PO_4 levels. However, serum Ca levels were significantly increased.

In another study, Martin et al. observed a decrease in both biointact and intact PTH levels in HD patients treated with cinacalcet by 38%, but the ratio of biointact to intact PTH was not affected. Thus, the study shows that PTH as measured by both assays can be used in HD patients to follow the response to cinacalcet.

Although the third-generation assay measures only biointact PTH, it was shown that it also can measure a new form of PTH with an intact N-terminus in patients with parathyroid carcinoma, and severe primary as well as secondary hyperparathyroidism. Although the function of this new N-PTH molecule is not known, it is secreted by enlarged parathyroid glands. An increase in biointact/intact PTH ratio was observed in a dialysis patient and this ratio was normalized after parathyroidectomy. Whether or not this new N-PTH molecule is biologically active is unknown.

Suggested Reading

Komaba H, Goto S, Fukagawa M. Critical issues of PTH assays. Bone. 2009;44:666–70.

Martin KJ, Jüppner H, Sherrard DJ, et al. First- and second-generation immunometric PTH assays during treatment of hyperparathyroidism with cinacalcet HCl. Kidney Int. 2005;68:1236–48.

Melamed ML, Eustace JA, Plantinga LC, et al. Third-generation parathyroid hormone assays and all-cause mortality in incident dialysis patients: the CHOICE study. Nephrol Dial Transpl. 2008;23:1650–8.

16. **Regarding calcium-sensing receptor (CaSR), which one of the following statements is FALSE?**

A. CaSR acts only in the kidney and parathyroid gland
B. Activation of CaSR leads to the release of intracellular Ca (Ca_i) and inhibition of PTH
C. Expression of CaSR gene is enhanced by active vitamin D in kidney and parathyroid cells
D. Activation of CaSR in the thick ascending limb of Henle's loop decreases paracellular transport of Ca
E. Activation of CaSR in the inner medullary collecting duct reduces vasopressin-stimulated waster reabsorption, causing polyuria in hypercalcemic conditions

The answer is A

CaSR senses changes in the extracellular Ca^{2+} levels and enables key tissues to maintain calcium homeostasis. It has been identified in many tissues, including the parathyroid glands, kidney, thyroid, intestine, bone, brain, and other organs. Therefore, option A is false.

The CaSR regulates three important functions of the parathyroid gland relevant to the kidney: (1) PTH synthesis, (2) PTH secretion, and (3) parathyroid cellular proliferation. In the kidney, activation of CaSR in the thick ascending limb of Henle's loop inhibits paracellular transport of Ca^{2+}, resulting in hypercalciuria. In the inner medullary collecting duct, CaSR is localized in the endosomes that contain vasopressin-regulated water channel, aquaporin 2. Activation of CaSR causes a reduction in vasopressin-stimulated water reabsorption, resulting in defective urinary concentration. As a result, polyuria ensues, particularly in conditions of hypercalcemia.

Ca^{2+} is not the only CaSR agonist. Other divalent and polyvalent cations such as Mg^{2+}, Be^{2+}, La^{3+}, and Gd^{3+} also function as CaSR agonists. These are called type 1 agonists, which activate CaSR even in the absence of extracellular Ca^{2+}. Type 2 agonists such as cinacalcet (Sensipar) require extracellular Ca^{2+} for activation.

Ca^{2+} is not the only CaSR agonist. Other divalent and polyvalent cations such as Mg^{2+}, Be^{2+}, La^{3+}, Gd^{3+} also function as CaSR agonists. These are called type 1 agonists, which activate CaSR even in the absence of extracellular Ca^{2+}. Type 2 agonists such as cinacalcet (Sensipar) require extracellular Ca^{2+} for activation.

Several factors upregulate the CaSR gene. These include Ca^{2+}, cinacalcet, vitamin D, interleukin 1β, and interleukin-6. Thus, options B through E are correct.

Suggested Reading

Brown EM, Hebert SC, Riccardi D, et al. The calcium-sensing receptor. In: Alpern RJ, Caplan MJ, Moe OW, editors. Seldin and Giebisch's the kidney. Physiology and pathophysiology. Wlatham: Academic Press; 2013. p. 2187–247.

Brown EM. Clinical lesions from the calcium-sensing receptor. Nature Clin Pract Endocrinol Metab. 2007;3:122–33.

Christov M, Sprague SM. Chronic kidney disease-mineral bone disorder. In: Yu ASL, Chertow GM, Luyckx VA, et al., editors. Brenner & Rector's the kidney. 11th ed. Philadelphia: Elsevier; 2020. p. 1805–37.

Hebert SC. Therapeutic use of calcimimetics. Annu Rev Med. 2006;57:349–64.

17. Since the identification of calcium-sensing receptor (CaSR), a number of inherited and acquired disorders of Ca-sensing have been reported. **Which one of the following disorders is NOT caused by abnormal Ca sensing?**

A. Familial hypocalciuric hypocalcemia (FHH)
B. Autoimmune hypocalciuric hypercalcemia
C. Autosomal dominant hypoparathyroidism
D. Type 5 Bartter syndrome
E. Type 1 Bartter syndrome

The answer is E

At least a dozen disorders of CaSR have been characterized. These disorders are either inherited or acquired. One of the well-documented inherited disorders is the FHH, which is due to inactivating mutations of the CaSR. Patients are generally young adolescents with mild elevations in serum calcium and magnesium concentrations. PTH levels are usually normal or mildly elevated. However, these patients are hypocalciuric. Despite hypercalcemia, these patients have normal urine concentrating ability. The patients with FHH do not require any treatment for hypercalcemia or mild hyperparathyroidism. Unlike patients with primary hyperparathyroidism, CaSRs in patients with FHH are resistant to Ca but normal in primary hyperthyroidism.

Autoimmune hypocalciuric hypercalcemia is an acquired disease due to inactivating antibodies to the CaSR in the setting of other autoimmune diseases (e.g., Hashimoto's diseases). Five patients presented with PTH-dependent hypercalcemia and relative hypocalciuria; however, parathyroidectomy in two patients did not abolish the antibodies. Thus, conservative management is sufficient in these patients.

Autosomal dominant hypoparathyroidism (also called autosomal dominant hypocalcemia) is due to activating mutations of the CaSR. Patients with this disease have symptomatic hypocalcemia. They also have hypomagnesemia, hyperphosphatemia, and PTH levels slightly higher than those with idiopathic hypoparathyroidism. Urinary Ca excretion is either inappropriately normal for a hypocalcemic patient or elevated. Aggressive treatment with oral Ca or vitamin D may not be necessary as some patients may develop nephrolithiasis and nephrocalcinosis. It is, therefore, advisable to raise serum Ca sufficient enough to improve signs and symptoms of hypocalcemia.

Type 5 Bartter syndrome is caused by activating mutations in CaSR located in the basolateral membrane of the thick ascending limb of Henle's loop. Patients with this disorder develop hypocalcemia, hypomagnesemia, low PTH levels, and hypercalciuria as well as hypermagnesuria. They also develop hypokalemia due to CaSR-mediated inhibition of Na/K/2Cl cotransporter in the apical membrane and loss of K in the urine.

Type 1 Bartter syndrome is due to mutations in the Na/K/2Cl cotransporter in the apical membrane of the thick ascending limb of Henle's loop, although hypokalemia, Na wasting, and hypercalciuria occur in this syndrome. Thus, option E is incorrect.

Suggested Reading

Brown EM, Hebert SC, Riccardi D, et al. The calcium-sensing receptor. In: Alpern RJ, Caplan MJ, Moe OW, editors. Seldin and Giebisch's the kidney. Physiology and pathophysiology. Wlatham: Academic Press; 2013. p. 2187–247.

Hannan FM, Babinsky VN, Thakker RV. Disorders of the calcium-sensing receptor and partner proteins: insights into the molecular basis of calcium homeostasis. J Mol Endocrinol. 2016;57:R127–42.

Nemeth EF, Goodman WG. Calcimimetic and calcilytic drugs: feats, flops, and futures. Calcif Tissue Int. 2016;98:341–58.

18. **Which one of the following physicochemical properties of cinacalcet is FALSE?**

A. After oral administration, the maximum plasma concentration of the drug is observed in 2–6 h
B. It is approximately 95% bound to plasma proteins with half-life of 30 to 40 h
C. Dose adjustment is necessary in renal failure patients
D. Ketoconazole increases cinacalcet levels
E. Nausea and vomiting are the major side effects of cinacalcet

The answer is C

Cinacalcet (Sensipar in the USA and Mimpara in Europe) is a second-generation calcimimetic. It lowers PTH levels by increasing the sensitivity of the calcium-sensing receptor to extracellular Ca. Except for option C, all other properties have been described with cinacalcet. Dose adjustment is not necessary in renal failure patients, but decreased dose is recommended in patients with moderate-to-severe liver failure.

Cinacalcet is metabolized by the enzyme CYP3A4, and ketoconazole is a strong inhibitor of this enzyme. Therefore, a decreased dose of ketoconazole is recommended in patients taking cinacalcet.

Suggested Reading

Nemeth EF, Goodman WG. Calcimimetic and calcilytic drugs: feats, flops, and futures. Calcif Tissue Int. 2016;98:341–58.

Torres PU. Cinacalcet HCl: a novel treatment for secondary hyperparathyroidism caused by chronic kidney disease. J Ren Nutr. 2006;16:253–8.

Vervloet MG, du Buf-Vereijken PW, Potter van Loon BJ, et al. Cinacalcet for secondary hyperparathyroidism: from improved mineral levels to improved mortality? Neth J Med. 2013;71:348–54.

19. **Regarding cinacalcet, which one of the following statements is INCORRECT?**

   A. Plasma levels of PTH fall after a single 100 mg oral dose of cinacalcet by 60–70% in 2–4 h with a gradual rise to a predose level in 24 h
   B. Serum Ca^{2+} level falls 12–14 h after cinacalcet treatment has begun and stabilizes within 12–24 h
   C. Cinacalcet is equally effective in patients with mild, moderate, or severe secondary hyperparathyroidism, although Ca-sensing receptor (CaSR) expression is diminished in secondary hyperparathyroidism
   D. Studies indicate that simultaneous use of cinacalcet and low dose of active vitamin D is effective in lowering PTH and FGF-23
   E. Cinacalcet therapy improves cardiovascular and all-cause mortality in all age-group hemodialysis (HD) patients

The answer is E

Cinacalcet (Sensipar) is a calcimimetic agent that sensitizes CaSR to lower PTH in a dose-dependent manner. PTH levels fall to 60–70% from baseline values after a single oral dose within 2–4 h. However, the PTH levels gradually reach the predose level within 24 h due to low circulating cinacalcet levels and associated decrease in CaSR activation.

Along with PTH, Ca^{2+} levels also decrease after 12–24 h with cinacalcet treatment. This decrease is due to an early decrease in PTH level. Interestingly, PO_4 levels also decrease. Thus, cinacalcet lowers PTH, Ca^{2+}, and PO_4 levels in dialysis patients.

Dose titration is necessary when treatment is started. The initial dose is 30 mg daily, and can be increased to 60 mg in 2- to 3-week intervals up to 180 mg per day. This escalated dose is dependent on the response of PTH and no hypocalcemia is present. Cinacalcet is effective in dialysis patients with varying degrees of secondary hyperparathyroidism, including severe form, even though CaSR expression is diminished. The available data indicate that the combination of cinacalcet with low doses of calcitriol analogues lowers not only PTH but also FGF-23 levels in dialysis patients. This combination may also avoid hypocalcemia induced by cinacalcet.

Cinacalcet treatment for 21.2 months in HD patients with moderate-to-severe secondary hyperparathyroidism did not significantly reduce the risk of death or major cardiovascular events. Also, a meta-analysis concluded that cinacalcet reduces the need for parathyroidectomy in HD patients, but does not reduce all-cause or cardiovascular mortality. A subsequent analysis of the EVOLVE study, however, showed a beneficial effect in patients ≥65 years of age with moderate-to-severe hyperparathyroidism. Cinacalcet decreased both the risk of death and also of major cardiovascular events. This beneficial effect was not observed in patients ≤65 years of age. This difference between the younger and older patients seems to be related to more cardiovascular risk factors in the younger patients. Thus, option E is incorrect.

Suggested Reading

Effect of cinacalcet on cardiovascular disease in patients undergoing dialysis. The EVOLVE Trial Investigators. N Engl J Med. 2011;367:2482–92.

Nemeth EF, Goodman WG. Calcimimetic and calcilytic drugs: feats, flops, and futures. Calcif Tissue Int. 2016;98:341–58.

Palmer SC, Nistor I, Craig JC, et al. Cinacalcet in patients with chronic kidney disease: a cumulative meta-analysis of randomized controlled studies. PLOS Med. 2013;10:e1001436.

Parfrey PS, Drüeke TB, Block GA, et al. Evaluation of Cinacalcet HCl Therapy to Lower Cardiovascular Events (EVOLVE) Trial Investigators. The effects of Cinacalcet in older and younger patients on hemodialysis: the Evaluation of Cinacalcet HCl Therapy to Lower Cardiovascular Events (EVOLVE) Trial. Clin J Am Soc Nephrol. 2015;10:791–9.

Strippoli GFM, Palmer S, Tong A, et al. Meta-analysis of biochemical and patient-level effects of calcimimetic therapy. Am J Kidney Dis. 2006;47:715–26.

Wetmore JB, Liu S, Krebill R, et al. Effects of cinacalcet and concurrent low-dose vitamin D on FGF-23 levels in ESRD. Clin J Am Soc Nephrol. 2010;5:110–6.

20. A 50-year-old man with hypertension and CKD 5 on hemodialysis is found to have a serum Ca^{2+} of 10.5 mg/dL, PO_4 of 7.2 mg/dL, and intact PTH (iPTH) of 700 pg/mL. He is on sevelamer 2400 mg three times daily with meals and paricalcitol 4 μg three times a week. The patient follows low phosphate diet. **Which one of the following options is CORRECT?**

   A. Increase paricalcitol to 10 μg three times a week
   B. Add calcium acetate (PhosLo) 667 mg three times a day
   C. Prepare the patient for parathyroidectomy
   D. Start cinacalcet at 30 mg/day with increasing dosage up to 180 mg/day
   E. Consult a dietician for vigorous control of PO_4 in diet

The answer is D

This patient has severe hyperparathyroidism with hypercalcemia and hyperphosphatemia despite on adequate dose of sevelamer. Increasing paricalcitol and adding calcium acetate will worsen hypercalcemia, but hyperphosphatemia may slightly improve. Further control of PO_4 in diet may not help in controlling Ca^{2+}. The best approach is to treat the patient with the starting dose of cinacalcet (30 mg daily with escalation of dose in 2–4 weeks). Surgical consult is too early for parathyroidectomy, and it may be necessary if cinacalcet fails to control Ca^{2+}, PO_4, and iPTH.

Suggested Reading

Nemeth EF, Goodman WG. Calcimimetic and calcilytic drugs: feats, flops, and futures. Calcif Tissue Int. 2016;98:341–58.
Torres PU. Cinacalcet HCl: a novel treatment for secondary hyperparathyroidism caused by chronic kidney disease. J Renal Nutr. 2006;16:253–8.
Vervloet MG, du Buf-Vereijken PW, Potter van Loon BJ, et al. Cinacalcet for secondary hyperparathyroidism: from improved mineral levels to improved mortality? Neth J Med. 2013;71:348–54.

21. **As per the position statement from Kidney Disease: Improving Global Outcomes (KDIGO) CKD-MBD Update Work Group, which one of the following target ranges for bone mineral metabolism in CKD 5 (eGFR <15 mL/min) is INCORRECT?**

A. Intact PTH (iPTH) levels up to 600 pg/mL
B. Albumin-adjusted Ca^{2+} of 8.4–9.5 mg/dL
C. Serum PO_4 level of 3.5–5.5 mg/dL
D. Ca and PO_4 (C × P) product <55 mg/dL
E. iPTH levels of 150–300 pg/dL

The answer is E

The term chronic kidney disease-mineral and bone disorder (CKD-MBD) has been introduced into nephrology practice to describe the systemic components of the clinical syndrome that includes bone abnormalities, Ca^{2+}, PO_4, PTH, vitamin D balance, and vascular calcification. Disturbed CKD-MBD gives rise to several systemic complications, including bone pain, bone fractures, parathyroid hyperplasia, parathyroidectomy, and vascular calcification. These complications lead to severe cardiovascular complications and morbidity as well as mortality. In 2003, the National Kidney Foundation Advisory Committee (the Kidney Disease Outcomes Quality Initiative, KDOQI) developed clinical guidelines that include recommendation targets for iPTH, Ca^{2+}, PO_4, and Ca × P product in patients with CKD to improve morbidity and mortality. Options B to E are the target ranges for Ca^{2+}, PO_4, Ca × P product, and iPTH as proposed by KDOQI guidelines.

As mentioned previously, iPTH determination is variable, and the range of PTH from 150 to 300 pg/mL may not be predictive of underlying bone histology. Therefore, the KDIGO guidelines proposed target iPTH levels to be three to nine times the normal levels of iPTH (65 pg/mL). Thus, option E is incorrect.

Suggested Reading

Kidney Disease Improving Global Outcomes. Clinical practice guidelines for the management of CKD-MBD. Kidney Int. 2009;76 (S113):S1–S130.
Kidney Disease: Improving Global Outcomes (KDIGO) CKD-MBD Update Work Group. KDIGO 2017 Clinical Practice Guideline Update for the Diagnosis, Evaluation, Prevention, and Treatment of Chronic Kidney Disease–Mineral and Bone Disorder (CKD-MBD). Kidney Int Suppl. 2017;7:1–59.
National Kidney Foundation. K/DOQI clinical practice guidelines for bone metabolism and disease in chronic kidney disease. Am J Kidney Dis. 2003;42(Suppl 3):S1–S201.

22. **Which one of the following metabolic abnormalities is NOT related to severe hypophosphatemia (<1.0 mg/dL)?**

A. Rhabdomyolysis
B. Metabolic acidosis
C. Increased susceptibility to infection
D. Decreased cardiac output
E. Metabolic alkalosis

The answer is E

Moderate hypophosphatemia is defined as serum phosphate level between 1.2 and 1.8 mg/dl, whereas severe hypophosphatemia constitutes serum phosphate level <1.0 mg/dl. Metabolic complications are clearly evident with severe hypophosphatemia. Muscle requires adequate amounts of ATP and creatine phosphate for its actions. Phosphate depletion leads to low intracellular phosphate and an increase in Na^+, Cl^-, and water, resulting in myopathy, weakness, and muscle injury. Rhabdomyolysis is a complication of low serum phosphate, which may present with acute kidney injury.

Metabolic acidosis due to severe hypophosphatemia is related to a decrease in net acid excretion (titratable acid and NH_3), resulting in retention of H^+. Also, hypophosphatemia decreases renal tubular reabsorption of HCO_3^-. Thus, metabolic acidosis in severe hypophosphatemia is due to the above mechanisms.

Increased susceptibility to infection is related to leukocyte dysfunction caused by decreased ATP production.

Severe hypophosphatemia is associated with cardiomyopathy and low cardiac output, which are due to low myocyte concentration of phosphate, ATP, and creatine phosphate. Metabolic alkalosis is not a complication of severe hypophosphatemia, and thus option E is incorrect.

Suggested Reading

Reddi AS. Disorders of phosphate: hypophosphatemia. In: Reddi AS, editor. Fluid, electrolyte, and acid-base disorders. Clinical evaluation and management. 2nd ed. New York: Springer; 2018. p. 259–72.

23. Both in hospitalized and clinic patients, hypophosphatemia is a common electrolyte disorder. **Which one of the following drugs does NOT cause hypophosphatemia?**

A. Imatinib
B. Tenofovir
C. Corticosteroids
D. Glucose
E. Bisphosphonates

The answer is E

Except for bisphosphonates, all other drugs cause hypophosphatemia. Imatinib, a tyrosine kinase inhibitor, is used in many malignant diseases. Long-term use of imatinib causes hypophosphatemia and secondary hyperparathyroidism. Tenofovir, a nucleotide reverses transcriptase inhibitor, causes transient hypophosphatemia with unknown mechanism.

Corticosteroids cause a decrease in intestinal absorption of PO_4 and they also promote renal excretion of phosphate (PO_4). Both these processes account for hypophosphatemia. Intravenous glucose or carbohydrate intake transports PO_4 into the cell, causing hypophosphatemia.

Bisphosphonates, as a class, cause an increase in renal tubular reabsorption without significant excretion of PO_4, resulting in hyperphosphatemia. Therefore, option E is incorrect.

Suggested Reading

Chonchol M, Smogorzewski MJ, Stubs JR, et al. Disorders of calcium, magnesium, and phosphate balance. In: Yu ASL, Chertow GM, Luyckx VA, et al., editors. Brenner & Rector's the kidney. 11th ed. Philadelphia: Elsevier Saunders; 2020. p. 580–613.
Jao J, Wyatt CM. Antiretroviral medications: adverse effects on the kidney. Adv Chronic Kidney Dis. 2010;17:72–82.
Osorio S, Noblejas AG, Duran A et al. Imatinib mesylate induces hypophosphatemia in patients with myeloid leukemia in late chronic phase, and this effect is associated with response. Am J Hematol. 2007;82:394–5.

24. **Which one of the following metabolic abnormalities is NOT related to severe hypophosphatemia (<1.0 mg/dL)?**

A. Rhabdomyolysis
B. Metabolic acidosis
C. Increased susceptibility to infection
D. Decreased cardiac output
E. Metabolic alkalosis

The answer is E

Moderate hypophosphatemia is defined as serum PO_4 level between 1.2 and 1.8 mg/dL, whereas severe hypophosphatemia constitutes serum PO_4 level <1.0 mg/dL. Metabolic complications are clearly evident with severe hypophosphatemia. Muscle requires adequate amounts of ATP and creatine PO_4 for its actions. PO_4 depletion leads to low intracellular PO_4 and an increase in Na^+, Cl^-, and water, resulting in myopathy, weakness, and muscle injury. Rhabdomyolysis is a complication of low serum PO_4, which may present with acute kidney injury (AKI).

Metabolic acidosis due to severe hypophosphatemia is related to a decrease in net acid excretion (titratable acid and ammonium), resulting in retention of H^+. Also, hypophosphatemia decreases renal tubular reabsorption of HCO_3^-. Thus, metabolic acidosis in severe hypophosphatemia is due to the above mechanisms.

Increased susceptibility to infection is related to leukocyte dysfunction caused by decreased ATP production.

Severe hypophosphatemia is associated with cardiomyopathy and low cardiac output, which are due to low myocyte concentration of PO_4, ATP, and creatine PO_4. Metabolic alkalosis is not a complication of severe hypophosphatemia, and thus option E is incorrect.

Suggested Reading

Chonchol M, Smogorzewski MJ, Stubs JR, et al. Disorders of calcium, magnesium, and phosphate balance. In: Yu ASL, Chertow GM, Luyckx VA, et al., editors. Brenner & Rector's the kidney. 11th ed. Philadelphia: Elsevier Saunders; 2020. p. 580–613.

Gassbeek A, Meinders E. Hypophosphatemia: an update on its etiology and treatment. Am J Med. 2005;118:1094–101.

25. A 67-year-old thin woman with colon cancer and colostomy is admitted for poor oral intake, weakness, dizziness, and weight loss. She is receiving chemotherapy. The oncologist starts her on total parenteral nutrition with 2000 calories a day. Serum chemistry is normal, including Ca^{2+}, Mg^{2+}, and PO_4. Two days later, the patient complains of worsening weakness. Repeat lab shows: K^+ 3.1 mEq/L, Ca^{2+} 7.8 mg/dL, Mg^{2+} 1.8 mEq/L, and PO_4 1.1 mg/dL. **Which one of the following describes the BEST for the above lab abnormalities?**

A. Metabolic acidosis
B. Respiratory alkalosis
C. Refeeding syndrome
D. Chemotherapy
E. None of the above

The answer is C

Refeeding syndrome (RFS) occurs in malnourished individuals following administration of oral, enteral, or parenteral nutrition. It is commonly seen in hospitalized patients, who are malnourished due to poor oral intake, starvation, anorexia nervosa, or systemic illness such as malignancy. Hypophosphatemia is the most commonly observed electrolyte abnormality induced by RFS. Many mechanisms contribute to hypophosphatemia: (1) a high carbohydrate meal causes intracellular shift of PO_4; (2) increased consumption of PO_4 during glycolysis; (3) depleted body stores of PO_4 during poor oral intake of food; and (4) consumption of PO_4 for formation of ATP and increased production of products such as creatine kinase and 2,3-diphosphoglycerate.

Sudden deaths also have been reported following RFS with high caloric diet due to hypophosphatemia. Almost all organ systems fail. To prevent hypophosphatemia, the feeding should consist of low calories with gradual increase to maintain the target caloric intake. Along with hypophosphatemia, other electrolyte abnormalities such as hypokalemia and hypomagnesemia also occur due to high glucose. Supplementation of K^+, Mg^{2+}, and PO_4 along with nutrition will prevent RFS.

Suggested Reading

Khan LUR, Ahmed J, Khan S, et al. Refeeding syndrome: a literature review. Gastroenterol Res Pract. 2011;2011:Article ID 410971, 6 pages. https://doi.org/10.1155/2011/410971.

Marinella MA. Refeeding syndrome and hypophosphatemia. J Intensive Care Med. 2005;20:155–9.

Marinella MA. Refeeding syndrome in cancer patients. Int J Clin Pract. 2008;62:460–5.

Reber E, Freidli N, Vasiloglou MF, et al. Management of refeeding syndrome in medical patients. J Clin. Med. 2019;8(12):2202. https://doi.org/10.3390/jcm8122202.

26. **Regarding treatment of hypophosphatemia, which one of the following statements is FALSE?**

A. In asymptomatic ambulatory patient, moderate hypophosphatemia (1.2 to 1.8 mg/dL) can be corrected by oral PO_4 repletion
B. Hyperalimentation-induced severe hypophosphatemia (<1 mg/dL) requires aggressive intravenous (IV) treatment with 1 mmol/kg over 10 h
C. IV PO_4 repletion depends on the severity of PO_4 deficiency and body weight
D. Moderate degree of hypophosphatemia after heavy carbohydrate meal does not require PO_4 repletion
E. Hypophosphatemia (>1 mg/dL) generally causes severe metabolic complications and requires vigorous IV replacement of PO_4

The answer is E

The treatment of hypophosphatemia depends on its signs and symptoms and the degree (severity) of PO_4 deficiency. Asymptomatic patients should be treated with oral preparations (Table 3.2). Serum PO_4 levels can rise by as much as 1.5 mg/dL, 60 to 120 min after oral intake of 1 g of elemental PO_4. In children and malnourished individuals, skim milk is an adequate repletion of PO_4 because each liter contains 1 g of elemental PO_4 and better tolerated than regular milk.

IV administration of PO_4 is reserved for patients with severe hypophosphatemia (<1 mg/dL) with symptoms and those receiving hyperalimentation and critically ill patients. In hyperalimentation-induced hypophosphatemic (<1.5 mg/dL) patients in an intensive care setting, an infusion of 1 mmol/kg (1 mmol = 3.1 mg/dL) phosphorus diluted in 100 or 250 mL of either normal saline or D5W at a rate not to exceed 7.5 mmol/h was sufficient to normalize serum PO_4 in 48 h.

In surgical intensive care patients, Taylor et al. used a weight- and serum PO_4-based protocol for IV PO_4 repletion (Table 3.3). Either sodium PO_4 or potassium PO_4, depending on serum K^+ levels, was dissolved in 250 ml of D5W and infused over 6 h as a single dose to severely hypophosphatemic (<1 mg/dL) or moderately hypophosphatemic (1.5-1.8 mg/dL) patients. Successful repletion occurred in 63% of severe and 78% of moderate hypophosphatemic patients. Thus, severe hypophosphatemic patients may benefit from more aggressive and tailored IV phosphorous regimens.

Transcellular distribution of PO_4 from ECF to ICF occurs after a carbohydrate load or glucose infusion, which does not require immediate treatment. Serum PO_4 level >1 mg/dL may not cause severe metabolic complications, and vigorous IV treatment is not necessary. Thus, option E is false. Be aware of complications such as hypocalcemia, hyperphosphatemia, AKI, and hyperkalemia with potassium PO_4 that are common with vigorous IV administration.

Table 3.2 Oral and intravenous phosphate preparations

Preparation	PO_4	Na (mEq/L)	K (mEq/L)
Oral			
Skim milk	1 g/L	28	38
Neutra-phos	250 mg/packet	7.1/packet	7.1/packet
Neutra-phos K	250 mg/capsule	0	14.25/capsule
Phospho-Soda	150 mg/mL	4.8	0
K-Phos Original	150 mg/capsule	0	3.65/capsule
K-Phos Neutral	250 mg/tablet	13	1.1
Intravenous			
Neutral Na/K PO_4	1.1 mmol/mL	0.2	0.02
Neutral Na PO_4	0.09 mmol/mL	0.2	0
Sodium PO_4	3 mmol/mL	4	0
Potassium PO_4	3 mmol/mL	0	4.4

Note: 1 mmol/L = 3.1 mg/dL

Table 3.3 Intravenous phosphorus (mmol) repletion protocol

Serum PO_4	Wt (40–60 kg)	Wt (61–80 kg)	Wt (81–120 kg)
<0.32 mmol/L (<1 mg/dL)	30	40	50
0.32–0.54 mmol/L (1–1.7 mg/dL)	20	30	40
0.58–0.7 mmol/L (1.8–2.2 mg/dL)	10	15	20

Adapted from Taylor et al. [1]

Reference

1. Taylor BE, Huey WY, Buchman T, et al. Treatment of hypophosphatemia using a protocol based on patient weight and serum phosphorus level in a surgical intensive care unit. J Am Coll Surg 198:198–204, 2004.

Suggested Reading

Brunelli SM, Goldfarb S. Hypophosphatemia: clinical consequences and management. J Am Soc Nephrol. 2007;18:1999–2003.

27. A 68-year-old woman with diabetes mellitus is admitted for mucormycosis of the left ear. She is started on high doses of liposomal amphotericin B (L-AMP). One week later, her serum PO_4 increased from 4.2 mg/dL to 10.8 mg/dL, and repeat PO_4 is 11.2 mg/dL. Her creatinine, Ca^{2+}, uric acid, and creatine kinase (CK) are normal. **Which one of the following is the MOST likely cause of her hyperphosphatemia?**

A. Rhabdomyolysis
B. Respiratory alkalosis
C. Liposomal amphotericin B
D. Tumor calcinosis
E. None of the above

The answer is C

The sudden increase in serum PO_4 in a patient who is not on PO_4 replacement is suspicious of laboratory error. Repeat analysis confirmed hyperphosphatemia. The patient was asymptomatic. Rhabdomyolysis was ruled out based on normal creatinine, Ca^{2+}, uric acid, and CK levels. ABG showed chronic respiratory alkalosis, which causes hypophosphatemia by transcellular distribution of PO_4. Tumor calcinosis is a rare genetic disorder that is characterized by hyperphosphatemia, elevated levels of $1,25(OH)_2D_3$, and decreased renal excretion of PO_4. Thus, options A, B, and D are incorrect.

L-AMP is an antifungal preparation that contains amphotericin B embedded in a phospholipid bilayer of unilamellar liposomes. Measurement of PO_4 from L-AMP-treated patients with a specific autoanalyzer called Synchron LX20 (Beckman Coulter) gives a high level with normal Ca^{2+} levels. This autoanalyzer measures the PO_4 at low pH (<1.0). At this acid pH, organic PO_4 contained in the lipid bilayer of the liposomes is hydrolyzed and gives falsely high levels of serum PO_4. Thus, high doses of L-AMP will give pseudohyperphosphatemia when measured with LX20 system. Other autoanalyzers measure the reaction at high pH, and do not give pseudohyperphosphatemia. Thus, option C is correct.

Other conditions such as hyperbilirubinemia, paraproteinemia, heparin, and hyperlipidemia also cause pseudohyperphosphatemia, which is due to assay interference.

Suggested Reading

Bailey HL, Chan EM. Liposomal Amphotericin B interferes with the phosphorus assay on the Synchron LX20 analyzer. Clin Chem. 2007;53:795–6.

Lane JW, Rehak NN, Hortin GL, et al. Pseudohyperphosphatemia associated with high-dose liposomal amphotericin B therapy. Clin Chim Acta. 2008;387:145–9.

Senthilkumaran S, Menezes RG, Jayaraman S, et al. Pseudohyperphosphatemia due to contamination with heparin: a case for caution. Indian J Nephrol. 2014;24:409–10.

Talebi S, Gomez N, Iqbal Z, et al. Spurious hyperphosphatemia: a diagnostic and therapeutic challenge. Am J Med. 2016;129:e215–6.

28. **Match the following serum values with the patient history.**

Option	Calcium	Phosphorus	Calcitriol ($1,25(OH)_2D_3$)	FGF-23	PTH
A	↑	↓	↑	N↑	↑
B	↑	↓	↓	↑	N↓
C	↑	N	↑	↓	↓
D	↓	↓	N↓	↑ (?)	↑
E	↓	↑	↓	↑	↑
F	N	↓	↓	↑	N

↑ Increase; ↓ decrease; and N normal

1. A 45-year-old African American woman with hilar adenopathy on CXR and decreased diffusing lung capacity on pulmonary function tests.
2. A 30-year-old obese woman with short-bowel resection and subsequent fat malabsorption.
3. A 60-year-old man with long history of smoking and a lung mass on CXR.
4. A 24-year-old female with bilateral flank pain, frequent urinary tract infections (UTIs) with hematuria, and envelope-like crystals on urine microscopy.
5. A 50-year-old housewife with joint pain, headache, hypertension, and nocturia, and a urinalysis revealing dysmorphic RBCs and 1+ proteinuria.
6. A 40-year-old man with anemia due to gastrointestinal bleeding who received IV iron (ferric) carboxymaltose.

Answers: A = 4; B = 3; C = 1; D = 2, E = 5, F = 6

The patient described in option 1 seems to have sarcoidosis. The patient with sarcoidosis usually has hypercalcemia due to elevated calcitriol secreted by the granuloma. PTH is generally low because of its inhibition by high levels of calcitriol and hypercalcemia. Phosphorus levels are normal. FGF-23 may be elevated or remains normal. Labs shown in option C are consistent with sarcoidosis.

Subjects with short bowel syndrome (option 2) develop vitamin D deficiency, which causes low calcitriol, hypocalcemia, and hypophosphatemia. Hypocalcemia and low calcitriol stimulate PTH secretion, resulting in elevated PTH levels. Low calcitriol stimulates FGF-23, which, in turn, causes phosphaturia and hypophosphatemia. High PTH may also contribute to hypophosphatemia. Labs shown in D are suggestive of vitamin D deficiency.

The patient with lung mass (option 3) seems to have lung cancer, which secretes PTH_{rp} (PTH-related protein) and causes hypercalcemia. Patients with humoral hypercalcemia also demonstrate hypophosphatemia, inappropriately low calcitriol, and low calcitriol-induced high FGF-23 levels; the latter causing hypophosphatemia. PTH may be either normal or slight low. Labs shown in B are consistent with lung malignancy.

The description of a young female (option 4) with UTIs and envelope-like crystals (ca oxalate) is suggestive of primary hyperparathyroidism, causing elevated PTH, hypercalcemia, and hypophosphatemia. FGF-23 levels have been shown to be either normal or elevated in primary hyperparathyroidism. Labs given in A are consistent with primary hyperthyroidism.

The clinical manifestations of the housewife (option 5) are suggestive of stages 3-4 CKD probably related to analgesic use. Hypocalcemia, hypophosphatemia hyperparathyroidism, and elevated FGF-23 levels are related to declining renal function. Values shown in E are suggestive of CKD.

The newly introduced IV iron preparation for iron deficiency anemia causes severe hypophosphatemia possibly by increasing FGF-23 levels. Values shown in F are consistent in a patient with iron deficiency anemia (option 6).

Suggested Reading

Bär L, Stournaras C, Lang, F, et al. Regulation of fibroblast growth factor 23 (FGF 23) in health and disease. FEBS Lett. 2019;593:1879–900.

Liu S, Quarles DI. How fibroblast growth factor 23 works. J Am Soc Nephrol. 2007;18:1637–47.

Razzaque MS, Lanske B. The emerging role of the fibroblast growth factor-23-Klotho axis in renal regulation of phosphate homeostasis. J Endocrinol. 2007;194:1–10.

29. **Which one of the following functions is NOT related to FGF-23?**

A. Inhibition of Na/Pi cotransporter in the proximal tubule
B. Stimulation of renal PO_4 excretion
C. Inhibition of renal 1,α-hydroxylase
D. Stimulation of renal Ca^{2+} excretion
E. Stimulation of osteoblast differentiation

The answer is D

FGF-23 was originally identified as one of the phosphatonins that was responsible for hypophosphatemia, renal Po_4 wasting, and reduced active vitamin D 1,25-dihydroxyvitamin D3 [$1,25(OH)_2D_3$ or calcitriol] in patients with tumor-induced osteomalacia. This hormone is secreted by osteoblasts and osteocytes. In the proximal tubule, FGF-23 inhibits Na-dependent PO_4 cotransporter, thus promoting PO_4 excretion. Also FGF-23 inhibits 1α-hydroxylase activity, leading to reduced levels of $1,25(OH)_2D_3$. Since $1,25(OH)_2D_3$ promotes intestinal PO_4

absorption, reduced level of this vitamin can cause hypophosphatemia. Interestingly, FGF-23 stimulates 24-hydroxylase, an enzyme that participates in the catabolism of 25 (OH)D and 1,25(OH)$_2$D$_3$.

Animal studies have shown that FGF-23 directly regulates osteoblast differentiation, while absence of FGF-23 impairs skeletal mineralization despite normal levels of PO$_4$ and vitamin D.

So far, FGF-23 has not been shown to have direct effect on renal Ca^{2+} excretion. On the other hand, low Ca^{2+} levels inhibit FGF-23 synthesis. Thus, option D is incorrect.

Suggested Reading

Erben RG. Physiological actions of fibroblast growth factor-23. Front Endocrinol. 2018. https://doi.org/10.3389/fendo.2018.00267.

Gutiérrez OM. Fibroblast growth factor 23, klotho, and phosphorus metabolism in chronic kidney disease. In: Turner N, Lameire N, Goldsmith DJ, et al., editors. Oxford textbook of clinical nephrology. 4th ed. Oxford: Oxford University Press; 2016. p. 947–56.

Ramon I, Kleynen P, Body J-J, et al. Fibroblast growth factor 23 and its role in phosphate homeostasis. Eur J Endocrinol. 2010;162:1–10.

Wesseling-Perry K. FGF-23 in bone biology. Pediatr Nephrol. 2010;25:603–8.

Wolf M. Fibroblast growth factor 23 and the future of phosphorus management. Curr Opin Nephrol Hypertens. 2009;18:463–8.

30. **Which one of the following factors LOWERS the levels of FGF-23?**

A. High PO$_4$ intake
B. Active vitamin D (1,25(OH)$_2$ D$_3$)
C. PTH
D. Low PO$_4$ intake
E. Hypoxia, anemia, iron deficiency, and erythropoietin

The answer is D

FGF-23 is regulated by PO$_4$, vitamin D, and possibly PTH. Studies have shown that high diet containing high PO$_4$ induces FGF-23 secretion, whereas low PO$_4$ diet suppresses FGF-23 secretion. Low PO$_4$ diet lowers FGF-23 secretion. Thus, option D is correct.

Exogenous administration of 1,25(OH)$_2$D$_3$ is shown to increase FGF-23 expression and secretion due to a direct effect of this vitamin on FGF-23 via a vitamin D response element located upstream of the FGF-23 promotor.

PTH also seems to increase FGF-23 levels by stimulating the skeletal release of FGF-23, but the mechanism is unclear. Studies have also shown that hypoxia, anemia, iron deficiency, and erythropoietin stimulate FGF-23 production by various mechanisms.

Suggested Reading

Bär L, Stournaras C, Lang F, et al. Regulation of fibroblast growth factor 23 (FGF23) in health and disease. FEBS Lett. 2019;593:1879–900.

Erben RG. Physiological actions of fibroblast growth factor-23. Front Endocrinol. 2018. https://doi.org/10.3389/fendo.2018.00267.

Gutiérrez OM. Fibroblast growth factor 23, klotho, and phosphorus metabolism in chronic kidney disease. In: Turner N, Lameire N, Goldsmith DJ, et al., editors. Oxford textbook of clinical nephrology. 4th ed. Oxford: Oxford University Press; 2016. p. 947–56.

Ramon I, Kleynen P, Body J-J, et al. Fibroblast growth factor 23 and its role in phosphate homeostasis. Eur J Endocrinol. 2010;162:1–10.

Wesseling-Perry K. FGF-23 in bone biology. Pediatr Nephrol. 2010;25:603–8.

Wolf M. Fibroblast growth factor 23 and the future of phosphorus management. Curr Opin Nephrol Hypertens. 2009;18:463–8.

31. **Which one of the following human phosphate wasting diseases is ASSOCIATED with high levels of active vitamin D (1,25 (OH)$_2$D$_3$)?**

A. Autosomal dominant hypophosphatemic rickets (ADHR)
B. Autosomal recessive hypophosphatemic rickets (ARHR)
C. X-linked hypophosphatemic rickets (XLH)

D. Tumor-induced osteomalacia (TIO)
E. Primary hyperparathyroidism

The answer is E

The etiology for hypophosphatemia in the above disorders other than primary hyperparathyroidism is elevated levels of FGF-23. In these disorders, the active vitamin D levels are generally low to normal, but in hyperparathyroidism they are elevated. Thus, option E is incorrect. Table 3.4 shows the levels of phosphorous (PO_4), calcium (CA), vitamin D, PTH, and FGF-23 in all of the above disorders.

ADHR is a rare disorder caused by activating mutations in the FGF-23 gene, and these mutations prevent proteolytic cleavage of FGF-23 with the resultant increase in circulating levels of this hormone. The disorder is characterized by hypophosphatemia due to renal excretion of PO_4, low 1,25$(OH)_2$D3, and rickets as well as osteomalacia.

ARHR is caused by inactivating mutations in the dentin matrix protein (DMP) 1 gene. DMP 1 is derived from osteoblasts and osteocytes and participates in bone mineralization of extracellular matrix. The deficiency of DMP 1 results in increased FGF-23 expression and levels and clinical manifestation similar to that of ADHR.

X-linked dominant disease is the most common form of inherited disorder. It is caused by inactivating mutations in the PHEX (phosphate-regulating gene with homologies to endopeptidases on the X chromosome) gene encoding a zinc-dependent endopeptidase. The clinical and laboratory findings are similar to ADHR/ARHR.

TIO is a mesenchymal tumor with clinical and biochemical findings similar to ADHR. In addition to FGF-23, three other phosphaturic factors, namely sFRP-4, MEPE, and FGF-7, have been identified with the tumor.

Primary hyperparathyroidism is characterized by elevated serum Ca, 1,25$(OH)_2D_3$, PTH, and near-normal FGF-23 levels. Serum PO_4 levels may be low or low normal.

Table 3.4 Serum chemistry in disorders of hypophosphatemia

Disorder	PO_4	Ca	1,25 $(OH)_2$D3	PTH	FGF-23
ADHR	↓	N	↓	N	↑
ARHR	↓	N	N	N	↑
XLH	↓	N	↓/N	N	↑
TIO	↓	N	↓/N	N	↑
1° hyperparathyroidism	↓	↑	↑	↑	↑/ N

Adapted from Ref. [1]
↑ = increase; ↓ = decrease; N = normal; and ↓/N = low normal

Reference

1. Ramon I, Kleynen P, Body J-J, et al. Fibroblast growth factor 23 and its role in phosphate homeostasis. Eur J Endocrinol 162:1–10, 2010.

Suggested Reading

Bär L, Stournaras C, Lang F, et al. Regulation of fibroblast growth factor 23 (FGF23) in health and disease. FEBS Lett. 2019;593:1879–900.

Razzaque MS, Lanske B. The emerging role of the fibroblast growth factor-23-Klotho axis in renal regulation of phosphate homeostasis. J Endocrinol. 2007;194:1–10.

32. **FGF-23 exerts its effects on the kidney by which ONE of the following mechanisms?**

A. Binding to PTH receptor
B. Binding to vasopressin receptor
C. Binding to other phosphatonins (sFRP-4)
D. Binding to FGF receptor with KLOTHO
E. None of the above

The answer is D

Most of the FGF family members exert their effects through interaction with FGF receptors (FGFRs). There are at least four FGFRs with various subtypes that have been identified. Studies have shown that FGF-23 can interact with FGFR1c, 3c, and 4c. However, FGF-23-mediated receptor activation requires a cofactor called klotho. The klotho gene is an aging-suppressor gene, and its deficiency causes premature aging. Overexpression of this gene

extends life span in animals. FGF-23 fails to exert its effects in the absence of klotho. Thus, klotho is required for phosphaturic and other effects of FGF-23. Thus, option D is correct. The interaction of FGF-23 with other receptors has not been described as yet.

Suggested Reading

Bär L, Stournaras C, Lang F, et al. Regulation of fibroblast growth factor 23 (FGF23) in health and disease. FEBS Lett. 2019;593:1879–900.

Liu S, Quarles DI. How fibroblast growth factor 23 works. J Am Soc Nephrol. 2007;18:1637–47.

Ramon I, Kleynen P, Body J-J, et al. Fibroblast growth factor 23 and its role in phosphate homeostasis. Eur J Endocrinol. 2010;162:1–10.

Razzaque MS, Lanske B. The emerging role of the fibroblast growth factor-23-Klotho axis in renal regulation of phosphate homeostasis. J Endocrinol. 2007;194:1–10.

33. **With regard to magnesium (Mg^{2+}) handling by the nephron, which one of the following statements is INCORRECT?**

A. Mg^{2+} reabsorption is only 25% of the filtered load in the proximal tubule
B. Both Na^{+} and Mg^{2+} are equally reabsorbed in the proximal tubule
C. About 70% of the filtered load of Mg^{2+} is reabsorbed in thick ascending limb of loop of Henle (TALH)
D. Only 10% of filtered load of Mg^{2+} is reabsorbed in the distal convoluted tubule (DCT)
E. Fractional excretion of Mg^{2+} is between 3% and 5%, and it can be decreased to <1% in hypomagnesemia

The answer is B

Mg^{2+} is the second most common intracellular cation next to K^{+} in the body. A 70- kg individual has approximately 25 g of Mg^{2+}. About 67% of this Mg^{2+} is present in bone, about 20% in muscle, and 12% in other tissues such as the liver. Only 1-2% is present in the extracellular space. In plasma, Mg^{2+} exists as free (60%) and in bound (40%) forms. About 10% is bound to HCO_3^-, citrate, and phosphate and 30% to albumin. Only the free and nonprotein-bound Mg^{2+} is filtered at the glomerulus.

Approximately 2,000 mg of Mg^{2+} is filtered and only 100 mg is excreted in the urine, which implies that 95% of the filtered Mg^{2+} is reabsorbed. The proximal tubule reabsorbs about 25% of the filtered Mg^{2+}. This amount is relatively low when compared to the reabsorption of Na^{+}, K^{+}, Ca^{2+}, or PO_4 at the proximal tubule. Thus, option B is incorrect.

The most important segment for Mg^{2+} reabsorption is the cortical (TALH). In this segment, about 70% of Mg^{2+} is reabsorbed. The transport of Mg^{2+} in the TALH is both passive and active. Passive transport is dependent on the lumen-positive voltage difference secondary to Na/K/2Cl cotransport and backleak of K^{+} into the lumen via ROMK. This positive voltage difference facilitates paracellular movement of Mg^{2+}. The Ca-sensing receptor inhibits paracellular transport of Mg^{2+}. Inhibition of the Na/K/2Cl cotransport by a loop diuretic diminishes Mg^{2+} reabsorption. A similar decrease in Mg^{2+} reabsorption is also observed with volume expansion. Both these situations lower the potential difference, and thus provide prompt passive transport of Mg^{2+} in this segment of the nephron.

Evidence also exists for active transport of Mg^{2+} in the cortical TALH. This mechanism has been suggested based on the observation that Mg^{2+} transport is stimulated by antidiuretic hormone and glucagon without any change in the potential difference.

The DCT reabsorbs about 10% of the filtered Mg^{2+}, and very little reabsorption occurs in the collecting duct. Thus, the DCT is the last site of Mg^{2+} reabsorption in the nephron. It occurs by an active transcellular mechanism. At the lumen, Mg^{2+} enters the cell via transient receptor potential melastatin 6 (TRPM6). Intracellular Mg^{2+} and thiazide diuretics inhibit TRPM6. Under steady-state conditions, the urinary excretion of Mg is about 3–5% of the filtered load.

Suggested Reading

Alexander RT, Hoenderop JG, Bindels RJ. Molecular determinants of magnesium homeostasis: insights from human disease. J Am Soc Nephrol. 2008;19:1451–8.

Chonchol M, Smogorzewski MJ, Stubs JR, et al. Disorders of calcium, magnesium, and phosphate balance. In: Yu ASL, Chertow GM, Luyckx VA, et al., editors. Brenner & Rector's the kidney. 11th ed. Philadelphia: Elsevier Saunders; 2020. p. 580–613.

Reddi AS. Intravenous fluids: composition and indications. In: Reddi AS, editor. Fluid, electrolyte, and acid-base disorders. Clinical evaluation and management. 2nd ed. New York: Springer; 2018. p. 35–49.

34. **Which one of the following drugs does NOT cause hypomagnesemia?**

   A. Cisplatin
   B. Amphotericin B (Amp B)
   C. Proton pump inhibitor (PPI)
   D. Alcohol
   E. Vancomycin

   The answer is E

   Except for vancomycin, all other drugs cause hypomagnesemia. Cisplatin and Amp B cause renal wasting of Mg. Both drugs also cause hypocalciuria. PPIs have been shown to induce hypomagnesemia with no proven etiology. Hoorn et al. reported not only hypomagnesemia but also hypokalemia and hypocalcemia with PPIs. Hypokalemia is due to renal wasting of K. Patients with chronic alcoholism may develop hypomagnesemia by several mechanisms, including inadequate dietary intake, steatorrhea, diarrhea, PO_4 deficiency, fatty acid or ATP-Mg complex formation, and alcohol-induced magnesuria. To date, vancomycin has not been shown to cause hypomagnesemia, making choice E incorrect.

   Suggested Reading

Chonchol M, Smogorzewski MJ, Stubs JR, et al. Disorders of calcium, magnesium, and phosphate balance. In: Yu ASL, Chertow GM, Luyckx VA, et al., editors. Brenner & Rector's the kidney. 11th ed. Philadelphia: Elsevier Saunders; 2020. p. 580–613.
Danziger J, William JH, Scott DJ, et al. Proton-pump inhibitor use is associated with low serum magnesium concentrations. Kidney Int. 2013;83:692–9.
El-Charabaty E, Saifan C, Abdallah M, et al. Effects of proton pump inhibitors and electrolyte disturbances on arrhythmias. Int J Gen Med. 2013;6:515–8.
Liao S, Gan L, Mei Z. Does the use of proton pump inhibitors increase the risk of hypomagnesemia an updated systematic review and meta-analysis. Medicine. 2019;98:13:e15011.

35. **Of the following, which one is the recently proposed mechanism for hypomagnesemia-induced hypokalemia?**

   A. Inhibition of Na/K/2Cl cotransporter
   B. Inhibition of Na/Cl cotransporter
   C. Blockage of ROMK channel by Mg in distal convoluted tubule (DCT)
   D. Inhibition of ENaC
   E. None of the above mechanisms

   The answer is C

   Combined Mg^{2+} and K^+ deficiency is seen in many conditions such as loop or thiazide diuretics, alcoholism, diarrhea, Bartter and Gitelman syndrome, aminoglycosides, amphotericin B, and cisplatin. Inhibition of Na/K/2Cl and Na/Cl cotransporters cause Bartter and Gitelman syndromes, respectively. However, hypokalemia can be to some extent corrected by administration of KCl. In contrast, hypokalemia induced by magnesium (Mg) deficiency is not corrected by KCl alone. The mechanism of hypokalemia in Mg deficiency remains unclear. However, several lines of evidence suggest that Mg administration decreases K secretion, and Mg deficiency promotes K^+ excretion. These effects occur independently of Na/K/2Cl, Na/Cl, and ENaC channels. It has been proposed that Mg^{2+} deficiency inhibits skeletal muscle Na/K-ATPase, causing efflux of K and secondary kaliuresis.

   The currently proposed mechanism is that changes in intracellular Mg^{2+} concentration affect K^+ secretion through ROMK channel in the DCT. At the physiologic intracellular Mg^{2+} concentration (e.g., 1 mM), K^+ entry through ROMK is more than its exit because the intracellular Mg^{2+} binds ROMK and blocks K^+ exit. According to Huang and Kuo proposal, Mg deficiency may lower intracellular Mg concentration which relieves the binding and promote K^+ secretion. Thus, option C is correct.

   Suggested Reading

Huang C-L, Kuo E. Mechanism of hypokalemia in magnesium deficiency. J Am Soc Nephrol. 2007;18:2649–52.
Mount DB. Disorders of potassium balance. In: Yu ASL, Chertow GM, Luyckx VA, et al., editors. Brenner and Rector's the kidney. 11th ed. Philadelphia: Elsevier; 2020. p. 537–79.

36. **Which one of the following facts about nephrolithiasis is CORRECT?**

A. Stones are the third most common disorders of the urinary tract after urinary tract infections and prostate conditions
B. Most common types of stones are calcium, uric acid, struvite (infection), and cystine
C. Approximately 80% of kidney stones contain calcium (Ca)
D. Nephrolithiasis is more common in men than in women in adults until sixth decade of life, after which the incidence rises in women
E. All of the above

The answer is E

All of the above statements regarding the epidemiology of nephrolithiasis are correct. Ca is the major component of approximately 80% of all stones (60% Ca oxalate, 20% hydroxyapatite, and 3% brushite). Uric acid stones comprise 8–10%, whereas struvite and cysteine stones account for 5% each. Thus, answer E is correct.

Suggested Reading

Moe OW. Kidney stones: pathophysiology and medical management. Lancet. 2006;367:333–44.
Pfau A, Knauf F. Core curriculum in nephrology. Update on nephrolithiasis: core curriculum 2016. Am J Kidney Dis. 2016;68:973–85.
Sohgaura A, Bigoniya P. A review on epidemiology and etiology of renal stone. Am J Drug Discov Develop. 2017;7:54–62.
Taylor EN, Curhan GC. Epidemiology of nephrolithiasis. In: Turner N, Lameire N, Goldsmith DJ, et al., editors. Oxford textbook of clinical nephrology. 4th ed. Oxford: Oxford University Press; 2016. p. 1631–6.

37. **Which one of the following statements regarding idiopathic hypercalciuria is FALSE?**

A. It has a strong family history of renal stones
B. Activating (gain-of-function) mutations in calcium-sensing receptor (CaSR) cause hypercalciuria
C. Mutations in claudin-16 cause hypercalciuria
D. Mutations in transient receptor potential vanilloid member 5 protein (TRPV5) cause hypercalciuria
E. Patients with Dent disease will never have hypercalciuria

The answer is E

Although the genetic factors underlying hypercalciuria remain unclear, some epidemiologic studies have shown an association between hypercalciuria and family history of stone disease. Gain-of-function mutations in CaSR result in type V Bartter syndrome with hypercalciuria and nephrolithiasis. Also, mutations in the gene claudin-16, a tight junction protein, cause a familial disorder that is characterized by hypomagnesemia, hypercalciuria, and nephrolithiasis. TRPV5 is a Ca^{2+} channel that promotes Ca reabsorption in the distal tubule, and mutation in TRPV5 gene causes hypercalciuria. Similarly, patients with Dent disease have hypercalciuria and nephrolithiasis. Thus, option E is false.

Suggested Reading

Arcidiacono T, Mingione A, Macrina L, et al. Idiopathic calcium nephrolithiasis: a review of pathogenic mechanisms in the light of genetic studies. Am J Nephrol. 2014;40:499–506.
Coe FL, Worcester EM, Evan AP. Idiopathic hypercalciuria and formation of calcium renal stones. Nat Rev Nephrol. 2016;12:519–33.
Devuyst O, Pirson Y. Genetics of hypercalciuric stone forming disease. Kidney Int. 2007;72:1065–72.
Policastro LJ, Saggi SJ, Goldfarb DS, et al. Personalized intervention in monogenic stone formers. J Urol. 2018;199:623–32.
Sayer JA. Progress in understanding the genetics of calcium-containing nephrolithiasis. J Am Soc Nephrol. 2017;28:748–59.
Stechman MJ, Loh NY, Thakkar RV. Genetic causes of hypercalciuric nephrolithiasis. Pediatr Nephrol. 2009;24:2321–32.

38. **Which one of the following mechanisms of uric acid stone formation is FALSE?**

A. Acid urine pH (<5.6)
B. Low urine volume
C. Hyperuricosuria
D. A and C
E. A, B, and C

The answer is D

Three major mechanisms for uric acid stone formation are acidic pH, low urine volume, and hyperuricosuria (>600 mg/day). Uric acid stone formers have a defect either in NH_4^+ production or its excretion. Also, they have increased net acid excretion. Therefore, patients with uric acid stones have acidic urine pH.

Normally, urine uric acid solubility is limited to 96 mg/L. If urinary uric acid excretion exceeds 600 mg/day, the urine is supersaturated with uric acid and in the presence of acidic pH and low urine volume, it precipitates and causes uric acid stones. Thus, option D is false.

Suggested Reading

Daudon M, Jungers P. Uric acid stones. In: Turner N, Lameire N, Goldsmith DJ, et al., editors. Oxford textbook of clinical nephrology. 4th ed. Oxford: Oxford University Press; 2016. p. 1661–5.

Ma Q, Fang L, Su R, et al. Uric acid stones, clinical manifestations and therapeutic considerations. Postgrad Med J. 2018;94:458–62.

Pfau A, Knauf F. Core curriculum in nephrology. Update on nephrolithiasis: core curriculum 2016. Am J Kidney Dis. 2016;68:973–85.

Sakhaee K, Moe OW. Urolithiasis. In: Yu ASL, Chertow GM, Luyckx VA, et al., editors. Brenner and Rector's the kidney. 11th ed. Philadelphia: Elsevier; 2020. p. 1277–326.

Sakhaee K. Recent advances in the pathophysiology of nephrolithiasis. Kidney Int. 2009;75:585–95.

39. **Which one of the following genetic diseases is NOT associated with nephrolithiasis?**

A. Dent disease
B. Oculocerebrorenal syndrome of Lowe (OCRL)
C. Gitelman syndrome
D. Bartter syndrome, type V
E. Distal renal tubular acidosis (RTA)

The answer is C

Except for Gitelman syndrome, all of the above hereditary diseases are associated with hypercalciuria and nephrolithiasis. Dent disease is an X-linked recessive disorder caused by inactivating mutations in the CLCN5 gene, which encodes a renal chloride channel, CLC-5. The disease is characterized by varying degrees of low-molecular-weight proteinuria, hypercalciuria, nephrolithiasis, hyperphosphaturia, and rickets. Renal failure gradually develops in patients with Dent's disease.

OCRL is also an X-linked recessive disorder that is characterized by congenital cataracts, mental retardation, rickets, muscle hypotonia, proximal tubular wasting of bicarbonate, phosphate, and amino acids. Some patients will have hypercalciuria and nephrolithiasis. Mutations in the gene that encodes inositol phosphate 5-phosphatase result in OCRL.

Type V Bartter syndrome is due to activating mutations of the calcium-sensing receptor (CaSR). The disease is characterized by hypokalemia, metabolic alkalosis, hypercalciuria, and nephrolithiasis.

Distal RTA is a condition with hypokalemia, nonunion gap metabolic acidosis, hypercalciuria, nephrocalcinosis, and nephrolithiasis.

Gitelman syndrome is characterized by hypocalciuria; therefore, nephrolithiasis does not occur. However, chondrocalcinosis is frequently seen in patients with Gitelman syndrome. Thus, option C is incorrect.

Suggested Reading

Bonnardeaux A, Bichet DG. Inherited disorders of the renal tubule. In: Yu ASL, Chertow GM, Luyckx VA, et al., editors. Brenner and Rector's the kidney. 11th ed. Philadelphia: Elsevier; 2020. p. 1450–89.

Stechman MJ, Loh NY, Thakkar RV. Genetic causes of hypercalciuric nephrolithiasis. Pediatr Nephrol. 2009;24:2321–32.

40. Transient receptor potential vanilloid member 5 (TRPV5) is the rate-limiting Ca entry channel in the distal convoluted tubule (DCT) and connecting tubule (CNT). **Which one of the following statements is FALSE regarding TRPV5?**

A. TRPV5 colocalizes with calbindin-D_{28k}, Na/Ca exchanger and Ca-ATPase
B. Klotho stabilizes the TRPV5 channel in the plasma membrane by deglycosylation of the protein
C. TRPV5 is regulated by $1,25(OH)_2D_3$ and PTH

D. TRPV5 knockout mice show hypercalciuria, elevated levels of 1,25$(OH)_2D_3$, increased intestinal Ca absorption, and decreased trabecular bone density
E. A link between TRPV5 mutations and idiopathic hypercalciuria has been well established in humans

The answer is E

Most of the Ca^{2+} reabsorption occurs passively in the proximal tubule and the thick ascending limb of Henle's loop. About 15% of Ca^{2+}reabsoprtion takes place transcellularly in the DCT and CNT. This transcellular process occurs in three steps. First, Ca^{2+} is transported across the apical membrane via TRPV5. Second, once Ca^{2+} is inside the cell, it combines with calbindin-D_{28k} and shuttled through the cytosol toward the basolateral membrane; and finally, Ca^{2+} is extruded via Na/Ca exchanger and Ca-ATPase into blood. Less than 3% of filtered Ca^{2+} is excreted in the urine.

TRPV5 is regulated by klotho, 1,25$(OH)_2D_3$, and PTH. Klotho enhances TRPV5 activity by hydrolyzing the sugar residue at the extracellular domain of TRPV5 by β-glucuronidase activity of klotho. This is confirmed by showing that klotho knockout mice have decreased expression of TRPV5. 1,25$(OH)_2D_3$ and PTH increase the expression of TRPV5, indicating increased transcellular Ca^{2+} transport in the DCT and CNT segments of the nephron.

TRPV5 knockout mice have been shown to have hypercalciuria, elevated levels of 1,25$(OH)_2D_3$, increased intestinal Ca^{2+} absorption, and decreased trabecular bone density. This suggests that TRPV5 plays an important role in the fine tuning of Ca^{2+} reabsorption in the DCT and CNT. However, screening of patients with hypercalciuria failed to detect significant mutations in TRPV5. Thus, option E is false.

Suggested Reading

Felsenfelda A, Rodriguezb M, and Levine B. New insights in regulation of calcium homeostasis. Curr Opin Nephrol Hypertens. 2013;22:371–6.
Mensenkamp AR, Hoenderop JGJ, Bindels RJM. Recent advances in renal tubular calcium reabsorption. Curr Opin Nephrol Hypertens. 2004;15:524–9.
Woudenberg-Vrenken TE, Bindels RJM, Hoenderop JGJ. The role of transient receptor potential channels in kidney disease. Nature Rev Nephrol. 2009;5:441–9.

41. Dietary factors play an important role in nephrolithiasis. **Which one of the following dietary factors promotes the formation of renal stones?**

A. High calcium intake
B. Low calcium intake
C. Low protein intake
D. Low sodium intake
E. High magnesium and potassium intake

The answer is B

The role of dietary factors in the formation and prevention of renal stones has been extensively studied. Until recently, high dietary calcium was thought to increase the risk of stone formation. However, a few studies showed that low dietary calcium (400 mg/day) rather than high dietary calcium (1200 mg/day) promotes stone formation. The mechanism seems to be that high calcium intake will bind dietary oxalate in the gut, and thereby reducing oxalate absorption and urinary excretion. Therefore, choice B is incorrect.

It has been shown that dietary calcium rather than supplemental calcium is important in lowering stone formation. This discrepancy between these two forms of calcium intake is related to the timing of calcium intake. It seems that supplemental calcium pills when taken in-between meals can reduce binding of oxalate in the gut. For this reason, diet rich in calcium rather than supplemental calcium reduces stone formation.

High sodium diet promotes calcium excretion; therefore, low sodium diet is recommended to decrease hypercalciuria.

A diet restricted in potassium can promote urinary calcium excretion. Furthermore, relative hypokalemia promotes citrate absorption. Diet rich in potassium promotes urinary excretion of citrate, which is an inhibitor of calcium oxalate stone formation.

Higher magnesium intake prevents supersaturation of calcium oxalate in the urine because magnesium combines with oxalate, and also magnesium reduces oxalate absorption in the gut.

Thus, a diet rich in calcium, potassium, and magnesium with low sodium is beneficial in preventing stone formation.

High protein intake generates acid load by metabolizing sulfur-containing amino acids to sulfuric acid, as well as organic acid production. This acid production induces an increase in urinary calcium and a decrease in citrate excretion. Thus, high protein intake promotes stone formation as well as osteopenia.

Suggested Reading

Sakhaee K, Moe OW. Urolithiasis. In: Yu ASL, Chertow GM, Luyckx VA, et al., editors. Brenner and Rector's the kidney. 11th ed. Philadelphia: Elsevier; 2020. p. 1277–326.

Southern ES. Nutrition management of hypercalciuria. In: Monga, M, Penniston KL, Goldfarb DS, editors. Pocket guide to kidney stone prevention. Switzerland: Springer; 2015. p. 29–36.

Taylor EN, Curhan GC. Diet and fluid prescription for stone disease. Kidney Int. 2006;70:835–9.

Taylor EN, Curhan GC. Epidemiology of nephrolithiasis. In: Turner N, Lameire N, Goldsmith DJ, et al., editors. Oxford textbook of clinical nephrology. 4th ed. Oxford: Oxford University Press; 2016. p. 1631–6.

42. **Match the following inhibitory urinary macromolecules with the pathogenic mechanisms of calcium oxalate crystallization:**

A. Nephrocalcin
B. Tamm-Horsfall protein
C. Uropontin (osteopontin)
D. Glycosaminoglycans (GAGs)

1. Inhibition of nucleation, growth, aggregation, and cell adhesion
2. Inhibition of aggregation only
3. Inhibition of nucleation, growth, and aggregation but not nucleation

Answers: A = 1; B = 2; C = 1; D = 3

The pathogenesis of stone formation involves several mechanisms, including urinary supersaturation of stone substances, nucleation, crystal growth, and aggregation as well as cell adhesion (cell-crystal interaction). Stone formation starts when crystals of the offending substance are excreted in the urine, and the urine is supersaturated with the stone-forming substances. The next step is the formation of a nucleus or nidus that has formed spontaneously (homogenous nucleation) or the crystal that has been formed on a preexisting crystal nidus of a different compound (heterogeneous nucleation). For instance, monosodium urate and uric acid form excellent heterogeneous nuclei for calcium oxalate stone formation. Also, calcium phosphate plaques found in the renal papilla (so-called Randall plaques) may act as a nucleating surface for calcium oxalate stones.

Crystal growth and aggregation are then critical steps in stone formation. Small crystals aggregate into large crystalline masses. These crystals must anchor to the renal tubular epithelium or urothelium (cell adhesion) to grow larger and become urinary calculi.

Urinary supersaturation alone is not sufficient to form a stone. Normal subjects have inhibitors of crystal growth, nucleation, as well as aggregation and cell adhesion. Pyrophosphate, citrate, and magnesium are the most important low-molecular-weight crystallization inhibitors. In addition, high-molecular-weight substances such as nephrocalcin, Tamm-Horsfall protein, uropontin, and glycosaminoglycans have been identified as inhibitors of calcium oxalate stone formation. Nephrocalcin has been shown to inhibit nucleation, growth, aggregation, and cell adhesion, whereas Tamm-Horsfall protein inhibits aggregation only. Uropontin, similar to nephrocalcin, inhibits all aspects of calcium oxalate crystallization. Also, glycosaminoglycans inhibit growth, aggregation, and cell adhesion with little effect on nucleation.

Three other macromolecular urinary protein inhibitors have been identified: prothrombin fragment 1, bikunin, and calgranulin.

Suggested Reading

Hruska KA, Beck AM. Nephrolithiasis. In: Coffman TM, Falk RJ, Molitoris BA, et al., editors. Schrier's diseases of the kidney. 9th ed. Philadelphia: Wolters Kluwer/Lippincott Williams & Wilkins; 2013. p. 642–72.

Robertson WG. Do "inhibitors of crystallisation" play any role in the prevention of kidney stones? A critique. Urolithiasis. 2017;45:43–56.

Sakhaee K, Moe OW. Urolithiasis. In: Yu ASL, Chertow GM, Luyckx VA, et al., editors. Brenner and Rector's the kidney. 11th ed. Philadelphia: Elsevier; 2020. p. 1277–326.

43. **Match the following low-molecular-weight urinary inhibitors with their mechanisms of action in reducing stone formation:**

A. Pyrophosphate
B. Magnesium
C. Citrate

1. Inhibition of both heterogeneous nucleation and growth of calcium oxalate
2. Binds calcium in the urine and increases the inhibitory activity of Tamm-Horsfall protein.

Answers: A = 1; B = 1; C = 2

It has been reported that pyrophosphate inhibits spontaneous calcium oxalate crystallization as well as heterogeneous nucleation of calcium oxalate by hydroxyapatite. Magnesium complexes with oxalate and decreases calcium oxalate supersaturation in the urine. Furthermore, magnesium was found to inhibit both nucleation and growth of calcium oxalate crystallization. Normally urine citrate complexes with calcium and reduces its ionic strength. As a result, oversaturation of urine with calcium oxalate or calcium phosphate is prevented. The significance of citrate in the prevention of stone formation is further strengthened by the observation that hypocitrituria is found in 15% to 60% stone formers. In addition, citrate has been shown to inhibit nucleation, growth, and aggregation of calcium oxalate crystals. Also, citrate potentiates the inhibitory effect of Tamm-Horsfall protein on calcium oxalate aggregation.

Urinary excretion of citrate is reduced by metabolic acidosis, hypokalemia, and carbonic anhydrate inhibitors. It has been suggested that estrogens, PTH, calcitonin, and vitamin D increase citrate excretion.

Suggested Reading

Hruska KA, Beck AM. Nephrolithiasis. In: Coffman TM, Falk RJ, Molitoris BA, et al., editors. Schrier's diseases of the kidney. 9th ed. Philadelphia: Wolters Kluwer/Lippincott Williams & Wilkins; 2013. p. 642–72.

Sakhaee K, Moe OW. Urolithiasis. In: Yu ASL, Chertow GM, Luyckx VA, et al., editors. Brenner and Rector's the kidney. 11th ed. Philadelphia: Elsevier; 2020. p. 1277–326.

Sinnott B, Maalouf N, SakhaeeK, et al. Medical management of nephrocalcinosis and nephrolithiasis. In: Turner N, Lameire N, Goldsmith DJ, et al., editors. Oxford textbook of clinical nephrology. 4th ed. Oxford: Oxford University Press; 2016. p. 1697–712.

44. **Which one of the following stones is LEAST likely dependent on urinary pH?**

A. Calcium phosphate
B. Calcium oxalate
C. Uric acid
D. Cystine
E. Magnesium ammonium phosphate (struvite)

The answer is B

Urinary pH is dependent on the intake of fluids and diet as well as metabolic state. It is the most important determinant of the urinary ionic product of calcium phosphate. High pH (>6.5) increases the availability of $PO4^{3-}$ and $HPO4^{2-}$ for formation of octacalcium phosphate (Ca_4H (PO4)3.2.5H_2O) and brushite (CaHPO4.2H_2O) stones, respectively. Thus, calcium phosphate crystals dominate in alkaline urine pH values. Also, struvite (infection) stones form in alkaline urine.

Uric acid and cystine stones form in acidic pH. At low pH, uric acid is least soluble, and it is highly soluble as urate at alkaline pH. Similarly, cystine is highly soluble at alkaline than acid pH. Thus, therapy of uric acid and cystine stones includes alkalanization of urine to a pH >6.5.

The ion activity product of calcium oxalate is least influenced by urinary pH, although crystals of calcium oxalate are found in acid urine. Thus, answer B is incorrect.

Suggested Reading

Hruska KA, Beck AM. Nephrolithiasis. In: Coffman TM, Falk RJ, Molitoris BA, et al., editors. Schrier's diseases of the kidney. 9th ed. Philadelphia: Wolters Kluwer/Lippincott Williams & Wilkins; 2013. p. 642–72.

Sakhaee K, Moe OW. Urolithiasis. In: Yu ASL, Chertow GM, Luyckx VA, et al., editors. Brenner and Rector's the kidney. 11th ed. Philadelphia: Elsevier; 2020. p. 1277–326.

Sinnott B, Maalouf N, SakhaeeK, et al. Medical management of nephrocalcinosis and nephrolithiasis. In: Turner N, Lameire N, Goldsmith DJ, et al., editors. Oxford textbook of clinical nephrology. 4th ed. Oxford: Oxford University Press; 2016. p. 1697–712.

45. **Select the appropriate therapeutic modality for patients with various forms of nephrolithiasis?**

A. Sodium cellulose phosphate, orthophosphate, and thiazide diuretics
B. Parathyroidectomy, calcimimetics, and bisphosphonates
C. Pyridoxine, dietary calcium and magnesium, and liver and kidney transplantation
D. Allopurinol
E. Dietary restriction of methionine, D-penicillamine, tiopronin, and captopril
F. Surgery and acetohydroxamic acid

1. Magnesium and ammonium phosphate (struvite) stones
2. Cystine stones
3. Uric acid stones
4. Increased hypercalciuria
5. Hyperoxaluria
6. Primary hyperparathyroidism

Answers: A = 4; B = 6; C = 5; D = 3; E = 2; F = 1

Hypercalciuria is the major reason for calcium (Ca) nephrolithiasis. A number of pathophysiologic mechanisms have been proposed for hypercalciuria including the involvement of kidney, gut, skeleton, PTH, and vitamin D. Hypercalciuria occurs by three mechanisms: (1) increased intestinal Ca absorption or absorptive hypercalciuria; (2) defective renal tubule Ca absorption; and (3) resorptive hypercalciuria. In patients with absorptive hypercalciuria, serum Ca levels are slightly above normal, reabsorption of Ca increases, resulting in hypercalciuria. In defective renal tubule, a renal leak of Ca would cause hypercalciuria. This results in secondary hyperparathyroidism and stimulation of 1,25(OH)$_2$D$_3$, causing increased intestinal calcium absorption. In resorptive hypercalciuria, increased release of Ca occurs from bone, which may be PTH dependent or PTH independent. Primary hyperparathyroidism or elevated PTH levels release Ca from bone. PTH-independent mechanism may involve 1,25(OH)$_2$D$_3$. Both mechanism cause filtration of Ca with resultant hypercalciuria.

Cellulose phosphate is a Ca-binding ion-exchange resin that is recommended for the treatment of absorptive hypercalciuria. It should be taken with meals when calcium is available. Secondary hyperoxaluria may develop due to calcium in the gut.

Orthophosphate (Neutra-phos) inhibits 1,25(OH)$_2$D$_3$ and should be taken after meals and before bedtime. A thiazide diuretic (HCTZ) is an alternative treatment for cellulose phosphate. It decreases renal secretion of calcium. Occasionally, cellulose phosphate may be alternated with a thiazide diuretic for an effective management.

Removal of hyperplastic parathyroid glands or adenoma is usually performed in patients with symptomatic hypercalcemia (>12 mg/dl), stone or bone disease, and other manifestations of hyperparathyroidism. Medical therapy, prior to surgery, includes bisphosphonates to improve bone disease and calcimimetics (cinacalcet) to lower circulating PTH and Ca levels can be tried. The effect of these agents on stone disease and hypercalciuria has not been studied.

Hyperoxaluria can result from excessive dietary intake, (dietary oxaluria), and gastrointestinal disorders causing malabsorption (enteric oxaluria) or primary hyperoxaluria. Dietary oxaluria can be treated with restriction of oxalate intake and calcium carbonate, the latter binds oxalate and prevents its absorption.

Malabsorptive disorders can be treated based on the cause of malabsorption. For example, gluten-free diet may be helpful in patients with sprue. In patients with bowel resection, low-fat diet, medium-chain triglycerides, and cholestyramine may reduce oxalate absorption.

Primary oxaluria is a rare hereditary disease and includes two types. Type I primary hyperoxaluria is due to complete or relative absence of alanine-glyoxylate aminotransferase (AGT) in the liver. AGT is a pyridoxal phosphate-dependent enzyme, which converts glyoxylate into glycine. Deficiency of AGT results in the conversion of glyoxylate to oxalate. Thus, patients with type 1 primary oxaluria develop calcium oxalate stones and subsequently renal failure.

Pyridoxine (25–1000 mg/day) reduces oxalate excretion in patients with partial deficiency of AGT. Also, the combination of pyridoxine and neutral orthophosphate is effective in reducing urine supersaturation of calcium oxalate during therapy.

Type 2 primary hyperoxaluria is due to a deficiency of glycolate reductase – hydroxypyruvate reductase (GRHPR) enzyme. Deficiency of this enzyme reduces the conversion of glyoxylate to glycolate, resulting in increased production of oxalate. Both types of primary hyperoxalurias are inherited as autosomal recessive

disorders. Once renal failure develops, a combined liver and kidney transplantation has cured this previously fatal disease.

Uric acid stones form in acid urine. Urine alkalinization to dissolve uric acid stones is achieved by oral potassium citrate (20–30 mEq, 2–3 times per day). Allopurinol, which is a xanthine oxidase inhibitor, is useful in patients with not only uric acid stones but also gout.

Cystinuria is a hereditary disorder of cystine and dibasic amino acids in the renal tubule and intestine. Cystine stones dissolve in alkaline pH, therefore, urine pH should be maintained >7.5, preferably with potassium salts because sodium-containing salts increase cystine excretion. Methionine is a precursor of cystine, and dietary restriction of this amino acid is used to reduce cystine production. However, chronic restriction of methionine diet causes clinically significant cystine deficiency.

Other medical therapy includes D-penicillamine, tiopronin, and captopril. These agents complex with cystine to form a thiolcysteine compound, which is more soluble than cystine.

Large cystine stones form staghorn calculi, which require surgical removal. Extracorporeal shock-wave lithotripsy (ESWL) and percutaneous lithotripsy can be tried prior to surgical therapy.

Magnesium ammonium phosphate (struvite) stones are more commonly found in women than men. These stones are caused by urea-splitting organism such as proteus and pseudomonas. *E. coli* does not possess urease. Urea-splitting organisms produce ammonium, which causes alkaline urine pH and promotes struvite stone formation. Therefore, acidification of urine is desirable. Oral acidifying agents are usually ineffective, but irrigation of the renal pelvis can be helpful. Surgical removal of the staghorn calculi is usually the treatment of choice because it prevents total nephrectomy.

Percutaneous nephrolithotomy as well as ESWL with ureteral stenting have also been shown to be effective for large-volume struvite stones.

Acetohydroxamic acid is a urease inhibitor, which reduces urinary saturation of struvite. It may prevent stone growth. However, it has several side effects, including hemolytic anemia, thrombophlebitis, headache, and disorientation.

Suggested Reading

Hruska KA, Beck AM. Nephrolithiasis. In: Coffman TM, Falk RJ, Molitoris BA, et al., editors. Schrier's diseases of the kidney. 9th ed. Philadelphia: Wolters Kluwer/Lippincott Williams & Wilkins; 2013. p. 642–72.

Pfau A, Knauf F. Core curriculum in nephrology. Update on nephrolithiasis: core curriculum 2016. Am J Kidney Dis. 2016;68:973–85.

Sakhaee K, Moe OW. Urolithiasis. In: Yu ASL, Chertow GM, Luyckx VA, et al., editors. Brenner and Rector's the kidney. 11th ed. Philadelphia: Elsevier; 2020. p. 1277–326.

Sinnott B, Maalouf N, Sakhaee K, et al. Medical management of nephrocalcinosis and nephrolithiasis. In: Turner N, Lameire N, Goldsmith DJ, et al., editors. Oxford textbook of clinical nephrology. 4th ed. Oxford: Oxford University Press; 2016, p. 1697–712.

46. **Which one of the following drugs does NOT cause nephrolithiasis?**

A. Xanthine
B. Indinavir
C. Ceftriaxone
D. Topiramate
E. Methanol

The answer is E

Drug-induced calculi represent 1–2% of all kidney stones. Except for methanol, all other drugs are reported to cause renal stones. Xanthine stones are formed in subjects with congenital deficiency of xanthine oxidase. These stones are radiolucent, and urine alkalinization is useful in the management of xanthine stones. Indinavir is a protease inhibitor, which causes radioluscent stones. Discontinuation of the drug and hydration allow the stone to pass in the urine. It was reported that children treated with high-dose ceftriaxone for 7 days may develop nephrolithiasis. This antibiotic, which is an anion, can combine with Ca to form an insoluble complex and precipitation of a stone.

Topiramate is a neuromodulatory drug used in the treatment of seizure disorder. It inhibits carbonic anhydrase type II, and causes metabolic acidosis, hypocitraturia, and alkaline urine pH. These changes result in calcium phosphate stones. Methanol has not been shown to cause nephrolithiasis. Therefore, choice E is incorrect.

Suggested Reading

Daudon M, Frochot V, Bazin D, et al. Drug-induced kidney stones and crystalline nephropathy: pathophysiology, prevention and treatment. Drugs. 2018;78:163–201.

Hruska KA, Beck AM. Nephrolithiasis. In: Coffman TM, Falk RJ, Molitoris BA, et al., editors. Schrier's diseases of the kidney. 9th ed. Philadelphia: Wolters Kluwer/Lippincott Williams & Wilkins; 2013. p. 642–72.

Sakhaee K, Moe OW. Urolithiasis. In: Yu ASL, Chertow GM, Luyckx VA, et al., editors. Brenner and Rector's the kidney. 11th ed. Philadelphia: Elsevier; 2020. p. 1277–326.

47. Many microorganisms have been implicated in the pathogenesis and prevention of nephrolithiasis. **Which one of the following microorganisms is able to prevent calcium oxalate stone formation?**

A. Nanobacteria
B. Proteus mirabilis
C. Oxalobacter formigenes
D. Ureaplasma urealyticum
E. Klebsiella pneumoniae

The answer is C

Except for Oxalobacter formigenes, other bacteria have been implicated in the genesis of kidney stones. O. formigenes is an obligate anaerobe colonized in the colon of humans and other mammalian species. It degrades dietary oxalate in the intestine to formate so that intestinal absorption and urinary excretion of oxalate is reduced. Therefore, formation of hyperoxaluria and calcium oxalate stone is prevented. It has been shown that antibiotic use may reduce colonization of O. formigenes, resulting in hyperoxaluria and stone formation. This suggests that O. formigenes may be important in the prevention of calcium oxalate stone formation. Thus, choice C is correct.

Nanobacteria are ubiquitous microorganisms that have been cultured from all forms of stones. It is suggested that nanobacteria can nucleate carbonate apatite on their surfaces and thereby provide the nidus for stone formation. *Proteus*, *Ureaplasma*, and *Klebsiella* forms struvite stones.

Suggested Reading

Kaufman DW, Kelly JP, Curhan GC, et al. Oxalobacter formigenes may reduce the risk of calcium oxalate stones. J Am Soc Nephrol. 2008;19:1197–203.

PeBenito A, Nazzal L, Wang C, et al. Comparative prevalence of Oxalobacter formigenes in three human populations. Sci Rep. 2019;9:574.

Sakhaee K. Recent advances in the pathophysiology of nephrolithiasis. Kidney Int. 2009;75:585–95.

48. A 30-year-old man presents to the Emergency Department with nausea, vomiting, severe flank pain, and hematuria. **Which one of the following diagnostic images is appropriate in this subject?**

A. A plain film of the abdomen (KUB)
B. An ultrasound of the kidneys
C. An intravenous urogram
D. An unenhanced helical (spiral) CT of abdomen
E. An MRI

The answer is D

Historically, the routine workup of a patient with renal colic includes a KUB, renal ultrasound, and an intravenous urography (IVU). The disadvantage with KUB is that it cannot detect radiolucent stones such as uric acid or xanthine stone, but it can show radiopaque stones such as calcium, cystine, or struvite. KUB is recommended during follow-up of patients. The ultrasound demonstrates hydronephrosis in the obstructed kidney as well as the calculus itself. However, ultrasonography has limited accuracy for determining stone size and in detecting ureteral calculi. Therefore, IVU is used to document obstructed kidney because it shows prolonged nephrogram phase, delayed excretion of contrast medium, and pelvicalyceal and ureteral dilation. Despite the routine use of IVU, recent studies have shown that unenhanced CT is the initial examination of choice because of high sensitivity and identification of hydronephrosis as well as small renal and ureteral stones.

Nonenhanced (no contrast) CT is superior in sensitivity and specificity to both ultrasound and IVU in depicting obstructing ureteral calculi regardless of their size, composition, or location. Furthermore, CT has the

advantage of shorter examination time, greater diagnostic accuracy, and detecting extrarenal diseases such as appendicitis or diverticulitis. Because of shorter examination time, the cost is much less than IVU. However, one disadvantage of unenhanced CT is that it uses a higher radiation dosage than conventional IVU. For this reason, low-dose CT is recommended. Thus, answer D is correct.

MRI is useful in pregnant women when ultrasound is not diagnostic or in patients allergic to contrast material. However, MRI is not sensitive in detecting small calculi and analyzing filling defects. Thus, MRI is not the test of choice in patients with renal colic.

Suggested Reading

Eisner BH, McQuaid JW, Hyams E, et al. Nephrolithiasis: what surgeons need to know. AJR Am J Roentgenol. 2011;196:1274–8.

Raynal G, Traxer O. Imaging and interventional treatment: urolithiasis from the surgeon's point of view. In: Turner N, Lameire N, Goldsmith DJ, et al., editors. Oxford textbook of clinical nephrology. 4th ed. Oxford: Oxford University Press; 2016. p. 1713–21.

49. The above patient had calcium oxalate stones, which recurred in 8 months. Serum chemistry is normal. **Which one of the following imaging studies is appropriate during follow-up of this patient?**

   A. Nonenhanced CT of abdomen
   B. Renal ultrasonography (US)
   C. KUB radiography
   D. B and C
   E. All of the above

   The answer is D

   Although nonenhanced CT of abdomen is the imaging study of choice, it should be avoided because of increased radiation exposure. In a prospective study, Ripollès et al. showed that the combination of US and KUB provides similar information as nonenhanced CT with low-radiation exposure. The combination also has higher sensitivity than either imaging study alone. Thus, option D is correct.

   Suggested Reading

Eisner BH, McQuaid JW, Hyams E, et al. Nephrolithiasis: what surgeons need to know. AJR Am J Roentgenol. 2011;196:1274–8.

Ripollès T, Agramunt M, Errando J, et al. Suspected ureteral colic: plain film and sonography vs unenhanced helical CT. A prospective study in 66 patients. Eur Radiol. 2004;14:129–36.

50. A 34-year-old man is referred to you for evaluation of recurrent nephrolithiasis. He has formed three stones in the last 5 years, requiring ureteral stent placement one time. Each time the stones were seen clearly on plain film of the abdomen. He says that he takes adequate amounts of dairy products, water, and lemon juice. He admits to consuming large amounts of meat and spinach. Serum chemistry is normal, including calcium, phosphorus, uric acid, and albumin. Twenty-four-hour urine shows:

   Volume: 1.8 L
   Creatinine: 1360 mg
   Calcium: 400 mg
   Oxalate: 42 mg
   Uric acid: 540 mg
   Citrate: 360 mg

   Which one of the following recommendations is FALSE?

   A. A thiazide diuretic
   B. Decrease intake of meat and spinach
   C. Increase water intake with the goal of producing about 2 L of urine daily
   D. Increase dairy products and recommend lettuce
   E. Cinacalcet 30 mg daily

The answer is E

All of the choices except for choice E are appropriate in the management of the patient who has recurrences of stone formation. Thiazides have been shown to reduce recurrence of stones by 50% and also help maintain bone density.

Decreased intake of meat reduces calcium excretion and increases citrate excretion. In addition, bone mineral dissolution is prevented by low meat consumption. Limited intake of spinach, but not lettuce, prevents oxalate formation.

High fluid intake to generate at least 2-L urine per day has been shown to reduce urinary supersaturation, and thus the risk for stone formation.

An increase in consumption of dairy products is associated with an increase in calcium intake, which results in decreased oxalate excretion.

Cinacalcet stimulates calcium-sensing receptor in the parathyroid gland with resultant decrease in PTH secretion. In rats with hereditary hypercalciuria, cinacalcet did not have any effect on either calciuria or uricosuria. Also, it has not been shown that cinacalcet prevents recurrence of stone formation.

Suggested Reading

Hruska KA, Beck AM. Nephrolithiasis. In: Coffman TM, Falk RJ, Molitoris BA, et al., editors. Schrier's diseases of the kidney. 9th ed. Philadelphia: Wolters Kluwer/Lippincott Williams & Wilkins; 2013. p. 642–72.

Sakhaee K, Moe OW. Urolithiasis. In: Yu ASL, Chertow GM, Luyckx VA, et al., editors. Brenner and Rector's the kidney. 11th ed. Philadelphia: Elsevier; 2020. p. 1277–326.

Taylor EN, Curhan GC. Diet and fluid prescription for stone disease. Kidney Int. 2006;70:835–9.

51. Medical expulsive therapy (MET) for ureteral calculi is in practice to reduce renal colic. **Which one of the following is CORRECT for MET?**

A. Tamsulosin (α1-blocker)
B. Nifedipine (a calcium channel blocker, CCB)
C. Corticosteroids
D. No benefit of MET
E. A and C

The answer is D

MET has gained popularity as a medical therapy to facilitate the passage of ureteral stones. A Cochrane review of 32 randomized trials evaluating α1-blockers found an improvement in stone-free rate in the α1-blocker group compared with standard management. Therapy with α1-bockers was found to reduce the number of painful episodes, analgesic use, and hospitalization rate as well as early expulsion of stone. Tamsulosin is commonly used to lower urinary tract symptoms due to benign prostatic hypertrophy. It inhibits ureteric tone and peristalsis frequency and contraction. Tamsulosin is the most studied α1-blocker for MET to reduce analgesic need in patients with ureteral colic. Terazosin and doxazosin have also been helpful in MET.

CCBs seem to have an inhibitory effect on ureteric function and reduce the ureterorenal distension that is responsible for pain. Corticosteroids have been used in MET with the assumption that they reduce ureteral inflammation and edema. However, α1-blockers have been suggested as a treatment for ureteral stones with least adverse effects.

Although MET is useful in selected patients, recent trials did not find any benefit of MET compared with standard therapy. Thus, answer D is correct. A recent review concludes by saying "Individual clinicians are required to decide for themselves which studies to believe. Alpha-blockers as MET may retain a role in a selective group of well-counselled patients with larger stones who understand the side effects and off-label use."

Suggested Reading

De Coninck V, Antonelli J , Chew B, et al. Medical expulsive therapy for urinary stones: future trends and knowledge gaps. Eur Urol. 2019;76:658–66.

Ludwig WW, Matlaga BR. Urinary stone disease diagnosis. Medical therapy, and surgical management. Med Clin N Am. 2018;102:265–77.

Seitz C, Liatsikos E, Porpiglia F, et al. Medical therapy to facilitate the passage of stones: what is the evidence? Eur Urol. 2009;56:455–71.

52. An association between specific beverages and risk for stone formation has been suggested by observational studies. **Which one of the following beverages causes increased risk for stone formation?**

    A. Alcohol
    B. Coffee and tea
    C. Milk
    D. Water intake with urine output of 2 L/day
    E. Grapefruit and orange juice

    The answer is E

    A few studies evaluated the effects of fluid and beverage intake on the risk of stone formation. It was shown that intake of alcohol, wine, coffee, tea, and milk reduced the risk for stone formation. Also, urine output >2 L/day was found to lower the risk for stone formation. The mechanism seems to be related to inhibition of antidiuretic hormone by alcohol and caffeine with increased urine output. Milk binds to oxalate in the gut and reduces its absorption. Thus, answers A–D are correct.

    It is of interest to note that tea has high oxalate content (14 mg/cup), but its impact on urine excretion is extremely low. Both grapefruit and orange juice provide citrate, but studies have shown that these juices were found to be associated with increased risk of stone formation. Grapefruit juice seems to increase urine excretion of both citrate and oxalate. Thus, answer E is correct.

    Suggested Reading

Curhan GC, Willett WC, Rimm EB, et al. Prospective study of beverage use and the risk of kidney stones. Am J Epidemiol. 1996;143:240–7.
Taylor EN, Curhan GC. Diet and fluid prescription for stone disease. Kidney Int. 2006;70:835–9.
Taylor EN, Curhan GC. Epidemiology of nephrolithiasis. In: Turner N, Lameire N, Goldsmith DJ, et al., editors. Oxford textbook of clinical nephrology. 4th ed. Oxford: Oxford University Press; 2016. p. 1631–6.

53. Highly active antiretroviral therapy (HAART) is effective in prolonging life in patients with HIV infection. **Which one of the following HAART medications does NOT cause nephrolithiasis?**

    A. Nelfinavir
    B. Amprenavir
    C. Saquinavir
    D. Atazanavir
    E. Tenofovir

    The answer is E

    Except for tenofovir, which is a nucleotide reverse transcriptase inhibitor, all other drugs (protease inhibitors) have been shown to cause nephrolithiasis. However, newer protease inhibitors such as tipranavir and darunavir are not associated with nephrolithiasis.

    Suggested Reading

Daudon M, Frochot V, Bazin D, et al. Drug-induced kidney stones and crystalline nephropathy: pathophysiology, prevention and treatment. Drugs. 2018;78:163–201.
Izzedine H, Harris M, Perazella MA. The nephrotoxic effects of HAART. Nature Rev Nephrol. 2009;5:563–73.
Jao J, Wyatt CM. Antiretroviral medications: adverse effects on the kidney. Adv Chronic Kidney Dis. 2010;17:72–82.

54. **Which one of the following factors does NOT cause hypocitraturia?**

    A. Distal renal tubular acidosis (dRTA)
    B. High protein diet
    C. Hypokalemia
    D. Diarrhea
    E. Consumption of fruits and vegetables

    The answer is E

    Hypocitraturia is a common metabolic disorder found in 20% to 60% of stone formers. Some of the causes include dRTA, high protein intake, hypokalemia, bowel dysfunction, and genetic factors.

It was reported that acidosis lowers and alkalosis increases citrate excretion. Acidosis increases renal tubular reabsorption of citrate, and also increases cellular metabolism. High protein intake causes acidosis, which in turn promotes citrate absorption and its metabolism. Similarly, hypokalemia causes both intracellular and renal tubular acidosis, thus promoting citrate absorption and metabolism. Diarrhea causes hypocitraturia by generating metabolic acidosis. Increased consumption of fruits and vegetables is associated with an increase in citrate excretion in hypocitraturic patients and increase in urine pH. Thus, option E is incorrect.

Suggested Reading

Sakhaee K, Moe OW. Urolithiasis. In: Yu ASL, Chertow GM, Luyckx VA, et al., editors. Brenner and Rector's the kidney. 11th ed. Philadelphia: Elsevier; 2020. p. 1277–326.
Zuckerman JM, Assimos DG. Hypocitraturia: pathophysiology and medical management. Rev Urol. 2009;11:134–44.

55. A 50-year-old obese woman with type 2 diabetes visits the Emergency Department for severe abdominal pain. A spiral CT of abdomen shows a kidney stone >10 mm in size. She is on metformin with A1c of 8.5%. **Which one of the following mechanisms accounts for her kidney stone formation?**

A. Insulin resistance with hyperinsulinemia
B. Low urine pH
C. Low urine NH_4 excretion
D. Excess dietary intake
E. All of the above

The answer is E

All of the above factors contribute to the formation of stone formation in obese individuals. It has been shown that risk of stone disease increases with an increase in body mass index. Obesity is usually associated with insulin resistance, hyperinsulinemia, and diabetes, a part of metabolic syndrome. Studies have shown that diabetic subjects develop uric acid stones than nondiabetic subjects. Also, urine studies in subjects with metabolic syndrome or diabetes alone showed low urine pH, higher levels of oxalate, sodium, uric acid, and phosphate than nonobese or nondiabetic subjects. These studies indicate that obese individuals had high dietary intake that contain lithogenic substances. Insulin resistance causes low NH_4 excretion with low urine pH, an important risk factors for uric acid stone formation. Thus, answer E is correct.

Suggested Reading

Ahmed MH, Barakat S, Almobarak AO. The association between renal stone disease and cholesterol gallstones: the easy to believe and not hard to retrieve theory of the metabolic syndrome. Ren Fail. 2014;36:957–62.
Asplin JR. Obesity and urolithiasis. Adv Chronic Kidney Dis. 2009;16:11–20.
Aune D, Mahamat-Saleh Y, Norat T, et al. Body fatness, diabetes, physical activity and risk of kidney stones: a systematic review and meta-analysis of cohort studies. Eur J Epidemiol. 2018;33:1033–47.
Carbone A, Al Salhi Y, Tasca A, et al. Obesity and kidney stone disease: a systematic review. Minerva Urol Nefrol. 2018;73:393–400.

56. **Infection (struvite) stones occur with repeated urinary tract infection. Which one of the following statements is CORRECT concerning struvite stones?**

A. Struvite stones develop into staghorn calculi, if untreated
B. Struvite stones are composed of magnesium ammonium phosphate (struvite) and calcium carbonate-apatite
C. Medical therapy alone is inadequate for management of staghorn calculi
D. Surgical therapy followed by antibiotic use is the most appropriate therapy for staghorn calculi
E. All of the above

The answer is E

As mentioned previously, struvite stones develop as a result of urinary tract infection with bacteria that produce the enzyme urease. This enzyme splits urea into NH_3 and CO_2, and NH_3 combines with water to form NH_4^+ OH^-. This hydroxyl moiety causes alkaline urine pH, as shown below:

$$\text{Urea} \rightarrow 2NH_3 + CO_2$$
$$NH_3 + H_2O \rightarrow NH_4^+ + OH^-$$

If the causative microorganism is not treated with appropriate antibiotics, the struvite stone develops into staghorn calculus, which is a large calculus that occupies most or all of the renal collecting system. The name staghorn is given to the struvite stone because it looks like the antlers of a deer or stag on renal imaging. Antibiotic use alone is not sufficient to treat struvite stone because the bacteria reside within (interstices) the stone, and antibiotics do not penetrate the stone. Therefore, removal of the entire stone by surgical approach is needed. Several surgical approaches, as shown below, have been tried:

1. **Open surgery**
2. **Laparoscopic surgery**
3. **Percutaneous nephrolithotomy (PCNL)**
4. **Shock-wave lithotripsy (SWL)**
5. **Combination of PCNL and SWL**
6. **Ureteroscopy**
7. **Combination of PCNL and ureteroscopy**

Of the above procedures, PCNL is suggested as the first line of treatment for most patients, and the combination of PCNL and SWL may be necessary in some patients. Thus, answer E is correct.

Suggested Reading

Espinosa-Ortiz EJ, Eisner BH, Lange D, et al. Current insights into the mechanisms and management of infection stones. Nat Rev Urol. 2019;16:35–53.
Flannigan R, Choy WH, Chew B, et al. Renal struvite stones-pathogenesis, microbiology, and management strategies. Nat Rev Urol. 2014;11:333–41.
Marien T, Miller NL. Treatment of the infected stone. Urol Clin N Am. 2015;42:459–72.

57. A 38-year-old woman visits Emergency Department for frequent urinary tract infections. She has history of infection stones. **On urine culture, which one of the following bacteria is LEAST likely to grow?**

   A. Pseudomonas
   B. Klebsiella
   C. Proteus
   D. Enterococcus
   E. E. coli

The answer is E

This patient has history of infection stones, which are usually caused by urease-producing organisms. Of all the above organisms, only *E. coli* does not have urease enzyme. Therefore, answer E is correct.

Suggested Reading

Espinosa-Ortiz EJ, Eisner BH, Lange D, et al. Current insights into the mechanisms and management of infection stones. Nat Rev Urol. 2019;16:35–53.
Flannigan R, Choy WH, Chew B, et al. Renal struvite stones-pathogenesis, microbiology, and management strategies. Nat Rev Urol. 2014;11:333–41.
Marien T, Miller NL. Treatment of the Infected Stone. Urol Clin N Am. 2015;42:459–72.

58. **Which one of the following empiric therapies for calcium kidney stone prevention is CORRECT?**

   A. Fluid intake 3 L/day
   B. Low salt, low protein, low oxalate, and calcium 100 mg/day
   C. Weight loss
   D. K-citrate and K-bicarbonate
   E. All of the above

The answer is C

It has been suggested that weight loss and diets, such as Borghi and dietary approaches to stop hypertension (DASH) diets, can prevent calcium stones formation. As discussed in one of the questions, obesity is a risk factor for stone formation, and weight loss prevents stone formation. The Borghi diet has high calcium intake with reduced sodium as well as reduced animal protein and oxalate intake, and this diet has been shown to prevent

stones in a randomized, controlled trial. The DASH diet includes fruits, vegetables, nuts and legumes, whole grains, and dairy products and low intake of red and processed meats. This diet caused increased urine volume and citrate excretion. Total fluid intake mostly water and other fluids such as coffee, juice, beer, and wine to a total of 3 L/day is recommended. Medications such as K-citrate (15–30 mEq twice daily or K-carbonate 25 mEq twice daily and chlorthalidone 25 mg once daily or indapamide 2.5 mg once daily and alendronate 70 mg once a week) are suggested. Thus, answer E is correct.

Suggested Reading

Borghi L, Schianchi T, Meschi T, et al. Comparison of two diets for the prevention of recurrent stones in idiopathic hypercalciuria. N Engl J Med. 2002;346:77–84.
Goldfarb DS. Empiric therapy for kidney stones. Urolithiasis. 2019;47:107–13.
Taylor EN, Stampfer MJ, Mount DB, et al. DASH-style diet and 24-hour urine composition. Clin J Amer Soc Nephrol. 2010;5:2315–22.

59. **Match the following case histories with the type of stones in the urine?**

A. A 24-year-old well-developed woman is seen for weakness. She has no history of weakness, shortness of breath, or abdominal pain. Her BP is normal. Laboratory findings: Na^+ 136 mEq/dL, K^+ 2.4 mEq/dL, Cl^- 110 mEq/dL, HCO_3^- 18 mEq/dL, and albumin 3.8 g/dL; urine pH 7.2
B. A 26-year-old, 7-week pregnant woman comes to the emergency department with a complaint of rapid breathing for 2 days without chest pain. An ABG reveals a high anion gap (AG) metabolic acidosis. Two hours later her breathing has improved, and repeat ABG is normal. A urinalysis shows needle-shaped crystals
C. A 30-year-old obese woman follows diet and some herbal medication to lose weight

She has no consistent effects on weight loss; therefore, her physician starts on Orlistat 120 mg twice daily, which was increased to 120 mg three times a day. Four months later, she visits the physician's office with a complaint of abdominal pain and KUB shows a renal stone

1. Calcium oxalate
2. Calcium phosphate
3. Hippurate

Answers: A = 2; B = 3; C = 1

The history and laboratory findings shown for patient A are consistent with distal (Type 1) RTA. Calcium phosphate stones are usually seen in such patients because of alkaline urine pH.

The patient described in choice B has toluene ingestion from paints and glues. At times, pregnant women crave for paint ingestion. Toluene is metabolized to hippurate, thereby generating a high AG metabolic acidosis. However, hippurate is excreted by the kidney within a few hours, and repeat ABG shows normal HCO_3^- levels. Hippurate appears as needle-shaped crystals in the urine.

Orlistat is a gastrointestinal lipase inhibitor and used in obese individuals. It has been that orlistat reduces free Ca^{2+}, thereby increasing oxalate absorption and calcium oxalate stone formation. The history presented in choice C is consistent with calcium oxalate stone formation.

Suggested Reading

Humayun Y, Ball KC, Lewin JR, et al. Acute oxalate nephropathy associated with orlistat. J Nephropathol. 2016;5:79–83.
Lumlertgul N, Siribamrungwong M, Jaber BL, et al. Secondary oxalate nephropathy: a systematic review. Kidney Int Rep. 2018;3:1363–72.
Singh A, Sarkar SR, Gaber LW, et al. Acute oxalate nephropathy associated with Orlistat, a gastrointestinal lipase inhibitor. Am J Kidney Dis. 2007;49:153–7.

Chapter 4
Chronic Kidney Disease

1. A 30-year-old African American female student is referred to you for evaluation of hematuria. Urinalysis shows >20 RBCs per high power field. There is no proteinuria. Repeat urinalysis 1 month later shows similar number of RBCs. There are no RBC casts. Her hematuria is unrelated to her menstrual cycle. BP is 120/78 mm Hg. Serum creatinine is 1.0 mg/dL. She weighs 60 kg. Renal ultrasound reveals large kidneys with multiple cysts. She wants to know whether or not she has kidney disease. **Regarding her kidney status, which one of the following statements is CORRECT?**

   A. She cannot be classified as having chronic kidney disease (CKD) because her serum creatinine is normal
   B. She cannot be classified as having CKD because she has no proteinuria
   C. She needs a renal biopsy to make the diagnosis of CKD
   D. She has CKD based on hematuria and abnormal renal imaging
   E. None of the above

   The answer is D

   In order to provide a uniform definition of CKD, the Kidney Disease Outcome Quality Initiative (KDOQI) of the National Kidney Foundation defined CKD as kidney damage (with or without decreased GFR) or decreased GFR <60 mL/min/1.73 m^2 for >3 months. .3Kidney damage is defined as pathological abnormalities or markers of damage including abnormalities in blood or urine tests or in imaging studies. Based on the above definition, the patient has microscopic hematuria and large kidneys with cysts. Thus, she is considered to have CKD. Therefore, option D is correct.

   The KDIGO (Kidney Disease Improving Global Outcomes) 2012 Clinical Practice Guideline for the Evaluation and Management of Chronic Kidney Disease also developed similar criteria to define CKD. In this guideline, CKD is defined as "abnormalities of kidney structure or function, present for >3 months with implications for health." Table 4.1 shows the KDIGO recommendations for CKD definition.

Table 4.1 Criteria for CKD (either of the following present for >3 months)

Criterion	Recommendation
Markers of kidney damage (one or more)	Albuminuria (AER ≥30 mg/24 h; ACR ≥30 mg/g [≥3 mg/mmol] Urine sediment abnormalities Electrolyte and other abnormalities due to tubular disorders Abnormalities detected by histology Structural abnormalities detected by imaging History of kidney transplantation
Decreased GFR	GFR <60 mL/min/1.73 m^2 (GFR categories G3a-G5)

AER albumin excretion rate, *ACR* albumin-creatinine ratio, *GFR* glomerular filtration rate

Suggested Reading

Kidney Disease Improving Global Outcomes. KIDIGO 2012 clinical practice guideline for the evaluation and management of chronic kidney disease. Kidney Int Suppl. 2013;3:1–150.

A. S. Reddi, *Absolute Nephrology Review*, https://doi.org/10.1007/978-3-030-85958-9_4

National Kidney Foundation. Chronic kidney disease. A guide to select NKF/KDOQI guidelines and recommendations (in association with Nephrology Pharmacy Associates). New York: National Kidney Foundation; 2006. p. 1–115.

National Kidney Foundation. K/DOQI clinical practice guidelines for chronic kidney disease: evaluation, classification and stratification. Am J Kidney Dis. 2002;39(Suppl 1):S1–266.

2. **Regarding the prevalence of CKD in the USA, which one of the following statements is INCORRECT?**

A. 15% of US adults (37 millions) are estimated to have CKD
B. The prevalence is higher in people aged 65 years or older than in people aged <64 years
C. The prevalence is higher in women than in men
D. Non-Hispanic blacks have higher prevalence than non-Hispanic whites
E. All of the above

The answer is E

According to the Centers for Disease Control and Prevention, all of the above answers are correct. Thirty-seven million (15%) US adults are estimated to have CKD. Of these 37 million, 38% of people aged 65 years or older have CKD, as compared with 13% aged 45–64 years and 7% aged 18–44 years. CKD is more common in women (15%) than in men (12%). The prevalence of CKD is more common in non-Hispanic blacks (16%) than in non-Hispanic whites (13%). Figure 4.1 shows these percentages.

Percentage* of CKD Among US Adults Aged 18 Years or Older,
By Age, Sex, and Race/Ethnicity

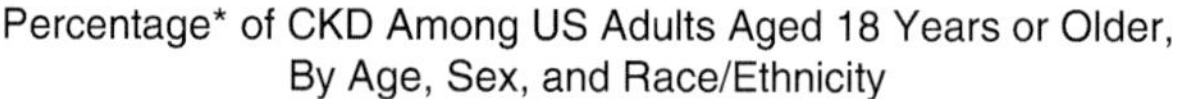

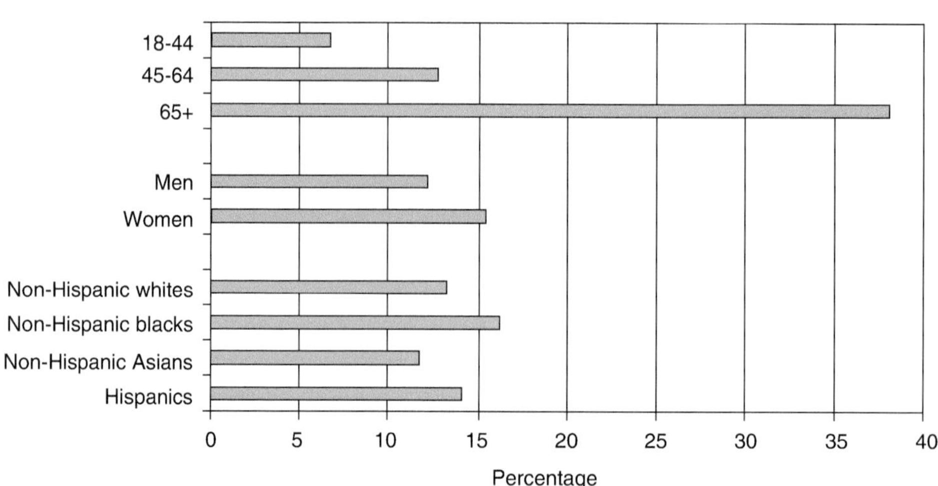

Fig. 4.1 Percentages of CKD among US adults

Suggested Reading

Centers for Disease Control and Prevention. Chronic kidney disease surveillance system website. https://nccd.cdc.gov/CKD. Accessed 7 Jan 2019.

3. **Which one of the following is NOT a traditional risk factor for cardiovascular disease (CVD)?**

A. HTN
B. Diabetes
C. Albuminuria
D. Smoking
E. Dyslipidemia

The answer is C

Except for albuminuria, the remaining factors have been reported as traditional risk factors, as suggested by the Framingham study. Table 4.2 lists both traditional and nontraditional risk factors for CKD as well as CVD, suggesting that both CKD and CVD share similar risk factors.

Table 4.2 Risk factors for CKD

Traditional risk factors	Nontraditional risk factors
Old age	Albuminuria
Male gender	Anemia
HTN	Oxidative stress
High LDL cholesterol	Inflammation
Low HDL cholesterol	Homocysteine
Diabetes	Thrombogenic factors
Smoking	
Physical inactivity	
Family history of CKD or CVD	

Suggested Reading

Kendrick J, Chonchol MB. Nontraditional risk factors for cardiovascular disease in patients with chronic kidney disease. Nat Clin Pract Nephrol. 2008;4:672–81.

Menon V, Gul A, Sarnak MJ. Cardiovascular risk factors in chronic kidney disease. Kidney Int. 2005;68:1413–18.

Menon V, Sarnak MJ, Levey AS. Risk factors and kidney disease. In: Brenner BM, editor. Brenner and Rector's the kidney. 8th ed. Philadelphia: Saunders; 2008. p. 633–53.

4. A 40-year-old man with hypertension is referred to you for evaluation of his risk for progression of kidney disease. His BP is 140/80 mm Hg. His serum creatinine is 1.8 mg/dL (eGFR 59 mL/min) and a 24-h urine albuminuria of 200 mg. He has no diabetes or other comorbid conditions. **According to 2012 KDIGO Guideline, how would you classify his risk of kidney progression?**

A. Low risk
B. Moderate risk
C. High risk
D. Very high risk
E. None of the above

The answer is C

The 2012 KDIGO Guideline recommends in any CKD patient to identify the cause of CKD, GFR category, albuminuria category, and other risk factors, including comorbid conditions in predicting prognosis of CKD. Tables 4.4 and 4.5 help predict the prognosis of this patient's kidney progression.

From Tables 4.3 and 4.4, this patient with CKD is at high risk for progression of his kidney disease. Thus, option C is correct.

Table 4.3 Albuminuria categories in CKD

ACR (approximate equivalent)				
AER				
Category	(mg/24 h)	(mg/mmol)	(mg/g)	Terms
A1	<30	<3	<30	Normal to mildly increased
A2	30–300	3–30	30–300	Moderately increased[a]
A3	>300	>30	>300	Severely increased[b]

AER albumin excretion rate, *ACR* albumin to creatinine ratio, *CKD* chronic kidney disease; [a]Relative to young adult level, [b]Including nephrotic syndrome

Table 4.4 Prognosis of CKD by GFR (G) and albuminuria categories

				Persistent albuminuria categories Description and range		
				A1	A2	A3
				<30 mg/g <3 mg/mmol	30–300 mg/g 3–30 mg/mmol	>300 mg/g >30 mg/mmol
GFR (mL/min/1.73 m²)	G1	Normal or high	≥90	Low	Moderate	High
	G2	Mildly decreased	60–89	Low	Moderate	High
	G3a	Mildly to moderately decreased	45–59	Moderate	High	Very high
	G3b	Moderately to severely decreased	30–44	High	Very high	Very high
	G4	Severely decreased	15–29	Very high	Very high	Very high
	G5	Kidney failure	<15	Very high	Very high	Very high

In all questions of this review book, CKD stages 1-5 rather than GFR (G) categories were used. Note that CKD stages 1-5 are equal to G categories G1-G5

Suggested Reading

Kidney Disease Improving Global Outcomes. KIDIGO 2012 clinical practice guideline for the evaluation and management of chronic kidney disease. Kidney Int Suppl. 2013;3:1–150.

5. **Regarding CKD awareness among patients, which one of the following statements is FALSE?**

   A. According to The Kidney Early Evaluation Program (KEEP), awareness of kidney disease is low for all stages of CKD from years 2000 to 2005
   B. According to the National Health and Nutrition Examination Survey (NHANES), awareness improved over time in those with CKD stage 3 only and not in those with stages 1 and 2
   C. According to an Italian study of general practitioners, awareness of kidney disease stages 3 to 5 is scarce because of limited availability of serum creatinine and difficulty recognizing eGFR in the absence of increased serum creatinine testing
   D. According to a survey of internal medicine residents in the USA, almost all residents knew the definition and stages of CKD as proposed by the National Kidney Foundation guidelines
   E. The KEEP observed more profound increase in awareness for CKD stages 4 to 5 compared to CKD stages 1 to 3 from 2000 to 2005

The answer is D

CKD is usually recognized incidentally in most of the subjects, and the management becomes rather difficult to prevent its progression to ESKD. One major problem is awareness of the disease. Several studies assessed awareness of CKD, which showed that the level of awareness by both patient and provider is unacceptably low. Although about 90% of patients with CKD had seen a physician within the previous year in the KEEP, awareness of their disease was low for all stages of CKD. However, awareness was profoundly increased among patients with CKD stages 4 to 5 compared to stages 1 to 3. Thus, options A and E are correct.

Plantinga et al. assessed awareness in participants of NHANES from 1999 to 2004 for CKD stages 1 to 4, and found that awareness improved over time in those with CKD stage 3 only from 4.7% to 9.2% (4.7% for 1999–2000; 8.9% for 2001–2002; 9.2% for 2003–2004). This survey also showed that patients with diabetes, hypertension, or proteinuria are more likely to be aware of their stage 3 kidney disease.

Awareness of CKD is also lacking among general practitioners in Italy. In a survey of 451,548 individuals, only 17.2% (77,630) had a serum creatinine testing, and only 15.2% were recognized as having CKD from billing. Referral to a nephrologist ranged from 4.9% for patients with stage 3 CKD (eGFR 59–30 mL/min) to 56% for patients with CKD stage 4 (eGFR <30 mL/min). Thus, the prevalence of CKD stages 3 to 5 is frequent but awareness of the disease among general practitioners is scarce. A study in 2014 reported self-awareness of CKD was only 8%, a much lower percentage compared to that of diabetes.

In a cross-sectional study using an online questionnaire survey among 479 PGY 1, PGY 2, and PGY 3 internal medicine residents of the USA, Agrawal et al. reported that half of the residents did not know that proteinuria for 3 or more months defines CKD, and one-third did not know the staging of CKD. However, most residents knew the traditional risk factors and goal BP for CKD. Also, most residents chose to refer a patient with eGFR <30 mL/min to a nephrologist. Thus, it is important to improve education among residents for better understanding of CKD and its management. Thus, option D is false.

Suggested Reading

Agrawal V, Ghosh AK, Barnes MA, et al. Awareness and knowledge of clinical practice guidelines for CKD among internal medicine residence: a national online survey. Am J Kidney Dis. 2008;52:1061–9.

Minutolo R, De Nocola L, Mazzaglia G, et al. Detection and awareness of moderate to advanced CKD by primary care practitioners: a cross-sectional study from Italy. Am J Kidney Dis. 2008;52:444–53.

Plantinga LC, Boulware E, Coresh J, et al. Patient awareness of chronic kidney disease. Trends and predictors. Arch Intern Med. 2008;168:2268–75.

Plantinga LC, Tuot DS, Powe NR. Awareness of chronic kidney disease among patients and providers. Adv Chronic Kidney Dis. 2010;17:225–36.

Saab G, McCullough PA, Bakris GL. CKD awareness in the United States: the Kidney Early Evaluation Program. Am J Kidney Dis. 2008;52:382–3.

Verhave JC, Troyanov S, Mongeau F, et al. Prevalence, awareness, and management of CKD and cardiovascular risk factors in publicly funded health care. Clin J Am Soc Nephrol. 2014;9:713–9.

6. Many edible plant products have been implicated in the development of CKD. **Match the following plant-derived compounds that are associated with the documented chronic kidney disease (CKD)?**

A. Aristolochic acid
B. Nordihydroguaiaretic acid
C. Salicin
D. Yohimbine
E. Anthraquinone

1. Chronic tubulointerstitial nephritis
2. Lupus nephritis
3. Renal papillary necrosis
4. Renal cysts and renal cell carcinoma

Answers: A = 1; B = 4; C =3; D = 2; E = 1

CKD has been described in association with ingestion of many plant-derived compounds, usually called herbal medicines. The use of herbal medicines has increased throughout the world, and accounts for approximately 20% of the overall drug market. These herbal medications produce a variety of tubular and tubulointerstitial diseases (TIDs).

Aristolochic acid is derived from the plant *Aristolochia* spp. This compound causes TID and acute and chronic kidney disease. Also, uroepithelial malignancies have been described with the ingestion of the *Aristolochia* spp.

Nordihydroguaiaretic acid is derived from the leaves of creosote bush, Larrea tridentate, which is a Native American shrub and used in tea. In addition, its roots and leaves are distributed in the pill form as chaparral. Nordihydroguaiaretic acid is an antioxidant and also inhibits cell division, and its long-term use is implicated in the development of renal cysts and renal cell carcinoma.

Salicin is the toxic component of the plant, Salix daphnoides, and metabolizes to salicylate. It is usually called willow bark and causes renal papillary necrosis. Yohimbine is derived from the plant, *Pausinystalia yohimbe*. Chronic ingestion of yohimbine causes lupus nephritis, which responds to steroids. Anthraquinone is a toxic product of the plant, *Rhizoma rhei*. It is commonly called rhubarb and causes chronic TID.

Suggested Reading

Jha V. Herbal medicines and chronic kidney disease. Nephrology. 2010;15:10–7.

Luyckx VA, Naicker S. Acute kidney injury associated with the use of traditional medicines. Nature Clin Pract Nephrol. 2008;4:664–71.

Yang B, Xie Y, Guo M, et al. Nephrotoxicity and Chinese herbal medicine. Clin J Am Soc Nephrol. 2018;13:1605–11.

7. Compared with the Modification of Diet in Renal Disease (MDRD) Study equation, the CKD-EPI (chronic kidney disease-epidemiology collaboration) equation has several advantages. **Which one of the following statements regarding the CKD-EPI equation is INCORRECT?**

A. CKD-EPI equation is more accurate in estimative GFR than MDRD study equation
B. CKD-EPI equation has higher false-positive diagnoses of CKD

C. CKD-EPI equation predicts lower prevalence of CKD
D. CKD-EPI equation may have more accurate prediction for adverse outcomes
E. Drug dosing using CKD-EPI equation may be more accurate than MDRD equation

The answer is B

Except for statement B, all other statements are correct. The CKD-EPI creatinine equation was developed using the same variables as the MDRD equation in a total of 8,254 participants in 10 studies (equation development data set) and 3,896 participants in 16 studies (validation data set). Using the CKD-EPI equation, the median estimated GFR was 94.5 mL/min/1.73 m^2 (simply referred to as mL/min) as compared with 85.0 mL/min using the MDRD study equation. Also, the prevalence of CKD with the CKD-EPI equation was 11.6% as compared with 13.1% using the MDRD study equation. Thus, the CKD-EPI equation has lower rather than higher false-positive diagnoses of CKD. Thus, the statement B is incorrect.

At least, two independent studies, namely, the ARIC (Atherosclerosis Research in Communities) and the AusDiab (Australian Diabetes, Obesity and Lifestyle Study), confirmed the observations of the CKD-EPI equation. In both studies 43.5% and 25% participants with CKD stage 3a (eGFR 45–59 mL/min) were reclassified as having no CKD. Thus, the CKD-EPI equation is more accurate than the MDRD study equation in classifying CKD.

Suggested Reading

Levey AS, Inker LA, Coresh J. GFR estimation: from physiology to public health. Am J Kidney Dis. 2014;63:820–34.
Levey AS, Stevens LA, Schmid CH, et al. A new equation to estimate glomerular filtration rate. Ann Intern Med. 2009;150:604–12.
Levey AS, Stevens LA. Estimating GFR using the CKD epidemiology collaboration (CKD-EPI) creatinine equation: more accurate GFR estimates, lower CKD prevalence estimates, and better risk predictions. Am J Kidney Dis. 2010;55:622–7.
Matsushita K, Selvin E, Bash LD, et al. Risk implications for the new epidemiology collaboration (CKD-EPI) equation compared with MDRD Study equation for estimated GFR: the Atherosclerosis Risk in Communities (ARIC) study. Am J Kidney Dis. 2010;55:648–59.
White SL, Polkinghorne KR, Atkins RC, et al. Comparison of the prevalence and mortality risk of CKD in Australia using the CKD epidemiology collaboration (CKD-EPI) and Modification of Diet in Renal Disease (MDRD) study GFR estimating equations: the AusDiab (Australian Diabetes, Obesity and Lifestyle) study. Am J Kidney Dis. 2010;55:660–70.

8. An 89-year-old cachectic woman is transferred from the Nursing Home for evaluation of fever and tachycardia. She weighs 50 kg. Her urine culture grows *Escherichia coli* that is sensitive to gentamicin only. Her lying and sitting BP and pulse rate are suggestive of orthostatic changes. Her serum creatinine is 0.9 mg/dL and eGFR is >60 mL/min. **Which one of the following equations/tests is more useful in adjusting the gentamicin dose?**

A. MDRD study equation
B. Cockcroft-Gault equation
C. 24-h creatinine clearance
D. Iothalamate clearance
E. Schwartz equation

The answer is B

The MDRD study equation has not been validated in the elderly and females (>70 years), and overestimates GFR in individuals with GFR >60 mL/min. Estimation of 24-h creatinine clearance is useful, but not practical at bed side. Iothalamate clearance involves radioisotopes and is expensive as well as time-consuming. Alo, it is not practical in drug dosing. Schwartz equation [GFR (mL/min/1.73 m^2) = 0.55 × Ht (cm)/serum creatinine (mL/dL)] is applicable to children but not adults. Therefore, the only formula that is useful for drug dosing at bed side is the Cockcroft-Gault equation, which provides approximate endogenous creatinine clearance in mL/min.

The formula to calculate creatinine clearance (C_{cr}) is as follows:

$$\text{Ccr}(\text{mL}/\text{min}) = \frac{(140 - \text{age}) \times \text{Body wt}(\text{kg})}{72 \times \text{Serum creatinine}(\text{mg}/\text{dL})}$$

For females, multiply by 0.85

For the above patients, the C_{cr} is: $\dfrac{(140-89)\times 50\times 0.85}{72\times 0.9}$

$$= \frac{51\times 50}{72\times 0.9} = \frac{2{,}550\times 0.85}{64.8} = 34\,\mathrm{mL/min}$$

Thus, the calculated C_{cr} is approximately 34 mL/min, which is much different from the reported eGFR of >60 mL/min. Thus, gentamicin dose needs to be reduced in this patient. Therefore, option B is correct.

Although it has been shown that the MDRD study equation is as good as Cockcroft-Gault equation in drug dosing by Stevens and Levey, a kinetic model by Spruill et al. demonstrated that the MDRD study equation in the elderly overestimates kidney function, leading to possible drug overdosing and drug toxicity. Also, dosing of many drugs was based on the Cockcroft-Gault equation prior to the introduction of MDRD study equation. Although determination of eGFR by CKD-EPI equation is as good or superior to Cockcroft-Gault equation in drug dosing, in this particular patient the eGFR by this equation would not give this low creatinine clearance. Therefore, Cockcroft-Gault equation has a role in drug dosing, particularly, in certain conditions.

Suggested Reading

Spruill WJ, Wade WE, Cobb HH III. Continuing the use of Cockcroft-Gault equation for drug dosing in patients with impaired renal function. Clin Pharmacol Ther. 2009;86:466–70.

Stevens LA, Levey AS. Use of the MDRD study equation to estimate kidney function for drug dosing. Clin Pharmacol Ther. 2009;86:465–7.

9. A 30-year-old obese woman is admitted for management of acute exacerbation of asthma. She weighs 400 lbs. Her serum creatinine is 0.8 mg/dL. **Which one of the following is the best method to assess her kidney function?**

   A. MDRD study equation
   B. Cockcroft-Gault equation
   C. Serum creatinine and BUN
   D. Serum creatinine and albuminuria
   E. Two or more 24-h urine creatinine clearances

The answer is E

The MDRD study equation can be used, but it has limited validation in extremely obese individuals. The Cockcroft-Gault equation overestimates creatinine clearance unless ideal body weight is calculated, which is difficult in many patients. Serum creatinine and BUN are not good markers of kidney function in obese individuals with low muscle mass. The presence of elevated creatinine and albuminuria reflects kidney disease rather than kidney function. Determination of two or more 24-h urine creatinine clearances is the better approach to evaluate kidney function in extremely obese individuals. However, this method can also overestimate GFR. Of all the above options, option E seems appropriate.

Suggested Reading

Glassock RJ, Winearls C. Screening for CKD with eGFR: doubts and dangers. Clin J Am Soc Nephrol. 2008;3:1563–8.

Jesudasan DR, Clifton P. Interpreting different measures of glomerular filtration rate in obesity and weight loss: pitfalls for the clinician. Int J Obes. 2012;36:1421–7.

10. **The MDRD study equation is a useful method to estimate GFR in which one of the following groups?**

    A. Southeast Asians
    B. Vegetarians
    C. Elderly females
    D. Malnourished and paraplegics
    E. CKD patients with lower levels of GFR regardless of CKD diagnosis

The answer is E

The widely accepted and approved serum creatinine-based method of estimated GFR is the MDRD study equation. Also, this equation has been adequately validated in CKD population, including African Americans,

diabetics, and kidney transplant recipients who have low GFRs (<60 mL/min). Despite its wide acceptance, the MDRD formula still has several limitations, as shown in Table 4.5, and suggests the use of clearance methods.

Table 4.5 Limitations of the MDRD study equation

Extreme age
Obesity
Malnutrition
Skeletal muscle disease
Paraplegia, quadriplegia
Vegetarians
AKI
Pregnancy
Dosing of renally excreted drugs
Asian population

Suggested Reading

Kidney Disease Improving Global Outcomes. KIDIGO 2012 clinical practice guideline for the evaluation and management of chronic kidney disease. Kidney Int Suppl. 2013;3:1–150.

Stevens LA, Lafayette RA, Perrone RD, et al. Laboratory evaluation of kidney function. In: Schrier RW, editor. Diseases of the kidney & urinary tract. 8th ed. Philadelphia: Lippincott Williams & Wilkins; 2007. p. 299–336.

Stevens LA, Padala S, Levey AS. Advances in glomerular filtration rate-estimating equations. Curr Opin Nephrol Hypertens. 2010;19:298–307.

11. **Measurement of serum cystatin C as a marker of GFR has been reported to be more accurate and precise than serum creatinine in which one of the following conditions?**

A. Children
B. Elderly
C. Diabetes
D. Pregnancy
E. All of the above

The answer is E

Cystatin C is a nonglycosylated cysteine proteinase inhibitor with a molecular weight of 13 KDa. It is secreted at a constant rate by all nucleated cells. Cystatin C is freely and totally filtered at the glomerulus without peritubular uptake. After filtration, the proximal tubules reabsorb and catabolize virtually all of cystatin C in lysosomes. Therefore, its secretion and presence in urine is negligible. Because of its absence in the urine, the clearance of Cystatin C cannot be measured but its serum concentration is considered a good measure of GFR. Unlike serum creatinine levels, cystatin C levels are not influenced by muscle mass or malnutrition.

Several studies reported that serum cystatin C levels have higher diagnostic accuracy and precision than serum creatinine levels, particularly in children, elderly, diabetics, pregnant women, and patients with cirrhosis. Thus, option E is correct.

It has been shown that determinations of both serum creatinine and cystatin C may be a better reflection of GFR than either measurement alone.

Suggested Reading

Chew JSC, Saleem M, Florkowski CM, et al. Cystatin C – a paradigm of evidence based laboratory medicine. Clin Biochem Rev. 2008;29:47–62.

Shlipak MG, Mattees MD, Peralta CA. Update on cystatin C: incorporation into clinical practice. Am J Kidney Dis. 2013;62:595–603.

Westhuyzen J. Cystatin C: a promising marker and predictor of impaired renal function. Ann Clin Lab Sci. 2006;36:387–94.

12. **Which one of the following factors is NOT associated with elevated levels of cystatin C?**

A. Older age and males
B. Neonates (1–30 days)

C. Glucocorticoids
D. Cyclosporine
E. Hyperthyroidism

The answer is D

A number of factors have been shown to influence cystatin C levels. Older age, male gender, glucocorticoids and hyperthyroidism, cigarette smoking, and elevated CRP levels were independently associated with elevated serum cystatin C levels. Also, greater weight and height, neonates under 30 days of age, and asthmatics were found to have high cystatin C levels. In contrast, cyclosporine has been shown to decrease cystatin C levels (D). Also, hypothyroidism causes low levels of cystatin C.

Suggested Reading

Chew JSC, Saleem M, Florkowski CM, et al. Cystatin C – a paradigm of evidence based laboratory based medicine. Clin Biochem Rev. 2008;29:47–62.
Kidney Disease Improving Global Outcomes. KIDIGO 2012 clinical practice guideline for the evaluation and management of chronic kidney disease. Kidney Int Suppl. 2013;3:1–150.
Westhuyzen J. Cystatin C: a promising marker and predictor of impaired renal function. Ann Clin Lab Sci. 2006;36:387–94.

13. A 50-year-old nonobese man with hypertension has eGFR of 30 mL/min/1.73 m^2, as calculated by the MDRD study equation. He wants to know how soon he needs renal replacement therapy. **Which one of the following statements is CORRECT regarding the slope of decline in kidney function?**

A. The eGFR tends to overestimate the decline in measured GFR by iothalamate clearance by approximately 28%
B. The eGFR tends to underestimate the decline in measured GFR by iothalamate clearance by approximately 28%
C. Compared to eGFR by the MDRD study equation the Cockcroft-Gault equation estimation of GFR is better in predicting the slope of decline in kidney function
D. 24-h urine creatinine clearance is a better way in estimating the decline in kidney function
E. None of the above methods is accurate in the above patient

The answer is B

The rate of GFR loss in CKD stages 3–5 patients remains unclear. However, a few studies addressed this issue in both diabetic and nondiabetic patients. A study by Xie et al. calculated the eGFR slope of decline in kidney function in the MDRD study participants with measured GFR between 25 and 55 mL/min and a median follow-up of 2.6 years. They found that the eGFR tended to underestimate measured decrements in GFR by 28%. For example, the mean of measured GFR slope was −3.9 mL/min/1.73 m^2 as compared with the mean eGFR slope of −2.8 mL/min/1.73 m^2, representing an underestimation of 28%. Thus, option B is correct. In some studies, both MDRD study equation and Cockcroft-Gault equation yielded similar slopes of decline in kidney function. The 24-h urine creatinine clearance is not a good indicator of GFR in CKD patients, as it overestimates GFR because of high rates of creatinine secretion by the proximal tubule in CKD patients.

Suggested Reading

Rule AD, Larson TS, Bergstralh EJ, et al. Using serum creatinine to estimate glomerular filtration rate: accuracy in good health and in chronic kidney disease. Ann Intern Med. 2004;141:929–37.
Xie D, Joffe MM, Brunelli SM, et al. A comparison of change in measured and estimated glomerular filtration rate in patients with nondiabetic kidney disease. Clin J Am Soc Nephrol. 2008;3:1332–8.

14. Since serum creatinine is influenced by muscle mass, diet, and other variables, it is believed that its measurement only or 24-h creatinine clearance may be incorrect in following the progression of kidney disease. Therefore, creatinine or cystatin C-based equations have been used to monitor GFR changes longitudinally over time in clinical and research practice. **Which one of the following statements is INCORRECT regarding these equations and progression of kidney disease in CKD patients from several studies?**

A. MDRD study equation (either 6 variable or 4 variable) underestimated eGFR compared to measured GFR in one Australian-New Zealand study
B. Cockcroft-Gault (CG) equation, either corrected or uncorrected for body surface area, overestimated GFR compared to measured GFR in the above study

C. Either hemoglobin (Hgb) or PTH levels are found to have no association with eGFR in the above study
D. In the AASK (African American Study of Kidney Disease), the outcomes between the eGFR-based equation by the MDRD study formula and the measured GFR by iothalamate clearance were similar over a period of 4-year follow-up
E. Serial measurements of serum cystatin C in type 2 diabetic patients accurately detect trends in kidney function over a period of 4-year follow-up

The answer is C

Serum creatinine or cystatin C-based equations are extremely important in assessing the decline in kidney function over a period of follow-up in CKD patients. This follow-up is important in making treatment decisions. Lee et al. conducted a multicenter trial in Australia and New Zealand and compared the slopes of decline in kidney function in 155 patients with CKD stages 3–5 using radionuclide-measured GFR and eGFR calculated from four equations (4- and 6-variable MDRD study equations and C-G equation with or without correction for body surface area) at baseline, 12 and 24 months. The data showed that the two MDRD equations initially underestimated GFR and the two C-G equations overestimated GFR. The MDRD study equations showed a sustained advantage in estimating kidney function longitudinally than the C-G equations.

Interestingly, an increase in Hgb concentration was associated with a modest but statistically significant overestimation of eGFR. On the other hand, an increase in the PTH level was associated with a small underestimation of GFR. The clinical significance of these observations is unclear. Thus, option C is incorrect.

In the AASK Study, the agreement of the eGFR-based outcomes with iothalamate clearance-based outcomes was similar when the MDRD study equation was used instead of the AASK equation.

Perkins et al. followed 30 type 2 diabetic patients with GFR >20 mL/min/1.73 m^2, and their GFR was measured by iothalamate clearance and serum cystatin C levels at baseline and yearly for 4 years. Both measures were concordant and had similar slopes (or annual percentage changes) in 20 patients who showed a decline in kidney function. In contrast, creatinine-based equations had poor correlations in slopes compared to iothalamate clearances. Thus, the authors concluded that serial determinations of serum cystatin levels, plotted as 1/cystatin C x 100, can detect accurately the level of decline in kidney function during follow-up of type 2 diabetic patients.

Suggested Reading

Lee D, Levin A, Roger LP, et al. Longitudinal analysis of performance of estimated glomerular filtration rate as renal function declines in chronic kidney disease. Nephrol Dial Transplant. 2009;24:109–16.
Perkins BA, Nelson RG, Ostrander BEP, et al. Detection of renal function decline in patients with diabetes and normal or elevated GFR by serial measurements of serum cystatin C concentration: results of a 4-year follow-up study. J Am Soc Nephrol. 2005;16:1404–12.
Wang X, Lewis J, Appel L, et al. Validation of creatinine-based estimates of GFR when evaluating risk factors in longitudinal studies of kidney disease. J Am Soc Nephrol. 2006;17:2900–9.

15. **Regarding late referral of CKD patients to nephrologists by primary care physicians or general practitioners, which one of the following patient and health system characteristics is INCORRECT?**

A. Old age
B. All ethnic groups, including Caucasians
C. Lack of insurance
D. Socioeconomic status
E. Level of education

The answer is B

Late referral is usually considered an appointment with a nephrologist <4 months of starting a renal replacement therapy. A number of studies have evaluated the pros and cons of late referral. There are several barriers that cause late referral, including old age, comorbidities, race other than Caucasians, lack of insurance, poverty, and lower level of education. Thus, option B is incorrect.

Additional factors have also been implicated in late referral. Lack of primary care physician's knowledge about appropriate time of referral, lack of communication between the referring physician and nephrologist, patients with nondiabetic kidney disease also accounted for late referrals. In one study, patient's age (>70 years), limited life expectancy, and patient refusal to go on dialysis influenced primary care physician referral. Special

attention should be paid for African Americans with a family history of ESKD because these individuals may be predisposed to have low GFRs than those without a family history of ESKD. These individuals require early rather than late referral.

Thus, patient-, healthcare system-, and physician-related factors were found to be potential barriers for early referral.

Suggested Reading

Black C, Sharma P, Scotland G, et al. Early referral strategies for management of people with markers of renal disease: a systematic review of the evidence of clinical effectiveness, cost-effectiveness and economic analysis. Health Technol Assess. 2010;14(21):1–184.

Kidney Disease Improving Global Outcomes. KIDIGO 2012 clinical practice guideline for the evaluation and management of chronic kidney disease. Kidney Int Suppl. 2013;3:1–150.

Navaneethan SD, Aloudat S, Singh S. A systematic review of patient and health system characteristics with late referral in chronic kidney disease. BMC Nephrol. 2008;9:3.

Navaneethan SD, Kandula P, Jeevanatham V, et al. Referral patterns of primary care physicians for chronic kidney disease in general population and geriatric patients. Clin Nephrol. 2010;73:260–7.

Navaneethan SD, Nigwekar S, Sengodan M, et al. Referral to nephrologists for chronic kidney disease care: is non-diabetic kidney disease ignored? Nephron Clin Pract. 2007;106:c113–8.

16. As an internist, you are following a 50-year-old man with hypertension for 10 years. Currently, the patient has stage 4 (GFR 15–29 mL/min) CKD. **You refer this patient to a nephrologist for consultation and co-management because of which one of the following reasons?**

A. To make a clinical action plan
B. To carry out the prescribed evaluation
C. To follow the recommended treatment plan
D. To avoid malpractice
E. A, B, and C

The answer is E

The K/DOQI Clinical Practice Guidelines for CKD suggest that "People with CKD should be referred to a specialist for consultation and co-management if the clinical action plan cannot be prepared, the prescribed evaluation of the patient cannot be carried out or the recommended treatment cannot be carried out. In general people with GFR <30 mL/min/1.73 m^2 should be referred to a nephrologist." The clinical action plan for stage 4 CKD is to prepare for kidney replacement therapy. This defines early referral.

Suggested Reading

National Kidney Foundation. K/DOQI clinical practice guidelines for chronic kidney disease: evaluation, classification and stratification. Am J Kidney Dis. 2002;39(Suppl 1):S1–266.

National Kidney Foundation. Chronic kidney disease. A guide to select NKF/KDOQI guidelines and recommendations (in association with Nephrology Pharmacy Associates). New York: National Kidney Foundation; 2006. p. 1–115.

17. A 20-year-old college student with a family history of adult polycystic kidney disease and her mother on hemodialysis seeks your advice and follow-up by you. Based on her family history, you consider her to be at increased risk for CKD. **Which one of the following appears to be the BEST protocols for this individual?**

A. Perform a good physical examination and obtain appropriate serum chemistry
B. Obtain an eGFR and assess her comorbid conditions
C. Test for markers of kidney damage
D. Advise to undergo repeat periodic evaluation and follow a program of risk factor reduction
E. All of the above

The answer is E

The Kidney Disease Outcome Quality Initiative (KDOQI) of the National Kidney Foundation recommends that individuals without kidney damage and with normal or elevated GFR, who are at increased risk for development of CKD should have: (1) routine heath examination; (2) estimation of their kidney function (eGFR); (3) testing

for markers of kidney damage; (4) periodic examination; and (5) follow-up in a program of risk factor reduction, if appropriate, as in the above case. Thus, option E is correct.

Suggested Reading

National Kidney Foundation. K/DOQI clinical practice guidelines for chronic kidney disease: evaluation, classification and stratification. Am J Kidney Dis. 2002;39(Suppl 1):S1–266.

National Kidney Foundation. Chronic kidney disease. A guide to select NKF/KDOQI guidelines and recommendations (in association with Nephrology Pharmacy Associates). New York: National Kidney Foundation; 2006. p. 1–115.

18. **Based on the history, blood pressure (BP), eGFR, and albuminuria, which one of the following patients requires referral to a nephrologist?**

History	BP (mm Hg)	eGFR (mL/min)	Albuminuria (mg/g creatinine)
A. A 50-year-old man with hypertension (HTN) and noncompliant with antihypertensive medications	152/98 Pulse rate 74 beats/min	22	262
B. A 40-year-old woman with diabetes and HTN	150/86 Pulse rate 68 beats/min	48	310
C. A 40-year-old man with diabetes and HTN	160/82 Pulse rate 64 beats/min	69	420
D. A 40-year-old woman with diabetes and HTN	136/80 Pulse rate 72 beats/min	50	24
E. A, B, and C			

The answer is E

The patient described in A seems to have a long-standing poorly controlled HTN with noncompliance to antihypertensive medications. Based on eGFR and albuminuria, the patient has CKD 4 and moderately increased albuminuria (category A2). He needs follow-up by a nephrologist because of severe renal dysfunction.

Patient B has CKD 3a and severely increased albuminuria (A3 category) and should be referred to a nephrologist for management of both kidney function and albuminuria. Patient C has CKD 2 but has severely increased albuminuria (A3 category) and needs to be referred to a nephrologist. The patient described in D has CKD 3a and normal to very mildly elevated albuminuria. Her CKD is a normal observation and does not need any referral to a nephrologist. Thus, answer E is correct.

Suggested Reading

Kidney Disease Improving Global Outcomes. KIDIGO 2012 clinical practice guideline for the evaluation and management of chronic kidney disease. Kidney Int Suppl. 2013;3:1–150.

19. A 56-year-old educated woman with type 2 diabetes and hypertension is referred to for follow-up of her kidney function. Her blood pressure is 134/80 mm Hg with a pulse rate of 64 beats/min. Pertinent labs: hemoglobin A1c is 7.1%, eGFR 50 mL/min (CKD 3a) and proteinuria 0.2 g/g creatinine. She is aware of the status of her kidney function. She asks you how many years approximately she can maintain the same eGFR or stay in CKD 3a. **Which one of the following answers is CORRECT?**

A. 5 years
B. 6 years
C. 7 years
D. 8 years
E. 9 years

The answer is D

One of the objectives of CKD management is to prevent the progression of kidney disease and delay the onset of end-stage kidney disease. Most studies evaluated progression of CKD either in the form of decline in eGFR or percentage loss of kidney function per year. In contrast, the study of Ku et al. provides estimates of the time spent in each stage from CKD 3a to CKD 5. These estimates were obtained from data from the Chronic Renal Insufficiency Cohort of 3682 adults with various stages of CKD followed for a median of 9.5 years. The amount

of time spent in each CKD stage was calculated in the presence or absence of individual risk factors of interest. The results of the study are shown in Table 4.6. When the effect of known risk factors such as diabetes with Hgb A1c ≥7.5%, systolic blood pressure ≥144 mm Hg, and proteinuria >1 g/g were evaluated, much less time was spent in each stage from CKD 3a to CKD 5, as compared with patients whose HgbA1c <7.5%, systolic blood pressure <144 mm Hg, and proteinuria <1 g/g. Based on this study, the correct answer is D.

Table 4.6 Median time (years with IQR) spent in each stage of CKD

Group	CKD 3a	CKD 3b	CKD 4	CKD 5
Whole group	7.9 (IQR 2.3->12)	5 (IQR 1.8–11.5)	4.2 (IQR 2.4–6.6)	0.8 (IQR 0.3–1.6)
Uncontrolled diabetes (years less in CKD stages)	1.8	1.4	–	0.1
Systolic BP ≥140 mm Hg (years less in CKD stages)	6.1	3.3	–	0.2
Proteinuria >1 g/g creatinine (years less in CKD stages)	8	5.6	–	0.6

IQR interquartile range

Suggested Reading

Ku E, Johansen KL, McCulloch CE. Time-centered approach to understanding risk factors for the progression of CKD. Clin J Am Soc Nephrol. 2018;13:693–701.

20. A 40-year-old African American woman is being followed by an internist for management of hypertension (HTN) for 10 years. Her eGFR is 28 mL/min. She has a good medical insurance. Despite a 4-drug regimen (Amlodipine 10 mg, hydrochlorothiazide (HCTZ) 50 mg, Bidil (combination of hydralazine and nitrate) 1 tablet twice daily, and Metoprolol 50 mg twice daily), her BP is >140/90 mm Hg. **Referral of this patient to a nephrologist may improve which one of the following conditions?**

A. Management of her HTN with appropriate antihypertensive agents
B. Cardiovascular risk factors and other comorbidities
C. Delay the need for urgent dialysis
D. Hospital stay and hospital cost
E. All of the above

The answer is E

One of the important aims of referral of CKD patients with 3–4 stages to a nephrologist is to implement interventions to slow the progression toward the initiation of renal replacement therapy. Studies have shown that early referral of CKD 3-4 patients to a nephrologist can have marked impact on all of the following patient outcomes:

1. **All the conditions stated in A to D**
2. **Delay the need for all forms of dialysis**
3. **Creation of an early A-V access**
4. **Improve patient survival**
5. **Better management of metabolic parameters at initiation of dialysis**

The impact of early referral on BP control was evaluated by only a few studies. These studies showed that a higher portion of patients in the nephrology care group had good BP control than the patients in the non-nephrology group.

This patient's BP should be <140/90 mm Hg or 130/80 mm Hg, if proteinuria is present) to prevent progression of her renal dysfunction. This will delay not only the initiation of renal replacement therapy but also maintain near normal quality of life. HCTZ has decreased BP-lowering effect in patients with GFR <30 mL/min.

Suggested Reading

Black C, Sharma P, Scotland G, et al. Early referral strategies for management of people with markers of renal disease: a systematic review of the evidence of clinical effectiveness, cost-effectiveness and economic analysis. Health Technol Assess. 2010;14(21):1–184.

Kidney Disease Improving Global Outcomes. KIDIGO 2012 clinical practice guideline for the evaluation and management of chronic kidney disease. Kidney Int Suppl. 2013;3:1–150.

Navaneethan SD, Kandula P, Jeevanatham V, et al. Referral patterns of primary care physicians for chronic kidney disease in general population and geriatric patients. Clin Nephrol. 2010;73:260–7.

21. A 30-year-old male student is seen for hematuria. Renal ultrasound shows multiple cysts. His BP is normal. He has no insurance. He is being followed by a primary care physician (PCP) who charges a small fee for each visit. The patient refused to see a nephrologist and says that he will see a specialist in a few years when he affords medical insurance. **Which one of the following statements is INCORRECT regarding referral of patients to a nephrologist?**

    A. Early referral had better renal outcomes than late referral
    B. Hospital physicians (other than nephrologists) referred patients with CKD later to nephrologists than general practitioners (GPs)
    C. Nondiabetics with CKD had earlier referral than diabetics with CKD
    D. Patients with congenital kidney disease were referred earlier than patients with HTN
    E. Patients with rapidly progressive renal disease were referred earlier than patients with gradual decline in kidney function

    The answer is C

    Mortality at 1 year was much higher in CKD patients who were referred late compared to those who were referred earlier. Also, long-term follow-up confirmed higher mortality in the late referral group.

    Several studies reported that hospital physicians (not nephrologists) rather than GPs were more likely to refer CKD patients later to nephrologists.

    Navaneethan et al. reported that patients with nondiabetic kidney disease were 1.4 times more likely to be referred later rather than earlier to nephrologists than patients with diabetic kidney disease. Thus, option C is incorrect.

    In contrast, patients with congenital kidney disease and rapidly progressive renal disease were referred earlier to nephrologists than patients with HTN and patients with gradual decline in kidney function, respectively.

    Suggested Reading

Black C, Sharma P, Scotland G, et al. Early referral strategies for management of people with markers of renal disease: a systematic review of the evidence of clinical effectiveness, cost-effectiveness and economic analysis. Health Technol Assess. 2010;14(21):1–184.

Heatley SA. Optimal referral is early referral. Perit Dial Int. 2009;29:S128–31.

Navaneethan SD, Kandula P, Jeevanatham V, et al. Referral patterns of primary care physicians for chronic kidney disease in general population and geriatric patients. Clin Nephrol. 2010;73:260–7.

22. Late referral of CKD 4 patients to a nephrologist has several adverse effects on renal outcomes. **Which one of the following consequences is FALSE regarding late referral?**

    A. Low prevalence of permanent dialysis access
    B. Anemia and left ventricular hypertrophy (LVH)
    C. Poor survival after initiation of dialysis
    D. Early and late referral have the same impact on cardiovascular morbidity and mortality in hemodialysis patients
    E. Delayed referral for kidney transplantation

    The answer is D

    Referral is usually considered late when a patient is seen by a nephrologist <4 months before the commencement of dialysis. The consequences of late referral are many, including the delay in creation of an A-V access for hemodialysis, anemia and low hematocrit, LVH, poor survival due to cardiovascular disease on dialysis, higher hospital stay and costs, and late referral to kidney transplantation. Thus, option D is false. However, the cost-effectiveness of early vs late referral is unclear.

    Suggested Reading

Black C, Sharma P, Scotland G, et al. Early referral strategies for management of people with markers of renal disease: a systematic review of the evidence of clinical effectiveness, cost-effectiveness and economic analysis. Health Technol Assess. 2010;14(21):1–184.

Heatley SA. Optimal referral is early referral. Perit Dial Int. 2009;29:S128–31.

Kidney Disease Improving Global Outcomes. KIDIGO 2012 clinical practice guideline for the evaluation and management of chronic kidney disease. Kidney Int Suppl. 2013;3:1–150.

Navaneethan SD, Kandula P, Jeevanatham V, et al. Referral patterns of primary care physicians for chronic kidney disease in general population and geriatric patients. Clin Nephrol. 2010;73:260–7.

23. You are consulted to see a 24-year-old pregnant African American woman at 18 weeks of gestation for proteinuria of 1.2 g/day. She has a history of hypertension. Her BP is 112/74 mm Hg. She was told that she may have a low birth weight baby (<2500 g). She says that she wants to know about complications of low birth weight. **Which one of the following statements is INCORRECT regarding low birth weight and kidney disease?**

A. Low birth weight is associated with low nephron number and increased glomerular volume
B. There is a good association between low birth weight and development of HTN later in life
C. Low birth weight is associated with albuminuria and kidney disease later in life
D. Low birth weight is associated with increasing risk for development of ESKD in the first 14 years of life compared to the risk at older age
E. Men and women with low birth weights equally develop albuminuria and low GFR

The answer is E

The fetus in utero, when exposed to an environmental insult, is predisposed to several adult chronic diseases such as diabetes, HTN, cardiovascular diseases, and kidney failure. This phenomenon of fetal programming is seen both in animals and humans. Predisposition to HTN and kidney damage is largely related to low birth weight. Both animal and human studies have shown that low birth weight is associated with smaller kidney size, low nephron number, and increased glomerular volume. HTN may be related to increased glomerular hyperfiltration and a defect in Na^+ excretion. The net result is glomerular structural damage and sclerosis, further elevation of BP, albuminuria, and renal failure.

An interesting study from Norway showed that low birth weight for gestational age was associated with a risk for development of ESKD. This risk was greatest in the first 14 years of life with less of a risk at older ages. This observation needs confirmation in other ethnic groups.

Li et al. provided evidence that individuals with low birth weight were more likely to be African American or females, but the incidence of albuminuria or low GFR (<60 mL/min) was higher in Caucasian men only. It is of interest to note that there was no association between low birth weight and subsequent kidney disease in women. Thus, option E is incorrect.

Suggested Reading

Li S, Chen SC, Shlipak M, et al. Low birth weight is associated with chronic kidney disease only in men. Kidney Int. 2008;73:637–42.
Luyckx VA, Moritz KM, Bertram JF. Developmental programming of blood pressure and renal function through the life course. In: Yu ASL, Chertow GM, Luyckx VA, et al., editors. Brenner & Rector's the kidney. 11th ed. Philadelphia: Elsevier, Saunders; 2020. p. 667–709.
Vikse BE, Irgens LM, Leivestad T, et al. Low birth weight increases risk for end-stage renal disease. J Am Soc Nephrol. 2008;19:151–7.

24. **Environmental insult to the fetus in utero seems to signal the fetal programming. Which one of the following factors is NOT associated with reduced nephron number?**

A. Poor maternal protein intake
B. Fetal exposure to glucocorticoids
C. Fetal exposure to hyperglycemia
D. Low socioeconomic status
E. All of the above

The answer is E

Low birth weight, and therefore, reduced nephron number is associated with poor maternal nutrition, fetal exposure to high levels of glucocorticoids or glucose, maternal socioeconomic status, smoking, alcohol ingestion, and infection as well as exposure to certain antibiotics. Thus, answer E is correct.

Experimental studies have shown that maternal protein restriction causes low birth weight as well as reduced kidney mass and nephron number. An associated observation is the development of HTN at 8 weeks of pups born to low protein-fed mothers during pregnancy. One of the proposed mechanisms is increased apoptosis in metanephrons and postnatal kidney.

Generally, the fetus is protected from high glucocorticoid exposure because of the placental 11β-hydroxysteroid dehydrogenase type 2 (11 β-HSD2), which converts the active cortisol into inactive cortisone. When fetus is exposed to an environmental insult such as low protein intake, the activity of placental 11 β-HSD2 activity is decreased. This causes increased steroid activity at the kidney level with resultant Na^+ reabsorption and HTN. However, the mechanism for reduced number of nephrons is unclear.

It is well known that maternal hyperglycemia during pregnancy causes several congenital abnormalities, including large for-date-babies. However, the number of nephrons is reduced, which is due to altered insulin-like growth factor-II activity.

Other factors that may cause low nephron number include exposure of fetus to low vitamin A, gentamicin, certain β-lactams, and cyclosporine.

Suggested Reading

Hoy WE, Hughson MD, Bertram JF, et al. Nephron number, hypertension, renal disease, and renal failure. J Am Soc Nephrol. 2005;16:2557–64.

Luyckx VA, Moritz KM, Bertram JF. Developmental programming of blood pressure and renal function through the life course. In: Yu ASL, Chertow GM, Luyckx VA, et al., editors. Brenner & Rector's the kidney. 11th ed. Philadelphia: Elsevier, Saunders; 2020. p. 667–709.

25. A 40-year-old menstruating woman with membranous nephropathy is referred to you for further management of her proteinuria. She tells you that one of her male cousins has the same kidney disease with rapid progression to ESKD. **Regarding gender differences in CKD, which one of the following statements is INCORRECT?**

A. Men with membranous nephropathy, polycystic kidney disease, and IgA nephropathy progress at a faster rate to ESKD than women
B. Estrogens are more protective of renal disease than testosterone in patients with lupus nephritis
C. Women have few glomeruli than men
D. Filtration traction is increased in response to angiotensin II infusion in young healthy men than women
E. Proteinuric type 1 diabetic males have a poor renal prognosis than proteinuric type 1 diabetic females

The answer is B

Gender influences the rate of renal disease progression. In a meta-analysis, it was found that renal disease in women with polycystic kidney disease, membranous nephropathy, and IgA nephropathy progresses at a much slower rate than men with similar disease states. The MDRD study also reported slower rate of decline in kidney function in women than in men. The prevalence of ESKD between the years 2000 and 2005 increased by 14% in men as compared to approximately 10% in women.

In contrast, the prevalence of lupus nephritis is slightly higher in women than in men. Androgens are immunosuppressive, whereas estrogens stimulate immune responsiveness. Accordingly, androgens are protective, and estrogens exacerbate disease activity. Thus, option B is incorrect.

Studies from autopsy findings showed that women have 10–15% fewer glomeruli than men possibly because of smaller body surface area.

The GFR may be similar in both men and women when corrected for body surface area. However, infusion of angiotensin II to healthy young men increased filtration fraction (FF) but women showed no change in their FF, suggesting increased glomerular capillary pressure in men. This increase in glomerular pressure may account for rapid progression of glomerular disease in men.

It was reported that proteinuric type 1 diabetic males have poorer renal prognosis than females. The DCCT/EDIC trial also showed that male gender was associated with higher urinary albumin excretion. Thus, men are at higher risk for progression than women.

Suggested Reading

Iseki K. Gender differences in chronic kidney disease. Kidney Int. 2008;74:415–7.

Neugarten J, Silbiger SR, Golestaneh L. Gender and kidney disease. In: Brenner BM, editor. Brenner and Rector's the kidney. 8th ed. Philadelphia: Saunders; 2008. p. 674–80.

Silbiger S, Neugarten J. Gender and human chronic renal disease. Gender Med. 2008;5(Suppl A):S3–10.

26. **The rate of progression of kidney disease is lower in premenopausal women than in postmenopausal women. Which one of the following effects of estrogen on mesangial cells in INCORRECT?**

A. It inhibits type IV collagen synthesis
B. It inhibits oxidation of LDL
C. It inhibits nitric oxide production
D. It inhibits TGF-β-induced apoptosis
E. It increases collagenase activity

The answer is C

Estrogens have several beneficial effects on mesangial cells. In vitro studies have shown that estrogens decrease type IV collagen synthesis by increasing collagenase activity, inhibit LDL oxidation, and reverse TGF-β-induced apoptosis. Also, estrogens inhibit mesangial cell proliferation.

Estrogens increase nitric oxide synthesis, PGE_2, and prostacyclin levels. Female rats have higher levels of nitric oxide than male rats, and ovariectomy abolishes these levels. Thus, option C is incorrect.

Suggested Reading

Neugarten J, Reckelhoff LF. Gender issues in chronic kidney disease. In: Kimmel PL, Rosenberg ME, editors. Chronic renal disease. 2nd ed. London: Academic Press, Elsevier; 2020. p. 91–107.
Neugarten J, Silbiger SR, Golestaneh L. Gender and kidney disease. In: Brenner BM, editor. Brenner and Rector's the kidney. 8th ed. Philadelphia: Saunders; 2008. p. 674–80.
Silbiger S, Neugarten J. Gender and human chronic renal disease. Gender Med. 2008;5(Suppl A):S3–10.

27. **Sex hormones play an important role in the development of HTN, which is a major risk factor for CKD. Of the following statements, which one is FALSE regarding sex hormones?**

A. Estrogens decrease renin, angiotensin-converting enzyme (ACE), and angiotensin II (AII) expression and levels
B. Estrogens decrease AT_1 receptors and increase AT_2 receptors
C. Estrogens stimulate ATP-sensitive potassium (K_{ATP}) channels via attenuation of Ca influx into vascular smooth muscle (VSM) cells of the endothelium
D. Estrogens increase renal Na^+ excretion and protect against salt-induced HTN
E. Testosterone decreases proximal tubular Na^+ reabsorption and renin activity

The answer is E

Estrogens cause vasodilation and lower BP. Several mechanisms are involved. First, estrogens downregulate the expression of renin, ACE, and AII and their levels. Second, estrogens upregulate the expression of angiotensinogen and AT_2 receptor density. Third, estrogens activate K_{ATP} channels, causing efflux of K^+ from VSM cells. As a result, these VSM cells become hyperpolarized, and entry of Ca^{2+} into these cells is inhibited. Also, estrogens may promote Ca^{2+} efflux or inhibit Ca^{2+} release from sarcoplasmic reticulum. Finally, estrogens have been shown to promote Na^{2+} excretion by the kidney and thus attenuate Na-dependent HTN. In contrast, testosterone increases renal Na^+ reabsorption with resultant HTN. Thus, option E is false.

Suggested Reading

Neugarten J, Reckelhoff LF. Gender issues in chronic kidney disease. In: Kimmel PL, Rosenberg ME, editors. Chronic renal disease. 2nd ed. London: Academic Press, Elsevier; 2020. p. 91–107.
Neugarten J, Silbiger SR, Golestaneh L. Gender and kidney disease. In: Brenner BM, editor. Brenner and Rector's the kidney. 8th ed. Philadelphia: Saunders; 2008. p. 674–80.
Silbiger S, Neugarten J. Gender and human chronic renal disease. Gender Med. 2008;5(Suppl A):S3–10.

28. **Both animal and human studies showed that uric acid is a risk factor for development of HTN and progression of CKD. Among the following mechanisms, which mechanism is LEAST implicated in the pathogenesis of HTN and CKD?**

A. Endothelial dysfunction and low NO production
B. Vascular smooth muscle (VSM) cell proliferation due to activation of mitogen-activated protein (MAP) kinases and nuclear transcription factors

C. Increased intrarenal renin expression and production
D. Increased renal plasma flow
E. Increased glomerular capillary pressure

The answer is D

In a rat model, it was demonstrated that serum uric acid levels that were 1.5 to threefold greater than normal levels induced HTN with afferent arteriolar thickening, glomerular hypertrophy, proteinuria, glomerulosclerosis (GS), and interstitial fibrosis. These lesions were similar to those with age-related GS and gouty nephropathy. However, the deposition of urate crystals as seen in gouty nephropathy was absent in the rat model of hyperuricemia.

The mechanisms causing HTN and renal lesions by uric acid include endothelial dysfunction with low NO production, stimulation of VSM cell proliferation via activation of MAP kinases, nuclear transcription factors (NF-kB and AP-1), and induction of inflammatory mediators.

Other mechanisms were found to be an increase in intrarenal renin expression and glomerular capillary pressure. Because of afferent arteriolar thickening, the renal plasma flow was found to be decreased rather than increased. Thus, option D is incorrect.

Suggested Reading

Feig DI. Uric acid: a novel mediator and marker of risk in chronic kidney disease? Curr Opin Nephrol Hypertens. 2009;18:526–30.

Giodano C, Karasik O, King-Morris K, et al. Uric acid as a marker of kidney disease: review of the current literature. Dis Markers. 2015;2015:382918, 6 pages.

Kang D-H, Johnson RJ. Uric acid metabolism and the kidney. In: Kimmel PL, Rosenberg ME, editors. Chronic renal disease. 2nd ed. London: Academic Press, Elsevier; 2020. p. 689–701.

Tangri N, Weiner DE. Uric acid, CKD, and cardiovascular disease: confounders, culprits, and circles. Am J Kidney Dis. 2010;56:247–50.

29. A 25-year-old African American female student with HTN and CKD (eGFR 58 mL/min) seeks your advice for further management of her HTN. Her last menstruation is 1 week ago. She is on losartan 100 mg/day. Her BP is 130/80 mm Hg. Her serum uric acid is 5.2 mg/dL. She read about allopurinol in the treatment of HTN and CKD. **Which one of the following suggestions is APPROPRIATE?**

A. Adding allopurinol 100 mg four times a day will slow progression of her kidney disease
B. Adding allopurinol 300 mg daily is sufficient at this time
C. Adverse effects of allopurinol are minimal and benefit of the drug outweighs the adverse effects
D. Advise her to take aspirin 325 mg daily to improve cardiovascular risk
E. Tell her that clinical trials on CKD progression and allopurinol are not conclusive

The answer is E

Although hyperuricemia is a modifiable risk factor for CKD and also cardiovascular disease (CVD), sufficient data from clinical trials using allopurinol are not available at the present time. The following three studies showed a beneficial effect of allopurinol on HTN and CKD progression.

Siu et al. reported on the effect of allopurinol on progression of CKD in 51 patients with hyperuricemia. Allopurinol (100 to 300 mg/day) was given to 25 patients with a mean serum creatinine of 1.64 mg/dL. The other group of 26 patients with serum creatinine levels of 1.86 mg/dL served as controls. At 12 months, serum uric acid dropped from 9.75 to 5.88 mg/dL. There was no difference in BP between the two groups. However, 4 of 25 (16%) in the allopurinol group and 12 of 26 (46%) in the control group had deterioration in their kidney function and dialysis dependency. Thus, allopurinol slowed the progression of CKD without improvement in BP.

In a study of Talaat and El-sheikh, 50 patients with CKD stages 3–4 (serum creatinine 3.35–3.41 mg/dL) had treatment with allopurinol (100–400 mg/day) for hyperuricemia (uric acid 9.5–9.8 mg/dL). The patients were divided into three groups. The first and second groups were on ACE-I and ARB, respectively. The third group was on antihypertensives other than ACE-I or ARB. In all groups, BP, serum creatinine, and uric acid were followed

for 12 months after withdrawal of allopurinol. In the third group, all of the above three parameters worsened. Also, in this group, the urinary excretion of TGF-β levels was increased. The authors concluded that treatment of asymptomatic hyperuricemia by allopurinol is beneficial only in patients on renin-angiotensin inhibitors.

Feig et al. reported that allopurinol (200 mg twice daily) reduced both systolic and diastolic BP by 6.9 mm Hg and 5.1 mm Hg in newly diagnosed adolescents with essential HTN as compared with a decrease of 2.0 mm Hg in systolic BP and 2.4 mm Hg in diastolic BP in the placebo group in 4 weeks. The mean serum uric acid levels prior to randomization were 6.90 mg/dL (range 6.5–7.4 mg/dL). Thus, allopurinol has a beneficial effect on BP.

Goicoechea et al. studied prospectively the effect of allopurinol (100 mg/day) in CKD patients with eGFR <60 mL/min for 2 years. At the end of the study, serum uric acid and CRP levels were significantly lower in allopurinol-treated than untreated patients. Also, GFR increased by 1.3 mL/min in the treated group compared to a decline of 3.3 mL/min in untreated group. Allopurinol treatment significantly reduced the cardiovascular events in 71% of the patients. Thus, allopurinol reduced the progression of kidney disease in CKD patients.

However, the study of Chonchol et al. did not suggest that uric acid is a major determinant of developing CKD or risk for CKD progression. Therefore, it is better for the patient to wait until other randomized studies are available that show the benefit of allopurinol on HTN and CKD progression.

Two meta-analyses were published on the relationship of allopurinol and CKD. The first one analyzed eight studies, of which five studies did not show any benefit of allopurinol on CKD. The other three studies reported a benefit of slowing the progression of CKD. The second meta-analysis included 18 randomized clinical trials (992 patients) with CKD 3-5 stages and reported a reduction in uric acid and blood pressure with preservation of GFR compared to control group. Thus, the beneficial effect of allopurinol on CKD progression is not uniform. Therefore, option E is correct.

A large number of adverse effects of allopurinol in CKD patients have been described. Dosage adjustment is necessary in patients with CKD to avoid adverse effects. Low dose aspirin is indicated in CKD patients without hyperuricemia. However, low dose aspirin increases serum uric acid levels, and its use should be carefully evaluated in a patient with hyperuricemia, as in the present case. It is of interest to note that African American race is associated with hyperuricemia. Therefore, options A–D are incorrect.

Suggested Reading

Bose B, Badve SV, Hiremath SS, et al. Effects of uric acid-lowering therapy on renal outcomes: a systematic review and meta-analysis. Nephrol Dial Transplant. 2014;29:406–23.

Chonchol M, Shlipak MG, Katz R, et al. Relationship of uric acid with progression of kidney disease. Am J Kidney Dis. 2007;50:239–47.

Feig DI, Soletsky B, Johnson RJ. Effect of allopurinol on blood pressure of adolescents with newly diagnosed essential hypertension. A randomized trial. JAMA. 2008;300:924–32.

Goicoechea M, Vinuesa SG, Verdalles U, et al. Effect of allopurinol in chronic kidney disease progression and cardiovascular risk. Clin J Am Soc Nephrol. 2010;5(8):1388–93.

Gois PH, Souza ER. Pharmacotherapy for hyperuricemia in hypertensive patients. Cochrane Database Syst Rev. 2013;31:1.

Kanji T, Gandhi M, Clase CM. Urate lowering therapy to improve renal outcomes in patients with chronic kidney disease: systematic review and meta-analysis. BMC Nephrol. 2015;16:58.

Siu Y-P, Leung K-T, Tang MK-H, et al. Use of allopurinol in slowing the progression of renal disease through its ability to lower serum uric acid level. Am J Kidney Dis. 2006;47:51–9.

Talaat KM, El-Sheikh AR. The effect of mild hyperuricemia on urinary transforming growth factor beta and the progression of chronic kidney disease. Am J Nephrol. 2007;27:435–40.

30. A 50-year-old man is referred to your CKD clinic for follow-up of his kidney disease due to hypertension. His eGFR is 50 mL/min, which is classified as CKD stage G3a (or CKD 3a). **Which one of the following laboratory tests you order to evaluate bone mineral disorder (BMD)?**

A. Calcium (Ca^{2+})
B. Phosphate
C. PTH
D. Alkaline phosphatase
E. All of the above

The answer is E

According to KDIGO CKD-MBD recommendations, all of the above laboratory tests need to be monitored beginning in CKD stage G3a. Thus, answer E is correct. Also, 25 $(OH)D_3$ levels should be measured. Frequent monitoring is required, if there are any abnormalities in any or all of the above laboratory tests. Therapeutic decisions are based on the trend rather than on a single laboratory value. Specifically, PTH and bone-specific alkaline phosphatase values are used to evaluate bone disease because high or low levels predict either high turnover or low turnover bone disease.

Suggested Reading

Kidney Disease: Improving Global Outcomes (KDIGO) CKD-MBD Update Work Group. KDIGO 2017 clinical practice guideline update for the diagnosis, evaluation, prevention, and treatment of chronic kidney disease–mineral and bone disorder (CKD-MBD). Kidney Int Suppl. 2017;7:1–59.

31. **Regarding monitoring recommendation of CKD-MBD biochemical abnormalities is concerned, which one of the following is FALSE?**

A. Calcium	CKD 3a-3b Every 6–12 months CKD 4 Every 3–6 months CKD 5-5D Every 1–3 months
B. Phosphate	CKD 3a-3b Every 6–12 months CKD 4 Every 3–6 months CKD 5-5D Every 1–3 months
C. PTH	CKD 3a-3b Base on baseline and CKD progression CKD 4 Every 6–12 months CKD 5-5D Every 3–6 months
D. Alkaline phosphatase	CKD 4-5D Every 12 months, or more frequently in the presence of elevated PTH
E. 25$(OH)D_3$ (calcidiol)	CKD 3a-5D Every month

The answer is E

The suggested monitoring schedule for calcium, phosphate, PTH, and alkaline phosphatase for various stages of CKD as recommended by the KDIGO-MBD guideline is presented in answers A–D. The guideline suggests that calcidiol should be measured at baseline in patients with CKD 3a-5D and if necessary for it should be repeated for therapeutic intervention. It is recommended to maintain calcidiol level >30 ng/mL in CKD patients. Thus, answer E is false.

Suggested Reading

Kidney Disease: Improving Global Outcomes (KDIGO) CKD-MBD Update Work Group. KDIGO 2017 Clinical Practice Guideline Update for the Diagnosis, Evaluation, Prevention, and Treatment of Chronic Kidney Disease–Mineral and Bone Disorder (CKD-MBD). Kidney Int Suppl 7:1-59, 2017.

32. A-55-year-old woman with CKD G3b is found to have serum phosphate level of 4.2 mg/dL. Since hyperphosphatemia is a risk factor for cardiovascular disease, the patient asks you whether she needs phosphate-binder to lower her phosphate level even further. **Which one of the following answers is APPROPRIATE for her question?**

A. She needs a small dose of Ca-containing binder (calcium acetate 667 mg with each meal)
B. She needs a small dose of nonCa-containing binder
C. She does need any phosphate binder at this time
D. She requires high intake of animal protein diet
E. None of the above

The answer is C

In nondialysis patients, serum phosphate levels should be maintained within normal limits. This can be achieved by two methods: (1) dietary restriction of phosphate, and (2) phosphate binders. Dietary restriction is very effective when properly executed; however, patients are usually noncompliant. Also, intestinal phosphate absorption

and its source are important aspects of dietary phosphate restriction. Inorganic phosphate (as found in food additives) is absorbed rapidly, as compared with less (40–60%) absorbed phosphate (derived from animal source) or phytate (derived from vegetables).

In a randomized controlled trial of patients with eGFR 20–45 mL/min and near normal serum phosphate levels (4.2 mg/dL), phosphate binders reduced phosphate levels to 3.9 mg/dL with no effect on FGF-23 levels. However, PTH levels remained stable compared to progression in placebo group. Patients on phosphate binders had increased vascular calcification compared to those on placebo. Phosphate binders are, thus, not indicated in CKD stages 3a-4 unless dietary restriction failed or serum phosphate level is >4.5 mg/dL. High intake of protein of animal origin delivers high phosphate. Thus, the patient does not require any phosphate binder or high protein intake at this time. Her phosphate level should be monitored closely and make a decision once its level is >4.5 mg/dL. Thus, answer C is correct.

Suggested Reading

Bacchetta J, Bernardor J, Garnier C, et al. Hyperphosphatemia and chronic kidney disease: a major daily concern both in adults and in children. Calcif Tissue Int. 2021;108(1):116–27. https://doi.org/10.1007/s00223-020-00665-8.

Block GA, Wheeler DC, Persky MS, et al. Effects of phosphate binders in moderate CKD. J Am Soc Nephrol. 2012;23:1407–15.

Kidney Disease: Improving Global Outcomes (KDIGO) CKD-MBD Update Work Group. KDIGO 2017 clinical practice guideline update for the diagnosis, evaluation, prevention, and treatment of chronic kidney disease–mineral and bone disorder (CKD-MBD). Kidney Int Suppl. 2017;7:1–59.

33. Hyperphosphatemia is not evident until the kidney disease progresses to CKD 4 or CKD 5 (eGFR <30 mL/min). **Which one of the following primary hormone actions is responsible for maintaining normal phosphate level in patients with CKD 3a to CKD 4?**

    A. FGF-23
    B. PTH
    C. Calcitriol
    D. A and B
    E. Insulin

    The answer is D

    Hyperphosphatemia is not clinically evident until eGFR <40 mL/min. This is related to increased phosphaturia caused by elevated levels of FGF-23 and PTH. Of these hormones, FGF-23 levels increase at much earlier stages of CKD than increase in PTH. Calcitriol promotes intestinal Ca^{2+} absorption, and its level decreases in CKD. Also, FGF-23 lowers calcitriol levels. Low calcitriol causes hypocalcemia, which stimulates the secretion of PTH, resulting in hyperparathyroidism. Thus, calcitriol has an indirect effect on phosphaturia. Insulin promotes uptake of phosphate into cells, and causes hypophosphatemia and hypophosphaturia. Thus, answer D is correct.

Suggested Reading

Cannata-Andia JB, Martin KJ. The challenge of controlling phosphorus in chronic kidney disease. Nephrol Dial Transplant. 2016;31:541–7.

Gutiérrez O, Isakova T, Rhee E, et al. Fibroblast growth factor-23 mitigates hyperphosphatemia but accentuates calcitriol deficiency in chronic kidney disease. J Am Soc Nephrol. 2005;16:2205–15.

Kidney Disease: Improving Global Outcomes (KDIGO) CKD-MBD Update Work Group. KDIGO 2017 clinical practice guideline update for the diagnosis, evaluation, prevention, and treatment of chronic kidney disease–mineral and bone disorder (CKD-MBD). Kidney Int Suppl. 2017;7:1–59.

34. High serum phosphate (PO_4) level is an independent risk factor for cardiovascular morbidity and mortality in CKD 4 and dialysis patients. **Which one of the following factors regarding hyperphosphatemia is FALSE?**

    A. Hyperphosphatemia stimulates PTH secretion independent of Ca levels
    B. Hyperphosphatemia may increase cell proliferation and growth of parathyroid through transforming growth factor-α (TGF-α)

C. Hyperphosphatemia reduces the expression of the calcium-sensing receptor (CaSR) and decreases the ability of the parathyroid gland to respond to changes in ionized calcium
D. Hyperphosphatemia indirectly increases PTH by inhibiting 1-α hydroxylase activity, thereby reducing the production of active vitamin D
E. Hyperphosphatemia alone is not sufficient to cause vascular calcification in the absence of hypercalcemia

The answer is E

Studies have shown that hyperphosphatemia can stimulate PTH secretion directly and indirectly. Regulation of PTH secretion by PO_4 alone was demonstrated in CKD animals with PO_4-restricted diet. In these studies, low PO_4 diet reduced PTH secretion independent of serum Ca^{2+} and $1,25(OH)_2D_3$ levels. These results were reproduced in CKD patients. It appears that the parathyroid gland responds to changes in serum PO_4 at the level of secretion, gene expression, and cell proliferation through phospholipase A_2-activated signal transduction mechanism. It was also shown that hyperphosphatemia may promote cell proliferation and growth of parathyroid via TGF-α and epidermal growth factor.

Hyperphosphatemia has also been shown to reduce the expression of CaSR, thereby decreasing the ability of the parathyroid gland to respond to changes in ionized Ca^{2+}. Restriction of PO_4 in diet restores the expression and sensitivity of the receptor.

Hyperphosphatemia stimulates PTH secretion indirectly by lowering Ca^{2+} via inhibition of 1-α hydroxylase in the kidney, thereby reducing the conversion of $25(OH)_3$ to $1,25(OH)_2D_3$. Also, several studies have shown that hyperphosphatemia alone can cause vascular calcification in CKD patients without the combination of hypercalcemia and vitamin D. Thus, option E is false.

Suggested Reading

Askar AM. Hyperphosphatemia. The hidden killer in chronic kidney disease. Saudi Med J. 2015;36:13–19.
Cozzolino M, Ciceri P, Galassi A. Hyperphosphatemia: a novel risk factor for mortality in chronic kidney disease. Ann Transl Med. 2019;7:55.
Giachelli CM. The emerging role of phosphate in vascular calcification. Kidney Int. 2009;75:890–7.
Kendrick J, Kestenbaum B, Chonchol M. Phosphate and cardiovascular disease. Adv Chronic Kid Dis. 2011;18:113–9.
McGovern AP, de Lusignan S, van Vlymen J, et al. Serum phosphate as a risk factor for cardiovascular events in people with and without chronic kidney disease: a large community based cohort study. PLoS One. 2013;8:e74996.
Silver J, Naveh-Many T. Phosphate and the parathyroid. Kidney Int. 2009;75:898–905.
Spasovski G, Massy Z, Vanholder R. Phosphate metabolism in chronic kidney disease: from pathophysiology to clinical management. Semin Nephrol. 2009;22:357–62.

35. A 45-year-old man with CKD 5 with eGFR 12 mL/min and not on dialysis is found to have serum phosphate level of 5.8 mg/dL. He wants you to suggest him the various methods to lower his phosphate to normal levels. **Which one of the following interventions is applicable to this patient?**

A. Dietary restriction of phosphate
B. Phosphate binders
C. Inhibition of intestinal phosphate
D. Dialysis, if the patient becomes uremic
E. All of the above

The answer is E

All of the above interventions lower serum phosphate level in patients with CKD 4-5D. Thus, answer E is correct.

Suggested Reading

Bacchetta J, Bernardor J, Garnier C, et al. Hyperphosphatemia and chronic kidney disease: a major daily concern both in adults and in children. Calcif Tissue Int. 2021;108(1):116–27. https://doi.org/10.1007/s00223-020-00665-8.
Barreto FC, Veit Barreto D, Massy ZA, et al. Strategies for phosphate control in patients with CKD. Kidney Int Rep. 2019;4:1043–56.
Cannata-Andia JB, Martin KJ. The challenge of controlling phosphorus in chronic kidney disease. Nephrol Dial Transplant. 2016;31:541–7.

Taketani Y, Koiwa F, Yokoyama K. Management of phosphorus load in CKD patients. Clin Exp Nephrol. 2017;21(suppl 1):s27–36.

Vervloet MG, van Ballegooijen AJ. Prevention and treatment of hyperphosphatemia in chronic kidney disease. Kidney Int. 2018;93:1060–72.

36. The 2017 KDIGO-MBD guideline suggests limiting phosphate in the diet alone or in combination with other treatments to control hyperphosphatemia in CKD 3a-5D. Your patient asks you to explain him the source of phosphate in the diet. **Which one of the following dietary sources is INCORRECT?**

A. Phosphate from animal-derived foods
B. Phosphate from vegetable-derived foods
C. Phosphate from food additives
D. Phosphate from medications
E. All of the above

The answer is E

Restriction of phosphate in the diet is not that easy to follow by the patient because a young to middle aged man consumes >1600 mg/day compared to similar aged woman who take in 1000 mg/day. The recommended phosphate intake in CKD patients is 800–1000 mg/day. Limiting phosphate also limits intake of other nutrients and protein. Therefore, a multiteam approach with extensive counseling is required to make the patient adhere to low phosphate diet.

Phosphorous in the diet is present as organic and inorganic phosphate. Organic phosphate derived from animal source is bound mostly to protein, whereas vegetable-derived phosphate is bound to phytic acid or phytate. The main sources of phosphate from animals are eggs, meat, fish, and dairy products. Cereals, nuts, and vegetable are some of nonanimal sources of phosphate combined with phytate. Organic phosphates need to be hydrolyzed before free phosphate is available for intestinal absorption.

It should be noted that all the phosphate is not absorbed, because absorption is based on the principle of bioavailability (i.e., a fraction of phosphate that is absorbed and delivered to circulation). For example, absorption is 40–60% for phosphate derived from animal origin compared to 20–50% absorption of phosphate derived from vegetable source. This suggests that bioavailability is the major determining factor in phosphate uptake from the diet, and consumption of vegetarian diet containing high protein may improve serum phosphate levels. Indeed, this has been shown to be the case from a small study of CKD 3b patients.

Several factors can modify bioavailability of phosphate. One such factor is boiling of food. Boiling sliced meat in soft water for 30 min reduced its phosphate content by 20–60% without any change in protein content.

Phosphate is present not only in raw food but also in processed foods. This is an added phosphate, which is in the inorganic form as sodium, potassium, and magnesium phosphate or phosphoric acid. The bioavailability of inorganic phosphate is much higher (90–100%) than organic phosphate in raw food.

Another source of unidentified phosphate is medications. Many antihypertensive medications are used to control blood pressure in both predialysis and dialysis patients. For example, amlodipine 10 mg has 7.9 mg to 165.6 mg of phosphorous depending on the manufacturer. Similarly, Lisinopril 40 mg has 26.2–30.8 mg of phosphorous.

Taken together, ingestion of phosphate from food additives and medications may amount to 40% of total phosphate intake. The total intake of phosphate is high, if the patient eats processed food in addition to the prescribed diet. This causes hyperphosphatemia despite strict dietary recommendations.

Phosphate intake is linked to protein intake. For example, high intake of animal-based protein is associated with high phosphate intake. Low phosphate diet with low protein intake may lead to protein energy wasting and possibly increased morbidity and mortality. To circumvent this, calculation of phosphate (mg) to protein (g) ratio was introduced. This ratio is useful in identifying which food supplies less phosphorous with the same amount of protein. A ratio of 12–16 mg/g was suggested to identify foods that are not associated with high mortality. Tables have been developed with phosphate to protein ratio in preparing proper menu for CKD patients. For example, egg white has a ratio of 1.4 compared to 22.8 for egg yolk. Egg yolk is a source of proteins with high biologic value and no cholesterol. However, this ratio does not take into account the exact intake of phosphate by the patient so that the daily intake of phosphate does not exceed 1000 mg/day. Thus, answer E is correct.

Suggested Reading

Bacchetta J, Bernardor J, Garnier C, et al. Hyperphosphatemia and chronic kidney disease: a major daily concern both in adults and in children. Calcif Tissue Int. 2021;108(1):116–27. https://doi.org/10.1007/s00223-020-00665-8.

Barreto FC, Veit Barreto D, Massy ZA, et al. Strategies for phosphate control in patients with CKD. Kidney Int Rep. 2019;4:1043–56.

Cannata-Andia JB, Martin KJ. The challenge of controlling phosphorus in chronic kidney disease. Nephrol Dial Transplant. 2016;31:541–7.

D'Alessandro C, Piccoli GB, Cupisti A. The "phosphorus pyramid": a visual tool for dietary phosphate management in dialysis and CKD patients. BMC Nephrol. 2015;16:9. http://www.biomedcentral.com/1471-2369/16/9.

Kalantar-Zadeh K, Gutekunst L, Mehrotra R, et al. Understanding sources of dietary phosphorus in the treatment of patients with chronic kidney disease. Clin J Am Soc Nephrol. 2010;5:519–30.

Li J, Wang L, Han M, et al. The role of phosphate-containing medications and low dietary phosphorusprotein ratio in reducing intestinal phosphorus load in patients with chronic kidney disease. Nutr Diabetes. 2019;9:14. https://doi.org/10.1038/s41387-019-0080-2.

Sinha A, Prasad N. Dietary management of hyperphosphatemia in chronic kidney disease. Clin Quer Nephrol. 2014;3:38–45.

Taketani Y, Koiwa F, Yokoyama K. Management of phosphorus load in CKD patients. Clin Exp Nephrol. 2017;21(suppl 1):s27–36.

37. A 45-year-old woman with CKD 3b (eGFR 30–44 mL/min) is found to have intact PTH level of 246 pg/mL and left ventricular hypertrophy (LVH). Her serum Ca^{2+}, phosphate, and $25(OH)D_3$ levels are normal. Repeat PTH level is 250 pg/mL. **Which one of the following answers is CORRECT in managing her hyperparathyroidism?**

A. Start vitamin $25(OH)D_3$
B. Start oral calcitriol
C. Start paricalcitol
D. Parathyroidectomy
E. None of the above

The answer is E

The optimal PTH level is not clearly identified in patients with CKD 3a-5 not on dialysis. The KDIGO-MBD guideline 2017 suggests that calcitriol and vitamin D analogs not be routinely used in adults with CKD 3a-5 who are not on dialysis. This suggestion is based on two randomized, controlled trials, which showed no difference between paricalcitol-treated and placebo groups. In both trials, the patients had PTH levels between 50 and 300 pg/mL. Also, LVH index did not improve in both study patients. One of the adverse effects was hypercalcemia. Thus, answers A–D are incorrect.

Suggested Reading

Thadhani R, Appelbaum E, Pritchett Y, et al. Vitamin D therapy and cardiac structure and function in patients with chronic kidney disease: the PRIMO randomized controlled trial. JAMA. 2012;307:674–84.

Wang AY, Fang F, Chan J, et al. Effect of paricalcitol on left ventricular mass and function in CKD--the OPERA trial. J Am Soc Nephrol. 2014;25:175–86.

38. **Which one of the following hormone combinations is found to DECREASE with progression of CKD?**

A. FGF-23 and α-Klotho
B. PTH and calcitriol ($1,25(OH)_2D_3$)
C. FGF-23 and PTH
D. Calcitriol and α-Klotho
E. FGF-23 and calcitriol

The answer is D

FGF-23 exerts its effects through interaction with its receptor, and activation of this receptor requires a cofactor called α-Klotho. Accordingly, FGF-23 fails to exert its effects in the absence of α-Klotho. α-Klotho is released from cellular membrane of the kidney into circulation as soluble α-Klotho.

As discussed previously, levels of FGF-23 increase prior to PTH elevation in CKD. Thus, the levels of both hormones are increased in CKD. Conversely, soluble α-Klotho levels start to decrease from CKD stage 2 and its deficiency occurs at CKD 5. Similarly, calcitriol levels also decrease early in CKD stages 1-2, and further decrease with progression of CKD. Thus, the levels of both calcitriol and α-Klotho decrease in CKD (answer D is correct).

Suggested Reading

Gutiérrez O, Isakova T, Rhee E, et al. Fibroblast growth factor-23 mitigates hyperphosphatemia but accentuates calcitriol deficiency in chronic kidney disease. J Am Soc Nephrol. 2005;16:2205–15.
Zou D, Wu W, He Y, et al. The role of klotho in chronic kidney disease. BMC Nephrol. 2018;19:285. https://doi.org/10.1186/s12882-018-1094-z.

39. **Which one of the following is NOT a complication of α-Klotho deficiency in CKD?**

A. Progression of CKD
B. Kidney fibrosis
C. Vascular calcification
D. Hyperphosphatemia
E. Decreased FGF-23 levels

The answer is E

As stated previously, soluble α-Klotho deficiency occurs in CKD. This deficiency of α-Klotho causes progression of CKD due to kidney fibrosis, vascular calcification, and hyperphosphatemia. Also, as α-Klotho level decreases, FGF-23 resistance ensues, and hyperphosphatemia develops. Multiple mechanisms have been implicated in the development of above complications. Thus, answers A–D are correct. Interestingly, α-Klotho deficiency stimulates FGF-23 levels (answer E is incorrect). Exogenous administration of α-Klotho improves all of the above complications.

α-Klotho expression is also downregulated by uremic toxins, inflammation, oxidative stress, low levels of calcitriol, hyperphosphatemia, and renin-AII-angiotensin axis.

Suggested Reading

Hu MC, Kuro-o M, Moe OW. Renal and extrarenal actions of klotho. Semin Nephrol. 2013;33:118–29.
Hu MC, Kuro-o M, Moe OW. Secreted klotho and chronic kidney disease. Adv Exp Med Biol. 2012;728:126–57.
Zou D, Wu W, He Y, et al. The role of klotho in chronic kidney disease. BMC Nephrol. 2018;19:285. https://doi.org/10.1186/s12882-018-1094-z.

40. A 52-year-old woman with CKD 4 has serum calcium level of 10.2 mg/dL and Phosphate level of 5.8 mg/dL. She takes 1000 mg of calcium daily and follows low phosphate diet. **In the evaluation of vascular calcification (VC), which one of the following diagnostic tests is suggested by the KDIGO-MBD guideline?**

A. CT of the abdomen
B. MRI of the abdomen
C. Lateral abdominal radiograph
D. Echocardiogram (ECHO)
E. C and D

The answer is E

Clinical practice needs a simple and cost-effective technique to provide useful information about VC. The 2017 KDIGO-MBD guideline suggests that a lateral abdominal radiograph (abdominal aorta), or chest (aortic arch) can be used to detect the presence or absence of VC, and an ECHO to detect valvular calcification as a reasonable alternative to CT-based imaging in CKD 3a-5. Thus, answer E is correct.

Suggested Reading

Kidney Disease: Improving Global Outcomes (KDIGO) CKD-MBD Update Work Group. KDIGO 2017 clinical practice guideline update for the diagnosis, evaluation, prevention, and treatment of chronic kidney disease–mineral and bone disorder (CKD-MBD). Kidney Int Suppl. 2017;7:1–59.

41. A 52-year-old man with CKD 5 due to hypertension and not on dialysis is found to have aortic valve calcification on ECHO. He has left ventricular hypertrophy but asymptomatic. **Which one of the following endogenous inhibitors of vascular calcification (VC) is DEFICIENT?**

A. Fetuin-A
B. Matrix γ-carboxyglutamate protein (MGP)
C. Osteoprotegerin
D. Pyrophosphate
E. All of the above

The answer is E

All of the above answers are correct. VC is a pathological deposition of calcium and phosphate with matrix in the vascular system. It is usually classified into four main categories according to location: (1) atherosclerotic intimal calcification; (2) arterial medial calcification (Mönckeberg's sclerosis); (3) cardiac valve calcification; and (4) calcific uremic arteriolopathy (calciphylaxis). The hemodynamic consequences of VC are the loss of arterial stiffness, increase in pulse pressure, development of left ventricular hypertrophy, decrease in coronary artery perfusion, and myocardial ischemia and failure. These changes eventually lead to cardiovascular morbidity and mortality.

The pathophysiology of VC is complex, involving an imbalance between inhibitors and promoters. One of the mechanisms is deficiency of endogenous inhibitors of VC. Feutin-A is a calcium-binding protein found in blood, which is synthesized by the liver. It is a potent inhibitor of hydroxyapatite formation. Fetuin-A molecules form stable colloidal spheres with calcium and phosphate to form insoluble calciprotein particles, which are removed by the reticuloendothelial system. Fetuin-A null mice develop VC and renal dysfunction. Thus, deficiency of fetuin-A causes VC.

Matrix γ-carboxyglutamate protein (MGP) was originally isolated from bone, but it is present in several tissues including kidney, lung, heart, cartilage, and vascular smooth muscle cells of the blood vessel wall. It is a vitamin K-dependent protein that acts locally to prevent VC. MGP null mice develop VC. It binds to calcium and inhibits its crystal growth. Vitamin K deficiency and warfarin cause undercarboxylation of glutamic acid residues of MGP and promote VC. An increase in circulating underglysylated MGP was reported in CKD and dialysis patients. Also, subclinical deficiency of vitamin K levels was also reported in CKD patients. Studies are underway to evaluate vitamin K supplementation on VC in dialysis patients.

Osteoprotegerin (OPG) inhibits osteoclast differentiation and is a crucial modulator of bone resorption. OPG functions as a soluble (decoy) receptor to prevent binding of RANKL (receptor activator of nuclear factor kB ligand) to RANK (an important system that is involved in bone resorption and VC), leading in turn to inhibition of osteoclast function and bone resorption. In other words, OPG specifically inhibits osteoclastic bone resorption by interfering with RANKL binding to RANK. It is released by endothelial cells as a protective mechanism for their survival in pathologic conditions. OPG null mice develop osteoporosis and medial calcification, suggesting that OPG is a link between bone and vascular disease. Thus, OPG functions as an in vivo inhibitor of VC. Blood OPG levels in conditions of VC are elevated, and these elevated levels represent biomarker of VC.

Pyrophosphate (PPi) is also another inhibitor of VC, which inhibits hydroxyapatite crystal formation. Only the circulating PPi that is primarily responsible for inhibiting calcification. PPi generates from ATP by the enzyme ectonucleotide pyrophosphatase/phosphodiesterase1 (eNPP1). Deficiency or inactivation of eNPP1 results in medial calcification in children. PPi is degraded into phosphate enzymatically by tissue-nonspecific alkaline phosphatase (TNAP). TNAP is an important enzyme that controls PPi production, and overexpression of this enzyme selectively in smooth muscle cells causes medial calcification.

It is reasonable to think that intake of oral PPi may prevent VC; however, PPi is hydrolyzed in the stomach and becomes ineffective. Intravenous administration of PPi may be helpful, if it remains in circulation for extended period of time. Alternatively, inhibitors of TNAP may improve VC in CKD patients. Thus, answer E is correct.

In addition to the above inhibitors, osteopontin is found to have an inhibitory effect on VC.

Suggested Reading

Chen N-C, Hsu C-Y, Chen C-L. The strategy to prevent and regress the vascular calcification in dialysis patients. BioMed Res Int. 2017;2017:9035193, 11 pages.

Chen NX, Moe SM. Pathophysiology of vascular calcification. Curr Osteoporos Rep. 2015;13:372–80.

Mizobuchi M, Towler D, Slatopolsky E. Vascular calcification: the killer of patients with chronic kidney disease. J Am Soc Nephrol. 2009;20:1453–64.
Proudfoot D, Shanahan CM. Molecular mechanisms mediating vascular calcification: role of matrix Gla protein. Nephrology. 2006;11:455–61.
Shea MK, Booth SL. Vitamin K, vascular calcification, and chronic kidney disease: current evidence and unanswered questions. Curr Dev Nutr. 2019;3:nzz077.
Villa-Bellosta R, O'Neill WC. Pyrophosphate deficiency in vascular calcification. Kidney Int. 2018;93:1293–7.

42. A 52-year-old woman on hemodialysis (HD) for 6 years develops the following necrotizing ulcer on her lower extremity (Fig. 4.2). **Which one of the following therapeutic interventions is APPROPRIATE at this time?**

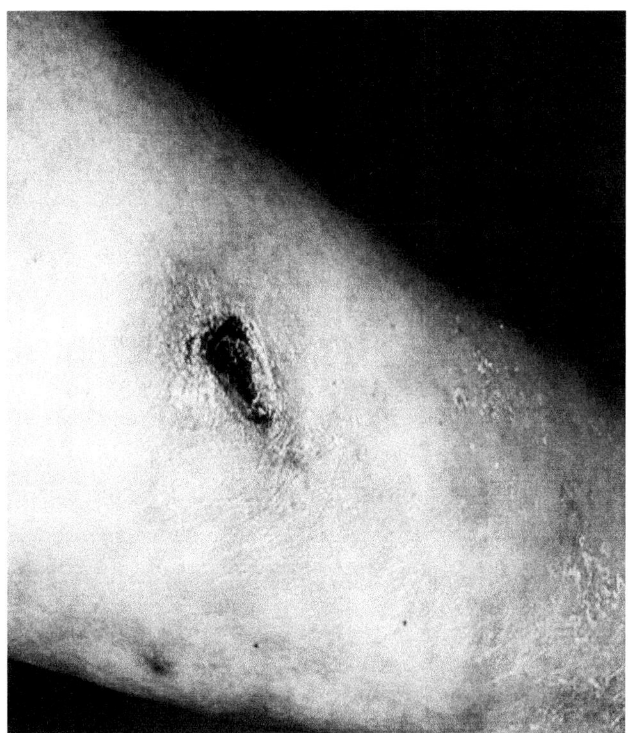

Fig. 4.2 Necrotizing lesion on lower extremity (with permission from Elsevier Ltd)

A. Lower serum PO_4 by Ca-based phosphate binder
B. Vitamin D therapy
C. Start warfarin to prevent thrombosis
D. Continue regular HD
E. Avoid Ca-based binder, vitamin D therapy, warfarin, and institute aggressive wound management and antibiotics, intensify HD (4 h a day for 7 days followed by 5–6 times weekly), and sodium thiosulfate with O_2 therapy and vitamin K_1

The answer is E

This patient has calciphylaxis (calcific uremic arteriolopathy) of her lower extremity. Calciphylaxis is characterized by painful skin ulceration with necrosis, and medial calcification. Calcification of subcutaneous tissue is also common. Clinically the lesions may manifest as discoloration of skin with induration and progression to ulceration. It occurs both in chronic HD and nondialysis CKD patients. The incidence varies from <1% to 4%. One

year mortality is 40–50% in nondialysis patients and 50–80% in HD patients. Traditional risk factors include secondary hyperparathyroidism, hypercalcemia, hyperphosphatemia, Ca-based phosphate binders, obesity, diabetes, protein C deficiency, female sex, warfarin use, vitamin K deficiency, and low levels of albumin as well as inhibitors of vascular calcification.

There is no definitive treatment, however, a multi-interventional treatment is recommended. First, use of Ca-based binder, vitamin D, and warfarin should be avoided. Second, institution of aggressive wound management and antibiotic use, intensification of HD (4 h a day for 7 days followed by 5–6 times weekly), and long-term sodium thiosulfate 25 g in 100 mL of saline iv in 30 min three times a week with O_2 therapy through a face mask should be started. An Australian retrospective study showed that sodium thiosulfate infusion (25 g three times a week) in HD patients for a median of 96 days resulted in complete remission in 14 of 27 (52%) of patients. Besides chelating Ca^{2+}, sodium thiosulfate may have other effects in improving calciphylaxis; and third, vitamin K_1 supplementation (phytonadione administered at a dose of 2 mg daily for 12 months) slowed the progression of aortic-valve calcification. Thus, option E is correct.

Other therapeutic modalities include vitamin K supplementation, lanthanum, bisphosphonates, cinacalcet, corticosteroids to improve inflammation, surgery of the wound, and hyperbaric oxygen. A few clinical trials are underway.

Suggested Reading

Baldwin C, Farah M, Leung M, et al. Multi-intervention management of calciphylaxis: a report of 7 cases. Am J Kidney Dis. 2011;58:988–91.

Nigwekar SU, Thadani R, Brandenburg VM. Calciphylaxis. N Engl J Med. 2018;378:1704–10.

Ross EA. Evolution of treatment strategies for calciphylaxix. Am J Nephrol. 2011;34:460–7.

Seethapathy H, Nigwekar SU. Revisiting therapeutic options for calciphylaxis. Curr Opin Nephrol Hypertens. 2019;28:448–54.

Vedvyas C, Winterfield LS, Vleugels RA. Calciphylaxis: a systematic review of existing and emerging therapies. J Am Acad Dermatol. 2012;67:e253–60.

Zitt E, König M, Vychytil A, et al. Use of sodium thiosulfate in a multi-interventional setting for the treatment of calciphylaxis in dialysis patients. Nephrol Dial Transplant. 2013;28:1232–40.

43. **Match the following bone biopsy findings with the clinical scenarios:**

1. Normal bone
2. Patient with secondary hyperparathyroidism
3. Patient with adynamic bone disease
4. Patient with aluminum toxicity
5. Patient with osteomalacia

Answers: 1= Fig. A; 2= Fig. B; 3= Fig. C; 4= Fig. D; 5= Fig. E

Bone biopsy in CKD 4-5 patients is the standard method of determining the bone disease. Fig. A shows normal bone histology with mineralized lamellar bone (blue) and cellular area between the two mineralized bone.

Figure B shows the bone histology of osteitis fibrosa due to severe secondary hyperparathyroidism. Note that the density of the mineralized bone is decreased and the cellular component is fibrosed (arrow). Osteitis fibrosa is characterized by an increased rate of bone formation and resorption with increased osteoclastic activity, resulting in unmineralized bone matrix and bone marrow fibrosis. Osteitis fibrosa is an example of high turnover bone disease.

Figure C is an example of adynamic (low turnover) bone disease. It is characterized by absence of osteoblasts and osteoclasts, increased osteoid formation and endosteal fibrosis. As a result of decreased cell number, bone formation and resorption are decreased.

Figure D is an example of aluminum deposition in bone. Villanueva and aurintricarboxylic acid stain gives red band at the osteoid-bone interface. Generally, aluminum disease is associated with osteomalacia (Fig. E), which is characterized by decreased mineralization with excess unmineralized osteoid. Decreased cell activity and absence of endosteal fibrosis also characterize osteomalacia.

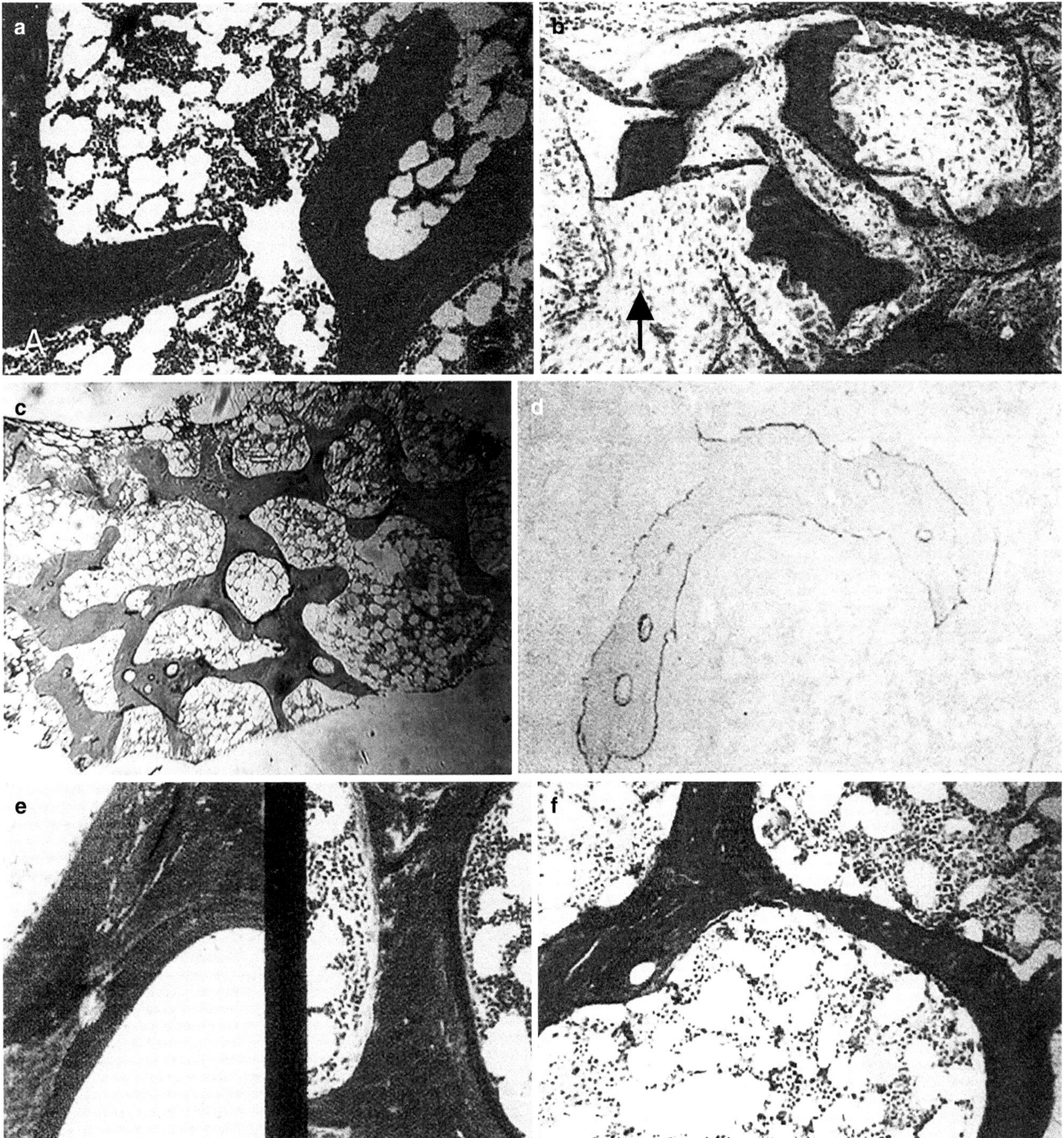

Fig. 4.3 Normal and abnormal bone biopsy findings. (With permission from Elsevier Ltd)

Suggested Reading

Christov M, Sprague SM. Chronic kidney disease-bone and mineral disease. In: Yu ASL, Chertow GM, Luyckx VA, et al., editors. Brenner & Rector's the kidney. 11th ed. Philadelphia: Elsevier, Saunders; 2020. p. 1805–37.

44. Fractures are common in CKD patients and increase in proportion to the severity of the disease. **According to the 2017 KDIGO-MBD guideline, which one of the following statements regarding bone examination in patients with CKD 3a-5D is FALSE?**

    A. Dual-energy X-ray absorptiometry (DXA) measures of bone mineral disorder (BMD), particularly lower femoral neck and total hip, predict a greater risk for fractures
    B. DXA BMD does not distinguish among types of renal osteodystrophy

C. Biochemical abnormalities (calcium, phosphate, PTH, and bone-specific alkaline phosphatase) can identify different types of renal osteodystrophy
D. Bone biopsy is recommended to identify various types of renal osteodystrophy
E. Bone biopsy should be considered in patients with unexplained fractures, resistant hypercalcemia, or suspicion of osteomalacia

The answer is C

Statement C is false because there are no prospective studies to demonstrate that circulating biomarkers alone are enough to predict changes in bone histology in CKD patient stages 3a-5D. However, only one study in hemodialysis patients that elevation in bone-specific alkaline phosphatase can predict incident fractures but not renal osteodystrophy. Other statements are correct. The 2017 KDIGO-MBD guideline provides evidence from four prospective cohort studies that DXA BMD can be used to predict fractures in CKD 3a-5D. However, DXA BMD does not differentiate various types of renal osteodistrophy, and the diagnostic utility of biochemical markers is limited by their poor sensitivity and specificity.

Kidney biopsy is the gold standard for the diagnosis and classification of renal osteodystrophy (high or low bone turnover). It should also be considered in several conditions such as: (1) unexplained fractures; (2) refractory hypercalcemia; (3) unexplained hypophosphatemia; (4) suspected osteomalacia; (5) worsening BMD despite standard therapy; and (6) to distinguish osteoporosis from suspected osteomalacia and unexplained osteosclerosis.

Suggested Reading

Kidney Disease: Improving Global Outcomes (KDIGO) CKD-MBD Update Work Group. KDIGO 2017 clinical practice guideline update for the diagnosis, evaluation, prevention, and treatment of chronic kidney disease–mineral and bone disorder (CKD-MBD). Kidney Int Suppl. 2017;7:1–59.

45. **Which one of the following medications is used to treat osteoporosis in CKD patients?**

A. 25-hydroxyvitamin D_3
B. Bisphosphonate
C. Denosumab
D. Teriparatide (recombinant PTH)
E. All of the above

The answer is E

The first-line therapy for the management of CKD-associated osteoporosis is treatment of biochemical abnormalities associated with CKD-MBD. Management of hyperparathyroidism, hyperphosphatemia, and vitamin D deficiency need to be evaluated before initiation of anti-osteoporosis medications. PTH levels should be <600 pg/mL and phosphate levels in the normal range. 25-hydroxy vitamin D_3 levels should be maintained >30 ng/mL with ergocalciferol or calcidiol.

Bisphosphonates prevent bone resorption by inhibiting osteoclast activity. Most of these drugs are taken up by the skeleton and retained in skeleton for years. The extraskeletal drug is excreted by the kidney. Therefore, they are not recommended in patients with eGFR <30 mL/min. Also, one study reported adynamic bone disease with the use of bisphosphonates. However, studies in postmenopausal women with decreased kidney function and CKD 3–5D patients showed improvement in bone mineral disorder (BMD) and fractures. Thus, evidence is accumulating for their safety in CKD patients. Renal biopsy prior to bisphosphonate use is not recommended to document adynamic bone disease.

Denosumab prevents bone resorption. It is a monoclonal antibody against the receptor activator of NF-κB ligand, and it inhibits osteoclast proliferation and development. Unlike bisphosphonates, denosumab is not excreted by the kidney, and can be used in CKD patients. The only complication of denosumab is hypocalcemia.

Teriparatide is a recombinant PTH. It consists of the first 34 amino-terminal residues of PTH. It was the first Food and Drug Administration (FDA)-approved osteoanabolic agent to treat osteoporosis and prevent fractures in both age-related and glucocorticoid-induced osteoporosis. In postmenopausal women with different severity of renal dysfunction, teriparatide improved increased BMD at the spine and femoral neck. Also, observational studies in dialysis patients improved BMD in the spine and hip. Thus, answer E is correct.

Suggested Reading

Khairallah P, Nickolas TL. Management of osteoporosis in CKD. Clin J Am Soc Nephrol. 2018;13:962–9.
Nitta K, Yazima A, Tsuchiya K. Management of osteoporosis in chronic kidney disease. Intern Med. 2017;56:3271–6.
Wilson LM, Rebholz CM, Jirru E, et al. Benefits and harms of osteoporosis medications in patients with chronic kidney disease: a systematic review and meta-analysis. Ann Intern Med. 2017;166:649–58.

46. **Targeting higher Hgb levels (>12 g %) in CKD 3–4 patients is associated with which one of the following complications?**

A. Hypertension and cardiovascular death
B. Stroke
C. Vascular access thrombosis
D. All of the above
E. None of the above

The answer is D

An early meta-analysis of nine randomized studies involving 5,143 patients with CKD 3–4 concluded that achieving higher Hgb (>12 g/dL) with erythropoiesis-stimulating agents (ESAs) was associated with increased risk for all-cause mortality, HTN, and A-V access thrombosis, as compared with low targeted Hgb (9.5–11.5 g/dL) levels. Subsequent meta-analysis of 27 trials with 10, 452 patients with CKD showed that higher Hgb levels are associated with increased risk for hypertension, stroke, and vascular access thrombosis as well as probable risk for cardiovascular events, ESKD, and death. Therefore, the appropriate Hgb levels in CKD patients should be between 10 and 11 g/dL.

Suggested Reading

Mimura I, Tanaka T, Nangaku M. How the target hemoglobin of renal anemia should be? Nephron. 2015;131:201–9.
Palmer SC, Navaneethan SD, Craig JC, et al. Meta-analysis: erythropoiesis-stimulating agents in patients with chronic kidney disease. Ann Intern Med. 2010;153:23–33.
Phrommintikul A, Haas SJ, Elsik M, et al. Mortality and target haemoglobin concentrations in anaemic patients with chronic kidney disease treated with erythropoietin: a meta-analysis. Lancet. 2007;369:381–8.

47. A 40-year-old female patient with CKD 3 is referred to you for evaluation of serum phosphate (PO_4) level of 5.6 mg/dL. The patient mother and father are alive and both have diabetes, HTN, and cardiomyopathy. The patient wants to know whether or not her elevated PO_4 is a risk factor for cardiovascular disease (CVD). **Which one of the following statements is FALSE regarding the association between high serum PO_4 and CVD?**

A. High serum PO_4 level is associated with CVD events and mortality
B. Each 1 mg/dL serum PO_4 level above 3.5 mg/dL is associated with a 27% increase in all-cause mortality
C. Each 1 mg/dL serum PO_4 level above 4 mg/dL is associated with a 31% increase in the first major CV event
D. High serum PO_4 levels are associated with increased incidence of stroke
E. High serum PO_4 levels are associated with an increased risk of myocardial infarction (MI), heart failure, and composite of coronary death

The answer is D

Several epidemiologic studies showed the serum PO_4 levels even within normal range are associated with CVD morbidity or even mortality in CKD 3–5 and dialysis patients (Table 4.7), although survival in dialysis patients seems to decrease at serum PO_4 levels >5.5 mg/dL. However, increased risk for stroke has not been reported. Thus, statement D is false.

Table 4.7 Association between serum PO_4 level and cardiovascular events

Study	Serum PO_4 (mg/dL)	Association
Tonelli et al. (1)	≥3.5	Each 1 mg/dL higher serum PO_4 is associated with a 27% increase in all-cause mortality Increased risk of new MI, heart failure, and the composite of coronary death, but not the risk of STROKE
Foley et al. (2)	3.5	Higher PO_4 levels are associated with higher CVD events and mortality
De Boer et al. (3)	>4.0	Each 1 mg/dL higher serum PO_4 is associated with a 31% increase in the first major CVD event

One should consider possible secondary hyperparathyroidism and elevated FGF-23 levels involvement in normal to high serum PO_4 levels in adverse CV events.

Suggested Reading

de Boer IH, Rue TC, Kestenbaum B. Serum phosphorus concentrations in the third National Health and Nutrition Examination Survey (NHANES III). Am J Kidney Dis. 2009;53:399–407.

Disthabanchong S. Phosphate and cardiovascular disease beyond chronic kidney disease and vascular calcification. Int J Nephrol. 2018;2018:3162806, 7 pages.

Foley RN, Collins AJ, Ishani A, et al. Calcium-phosphate levels and cardiovascular disease in community-dwelling adults: the Atherosclerosis in Communities (ARIC) Study. Am Heart J. 2008;156:556–63.

Tonelli M, Sacks F, Pfeffer M, et al. Relation between serum phosphate level and cardiovascular event rate in people with coronary disease. Circulation. 2005;112:2627–33.

48. A 45-year-old type 2 diabetic African American woman with HTN, diastolic dysfunction, proteinuria, and CKD 2 is referred to you by a primary care physician for possible prevention of cardiovascular disease (CVD) events. She is on enalapril 10 mg/day and losartan 100 mg/day. Her BP is 142/88 mm Hg, and proteinuria is 2.2 g/24 h. Her serum potassium is normal. Her glycated HbA1c is 10.2%. **Based on the available evidence, which one of the following recommendations is INCORRECT?**

A. Continue either enalapril or losartan and not both
B. Maintain glycated HbA1c ~7%
C. Maintain glycated HbA1c <6.5% as suggested for type 1 diabetic patients
D. Add chlorthalidone 25 mg/day to either enalapril or losartan
E. Combination of an ACE-I and an ARB (angiotensin receptor blocker) is less renoprotective than either drug alone

The answer is C

The available evidence shows that strict glycemic control (HbA1c <6.5%) is a risk factor for CVD events in type 2 diabetic patients. The recommended HgA1c is between 6.5 and 7.5%. Thus, option C is incorrect.

Although earlier studies reported that the combination of an ACE-I and an ARB reduces proteinuria compared to either drug alone, a large study showed that such a combination may cause worsening kidney function, hypotension, and hyperkalemia. The ONTARGET study found that combination of ramipril and telmisartan increased the risk for renal failure than either drug alone. This was confirmed in a recent study on type 2 diabetic patients.

The patient needs glucose and BP control, which would improve proteinuria.

Maintaining HbA1c ~7% and BP <130/80 mm Hg is advisable. Adding a thiazide diuretic such as chlorthalidone or hydrochlorothiazide 25 mg/day may help control BP. If BP is not within target range, adding aldosterone antagonist to the existing BP medications has an additive effect in lowering BP and proteinuria. However, the diabetic patient on a combination of RAAS inhibitors and aldosterone antagonists needs close monitoring for hyperkalemia.

Suggested Reading

Bomback AS, Kshirsagar AV, Amamoo MA, et al. Change in proteinuria after adding aldosterone blockers in ACE inhibitors or angiotensin receptor blockers in CKD: a systematic review. Am J Kidney Dis. 2008;51:199–211.

Gerstein HC, Miller ME, Byington RP, et al. Effects of intensive glucose lowering in type 2 diabetes. N Engl J Med. 2008;358:2545–59.

Mann JF, Schmieder RE, McQueen M, et al. Renal outcomes with telmisartan, ramipril, or both, in people at high vascular risk (the ONTARGET study): a multicentre, randomized, double-blind, controlled trial. Lancet. 2008;372:547–53.

49. **According to the Chronic Renal Insufficiency Cohort (CRIC) study, which one of the following options regarding cardiovascular disease (CVD) is INCORRECT?**

A. Prevalence of left ventricular hypertrophy (LVH) in those with eGFR <30 mL/min is 75%
B. Low eGFR (<30 mL/min) is strongly associated with higher LV mass and LVH

C. There is a strong and graded relationship between coronary artery calcification (CAC) and severity of CKD independent of traditional risk factors
D. No difference in LV mass index was observed between advanced CKD (eGFR <20 mL/min) and newly started hemodialysis or peritoneal dialysis patients
E. There is a strong relationship between cardiac troponin and diastolic dysfunction

The answer is E

The CRIC is a multicenter observational study that enrolled approximately 4,000 patients with a mean eGFR of 43.4 ± 13.5 mL/min. It is an ethnically and racially diverse study. Patients with polycystic kidney disease, bone marrow or solid organ transplant, and New York Heart Association Classification III/IV heart failure were excluded from the study. The CRIC Study was designed to examine the various risk factors for the progression of CKD and CVD in CKD patients.

With regard to eGFR and CVD, the prevalence of LVH in patients with eGFR <30 mL/min was 75%, but in the entire CRIC Study patients the prevalence was 50%. This indicates that LVH is a common abnormality in patients with CKD.

The CRIC Study found a strong relationship between GFR and LV mass. Low GFR (<30 mL/min) was found to be independently associated with excess concentric and eccentric hypertrophy, and remodeling of the heart. Also, the study showed a graded relationship between the decline in GFR and higher degrees of CAC independent of traditional risk factors.

Although low GFR is associated strongly with abnormal LV structure, there was no difference in LV mass index between those patients with eGFR <20 mL/min and those on newly started dialysis patients, suggesting that GFR <20 mL/min has no additional effect on LV structure. However, the study found that LV ejection fraction is substantially reduced in those on dialysis. This indicates that dialysis patients are at higher risk for heart failure compared to predialysis patients.

The CRIC study also showed that cardiac troponin was strongly associated with LVH and moderately associated with systolic dysfunction; however, there was no association with diastolic dysfunction. Thus, option E is incorrect.

Suggested Reading

Bansal N, Keane M, Delafontaine P, et al. A longitudinal study of left ventricular function and structure from CKD to ESRD; The CRIC Study. Clin J Am Soc Nephrol. 2013;8:355–62.

Budoff MJ, Rader DJ, Reilly MP, et al. Relationship of estimated GFR and coronary artery calcification in the CRIC (Chronic Renal Insufficiency Cohort) Study. Am J Kidney Dis. 2011;58:519–26.

Lash JP, Go AS, Appel LJ, et al. Chronic Renal Insufficiency Cohort (CRIC) Study: Baseline characteristics and associations with kidney function. Clin J Am Soc Nephrol. 2009;4:1302–11.

Mishra RK, Li Y, DeFilippi C, et al. Association of cardiac troponin T with left ventricular structure and function in CKD. Am J Kidney Dis. 2013;61:701–9.

Park M, Hsu C-Y, Li Y, et al. Associations between kidney function and subclinical cardiac abnormalities in CKD. J Am Soc Nephrol. 2012;23:1725–34.

50. A 54-year-old African American woman with CKD 4 is admitted for chest pain without EKG changes. **With regard to cardiac troponin T (cTnT), which one of the following statements is INCORRECT?**

A. Increase in cTnT identifies a subgroup of patients at increased risk for major cardiac events
B. Elevated cTnT has a significant effect on survival in predialysis patients
C. Can't is really excreted and its elevated levels in CKD 4 patients has no prognostic significance
D. In patients with eGFR <60 mL/min, cTnT levels should be interpreted with caution with regard to the diagnosis of acute coronary syndrome (ACS)
E. Detectable cTnT levels were found to be associated strongly with LVH, a modest association with systolic dysfunction, and no association with diastolic Dysfunction in a cohort of CKD 2-4 patients without heart failure

The answer is C

Cardiac troponins T and I are involved in myocardial contractility. Their elevated serum levels have been reported to be specific markers of myocardial injury. Both troponins are excreted by the kidney; therefore, an elevation in these markers is expected in patients with renal failure. Troponin increase occurs early in CKD, and its interpretation in the evaluation of ACS is difficult in asymptomatic patients. However, detectable levels of cardiac

troponins are associated with structural heart disease, such as LVH, increased cardiovascular events, and survival in CKD patients.

As stated above, circulating levels of cTnT are high in CKD stages 2–4, and their levels should be interpreted cautiously in these patients. In the absence of ACS, however, elevated levels of cardiac troponins can identify a subgroup of patients at increased risk for major cardiac events. Thus, elevated levels of cTnT can have a prognostic significance. Therefore, option C is incorrect, and all other statements are correct.

Suggested Reading

de Lemos JA, Drazner MH, Omland T, et al. Association of troponin T detected with a highly sensitive assay and cardiac structure and mortality risk in the general population. JAMA. 2010;304:2503–12.

deFilippi CR, de Lemos JA, Christenson RH, et al. Association of serial measures of cardiac troponin T using a sensitive assay with incident heart failure and cardiovascular mortality in older adults. JAMA. 2010;304:2494–502.

Mishra RK, Li Y, deFilippi C, et al. on behalf of the CRIC Study Investigators. Association of cardiac troponin T with left ventricular structure and function in CKD. Am J Kidney Dis. 2013;61:701–9.

51. A 55-year-old woman with CKD due to type 2 diabetes is admitted for shortness of breath. Other than trace pedal edema, the physical examination is otherwise normal. Chest x-ray shows pulmonary congestion. **Which one of the following statements is INCORRECT regarding serum brain natriuretic peptide (BNP) and N-terminal proB-type natriuretic peptide (NT-proBNP) level in this patient?**

   A. Serum NT-proBNP levels should be interpreted cautiously in CKD patients with regard to heart failure and volume status
   B. Concentrations of NT-proBNP are elevated proportionately to the degree of LV mass increase
   C. NT-proBNP has longer half-life than BNP
   D. BNP predicts reliably the volume status and heart failure in CKD 4-5 stages
   E. Higher levels of NT-proBNP predict the future cardiovascular events (CVEs) in CKD patients

   The answer is D

   Natriuretic peptides, particularly, atrial natriuretic peptide (ANP), and BNP have been extensively studied because of their involvement in salt and water homeostasis. Of these natriuretic peptides, concentrations of BNP have been used for detection and stratification of CHF. BNP has been shown to be superior to ANP as a biomarker for CHF and LV dysfunction.

   BNP is synthesized in the ventricle as preprohormone with 134 amino acids. This preprohormone is cleaved to proBNP with 108 amino acids. Further breakdown of this proBNP leads to the formation of the active BNP (32 amino acids) and the inactive 76-amino acid-containing NT-proBNP. Compared to BNP, the half-life of NT-proBNP is longer, and both of these biomarkers of cardiac disease replaced the combination of ANP and BNP in patients with normal kidney function.

   Both BNP and NT-proBNP are cleared by the kidneys; therefore, their serum levels should be interpreted with caution in patients with eGFR <60 mL/min. Thus, option D is incorrect. Despite the difficulty in diagnosing CHF in CKD patients, studies have shown that elevated levels of BNP, NT-proBNP, and troponins are associated with increased CVEs. Both the PREVEND (The Prevention of Renal and Vascular End-Stage Disease) and TREAT (The Trial to Reduce Cardiovascular Events with Aranesp Therapy) have reconfirmed the previous observations of strong association between elevation in cardiac biomarkers and CVEs.

Suggested Reading

Landry MJ, Emberson JR, Blackwell L, et al. Prediction of ESKD and death among people with CKD: the Chronic Renal Impairment in Birmingham (CRIB) prospective cohort study. Am J Kidney Dis. 2010;56:1082–94.

McMurray JJ, Uno H, Jarolim P, et al. Predictors of fatal and nonfatal cardiovascular events in patients with type 2 diabetes mellitus, chronic kidney disease, and anemia: an analysis of the Trial to Reduce cardiovascular Events with Aranesp (darbepoietin-alfa) Therapy (TREAT). Am Heart J. 2011;162:748–55.e3.

Scheven L, de Jong PE, Hillege HL, et al. PREVEND study group: High-sensitive troponin T and N-terminal pro-B type natriuretic peptide are associated with albuminuria and glomerular filtration rate. Eur Heart J. 2012;33:2272–81.

52. A 60-year-old man with hypertensive nephrosclerosis and CKD 4 is admitted to cardiac critical care unit with acute chest tightness and shortness of breath. An EKG shows acute ischemic changes. The diagnosis of acute coronary syndrome (ACS) is made. **Regarding ACS in CKD patients, which one of the following statements is CORRECT?**

   A. The clinical presentation of ACS in patients with CKD is different from that of non-CKD patients
   B. The prevalence of chest pain decreases with increasing CKD stages
   C. Patients with advanced CKD (CKD 4-5) are less likely to have ST-segment elevation than non-CKD patients
   D. The EKG changes on presentation vary according to kidney function where STEMI is common in early stages and NSTEMI in advanced stages of CKD
   E. All of the above

   The answer is E

   Studies have shown that CKD patients have atypical clinical presentation than non-CKD patients. Nondialysis CKD patients with stages 4–5 (40.4%) and dialysis patients (41.1%) were less likely to have chest pain at the time of admission compared to non-CKD patients (61.6%). Because of atypical presentation, the diagnosis of ACS was missed in 54% of the time in patients with advanced CKD and 52% of the time in dialysis patients. The pattern of EKG changes is also different in CKD patients. Advanced CKD patients are less likely to have ST-segment elevation compared to non-CKD patients (15.9% versus 32.5%, respectively), but more likely to have heart failure and in-hospital mortality than non-CKD patients. Among CKD patients, STEMI is more common in patients with CKD 2–3b than patients with CKD 4–5D. In contrast, the frequency of NSTEMI is relatively higher in patients with CKD 4–5D compared to patients with CKD stages 2–3b. Thus, ACS is distinctly different in CKD patients compared to non-CKD patients. Therefore, all the above statements about ACS are correct.

   Suggested Reading

Roberts JK, McCullough PA. The management of acute coronary syndromes in patients with chronic kidney disease. Adv Chronic Kidney Dis. 2014;21:472–9.

Washam JB, Herzog CA, Beitelshees AL, et al. Pharmacotherapy in chronic kidney disease patients presenting with acute coronary syndrome. A scientific statement from the American Heart Association. Circulation. 2015;131:1123–49.

53. A 68-year-old man with type 2 diabetes and CKD 3 is seen in your office as a follow-up visit. He is on oral hypoglycemic agents, and his recent HbA1c is 6%. His only complaint is infrequent shivering 4–6 hours after taking his oral hypoglycemic agents. You suspect hypoglycemia. **Regarding hypoglycemia (<50 mg/dL) and cardiovascular events (CVEs), which one of the following statements is CORRECT?**

   A. No relationship between hypoglycemia and CVEs
   B. Hypoglycemia increases the risk of CVEs and all-cause hospitalization, and all-cause mortality
   C. CKD patients are at higher risk for CVEs than non-CKD patients
   D. Younger patients (<65 years) develop severe hypoglycemia than older patients (>65 years)
   E. None of the above

   The answer is B

   Hypoglycemia is a common complication of glucose-lowering drugs (insulin and oral hypoglycemic agents), which is more common in patients with both diabetes and CKD 4–5. In clinical practice, this is unavoidable in both types of diabetic patients. Several studies have shown that hypoglycemia is associated with both cardiovascular and non-cardiovascular complications, including all-cause hospitalizations and mortality. Thus, option B is correct.

   Although CKD patients are at higher risk for hypoglycemia, hypoglycemia-induced CVEs are equally present in both CKD and non-CKD patients. Older patients are at higher risk than younger patients for hypoglycemia and predisposition to CVEs.

   Hypoglycemia-induced CVEs may be due to increasing (1) thrombogenic tendency, (2) sympathetic overactivity, (3) inflammation and oxidative stress, and (4) abnormal cardiac repolarization and accelerating atherosclerosis.

   In this patient, the use of oral hypoglycemic agents should be reevaluated, and his HbA1c should be maintained between 7 and 7.5% to avoid hypoglycemia and CVEs.

Suggested Reading

Hanefeld M, Duetting E, Bramlage P. Cardiac implications of hypoglycaemia in patients with diabetes-a systematic review. Cardiovasc Diabetol. 2013;12:135.

Hanefeld M, Frier BM, Pistrosh F. Hypoglycemia and cardiovascular risk: is there a major link? Diabetes Care. 2016;39(Suppl 2):S205–9.

Hsu P-F, Sung S-H, Cheng H-M, et al. Association of clinical symptomatic hypoglycemia with cardiovascular events and total mortality in type 2 diabetes. A nationwide population-based study. Diabetes Care. 2013;36:894–990.

Yakubovich N, Gerstein HC. Serious cardiovascular outcomes in diabetes: the role of hypoglycemia. Circulation. 2011;123:342–8.

Zoungas S, Patel A, Chalmers J, et al. Severe hypoglycemia and risks of vascular events and death. N Engl J Med. 2010;363:1410–8.

54. A 54-year-old African American male executive with hypertension and CKD 3 is referred to you for management of his kidney function and new-onset asymptomatic atrial fibrillation (AF). The patient refuses warfarin therapy because the heart rate does not bother him, and he wants to gather more information about anticoagulation. **Regarding CKD and AF, which one of the following statements is INCORRECT?**

A. Approximately 18 to 21% of predialysis patients are at risk of developing AF
B. Prevalence of AF is higher in African Americans in CRIC study population
C. Incident AF increases with an increase in CKD stages
D. Predialysis patients are protected from thromboembolic events than dialysis patients
E. Albuminuric patients are at higher risk for AF than normoalbuminuric patients

The answer is D

All of the above statements except for D are correct. Patients with CKD stages 3–5 are at high risk for developing AF. CKD is an independent risk factor for AF. In the ARIC (Atherosclerosis Risk in Communities) Study, patients with eGFR of 60–89 (CKD 2), 30–59 (CKD 3), and 15–29 mL/min (CKD 4) had hazards ratios of 1.3, 1.6, and 3.2, respectively, of developing new-onset AF during a median follow-up of 10.1 years compared to those with an eGFR >90 mL/min. Also, micro- (A2 albuminuric category) and macroalbuminuric (A3 albuminuric category) patients were at higher risk for AF than normoalbuminuric (ACR<30 mg/g; A1 albuminuric category)) patients. Risk of AF was elevated in those with low eGFR and macroalbuminuria. Also, REGARDS (Reasons for Geographic and Racial Differences in Stroke) study showed that the odds ratios for prevalent AF were significantly higher in CKD than in non-CKD patients. The CRIC study showed increased prevalence of AF in African Americans. Both predialysis and dialysis patients are equally at risk for AF and thrombotic events. Thus, CKD 3–5 patients, whether or not on dialysis, are at higher risk for AF and thromboembolic events.

Suggested Reading

Alonso A, Lopez FL, Matsushita K, et al. Chronic kidney disease is associated with the incidence of atrial fibrillation: the Atherosclerosis Risk in Communities (ARIC) study. Circulation. 2011;123:2446–53.

Baber U, Howard VJ, Halperin JL, et al. Association of chronic kidney disease with atrial fibrillation among adults in the United States: REasons for Geographic and Racial Differences in Stroke (REGARDS) Study. Circ Arrhythm Electrophysiol. 2011;4:26–32.

Ng KP, Edwards NC, Lip GYH, et al. Atrial fibrillation in CKD: balancing the risks and benefits of anticoagulation. Am J Kidney Dis. 2013;62:615–32.

Nimmo C, Wright M, Goldsmith D. Management of atrial fibrillation in chronic kidney disease: double trouble. Am Heart J. 2013;166:230–9.

Soliman EZ, Prineas RJ, Go AS, et al. Chronic kidney disease and prevalent atrial fibrillation: the Chronic Renal Insufficiency Cohort (CRIC). Am Heart J. 2010;159:1102–7.

55. The above patient returns to you 2 weeks later and asks you about anticoagulation and the drugs you want to use in him. **Which one of the following statements regarding anticoagulation is CORRECT?**

A. Anticoagulation is not required at this time because of increased risk for bleeding
B. Anticoagulation is required with FDA approved drugs (warfarin and apixaban)
C. Anticoagulation is required with fixed dose warfarin and aspirin

D. Bleeding with an adjusted dose warfarin is much higher than fixed dose warfarin and aspirin
E. Aspirin alone is sufficient to prevent stroke in CKD patients not on dialysis

The answer is B

Ischemic stroke is the major complication of AF in both predialysis and dialysis patients. However, controversy exists whether anticoagulation protects stroke in these patients. An initial retrospective study reported that stroke was more common in hemodialysis patients with sinus rhythm than those with AF, suggesting that AF in CKD patients does not increase the incidence of stroke. However, subsequent retrospective and prospective studies have shown an association between AF and stroke in CKD patients. Thus, anticoagulation is indicated in both predialysis and dialysis patients.

Of the five oral anticoagulant drugs (warfarin, dabigatran, apixaban, rivaroxaban, and edoxaban), only warfarin and apixaban are approved by the Food and Drug Administration for use in nondialysis CKD and dialysis patients. Of these two drugs, apixaban is expensive. Both drugs cause bleeding, and hemodialysis does not reverse bleeding. Thus, answer B is correct.

In a study by Hart et al., treatment of CKD 3 patients with AF with adjusted dose of warfarin reduced the risk of stroke or thromboembolism by 76% compared to those with fixed low dose warfarin (1–3 mg/day) and aspirin (325 mg/day). However, the frequency of major bleeding was not different between the two groups of patients with CKD 3. Adjusted dose warfarin is, therefore, indicated in stage 3 patients.

Also, the study of Arnson et al. suggested that oral anticoagulant use was associated with reduced stroke and intracranial bleeding risk regardless of CKD stage. They also reported reduced mortality risk in CKD stages 1–3.

The use of aspirin alone to prevent stroke is inferior to warfarin. Also, there is no evidence that aspirin prevents stroke in CKD 3 patients. Except for option B, other statements are incorrect.

Suggested Reading

Arnson Y, Hoshen M, Berliner-Sendrey A, et al. Risk of stroke, bleeding, and death in patients with nonvalvular atrial fibrillation and chronic kidney disease. Cardiology. 2010;145:178–86.

Aursulesei V, Costache II. Anticoagulation in chronic kidney disease: from guidelines to clinical practice. Clin Cardiol. 2019;42:774–82.

Hart RG, Pearce LA, Asinger RW, et al. Warfarin in atrial fibrillation patients with moderate chronic kidney disease. Clin J Am Soc Nephrol. 2011;6:2599–604.

Jain N, Reilly RF. Clinical pharmacology of oral anticoagulants in patients with kidney disease. Clin J Am Soc Nephrol. 2019;14:278–87.

Ng KP, Edwards NC, Lip GYH, et al. Atrial fibrillation in CKD: balancing the risks and benefits of anticoagulation. Am J Kidney Dis. 2013;62:615–32.

Nimmo C, Wright M, Goldsmith D. Management of atrial fibrillation in chronic kidney disease: double trouble. Am Heart J. 2013;166:230–9.

Olesen JB, Lip GY, Kamper AL, et al. Stroke and bleeding in atrial fibrillation with chronic kidney disease. N Engl J Med. 2012;367:625–35.

56. One of the cited reasons against the use of warfarin is progression of renal disease in CKD patients. **Which one of the following mechanisms is implicated in warfarin-related nephropathy (WRN)?**

A. Vascular calcification
B. Glomerular hemorrhage
C. Renal tubular obstruction by red blood cell casts
D. Inhibition of vitamin K-dependent factors
E. All of the above

The answer is E

All of the above mechanisms have been implicated in the progression of renal disease in WRN. Several case reports have been published relating high INR and acute kidney injury. Also, some clinical studies reported the development of WRN in more CKD patients on warfarin than those patients without CKD. In addition, warfarin therapy increased 1-year mortality. Vitamin-activated matrix GIa protein inhibits vascular calcification, and warfarin inhibition of vitamin K accelerates vascular calcification. Because of these effects of warfarin, many nephrologists use anticoagulation judiciously in patients with CKD.

Suggested Reading

Brodsky SV, Eikelbloom J, Hebert LA. Anticoagulant-related nephropathy. Am Soc Nephrol. 2018;29:2787–93.
Brodsky SV, Nadasdy T, Rovin BH, et al. Warfarin-related nephropathy occurs in patients with and without chronic kidney disease and is associated with an increased mortality rate. Kidney Int. 2011;80:181–9.
Brodsky SV, Satoskar A, Chen J, et al. Acute kidney injury during warfarin therapy associated with obstructive tubular red blood cell casts: a report of 9 cases. Am J Kidney Dis. 2009;54:1121–6.
Glassock, RJ. Anticoagulant-related nephropathy. It's the real McCoy. Clin J Am Soc Nephrol. 2019;14:935–7.

57. A 40-year-old type 2 diabetic woman with CKD 3 is found to have Hgb of 10.4 g/dL. She is on ACE-I. Despite on erythropoietin (100 U/kg subcutaneously once a wk) and iron, her Hgb did not improve. Her serum iron is 28 μg/dL and ferritin 800 ng/mL. It is felt that the patient's functional iron deficiency, anemia, and erythropoietin resistance are related to high hepcidin levels. **Which one of the following statements is INCORRECT in this patient?**

A. Diabetic patients develop anemia more frequently at earlier stages of CKD than nondiabetic patients
B. ACE-Is cause erythropoietin resistance in all patients irrespective of the etiology of renal disease
C. Iron stimulates hepatic hepcidin expression
D. Hepcidin excess is the underlying cause for low circulating iron, and ferritin levels during inflammation
E. Hypoxia is a potent stimulator of hepcidin expression via hypoxia-inducible factor (HIF)

The answer is E

The cause of anemia in CKD is multifactorial, including relative erythropoietin deficiency, decreased erythrocyte survival, and several uremic toxins inhibiting erythropoiesis. Anemia can be corrected with erythropoiesis-stimulating agents (ESAs). However, 10–20% of patients are poorly responsive to ESAs. There are several causes for poor response to ESA therapy. These include iron deficiency, inflammation, infection, hyperparathyroidism, ACE-I therapy, carnitine deficiency, increased hepcidin levels, and anti-EPO antibodies causing pure red cell aplasia. Angiotensin II (AII) stimulates erythropoiesis, and inhibition of AII causes hyporesponsiveness to ESA therapy. Thus, option B is correct.

Anemia develops in all CKD patients irrespective of the etiology of renal disease. However, in diabetics Hb levels are much lower than nondiabetics at any degree of renal impairment. Several studies have confirmed this observation. Several mechanisms for low Hb levels have been proposed, including hyporeninism, glycation of EPO receptor, impairment of HIF, and cytokine inhibition of erythropoiesis. Thus, option A is correct.

Hepcidin is a hormone with 25 amino acids. It is predominantly secreted by hepatocytes and excreted by the kidney. It inhibits gastrointestinal absorption of iron, and also inhibits iron release from reticuloendothelial cells. Thus, hepcidin regulates systemic iron homeostasis. Mice that lack hepcidin and hepcidin mutations in humans develop severe iron load. Iron administration stimulates hepcidin levels, thus providing a feedback mechanism to prevent iron absorption and load. Thus, option C is correct. In inflammation, hepcidin synthesis is increased to limit iron absorption and its use for erythropoiesis. Thus, option D is correct. On the other hand, anemia and hypoxia inhibit hepcidin synthesis thereby increasing iron availability for erythropoiesis. Thus, option E is incorrect.

Suggested Reading

Babitt JL, Lin HY. Molecular mechanisms of hepcidin regulation: implications for the anemia of CKD. Am J Kidney Dis. 2010;55:726–41.
Deray G, Heurtier A, Grimaldi A, et al. Anemia and diabetes. Am J Nephrol. 2004;24:522–6.
Ganz T, Nemeth E. Iron balance and the role of hepcidin in chronic kidney disease. Semin Nephrol. 2016;36:87–93.
Santos-Silva A, Ribeiro S, Reis F, et al. Hepcidin in chronic kidney disease anemia. Vitam Horm. 2019;110:243–64.

58. A 52-year-old hypertensive man with CKD 3 (eGFR 40 mL/min) is referred to you for evaluation of anemia. Past medical history is significant for occasional use of alcohol. The primary care physician ruled out other causes of anemia, such as GI bleeding and hemoglobinopathies. He is not on iron therapy. His medications include hydrochlorothiazide and lisinopril. His blood pressure is controlled; however, left ventricular hypertrophy (LVH) was documented on echocardiography His hemoglobin (Hgb) is 9.4 g/dL. **Regarding the pathogenesis of his anemia, which one of the following statements is CORRECT?**

A. Decreased production of erythropoietin (EPO)
B. Nutritional deficiency

C. Subclinical inflammation
D. Elevated levels of hepcidin
E. All of the above

The answer is E

According to the KDIGO Guidelines, anemia of CKD is defined as Hgb level <13 g/dL in males and <12 g/dL in females. The prevalence of anemia increases with increases in CKD stages. According to one report, the prevalence of anemia varies from 1.3% in CKD 3, 5.2% in CKD 4–44.1% in CKD 5 stages.

The pathogenesis of anemia in CKD is multifactorial: (1) decreased production of EPO due to decreased renal mass; (2) diet poor in vitamins such as folate, B12, or iron, causing reduced red cell mass and anemia; (3) increased production of proinflammatory cytokines, causing a state of chronic subclinical inflammation; and (4) increased production and decreased excretion of hepcidin, resulting in elevated level of this iron-regulating hormone. Thus, option E is correct.

Suggested Reading

Batchelor EK, Kapitsinou P, Pergola PE, et al. Iron deficiency in chronic kidney disease: updates on pathophysiology, diagnosis, and treatment. J Am Soc Nephrol. 2020;31:456–68.
Gafter-Gvilia A, Schechter A, Rozen-Zvic B. Iron deficiency anemia in chronic kidney disease. Acta Haematol. 2019;142:44–50.
Kidney Disease Improving Global Outcomes. KDIGO clinical practice guideline for anemia in chronic kidney disease. Kidney Int Suppl. 2012;2(4):283–335.

59. The patient's repeat hemoglobin and iron studies became available, and are as follows:

- Hgb= 9.2 g/dL
- Mean corpuscular volume (MCV) = 102 fL (elevated)
- Iron= 30 μg/dL (normal 45–160 μg/dL)
- Total iron-binding capacity (TIBC) = 220 μg/dL (normal 228–428 μg/dL)
- Ferritin= 90 μg/L (normal 15–300 μg/L)
- Transferrin saturation (TSAT) = 13% (normal 20–50%)

Based on the above laboratory values, which one of the following treatment strategies is APPROPRIATE?

A. Oral iron
B. Oral iron and erythropoiesis-stimulating agent (ESA)
C. Intravenous (iv) iron and ESA
D. Oral iron and folate and/or vitamin B12
E. Blood transfusion and folate

The answer is D

The patient has iron deficiency anemia of chronic disease; however, the MCV is high due to deficiency of folate, B12, or both deficiencies. The deficiency of these vitamins and iron seems to be related to insufficient nutrition. Measurement of folate and B12 in this patient with alcohol use is indicated. On the other hand, iron deficiency in CKD patients is common due to a variety of causes, including blood loss, poor iron absorption, inflammation, and elevated levels of hepcidin. Oral iron use alone may not be adequate in this patient (option A).

Oral iron therapy has not been tried in this patient. Therefore, oral iron (ferrous sulfate 325 mg three times daily) to deliver approximately 200 mg of elemental iron should be tried first with 5 mg of folate and/or 100 μg of B12 injection. Oral iron (325 mg equals 65 mg elemental iron) therapy should be continued for 1–3 months with measurement of iron indices. Thus, option D is correct. IV iron can be considered once oral therapy fails. ESA therapy is not indicated at this time (option C). Also, blood transfusion is not indicated (option E).

Suggested Reading

Brugnara C, Eckardt K-U. Hematological aspects of kidney disease. In: Yu ASL, Chertow GM, Luyckx VA, et al., editors. Brenner & Rector's the kidney. 11th ed. Philadelphia: Elsevier, Saunders; 2020. p. 1861–1900.
Kidney Disease Improving Global Outcomes. KDIGO clinical practice guideline for anemia in chronic kidney disease. Kidney Int Suppl. 2012;2(4):283–335.

Macdougall IC, Eckardt K-W. Anemia in chronic kidney disease. In: Feehally J, Floege J, Tonelli M, et al., editors. Comprehensive clinical nephrology. 6th ed. Philadelphia: Elsevier; 2019. p. 958–66.

Pergola PE, Fishbane S, Ganz T. Novel oral iron therapies for iron deficiency anemia in chronic kidney disease. Adv Chronic Kidney Dis. 2019;26:272–91.

Roger SD. Practical considerations for iron therapy in the management of anaemia in patients with chronic kidney disease. Clin Kidney J. 2017;10(Suppl 1):i9–15.

60. The patient comes back 3 months later, and the following laboratory values are available:

- Hemoglobin (Hgb) = 9.5 g/dL
- Mean corpuscular volume (MCV) = 82 fL
- Iron= 32 μg/dL (normal 45–160 μg/dL)
- Total iron-binding capacity (TIBC) = 140 μg/dL (normal 228–428 μg/dL)
- Ferritin= 250 μg/L (normal 15–300 μg/L)
- Transferrin saturation (TSAT) = 23% (normal 20–50%)

Which one of the following treatment strategies is APPROPRIATE to maintain Hgb level between 10.5 and 11.5 g/dL?

A. Continue oral iron only for 6 months
B. Start iv iron and ESA
C. Oral iron and ESA
D. ESA only
E. ESA and antibiotics to improve subclinical infection

The answer is B

The patient has failed on oral iron. Despite normalization of MCV, there is no improvement either in iron or Hgb status. This warrants IV iron therapy, which may increase Hgb concentration, decrease ESA dose, or both. In this patient, the use of both IV iron and ESA administration is justified. Three ESAs are available: (1) epoetin-α or epoetin-β; (2) darbepoetin-α or Aranesp; and (3) methoxy polyethylene glycol epoetin-β or continuous erythropoietin receptor activator (CERA or Mercera). The initial dosage schedule is as follows:

Epoetin-α: 20–50 IU/kg 3 times a week subcutaneously
darbepoetin-α: starting dose 0.45 μg/kg once a week subcutaneously or IV or 0.75 μg/kg every 2 weeks
Mercera: 30–50 μg every 2 weeks or 75 μg every 4 weeks subcutaneously or IV

The dose of each one of these ESAs may change depending on the HgB level. The goal of ESA therapy is to increase Hgb by 1–2 g/dL a month until target level is reached. Avoid correction of Hgb >13 g/dL. Thus, option B is correct. Other options are incorrect.

Suggested Reading

Abramovitz B, Berns JS. Management of anemia in chronic kidney disease. In: Kimmel PL, Rosenberg ME, editors. Chronic renal disease. 2nd ed. London: Academic Press, Elsevier; 2020. p. 991–1000.

Alsalimy N, Awaisu A. Methoxy polyethylene glycol-epoetin beta versus darbepoetin alfa for anemia in non-dialysis-dependent CKD: a systematic review. Int J Clin Pharm. 2014;36:1115–25.

Kidney Disease Improving Global Outcomes. KDIGO clinical practice guideline for anemia in chronic kidney disease. Kidney Int Suppl. 2012;2(4):283–335.

Macdougall IC. Intravenous iron therapy in patients with chronic kidney disease: recent evidence and future directions. Clin Kidney J. 2017;10(Suppl 1):i16–24.

Roger SD. Practical considerations for iron therapy in the management of anaemia in patients with chronic kidney disease. Clin Kidney J. 2017;10(Suppl 1):i9–15.

61. The above patient's Hgb is 12 g/dL after 6 weeks of darbepoetin therapy and says that he read from internet that higher Hgb concentrations are "bad for the heart." **Regarding higher concentration of Hgb (>13 g/dL), which one of the following statements is CORRECT in CKD 3–5 patients?**

A. Hgb >13 g/dL is associated with high cardiovascular events and death
B. Hgb >13 g/dL is associated with high incidence of strokes

C. Hgb >13 g/dL does not improve left ventricular hypertrophy
D. Hgb >13 g/dL is always associated with improvement of quality of life (QOL)
E. A, B, C only

The answer is E

Anemia is a risk factor for cardiovascular disease in CKD patients. Also, poor QOL has been reported in anemic patients. With the introduction of ESAs, it was felt that cardiovascular events and QOL would greatly improve with normalization of Hgb. This assumption was based on improvement of "better feeling" when Hgb was raised to a level of 10 g/dL from severe anemic level (<8 g/dL). However, clinical trials in both predialysis and dialysis patients do not support a cardiovascular benefit with normal or near normalization of Hgb. There are three clinical trials in predialysis patients. In the CHOIR (the Correction of Hemoglobin and Outcomes in Renal Insufficiency) trial, 1,432 patients with CKD (eGFR between 15 and 50 mL/min) and a Hgb <11 g/dL were randomly assigned to a high (13.5 g/dL) or low (11.3 g/dL) using epoetin-α. However, the achieved Hgb level in the higher group was 12.6 g/dL and 11.3 g/dL in the lower group. The primary endpoint was the composite of death, myocardial infarction, stroke, and hospitalization for heart failure. The study had to be terminated early (median of 16 months) because of significant higher number of all cardiovascular events in the higher Hgb group. No difference in the rate of progression to ESKD was observed between the two Hgb target groups. Also, no improvement in QOL was noted in the higher Hb group.

The CREATE (the Cardiovascular risk Reduction by Early Treatment with Epoetin-beta) trial randomized 603 patients with eGFR between 15 and 35 mL/min to either a higher Hgb (13 to 15 g/dL) or a lower Hgb (10.5 to 11.5 g/dL) groups. The achieved Hgb levels were 13.5 and 11.5 g/dL, respectively. The primary endpoint was a composite of 8 cardiovascular events. At 3 years, there was no difference in the primary endpoint between the groups, although a trend toward the higher event rate was observed in the higher Hb group. In contrast to the CHOIR trial, an improvement in the QOL was observed in the higher Hgb arm.

In the TREAT (the Trial of Reduction of End points with Aranesp Therapy) study, 4,038 type 2 diabetic patients with eGFR between 20 and 60 mL/min and anemia (≤11 g/dL) were randomly assigned to receive darbepoetin-α to achieve a Hgb level of 13 g/dL or placebo. Darbepoetin was used as a rescue therapy in the placebo group if Hgb is <9 g/dL until Hb reached >9 g/dL and then stopped. The mean achieved Hgb levels were 12.5 g/dL and 10.6 g/dL in the treated and placebo groups, respectively. The primary endpoint was the composite of death or a cardiovascular event and of death and ESKD. At a median of 29 months follow-up, there was no difference in deaths or cardiovascular events between the groups. However, an increase in fatal or nonfatal stroke was observed in darbepoetin group (101 versus 53 patients). Also, an increase in the risk of death due to malignancy, primarily in patients with history of malignancy, was observed in darbepoetin group. QOL in terms of fatigue was better in higher Hb group. Blood transfusion was more common in placebo arm (496 versus 297 patients.

These three important trials had different results with high Hgb levels, although all of them point to better adverse events with low Hgb levels (10.5–11.5 g/dL). Also, the evaluation of QOL measures was not uniform. Several meta-analyses have arrived at similar conclusions. Thus, option D is incorrect.

Although several small studies in hemodialysis patients have shown regression of LVH with improvement in anemia, many large studies failed to confirm this observation in CKD patients. Thus, option E is correct.

Suggested Reading

Drüeke TB, Locatelli F, Clyne N, et al. Normalization of hemoglobin level in patients with chronic kidney disease and anemia. N Engl J Med. 2006;355:2071–84.
Kidney Disease Improving Global Outcomes. KDIGO clinical practice guideline for anemia in chronic kidney disease. Kidney Int Suppl. 2012;2(4):283–335.
Palmer SC, Navaneethan SD, Craig JC, et al. Meta-analysis: erythropoiesis-stimulating agents in patients with chronic kidney disease. Ann Intern Med. 2010;153:23–33.
Pfeffer MA, Burdmann EA, Chen CY, et al. A trial of darbepoetin alfa in type 2 diabetes and chronic kidney disease. N Engl J Med. 2009;361:2019–32.
Singh AK, Szczech L, Tang KL, et al. Correction of anemia with epoetin alfa in chronic kidney disease. N Engl J Med. 2006;355:2085–98.

62. The above patient received iron sucrose (1 g in 8 weeks) and darbepoetin (60 μg subcutaneously once in 2 weeks for 8 weeks), and Hgb as well as iron indices improved. He had pneumonia 1 week after completion of his Hgb protocol. Laboratory values in the hospital show the following:

White blood cell count= 14,000
Hgb= 10.4 g/dL (11.5 g/dL 1 week ago)
Iron= 42 μg/dL (normal 45–160 μg/dL)
Total iron-binding capacity (TIBC)= 240 μg/dL (normal 228–428 μg/dL)
Ferritin= 650 μg/L (normal 15–300 μg/L)
Transferrin saturation (TSAT)= 17% (normal 20–50%)

The above laboratory values suggest which one of the following types of iron deficiency?

A. Absolute iron deficiency
B. Functional iron deficiency
C. Reticuloendothelial blockade
D. All of the above
E. None of the above

The answer is C

Iron deficiency in CKD 3–5 patients can be classified into three categories: (1) absolute (true) iron deficiency; (2) functional iron deficiency; and (3) reticuloendothelial blockade. Absolute iron deficiency results from blood loss, which requires evaluation for occult blood loss from GI tract and other sources. This type of deficiency is characterized by low serum iron, low ferritin levels, and low TSAT. Hepcidin levels are also low, and anemia responds to iron and ESA. Another distinct entity of iron deficiency, called functional iron deficiency, is characterized by low serum iron, low TSAT with normal to high iron (ferritin) stores. ESA treatment is the most important cause of functional iron deficiency. The third type of iron deficiency is called reticuloendothelial blockade. It is characterized by low serum iron, increased ferritin, normal TSAT, and increased hepcidin levels. Reticuloendothelial blockade occurs in patients with inflammation and/or infection. Infection or inflammation also lowers transferrin levels (TIBC), causing normal to high TSAT. Hepcidin blocks the release of stored iron from hepatocytes and macrophages (reticuloendothelial system) by reducing ferroportin action. This type of iron deficiency does not respond to either iron or ESA. Therefore, lowering hepcidin levels and elimination of the cause of infection or inflammation may improve anemia. This patient has reticuloendothelial blockade (see Table 4.8) due to infection. Therefore, option C is correct.

Table 4.8 Types of iron deficiency in CKD patients

Deficiency state	Serum iron	TSAT	Serum ferritin	ESA response	Iron response	Serum hepcidin	Clinical setting
Absolute deficiency	↓	↓	↓	↑	↑	↓*	Blood loss
Functional deficiency	↓	↓	N↑	↓	N	↑	ESA treatment
Reticuloendothe-lial blockade	↓	N	↑	↓	↓	↑	Inflammation

↑ increase ↓ decrease N normal ESA erythropoiesis-stimulating agents; * decreased relative to functional deficiency.

Suggested Reading

Gafter-Gvilia A, Schechter A, Rozen-Zvic B. Iron deficiency anemia in chronic kidney disease. Acta Haematol. 2019;142:44–50.

Macdougall IC. Anemia. In: Daugirdas JT, editor. Handbook of chronic kidney disease management. 2nd ed. Philadelphia: Lippincott Williams & Wilkins; 2019. p. 365–89.

63. **Hyporesponsiveness to ESA therapy has been described not only in infectious (inflammation) state, but also in other conditions. Which one of the following conditions is associated with ESA hyporesponsiveness?**

A. Iron deficiency
B. Pure red cell aplasia
C. Use of ACE-Is (angiotensin-converting enzyme inhibitors)
D. Hyperparathyroidism
E. All of the above

The answer is E

Hyporesponsiveness to ESA therapy is considered when the Hgb concentration remains below 11 g/dL despite increasing doses of ESA. Approximately 5–10% of patients with CKD develop hyporesponsiveness to ESAs. The major causes of ESA resistance are iron deficiency and infection or inflammation in CKD 3–5 patients. In addition, underdialysis in hemodialysis patients is a major reason for ESA resistance. Other causes include primary bone marrow failure (pure red cell aplasia), ACE-Is or angiotensin receptor blockers (ARBs), hyperparathyroidism, folate and B12 deficiency, aluminum toxicity, and hemolysis. Option E, therefore, is correct.

Angiotensin II seems to stimulate red cell production. Therefore, ACE-Is or ARBs may cause ESA resistance. These drugs should not be stopped in view of their several beneficial effects in both predialysis and hemodialysis patients. Increasing the ESA dose may be sufficient, if anemia does not improve due to ACE-Is or ARBs.

It has been suggested that administration of pentoxifylline, 400 mg daily, may improve Hgb during states of infection or inflammation.

Suggested Reading

Johnson DW, Pollock CA, Macdougall IC. Erythropoiesis-stimulating agent hyporesponsiveness. Nephrology. 2007;12:321–30.

Kidney Disease Improving Global Outcomes. KDIGO clinical practice guideline for anemia in chronic kidney disease. Kidney Int Suppl. 2012;2(4):283–335.

Ogawa T, Nitta K. Erythropoiesis-stimulating agent hyporesponsiveness in end-stage renal disease patients. Contrib Nephrol. Basel, Karger. 2015;185:76–86.

64. A 54-year-old diabetic man is referred to you for evaluation of increasing serum creatinine levels. He has history of hypertension and hyperlipidemia. His medications are lisinopril (40 mg/day), hydrochlorothiazide (25 mg/day), and atorvastatin (80 mg). He complains of weakness and muscle ache. His liver function tests are normal, but creatine kinase is mildly elevated. His primary care physician attributes this weakness and myopathy to statin. His current eGFR is 40 mL/min, which decreased from 44 mL/min 3 months ago. **With regard to statin use in this patient, which one of the following statements is FALSE?**

A. Lower the dose of atorvastatin to 40 mg/day
B. Statins have been shown to improve cardiovascular morbidity and mortality in CKD
C. Discontinue atorvastatin as his eGFR is decreasing
D. Statins do not have any cardioprotection in hemodialysis patients
E. Change atorvastatin to another statin will not help his myopathy

The answer is C

CKD 3–5 stages are associated with lipid abnormalities. All CKD guidelines suggest monitoring of total cholesterol, LDL-cholesterol, HDL-cholesterol, and triglycerides in all patients. The KDIGO guideline for lipid management in CKD recommends statin or statin/ezetimibe to the following subjects, who are not on dialysis or received transplantation:

1. **Adults aged ≥50 years with eGFR < 60 mL/min.**
2. **Adults aged ≥50 years with CKD and eGFR ≥60 mL/min.**
3. **Adults aged 18–49 years with CKD should have statin treatment, if they have one or more of the following conditions:**

A. **Known coronary disease (myocardial infarction or coronary revascularization)**
B. **Diabetes mellitus**
C. **Prior ischemic stroke**
D. **Estimated 10-year incidence of coronary death or nonfatal myocardial infarction >10%**

4. **Patients on dialysis should not receive either statin or statin/ezetimibe unless they have been receiving these drugs prior to initiation of dialysis.**
5. **Adults with kidney transplantation should receive statin.**

A number of studies have shown that predialysis patients benefit from statin use. Several meta-analyses suggested that statins decrease all-cause and cardiovascular mortality in CKD 3–5 patients not on dialysis. Statins do not prevent cardiovascular morbidity and mortality in hemodialysis patients. Although statins are beneficial in transplant patients, a meta-analysis evaluation showed uncertain effects.

Myopathy and an increase in creatine kinase levels are rather common in statin users. These abnormalities will improve with discontinuation of statin. However, the risk-benefit ratio should be evaluated before discontinuation of the drug in patients with risk factors. Dose should be reduced in those with severe kidney insufficiency. Changing one statin to another will not help myopathy in many patients. In the above patient reducing atorvastatin to 40 mg/day is appropriate, but discontinuation of a statin is inappropriate. Thus, option C is false.

The cost-effectiveness of statins for primary cardiovascular prevention in CKD patients has recently been evaluated. Patients at lower risk for cardiovascular disease, statins obtained at average retail prices are less cost-effective than generic statins obtained at $4 a month. Thus, judicious use of statins is advised in patients at low risk for cardiovascular disease.

Suggested Reading

Barylski M, Nikfar S, Mikhalidis DP, et al. Statins decrease all-cause mortality only in CKD patients not requiring dialysis therapy: a meta-analysis of 11 randomized controlled trials involving 21,295 patients. Pharmacol Res. 2013;72:35–44.

Cholesterol Treatment Trialists' (CTT) Collaboration, Herrington WG, Emberson J, Mihaylova B, et al. Impact of renal function on the effects of LDL cholesterol lowering with statin-based regimens: a meta-analysis of individual participant data from 28 randomised trials. Lancet Diabetes Endocrinol. 2016;4:829–39.

Erickson KF, Japa S, Owens DK, et al. Cost-effectiveness of statins for primary cardiovascular prevention in chronic kidney disease. J Am Coll Cardiol. 2013;61:1250–8.

Kalaitzidis RG, Elisaf M. The role of statins in chronic kidney disease. Am J Nephrol. 2011;34:195–202.

Kidney Disease Improving Global Outcomes. KDIGO clinical practice guideline for lipid management in chronic kidney disease. Kidney Int Suppl. 2013;3:259–305.

Navaneethan SD, Hegbrant J, Strippoli GFM. Role of statins in preventing adverse cardiovascular outcomes in patients with chronic kidney disease. Curr Opin Nephrol Hypertens. 2011;20:146–52.

Palmer SC, Craig JC, Navaneethan SD, et al. Benefits and harms of statin therapy for persons with chronic kidney disease. A systematic review and meta-analysis. Ann Intern Med. 2012;157:263–75.

65. A 62-year-old woman with CKD 4 with an eGFR of 18 mL/min is found to have prolonged bleeding (10 min) following blood drawing. Her hemoglobin is 9.2 g/dL. You tell her that her platelet function is not normal because of kidney failure. **Which one of the following abnormalities accounts for her platelet dysfunction?**

A. Dysfunction of glycoprotein IIb/IIIa
B. Reduced platelet release of ADP and serotonin
C. Decreased platelet release of thromboxane A_2
D. Abnormal interaction between platelets and endothelium of the vessel wall
E. All of the above

The answer is E

Abnormal bleeding is common in advanced CKD stages. It has been reported in 24–50% of patients with CKD or on hemodialysis. Bleeding occurs in the presence of normal platelet count and other coagulation factors. Therefore, bleeding diathesis is due to platelet dysfunction.

Platelet dysfunction is caused by both intrinsic platelet abnormalities and extrinsic factors (Table 4.9). Evidence for platelet dysfunction includes elevated bleeding time, and diminished aggregation in response to ADP and epinephrine as well as abnormal interaction between platelets and endothelium of blood vessel wall.

Table 4.9 Intrinsic and extrinsic contributors of bleeding in CKD

Intrinsic	Extrinsic
Dysfunction of glycoprotein IIb/IIIa	Anemia
Reduced platelet release of ADP and serotonin	Uremic toxins
Abnormal prostaglandin metabolism and decreased thromboxane A2 generation	Abnormal interaction between platelets and endothelium of vessel wall
Abnormal platelet cytoskeleton assembly and function	Abnormal vWF function
	Increased NO production

The levels of platelet aggregation agonists such as serotonin and ADP are reduced in CKD. Platelet Ca^{2+} is increased in CKD 5–5D, but its mobilization is decreased in response to stimulants, causing less aggregation. Prostaglandin metabolism is altered in CKD, causing an increase in vasodilatory prostacyclin and a decrease in thromboxane A_2 with resultant platelet dysfunction. Also, there is an increase in NO levels, causing decreased platelet aggregation.

The quantity of platelet cytoskeleton proteins and their assembly are reduced in CKD, causing less cellular mobility and contraction. In addition, defects in adhesion receptors, namely, glycoprotein (Gp) Ib and Gp IIb/IIIb complex, have been described. As a result, the adhesion of platelets to vascular endothelium is disturbed.

Anemia plays an important role in platelet function and bleeding. During normal circulation, red blood cells (RBCs) tend to distribute toward the endothelial surface. When there is endothelial injury, platelets that are close to the vessel wall are activated, and subsequently aggregated to form a hemostatic plug. RBCs also participate in activation of platelets by releasing ADP and thromboxane A_2. With anemia, more platelets circulate in the center and away from the endothelial surface. As a result, platelet activation in hindered and prolonged bleeding occurs. Correction of anemia improves bleeding in CKD 5–5D.

Uremic toxins are shown to cause platelet dysfunction. When normal plasma was mixed with uremic platelets, platelet function improved. On the other hand, when uremic plasma was mixed with normal platelets, platelet dysfunction was observed. These studies suggest that uremic toxins play an important role in uremic bleeding. Thus, answer E is correct.

Suggested Reading

Dager WE, Kiser TH. Systemic anticoagulation considerations in chronic kidney disease. Adv Chronic Kidney Dis. 2010;17:420–7.

Kaw D, Malhotra D. Platelet dysfunction and end-stage renal disease. Semin Dial. 2006;19:317–22.

Lutz J, Menkel J, Sollinger D, et al. Haemostasis in chronic kidney disease. Nephrol Dial Transplant. 2014;29:29–40.

Pavord S, Myers B. Bleeding and thrombotic complications of kidney disease. Blood Rev. 2011;25:271–8.

66. **In the above patient, which one of the following is APPROPRIATE in the management of her bleeding?**

A. Blood transfusion
B. Desmopressin (DDAVP) 0.3–0.4 μg/kg iv or subcutaneously (sc)
C. Cryoprecipitate
D. Start hemodialysis
E. Start erythropoietin

The answer is B

This patient has prolonged bleeding time without uremic symptoms, which can be corrected by administration DDAVP, which is a synthetic product of vasopressin. One dose either iv or sc can correct her bleeding time. Intranasal form also is available. The mechanism of action of DDAVP is related to a reduction of protein C and PAI-1 and an increase of vWF and factor VIII. Thus, answer B is correct.

Blood transfusion and cryoprecipitate (contains substantial amounts of vWF, factor VIII, and fibrinogen) can be reserved for acute bleeding or the patient requires surgery (A and C are incorrect). Although hemodialysis can improve uremic bleeding, it is not a good option for this patient at this time (D is incorrect). Starting erythropoietin after checking iron and ferritin levels is an ideal option for this patient; however, it takes 2–3 weeks to achieve Hgb concentration above 10.0 g/dL (E is incorrect). Maintaining Hgb between 10.0 and 11.5 g/dL improves bleeding time.

Other options for improving chronic bleeding are tranexamic acid and conjugated estrogens. Tranexamic acid inhibits fibrinolysis by forming a reversible complex with plasminogen and preventing its conversion to plasmin. It can be given orally or iv. Conjugated estrogens can be given iv, orally, or transdermally.

Suggested Reading

Hedges SJ, Dehoney SB, Hooper JS, et al. Evidence-based treatment recommendations for uremic bleeding. Nat Clin Pract Nephrol. 2007;3:138–53.

Lutz J, Menke J, Sollinger D, et al. Haemostasis in chronic kidney disease. Nephrol Dial Transplant. 2014;29:29–40.

67. A 38-year-old Caucasian woman with type 2 diabetes and proteinuria (500 mg/day) is on an angiotensin receptor blocker (ARB). She could not tolerate ACE-I because of cough and rash. She has no adverse effects with any ARB, and her proteinuria decreased to 150 mg/day. She found from the internet that ARBs cause cancer and says that she has a family history of breast cancer. **Which one of the following statements is INCORRECT regarding the association between ARBs and cancer?**

    A. Initial study with candesartan showed increased risk for all types of cancer
    B. Activation of AT2 receptors may play a role in carcinogenesis
    C. Both ARBs and ACE-Is were found to decrease cancer risk in experimental animals
    D. The FDA reports no increased risk of new cancer with ARB treatment
    E. All meta-analyses to date show an association between ARB use and cancer

    The answer is E

    In 2003, Pfeffer et al. observed an increased number of new cancers in patients treated with candesartan for chronic heart failure compared to placebo group. Subsequent studies also showed an association between ARBs and cancer. This prompted Sipahi et al. to analyze several studies in a meta-analysis and concluded that ARB use is associated with increased risk of new cancer. Subsequent meta-analysis by the FDA, which included 31 randomized trials concluded that ARBs are not associated with increased risk of new cancer. Thus, the FDA drug safety communication states that "treatment with an ARB medication does not increase a patient's risk of developing cancer." Another meta-analysis concluded that ARBs are not associated with increased risk of cancer. The FDA will continue to monitor ARBs for emerging safety issues. Thus, only one meta-analysis showed an association, but the remaining two meta-analyses did not show any association between ARBs and cancer. Therefore, option E is incorrect.

    Angiotensin is a growth factor, causing cell proliferation and angiogenesis. Blockade of renin-angiotensin-aldosterone axis in experimental animals with ARBs or ACE-Is has suggested decreased risk of cancer (option C). Also, it was suggested that blockade of AT1 receptor by ARBs would preferentially activate AT2 receptor, which may promote tumor growth (option B). The available data do not support the role of ARBs in the development of new cancer.

    Suggested Reading

Pfeffer MA, Swedberg K, Granger CB, et al. Effects of candesartan on mortality and morbidity in patients with chronic heart failure: the CHARM-Overall programme. Lancet. 2003;362:759–66.

Sipahi I, Debanne SM, Rowland DY, et al. Angiotensin-receptor blockade and risk of cancer: meta-analysis of randomised controlled trials. Lancet Oncol. 2010;11:627–36.

US Food and Drug Administration: FDA drug safety communication: no increase in risk of cancer with certain BP drugs – angiotensin receptor blockers (ARBs). Available at: http://www.fda.gov/Drugs/Drug Safety/ucm257516.htm.

68. A 44-year-old man with history of hypertensive nephrosclerosis and CKD 3b (eGFR 30–44 mL/min) is found to have hyperchloremic metabolic acidosis with serum [HCO_3^-] of 18 mEq/L. He asks you about his renal progression due to his chronic acidosis. **Which one of the following mechanisms is implicated in the pathogenesis of metabolic acidosis-related renal progression?**

    A. Increased NH_3 genesis
    B. Endothelin-induced H^+ secretion and tubulointerstitial fibrosis
    C. Enhanced HCO_3^- generation with subsequent alkalinization of interstitium and precipitation of Ca^{2+} salts
    D. Activation of renin-angiotensin (AII)-aldosterone system
    E. All of the above

    The answer is E

    All of the above mechanisms contribute to the progression of renal disease in CKD. Hyperchloremic metabolic acidosis is rather common in patients with CKD 3–5 with serum [HCO_3^-] in the range of 12–23 mEq/L. Although many patients are asymptomatic, even slightly lower than normal serum [HCO_3^-] of 24 mEq/L may have profound adverse effects on several organs, including the kidney. First, metabolic acidosis stimulates the production of NH_3, which activates the alternative complement pathway and causes tubulointerstitial fibrosis. Second, metabolic acidosis increases endothelin production, which promotes tubulointerstitial fibrosis (via ET-A receptor) as

well as H^+ secretion (ET-B receptor). Third, it has also been suggested that new HCO_3^- is generated in response to metabolic acidosis, and this new HCO_3^- alkalinizes the interstitium, promoting the precipitation of Ca^{2+} salts and fibrosis. Finally, metabolic acidosis activates renin-AII-aldosterone system with resultant proteinuria, kidney damage, and deterioration in GFR. Thus, option E is correct.

Suggested Reading

Goraya N, Wesson DE. Does correction of metabolic acidosis slow chronic kidney disease progression? Curr Opin Nephrol Hypertens. 2013;22:193–97.

Kovesdy CP. Metabolic acidosis and kidney disease: does bicarbonate therapy slow the progression of CKD? Nephrol Dial Transplant. 2012;27:3056–62.

Kraut JA, Madias NE. Consequences and therapy of metabolic acidosis of chronic kidney disease. Pediatr Nephrol. 2011;26:19–28.

Navaneethan SD, Shao J, Buysse J, et al. Effects of treatment of metabolic acidosis in CKD. A systematic review and meta-analysis. Clin J Am Soc Nephrol. 2019;14:1011–20.

69. Besides kidney damage, chronic metabolic acidosis induces several other adverse effects in CKD patients. **Which one of the following is NOT an observed adverse effect of metabolic acidosis?**

A. Growth retardation in children
B. Exacerbation of bone disease
C. Reduced albumin synthesis
D. Stimulation of proinflammatory cytokine production
E. Maintenance of normal muscle protein

The answer is E

It has been clearly established that renal tubular acidosis causes growth retardation in children. Both bone mineralization and density are reduced in children with acidosis, and base therapy improves bone growth. Chronic acidosis stimulates PTH secretion and reduces vitamin D levels. At the same time, acidosis counteracts the effects of PTH. It is this counterbalance that may be responsible for changes in bone histomorphometry in acidosis. Animal studies have shown that chronic acidosis produces osteoporosis and exacerbates osteitis fibrosa cystica.

Reduced albumin synthesis has been reported in humans with acidosis, causing hypoalbuminemia. Supply of base either orally or during hemodialysis improved albumin levels and protein catabolic rate. Increased production of TNF-α has been reported in chronic metabolic acidosis, and treatment of acidosis reduced levels of this proinflammatory cytokine.

Muscle wasting in patients with metabolic acidosis and CKD is well known. This is due to decreased protein synthesis and increased protein degradation (see Table 4.10 for detailed mechanisms of adverse effect of metabolic acidosis). Thus, option E is incorrect.

Table 4.10 Mechanisms of adverse effects of metabolic acidosis

Adverse effect	Mechanism
Muscle wasting	Due to muscle protein degradation mediated by upregulation of ubiquitin-proteosome pathway and caspase-3 protease. Acidosis activates glucocorticoid effect on protein degradation. However, total protein synthesis is not affected. Administration of base improves lean body mass
Hypoalbuminemia	Chronic acidosis was found to decrease albumin synthesis as opposed to muscle total protein synthesis. Hypoalbuminemia has been reported in CKD patients with low GFR and HCO_3^- levels. Administration of base to CKD patients improves albumin levels
Progression of kidney disease	Several studies have shown progression of kidney disease in patients with lower serum HCO_3^- levels. Potential mechanisms include an increase in AII, aldosterone, and endothelin levels, which promote renal fibrosis. Increased NH_4^+ genesis by the surviving nephrons activate complement and inflammation with resultant fibrosis. Chronic acidosis may activate growth factors, cytokines, and chemokines that promote renal fibrosis. It should be noted that renal tubular acidosis may not be associated with progression of kidney disease
Bone disease	Not only abnormal vitamin D metabolism but also chronic acidosis causes bone disease in CKD. Kidney disease alone increases PTH and decreases calcitriol levels. Both cause release of Ca^{2+} salts from bone with resultant development of osteomalacia and renal osteodystrophy. Acidosis also stimulates PTH secretion. Bone buffers H^+ in CKD with resultant decrease in bone minerals. Thus, chronic metabolic acidosis contributes to bone disease

(continued)

Table 4.10 (continued)

Adverse effect	Mechanism
Insulin resistance	Insulin action is decreased in metabolic acidosis because of decreased insulin binding to its receptor. Thus, glucose intolerance is common in CKD
Growth hormone, IGF-1 and thyroid hormones	Chronic acidosis lowers levels of these hormones in CKD. Blunted IGF-1 response to growth hormone has been reported
Increased inflammation	Acidosis stimulates the release of proinflammatory cytokines from macrophages
Cardiac contractility	Severe acidosis impairs cardiac contractility via less Ca^{2+} binding to troponin and disturbed interaction between actin and myosin

Suggested Reading

Goraya N, Wesson DE. Clinical evidence that treatment of metabolic acidosis slows the progression of chronic kidney disease. Curr Opin Nephrol Hypertens. 2019;98:267–77.

Kraut JA, Madias NE. Metabolic acidosis of CKD: an update. Am J Kidney Dis. 2016;67:307–17.

Wesson DE, editor. Metabolic acidosis. A guide to clinical assessment and management. New York: Springer; 2016.

70. **Which one of the following drugs improves serum [HCO3$^-$] by binding intestinal HCl in the patient with metabolic acidosis?**

A. $NaHCO_3$
B. Na citrate
C. Na phosphate
D. Veverimer
E. K citrate

The answer is D

Veverimer is a novel, non-absorbed polymer that is introduced to treat metabolic acidosis. It binds HCl in the gastrointestinal tract and removes it from the body in the feces. As a result, serum [HCO_3^-] increases and acid load decreases in a CKD patient with metabolic acidosis. Veverimer is given orally as a suspension in water.

In a multicenter, randomized, blinded, placebo-controlled study, Wesson et al. evaluated the effect of veverimer (6 g/day) in CKD patients with eGFR of 20–40 mL/min/1.73 m^2 and serum [HCO_3^-] of 12–20 mEq/L, and reported a mean increase of 4 mEq/L in serum [HCO_3^-] over a 52-week period, as compared with placebo group. All patients tolerated the drug well with minimal adverse effects. Thus, veverimer seems to be a useful drug to improve metabolic acidosis in patients with CKD 3b-4. Thus, answer D is correct.

Other drugs do not bind HCl in the gastrointestinal tract. Thus, answers A, B, C, and E are incorrect.

Suggested Reading

Wesson DE, Mathur V, Tangri N, et al. Long-term safety and efficacy of veverimer in patients with metabolic acidosis in chronic kidney disease: a multicentre, randomised, blinded, placebo-controlled, 40-week extension. Lancet. 2019;394:396–406.

Wesson DE, Mathur V, Tangri N, et al. Veverimer versus placebo in patients with metabolic acidosis associated with chronic kidney disease: a multicentre, randomised, double-blind, controlled, phase 3 trial. Lancet. 2019;393:1417–27.

71. **A 56-year-old woman with CKD 4 due to hypertension and serum [HCO_3^-] of 18 mEq/L would benefit from which one of the following interventions?**

A. Protein intake of 1 g/kg/day
B. Reduction in total calorie intake
C. $NaHCO_3$ 650 mg/day
D. $NaHCO_3$ and fruits to raise serum [HCO_3^-] to >30 mEq/L
E. Fruit and vegetable diet to raise serum [HCO_3^-] to 23–26 mEq/L

The answers is E

Several studies have shown that treatment of metabolic acidosis with alkali ($NaHCO_3$, Na or K citrate, $CaCO_3$) slows kidney progression and GFR decline rate. Protein intake of 1 g/kg/day provides acid load and lowers serum

[HCO_3^-] even further. Reducing calorie intake does not improve mild acidosis in this patient. $NaHCO_3$ 600 mg/day may be insufficient to raise serum [HCO_3^-] to the desired level of 23–26 mEq/L Raising serum [HCO_3^-] to >30 mEq/L is not advisable because of development of metabolic alkalosis and its consequences. Thus, options A to D are incorrect.

Studies from Wesson et al. have suggested that ad libitum intake of base-inducing fruits (oranges, apples, apricots, peaches, pears, strawberries, raisins) and vegetables (potatoes, tomatoes, carrots, cauliflower, eggplant, lettuce, spinach) raised serum [HCO_3^-] and improved metabolic acidosis after 1 year of treatment. Also, markers of kidney injury were lower after fruit and vegetable diet. Serum [K^+] was not affected. Thus, fruit and vegetable diet improves metabolic acidosis and reduces kidney damage in CKD 4 patients without producing hyperkalemia.

Suggested Reading

Goraya N, Simoni J, Jo C, et al. Dietary acid reduction with fruits and vegetables or bicarbonate attenuates kidney injury in patients with a moderately reduced glomerular filtration rates due to hypertensive nephropathy. Kidney Int. 2012;81:86–93.

Goraya N, Wesson DE. Does correction of metabolic acidosis slow chronic kidney disease progression? Curr Opin Nephrol Hypertens. 2013;22:193–7.

Goraya N, Simoni J, Jo C, et al. A comparison of treating metabolic acidosis in CKD stage 4 hypertensive kidney disease with fruits and vegetables or sodium bicarbonate. Clin J Am Soc Nephrol. 2013;8:371–81.

72. Low dietary Na^+ or salt intake (<90 mEq/day) has been shown to prevent progression of kidney disease. **Which one of the following effects is NOT related to Na^+ restriction?**

A. Reduction in blood pressure
B. Reduction in proteinuria
C. Improvement in renin-AII-aldosterone system
D. Potentiation of diuretic and ACE-I effect
E. Reduction in "salt sensitivity" in CKD patients

The answer is C

Salt restriction stimulates renin-AII-aldosterone system probably related to mild volume depletion. Therefore, option C is incorrect. Salt restriction has several benefits. It lowers blood pressure, proteinuria, potentiates the diuretic and ACE-I activity, and improves the so-called salt sensitivity of CKD patients. Restriction of dietary Na^+ to <90 mEq/day is recommended for CKD 1–4. Note that 1 g Na^+ equals 44 mEq, whereas 1 g salt (NaCl) diet equals 17 mEq.

Suggested Reading

Goraya N, Wesson DE. Dietary approaches to kidney diseases. In: Yu ASL, Chertow GM, Luyckx VA, et al., editors. Brenner & Rector's the kidney. 11th ed. Philadelphia: Elsevier, Saunders; 2020. p. 1977–88.

Humalda JK, Navis G. Dietary sodium restriction: a neglected therapeutic opportunity in chronic kidney disease (review). Curr Opin Nephrol Hypertens. 2014;23:533–40.

Turban S, Miller ER III. Sodium and potassium intake. In: Daugirdas JT, editor. Handbook of chronic kidney disease management. 2nd ed. Philadelphia: Lippincott Williams & Wilkins; 2019. p. 74–86.

Wilcox CS. Dietary salt intake for patients with hypertension or kidney disease. In: Mitch WE, Ikizler TA, editors. Handbook of nutrition and the kidney. 6th ed. Philadelphia: Lippincott Williams & Wilkins; 2010. p. 233–42.

73. **With regard to K^+ intake and CKD, which one of the following statements is INCORRECT?**

A. High K^+ diet lowers blood pressure
B. High K^+ diet prevents progression of kidney disease
C. Chronic hypokalemia promotes kidney disease and renal cyst formation
D. Restriction of K^+ in diet to <30 mEq/day is recommended in CKD patients to prevent hyperkalemia.
E. High K^+ diet reduces kidney stone formation

The answer is D

There is no upper limit of K^+ intake in healthy subjects with normal kidney function, as almost all ingested K^+ is excreted in the urine. The KDOQI group recommends at least 4 g (102 mEq) of K^+ for CKD 1–2 patients (note that 1 g K equals 25.5 mEq). In CKD 3–4 patients, the recommended K^+ intake is 50–102 mEq/day. K^+ is usually restricted in patients with GFR <20 mL/min or in patients with type 4 RTA with hyperkalemia. Thus, option D is incorrect.

High K^+ diet lowers blood pressure and prevents kidney damage. The diet rich in K^+ reduces the risk for stroke and other cardiovascular disease. The risk for stone formation is also reduced with intake of high dietary K^+ intake. Low K^+ diet promotes kidney disease and cyst formation, probably due to increased oxidative stress and inflammation. K^+ supplementation has been shown to improve these abnormalities.

Suggested Reading

Mandayam SA, Mitch WE, Kopple JD. Dietary factors in the treatment of chronic kidney disease. In: Coffman TM, Falk RJ, Molitoris BA, et al., editors. Schrier's diseases of the kidney. 9th ed. Philadelphia: Wolters Kluwer/Lippincott Williams & Wilkins; 2013. p. 2506–44.

Staruschenko A. Beneficial effects of high potassium. Contribution of renal basolateral K+ channels. Hypertension. 2018;71:1015–22.

Turban S, Miller ER III. Sodium and potassium intake. In: Daugirdas JT, editor. Handbook of chronic kidney disease management. 2nd ed. Philadelphia: Lippincott Williams & Wilkins; 2019. p. 74–86.

74. A 27-year-old Caucasian man with type 1 diabetes for 20 years and progressive CKD with serum creatinine of 2.2 mg/dL (eGFR 44 mL/min) and proteinuria of 3.5 g/day is referred to you for evaluation and management of his nephrotic syndrome. His glycated HbA1c is 6.5% with a blood pressure of 130/80 mm Hg. He is on an ACE-I. He has normal dietary protein intake (>1.5 g/kg/day) and weighs 70 kg. **Regarding his proteinuria and kidney function, which one of the following statements is CORRECT?**

A. Advise the patient to have an A-V access for early dialysis
B. Increase dietary protein intake to compensate for worsening proteinuria
C. No adjustment in dietary protein intake at this time
D. Restrict his dietary protein intake to 0.6 g/kg/day
E. Add an angiotensin receptor blocker (ARB) to his ACE-I

The answer is D

There is substantial evidence that high protein diet induces renal vasodilation, resulting in an increase in renal blood flow, GFR, and proteinuria in diabetic patients. Thus, high protein diet in this patient increases his proteinuria. On the other hand, several studies and meta-analyses have shown that low protein diet reduces renal blood flow, GFR, and proteinuria in both diabetic and nondiabetic patients. The recommended dietary protein intake in patients with nephrotic syndrome is 0.6 g/kg/day. Thus, option D is correct. Creating an A-V access at this time is premature and not warranted. Also, adding an ARB to an ACE-I is not suggested at this time because of high incidence of acute kidney injury and hyperkalemia.

Suggested Reading

Fried L, Emanuele N, Zang JH, et al. Combined angiotensin inhibition for the treatment of diabetic nephropathy. N Engl J Med. 2013;369:1892–1903.

Goraya N, Wesson DE. Dietary approaches to kidney diseases. In: Yu ASL, Chertow GM, Luyckx VA, et al., editors. Brenner & Rector's the kidney. 11th ed. Philadelphia: Elsevier, Saunders; 2020. p. 1977–88.

Mandayam SA, Mitch WE, Kopple JD. Dietary factors in the treatment of chronic kidney disease. In: Coffman TM, Falk RJ, Molitoris BA, et al., editors. Schrier's diseases of the kidney. 9th ed. Philadelphia: Wolters Kluwer/Lippincott Williams & Wilkins; 2013. p. 2506–44.

75. You instructed the above patient to follow a low protein diet of 0.6 g/kg/day (42 g/day). He comes back for a follow-up visit in 3 months. His blood pressure is 132/78 mm Hg, and his weight remains at 70 kg. Repeat labs:

- Serum creatinine = 2.8 mg/dL (eGFR 38 mL/min)
- Serum albumin = 3.5 g/dL (no change from previous visit)

- Urine urea nitrogen = 8.5 g/day
- 24-h urine protein = 4.0 g

Based on his calculated daily protein intake, what would you do next?

A. Insist the patient to have an A-V access for dialysis in 6 months
B. Refer the patient to a dietician for further instruction on dietary protein intake
C. Lower dietary protein intake to <0.3 g/kg/day
D. Increase antiproteinuric medications
E. Continue current management

The answer is B

In this patient, it is important to calculate the dietary intake of protein prior to consideration of progressive diabetic nephropathy. Dietary protein intake can be estimated from 24-h urine urea nitrogen excretion or appearance rate. It is assumed that nitrogen is derived from protein and excreted as urea nitrogen and nonurea nitrogen (NUN). Since urea is the degradative product of protein, the urea appearance rate or urinary nitrogen appearance (UNA) parallels protein intake. NUN excretion (nitrogen in feces, urinary creatinine, amino acids, ammonia, uric acid) averages 0.031 g nitrogen/kg/day. The following formula can be used to calculate protein intake:

$$\textbf{Nitrogen intake}\left(\textbf{g / day}\right) = \textbf{UNA} + \left(\textbf{NUN} \times \textbf{Body weight in kg}\right)$$

where UNA represents urine urea nitrogen and NUN represents 0.031.

Using the patient values, we obtain

$$\mathbf{8.5 + \left(0.031 \times 70\right) 2.17 = 10.67\,g / day}$$

1 g urine urea nitrogen = 6.25 g of protein (or protein is 16% of nitrogen)

Protein intake = 10.67 g = 10.67 x 6.25 = 66.7 g/day or 0.95 g/kg/day

Based on the above calculation, the patient's dietary protein intake is 0.95 g/kg/day instead of 0.6 g/kg/day. Therefore, the most appropriate recommendation at this stage would be to refer the patient to the dietician for further instruction on dietary protein restriction. Thus, option B is correct. Considerations in other options are not warranted at this time.

Suggested Reading

Masud T, Manatunga A, Costonis G, et al. The precision of estimating protein intake of patients with chronic renal failure. Kidney Int. 2002;62:1750–6.

Shah M, Mitch WE. Nutritional management of kidney disease. In: Kimmel PL, Rosenberg ME, editors. Chronic renal disease. 2nd ed. London: Academic Press, Elsevier; 2020. p. 975–89.

76. A 60-year-old man with hypertensive nephrosclerosis with CKD 5 and an eGFR of 15 mL/min comes to you for a second opinion about initiation of hemodialysis (HD). He has no signs or symptoms of uremia or fluid overload. His appetite is good. His blood pressure is well controlled. Examination of heart and lungs is normal. His nephrologist created an A-V fistula 6 months ago, which is functional. He has renal residual function of 8 mL/min. **Which one of the following recommendations is APPROPRIATE for this patient?**

A. Tell him that he needs HD in a week
B. Suggest a low protein (0.6 g/day) and low salt (88 mEq/day) diet with follow-up in 4 weeks
C. Limit fluid intake to 500 mL/day
D. Ask him to see you in 4 months for specific recommendations
E. None of the above

The answer is B

This patient has no signs or symptoms of uremia or fluid overload. Also, he has some preserved residual kidney function. Early initiation of HD did not show significant benefits over late start of HD. Medical management with low protein and low salt diet is appropriate for this patient than starting HD. Supplementation of keto acids to low protein diet improves compliance to diet. Thus, answer B is correct. Frequent follow-ups by his nephrologist are needed to assess signs and symptoms of uremia. Other options are not appropriate at this time.

Suggested Reading

Cooper BA, Branley P, Bulfone L, et al. for the IDEAL Study. A randomized, controlled trial of early versus late initiation of dialysis. N Engl J Med. 2010;363:609–19.

Goraya N, Wesson DE. Dietary approaches to kidney diseases. In: Yu ASL, Chertow GM, Luyckx VA, et al., editors. Brenner & Rector's the kidney. 11th ed. Philadelphia: Elsevier, Saunders; 2020. p. 1977–88.

Rosansky S, Glassock RJ, Clark WF. Early start of dialysis: a critical review. Clin J Am Soc Nephrol. 2011;6:1222–8.

Shah M, Mitch WE. Nutritional management of kidney disease. In: Kimmel PL, Rosenberg ME, editors. Chronic renal disease. 2nd ed. London: Academic Press, Elsevier; 2020. p. 975–89.

77. Diet plays an important role in the prevention of CKD progression. **Which one of the following components of diet is associated with prevention of kidney disease and mortality?**

A. Low salt diet
B. Plant-based protein intake
C. Ingestion of vegetables and fruits
D. Less intake of red meat
E. All of the above

The answer is E

Several studies have shown that healthy dietary patterns are associated with lower mortality in people with kidney disease. Consumption of vegetables, fruits, fish, legume, whole grain, fiber, and reduced red meat, sodium, and refined sugar intake comprise healthy diet, which is effective in lowering mortality in patients with kidney disease. Also, plant-based rather than animal-based protein preserves kidney function. Healthy diet improves not only albuminuria but also hypertension, the two most important risk factors for kidney disease and associated complications. Thus, answer E is correct.

Suggested Reading

Bach KE, Kelly JT, Palmer SC, et al. Healthy dietary patterns and incidence of CKD: a meta-analysis of cohort studies. Clin J Am Soc Nephrol. 2019;14:1441–9.

Kelly JT, Palmer SC, Wai SN, et al. Healthy dietary patterns and risk of mortality and ESRD in CKD: a meta-analysis of cohort studies. Clin J Am Soc Nephrol. 2017;12:272–9.

Rysz J, Franczyk B, Ciałkowska-Rysz A, et al. The effect of diet on the survival of patients with chronic kidney disease. Nutrients. 2017;9(5):pii:E495. https://doi.org/10.3390/nu9050495.

78. Insomnia is a common complaint of many nondialysis and dialysis patients. **Which one of the following statements about insomnia in CKD is correct?**

A. The prevalence of insomnia varies from 14 to 85% in CKD patients
B. Insomnia is independently associated with depression, obstructive sleep apnea, and restless leg syndrome (RLS)
C. Insomnia decreases health-related quality of life (HRQOL)
D. Insomnia increases costs of medical care
E. All of the above

The answer is E

Sleep disorders are very common in both nondialysis and dialysis patients. Insomnia is one of the components of sleep disorder. The International Classification of Sleep Disorders, Third Edition (ICSD-3) defines insomnia as "a complaint of difficulty initiating sleep, difficulty maintaining sleep, or waking up too early, sleep that is chronically nonrestorative or poor in quality, or (in children) resistance to an inappropriate bedtime or difficulty falling asleep without adult intervention." Insomnia can be either short-term or chronic insomnia. Both types of insomnia cause disturbances in daytime function.

The prevalence of insomnia in CKD is variable. Different sources reported the prevalence from 14% to 85% in CKD patients. Impaired daytime functions may lead to fatigue, mood disturbances or irritability, reduced motivation, or reduced energy, and social and educational dysfunction.

Associated comorbidities include depression, RLS, and obstructive sleep apnea. RLS and insomnia are important risk factors for cardiovascular disease. The association between insomnia and depression is bidirectional.

Chronic insomnia may cause depression and the presence of depression may lead to insomnia. Daytime dysfunction, depression, and RLS may worsen HRQOL.

It has been reported that clinic visits, procedural costs, and hospitalizations increase the costs for medical care for patients with insomnia. Thus, answer E is correct.

The pathogenesis of insomnia is not completely understood. However, hypercalcemia, hyperparathyroidism, hyperphosphatemia, and anemia are implicated in causing insomnia. Interestingly, insomnia due to hyperparathyroidism improved following parathyroidectomy.

Suggested Reading

Lindner AV, Novak M, Bohra M, et al. Insomnia in patients with chronic kidney disease. Semin Nephrol. 2015;35:359–72.
Maung SC, El Sara A, Chapman C, et al. Sleep disorders and chronic kidney disease. World J Nephrol. 2016;5:224–32.
Nigam G, Camacho M, Chang ET, et al. Exploring sleep disorders in patients with chronic kidney disease. Nat Rev Sleep. 2018;10:35–42.

79. Sexual dysfunction is extremely prevalent in patients with CKD 4-5D. **Which one of the following causes is implicated in the development of sexual dysfunction?**

A. Vascular disease
B. Endocrine dysfunction
C. Autonomic neuropathy
D. Hyperparathyroidism
E. All of the above

The answer is E

The clinical manifestations of sexual dysfunction include erectile dysfunction (ED) in men, disturbances in menstruation in women, and decreased libido and infertility in both men and women. Atherosclerosis is a complication of CKD, which does not spare even penis. Studies have shown cavernosal artery occlusive disease in 78% of patients with CKD 5–5D. This results in decreased penile blood flow, causing ED in men. Disturbances in hypothalamic-pituitary-gonadal axis occur in CKD. Disturbances in various hormones were reported in both men and women. Table 4.11 shows some of the changes.

Table 4.11 Hormonal changes in CKD

Men	Women
Low testosterone level	High prolactin level
High prolactin level	Diminishes midcycle LH surge
Basal luteinizing hormone (LH) levels high due to feedback from low testosterone and also less renal clearance	Abnor
Diminished amplitude of LH	
Variable levels of follicle-stimulating hormone	

Autonomic neuropathy is another reason for decreased libido. Erection occurs through parasympathetic activity, release of NO, smooth muscle relaxation, and increased blood flow to the penis. When these processes are disturbed, ED develops. Thus, adequate parasympathetic outflow is essential for cavernous sinusoidal relaxation and hence increased cavernosal blood flow. In autonomic neuropathy, the parasympathetic nervous system is impaired with resultant ED.

Hyperparathyroidism contributes to ED by an unknown mechanism. Parathyroidectomy improved sexual dysfunction and lowered prolactin levels in dialysis patients. Thus, answers A–D are correct.

Other causes such as anemia, diabetes mellitus, hypertension, antihypertensive medications, and opioid use may account for sexual dysfunction in CKD patients.

Suggested Reading

Anantharaman P, Schmidt RJ. Sexual function in chronic kidney disease. Adv Chronic Kidney Dis. 2007;14:119–25.
Edey MM. Male sexual dysfunction and chronic kidney disease. Front Med (Lausanne). 2017;4:32.
Johansen K. Sexual dysfunction in chronic kidney disease. In: Kimmel PL, Rosenberg ME, editors. Chronic renal disease. 2nd ed. London: Academic Press, Elsevier; 2020. p. 593–611.

80. A 42-year-old woman with type 2 diabetes and hypertension is referred to you for evaluation of CKD with an eGFR of 70 mL/min. Her urine albumin is 24 mg/24 h. She drinks two cups of coffee and two diet sodas (12 oz each) a day. Her endocrinologist told her to drink 2 L of water in addition to coffee and sodas. She smokes marijuana twice a week. **Which one of the following is implicated as a risk factor for progression of kidney disease?**

    A. Coffee
    B. Diet soda
    C. Marijuana
    D. Water
    E. None of the above

    The answer is B

    Studies have shown that coffee exerts some beneficial effects on kidney. Not caffeine but chlorogenic acid, a component of coffee, has antioxidative and anti-inflammatory effects on the kidney. Thus, coffee lowers CKD risk. Unlike heroin or cocaine, marijuana seems to have no effect either on kidney disease or its progression. Also, drinking 2 L of water a day may not have any beneficial effect in this patient. However, water intake of >2 L per day is beneficial in patients with kidney stones and polycystic kidney disease.

    Drinking diet sodas may affect kidneys. Rebholz et al. examined prospectively the relationship between the consumption of diet soda and incident ESKD in the Atherosclerosis Risk in Communities study (n=15,368). Over a median follow-up of 23 years, 357 incident ESKD cases were observed. The risk of ESKD increased with increased consumption of soda. This study confirms earlier studies of the relationship between the consumption of artificially sweetened beverages and declining in eGFR of ≥3 mL/min per year. One of the mechanisms is phosphorous, which is added for color and flavor. This phosphorous may increase acid load to the body and thereby increasing additional risk for progression of CKD. Also, diet soda may induce glucose intolerance and associated metabolic consequences. Thus, consumption of diet soda is a risk factor for kidney disease in this patient, and answer B is correct.

    Suggested Reading

Lin J, Curhan GC. Associations of sugar and artificially sweetened soda with albuminuria and kidney function decline in women. Clin J Am Soc Nephrol. 2011;6:160–6.

Rebholz CM, Grams ME, Steffen LM, et al. Diet soda consumption and risk of incident end stage renal disease. Clin J Am Soc Nephrol. 2017;12:79–86.

81. Advanced glycation end products (AGEs) are implicated in the generation of several complications in both diabetic and nondiabetic subjects. AGEs are derived endogenously and exogenously. Exogenous AGEs come from daily food intake. **Which one of the following statements regarding AGEs is INCORRECT?**

    A. AGEs are formed by nonenzymatic process
    B. AGEs are cleared by renal excretion
    C. High temperature cooking enhances dietary AGE formation
    D. Tobacco smoking is a source of enhanced AGE formation
    E. Low temperature cooking enhances dietary AGE formation

    The answer is E

    Nonenzymatic glycation is a reaction between aldehyde group of glucose or other sugars and free amino groups at the N-terminus or ε-amino groups of lysine residues of various proteins without the aid of enzymes. It is a slow process in which glucose reacts with an amino group to form a labile Schiff base (or aldime), which subsequently undergoes a chemical rearrangement over a period of weeks to form a stable but reversible adduct called the ketoamine or Amadori product. The Schiff base and Amadori product constitute the early gycation products. However, some of these early glycation products undergo slow and complex chemical rearrangement to form AGEs and accumulate on matrix proteins or blood vessels. In the laboratory, some of the AGEs are determined as carboxymethyllysine, pentosidine, and methyglyoxal derivatives, and serve as AGE markers. The amount of AGEs does not always return to normal even after correction of hyperglycemia, and thus continue to accumulate over the lifetime of the matrix proteins or the vessel wall. Studies have shown that AGEs are responsible for

chronic micro- and macrovascular complications of diabetes. The following figure shows the mechanism of formation of early and AGEs.

Glucose + protein
Schiff bases
Amadori products
AGEs
Covalent bonds with amino groups

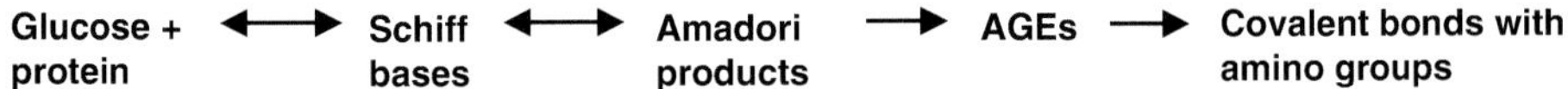

The level of circulating AGEs depends on the balance between endogenous formation and exogenous input from diet and smoking. Thus, it is evident that AGEs can be introduced into the circulation even in the absence of diabetes. High-temperature cooking foods (baking, roasting, frying) are the most important exogenous source of AGEs. AGEs are degraded into small AGE peptides and excreted by the kidneys. Renal failure causes an increase in circulating AGEs.

Proteins of animal origin and high fat diet have high amount of AGEs, whereas nonmeat proteins provide low amounts of AGEs. Foods cooking at low temperatures provide low amounts of AGEs. Thus, option E is incorrect.

Suggested Reading

Mark AB, Poulsen MW, Andersen S, et al. Consumption of a diet low in advanced glycation end products for 4 weeks improves insulin sensitivity in overweight women. Diabetes Care. 2014;37:88–95.

Nowotny K, Schröter D, Schreiner M, et al. Dietary advanced glycation end products and their relevance for human health. Ageing Res Rev. 2018;47:55–66.

Vlassara H, Uribarri J. Advanced glycation end products (AGE) and diabetes: cause, effect, or both? Curr Diab Rep. 2014;14:453.

82. A 52-year-old woman with type 2 diabetes is followed by you for CKD 2 and albumin:creatinine (ACR) ratio of 140 mg/g. She asks you about the importance of albuminuria and progression of kidney disease. **Which one of the following statements regarding the relationship between albuminuria and progression of kidney disease to ESKD is CORRECT?**

A. Only a decline in eGFR but not increase in albuminuria accounts for progression of kidney disease
B. A decline is albuminuria but not in EGFR decline accounts for progression of kidney disease
C. A fourfold increase in albuminuria from stable ACR carries a higher risk for progression of kidney disease
D. A decrease in albuminuria from stable ACR is protective of kidney disease progression
E. C and D

The answer is E

Albuminuria is a risk factor for not only kidney disease but cardiovascular disease as well. CKD guideline identifies only a decline in eGFR as a risk factor for progression of kidney disease. An observational study from the Stockholm CREAtinine Measurements (SCREAM) project, a healthcare utilization cohort from Stockholm, Sweden, reported a fourfold increase in ACR from stable ACR was associated with a 3.08-times higher risk of ESKD while a fourfold decrease in ACR was associated with a 0.34 times (0.26 to 0.45) lower risk of ESKD. Similar associations were found in diabetics, nondiabetics, hypertensives, and nonhypertensives. Thus, answer E is correct.

Suggested Reading

Carrero JJ, Grams ME, Sanao Y, et al. Albuminuria changes are associated with subsequent risk of end-stage renal disease and mortality. Kidney Int. 2017;91:244–51.

Coresh J, Heerspink HJL, Sang Y, et al. Chronic Kidney Disease Prognosis Consortium and Chronic Kidney Disease Epidemiology Collaboration. Change in albuminuria and subsequent risk of end-stage kidney disease: an individual participant-level consortium meta-analysis of observational studies. Lancet Diabetes Endocrinol. 2019;7:115–27.

Sumida K, Molnar MZ, Potuguchi PK, et al. Changes in albuminuria and subsequent risk of incident kidney disease. Clin J Am Soc Nephrol. 2017;12:1941–9.

83. **Regarding ethnicity and gender in the USA, which one of the following statements is CORRECT?**

A. Lifetime of ESKD is higher in men than women
B. Lifetime risk of ESKD in non-Hispanic and Hispanic men is higher in men than white men
C. Non-Hispanic and Hispanic women are at higher risk for development of ESKD than white women

D. The number of CKD-attributable deaths increased by 58.3% between 2002 and 2016
E. All of the above

The answer is E

Disparities in CKD prevalence and incidence rates continue in the USA. Lifetime risk of ESKD is also higher among Native American Indians. Thus, all of the above statements are correct.

Suggested Reading

Albertus P, Morgenstern H, Robinson B, et al. Risk of ESRD in the United States. Am J Kidney Dis. 2016;68:862–72.
Bowe B, Xie Y, Li T, et al. Changes in the US burden of chronic kidney disease from 2002 to 2016: an analysis of the global burden of disease study. JAMA Netw Open. 2018;1:e184412.

84. CKD management includes prevention of its progression to ESKD and improves cardiovascular outcomes. It requires multidisciplinary participation, including the patient. The goal of patients' involvement, called self-management, is to identify strategies that would help them to control their medical conditions and lead good quality of life. **Which one of the following statements regarding self-management of patient's health-related conditions is CORRECT?**

A. Self-management decreases HbA1c in diabetic patients with CKD compared to standard care
B. Self-management groups had a significant drop in blood pressure and 24-h urinary protein excretion
C. Patients in self-management programs experience improved exercise capacity and functional status
D. Self-management program reduces inflammatory markers such as CRP in CKD
E. All of the above

The answer is E

Self-management refers to the active participation in one's care. In CKD, it includes long-term behavior change and commitment to dietary, fluid intake, blood pressure, glucose, and medication management. Several studies have shown improvements in many health-related conditions, including glycemic and blood pressure control, proteinuria, and exercise tolerance in nondialysis and dialysis patients. Also, self-management lowered CRP levels, suggesting reduced inflammation. Self-management also reduced emergency department visits and medical costs, particularly in elderly people with multiple medical conditions. Thus, all of the above statements (answer E) are correct.

Suggested Reading

Peng S, He J, Huang J, et al. Self-management interventions for chronic kidney disease: a systematic review and meta-analysis. BMC Nephrol. 2019;20:142.
Washington T, Hilliard T, McGill T. The chronic disease self-management program: a resource for use with older CKD patients. National Kidney Foundation J Nephrol Soc Work. 2013;37:8–12.

85. **Which one of the following statements regarding CKD is CORRECT?**

A. Chronic glomerulonephritis (GN) is leading cause of CKD in Southeast Asia
B. Nephrolithiasis is the major cause of CKD in Thailand
C. Diabetes remains the leading cause of CKD in Latin America
D. The prevalence of CKD is lower in China Mainland than in South Korea, Japan, and Thailand
E. All of the above

The answer is E

In Southeast Asia, chronic GN is the most common cause of CKD in Singapore, Indonesia, Cambodia, and Vietnam (A is correct). In Thailand, nephrolithiasis is the cause for CKD (B is correct). Diabetes remains the leading cause of CKD in Latin American countries. Among ESKD patients, diabetes accounts for 65% in Puerto Rico, 51% in Mexico, 42% in Venezuela, and 42% in Columbia (C is correct). Interestingly, lower rates were reported in Brazil (26%), Uruguay (22%), Costa Rica (20%), and Paraguay (15%). The reason for this disparity remains unclear.

The prevalence of CKD is lower in China Mainland (10.8%) compared to South Korea (13.7%), Japan (12.9%), and Taiwan (11.9%). Thus, answer D is correct.

Suggested Reading

Correa-Rotter R, García-García G, Chăvez-Iñiguez J, et al. Ethnicity and chronic kidney disease in disadvantaged populations: an international perspective. In: Kimmel PL, Rosenberg ME, editors. Chronic renal disease. 2nd ed. London: Academic Press, Elsevier; 2020. p. 121–38.

Correa-Rotter R. Renal replacement therapy in the developing world: are we on the right track, or should there be a new paradigm? J Am Soc Nephrol. 2007;18:1635–6.

Kanno H, Kanno Y. Ethnicity and chronic kidney disease in Japan. In: Kimmel PL, Rosenberg ME, editors. Chronic renal disease. 2nd ed. London: Academic Press, Elsevier; 2020. p. 139–148.

86. **Which one of the following statements regarding global burden of CKD from 1990 to 2016 is CORRECT?**

A. The prevalence increased by 86.9%
B. The incidence increased by 88.8%
C. Deaths related to CKD increased by 98%
D. Disability-adjusted life years (years of life lost and years of poor health or disability) increased by 62.2%
E. All of the above

The answer is E

Xie et al. provided data from the Global Burden of Disease Study regarding the prevalence, incidence, deaths, and disability-adjusted life years (DALY) of CKD from 1990 to 2016. During these 26 years, the epidemiology of CKD changed dramatically. Table 4.12 shows these changes.

Table 4.12 Global CKD burden

Category of burden	1990 (millions)	2016 (millions)	Increase (%)
Prevalence	147.60	275.93	87
Incidence	11.29	21.33	89
Deaths	0.60	1.19	98
DALY	21.62	35.03	62

DALY disability-adjusted life years

DALY represents the sum of years lost due to premature death and also years living with disability due to the disease. As shown in the above table, the prevalence increased by 87%, incidence increased by 89%, death rate increased by 98%, and DALY increased by 62% from 1990 to 2016. From these increases, CKD may be an important noncommunicable disease, which requires more attention from healthcare workers. Thus, answer E is correct.

Suggested Reading

Jha V, Modi GK. Getting to know the enemy better – the global burden of chronic kidney disease. Kidney Int. 2018;94:462–4.

Xie Y, Bowe B, Mokdad AH, et al. Analysis of the Global Burden of Disease study highlights the global, regional, and national trends of chronic kidney disease epidemiology from 1990 to 2016. Kidney Int. 2018;94:567–81.

87. The sodium glucose cotransporter2 (SGLT2) inhibitors have been shown to improve both cardiovascular and renal outcomes in type 2 diabetic patients with various stages of CKD. **Which one of the following statements regarding SGLT2 inhibitors and renal outcomes is CORRECT?**

A. The BI 10773 (Empagliflozin) Cardiovascular Outcome Event Trial in Type 2 Diabetes Mellitus Patients (EMPA-REG OUTCOME) trial and the Canagliflozin Cardiovascular Assessment Study (CANVAS) Program were the original large studies that evaluated both cardiovascular and kidney outcomes in type 2 diabetic patients
B. SGLT2 inhibitors reduced eGFR initially (measured at 4 weeks) with stabilization or returning to baseline during follow-up
C. Overall, SGLT2 inhibitors improved both eGFR and albuminuria in type 2 diabetic patients
D. SGLT2 inhibitors can also be used patients with eGFR <30 mL/min
E. All of the above

The answer is E

The BI 10773 (Empagliflozin) Cardiovascular Outcome Event Trial in Type 2 Diabetes Mellitus Patients Trial was the first study to report improvements in cardiovascular and kidney outcomes with empagliflozin. Subsequently, the Canagliflozin Cardiovascular Assessment Study (CANVAS) program and the Dapagliflozin Effect on Cardiovascular events-Thrombosis in Myocardial Infarction 58 trial also reported improved cardiovascular and kidney outcomes for canagliflozin and dapagliflozin, respectively (A is correct). These studies showed an initial drop in eGFR followed by stabilization or returning to baseline in subsequent weeks of follow-up (B is correct). However, these studies were not primarily designed to evaluate kidney end points but evaluated as secondary kidney outcomes because of small number of CKD patients. The primary end points in the above studies were cardiovascular outcomes.

This led to continuation of other studies by the same drugs addressing the primary or prespecified kidney outcomes. One of the studies is EMPA-REG OUTCOME trial, the second one is Canagliflozin and Renal Events in Diabetes with Established Nephropathy Clinical Evaluation (CREDENCE) trial, which was designed to assess the effects of canagliflozin primarily on kidney outcomes in participants with type 2 diabetes, who had CKD and albuminuria, and the third study is DECLARE-TIMI 58 randomized trial.

In the EMPA-REG OUTCOME trial, the patients were randomly assigned to receive either empagliflozin (Empa) or placebo once daily. Prespecified renal outcomes included incident or worsening nephropathy (progression to macroalbuminuria, doubling of the serum creatinine level, initiation of renal-replacement therapy, or death from kidney disease) and incident albuminuria. Worsening nephropathy occurred in 12.7% of Empa group compared to 18.8% in placebo group (hazard ratio in the Empa group, 0.61; 95% confidence interval, 0.53 to 0.70; p<0.001). Doubling of the serum creatinine level occurred in 1.5% in the Empa group and 2.6% in the placebo group, suggesting a significant 44% risk reduction in the Empa group. Only 0.3% in the Empa group required renal replacement therapy compared to 0.6% in the placebo group, representing a 55% lower relative risk in the Empa group. However, there was no significant incident albuminuria was observed between the groups. Thus, Empa was associated with slower progression of kidney disease with hazard ratios <1.0.

In the CREDENCE trial, patients with eGFR 30 and 90 mL/min and ACR >300 mg/g were randomly assigned to receive either canagliflozin (Cana) or placebo. The primary outcome was a composite of ESKD (dialysis, transplantation, or a sustained eGFR of <15 mL/min), a doubling of serum creatinine level, or death from renal or cardiovascular causes. The results show that the relative risk of the primary outcome was 30% lower in the Cana group than in the placebo group (event rates of 43.2 and 61.2 per 100-patient years, respectively). Doubling of creatinine level or death from renal causes was lower by 34%, and the risk of ESKD was lower by 32% in the Cana group. ACR was low in the Cana group. These data suggest that Cana treatment is renoprotective. It should be noted that all the patients were on renin-angiotensin blockade.

In DECLARE–TIMI 58, patients were randomly assigned to either dapagliflozin (Dapa) or placebo. A prespecified secondary kidney composite outcome was defined as a sustained decline of at least 40% in eGFR to <60 mL/min, ESKD (defined as dialysis for at least 90 days, kidney transplantation, or confirmed sustained eGFR <15 mL/min), or death from renal cause. Sustained decline in eGFR by 40% to <60 mL/min was observed in 1.4% in the Dapa group compared to 2.4% in the placebo group. Also, the risk of ESKD or renal death was lower (0.1%) in the Dapa group than (0.3%) in the placebo group. Urine ACR also improved in the Dapa group. These results suggest that Dapa prevents progression of kidney disease in type 2 diabetic patients.

All of the above studies enrolled patients with a mean eGFR >50 mL/min. However, a more recent study, called DAPA-CKD study, included both type 2 diabetic and nondiabetic patients with an eGFR of 25–75 mL/min, and found that the composite outcome of sustained decline in eGFR of at least 50%, ESKD, or death from renal or cardiovascular causes was significantly lower with Dapa than with placebo. In this study, 13.6% of patients had an eGFR <30 mL/min in the Dapa group. Thus, SGLT2 inhibitors can improve kidney function in even in those with very low eGFR (<30 mL/min).

Of the above four studies, three studies included CKD patients with eGFR greater than 30 mL/min, and the most recent study included some patients with <30 mL/min. Therefore, use of SGLT2 inhibitors is recommended in patients with CKD 4. Thus, answer E is correct. Other details of these studies are summarized in Table 4.13.

Table 4.13 Summary of various studies of SGLT2 inhibitors on kidney outcomes

Variables	EMPA-REG outcome (1)	CREDENCE (2)	DECLAR E-TIMI 58 (3)	DAPA-CKD (4)
No.	7,018	4,401	17,160	4,304 (67.6% diabetics)
SGLT2 inhibitor	Empagliflozin	Canagliflozin	Dapagliflozin	Dapagliflozin
Median follow-up (yr)	2.6	2.62	4.2	2.4
HbA1c	8.03–8.10%	6.5–12%	7.1–9.5	ND
Mean eGFR (mL/min)	65.7	50.4	85.3	43 (25–75)
Urine ACR (mg/g)	<30 (55%) 30–300 (31%) >300 (14%)	<30 (1%) 30–300 (11%) >300 (88%)	<30 (69%) 30–300 (24%) >300 (7%)	Median 965 (Dapa) 934 (nondiabetics)
Kidney outcomes				
Primary		Composite of ESKD, doubling of creatinine or death from renal cause: 34% lower in Cana group compared to placebo group Decline in eGFR/ yr: Cana 1.85 mL/min vs placebo 4.59 mL/min Relative risk of ESKD: 32% lower in Cana group compared to placebo group Urine ACR: More patients in placebo group had higher ratio than in Cana group		Composite of decline in eGFR of 50%, ESKD or death from renal or cardiovascular cause: 9.2% in Dapa versus 14.5% in placebo (p<0.001)
Secondary (prespecified)	Doubling of creatinine: Empa 1.5% vs placebo 2.6% (reduction 44%) RRT started: Empa 0.3% vs placebo 0.6% (reduction 50%) Urine ACR: no difference		eGFR decline to <60 mL/min: Dapa 1.4% vs placebo 2.6% p <0.0001 ESKD or renal death: Dapa 0.1% vs 0.3% placebo p<0.012 UACR (mg/g) increase: < 30=Dapa 0.9% vs placebo 1.6% 30–300=Dapa 1.9% vs Placebo 3.3% >300=Dapa 5.2% vs Placebo 13% (all significant)	

References

1. Wanner C, Inzucchi SE, Lachin JM, et al. for the EMPA-REG OUTCOME Investigators. Empagliflozin and progression of kidney disease in type 2 diabetes. N Engl J Med 375:323-334, 2016.
2. Perkovic V, Jardine MJ, Neal B, et al. for the CREDENCE Trial Investigators. Canagliflozin and renal outcomes in type 2 Diabetes and nephropathy. N Engl J Med 380:2295-2306, 2019.
3. Mosenzon O, Wiviott SD, Cahn A, et al. Effects of dapagliflozin on development and progression of kidney disease in patients with type 2 diabetes: an analysis from the DECLARE–TIMI 58 randomised trial. Lancet Diabetes Endocrinol 7:606-617, 2019.
4. Heerspink HJL, Stefánsson BV, Correa-Rotter R, et al. for the DAPA-CKD Trial Committees and Investigators. Dapagliflozin in patients with chronic kidney disease. N Engl J Med 383:1436-1446, 2020.

Suggested Reading

Neal B, Perkovic V, Mahaffey KW, et al. CANVAS Program Collaborative Group. Canagliflozin and cardiovascular and renal events in type 2 diabetes. N Engl J Med. 2017;377:644–57.

Wiviott SD, Raz I, Bonaca MP, et al. DECLARE-TIMI 58 Investigators. Dapagliflozin and cardiovascular outcomes in type 2 diabetes. N Engl J Med. 2019;380:347–57.

Zinman B, Wanner C, Lachin JM, et al. EMPA-REG OUTCOME Investigators. Empagliflozin, cardiovascular outcomes, and mortality in type 2 diabetes. N Engl J Med. 2015;373:2117–28.

88. **SGLT2 inhibitors were found to have protective effects on the kidney by which one of the following pathophysiologic mechanisms?**

A. Activation of tubuloglomerular feedback (TGF) mechanism
B. Blood pressure (BP) reduction
C. Increased natriuresis
D. Reducing inflammation in the kidney
E. All of the above

The answer is E

All of the above mechanisms have been implicated in renoprotection by SGLT2 inhibition. Thus, answer E is correct. TGF is an adaptive mechanism through which renal blood flow and GFR are autoregulated. In moderate hyperglycemia, glomerular hyperfiltration occurs. When GFR increases, more glucose, Na^{+}, and Cl^{-} is delivered to the proximal tubule. This causes increased reabsorption of these solutes in the proximal tubules due to activation of SGLT 2 cotransporters and also Na/H cotransporter and less delivery of Na^{+} and Cl^{-} to the macula densa. Adenosine, a mediator of TGF mechanism, plays an important role in regulating afferent arteriolar resistance. High levels of adenosine cause vasoconstriction and low levels cause vasodilation of afferent arteriole. Decreased delivery of Na^{+} and Cl^{-} to macula densa causes decreased release of adenosine, which maintains renal vasodilation, increased renal blood flow, and GFR (hyperfiltration) in diabetes. Hyperfiltration is one of the mechanisms for glomerular fibrosis.

When delivery of Na^{+} and Cl^{-} is increased to macula densa by SGLT2 inhibition, adenosine release is increased, which causes an increase in afferent arteriolar resistance and a decrease in renal blood flow. As a result, glomerular hyperfiltration is reduced. Thus, activation of TGF mechanism by SGLT2 inhibition provides renoprotection (answer A is correct).

SGLT2 cotransporter inhibitors cause natriuresis and glucosuria, causing mild volume depletion and low body weight. These changes were found to lower systolic BP by approximately 5 mm Hg and diastolic BP by 2 mm Hg. Blood pressure control reduces glomerular fibrosis (answers B and C are correct).

By lowering HbA1c, SGLT2 inhibition reduces glucose toxicity with improvement in oxidative stress and inflammation. Indeed, it was shown that SGLT2 inhibition by dapagliflozin decreased urinary excretion of inflammatory markers in type 2 diabetic subjects. Both oxidative stress and inflammation contribute to progression of kidney disease in diabetic patients. Reducing these two pathways improves kidney function. Thus, answer D is correct.

Suggested Reading

Alicic RZ, Neumiller JJ, Johnson E, et al. Sodium-glucose cotransporter 2 inhibition and diabetic kidney disease. Diabetes. 2019;68:248–57.

Davidson JA. SGLT2 inhibitors in patients with type 2 diabetes and renal disease: overview of current evidence. Postgrad Med. 2019;131:251–60.

Rangaswami J, Bhalla V, de Boer IH, et al. Cardiorenal protection with the newer antidiabetic agents in patients with diabetes and chronic kidney disease. A scientific statement from the American Heart Association. Circulation. 2020;142:e265–86.

Vallon V, Thomson SC. Targeting renal glucose reabsorption to treat hyperglycaemia: the pleiotropic effects of SGLT2 inhibition. Diabetologia. 2017;60:215–25.

Chapter 5
Acute Kidney Injury and Critical Care Nephrology

1. **Several definitions of acute kidney injury (AKI) exist in the literature. Of all the definitions of AKI, which one of the following definitions has been validated and is considered most useful for epidemiological studies of AKI?**

   A. Increase in serum creatinine of 0.5 mg/dL in patients with baseline creatinine <1.9 mg/dL
   B. Increase in serum creatinine of 1.0 mg/dL in patients with baseline creatinine >2.0 mg/dL
   C. RIFLE (Risk, Injury, Failure, Loss, End-stage kidney disease) classification
   D. AKIN (Acute Kidney Injury Network) classification
   E. C and D

   The answer is E

   Before 2004, at least 30 different definitions have been reported in the literature, which were not validated or standardized. The definitions of AKI reported in options A and B were chosen by the study investigators and were not validated. In 2004, the RIFLE classification was introduced by the Acute Dialysis Quality Initiative (ADQI) group, which was subsequently validated. The definition of AKI was further refined by the AKIN investigators. Both classifications are based on serum creatinine and urine output. Changes that were made in AKIN classification were: (1) adding an increase in serum creatinine of at least 0.3 mg/dL even this increase may not reach 50% threshold to R in RIFLE criteria; (2) the increase in creatinine should occur within 48 h to make the diagnosis of AKI; (3) patients are included under F if they are on RRT irrespective of their creatinine or urine output at time of initiation of RRT; and (3) elimination of Loss and ESKD categories. Thus, option E is correct. Table 5.1 shows **both the RIFLE and AKIN classification (criteria) of AKI.**

Table 5.1 RIFLE and AKIN classification of AKI

RIFLE (criteria)	Serum creatinine (mg/dL)	Urine output[a]	AKIN criteria (Stages)	Serum creatinine (mg/dL)
R (Risk)	Increase in creatinine 1.5 times or GFR decrease >25%	<0.5 mL/kg/h for >6 h	1	1.5–1.9 times increase in creatinine from baseline or increase in creatinine ≥0.3 mg/dL)
I (Injury)	Increase in creatinine × 2 or GFR decrease >50%	<0.5 mL/k/h for ≥12 h	2	2–2.9 times increase in creatinine from baseline
F (Failure)	Increase in creatinine × 3 or creatinine >4 mg/dL or GFR decrease >75%	<0.3 mL/kg/h for ≥24 h or anuria for ≥12 h	3	3 times increase in creatinine from baseline or creatinine ≥4.0 mg/dL or initiation of renal replacement therapy
L (Loss)	Complete loss of renal function >4 weeks			
E (End-stage kidney disease)	ESKD >3 months			

[a]applies to both RIFLE and AKIN classification

A. S. Reddi, *Absolute Nephrology Review*, https://doi.org/10.1007/978-3-030-85958-9_5

Suggested Reading

Kidney Disease: Improving Global Outcomes (KDIGO) Acute Kidney Injury Work Group. KDIGO Clinical Practice Guideline for Acute Kidney Injury. Kidney Int (Suppl). 2012;2:1–138.

Singbartl K, Kellum JA. AKI in the ICU: definition, epidemiology, risk stratification, and outcomes. Kidney Int. 2012;81:819–25.

2. A 32-year-old woman is admitted to the intensive care unit (ICU) for sepsis due to pyelonephritis. Her serum creatinine is 0.5 mg/dL at time of admission. Twenty-four hours later her urine output started to decline, but her creatinine remains stable. The intensivist feels that the patient is in the process of developing acute kidney injury (AKI). The above patient had decreased urine output (<0.5 mL/kg/h) for 6 h, and her creatinine is gradually increasing. **Which one of the following statements is TRUE regarding decreased urine output (oliguria) and AKI in this patient?**

A. Oliguria is defined as urine output <0.3 mL/kg/h for at least 24 h by the Acute Dialysis Quality Initiative (ADQI) group
B. Oliguria may be an expression of either normal response of the kidneys to hypovolemia, or an expression of an underlying kidney disease
C. Approximately 69% of ICU patients who developed AKI were oliguric in one study
D. Oliguria in AKI patients is an independent predictor of mortality
E. All of the above

The answer is E

Generally, oliguria is defined as urine volume <500 mL/24 h. This definition was proposed on the concept that a healthy individual with normal kidney function can concentrate his/her urine to a maximum of 1200 mOsm/kg H_2O, assuming the daily intake of 600 mOsm/24 h. Therefore, the minimal amount of urine volume to excrete these 600 mOsm is 500 mL/24 h (600 mOsm/500 mL = 1200 mOsm). Any urine volume <500 mL is considered oliguria. However, this definition of oliguria has changed after the introduction of RIFLE (Risk, Injury, Failure, Loss, End-stage kidney disease) and AKIN (Acute Kidney Injury Network) classification system. This classification system defines oliguria in progressive stages as <0.5 mL/kg/h for >6 h, <0.5 mL/kg/h for >12 h, and <0.3 mL/kg/h for >24 h. Therefore, <0.5 mL/kg/h indicates decreased urine output and necessitates evaluation for oliguria.

Oliguria may be due to hypovolemia or hypotension. In these conditions, vasopressin secretion is increased with resultant reabsorption of filtered water in the kidney. Also, oliguria may be related to intrinsic disease of the kidney. Urine osmolality distinguishes these two conditions, where maximal urine concentration (osmolality >500 mOsm/kg H_2O) is observed with hypovolemia and isosthenuria (~300 >500 mOsm/kg H_2O) with diseased kidney. In one study, about 69% of ICU patients who developed AKI were found to be oliguric, and oliguria was found to be an independent risk factor for prolonged length of hospital stay and mortality. Furthermore, there seems to be a good correlation of poor outcomes with progressive stages of oliguria. Thus, E is correct.

Suggested Reading

Ricci Z, Cruz D, Ronco C. The RIFLE criteria and mortality in acute kidney injury: a systematic review. Kidney Int. 2008;73:538–46.

Rimmelė T, Kellum JA. Oliguria and fluid overload. In: Ronco C, Costanzo MR, Bellomo R, Maisel AS, editors. Fluid overload: diagnosis and management. Contrib Nephrol, Basel: Karger; 2010. Vol. 164. p. 39–45.

3. **Which one of the following is NOT a kidney injury biomarker for the early diagnosis of AKI?**

A. Neutrophil gelatinase-associated lipocalin (NGAL)
B. N-acetyl-β-D-galactosaminidase (NAG)
C. Kidney injury molecule-1 (KIM-1)
D. Interleukin-18 (IL-18)
E. Lactate dehydrogenase

The answer is E

AKI is common in ICUs. Serum creatinine is the only marker of kidney function besides urine output. The increase in serum creatinine does not occur until approximately 50% of kidney function is lost. It may take hours to days to see an increase in serum creatinine levels. Therefore, it is not possible to have therapeutic intervention prior to an increase in serum creatinine. This results in high morbidity and mortality.

Recent studies have focused on diagnosing AKI from tubular injury prior to detectable increase in serum creatinine using novel biomarkers. These biomarkers can be broadly divided into three categories:

1. **Low molecular weight biomarkers. These are filtered at the glomerulus and reabsorbed by the proximal tubule. These are secreted into the urine only when the proximal tubule epithelial cells are injured. Examples include β_2-microglobulin, cystatin C, and lysozyme.**
2. **Biomarkers that are upregulated in renal tubular cells in response to injury. These include NGAL and KIM-1.**
3. **Markers that are expressed by tubular cells and excreted into the urine following an acute injury to these cells. An example is N-acetyl-β-D-glucosaminidase.**

Other biomarkers include tissue inhibitor of metalloproteinases-2 (TIMP-2), insulin-like growth factor-binding protein 7 (IGFBP7) and liver fatty acid binding protein. In addition, interleukin-18 (IL-18) is released by macrophages and neutrophils during AKI. Of these biomarkers, NGAL has been studied extensively in both children and adults, and its serum and urine levels have been shown to increase prior to the increase in serum creatinine in the diagnosis of AKI. However, lactate dehydrogenase has not been studied. Thus, choice E is correct.

Suggested Reading

Oh D-J. A long journey for acute kidney injury biomarkers. Renal Fail. 2020;42:154–65.
Parikh CR, Mansour SG. Perspective on clinical application of biomarkers in AKI. J Am Soc Nephrol. 2017;28:1677–85.
Srisawat N, Kellum JA. The role of biomarkers in acute kidney injury. Crit Care Clin. 2020;36:125–140.

4. The study of kidney biomarkers for the early diagnostic and prognostic purposes of AKI is rapidly expanding. **The clinical utility of these biomarkers has been investigated in which one of the following conditions?**

   A. To distinguish between prerenal AKI or azotemia from acute tubular necrosis (ATN) in normal individuals
   B. To predict renal recovery following AKI
   C. To distinguish hepatorenal syndrome (HRS) from prerenal AKI and ATN in cirrhosis
   D. To guide therapeutic management in cardiorenal syndrome
   E. All of the above

The answer is E

One of the biomarkers that have been extensively studied is neutrophil gelatinase-associated lipocalin (NGAL). It has been shown that urine levels of this biomarker can distinguish prerenal AKI from acute tubular necrosis (ATN). In prerenal AKI, urine NGAL levels are low (<104 ng/mL) compared to much higher levels in ATN (>104 ng/mL). Similarly, levels of kidney injury molecule-1 (KIM-1) and interleukin-18 (IL-18) are high in kidney injury than in prerenal AKI.

Biomarkers have been used to predict renal recovery following AKI. For example, the role of plasma NGAL was tested for renal recovery in patients with stage 3 AKI. Patients with low levels had renal recovery compared to patients with no renal recovery. Thus, plasma NGAL levels can be used to make a therapeutic decision in patients with severe AKI.

It is always difficult to identify the cause of AKI in patients with decompensated cirrhosis. Creatinine has its own limitations as a marker of kidney function in cirrhosis. For this reason, the utility of biomarkers has been explored in the differential diagnosis of AKI in cirrhosis. Urine NGAL and IL-18 were found to be useful in differentiating ATN from HRS and prerenal AKI. The levels of these biomarkers were highest in ATN, intermediate in HRS, and low in prerenal AKI. Using cut-off values for these biomarkers, it was found that those patients who had above cut-off values of each marker had ATN rather than HRS or prerenal AKI. Thus, these biomarkers help the clinician to choose appropriate therapeutic regimen for AKI without causing harm to the patient.

Another area that has been extensively studied is cardiorenal syndrome. Elevated urine levels of NGAL, KIM-1, and N-acetyl-β-D-galactosaminidase were found to be elevated in patients with chronic heart failure with a mean eGFR of 78 mL/min, suggesting tubular injury. A therapeutic decision can be made for continuation of diuretics based on the levels of these biomarkers. If the patient has very low levels, diuretics can be continued, and if the levels are above the cut-off values the diuretics may be held.

The association of kidney biomarkers and long-term mortality was evaluated by Coca et al. in patients with cardiac surgery. These investigators measured five urinary biomarkers 1–3 days after cardiac surgery (coronary artery bypass graft and valve surgery) in 1199 patients and followed them for a median 3 years. Mean serum creatinine level and eGFR were 1.0 mg/dL and 68 mL/min, respectively. When data were analyzed by severity of

AKI, the highest tertiles of peak urinary NGAL, IL-18, KIM-1, liver fatty acid binding protein, and albumin associated independently with a 2.0- to 3.2-fold increased risk for mortality as compared with the lowest tertiles. In patients without clinical AKI, the highest tertiles of peak IL-18 and KIM-1 also associated independently with long-term mortality with hazard ratio of 1.2. Thus, kidney biomarkers, particularly IL-18 and KIM-1, provide additional prognostic information for 3-year mortality risk in patients with and without clinical AKI. Thus, answer E is correct.

Another interesting observation is the clinical utility of urine tissue inhibitor of metalloproteinases-2 (TIMP-2) and insulin-like growth factor-binding protein 7 (IGFBP7) in critically ill patients. These biomarkers induce cell cycle arrest in G1 phase, which is a consequence of AKI. When these two biomarker values are multiplied together, the resultant value has a better predictive power for assessing the development of severe AKI (stage 2–3) than either biomarker. For this reason, the FDA approved TIMP-2 x IGFBP7 test that can identify patients at high risk for severe AKI. A value of >0.3 identifies patients with a high likelihood to have moderate to severe AKI within 12 h, while a value of ≤0.3 suggests patients with a low risk to develop moderate to severe AKI within 12 h. This test is also approved in Europe. Appropriate patient population for this test include those undergoing major surgery (cardiac and noncardiac), those who are hemodynamically unstable, and those with sepsis.

Suggested Reading

Coca SG, Garg AX, Thiessen-Philbrook H, et al. TRIBE-AKI Consortium. Urinary biomarkers of AKI and mortality 3 years after cardiac surgery. J Am Soc Nephrol. 2014;25:1063–71.

Guzzi LM, Bergler T, Binnall B, et al. Clinical use of [TIMP-2]•[IGFBP7] biomarker testing to assess risk of acute kidney injury in critical care: guidance from an expert panel. 2019;Crit Care.23:225. https://doi.org/10.1186/s13054-019-2504-8.

Oh D-J. A long journey for acute kidney injury biomarkers. Renal Fail. 2020;42:154–65.

Parikh CR, Mansour SG. Perspective on clinical application of biomarkers in AKI. J Am Soc Nephrol. 2017;28:1677–85.

Srisawat N, Kellum JA. The role of biomarkers in acute kidney injury. Crit Care Clin. 2020;36:125–40.

Vijayan A, Faubel S, Askenazi DJ, et al. on behalf of the American Society of Nephrology Acute Kidney Injury Advisory Group.*Clinical use of the urine biomarker [TIMP-2] × [IGFBP7] for acute kidney injury risk assessment. Am J Kidney Dis. 2016;68:19–28.

5. A 55-year-old woman with type 2 diabetes, hypertension (HTN), serum creatinine of 1.4 mg/dL (eGFR 48 mL/min), and proteinuria of 800 mg/24 h is referred to you for further management of her kidney disease and HTN. **Which one of the following novel risk factors is associated with an increased susceptibility to AKI?**

   A. Hyperuricemia
   B. Hypoalbuminemia
   C. Obesity
   D. Genetic polymorphism
   E. All of the above

   The answer is E

   The above patient has four important traditional risk factors for AKI (diabetes, HTN, CKD, and proteinuria). However, several nontraditional factors, including hyperuricemia, hypoalbuminemia, certain genetic polymorphism, and obesity, have been implicated in the genesis and aggravation of AKI. Also, other risk factors that were found to be associated with higher incidence of AKI are chloride-rich solutions, hetastarches, and mechanical ventilation. Thus, careful management of patients with nontraditional risk factors is necessary to improve patient care and healthcare costs.

Suggested Reading

Fuhrmqan DY, Kane-Gill S, Goldstein SL, et al. Acute kidney injury epidemiology, risk factors, and outcomes in critically ill patients 16–25 years of age treated in an adult intensive care unit. Ann Intensive Care. 2018;8:26.

Nie S, Tang L, Zhang W, et al. Are there modifiable risk factors to improve AKI?. Biomed Res Int. 2017:pages 9.

Varrier M, Ostermann M. Novel risk factors for acute kidney injury. Curr Opin Nephrol Hypertens. 2014;23:560–9.

6. **Regarding the incidence of AKI, which one of the following statements is CORRECT?**

   A. The incidence of AKI varies depending on the definition of AKI, community population, and hospitalized patients

B. The incidence of AKI is 5–10 times higher in hospitalized patients than the incidence in community population
C. The incidence of AKI is lower in high-income countries than in low-to-middle income countries
D. A multinational study reported that AKI occurred in 57.3% of critically ill patients
E. All of the above

The answer is E

All of the above statements are correct. A number of population-based studies have shown that the incidence of AKI varies depending on the definition of AKI, and among community population as well as hospitalized patients. Because of these reasons, estimates of AKI prevalence varies from <1 to 66%. Lower incidence of AKI has been reported in high-income countries compared to low-to-middle-income countries. Water contamination and infections seem to account for higher incidence in low-to-middle-income countries. The incidence also increases with age until 9th ninth decade. Among hospitalized patients, the incidence of AKI is higher in critically ill patients admitted to the intensive care units. A multinational study reported that 57.3% of critically ill patients developed AKI. Thus, answer E is correct.

Suggested Reading

Hoste EJ, Bagshaw S, Bellomo R, et al. Epidemiology of acute kidney injury in critically ill patients: the multinational AKI-EPI study. Intensive Care Med. 2015;41:1411–23.
Hoste EA, Kellum JA, Selby NM, et al. Global epidemiology and outcomes of acute kidney injury. Nat Rev Nephrol. 2018;14:607–27.
Holmes J, Rainer T, Geen J, et al. on behalf of the Welsh AKI Steering Group. Acute kidney injury in the era of the AKI E-Alert. Clin J Am Soc Nephrol. 2016;11:2123–31.

7. **AKI is associated with which one of the following conditions?**

A. Increased in-hospital mortality
B. Increased hospital stay and cost
C. Increased need for renal replacement therapy (RRT)
D. Increased risk for progression to CKD and also ESKD
E. All of the above

The answer is E

AKI is not a benign condition. It has several complications, including higher morbidity and mortality, prolonged hospital stay and resource utilization, requirement for RRT, and progression to CKD and ESKD, as compared to non-AKI patients. The financial burden was much higher for AKI patients due to longer hospital stay. The cost is higher in patients requiring RRT than uncomplicated AKI patients without RRT. Thus, E is correct.

Suggested Reading

Faubel S, Shah PB. Immediate consequences of acute kidney injury: the impact of traditional and nontraditional complications on mortality in acute kidney injury. Adv Chronic Kidney Dis. 2016;23:179–85.
Kidney Disease: Improving Global Outcomes (KDIGO) Acute Kidney Injury Work Group. KDIGO clinical practice guideline for acute kidney injury. Kidney Int (Suppl). 2012;2:1–138.
Zeng X, McMahon GM, Brunelli SM, et al. Incidence, outcomes, and comparisons across definitions of AKI in hospitalized individuals. Clin J Am Sco Nephrol. 2014;9:12–20.

8. **Which one of the following statements is CORRECT regarding the epidemiology of AKI in critically ill patients globally?**

A. Severe AKI requiring ICU admissions occurs in 11 patients per 100,000 population per year
B. Using RIFLE criteria, one study reported the occurrence of AKI in 36.1% with 16.3% in RIFLE-R category, 13.6% in RIFLE-I, and 6.3% in RIFLE-F categories
C. Up to 20% of bacteremic patients develop AKI, and increases to 50% in patients with septic shock
D. The mortality in sepsis-related AKI is approximately 70% compared to approximately 45% in non-sepsis-related AKI patients
E. All of the above

The answer is E

All of the above statements are correct (E). The incidence of AKI is much higher in ICU than in non-ICU patients. Bacteremia/sepsis seems to be the underlying etiology for most of the patients admitted to ICU. It appears that the majority of patients admitted to ICU with AKI had previous kidney dysfunction.

Suggested Reading

Kidney Disease: Improving Global Outcomes (KDIGO) Acute Kidney Injury Work Group. KDIGO clinical practice guideline for acute kidney injury. Kidney Int (Suppl). 2012;2:1–138.

Singbartl K, Kellum JA. AKI in the ICU: definition, epidemiology, risk stratification, and outcomes. Kidney Int. 2012;81:819–25.

9. A 50-year-old woman with type 2 diabetes is admitted to ICU for hypotension, shortness of breath, and dysuria. Her admission creatinine is 1.6 mg/dL, which increased from 1.2 mg/dL from the last admission. Her HbA1c is 9.8%. **Which one of the following acute complications decreases overall survival in this patient?**

A. Volume overload
B. Hyperkalemia
C. Lactic acidosis
D. Respiratory failure
E. All of the above

The answer is E

This patient seems to have sepsis from urinary tract infection. She requires fluid management, pressor support, and antibiotic administration. All of the above complications are likely to develop in this patient, requiring renal replacement therapy and mechanical ventilation, and places her as a high risk patient to increased morbidity and mortality. Thus, answer E is correct.

The complications of AKI that increase morbidity and mortality can be divided into two groups: traditional and nontraditional, as suggested by Faubel and Shah (1). These are shown in Table 5.2.

Table 5.2 Traditional and nontraditional complications of AKI

Traditional	Nontraditional
Fluid overload	Systemic inflammatory response syndrome (SIRS)
Electrolyte and acid-base disturbances	Compensatory anti-inflammatory response syndrome (CARS)
Hyperkalemia	Immune dysregulation
Hyperphosphatemia	Sepsis
Hypocalcemia	Respiratory failure
Metabolic acidosis	Cardiogenic and noncardiogenic pulmonary edema
Uremic complications	Cardiac complications
Altered mental status	Type 3 cardiorenal syndrome
Pericarditis	
Bleeding	

Reference

Faubel S, Shah PB. Immediate consequences of acute kidney injury: the impact of traditional and nontraditional complications on mortality in acute kidney injury. Adv Chronic Kidney Dis. 2016;23:179–85.

10. **AKI is a common complication following cardiac surgery. Regarding cardiac surgery-related AKI, which one of the following statements is CORRECT?**

A. Based on the need for renal replacement therapy (RRT), rates of AKI range from 0.33 to 9.5%
B. According to a study that used the RIFLE classification, the incidence of AKI for R, I, and F were 9%, 5%, and 2%, respectively
C. Factors such as renal insufficiency, congestive heart failure, female gender, predispose patients to AKI following cardiac surgery
D. Exposure to nephrotoxic drugs such as nonsteroidal anti-inflammatory drugs increases the risk of AKI following cardiac surgery
E. All of the above

The answer is E

All of the above statements are correct (E). Although most of the risk factors are the same for both cardiac surgery-related and other forms of AKI, additional patient-related and procedure-related factors have been identified for AKI during and after cardiac surgery. Table 5.3 **shows these risk factors.**

Table 5.3 Cardiac surgery-related risk factors for AKI

Patient-related	Procedure-related	Postoperative
Diabetes (insulin-requiring) COPD Renal dysfunction (preoperative creatinine 1.2 to <2.1 mg/dL) Peripheral vascular disease CHF Ejection fraction <35% Left main coronary artery disease Cardiogenic shock (preoperative use of intra-aortic balloon pump) Emergency surgery Females Advanced age Liver disease Smoking	Length of cardiopulmonary bypass Cross-clamp time Off-pump versus on-pump Nonpulsatile flow Hemolysis Hemodilution Inotropic use Venous congestion Emboli (cholesterol)	Vasopressor use Hypovolemia Diuretic use Venous congestion Cardiogenic shock Anemia

Suggested Reading

Fuhrman DY, Kellum JA. Epidemiology and pathophysiology of cardiac surgery-associated acute kidney injury. Curr Opin Anesthesiol. 2017;30:60–5.

Rosner MH, Portilla D, Okusa MD. Cardiac surgery as a cause of acute kidney injury: pathogenesis and potential therapies. J Intensive Care Med. 2008;23:3–18.

Yi Q, Li K, Jian Z, et al. Risk factors for acute kidney injury after cardiovascular surgery: evidence from 2157 cases and 49 777 controls: a meta-analysis. Cardiorenal Med. 2016;6:237–50.

11. **Which one of the following pathophysiologic mechanisms is implicated in cardiac surgery-associated AKI?**

A. Nephrotoxins
B. Increased systemic venous congestion
C. Cardiopulmonary bypass-induced oxidative stress
D. Ischemia-reperfusion injury
E. All of the above

The answer is E

AKI complicates recovery from cardiac surgery in approximately 30% of patients. Also, it impairs the functions of the lung, brain, and gut, and causes a fivefold risk for morbidity and mortality during hospitalization. Therefore, it is extremely important to understand the pathophysiology of AKI in these patients for appropriate management of organ dysfunction.

The pathophysiology of cardiac surgery-associated is multifactorial that include all of the above listed mechanisms, making E as the correct answer. Nephrotoxins include antibiotics, released hemoglobin (iron) from hemolysis of blood during cardiopulmonary bypass, and high levels of myoglobin released during surgery or from rhabdomyolysis.

Systemic or renal venous congestion (systemic venous hypertension) has been proposed as one of the mechanisms causing AKI. High central venous pressure (CVP) due to right heart failure and other low cardiac output conditions seem to precipitate postoperative AKI. When CVP reaches the threshold of 14 mm Hg in postoperative period, the risk of AKI increases twofold with an odds ratio of 1.9. Venous congestion due to CHF increases renal vein pressure, which causes reduced renal perfusion and AKI. Fluid management of AKI is extremely important as fluid overload may worsen AKI.

The use of cardiopulmonary bypass (CPB) pump has been shown to activate proinflammatory cytokines compared to operative procedures done off-CPB pump. It seems that exposure of blood to the extracorporeal circuit

may activate alternative complement cascade and predispose to AKI. Also, hemolysis of blood with release of hemoglobin and iron-induced oxidative stress may play a role in causing AKI. Thus, CPB pump is an important risk factor for AKI.

Ischemia and reperfusion injury is another mechanism for cardiac surgery-induced AKI. Reperfusion injury is related to duration of ischemia. Renal ischemia is rather common in patients with low cardiac output because of compensatory increase in sympathetic and renin-angiotensin II-aldosterone systems. During reperfusion, reoxygenation occurs and causes production of reactive oxygen species (ROS). These ROS products induce several deleterious cellular responses, which lead to inflammation, cell death, and AKI. Thus, answer E is correct.

Suggested Reading

Bellomo R, Auriemma S, Fabbri A, et al. The pathophysiology of cardiac surgery-associated acute kidney injury (CSA-AKI). Int J Artif Organs. 2008;31:166–78.

Fuhrman DY, Kellum JA. Epidemiology and pathophysiology of cardiac surgery-associated acute kidney injury. Curr Opin Anesthesiol. 2017;30:60–5.

Gambardella I, Gaudino M, Ronco C, et al. Congestive kidney failure in cardiac surgery: the relationship between central venous pressure and acute kidney injury. Interact Cardiovas Thoracic Surg. 2016;23:800–5.

O'Neal JB, Shaw AD, Billings FT. Acute kidney injury following cardiac surgery: current understanding and future directions. Crit Care. 2016;20:187.

12. A 55-year-old African American man with diabetes and severe coronary artery disease (CAD) is admitted for acute coronary syndrome. He is on several medications for his CAD, and cardiac bypass surgery (CABG) has been suggested. **Which one of the following drugs needs to be discontinued before CABG to reduce the incidence of AKI?**

A. Hydralazine
B. Carvedilol
C. Ramipril/Losartan
D. Nitrates
E. None of the above

The answer is C

Besides drugs such as nonsteroidal anti-inflammatory drugs, many other drugs have been shown to cause AKI. Of these drugs, the clinical implications of ACE-Is and ARBs alone have been explored in patients who require cardiac surgery because these drugs are extensively used in patients with diabetes, hypertension, and heart disease. In a meta-analysis, Yacoub et al. concluded that preoperative use of either ACE-Is or ARBs is associated with increased incidence of postoperative AKI and mortality in patients undergoing cardiac surgery. These authors suggested to discontinue ACE-Is or ARBs prior to cardiac surgery. Thus, C is correct. The effect of other drugs is little understood.

Suggested Reading

Shiffermiller JF, Monson BJ, Vokoun CW, et al. Prospective randomized evaluation of preoperative angiotensin-converting enzyme inhibition (PREOP-ACEI). J Hosp Med. 2018;13:661–7.

Yacoub R, Patel N, Lohr JW, et al. Acute kidney injury and death associated with renin angiotensin system blockade in cardiothoracic surgery: a meta-analysis of observational studies. Am J Kidney Dis. 2013;62:1077–86.

13. You are asked to see a 22-year-old man with congestive heart failure (CHF) with ejection fraction of 12% for increasing serum creatinine from 1.2 mg/dL to 2.6 mg/dL in 3 days. Pulmonary artery pressure is 72 mm Hg. He has anasarca with increasing ascites despite adequate management of his CHF for the last 10 days. He did not receive any nephrotoxins, although he had cardiac catheterization 4 months ago. His urine output is slowly decreasing. **Which one of the following BEST describes his acute rise in creatinine and decrease in urine output?**

A. Possible hepatic congestion with further decrease in kidney function
B. Contrast-induced late acute kidney injury (AKI)
C. Increased intra-abdominal pressure (IAP)
D. Pulmonary hypertension precipitating AKI
E. None of the above

The answer is C

Of all the choices, choice C best describes his acute rise in serum creatinine and a decrease in urine output. IAP, also called intra-abdominal hypertension, affects many organs, including the kidneys. Although the mechanisms for AKI are not completely understood, renal vein compression with increased venous resistance and impaired venous drainage seems to be the most important mechanism for AKI. Renal blood flow decreases even further in a decompensated CHF patient by the presence of ascites. IAP should be considered in such a patient for acute rise in serum creatinine. IAP >15 may cause oliguria, but anuria develops at a pressure >30 mm Hg. Lowering IAP improves both creatinine and urine output. Other options are unlikely causes of AKI in this patient.

Suggested Reading

Hunt L, Frost SA, Hillman K, et al. Management of intra-abdominal hypertension and abdominal compartment syndrome: a review. J Trauma Manag Outcomes. 2014;8:2.

De Laet IE, Malbrain MLNG, De Waele JJ. A clinician's guide to management of intraabdominal hypertension and abdominal compartment syndrome in critically ill patients. Crit Care. 2020;24:97.

De Waele JJ, De Laet I, Kirkpatrick AW, et al. Intra-abdominal hypertension and abdominal compartment syndrome. Am J Kidney Dis. 2011;57:159–69.

14. A 62-year-old woman with type 2 diabetes and coronary heart disease is admitted with shortness of breath and palpitations. Pertinent medications include furosemide 40 mg once daily, ramipril 10 mg once daily, and glipizide 10 mg once daily. CXR shows pulmonary congestion. On physical exam, she has increased JVD, an S_3 and 2+ pitting edema of lower extremities. The ECHO showed an ejection fraction of 20%, and a diagnosis of acute decompensated heart failure (ADHF) was made. Labs: Na^+ 134 mEq/L, K^+ 3.8 mEq/L, Cl^- 90 mEq/L, HCO_3^- 28 mEq/L, BUN 46 mg/dL, creatinine 1.8 mg/dL (creatinine 1 week ago was 1.2 mg/dL), eGFR <60 mL/min, glucose 100 mg/dL, and $HbA1_c$ 7%. **Which one of the mechanisms is contributing to her decreased kidney function?**

A. Increased central and renal venous pressure
B. Activation of renin-AII-aldosterone system (RAAS)
C. Decreased renal perfusion
D. RAAS inhibitor use
E. All of the above

The answer is E

This patient has type 1 cardiorenal syndrome (CRS). CRS is an entity that refers to the interactivity between the heart and kidney. Both organs have a cross talk between them in health and disease. Renal dysfunction carries poor prognosis in hospitalized patients with acute decompensated heart failure. Thus, the relationship between the heart and the kidney is intricate and unavoidable. A classification of CRS has been developed to enhance our understanding of the pathophysiology of this syndrome. As shown in Table 5.4, **CRS has been classified into five types.**

Table 5.4 Classification of cardiorenal syndrome

Type	Description	Recommended treatment
Type 1	Abrupt worsening of cardiac function (e.g., cardiogenic shock, acute decompensated heart failure) leading to acute kidney injury (AKI)	A combination of a loop diuretic, a thiazide diuretic and aldosterone antagonist seems appropriate at this time. If creatinine increases due to diuretic therapy, ultrafiltration therapy seems justified
Type 2	Chronic heart failure leading to progressive CKD	Loop and K^+-sparing diuretics, vasodilators, including ACE-Is
Type 3	AKI leading to acute cardiac disorders (fluid overload, CHF, arrhythmias due to hyperkalemia)	Treat cardiac disorders appropriately
Type 4	CKD leading to chronic heart failure due to fibrosis, anemia, etc.	Loop diuretics, ACE-Is, ARBs, correction of anemia, and other drugs as indicated
Type 5	Systemic diseases (e.g., diabetes, lupus) leading to both cardiac and kidney dysfunction	Treat the underlying disease and institute appropriate management to prevent cardiac and kidney disease

The mechanisms for AKI in type 1 CRS include all of the above mechanisms (E). Of these mechanisms, a recently proposed mechanism, right-sided heart failure and renal congestion, is receiving much attention in the pathogenesis of AKI in type 1 CRS. The rise in venous pressure lowers the arteriovenous pressure gradient across the kidney, increases the renal interstitial pressure, and reduces renal blood flow, leading to decreased GFR. Use of diuretics and RAAS inhibitors also precipitates AKI. Although diuretics have been shown to activate RAAS and sympathetic tone, they are useful in improving symptoms of congestion. For this reason, loop diuretics are used in type 1 CRS.

Suggested Reading

Palazzuoli A, Ruocco C. Heart–kidney Interactions in cardiorenal syndrome type 1. Adv Chronic Kidney Dis. 2018;25:408–17.

Rangaswami J, Bhalla V, Blair JEA, et al. On behalf of the American Heart Association Council on the Kidney in Cardiovascular Disease and Council on Clinical Cardiology. Cardiorenal syndrome: classification, pathophysiology, diagnosis, and treatment strategies: a scientific statement from the American Heart Association. Circulation. 2019;139:e840–e878.

Ronco C, Haapio M, House AA, et al. Cardio-renal syndrome. J Am Coll Cardiol. 2008;52:1527–39.

15. A 56-year-old man with history of hypertension and coronary heart disease is admitted for acute decompensated heart failure (ADHF). His admission creatinine is 2.9 mg/dL, BUN 54 mg/dL. His blood pressure is 112/72 mm Hg with a heart rate of 76 beats per min. **Which one of the following variables is predictive of higher in-hospital mortality in patients with ADHF?**

    A. Creatinine >2.8 mg/dL
    B. BUN >43 mg/dL
    C. Systolic blood pressure (SBP) <115 mm Hg
    D. SBP >120 mm Hg
    E. A, B, and C

    The answer is E

    Renal dysfunction carries poor prognosis in hospitalized patients with acute decompensated heart failure. The Acute Decompensated Heart Failure National Registry (ADHERE) database study reported that of all the 39 variables the study evaluated, only high admission levels of BUN (≥43 mg/dL) followed by a systolic blood pressure <115 mm Hg, and creatinine levels ≥2.75 mg/dL predicted high mortality in hospitalized patients with heart failure. Among the three variables only the admission BUN levels ≥43 mg/dL remained as the single determinator between hospital survivors and nonsurvivors. Thus, option E is correct.

    Suggested Reading

    Fonarow GC, Adams Jr. KF, Abraham WT, et al. Risk stratification for in-hospital mortality in acutely decompensated heart failure. Classification and regression tree analysis. JAMA. 2005;293:572–80.

16. A 62-year-old man with history of hypertension and type 2 diabetes is admitted for fever and acute abdominal pain. CT of abdomen with contrast is negative. He receives 2 g of vancomycin, and 4 days later his creatinine increases to 1.9 mg/dL (admission creatinine 1.2 mg/dL). His urine output started to decrease to 300 mL/day, and subjectively developed shortness of breath (SOB). On physical exam, he has JVD and 1+ edema of his legs. He was given 40 mg of furosemide, but his urine output did not improve. **Which one of the following mechanisms is responsible for cardiac dysfunction in patients with AKI?**

    A. Altered cardiac hemodynamics following AKI
    B. Myocardial neutrophil invasion and apoptosis
    C. Fluid overload and hyperkalemia
    D. Metabolic acidosis
    E. All of the above

    The answer is E

    This patient has acute renocardiac syndrome (Type 3 CRS), which is characterized by sudden onset of AKI, leading to acute cardiac dysfunction. AKI in this patient is due to contrast and also probably vancomycin use.

Decreased urine output may cause fluid overload, SOB, and edema. Hyperkalemia is rather common in patients with AKI, which may induce arrhythmias, further decreasing kidney function. Severe metabolic acidosis reduces cardiac contractility. Type 3 CRS is rather uncommon than type 1 CRS.

AKI has several effects on the heart besides fluid overload and occasional hyperkalemia. In ischemia-reperfusion injury rat model of AKI, several hemodynamic changes in the heart were observed on ECHO, including left ventricular (LV) dilatation, increased LV end systolic and diastolic diameter, increased relaxation time, and decreased fractional shortening. These cardiac changes may be due to invasion of neutrophil and release of inflammatory cytokines. The neuroendocrine system may also play a role in altered cardiac function in type 3 CRS. Thus, option E is correct.

Suggested Reading

Damman K, Tang WH, Felker GM, et al. Current evidence on treatment of patients with chronic systolic heart failure and renal insufficiency: practical considerations from published data. J Am Coll Cardiol. 2014;63:853–71.

Kelly KJ. Distant effects of experimental renal ischemia/reperfusion injury. J Am Soc Nephrol. 2003;14:1549–58.

Rangaswami J, Bhalla V, Blair JEA, et al. On behalf of the American Heart Association Council on the Kidney in Cardiovascular Disease and Council on Clinical Cardiology. Cardiorenal syndrome: classification, pathophysiology, diagnosis, and treatment strategies: a scientific statement from the American Heart Association. Circulation. 2019;139:e840–78.

Ronco C, Haapio M, House AA, et al. Cardio-renal syndrome. J Am Coll Cardiol. 2008;52:1527–39.

17. The urine output of the above patient started to decrease and urine sediment showed numerous muddy brown casts. You made the diagnosis of acute tubular necrosis (ATN), and you are concerned about worsening of his kidney function and the need for renal replacement therapy (RRT). **Which one of the following tests is MOST likely to predict the development of stage 3 AKI and the need for RRT?**

A. Urinary Na^+ excretion >20 mEq/L
B. Urine neutrophil gelatinase-associated lipocalin (NGAL) level 140 ng/mL
C. Urine kidney injury molecule-1 (KIM-1)
D. Urine output <200 mL over a period of 2 h following i.v. furosemide at 1.5 mg/kg
E. None of the above

The answer is D

This patient has ATN, but it is difficult to predict whether his tubular function will worsen and require RRT or improve. AKI biomarkers, including urine Na^+, will help to some extent but do not forecast the need for RRT (answers A–C are incorrect). In the past, it was the practice to give i.v. furosemide to convert anuria into oliguria. However, this practice is currently not recommended because of adverse effects. Chawla and colleagues reintroduced the use of i.v. furosemide with a different concept of assessing renal tubular function in a prospective study, and called it "furosemide stress test (FST)." This test involves i.v. administration of furosemide at a dose of 1 mg/kg for those who did not receive furosemide in the past and 1.5 mg/kg for those who received furosemide, and follow urine output for a period of 2 h. If urine output is <200 mL, it predicted the progression of stages 1 and 2 AKI to stage 3 AKI, the need for RRT and in-hospital mortality. Urine out >200 mL is indicative of recovery of tubular function. Thus, answer D is correct.

In the following publication of the previous cohort, it was shown that 2-h urine output after FST was significantly better than each urinary biomarker tested in predicting progression to stage 3. When FST urine output was assessed in patients with increased biomarker levels, the predictive value for progression to stage 3, initiation of RRT and inpatient mortality was much improved. Thus, FST seems to be a useful test in critically ill patients for the assessment of severity of AKI.

Suggested Reading

Chawla LS, Davison DL, Brasha-Mitchell E, et al. Development and standardization of a furosemide stress test to predict the severity of acute kidney injury. Crit Care. 2013;17:R207.

Chen J-J, Chang C-H, Huang Y-T, et al. Furosemide stress test as a predictive marker of acute kidney injury progression or renal replacement therapy: a systemic review and meta-analysis. Crit Care. 2020;24:202.

Koyner JL, Davison DL, Brasha-Mitchell E, et al. Furosemide stress test and biomarkers for the prediction of AKI severity. J Am Soc Nephrol. 2015;26:2023–31.

18. You are called by a cardiologist for evaluation of creatinine of 2.2 mg/dL (eGFR 40 mL/min) in a 58-year-old woman who is admitted for management of CHF with ejection fraction (EF) of 40%. She is on enalapril, metoprolol, and spironolactone. She denies chest pain, shortness of breath, or palpitations. **Which one of the following appropriate therapeutic managements you recommend for the patient that would not affect kidney function?**

   A. Add an angiotensin receptor blocker (ARB)
   B. Strat ultrafiltration (UF)
   C. Discontinue enalapril and start sacubitril/valsartan
   D. Increase metoprolol dose
   E. Continue current management

   The answer is C

   Angiotensin converting enzyme inhibitors (ACE-Is) have been used for several years in the management of patients with severe heart failure with good results. Some patients on ACE-Is had some adverse effects. For this reason, ARBs were used. However, ARBs had inconsistent results. For this reason, a combination of neprilysin inhibitor (sacubitril) and valsartan (an ARB) was studied in patients with EF <40%.

   Neprilysin is a neutral endopeptidase. It degrades endogenous vasoactive peptides, such as natriuretic peptides, bradykinin, and adrenomedullin. Inhibition of neprilysin increases the levels of these substances, which counteract the neurohormonal overactivation that contributes to vasoconstriction, Na^+ retention, and maladaptive remodeling.

   The combination of sacubitril/valsartan was studied in patients with EF <40% and compared its effects with enalapril. In this PARADIGM-HF (The Prospective Comparison of ARNI [Angiotensin Receptor–Neprilysin Inhibitor] with ACE-I to Determine Impact on Global Mortality and Morbidity in Heart Failure) trial, the combination of sacubitril/valsartan was found to be superior in reducing the risk of death and hospitalization without any significant change in creatinine in patients with heart failure. Thus, answer C is correct. Other options are not appropriate for this patient, as adding an ARB induces AKI and hyperkalemia, UF is not warranted, and increasing metoprolol dose is not more advantageous because the patient is stable.

   Suggested Reading

McMurray JJV, Packer M, Desai AS, et al. PARADIGM-HF Investigators and Committees. Angiotensin-neprilysin inhibition versus enalapril in heart failure. N Engl J Med. 2014;371:993–1004.

19. The above patient gradually became edematous and became more short of breath, and did not respond to either bolus or continuous intravenous (IV) furosemide and metolazone. Also, no further improvement with nesiritide, dobutamine, and milrinone. Ultrafiltration with the Aqadex System 100 (CHF solutions, Minneapolis, MN) was started. **Which one of the following statements is CORRECT regarding ultrafiltration (UF) with Aquadex System 100 compared to IV diuretic therapy in patients with CHF?**

   A. UF group had a 38% greater weight loss and 28% fluid loss compared to diuretic group
   B. UF had a 50% reduction in rehospitalizations for heart failure at 90 days after discharge compared to diuretic group
   C. UF group had a nonsignificant lower mortality rate (9.6%) compared to 19.4% of diuretic group
   D. Removal of Na^+ by UF was greater than the removable by diuretic use
   E. All of the above

   The answer is E

   All of the above statements are correct. Diuretic resistance is not uncommon in some patients with CHF. UF is recommended when pharmacologic treatment fails. In the UNLOAD (Ultrafiltration versus Intravenous Diuretics for Patients Hospitalized for Acute Decompensated Congestive Heart Failure) study, those participants who received UF for 48 h lost more weight, more volume, and more Na^+ loss than participants treated with diuretics. Also, 90-day rehospitalization rates were significantly reduced in UF than diuretic group. However, the mortality at 90 days was not significant between the groups (9 deaths in UF group and 11 in diuretic group). Thus, option E is correct.

   However, it should be noted that the CARRESS-HF (The Cardio Rescue Study in Acute Decompensated Heart Failure) study reported that stepped care diuretic therapy is superior to UF in patients with acute decompensated heart failure patients. Further studies comparing UF with diuretic therapy in these patients may resolve some of these controversial issues.

A systematic review and meta-analysis of seven studies on UF versus pharmacologic therapy concluded that "UF is more efficient with regard to reduction in weight and fluid removal in patients with ADHF without an apparent untoward impact on kidney function. UF is also associated with reduction in the HF rehospitalization rate but does not portend any survival benefit" (Jain, Agrawal, Kajory, 2016).

Suggested Reading

Bart BA, Goldsmith SR, Lee KL, et al. for the Heart failure Clinical Research Network. Ultrafiltration in decompensated heart failure with cardiorenal syndrome. N Engl J Med. 2012;367:2296–304.

Costanzo MR, Guglin ME, Saltzberg MT, et al. For the UNLOAD Trial Investigators. Ultrafiltration versus intravenous diuretics for patients hospitalized for acute decompensated heart failure. J Am Coll Cardiol. 2007;49:675–83.

Dahle TG, Sabotka PA, Boyle AJ. A practical guide for ultrafiltration in acute decompensated heart failure. Congest Heart Fail. 2008;14:83–8.

Jain A, Agrawal N, Kazory A. Defining the role of ultrafiltration therapy in acute heart failure: a systematic review and meta-analysis. Heart Fail Rev. 2016;21:21:611–17.

20. In the above patient, the creatinine did not improve. Also, his serum [$HC0_3^-$] is decreasing. His blood pressure (BP) is 110/70 mm Hg. **Based on BP, fluid status, and electrolyte abnormalities, which one of the following renal replacement therapies (RRTs) is appropriate for this patient?**

    A. Intermittent hemodialysis (IHD)
    B. Slow continuous ultrafiltration (SCUF)
    C. Continuous venovenous ultrafiltration (CVVH)
    D. Peritoneal dialysis (PD)
    E. Continuous venovenous diafiltration (CVVHDF)

    The answer is E

    The choice of RRTs is usually based on the patient's hemodynamics, fluid status, electrolyte abnormalities, and solute removal. Based on BP, IHD is not appropriate in this patient because it may lower BP even further without sufficient removal of fluid (A is incorrect). SCUF and CVVH may improve fluid, but do not improve electrolyte abnormalities sufficiently (B and C are incorrect). PD is a slow process, and may compromise breathing, and D is, therefore, incorrect. In this patient, CVVHDF seems appropriate because it will improve volume status, creatinine, and electrolyte abnormalities. Therefore, E is correct. It should be noted that fluid overload at the initiation of dialysis is associated with increased risk of death.

Suggested Reading

Claure-Del Granado R, Macedo E, Mehta RL. Indications for continuous renal replacement therapy. Renal replacement versus renal support. In: Ronco C, Bellomo R, Kellum JA, et al. editors. Critical care nephrology. 3rd ed. Philadelphia: Elsevier; 2019, pp. 987–92.

Ricci Z, Ronco C. Timing, dose and mode of dialysis in acute kidney injury. Curr Opin Crit Care. 2011;17:558–61.

21. In preparation for CVVHDF, placement of a temporary catheter was ordered. **Which one of the following sites is associated with least bacteremia and catheter dysfunction?**

    A. Left internal jugular vein
    B. Right internal jugular vein
    C. Femoral vein
    D. Subclavian vein
    E. B and C

    The answer is E

    Studies have shown that left jugular vein catheter placement is associated with catheter dysfunction compared to right jugular vein. Also, the blood flow in left jugular and subclavian veins is erratic and lower than other sites. Earlier studies have also shown that femoral vein catheters were associated with bacteremia. However, randomized and cross-over studies showed that both femoral and jugular vein catheter placement in critically ill patients yielded similar results. Therefore, either femoral vein or jugular vein catheter placement is acceptable in the

above patient (E is correct). According to KDIGO guidelines, the following are the preference sites for catheter placement:

- **First choice – right jugular vein**
- **Second choice = femoral vein**
- **Third choice = left jugular vein**
- **Last choice = subclavian vein with preference to the dominant side**

Suggested Reading

Brain M, Winson E, Roodenburg O, et al. Non anti-coagulant factors associated with filter life in continuous renal replacement therapy (CRRT): a systematic review and meta-analysis. BMC Nephrol. 2017;18:69.

Duguè AE, Levesque SP, Fischer M-O, et al. Vascular access sites for acute renal replacement in intensive care units. Clin J Am Soc Nephrol. 2012;7:70–7.

Kidney Disease: Improving Global Outcomes (KDIGO) Acute Kidney Injury Work Group. KDIGO clinical practice guideline for acute kidney injury. Kidney Int (Suppl). 2012;2:1–138.

Parienti JJ, Megabane B, Lautrette A, et al. Catheter dysfunction and dialysis performance according to vascular access among 736 critically ill adults requiring renal replacement therapy. A randomized controlled study. Crit Care Med. 2010;38:1118–25.

22. **CVVHDF was started. Which one of the following effluent volume flow rate is recommended in patients undergoing CVVHDF?**

A. 45 mL/kg/h
B. 40 mL/kg/h
C. 35 mL/kg/h
D. 30 mL/kg/h
E. 20–25 mL/kg/h

The answer is E

A study in 2000 first demonstrated an improved survival in patients with AKI who received CVVH with effluent flow rate of 35 mL/kg/h compared to those who received 20 mL/kg/h. This study led to two prospective studies that evaluated the effect of high effluent flow rate versus low effluent flow rate. In the ATN (Acute Renal Failure Trial Network) study, there was no difference in mortality at 60 days between patients who received 35 mL/kg/h and 20 mL/kg/h. The other study, RENAL (Randomized Evaluation of Normal versus Augmented Level of Replacement Therapy), also showed no survival benefit at 90 days in patients who received effluent flow rate of either 40 mL/kg/h or 25 mL/kg/h during CVVHDF. Thus, no survival benefit could be achieved above 25 mL/kg/h (E is correct). Interruptions to either CVVHDF or CVVH do occur and may compromise dose, and therefore, the effluent flow rate is usually recommended between 25 and 30 mL/kg/h.

Suggested Reading

Bellomo R, Cass A, Cole L, et al. RENAL Replacement Therapy Study Investigators. Intensity of continuous renal-replacement therapy in critically ill patients. N Engl J Med. 2009;361:27–38.

Palevsky PM, Zang JH, O'Connor TZ, et al. The VA/NIH Acute Renal Failure Trial Network. Intensity of renal support in critically ill patients with acute kidney injury. N Engl J Med. 2008;359:7–20.

Ronco C, Bellomo R, Homel P, et al. Effect of different doses in continuous veno-venous haemofiltration on outcomes of acute renal failure: a prospective randomized trial. Lancet. 2000;356:26–30.

23. You started CVVHDF in a 70-kg man for AKI and fluid overload. His INR is 2.2, and not on any anticoagulation. Both arterial and venous pressures are normal. There is no kinking of the femoral access. Twenty-four hours later, the nurse reports to you that the filter is clotted and you want to verify your orders. She gives you the following values:

Blood flow 190 mL/min (Q_B)
Replacement (prefilter) 2500 mL/h
Fluid removal 150 mL/h
Hematocrit (Hct) 26%

Which one of the following is the MOST likely explanation for clotting of the filter?

A. Low blood flow
B. Low replacement fluid
C. Lack of anticoagulation
D. High filtration fraction (FF)
E. None of the above

The answer is D

Several factors can promote clotting of the filter (hemofilter). These include hemoconcentration (high blood viscosity), very high blood flows, high arterial and venous pressures, kinking of the catheter (subclavian catheter has increased risk of kinking), blood-air contact in the machine due to activation of coagulation, and high FF (>0.25–0.3 or 25–30%).

This patient does not need anticoagulation, as his INR is 2.2. Blood flow is sufficient, and not low. Also, the replacement fluid is approximately 35 mL/kg/h, which is higher than the recommended dose (20–25 mL/kg/h), making options A, B, and C incorrect. High FF is the most likely cause of his filter clotting (correct answer), although replacement fluid is given before the filter (predilution).

Simply FF describes a relationship between the amount of blood flow through the filter and the rate of removal of water from blood in the filter. The FF can be calculated by the values given above and using the following formula:

$$FF = \frac{Q_{UF}}{Q_B(1 - Hct)}$$

where Q_{UF} is ultrafiltration rate (replacement volume plus fluid removal rate), which equals 2500 mL plus 150 mL = 2650 mL. Q_B is blood flow rate (190 mL/min or 11,400 mL/h) and Hct 26% (1–0.26 = 0.74). Total denominator equals 11,400 x 0.74 = 8436 mL/h.

$$FF = \frac{2,650}{8,436} = 0.31 \text{ or } 31\%$$

or simply FF = Q_{UF}/Plasma flow rate (1-Hct) $= \frac{2650}{8436} = 0.31 \text{ or } 31\%$

Therefore, increased FF is the explanation for clotting of the hemofilter. It should be noted that not only postdilution but also predilution causes increased FF. In order to lower FF, either a decrease in the dose of replacement fluid to 25–30 mL/kg/h or an increase in blood flow to 200 mL/min can lower FF to <31%. Based on his weight of 70 kg, his replacement fluid should be 1750 to 2100 mL/kg/h.

Suggested Reading

Hatamizadeh P, Tolwani A, Palevsky P. Revisiting filtration fraction as an index of the risk of hemofilter clotting in continuous venovenous hemofiltration. Clin J Am Soc Nephrol. 2020;15:ccc–ccc. https://doi.org/10.2215/CJN.024.
Joannidis M, Oudermanns-van Straaten HM. Clinical review: patency of the circuit in continuous renal replacement therapy. Crit Care. 2007;11:218.
Ricci Z, Baldwin I, Ronco C. Alarms and troubleshooting. In: Kellum JA, Bellomo R, Ronco C, editors. Continuous renal replacement therapy. 2nd ed. Oxford: Oxford University Press; 2016, p. 131–8.
Tolwani A. Continuous renal-replacement therapy for acute kidney injury. N Engl J Med. 2012;367:2505–14.

24. Despite several adjustments during CVVHDF in the above patient, the hemofilter clotted several times. His blood pressure is 130/80 mm Hg. You decide to do intermittent HD (IHD) in view of clotting and also shortage of nursing staff. **Which one of the following statements is CORRECT regarding the renal replacement therapies (RRTs) on patient and renal survival?**

A. IHD is better than CVVH
B. CVVHD is better than CVVH
C. CVVHDF is better than CVVHD
D. Daily HD is better than high volume peritoneal dialysis (PD)
E. No difference among the above RRT modalities

The answer is E

Several studies have addressed the issue of RRTs and their effect on patient and kidney survival with different results. However, meta-analyses of these studies showed that the recovery of kidney function and survival rates were similar among various RRTs. Also, a randomized study showed no difference in metabolic control, mortality, and kidney function between high volume PD and daily HD. Therefore, a real benefit of one modality over the other has not been confirmed. Thus, option E is correct.

Suggested Reading

Bagshaw SM, Berthiaume LR, Delaney A, et al. Continuous versus intermittent therapy for critically ill patients with acute kidney injury: a meta-analysis. Crit Care Med. 2008;36:610–17.

Nash DM, Przech S, Wald R, et al. Systematic review and meta-analysis of renal replacement therapy modalities for acute kidney injury in the intensive care unit. J Crit Care. 2017;41:138–44.

Pannu N, Klarenbach S, Wiebe N, et al. Renal replacement therapy in patients with acute renal failure: a systematic review. JAMA. 2008;299:793–805.

25. **Regarding anticoagulation in CRRT in critically ill patients, which one of the following KDIGO guideline recommendations is CORRECT?**

    A. Regional citrate anticoagulation rather than heparin in patients who do not have contraindications for citrate
    B. Unfractionated or low molecular weight heparin for patients with contraindication to citrate
    C. Regional citrate anticoagulation, rather than no anticoagulation, in a patient with increased bleeding risk
    D. Avoidance of regional heparinization in a patient with increased bleeding risk
    E. All of the above

The answer is E

All of the above statements are correct. Regarding the selection of anticoagulant, regional citrate anticoagulation is recommended by most of the nephrologists and intensivists in order to avoid heparin-induced bleeding and thrombocytopenia as well as preventing heparin resistance.

Suggested Reading

Kidney Disease: Improving Global Outcomes (KDIGO) Acute Kidney Injury Work Group. KDIGO clinical practice guideline for acute kidney injury. Kidney Int (Suppl). 2012;2:1–138.

Liu C, Mao Z, Kang H, et al. Regional citrate versus heparin anticoagulation for continuous renal replacement therapy in critically ill patients: a meta-analysis with trial sequential analysis of randomized controlled trials. Crit Care. 2016;20:144.

Oudemans-van Straaten HM, Kellum JA, Bellomo R. Clinical review: Anticoagulation for continuous renal replacement therapy-heparin or citrate?. Crit Care. 2011;15:202.

26. A 54-year-old obese African American woman with history of hypertension is admitted for acute coronary syndrome, requiring coronary catheterization and emergent CABG (coronary artery bypass grafting). She became hypotensive during surgery with decreased urine output. Her preoperative serum creatinine was 1.4 mg/dL, which increased to 3.2 mg/dL. Over the next several days, she improved her serum creatinine with fluids and inotropes. She was discharged with creatinine of 1.6 mg/dL. **Which one of the following statements is CORRECT regarding AKI following CABG?**

    A. She is at increased risk for CKD and ESKD
    B. She is at increased risk for further cardiovascular disease
    C. CKD is a major risk factor for AKI after contrast use
    D. All of the above
    E. None of the above

The answer is D

There are several studies addressing the prognostic significance of community and in-hospital acquired AKI. Coca et al. evaluated 13 cohort studies of AKI leading to CKD, ESKD, and death, and reported the incidence of CKD and ESKD after AKI was 25.8 and 8.6 per 100 person-years, respectively. The pooled adjusted hazard ratio for mortality was 2 (CI 1.3–3.1). Also, AKI was independently associated with cardiovascular disease and congestive heart failure. Thus, D is correct.

Suggested Reading

Chawla LS, Eggers PW, Star RA, et al. Acute kidney injury and chronic kidney disease as interconnected syndromes. N Engl J Med. 2014;371:58–66.

Coca SG, Singanamala S, Parikh CR. Chronic kidney disease after acute kidney injury: a systematic review and meta-analysis. Kidney Int. 2012;81:442–8.

27. A 63-year-old man develops AKI following knee surgery and antibiotic use. The creatinine rose from 0.9 mg/dL to 6.4 mg/dL. His urine output is <200 mL in 12 h, and his serum [K^+] is 5.5 mEq/L. **Which one of the following is an absolute indication for RRT?**

A. Serum BUN 100 mg/dL
B. Serum [K^+] >6 mEq/L with EKG changes
C. Serum pH <7.15
D. Urine output <200 mL for 12 h or anuria
E. All of the above

The answer is E

All of the above choices are absolute indications for initiating RRT in patients with AKI. (E is correct.) In this patient, urine output <200 mL in 12 h is an indication for RRT. Using the RIFLE classification, a consensus statement was published regarding the absolute and relative indications of RRT for patients with AKI, as shown in Table 5.5**:**

Table 5.5 Indications for RRT in patients with AKI

Indication	Characteristics	Absolute	Relative
Metabolic abnormality	BUN >76 mg/dL		X
	BUN >100 mg/dL	X	
	Hyperkalemia >6 mEq/L		X
	Hyperkalemia >6 mEq/L with EKG changes	X	
	Dysnatremia		X
	Hypermagnesemia >8 mEq/L		X
	Hypermagnesemia >8 mEq/L with anuria and absent deep tendon reflexes	X	
Acidosis	pH >7.15		X
	pH <7.15	X	
	Lactic acidosis due to metformin		X
Anuria/oliguria	RIFLE class R		X
	RIFLE class I		X
	RIFLE class F		X
	Urine output <200 mL for 12 h or anuria	X	
Fluid overload	Diuretic-responsive		X
	Diuretic-resistant	X	

Absolute indications for RRT also include uremic signs and symptoms such as encephalopathy, pericarditis, bleeding, neuropathy, and myopathy. It should be noted that neuropathy is a complication of CKD rather AKI. Some patients with rhabdomyolysis-induced AKI may present with myopathy.

Suggested Reading

Küllmar M, Zarbock A. Renal replacement therapy in acute kidney injury: from the indications to cessation. Anaesthetist. 2019;68:485–96.

Mendu ML, Ciociolo GR Jr, McLaughlin SR, et al. A decision-making algorithm for initiation and discontinuation of RRT in severe AKI. Clin J Am Soc Nephrol. 2017;12:228–36.

Ricci Z, Ronco C. Timing, dose and mode of dialysis in acute kidney injury. Curr Opin Crit Care. 2011;17:558–61.

28. The above patient was started on CVVHDF because of sepsis, hypotension, and a slight increase in body weight due to fluid infusion. **Regarding timing of initiation of RRT, which one of the following statements is CORRECT?**

 A. Initial studies showed that early initiation of RRT in critically ill patients with AKI reduced mortality over the first 90 days compared to delayed initiation of RRT
 B. Early RRT initiation is justified when life-threatening changes in metabolic control, fluid, or acid-base balance are seen to improve morbidity
 C. Recent studies have shown no difference between early and late initiation of RRT
 D. All of the above
 E. None of the above

 The answer is D

 The issue of the optimal timing for initiation of RRT in critically ill patients with AKI had been the subject of controversy for many years. Initially, a few observational studies and a meta-analysis showed reduced mortality with early initiation of RRT in critically ill patients. This was supported by the study of Zarbock and associates (A is correct). In order to improve fluid, electrolyte and acid-base disorders, early RRT is justified (B is correct).

 When long-term outcomes (>60 days mortality) are concerned, other studies did not substantiate the observations of Zarbock and associates. For example, the study of Gaudry et al. showed that RRT is a risk factor for increased mortality compared to conservative management. Further observations by Gaudry et al. also showed no benefit of early versus late initiation of RRT regarding a 60-day mortality.

 The STARRT-AKI Investigators conducted a multinational, randomized, controlled trial involving critically ill patients with severe AKI. Patients were randomly assigned to receive either an early (12-h) or late (>72-h) RRT with the primary outcome of death from any cause at 90 days. The study showed that early initiation of RRT in critically ill patients with AKI was not associated with a lower risk of death at 90 days as compared with late initiation of RRT (C is correct).

 Suggested Reading

Bagshaw SM, Wald R, Adhikari NKJ, et al. The STARRT-AKI Investigators, for the Canadian Critical Care Trials Group, the Australian and New Zealand Intensive Care Society Clinical Trials Group, the United Kingdom Critical Care Research Group, the Canadian Nephrology Trials Network, and the Irish Critical Care Trials Group. Timing of initiation of renal-replacement therapy in acute kidney injury. N Engl J Med. 2020;383:240–51.

Gaudry S, Ricard J-D, Leclaire C, et al. Acute kidney injury in critical care: Experience of a conservative strategy. J Crit Care. 2014;29:1022–7.

Gaudry S, Hajage D, Schortgen F, et al. for the AKIKI Study Group. Initiation strategies for renal-replacement therapy in the intensive care unit. N Engl J Med. 2016; 375:122–33.

Zarbock A, Kellum JA, Schmidt C, et al. Effect of early vs delayed initiation of renal replacement therapy on mortality in critically ill patients with acute kidney injury: the ELAIN randomized clinical trial. JAMA. 2016;315:2190–9.

29. CVVHDF was continued in the above patient for 14 days, and the intensivist decides to discontinue it. **Regarding discontinuation of CVVHDF, which one of the following criteria is CORRECT?**

 A. Discontinue when intermittent HD (IHD) is indicated
 B. Discontinue when life support is withdrawn
 C. Discontinue when spontaneous urine output >400 mL/24 h and creatinine clearance >15 mL/min
 D. >2400 mL/24 h following diuretic use
 E. All of the above

 The answer is E

 The criteria for discontinuation of RRT in critically ill patients are not either validated or standardized. However, the intensivist and the nephrologist can decide when to stop RRT. A patient who was on CVVHDF for several days improves both blood pressure and metabolic status can go on IHD in order to allow the patient's own kidneys to get better during nondialysis days (A is correct). Also, discontinuation is preferred when care is withdrawn, or in multiorgan failure due to no return of function (B is correct). Studies have shown that improvement in spontaneous urine output or in response to diuretics has been shown to be an important predictor of discontinuation of RRT (C and D are correct). Thus, option E is correct.

It should be noted that some physician use diuretics to improve urine output following RRT. Although diuretics can improve urine output, their use is of no benefit either in improving renal recovery from AKI or the need for restarting RRT.

Suggested Reading

Kelly YP, Waikar SS, Mendu ML. When to stop renal replacement therapy in anticipation of renal recovery in AKI: the need for consensus guidelines. Sem Dial. 2019;32:205–9.

Kidney Disease: Improving Global Outcomes (KDIGO) Acute Kidney Injury Int (Suppl). 2012;2:1–138.

Romagnoli S, Clark WR, Ricci Z, et al. Renal replacement therapy for AKI: when? how much? when to stop?. Best Prat Anaesthel. 2017;31:371–85.

30. You are consulted on a patient with AKI following off-pump coronary artery bypass surgery (CABG). **Based on current evidence of off-pump versus on-pump CABG, which one of the following choices is CORRECT?**

    A. On-pump CABG causes higher incidence of AKI the off-pump CABG
    B. Off-pump CABG is likely to reduce the incidence of AKI
    C. Off-pump CABG is associated with a nonsignificant reduction in dialysis requirement
    D. Off-pump CABG is not associated with a significant reduction in mortality
    E. All of the above

    The answer is E

    AKI following CABG prolongs hospital stay, and increases the need for RRT. Traditionally, CABG is performed with extracorporeal cardiopulmonary bypass (CPB) machine. This procedure is called on-pump CABG. A meta-analysis reported that on-pump CABG was associated with increased incidence of AKI (4%), dialysis requirement (2.4%), and mortality of 2.6%. On the other hand, off-pump CABG was associated with a 40% lower odds of postoperative AKI, and a nonsignificant 33% lower odds of dialysis requirements. However, no reduction in mortality was observed. Thus, choice E is correct.

    The reasons that were proposed for higher incidence of AKI in on-pump CABG patients include renal hypoperfusion, hypotensive episodes, inflammation, and oxidant stress. Compared to on-pump surgery, off-pump surgery has potential benefits of reduced risk of AKI, reduced cerebral dysfunction, reduced ICU stay, and reduced mortality. However, KIDIGO guideline suggests that "off-pump coronary artery bypass graft surgery not be selected solely for the purpose of reducing perioperative AKI or need for RRT."

Suggested Reading

Kidney Disease: Improving Global Outcomes (KDIGO) Acute Kidney Injury Work Group. KDIGO Clinical practice guideline for acute kidney injury. Kidney Int (Suppl). 2012;2:1–138.

Seabra VF, Alobaidi S, Balk E, et al. Off-pump coronary artery bypass surgery and acute kidney injury: a meta-analysis of randomized controlled trials. Clin J Am Soc Nephrol. 2010;5:1734–44.

31. You are asked by a thoracic surgeon for an advice regarding prevention of AKI in a 52-year-old woman who had CABG with the use of atrial natriuretic peptide (ANP). Her serum creatinine is 0.8 mg/dL. **Which one of the following advices is MOST appropriate for this patient?**

    A. ANP reduces diuresis and GFR
    B. ANP reduces natriuresis
    C. ANP reduces mortality
    D. There are no definitive studies to support any natriuretic peptide use for prevention, or treatment of AKI
    E. There are several studies to support the use of natriuretic peptides for prevention, or treatment of AKI

    The answer is D

    ANP is a 28-amino acid peptide that is produced by atrial myocytes in response to atrial stretch. It has diuretic, natriuretic, and vasodilatory properties. It increases GFR (A and B are incorrect). ANP treatment has no effect on mortality (C is incorrect). Although several studies have shown renal beneficial effects of low-dose ANP infusion, many other studies have not shown any beneficial effects (E is incorrect). However, a Japanese study used preoperatively human ANP in CKD patients who underwent CABG, and compared renal outcomes with saline.

The infusion of ANP was continued 12 h into postoperative period. The results showed that the incidence of acute/early dialysis was higher in the saline group (5.5%) than the ANP group (0.7%). Despite this positive trial, the KIDIGO guideline suggests not to use either ANP, or nesiritide (brain natriuretic peptide) to prevent or treat AKI until the results of definitive studies are available (D is correct).

Suggested Reading

Kidney Disease: Improving Global Outcomes (KDIGO) Acute Kidney Injury Work Group. KDIGO clinical practice guideline for acute kidney injury. Kidney Int (Suppl). 2012;2:1–138.

Sezai A, Hata M, Niino T, et al. Continuous low-dose infusion of human natriuretic peptide in patients with left ventricular dysfunction undergoing coronary artery bypass grafting: The NU-HIT (Nihon University working group study of low-dose human ANP Infusion Therapy during cardiac surgery) for left ventricular dysfunction. J Am Coll Cardiol. 2010;55:1844–51.

32. A 55-year-old woman is transferred to ICU for hypotension and AKI following prolonged hip surgery. Her blood pressure is 70/40 mm Hg with heart rate of 92 BPM. She received Ringer's lactate during surgery and in ICU. Clinically she is adequately fluid resuscitated (trace edema). The intensivist started vasopressors. **Regarding vasopressors and shock, which one of the following statements is CORRECT?**

A. Dopamine use is associated with an increased risk of death in patients with cardiogenic shock
B. Norepinephrine (NE) is the drug of choice in patients with septic shock
C. Vasopressin is the most cost-effective second-line vasopressor in both the short- and long-term evaluations
D. Compared to NE, vasopressin is associated with lower progression of RIFLE-R category to F or L categories in adults with septic shock
E. All of the above

The answer is E

All of the above statements are correct (E). The use of vasopressors, dopamine, NE, and vasopressin has been recommended in vasomotor shock in patients at risk for AKI or in patients with AKI. The rationale is an increase in mean arterial blood pressure ≥65 mm Hg to improve not only renal but also perfusion to other organs. A meta-analysis showed that dopamine is associated with increased arrhythmias and mortality compared to NE. NE is usually the preferred first-line vasopressor used throughout the world. However, vasopressin has gained widespread popularity in conditions of NE resistance and alleviation of high doses of NE.

As a second-line vasopressor, vasopressin not only reduces the dose but also enhances the action of NE. A post-hoc analysis of the VASST (Vasopressin and Septic Shock Trial), which is a randomized study comparing vasopressin with NE in adults with septic shock showed that vasopressin, has an added advantage in reducing the progression of RIFLE-R category to F or L categories. Thus, NE and vasopressin are used to support blood pressure in ICUs.

Suggested Reading

Chawla LS, Ostermann M, Forni L, et al. Broad spectrum vasopressors: a new approach to the initial management of septic shock?. Crit Care. 2019;23:124.

De Backer D, Aldecoa C, Njimi H, et al. Dopamine versus norepinephrine in the treatment of septic shock. Crit Care Med. 2012;40:725–30.

Gelinas JP, Russell JA. Vasopressors during sepsis. Selection and targets. Clin Chest Med. 2016;37:251–62.

Gordon AC, Russell JA, Walley KR, et al. The effects of vasopressin on acute kidney injury in septic shock. J Intensive Care Med. 2010;36:83–91.

Lam SW, Barreto EF, Scott R, et al. Cost-effectiveness of second-line vasopressors for the treatment of septic shock. J Crit Care. 2020;55:48–55.

Ukor I-F, Walley KR. Vasopressin in vasodilatory shock. Crit Care Clin. 2019;35:247–61.

33. The above patient, who is not a diabetic, develops hyperglycemia with serum glucose level of 242 mg/dL. **Based on clinical studies, which one of the following glucose levels is considered appropriate?**

A. 90–105 mg/dL
B. 110–149 mg/dL
C. 150–180 mg/dL

D. 90–110 mg/dL
E. 100–160 mg/dL

The answer is B

In ICU patients with sepsis and other conditions, hyperglycemia develops due to stress-induced insulin resistance. Intensive insulin therapy lowers glucose. Studies have shown that intensive glucose control reduces the intensity and severity of AKI. However, the degree of intensity that avoids severe hypoglycemia has not been established. Following an extensive review of literature, the KDIGO guideline recommends maintenance of serum glucose between 110 and 149 mg/dL. Thus, B is correct.

Suggested Reading

Kidney Disease: Improving Global Outcomes (KDIGO) Acute Kidney Injury Work Group. KDIGO clinical practice guideline for acute kidney injury. Kidney Int (Suppl). 2012;2:1–138.

34. A 60-year-old man is admitted to the neuro ICU following subarachnoid hemorrhage. He has an intracranial pressure (ICP) of 22 mm Hg. The patient creatinine increases from 0.8 to 1.4 mg/dL and serum [K^+] 5.9 mEq/L due to Ringer's lactate. The creatinine did not improve with adequate fluid administration, and the patient is not fluid overloaded. The neurosurgeon calls you to consider dialysis. **Which one of the following is a reasonable RRT modality for this patient?**

A. Intermittent hemodialysis (IHD)
B. Slow continuous ultrafiltration (SCUF)
C. CVVH
D. CVVHDF
E. Peritoneal dialysis (PD)

The answer is D

IHD increases ICP and may worsen neurological status. Dialysis disequilibrium syndrome has also been reported with HD. SCUF and CVVH may be appropriate for patients with fluid overload. With these techniques, removal of creatinine is minimal, and acidosis, if any, will not improve. CVVHDF will improve AKI without raising too much ICP. Thus, D is correct. Comparative studies of PD with CVVHDF on changes in ICP are lacking. In this patient with relatively high [K^+], PD may not be sufficient even after discontinuation of Ringer's lactate.

Suggested Reading

Bagshaw SM, Peets AD, Hameed M, et al. Dialysis disequilibrium syndrome: Brain death following hemodialysis for metabolic acidosis and acute renal failure – a case report. BMC Nephrol. 2004;5:9.
Davenport A. Continuous renal replacement therapies in patients with acute neurological injury. Semin Dial. 2009;22:165–8.

35. CVVHDF was started in the above patient with ICP monitoring. There was only a 2 mm Hg increase in ICP. The patient is unable to have oral intake of food because of dysphagia due to prolonged intubation. **Regarding nutritional support, which one of the following choices is FALSE in this patient?**

A. A total energy intake of 20–30 kcal/kg/d is adequate in patients at any stage of AKI
B. Dietary prescription should be composed of 3–5 g/kg/d carbohydrate and 0.8–1.0 g/kg/d
C. Protein intake up to 1.7 g/kg/d needs to be recommended in patients on continuous renal replacement therapy (CRRT) or hypercatabolic
D. Enteral feeding is the preferred route of nutrition support than early parenteral route
E. Protein intake should be restricted in all AKI patients, including this patient

The answer is E

Except for E, all other choices are correct. Restriction of protein should be avoided. Hypercatabolic patients and patients on CRRT require high protein (1.7 g/kg/d). Enteral feeding is recommended because it maintains gut integrity, decreases gut atrophy as well as bacterial translocation, and may protect bleeding from stress ulcers. Early parenteral nutrition (within 48 h of ICU admission) support was found to cause more complications such as fever than late (before 8 days) nutrition support. Choice E is, therefore, false.

Suggested Reading

Casaer MP, Mesotten D, Hermans G, et al. Early versus late parenteral nutrition in critically ill patients. N Engl J Med. 2011;365:506–17.

Kidney Disease: Improving Global Outcomes (KDIGO) Acute Kidney Injury Work Group. KDIGO clinical practice guideline for acute kidney injury. Kidney Int (Suppl). 2012;2:1–138.

36. You are asked by your colleague, a cardiothoracic surgeon, about a patient who is scheduled for a valve replacement and the use of N-acetylcysteine (NAC) as a prophylactic agent to prevent postsurgical AKI. **Based on current evidence, which one of the following advices you would give to you colleague?**

A. Only oral NAC prevents postsurgical AKI
B. Only intravenous (IV) NAC prevents postsurgical AKI
C. Neither oral nor IV NAC has any effect on postsurgical AKI
D. Current evidence is not enough to make any decision
E. Enough evidence exists to support the use of NAC

The answer is C

NAC is an amino acid that replenishes the stores of reduced glutathione (GSH), which is an antioxidant and also a vasodilator. NAC has been shown to prevent or improve ischemic as well as nephrotoxic AKI in animals. Based on these studies, several investigators have tested in humans the protective effect of NAC in the prevention of AKI before and after contrast use, and cardiothoracic as well as abdominal vascular procedures. Although the results are mixed, many meta-analyses have not shown any beneficial effects of NAC either in prevention of AKI, or improving mortality. Based on the evidence, the KDIGO working group does not suggest either oral or IV NAC to prevent postsurgical AKI (C is correct). All other choices are, therefore, incorrect.

Suggested Reading

Kidney Disease: Improving Global Outcomes (KDIGO) Acute Kidney Injury Work Group. KDIGO clinical practice guideline for acute kidney injury. Kidney Int (Suppl). 2012;2:1–138.

37. A 65-year-old man undergoes transcatheter aortic valve implantation (TAVI) received 2 units of packed RBC (pRBC) and 1 unit postsurgically. His creatinine increased from 0.8 mg/dL to 1.2 mg/dL. **Regarding pRBC transfusion and AKI, which one of the following statements is CORRECT?**

A. The incidence of AKI from two studies has been reported to be 21 and 29%, respectively, following TAVI
B. There is a relationship between the number of units administered and the incidence of AKI
C. Transfusion of shorter storage time RBCs is much safer than longer storage time RBCs
D. RBCs of shorter storage time release less inflammatory cytokines and free iron than RBCs of longer storage time
E. All of the above

The answer is E

In recent years, interest in pRBC transfusion and AKI following cardiopulmonary bypass and TAVI is gaining popularity. Following TAVI, transfusion of pRBCs remains one of the strongest predictors of AKI, and an incidence of 21 and 29% has been reported in two studies. Also, a study has shown a relationship between the number of units and relative risk (RR) of AKI, as shown in Table 5.6.

Table 5.6 Relationship between the number of units and RR (relative risk) following TAVI

No. of units	RR (95% confidence interval)
1–2	1.43 (0.98–2.22)
3–4	3.05 (1.24–7.53)
≥5	4.81 (1.45–15.95)

Another concern of transfusion is the storage time of pRBCs. Currently, pRBCs are stored up to 42 days, and during prolonged storage changes in RBC structure with subsequent release of many inflammatory cytokines, free heme, and lipid peroxides. These released products seem to play an important role in the development of AKI. Thus, transfusion of pRBCs with shorter duration of storage is preferred to those stored for longer time. Thus, all of the above statements are correct (E).

Suggested Reading

Heddle NM, Cook RJ, Arnold DM, et al. The effect of blood storage duration on in-hospital mortality: a randomized controlled pilot feasibility trial. Transfusion. 2012;52:1203–12.

Karkouti K. Transfusion and acute kidney injury in cardiac surgery. Br J Anaesthesia. 2012;109:129–38.

Nuis RJ, Rodės-Cabau J, Sinning JM, et al. Blood transfusion and the risk of acute kidney injury after transcatheter aortic valve implantation. Circ Cardiovasc Interv. 2012;5:680–8.

38. You are consulted on a 60-year-old man who was intubated 3 days ago for evaluation of AKI. His creatinine increased from 0.8 to 1.4 mg/dL. He is euvolemic and his BP is 120/80 mm Hg. He is not on any nephrotoxic drugs. You believe that his AKI is related to mechanical ventilation (MV). **Which one of the following mechanisms is IMPLICATED in mechanical ventilation (MV)-induced AKI?**

    A. Hypoxemia
    B. Hypercapnia
    C. Reduced cardiac output
    D. Barotrauma
    E. All of the above

The answer is E

Several studies have shown that MV can cause AKI by all of the mechanisms (E is correct). Hypoxemia, either low PO_2 (<40 mm Hg) or high PCO_2 (>60 mm Hg), can decrease renal blood flow (RBF), and decrease GFR, by causing renal vasoconstriction. Hypercapnia has been shown to directly stimulate norepinephrine levels, which causes renal vasoconstriction. MV can reduce renal perfusion by reducing cardiac output. Reduction in cardiac output is due to decreased preload and increased right ventricular afterload. Barotrauma due to MV seems to stimulate the release of inflammatory cytokines in the lung, which then are released into the circulation, causing AKI. Thus, all of the above mechanisms seem to play in MV-induced AKI.

Suggested Reading

Hepokoskia ML, Atul Malhotra A, Singh P, et al. Ventilator-induced kidney injury: are novel biomarkers the key to prevention?. Nephron. 2018;40:90–3.

Koyner JL, Murray PT. Mechanical ventilation and lung-kidney interactions. Clin J Am Soc Nephrol. 2008;3:562–70.

Kuiper JW, Groeneveld ABJ, Slutsky AR, et al. Mechanical ventilation and acute renal failure. Crit Care Med. 2005;33:1408–15.

va den Akker JPC, Egal M, Grovenveld ABJ. Invasive mechanical ventilation as a risk factor for acute kidney injury in the critically ill: a systematic review and meta-analysis. Crit Care. 2013;17:R98.

39. The above patient slowly developed ARDS (acute respiratory distress syndrome). **Regarding nutrition and ventilation of this ARDS patient, which one of the following statements is CORRECT?**

    A. Routine use of omega-3 fatty acid/γ-linolenic acid supplementation is not necessary in patients with ARDS
    B. Aerosolized β-agonist therapy is contraindicated in patients with ARDS
    C. High-frequency oscillatory ventilation (HFOV) is not beneficial and may increase in-hospital mortality
    D. Prone positioning is beneficial in reducing mortality
    E. All of the above

The answer is E

All of the above statements are correct (E). ARDS is classified into mild (PO_2/FiO_2 ratio between 201 and 300), moderate (PO_2/FiO_2 ratio between 101 and 200), and severe (PO_2/FiO_2 ratio $\leq$100). In ARDS patients, low levels of omega-3 fatty acids have been reported, causing increased inflammation, and γ-linolenic acid also seems to reduce neutrophil leukotriene production and predisposes to inflammation. Replacement of diet containing both acids is believed to improve inflammation. However, studies have shown no benefit of omega-3 fatty acid/γ-linoleic acid supplementation. Indeed, this diet increased mortality (A is correct).

Studies on aerosolized β-agonist therapy is contraindicated in patients with ARDS because the use of solbutamol was associated with lactic acidosis, tachycardia, and arrhythmias (B is correct). Another study also had negative results.

A study published in 2013 reported that the use of HFOV in patients with moderate to severe ARDS was associated with increased in-hospital mortality (C is correct). Another study reported similar results. Early application

of prolonged prone positioning significantly reduced 28-day and 90-day mortality in patients with severe ARDS (D is correct).

Suggested Reading

Ferguson ND, Cook DJ, Guyatt GH, et al., for the OSCILLATE Trial Investigators and the Canadian Critical Care trial Group. High-frequency oscillation in early acute respiratory distress syndrome. N Engl J Med. 2013;368:795–805.

Gao Smith F, Perkins GD, Gates S, et al. Effect of intravenous beta-2-agonist treatment on clinical outcomes in acute respiratory distress syndrome (BALT1-2): a multicentre, randomized controlled trial. Lancet. 2012;379:229–35.

Guérin C, Reignier J, Richard J-C, et al. Prone positioning in severe acute respiratory distress syndrome. N Engl J Med. 2013;368:2159–68.

Rice TW, Wheeler AP, Thompson BT, et al. Enteral omega-3 fatty acid, gamma-linolenic acid, and antioxidant supplementation in acute lung injury. JAMA. 2011;306:1584–1.

40. **Hypoxemia may precipitate AKI. In patients with ARDS, which one of the following maneuvers is safe in improving oxygenation and outcomes in patients with ARDS?**

A. Low tidal volume
B. High levels of positive end-expiratory pressure (PEEP)
C. Neuromuscular blockade
D. Sedation
E. All of the above

The answer is E

Patients with acute lung injury and ARDS may benefit from low tidal volume, which was associated with lower mortality rate. High levels of PEEP may reduce refractory hypoxemia, and improve ventilator-free days. Studies on neuromuscular blockade with agents such as cisatracurium improved not only oxygenation but also 90-day mortality rate. Use of cisatracurium is safe in critically ill patients, as this neuromuscular blockade is not metabolized either by the kidney or liver. With neuromuscular blockade, it is better to use sedation (with lorazepam) and pain medications as well to make the patient comfortable because paralytics have no sedative or analgesic effects. Thus, E is correct.

Suggested Reading

Briel M, Meade M, Mercat A, et al. Higher vs lower positive end-expiratory pressure in patients with acute lung injury and acute respiratory distress syndrome: systematic review and meta-analysis. JAMA. 2010;303:865–73.

Papazian L, Forel JM, Gacouin A, et al. Neuromuscular blockers in early acute respiratory distress syndrome. N Engl J Med. 2010;363:1107–16.

The ARDS Network Ventilation with lower tidal volumes as compared with traditional tidal volumes for acute lung injury and the acute respiratory distress syndrome. N Engl J Med. 2000;342:1301–8.

41. Acute kidney injury (AKI) is an extrapulmonary complication of ARDS. **Which one of the following is the risk factor for AKI?**

A. Diabetes mellitus
B. Heart failure
C. Metabolic acidosis
D. Higher sequential organ failure assessment (SOFA) score
E. All of the above

The answer is E

In a retrospective study of 357 patients with ARDS and no Prior history of either AKI or CKD, 244 (68.3%) patients developed AKI. Of these 244 patients, 60 (24.6%) had stage 1 AKI, 66 (27%) had stage 2 AKI, and 118 (48.4%) had stage 3 AKI. The median time for AKI development was 2–4 days. All of the above answers were risk factors for AKI (answer E is correct). In addition, higher age, higher BMI, and peak airway pressure were associated with the development of AKI. Thus, AKI is a serious complication of ARDS and mechanical ventilation.

Suggested Reading

Panitchote A, Mehkri O, Hastings A, et al. Factors associated with acute kidney injury in acute respiratory distress syndrome. Ann Intensive Care. 2019;9:74. https://doi.org/10.1186/s13613-019-0552-5.

42. A 62-year-old type 2 diabetic woman is admitted with urosepsis develops AKI 3 days after admission. Her systolic BP is 100 mm Hg. The patient receives several liters of normal saline, and currently on norepinephrine. Her creatinine increased from 0.6 to 1.6 mg/dL. Her admission weight was 62 kg, and at time of consultation the weight was 70 kg (a gain of 8 kg). **Regarding her creatinine level and AKI, which one of the following statements is CORRECT?**

A. Her creatinine increase is only 1.0 mg/dL, and additional volume administration is needed to improve AKI
B. She needs 5% albumin to improve creatinine levels and AKI
C. Her elevation in creatinine is actually an underestimation in view of her weight gain
D. There is no relationship between volume expansion and creatinine level
E. None of the above

The answer is C

Several studies have shown that volume expansion (fluid overload) underestimates serum creatinine levels, and delay the initiation of diagnosing AKI and renal replacement therapies. Positive fluid balance increases the volume of creatinine distribution, and lowers its levels. Both in children and adults, fluid overload (>10%) was found to be associated with increased mortality. This patient gained 8 kg (>10%), which underestimates her serum creatinine. Thus, C is correct.

Suggested Reading

Godin M, Bouchard J, Mehta RL. Fluid balance in patients with acute kidney injury: emerging concepts. Nephron Clin Pract. 2013;123:238–45.
Payen D, de Pont AC, Sakr Y, et al. A positive fluid balance is associated with a worse outcome in patients with acute renal failure. Crit Care. 2008;12:R74.

43. In order to obtain real serum creatinine concentration in critically ill patients with fluid overload, fluid-adjusted serum creatinine concentration has been developed. The net cumulative fluid balance is 8 L in 3 days. **Based on the formula, which one of the following fluid-adjusted serum creatinine is CORRECT?**

A. 1,74 mg/dL
B. 1.84 mg/dL
C. 1.94 mg/dL
D. 2.04 mg/dL
E. 2.54 mg/dL

The answer is C

Macedo et al. developed a formula to calculate fluid-adjusted serum creatinine concentration as follows:

$$\text{Adjusted serum creatinine} = \text{serum creatinine} \times \text{correction factor}$$

where correction factor is:

$$[\text{hospital admission weight}\left(\text{kg} \times 0.6\right] + \Sigma\left(\begin{array}{l}\text{daily cumulative fluid balance}\left(\text{L}\right)/\\ \text{hospital admission weight} \times 0.6\end{array}\right)$$

$$\text{Serum creatinine} = 1.6\,\text{mg}/\text{dL}$$

Applying the patient's values, we obtain

$$\text{Weight} = 62\,\text{kg} \times 0.6 = 37.2\,\text{L}$$

$$\text{Cumulative fluid balance} = 8\,\text{L}, \text{or}$$

$$37.2 + 8 = 45.2/37.2 = 1.21$$

$$\text{Adjusted serum creatinine} = 1.6 \times 1.21 = 1.94\,\text{mg}/\text{dL}$$

Therefore, the actual creatinine is 1.94 mg/dL, and fluid gain decreased creatinine by 0.34 mg/dL. Thus, option C is correct.

Suggested Reading

Macedo E, Bouchard J, Soroko SH, et al. for Program to improve care in acute renal disease study: fluid accumulation, recognition and staging of acute kidney in critically ill patients. Crit Care. 2010;14:R82.

44. Her urinalysis showed 1+ proteinuria, 2–3 RBCs, and 10 WBCs. Urine sediment had 3–4 granular casts and 5 renal tubular cells. **Based on the current evidence, what would be her prognosis of AKI?**

A. She needs additional urine studies to evaluate her renal prognosis
B. She is at risk for progression to AKI stages 2–3
C. The urine microscopy findings have no relevance to AKI prognosis
D. Renal ultrasonography is useful in assessing AKI prognosis
E. Her creatinine will return to baseline, once her sepsis and BP improve without any future complications

The answer is B

Urinalysis (dipstick and sediment analysis) differentiates prerenal AKI from acute tubular necrosis (ATN). In prerenal AKI, the urinalysis is "bland" with few hyaline casts. However, the urinalysis is abnormal in ATN. The presence of "muddy brown" casts and renal tubular cells is indicative of ATN (mostly due to rhabdomyolysis). Recently, the urine microscopy has gained great importance in assessing renal prognosis in hospitalized patients with AKI. Perazella et al. developed a scoring system based on granular casts and renal tubular cells to differentiate ATN from prerenal AKI. The scoring system is as follows:

Score (points)	Renal tubular cells (per HPF)	Granular casts (per LPF)
1	0	0
2	0 or 1–5	1–5 or 0
3	1–5 or 0	1–5 or 6–10

HPF high power field, *LPF* low power field

It is clear from the above table that score 1 point favors prerenal stage 1 AKI and score points 2–3 favor ATN. Further analysis of the scoring system ≥2 revealed worsening of AKI (progression to higher stages of AKI, dialysis, or death) during hospitalization. Thus, urine microscopy is a valuable diagnostic tool in the diagnosis of ATN with good prognostic significance (B is correct).

Renal ultrasonography is useful in making the diagnosis of AKI due to obstruction, and it may have prognostic significance in CKD patients whose cortical thickness is <2 cm (C is incorrect). Even if her creatinine returns to baseline at discharge, she is at increased risk for CKD (D is incorrect).

Suggested Reading

Perazella MA, Coca SG, Kanbay M, et al. Diagnostic value of urine microscopy for differential diagnosis of acute kidney injury in hospitalized patients. Clin J Am Soc Nephrol. 2008;3:1615–9.
Perazella MA, Coca SG, Hall IE, et al. Urine microscopy is associated with severity and worsening of acute kidney injury in hospitalized patients. Clin J Am Soc Nephrol. 2010;5:402–8.
Perazella MA, Coca SG. Traditional urinary biomarkers in the assessment of hospital-acquired AKI. Clin J Am Soc Nephrol. 2012;7:167–74.

45. A 48-year-old woman is admitted to ICU with sepsis due to pneumonia. She has been vomiting for 4 days without any food intake. She stopped taking chlorthalidone 25 mg 2 days ago. Her BP is 80/60 mm Hg with a heart rate of 114 BPM. Her labs: Na^+ 130 mEq/L, K^+ 4.9 mEq/L, Cl^- 87 mEq/L, HCO_3^- 18 mEq/L, creatinine 1.6 mg/dL, BUN 36 mg/dL, and glucose 74 mg/dL. Lactate is 6 mmol/L. Hemoglobin is 9 g/dL. There is no peripheral edema. **Which one of the following resuscitation fluids is MOST appropriate for this patient?**

A. Ringer's lactate
B. Normal saline (0.9%)
C. 5% albumin
D. 6% hydroxyethyl starch (hetastarch)
E. 10% hetastarch

The answer is B

Of all the above fluids, normal saline seems appropriate to improve volume status, urine output, and BP. However, fluid overload with normal saline should always be avoided, as it may mask the recognition of further increase in serum creatinine, and delay the initiation of RRT. Also, serum Cl^- and HCO_3^- levels have to be followed to avoid hyperchloremia (>110 mEq/L) and dilutional acidosis.

Ringer's lactate is not appropriate at this time because of elevated lactate levels and slight elevation in K^+. Albumin was found to be no effective than isotonic saline in ICU patients [Saline vs Albumin Fluid Evaluation (SAFE) study]. Six percent hetastarch is isotonic, whereas 10% hetastarch is a hyperoncotic fluid. Several randomized trials using hetastarches for volume resuscitation in ICU patients with sepsis have shown increased incidence of AKI compared to crystalloids. Therefore, the use of all hetastarches in ICU patients is NOT recommended for initial fluid resuscitation. Thus, B is correct.

Suggested Reading

Casey JD, Brown RM, Semler MW. Resuscitation of fluids. Curr Opin Crit Care. 2018;24:512–8.
Godin M, Bouchard J, Mehta RL. Fluid balance in patients with acute kidney injury. Nephron Clin Pract. 2013;123:238–45.
Kidney Disease: Improving Global Outcomes (KDIGO) Acute Kidney Injury Work Group. KDIGO clinical practice guideline for acute kidney injury. Kidney Int (Suppl). 2012;2:1–138.
Kumar G, Walker E, Stephens R. Intravenous fluid therapy. Trend Anaesth Crit Care. 2014;4:55–9.
Reddy S, Weinberg L, Young P. Crystalloid fluid therapy. Critical Care. 2016;20:59.
van Haren F, Zacharowski K. What is new in volume therapy in intensive care unit?. Best Pract Clin Anaesthesiol. 2014;28:275–83.

46. The above patient received a total of 10 L normal saline. There is trace peripheral edema. Her serum [Cl^-] is 115 mEq/L. **Which one of the following statements about hyperchloremia is CORRECT?**

A. Hyperchloremia causes renal vasoconstriction
B. Chloride-restrictive fluids decrease the incidence of AKI and the need for RRT in critically ill patients
C. Hyperchloremic acidosis from saline causes systemic hypotension
D. Saline infusion is associated with longer time to first micturition compared to Ringer's lactate infusion
E. All of the above

The answer is E

All of the above statements are correct (E). Although crystalloid rather than colloids are recommended as initial choices of fluid resuscitation in ICU patients, hyperchloremia resulting from large volume infusion of saline may have several adverse effects on kidney function. Initial studies in animals showed renal vasoconstriction, resulting in decreased renal blood flow and GFR (A is correct). Clinically, chloride-rich fluid administration to ICU patients caused higher incidence of AKI and requirement for RRT than chloride-restrictive fluids (B is correct). Induction of hyperchloremia in animals led to a dose-dependent systemic hypotension (C is correct). In human volunteers and patients, high-chloride fluids caused longer time to first urination compared to low-chloride fluids. In noncardiac surgery patients, hyperchloremia was associated with poor postoperative outcomes. (D is correct.)

It is of interest to note that normal saline caused hyperkalemia and more acidosis than Ringer's lactate during kidney transplantation.

Suggested Reading

Casey JD, Brown RM, Semler MW. Resuscitation of fluids. Curr Opin Crit Care. 2018;24:512–8.
McCluskey SA, Karkouti K, Wijeysundera D, et al. Hyperchloremia after noncardiac surgery is independently associated with increased morbidity and mortality: a propensity-matched cohort study. Anesth Analg. 2013;117:412–21.
Myburgh JA, Mythen MG. Resuscitation fluids. N Engl J Med. 2013;369:1243–51.
Yunos NM, Bellomo R, Story D, et al. Bench-to-bedside: chloride in critical illness. Crit Care. 2010;14:226.
Yonos NM, Bellomo R, Hegarty C, et al. Association between a chloride-liberal vs chloride-restrictive intravenous fluid administration strategy and kidney injury in critically ill adults. JAMA. 2012;308:1566–72.

47. A 50-year-old woman is admitted to ICU with urosepsis and severe abdominal pain, requiring intubation for airway protection. She has history of hypertension, and her current BP is 110/80 mm Hg with a heart rate of 112 BPM. Her

serum creatinine is 1.6 mg/dL (her creatinine 2 weeks ago was 0.8 mg/dL). She requires fluids. **Which one of the following measures of intravascular volume is MOST appropriate for fluid responsiveness?**

A. Central venous pressure (CVP)
B. Pulmonary capillary wedge pressure (PCWP)
C. Pulse pressure variation (PPV) and stroke volume variation (SVV)
D. Inferior vena cava diameter
E. Right ventricular end-diastolic volume (RVEDV)

The answer is C

Fluid resuscitation is the most important initial management in critically ill and injured patient. Studies have shown that CVP and PCWP measurements, which are static measures of intravascular volume, are no longer recommended in critically ill patients for fluid responsiveness in these patients. Other static measures, such as (RVEDV) is also not recommended. Similarly, measurements of inferior vena-caval diameter require experienced intensivists and are difficult to measure in obese patients and those with laparotomy. Also, changes in inferior vena cava occur with changes in intra-abdominal pressures. Thus, this technique is not applicable to all patients.

Studies have shown that PPV, which is derived from analysis of the arterial waveform, and SVV derived from analysis of pulse contour can be highly predictive of fluid responsiveness. In this patient with abdominal pain PPV and SVV are most appropriate dynamic measures of intravascular measures of volume responsiveness, and, therefore, C is correct.

Suggested Reading

Frazee E, Kashani K. Fluid management for critically Ill patients: a review of the current state of fluid therapy in the intensive care unit. Kidney Dis. 2016;2:64–71.

Marik PE, Baram M, Vahid B. Does the central venous pressure predict fluid responsiveness? a systematic review of the literature and the tale of seven mares. Chest. 2008;134:172–8.

Marik PE. Fluid resuscitation and volume assessment. In: Marik PE, editors. Handbook of evidence-based critical care. New York: Springer; 2010, p. 55–77.

48. The above patient has difficulty in weaning because of mild pulmonary congestion, although her saturation is 92% on 50% FIO_2. **Which one of the following fluid management strategies will decrease ventilator-free days (VFD)?**

A. Administration of furosemide 10 mg/h intravenously
B. Fluid restriction increases VFD, but may increase serum creatinine
C. Liberal fluid administration decreases both VFD and serum creatinine
D. Ringer's lactate rather than normal saline (0.9%) may decrease VFD
E. High PEEP may expedite her weaning

The answer is B

In a study of 1000 patients with lung injury (ARDS), the effect of two fluid management strategies (conservative vs liberal) on mortality at 60 days and ventilator-free days (VFD) and measures of lung physiology was reported. In the first 7 days, the average fluid balance was −136 mL in the conservative-strategy group and 6992 mL in the liberal-strategy group. At 60 days, there was no difference in mortality between the two groups. However, the conservative strategy group improved oxygenation index, the lung injury score (lung function), and increased the number of VFDs (14.6 vs 12.1 days) compared to liberal-strategy group. Serum creatinine was insignificantly elevated in the conservative group. Thus, B is correct.

Diuretic use should be avoided in patients with AKI (A is incorrect). Options D and E are not applicable to this patient.

Suggested Reading

The National Heart, Lung, and Blood Institute Acute Respiratory Distress Syndrome (ARDS) Clinical Trials Network. Comparison of two fluids-management strategies in acute lung injury. N Engl J Med. 2006;354:2564–75.

49. **Regarding fluid overload, which one of the following statements is CORRECT?**

   A. Patients with fluid overload defined as an increase in body weight of over 10% had significantly more respiratory failure, need of mechanical ventilation, and more sepsis
   B. Increased renal interstitial fluid may reduce capillary blood flow and lead to renal ischemia, which can cause or worsen AKI
   C. The Vasopressin in Septic Shock Trial study investigators found that higher positive fluid balance correlated significantly with increased mortality and the highest mortality rate was observed in those with central venous pressure >12 mm Hg
   D. Fluid overload is associated with a lower likelihood of renal recovery in patients with AKI
   E. All of the above

   The answer is E

   Fluid overload is usually defined as either positive fluid balance or weight gain exceeding 10% of admission weight to the intensive care unit. It has been shown to affect functions of various organs, resulting in longer lengths of stay, higher mortalities, and decreased rates of recovery from AKI. Thus, all of the above statements are correct (answer E is correct).

   Fluid overload is associated with increased intra-abdominal pressure, predisposition to sepsis, pulmonary edema, and gut edema. Increased intra-abdominal pressure may cause delay in kidney function recovery, pulmonary edema may predispose to lung inflammation and pneumonia, and gut edema may predispose to sepsis. However, the pathophysiologic mechanisms for these adverse effects are poorly understood.

   Suggested Reading

Bouchard J, Soroko SB, Chertow GM, et al. Fluid accumulation, survival and recovery of kidney function in critically ill patients with acute kidney injury. Kidney Int. 2009;76:422–7.
Boyd JH, Forbes J, Nakada TA, et al. Fluid resuscitation in septic shock: a positive fluid balance and elevated central venous pressure are associated with increased mortality. Crit Care Med. 2011;39:259–65.
Claure_Del Granado R, Mehta RL. Fluid overload in the ICU: evaluation and management. BMC Nephrol. 2016;17:109.
Colbert GB, Szerlip HM. Euvolemia – a critical target in the management of acute kidney injury. Sem Dial. 2019;32:30–4.
Faubel S, Shah PB. Immediate consequences of acute kidney injury: the impact of traditional and nontraditional complications on mortality in acute kidney injury. Adv Chronic Kidney Dis. 2016;23:179–85.
McGuire MD, Heung M. Fluid as a drug: balancing resuscitation and fluid overload in the intensive care setting. Adv Chronic Kidney Dis. 2016;23:152–9.

50. You are asked to see a patient in CCU for evaluation of AKI. The patient is a 74-year-old woman with diabetes, hypertension, and congestive heart failure (CHF), who was admitted for progressively increasing edema and pain. Despite adequate doses of furosemide, his edema did not improve. He took ibuprofen 400 mg twice daily for a week. His serum creatinine increased from 1.4 to 2.4 mg/dL. **Which one of the following statements is FALSE regarding the relationship between nonsteroidal anti-inflammatory drugs (NSAIDs) and AKI?**

   A. NSAIDs cause renal vasoconstriction in patients with decreased effective arterial blood volume (EABV)
   B. NSAIDs may exert deleterious effects on kidney function in patients or healthy individuals who are on diuretics
   C. NSAIDs induce oliguric AKI
   D. Eosinophiluria is characteristic feature of NSAID-induced AKI
   E. Fractional excretion of Na^+ (FE_{Na}) is low in NSAID-induced AKI

   The answer is D

   Vasodilatory prostaglandins (PGs) counteract the effects of norepinephrine (NE) and maintain normal renal blood flow and GFR. When these PGs are inhibited by NSAIDs, the unopposed vasoconstrictive effects of NE prevail, and renal blood flow decreases with resultant AKI. NSAID-induced AKI is usually oliguric and urine output improves with time. Volume depletion with diuretics either in healthy individuals or patients with decreased EABV are prone to develop AKI after a few days of NSAID use. Decreased EABV is common in CHF and cirrhotic patients, and these patients are at increased risk for AKI. Also, the elderly are at increased risk for AKI due to NSAIDs.

FE_{Na} is usually low in NSAID-induced vasomotor AKI. However, eosinophiluria is not that common either in NSAID-induced AKI or tubulointerstitial disease. Less than 5% of patients with acute tubulointerstitial disease present with eosinophiluria. Thus, option D is false.

Suggested Reading

Abdel-Kader K, Palevsky P. Acute kidney injury in the elderly. Clin Geriatr Med. 2009;25:331–58.

Antunes Caires R, Torres da Costa e Silva V, Burdmann EA, et al. Drug-induced acute kidney injury. In: Ronco C, Bellomo R, Kellum JA, et al. editors. Critical care nephrology. 3rd ed. Philadelphia: Elsevier; 2019. p. 214–24.

Palmer B. Nephrotoxicity of nonsteroidal anti-inflammatory agents, analgesics, and inhibitors of the renin-angiotensin system. In: Coffman TM, Falk RJ, Molitoris BA, et al. editors. Schrier's diseases of the kidney. 9th ed. Philadelphia: Wolters Kluwer/Lippincott Williams & Wilkins; 2013. p. 943–958.

51. A 74-year-old obese man is admitted for fever and prostatitis. Blood cultures grew Gram negative rods, which are sensitive to all aminoglycosides. He was started on gentamicin, and 4 days later his serum creatinine increased from 0.7 to 1.4 mg/dL. **Which one of the following risk factors for aminoglycoside (AG)-induced AKI is CORRECT?**

    A. Older age
    B. Intravascular volume depletion
    C. Age-related decline in kidney function
    D. Continuous infusion or multiple daily doses of AG administration
    E. All of the above

The answer is E

There are several risk factors for AG-induced AKI. AGs cause nonoliguric AKI. Some of these risk factors can be controlled by the clinician and some are not modifiable. For example, old age and age-related decline are not modifiable risk factors. Others such as hypovolemia, and drug delivery are modifiable risk factors. Volume resuscitation with normal saline and single daily intravenous dose of AG can reduce the incidence of AG-induced AKI. Continuous infusion and multiple (frequent) daily doses should be avoided, as these practices can cause accumulation of AG, particularly gentamicin, in the renal cortex, and can take several days to wash out the drug out of the tissue with appropriate volume replacement. Thus, E is correct.

Other risk factors include recent AG exposure, sepsis syndrome, obesity, and concomitant use of other drugs such as vancomycin, amphotericin B, and contrast agents.

In critically ill patients with sepsis, the pharmacokinetics of AGs is altered. Therefore, following serum concentrations of AGs is recommended when a single daily dosing is used.

Suggested Reading

Antunes Caires R, Torres da Costa e Silva V, Burdmann EA, et al. Drug-induced acute kidney injury. In: Ronco C, Bellomo R, Kellum JA, et al., editors. Critical care nephrology. 3rd ed. Philadelphia: Elsevier; 2019, pp. 214–24.

De Broe ME. Antibiotic-and immunosuppression-related renal failure. In: Coffman TM, Falk RJ, Molitoris BA, et al. editors. Schrier's diseases of the kidney. 9th ed. Philadelphia: Wolters Kluwer/Lippincott Williams & Wilkins; 2013. p. 901–42.

Morales-Alvarez MC. Nephrotoxicity of antimicrobials and antibiotics. Adv Chronic Kidney Dis. 2020;27:31–37.

Verpooten GA, Tulkens PA, Molitoris BA. Aminoglycosides and vancomycin. In: De Broe ME, Porter GA, Bennett VM, editors. Clinical nephrotoxins-renal injury from drugs and chemicals. 2nd ed. Dordrecht: Kluwer Academic Publishers. p. 151–70.

52. **Regarding vancomycin-induced AKI or nephrotoxicity, which one of the following statements is FALSE?**

    A. Vancomycin is excreted mostly by the kidneys, and dose adjustment is necessary in renal failure
    B. The incidence of nephrotoxicity varies between 0% and 7% when vancomycin used alone
    C. There is no increased nephrotoxicity when vancomycin is used with aminoglycosides
    D. The incidence of nephrotoxicity increases with increasing trough levels of vancomycin
    E. Nephrotoxicity increases with combined use of vancomycin and pipercillin-tazobactam compared to either drug alone

The answer is C

All of the above statements are correct except C. Indeed, a meta-analysis reported 13.3% increase in nephrotoxicity in combination therapy compared vancomycin therapy alone. Thus, C is false.

Suggested Reading

Antunes Caires R, Torres da Costa e Silva V, Burdmann EA, et al. Drug-induced acute kidney injury. In: Ronco C, Bellomo R, Kellum JA, et al., editors. Critical care nephrology. 3rd ed. Philadelphia: Elsevier; 2019. p. 214–24.

Bilal A, Abu-Romeh A, Rousan TA, et al. Vancomycin-induced nephrotoxicity. In: Sahay M, editor. Basic nephrology and acute kidney injury. InTech; 2012. p. 183–226.

De Broe ME. Antibiotic-and immunosuppression-related renal failure. In: Coffman TM, Falk RJ, Molitoris BA, et al. editors. Schrier's diseases of the kidney. 9th ed. Philadelphia: Wolters Kluwer/Lippincott Williams & Wilkins; 2013. p. 901–42.

53. A 48-year-old woman with HIV and diabetes is admitted following surgery of spinal abscess. She is on appropriate antibiotics for Gram positive and Gram negative organisms. Her fever subsided, but 3 weeks later she started spiking fevers with elevated WBCs. Blood culture grew fungus for which she is started on liposomal amphotericin (AMP) B. **Regarding AMP B use and AKI, which one of the following statements is CORRECT?**

    A. Lipid formulations of AMP B cause less nephrotoxicity than conventional formulation (deoxycholate as a solvent) of AMP B
    B. Conventional AMP B causes afferent arteriolar vasoconstriction, resulting in decreased renal blood flow and GFR
    C. Hypokalemia and hypovolemia due to Na^+ loss are important risk factors for AMP B
    D. Azole (voriconazole, fluconazole, itraconazole) and echinocandin (caspofungin, micafungin) antifungal agents are less nephrotoxic than AMP B deoxycholate agent
    E. All of the above

The answer is E

Nephrotoxicity (AKI) was very common with AMP B deoxycholate preparations, and nephrotoxicity was found to be due to deoxycholate. Renal vasoconstriction is one of the mechanisms for AMP B-induced AKI. Subsequently released lipid formulations were found to be less nephrotoxic. Several risk factors have been identified for AKI, including drug dose, duration of therapy, volume and Na^+ depletion, preexisting kidney disease, and concomitant use of drugs (diuretics, aminoglycosides). Observational studies reported less nephrotoxicity with azole/echinocandin antifungals than conventional AMP B formulations. Thus, E is correct.

When equal efficacy is expected, the KIDIGO guideline recommends use of either azole or echinocandin antifungals for systemic mycoses or parasitic infections than conventional AMP B.

Suggested Reading

Antunes Caires R, Torres da Costa e Silva V, Burdmann EA, et al. Drug-induced acute kidney injury. In: Ronco C, Bellomo R, Kellum JA, et al. editors. Critical care nephrology. 3rd ed. Philadelphia: Elsevier; 2019. p. 214–24.

De Broe ME. Antibiotic-and immunosuppression-related renal failure. In: Coffman TM, Falk RJ, Molitoris BA, et al. editors. Schrier's diseases of the kidney 9th ed. Philadelphia: Wolters Kluwer/Lippincott Williams & Wilkins; 2013. p. 901–42.

Kidney Disease: Improving Global Outcomes (KDIGO) Acute Kidney Injury Work Group. KDIGO clinical practice guideline for acute kidney injury. Kidney Int (Suppl). 2012;2:1–138.

54. A 32-year-old woman with AIDS (CD 4 120) is admitted for headache followed by seizure activity. CT head showed a lesion suggestive of toxoplasmosis. She was started on sufadiazine and an antiepileptic, in addition to her regular HAART medications. She was treated for herpes zoster with acyclovir 4 months ago, and also for UTI with ciprofloxacin 6 months ago. Seven days later, her urine output started to decrease on 2 L of normal saline, and her serum creatinine rose from 0.4 to 1.1 mg/dL. Blood pressure is 140/80 mm Hg. Urinalysis showed hematuria, pyuria, and crystals. A representative crystal is shown in Fig. 5.1 (obtained from Renal Fellow Network). Her urine pH is 5.5. **Based on the above history, which one of the following is the MOST likely cause of her AKI?**

Fig. 5.1

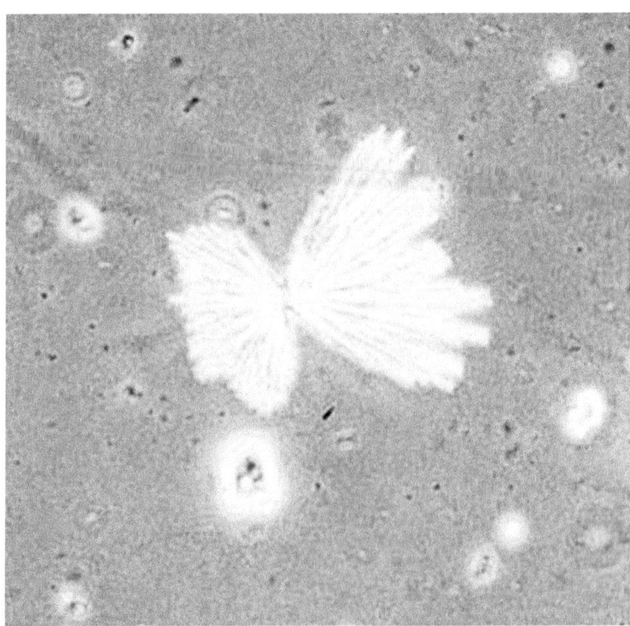

A. Acyclovir-induced crystalluria
B. Ciprofloxacin-induced crystalluria
C. Sulfadiazine-induced crystalluria
D. Prerenal azotemia
E. AKI due to HAART medications

The answer is C

The clinical picture and "shocks of wheat" appearing crystal is suggestive of sulfadiazine-induced crystalluria and tubular obstruction as the most likely cause of AKI in this patient (C is correct). Based on urinalysis, prerenal azotemia is unlikely. Also, the patient has been on HAART medication for long time, and sudden increase in creatinine is unlikely due to these medications (D and E are incorrect). The only medication that was started 1 week ago was sulfadiazine, which is known to cause AKI due to crystal deposition in renal tubules.

Drug-induced AKI is rather common in several situations. Examples include acyclovir, sulfadiazine, indinavir, and ciprofloxacin. Acyclovir crystals are birefringent needle-shaped crystals Sulfadiazine crystals are also birefringent and appear as "shocks of wheat" or shells with striations. Indinavir crystals are strongly birefringent, and have various appearances such as fan-shaped or starburst form. Ciprofloxacin crystals have star-like appearance. These drugs are commonly used in patients with HIV/AIDS.

In the above patient, hydration with normal saline or preferably 3 L of 0.45% saline with 75 mEq of $NaHCO_3$ a day will improve not only volume status but also wash out sulfadiazine crystals and alkalinize urine. Usually renal recovery occurs within a week with hydration and $NaHCO_3$ administration.

Suggested Reading

Dong BJ, Rodriquez RA, Goldschmidt RH. Sulfadiazine-induced crystalluria and renal failure in a patient with AIDS. J Am Board of Fam Pract. 1999;12:243–8.

Mulay SR, Shi C, Ma X et al. Novel insights into crystal-induced kidney injury. Kidney Dis. 2018;4:49–57.

Zarjou A, Agarwal A. Acute kidney injury associated with pigmenturia or crystal deposits. In: Coffman TM, Falk RJ, Molitoris BA, et al. editors. Schrier's diseases of the kidney 9th ed. Philadelphia: Wolters Kluwer/Lippincott Williams & Wilkins; 2013. p. 1018–44.

55. A 26-year-old man is admitted for confusion and AKI. He required intubation for air-way protection. In the Emergency Department, his vital signs are stable. He has a history of hypertension and suicidal ideation. He was unable to give any history prior to intubation. His physical exam is normal. His blood pressure is 130/82 mm Hg with heart rate of 110 BPM. Labs:

Serum	Urine
Na^+ = 141 mEq/L K^+ = 4.2 mEq/L Cl^- = 110 mEq/L HCO_3^- = 7 mEq/L BUN = 28 mg/dL Creatinine = 4.8 mg/dL Glucose = 72 mg/dL Albumin = 3.6 g/dL Serum osmolality = 312 mOsm/kg H_2O ABG = pH 7.21, pCO_2 17 mm Hg, pO_2 94 mm Hg, calculated HCO_3^- 6 mEq/L	Osmolality = 320 mOsm/kg H_2O pH = 5.4 Protein = trace Blood = negative Urine sediment = envelope-like crystals (Fig. 5.2)

Based on the above history and lab values, which one of the following is the MOST likely diagnosis in this patient?

A. Ethanol intoxication
B. Methanol ingestion
C. Ethylene glycol (EG) ingestion
D. Pyroglutamic acidosis
E. Isopropyl alcohol ingestion

The answer is C

It is extremely important to calculate the osmolal gap in this patient. Except for pyroglutamic acidosis, ingestion of any one of the above alcohol can give high osmolal gap. However, ingestion of isopropyl alcohol does not cause severe metabolic acidosis unless the patient has other acid-producing condition (lactic acidosis). Ethanol ingestion may give mild metabolic acidosis, but the labs do not suggest ethanol as a cause of his severe metabolic acidosis and AKI. Methanol and EG can give severe altered mental status and metabolic acidosis. However, the urinary sediment finding of calcium oxalate crystals (Fig. 5.2; **envelope-like crystals) is suggestive of EG ingestion. One of the final products of EG is oxalic acid. Thus, C is correct.**

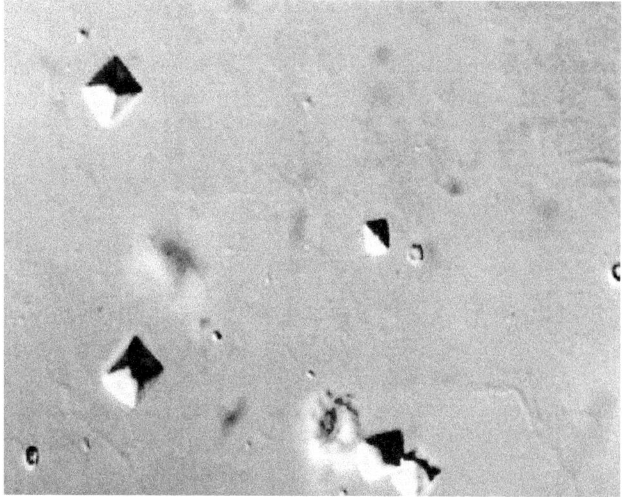

Fig. 5.2 Caption

Suggested Reading

Kraut JA, Xing SX. Approach to the evaluation of a patient with an increased serum osmolal gap and high-anion gap metabolic acidosis. Am J Kidney Dis. 2011;58:480–4.

Reddi AS. Toxin-induced acid-base disorders. In: Acid-base disorders. Clinical evaluation and management. New York: Springer; 2020. p. 103–26.

56. **Regarding treatment of the above patient, which one of the following initial strategies is MOST appropriate?**

    A. Start hemodialysis (HD) immediately
    B. Start fomepizole
    C. HD and fomepizole
    D. Hydration with D5W and 150 mEq $NaHCO_3$ to improve volume status, fomepizole, and preparation for HD
    E. Wait until BP reaches 140/90 mm Hg to start HD

    The answer is D

    Most of the patients are volume depleted, as in the above patient. This patient has history of HTN, and the BP on admission may reflect relative volume depletion. Therefore, hydration with D5W and 3 ampules (150 mEq) of $NaHCO_3$ to run at 100–120 mL/h to improve volume status should be started. At the same time, the antidote for ethylene glycol (EG) is fomepizole, which inhibits alcohol dehydrogenase and prevents further metabolism of EG. The initial dose is 15 mg/kg followed by 10 mg/kg every 12 h for 4 doses. Continue fomepizole, if EG levels are >20 mg/dL. Although serum [HCO_3^-] may improve with $NaHCO_3$ administration, the patient may benefit from HD to improve acidosis and creatinine. Thus, option D is correct. Other options are not appropriate in this patient.

    It is not inappropriate to start the patient on thiamine and riboflavin to improve lactate levels, as EG can be metabolized to lactate in the absence of hypoxia.

    Suggested Reading

Barceloux DG, Krenzelok EP, Olson K, et al. American academy of clinical toxicology practice guidelines on the treatment of ethylene glycol poisoning. J Toxicol Clin Toxicol. 1999;37:537–60.
Kraut JA, Xing SX. Approach to the evaluation of a patient with an increased serum osmolal gap and high-anion gap metabolic acidosis. Am J Kidney Dis. 2011;58:480–4.
Reddi AS. Toxin-induced acid-base disorders. In: Acid-base disorders. Clinical evaluation and management. New York: Springer; 2020, p. 103–26.

57. A 28-year-old man was admitted to neuro ICU following head injury during motor vehicle accident. In order to reduce intracranial pressure, he was started on mannitol. His creatinine on admission was 0.8 mg/dL. Four days later, his creatinine rose to 2.1 mg/dL. He is on antibiotics for fever. **Which one of the following choice is CORRECT regarding the acute rise in creatinine (AKI)?**

    A. Volume depletion
    B. Proximal tubule injury with vacuolization
    C. Concomitant use of nephrotoxins
    D. Higher doses of mannitol
    E. All of the above

    The answer is E

    Administration of hyperosmolar substances such as mannitol, sucrose, dextrans, immunoglobulin G, including high osmolar contrast agents, has been shown to cause AKI, a phenomenon called osmotic nephropathy. Mannitol is an osmotic diuretic. It extracts water from the intracellular compartment to the extracellular compartment, and expands the extracellular fluid volume. Initially mannitol and other osmotic diuretics dilate the afferent arteriole. As a result of these effects, the RBF is increased. A slight increase in GFR is also observed due to an increase in glomerular hydrostatic pressure. However, following excretion of water and salt, intravascular volume decreases with an increase in serum creatinine (prerenal azotemia). Furthermore, as the dose of mannitol increases and serum level is ~1000 mg/dL, the proximal tubule dilates and develop uniformly distributed vacuoles. Both animal and human renal biopsy studies have shown similar pathologic processes.

    Certain risk factors potentiate the nephrotoxicity of mannitol. These include volume depletion, concomitant use of nephrotoxins (antibiotics, contrast, cyclosporine), and preexisting kidney disease. Thus, E is correct.

    Suggested Reading

Ahsan N. Intravenous immunoglobulin-induced nephropathy: a complication of IVIG therapy. J Nephrol. 1998;1:157–61.
Visweswaran P, Massin EK, DuBose TD Jr. Mannitol-induced acute renal failure. J Am Soc Nephrol. 1997;8:1028–33.

58. A 43-year-old woman with type 2 diabetes is admitted for acute coronary syndrome. She is hypertensive and CKD 2 (creatinine 1.6 mg/dL) with albuminuria (150 mg). She is on low dose diuretic, lisinopril, glyburide, and atorvastatin. She receives 120 mL of contrast for coronary angiogram. **Which one of the following risk factors this patient has for contrast-associated AKI (CA-AKI)?**

   A. Diabetes
   B. Albuminuria
   C. CKD
   D. Acute MI
   E. All of the above

   The answer is E

   This patient is at high risk for CI-AKI. All of the conditions listed above are risk factors for C-AKI. Thus, E is correct. Table 5.7 **shows non-modifiable and modifiable risk factors for C-AKI.**

Table 5.7 Risk factors for contrast-associated AKI

Non-modifiable factors	Modifiable factors
Chronic kidney disease (eGFR <60 mL)	Contrast media volume
Diabetes mellitus (type 1 and type 2)	Volume depletion
Age >70 yr.	Hypotension
Emergent situations (benefit outweighs risk)	Anemia (hematocrit <35 g/L)
Left ventricular ejection fraction <40%	Intra-aortic balloon pump
Acute myocardial infarction	Hypoalbuminemia (<3.5 g/dL)
Severe hypertension	Drugs (diuretics, NSAIDs, antibiotics or anti-infectives)
Conditions with decreased effective arterial blood volume (congestive heart failure, cirrhosis, nephrotic syndrome)	<72 h between first and second study
Renal transplant	Intra-arterial injection

Suggested Reading

Kidney Disease: Improving Global Outcomes (KDIGO) Acute Kidney Injury Work Group. KDIGO clinical practice guideline for acute kidney injury. Kidney Int (Suppl). 2012;2:1–138.

Leisman S. Radiocontrast toxicity. Adv Chronic Kidney Dis. 2020;27:50–5.

Mehran R, Nikolsky E. Contrast-induced nephropathy: definition, epidemiology, and patients at risk. Kidney Int. 2006;69:S11–S15.

Weisbord SD, Palevsky PM. Contrast-induced acute kidney injury. In: Coffman TM, Falk RJ, Molitoris BA, et al., editors. Schrier's diseases of the kidney. 9th ed. Philadelphia: Wolters Kluwer/Lippincott Williams & Wilkins; 2013, p. 959–80.

59. The above patient is admitted and referred to you for evaluation of contrast-associated AKI (CA-AKI) and its prevention. **Which one of the following strategies you would recommend to prevent CI-AKI?**

   A. Intravenous (i.v.) furosemide
   B. i.v. dopamine
   C. i.v. N-acetylcysteine (NAC)
   D. 0.9% saline (1 mL/kg/h 6–12 h before and 6–12 h after procedure) or 3 mL/kg/h 1 h before and 1.5 mL/kg/h for 4 to 6 h postprocedure
   E. i.v. $NaHCO_3$ and NAC

   The answer is D

   The first step in the prevention of CI-AKI is the assessment of risk factors in the patient. The second step is the discontinuation of certain medications such as diuretics, and renin-AII-aldosterone inhibitors. The third step is assessment of volume status and choice of IV fluids to be given. According to KIDIGO guideline, the choice of i.v. fluid is either 0.9% saline or $NaHCO_3$. In a study by Weisbord and colleagues, no benefit of iv saline over iv

$NaHCO_3$ was found in the prevention of CI-AKI. Also, the same investigators reported that NAC has no protective effect over placebo in CI-AKI. In this study, the primary outcome was prevention of death, need for dialysis or persistent decline in kidney function at 90 days, which not different between saline and $NaHCO_3$ or between NAC and placebo groups. In this patient, normal saline is the fluid of choice, and, therefore, D is correct. Use of normal saline is also recommended by the authors of core curriculum 2018. However, Nijssen et al. reported no benefit of hydration over no hydration in the prevention of CI-AKI in patients with mean GFR of 47 mL/min. If this study is confirmed by other studies, hydration is not recommended for contrast studies and is cost-effective as well.

Administration of furosemide, dopamine, and NAC is inappropriate. Also, $NaHCO_3$ and NAC are not recommended, as these prophylactic agents are not superior to placebo in preventing CI-AKI (E is incorrect). Also, a large meta-analysis on CI-AKI showed no difference between low-osmolar contrast and iso-osmolar contrast agents in the development of CI-AKI.

Suggested Reading

Leisman S. Radiocontrast toxicity. Adv Chronic Kidney Dis. 2020;27:50–5.

Moore PK, Hsu RK, Liu KD. Management of acute kidney injury: core curriculum. Am J Kidney Dis. 2018;72:136–48.

Nijssen EC, Rennenberg RJ, Nelemans PJ, et al. Prophylactic hydration to protect renal function from intravascular iodinated contrast material in patients at high risk of contrast-induced nephropathy (AMACING): a prospective, randomised, phase 3, controlled, open-label, non-inferiority trial. Lancet. 2017;389:1312–22.

Weisbord SD, Gallagher M, Jneid H, et al. PRESERVE Trial Group: outcomes after angiography with sodium bicarbonate and acetylcysteine. N Engl J Med. 2018;378:603–14.

60. A 64-year-old type 2 diabetic woman with CKD 4 (eGFR <30 mL/min) is admitted with stroke, and an MRI without contrast showed ischemia as a cause for her stroke. Because of persistence of symptoms, a second MRI with contrast (with permission from the family) showed an extension of ischemia. **Which one of the following statements regarding gadolinium (Gd^{3+}) and CKD 4-5 is CORRECT?**

A. Gd^{3+} is deposited in skin, bone, heart, lungs, lymph nodes, liver, and other organs
B. Gd^{3+} is excreted by the kidneys
C. Nephrogenic systemic fibrosis (NSF) develops anywhere from 2 days to 18 months in patients with AKI, CKD 4-5, and dialysis patients
D. Gd^{3+}-based contrast agents such as Omniscan (Gadodiamide), Magnevist (Gadopentate), and Optimark (Gadoversetamide) are contraindicated in patients with AKI and patients on hemodialysis
E. All of the above

The answer is E

All of the above statements are correct (E). Gd^{3+}-based contrast agents are more nephrotoxic than iodinated contrast agents in equimolar concentrations. Because of the use of low volume for MRI and other studies, the incidence of nephrotoxicity with MRI agents is much lower than iodinated contrast agents. However, in diabetics, nondialysis patients with CKD stages 4-5 and dialysis patients, Gd^{3+}-based contrast agents induce nephrotoxicity called NFS even at standard doses.

NSF was originally identified as a cutaneous lesion with indurated plaques and papules on the extremities and trunk in patients on hemodialysis (HD) and failed renal transplant patients. Thickening of the skin, resembling scleroderma, is a common feature. In 2006, a relationship between NSF and Gd^{3+}-based contrast agents has been suggested.

NSF is not limited to skin only, but it involves muscles, diaphragm, heart, lungs, and liver of the body as well. Thus, it is a systemic disorder. The prevalence of NSF varies between 1.5 and 5% in biopsy-proven HD patients. It is even higher when clinical criteria are used. NSF develops anywhere from days to months (2 days to 18 months). Not only HD patients but also patients with CKD 4-5 and patients with AKI are prone to develop NSF The risk of NSF is related to dose and the type of Gd^{3+}-based contrast agents. Most of the cases were reported with the use of Omniscan, Magnevist, and Optimark.

Any patient with eGFR <30 mL/min, whether on dialysis or not, is at risk for NSF. Also, AKI is another risk factor. Many other risk factors such as metabolic acidosis, higher serum levels of iron, Ca^{2+}, phosphate, inflammation, and high doses of erythropoietin have been identified. However, the role of these factors has not been firmly established.

Gd^{3+} is extremely toxic because of its deposition in skin, lungs, lymph nodes, bone, and other organs. It may stimulate many cytokines that promote fibrosis. Joint contractures and limitations in mobility are common. Deep vein thrombosis, pulmonary embolism, atrial thrombus, and clotting of arterio-venous fistulas have been reported in patients with NSF. These patients seem to have antiphospholipid antibody syndrome. Fibrosis of several organs, including lungs, muscle, and diaphragm, may lead to morbidity and mortality. Sudden death from respiratory failure has been reported.

There is no proven treatment for NSF. Plasma exchange, ultraviolet light therapy, sodium thiosulfate, high dose immunoglobulin, and ACE-inhibitors have been tried with variable successes. Physical therapy improves joint mobility.

The following measures are suggested to prevent NSF in patients with AKI and different kidney function.

- **CKD stage 1 (eGFR .90 mL/min): No NSF has been reported.**
- **CKD stage 2 (eGFR 60–89 mL/min): The risk is low and lowest dose is recommended.**
- **CKD stage 3a (eGFR 45–59 mL/ min) and CKD stage 3b (eGFR 30–44 mL/min): The risk is low and the lowest dose is recommended.**
- **CKD stage 4 (eGFR 15–29 mL/min) and stage 5 (eGFR <15 mL/min): Patients who are not on HD are at high-risk for NSF.**

HD patients as well as patients with AKI:

1. **Identify the indication and risk-benefit ratio**
2. **Consider alternative study**
3. **If benefit outweighs the risk, explain the patient the risks and advantages of the procedure**
4. **Obtain consent**
5. **Use lowest possible dose of contrast agent**
6. **Use preferably macrocyclic low molecular weight agent**
7. **DO NOT use Omiscan, Magnevist, and Optimark (contraindicated)**
8. **Avoid multiple exposure, as cumulative dose is a risk factor**
9. **Provide HD 2–3 times after study, if possible or perform the study just before dialysis and HD later**

Suggested Reading

Cohan R, Chovke P, Cohen M, et al. Nephrogenic systemic fibrosis. American College of Radiology Manual on Contrast Media. Version 7. 2010;49–55.

Kidney Disease: Improving Global Outcomes (KDIGO) Acute Kidney Injury Work Group. KDIGO clinical practice guideline for acute kidney injury. Kidney Int (Suppl). 2012;2:1–138.

Leisman S. Radiocontrast toxicity. Adv Chronic Kidney Dis. 2020;27:50–55.

61. A 70-year-old man is admitted for abdominal pain and hematuria, and CT of abdomen is suggestive of renal cancer. His serum creatinine is 0.9 mg/dL. **Regarding cancer and AKI, which one of the following statements is FALSE?**

A. The incidence of AKI in patients with renal cancer is approximately 44%
B. The incidence of AKI is at least threefold higher in patients with cancer compared to those without cancer
C. Sepsis is the most common cause of AKI in critically ill patients with cancer
D. Chemotherapeutic agents are least likely causes of AKI
E. Medication-induced mucositis may limit oral intake and may precipitate prerenal AKI

The answer is D

All of the above statements are correct except for D. Indeed, most of the chemotherapeutic agents do cause AKI by a variety of mechanisms. A large Danish study reported the highest incidence of AKI in patients with renal cancer at 44% (A is correct), followed by 33% in patients with multiple myeloma, 31.8% in liver cancer patients. A number of studies reported the incidence of AKI is at least threefold higher in cancer patients than in patients without cancer (B is correct). Sepsis seems to be the leading cause of AKI in critically ill cancer patients (C is correct). Volume depletion due to poor oral intake causes prerenal azotemia in those with mucositis due to chemotherapeutic drugs (E is correct).

Suggested Reading

Campbell GA, Hu D, Okusa MD. Acute kidney injury in the cancer patient. Adv Chronic Kidney Dis. 2014;21:64–71.
Lahoti A, Chen S. Acute kidney injury incidence, pathogenesis, and outcomes. In: Finkel KW, Perazella MA, Cohen EP, editors. Onco-nephrology. St Louis: Elsevier;2020. p. 270–74.
Perazella MA. Onco-nephrology: renal toxicities of chemotherapeutic agents. Clin J Am Soc Nephrol. 2012;7:1713–21.
Sahni V, Choudhury D, Ahmed Z. Chemotherapy-associated renal dysfunction. Nature Rev Nephrol. 2009;5:451–62.

62. A 65-year-old man with long history of smoking was admitted initially for treatment of non-small cell lung cancer (NSCLC) and chemotherapy. His chemotherapy regimen includes cisplatin, gemcitabin, paclitaxel, and bevacizumab. He started having polyuria, and 10 days later, his creatinine increased from 0.9 to 2.1 mg/dL. He was found to be hyponatremic, hypokalemic, hypomagnesemic, hypophosphatemic, and hypocalcemic. He developed hypertension as well. He has no complaints other than weakness, and his urine has no hematuria. **Which one of the following is the MOST likely cause of his AKI?**

A. Cisplatin
B. Gemcitabin
C. Paclitaxel
D. Bevacizumab
E. Volume depletion

The answer is A

This patient developed cisplatin-induced nephrotoxicity (A is correct). Polyuria develops 24–48 h after cisplatin dose, which is related to defective concentrating ability of the kidneys. AKI develops 7–10 days later, and may persist for very long period of time. Cisplatin induces: (1) volume depletion by urinary excretion of Na^+ and hyponatremia, (2) Fanconi syndrome with urinary loss of Mg^{2+} and severe hypomagnesemia; (3) hpokalemia and hypocalcemia due to hypomagnesemia and urinary losses of these ions; and (4) AKI due to acute tubular necrosis. Thus, A is correct. Gemcitabin is a pyrimidine antagonist, and causes AKI due to thrombotic microangiopathy, and this patient does not have any clinical and laboratory findings suggestive of thrombotic microangiopathy (B is incorrect). Paclitaxel does not cause so many electrolyte problems (C is incorrect). B, Bevacizumab, antiangiogenic factor, is known to cause hypertension and AKI due to thrombotic microangiopathy. Severe electrolyte abnormalities are uncommon (D is incorrect). Although volume depletion causes prerenal AKI, it does not cause these electrolyte abnormalities (E is incorrect).

Suggested Reading

Campbell GA, Hu D, Okusa MD. Acute kidney injury in the cancer patient. Adv Chronic Kidney Dis. 2014;21:64–71.
Jhaveri KD, Wanchool R, Sakhiya V, et al. Adverse renal effects of novel molecular oncologic targeted therapies: a narrative review. Kidney Int Rep. 2017;2:108–27.
Perazella MA. Onco-nephrology: renal toxicities of chemotherapeutic agents. Clin J Am Soc Nephrol. 2012;7:1713–21.
Sahni V, Choudhury D, Ahmed Z. Chemotherapy-associated renal dysfunction. Nature Rev Nephrol. 2009;5:45–462.

63. **Which one of the following measures you would take to prevent cisplatin-induced nephrotoxicity in the above patient?**

A. Hydration with normal saline
B. Avoidance of diuretics
C. Reduction of cisplatin dose
D. Amifostine
E. All of the above

The answer is E

The major preventive measure of cisplatin-induced nephrotoxicity is hydration with normal saline 24 h before cisplatin infusion with continuation of saline for several days after cisplatin therapy. Some advocate forced diuresis with electrolyte replacement at 100 mL/hr 12 h before, during, and 2 days after cisplatin therapy (A is correct). Complete volume replacement has been shown to prevent cisplatin toxicity.

Diuretics should be stopped (B is correct). Forced diuresis with loop diuretics exacerbates not only AKI but also electrolyte abnormalities. Reduction in cisplatin dosage is suggested in patients with eGFR <60 mL/min (C is correct). Amifostine is an inorganic thiophosphate, which is cytoprotective. It has been used to prevent cisplatin

nephrotoxicity (D is correct). However, it is expensive and has several adverse reactions such as nausea, vomiting, flushing, and transient hypotension. Therefore, its use is restricted to only some patients. In addition, antioxidants such as N-acetylcysteine have been shown to have some preventative effect on cisplatin nephrotoxicity.

Suggested Reading

Lameire N. Nephrotoxicity of recent anti-cancer agents. Clin Kidney J. 2014;7:11–22.

Sahni V, Choudhury D, Ahmed Z. Chemotherapy-associated renal dysfunction. Nature Rev Nephrol. 2009;5:451–62.

Saly DE, Perazella MA. Adverse kidney effects of immunotherapies. In: Finkel KW, Perazella MA, Cohen EP, editors. Onco-nephrology. St Louis: Elsevier;2020. p. 168–83.

64. A 48-year-old man receives myeloablative allogenic hematopoietic cell transplantation (HCT) for acute myelogenic leukemia. He has no history of hypertension, liver disease, or kidney disease. Three weeks after discharge, he was readmitted for severe right upper quadrant (RUQ) pain, jaundice, and weight gain of 6 kg. He denies diarrhea, skin rash, photophobia, or pruritis. His BP is 148/86 mm Hg, which is elevated compared to pre-HCT. There are no orthostatic BP and pulse changes. Pertinent physical findings include normal eye, skin, lung, and heart examination. Abdominal examination is positive for RUQ pain, hepatomegaly, and ascites. There is 2+ pitting edema of both lower extremities. Labs: Na^+ 134 mEq/L, K^+ 4.1 mEq/L, Cl^- 100 mEq/L, HCO_3^- 24 mEq/L, BUN 36 mg/dL, creatinine 2.4 mg/dL (0.9 mg/dL prior to HCT), and total bilirubun 3.4 mg/dL. Urinalysis is normal except for bilirubinogen and proteinuria of 60 mg/dL. **Based on the above clinical findings and lab data, which one of the following is the MOST likely cause of AKI?**

A. Prerenal AKI
B. Hepatorenal syndrome (HRS)
C. Sinusiodal obstruction syndrome
D. Rapidly progressive glomerulonephritis (RPGN)
E. Acute graft versus host disease (aGVHD)

The answer is C

AKI is a complication of HCT. In one study, AKI occurred in 53% of patients at a median of 14 days. In this patient, there are no orthostatic BP and pulse changes, making prerenal AKI unlikely (A is incorrect). HRS is a strong consideration; however, RUQ pain, and no history of cirrhosis prior to HCT rules out this possibility of AKI (B is incorrect). RPGN is also unlikely in the absence of hematuria, and the clinical findings do not suggest this diagnosis (D is incorrect). aGVHD usually presents with skin rash, eye pain, and most importantly diarrhea. There will be orthostatic changes and electrolyte abnormalities in patients with aGVHD (E is incorrect)

The correct answer is C. This patient developed sinusoidal obstruction syndrome (SOS), also called veno-occlusive disease. This syndrome occurs in patients following HCT due to conditioning regimens, commonly cyclophosphamide, busulfan, and/or total body irradiation. AKI is the complication of SOS.

SOS is characterized by severe RUQ pain due to liver swelling, weight gain due Na^+ reabsorption, and jaundice. This patient has all the characteristics of SOS. Liver biopsy is necessary to rule out other causes of hepatic dysfunction. SOS is characterized by hepatic necrosis, deposition of extracellular matrix in the sinusoids, and sinusoidal hemorrhage.

Management of AKI in SOS includes volume repletion, diuretics to improve edema, and pain control. The prognosis of SOS depends on the extent of liver failure and involvement of other organs. Generally, SOS resolves completely. AKI may also resolve, but severe AKI may lead to CKD and dialysis dependency.

Suggested Reading

Belcher JM, Parikh CR. Acute kidney injury following hematopoietic cell transplantation and severe burns. In: Coffman TM, Falk RJ, Molitoris BA, et al., editors. Schrier's diseases of the kidney. 9th ed. Philadelphia: Wolters Kluwer/Lippincott Williams & Wilkins; 2013. p. 1057–85.

Joseph C, Angelo JR, Laskin BL, et al. Hematopoietic cell transplant associated kidney injury. In: Finkel KW, Perazella MA, Cohen EP, editors. Onco-nephrology. St Louis: Elsevier; 2020. p. 90–99.

Weiss BM, Sawinski D. Sinusoidal obstruction syndrome. In: Finkel KW, Perazella MA, Cohen EP, editors. Onco-nephrology. St Louis: Elsevier; 2020. p. 102–5.

65. A 36-year-old woman with lymphoma is treated with chemotherapy, and you are consulted to evaluate AKI. Her serum uric acid is 12.4 mg/dL. **Which one of the following is a risk factor for uric acid nephropathy?**

A. Urine pH <5.0

B. Volume depletion
C. Preexisting kidney disease
D. Increased uric acid excretion
E. All of the above

The answer is E

All of the above choices are correct (E). Uric acid is the end product of purine metabolism. It has a pK_a of 5.75. At a physiologic pH of 7.4, uric acid exists as urate anion. In clinical setting, the importance of uric acid lies in its solubility. In general, uric acid is less soluble than urate, and an acidic environment reduces uric acid solubility. At a pH of 5.0, the saturation of uric acid occurs at a concentration of <10 mg/dL, whereas at a pH >7.0, the saturation occurs at a concentration of >150 mg/dL. In the distal renal tubule, the pH is <7.0. During treatment of uric acid nephropathy, it is important to alkalinize the urine pH above 7.0, so that uric acid will not precipitate in renal tubules. Volume depletion or dehydration causes tubular deposition of urate. Therefore, adequate volume repletion is necessary. Preexisting kidney disease is an important precipitating factor for uric acid nephropathy. To alkalinize the urine 100 mEq of $NaHCO_3$ in 1 L of D5W can be used until the urine pH reaches 7 or above, and $NaHCO_3$ infusion can be discontinued once serum uric acid returns to normal.

Uric acid crystal deposition increases the tubular pressure, which opposes glomerular hydrostatic pressure with resultant increase in serum creatinine levels. Also, increased uric acid reduces renal blood flow, causing AKI.

Suggested Reading

Gupta A, Moore JA. Tumor lysis syndrome. JAMA Oncol. 2018;4:895.
Howard SC, Jones DP, Pui CH. The tumor lysis syndrome. N Engl J Med. 2011;364:1844–54.
Rastegar M, Kitchlu A, Shirali AC. Tumor lysis syndrome. In: Finkel KW, Perazella MA, Cohen EP, editors. Onconephrology. St Louis: Elsevier; 2020. p. 275–80.

66. **Rasburicase is used to treat hyperuricemia. Which one of the following steps is catalyzed by rasburicase?**

A. Conversion of adenosine to inosine
B. Conversion of hypoxanthine to xanthine
C. Conversion of xanthine to uric acid
D. Conversion of uric acid to allantoin
E. Conversion of guanine to xanthine

The answer is D

Uric acid is formed from purine metabolism. The two purine ribonucleosides are adenosine and guanosine (Fig. 5.3). **Adenosine deaminase converts adenosine to inosine, which is subsequently converted to hypoxanthine. Guanosine is converted to guanine, which is then formed to xanthine by guanine deaminase. Hypoxanthine is also converted to xanthine by xanthine oxidase, and the same enzyme converts xanthine to uric acid. In humans, uric acid is excreted in the urine, as it is not further degraded. However, animals convert uric acid to a more soluble form called allantoin by uricase or urate oxidase.**

Rasburicase is a recombinant uricase. It converts uric acid to allantoin, which is readily excreted in the urine. Thus, answer D is correct. Xanthine oxidase is inhibited by allopurinol and febuxostat. The following diagram (Fig. 5.3) **shows the production of uric acid and allantoin from purines.**

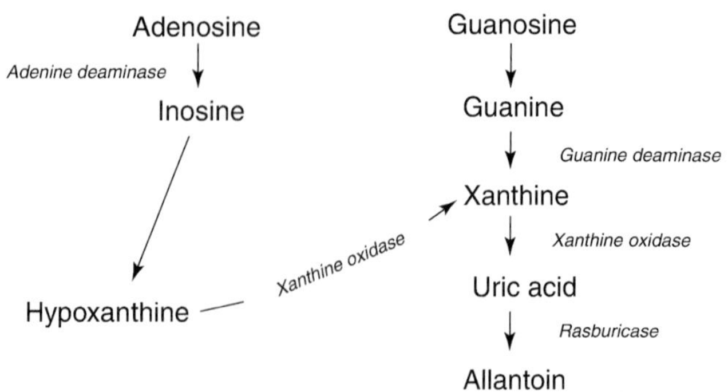

Fig. 5.3 Formation of uric acid and allantoin from purine ribonucleosides

Suggested Reading

Gupta A, Moore JA. Tumor lysis syndrome. JAMA Oncol. 2018;4:895.

Howard SC, Jones DP, Pui CH. The tumor lysis syndrome. N Engl J Med. 2011;364:1844–54.

Rastegar M, Kitchlu A, Shirali AC. Tumor lysis syndrome. In: Finkel KW, Perazella MA, Cohen EP, editors. Onco-nephrology. St Louis: Elsevier; 2020, p. 275–80.

67. A 26-year-old woman with HIV and alcoholism is brought to the emergency department in comatose condition by her boyfriend. She was found lying in bed for >24 h. She is electively intubated. Initial labs:

Serum	Urine
Na^+ = 134 mEq/L	Color = reddish-brown
K^+ = 3.0 mEq/L	pH = 5.2
Cl^- = 100 mEq/L	Blood = large
HCO_3^- = 16 mEq/L	RBCs = 10
BUN = 62 mg/dL	Protein = 2+
Creatinine = 3.6 mg/dL	Sediment = muddy-brown casts
Glucose = 80 mg/dL	FE_{Na} = <1%
Ca^{2+} = 6.9 mg/dL	Toxicology = cocaine, heroin
Phosphate = 2.1 mg/dL	
Uric acid = 12.6 mg/dL	
Albumin =3.2 g/dL	

Which one of the following serum tests is MOST appropriate in this patient?

A. Aldolase
B. Lactate dehydrogenase (LDH)
C. Plasma myoglobin
D. Creatine kinase (CK)
E. Complement levels

The answer is D

Elevated levels of aldolase and LDH are common in the above patient; however, they lack sensitivity and specificity because several other conditions are associated with elevation of these enzymes (A and B are incorrect). Plasma myoglobin has a very short half-life (2–3 h, and its levels are normal once myonecrosis is stopped. Also, it is rapidly excreted by the kidneys, if the patient is not anuric, or it is metabolized to bilirubin. It is crucial to determine myoglobin levels within 24 h of myonecrosis (C is incorrect). Complement levels may not be appropriate based on the above lab findings (E is incorrect).

The correct answer is D. Determination of serum CK levels is the most important test in this patient, which is elevated within 12 h after skeletal muscle injury, and persistent elevation is seen up to 3–4 days. CK levels start declining after cessation of myonecrosis.

Urine color is generally reddish-brown (tea-colored urine) due to myoglobin/hemoglobin. The pH is usually acidic. The presence of large blood with few red cells is due to myoglobin. Proteinuria is generally due to myoglobin and other muscle proteins. Urinary sediment shows muddy-brown casts and renal tubular cells. Low FE_{Na} is usually seen because of low intravascular volume, mimicking prerenal azotemia. Low albumin is related to capillary leak and extravasation to interstitium and other extravascular spaces.

Suggested Reading

Bosch X, Poch E, Grau JM. Rhabomyolysis and acute kidney injury. N Engl J Med. 2009;361:62–72.

Giannoglou GD, Chatzizisis Y, Misirli G. The syndrome of rhabdomyolysis: Physiology and diagnosis. Eur J Intern Med. 2007;18:90–100.

Torres PA, Helmstetter JA, Kaye AM, et al. Rhabdomyolysis: pathogenesis, diagnosis, and treatment. Ochsner J. 2015;15:58–69.

Zarzou A, Agarwal A. Acute kidney injury associated with pigmenturia or crystal deposits. In: Coffman TM, Falk RJ, Molitoris BA, et al. editors. Schrier's diseases of the kidney. 9th ed. Philadelphia: Wolters Kluwer/Lippincott Williams & Wilkins; 2013. p. 1018–44.

68. The urine myoglobin was 400 mg/mL (normal <50 mg/mL) and CK levels 120,000 U/L (normal <300 U/L). **In the above patient, which one of the following is the MOST likely cause of her rhabdomyolysis?**

A. Hypokalemia
B. Hypophosphatemia
C. Cocaine and heroin
D. HIV
E. All of the above

The answer is E

There are several causes for rhabdomyolysis: trauma, metabolic (hypokalemia, hypophosphatemia), drugs (alcohol, cocaine, heroin, statin), infections (viral, bacterial), exertion, genetic, and idiopathic (recurrent episodes). Generally rhabdomyolysis causes hyperkalemia and hyperphosphatemia, which are serious electrolyte abnormalities and require close monitoring. On the other hand, hypokalemia causes muscle injury by decreasing skeletal muscle blood flow. Hypophosphatemia causes rhabdomyolysis due depletion of ATP and energy.

Cocaine inhibits reuptake of norepinephrine at the nerve endings, resulting in continuous vasoconstriction and ischemia of muscle cells. Also, cocaine may have a direct effect on muscles, causing reduced excitability of the muscle fibers with resultant muscle weakness. Heroin may cause vasoconstriction and decreased blood flow to the skeletal muscle. An immunologic mechanism has also been suggested. Among infectious causes, HIV is also an offending agent that causes rhabdomyolysis. Thus, E is correct.

Suggested Reading

Huerta-Alardin A, Varon J, Marik PE. Bench-to-bedside review: rhabdomyolysis-an overview for clinicians. Crit Care. 2005;9:2.

Torres PA, Helmstetter JA, Kaye AM, et al. Rhabdomyolysis: pathogenesis, diagnosis, and treatment. Ochsner J. 2015;15:58–69.

Zarzou A, Agarwal A. Acute kidney injury associated with pigmenturia or crystal deposits. In: Coffman TM, Falk RJ, Molitoris BA, et al. editors. Schrier's diseases of the kidney. 9th ed. Philadelphia: Wolters Kluwer/Lippincott Williams & Wilkins; 2013. p. 1018–44.

69. Repeat chemistry is as follows: Na^+ 138 mEq/L, K^+ 4 mEq/L, phosphate 4.2 mg/dL, HCO_3^- 14 mEq/L, BUN 54 mg/dL, and creatinine 3.2 mg/dL. Her urine output is 30 mL/h. **Which one of the following management strategies is appropriate for this patient?**

A. $NaHCO_3$ 100 mEq/L of D5W to run at 200 mL/h
B. Initially normal saline followed by $NaHCO_3$ 100 mEq/L in D5W to run at 150–200 mL/h
C. D5W at 200 mL/h
D. Normal saline at 200 mL/h followed by furosemide 80 mg
E. Mannitol 12.5 g every 6 h

The answer is B

Generally the patients with rhabdomyolysis are hypovolemic because of sequestration of fluids into the injured muscle cells. Therefore, the initial management is fluid resuscitation with normal saline at 150–200 mL/h to improve urine output and renal blood flow. Subsequently, the use of $NaHCO_3$ to alkalinize the urine is based on urine pH and serum HCO_3^- concentration. As myoglobin is converted into ferrihemate in the presence of acidosis, which is toxic to renal tubules, it is necessary to raise serum HCO_3^- concentration to a level above 22 mEq/L. In this patient, serum HCO_3^- concentration is 14 mEq/L, and she requires a combination of both normal saline to improve volume status and $NaHCO_3$ to improve not only serum HCO_3^- concentration but also to raise her urine pH >6.5. Thus, choice B is correct. It should be noted that $NaHCO_3$ may cause metabolic alkalosis, which lowers ionized Ca^{2+} and may precipitate tetany. Therefore, monitoring serum HCO_3^- concentration is extremely important.

Either D5W or D5W with $NaHCO_3$ may not be adequate to improve volume status (A and C are incorrect). Forced diuresis with furosemide has been suggested; however, furosemide can acidify the urine and also induce volume depletion. Furthermore, the combination of furosemide and normal saline was not found to be superior to normal saline alone. Therefore, use of furosemide is not suggested (D is incorrect).

The use of mannitol with $NaHCO_3$ has been suggested by case studies to prevent or improve renal failure. However, studies have shown that mannitol may worsen renal failure by a process of osmotic nephropathy, and the mannitol-$NaHCO_3$ combination in D5W is not suggested until clinical trials are done (E is incorrect).

Daily hemodialysis or continuous venovenous diafiltration is required in patients with rapid increase in serum creatinine, hyperkalemia, or hyperphosphatemia.

Suggested Reading

Bosch X, Poch E, Grau JM. Rhabdomyolysis and acute kidney injury. N Engl J Med. 2009;361:62–72.

Torres PA, Helmstetter JA, Kaye AM, et al. Rhabdomyolysis: pathogenesis, diagnosis, and treatment. Ochsner J. 2015;15:58–69.

70. The above patient improves her serum electrolytes, creatinine, and CK. **Which one the following electrolyte abnormalities is seen MOST frequently during the recovery phase of AKI or cessation of rhabdomyolysis?**

A. Hypernatremia
B. Hyperkalemia
C. Hypercalcemia
D. Hyperuricemia
E. Hyperphosphatemia

The answer is C

In a patient with rhabdomyolysis, hypocalcemia is commonly seen due to: (1) hyperphosphatemia inhibits 1α-hydroxylase in the kidney with less formation of calcitriol. Also, renal failure causes low production of 1α-hydroxylase and low calcitriol synthesis; (2) formation and deposition of calcium phosphate crystals in injured muscles and other soft tissues; and (3) tentative skeletal resistance to PTH with resultant hypocalcemia. Once kidney function improves and muscle injury stabilizes, all of the above processes of hypocalcemia are reversed, and severe hypercalcemia occurs (C is correct). At times, it is necessary to use bisphosphonates and/or HD with low Ca^{2+} bath to improve sustained hypercalcemia. Most of the other electrolyte abnormalities correct themselves once renal failure and rhabdomyolysis improve.

Suggested Reading

Bosch X, Poch E, Grau JM. Rhabdomyolysis and acute kidney injury. N Engl J Med. 2009;361:62–72.

Torres PA, Helmstetter JA, Kaye AM, et al. Rhabdomyolysis: pathogenesis, diagnosis, and treatment. Ochsner J. 2015;15:58–69.

71. A 40-year-old man with long-standing cirrhosis due to hepatitis C develops refractory ascites requiring large volume (5–7 L) paracentesis every 2 weeks with albumin infusion. He is on furosemide and spironolactone at the maximum doses, but not on any prophylactic antibiotics. He has been stable for over 6 months. This time, he comes to the clinic with complaint of abdominal discomfort and pain. Following a large volume (6 L) paracentesis, he is admitted for possible spontaneous bacterial peritonitis (SBP) and antibiotic therapy. His [Na^+] is 130 mEq/L and creatinine 1.3 mg/dL, and bilirubin of 8 mg/dL. His urinalysis is benign other than bilirubin. His urine [Na^+] is <10 mEq/L. Ascitic fluid WBC count is 500, and culture result is pending. **In order to prevent AKI, which one of the following therapeutic measures you would take at this time?**

A. Discontinue diuretics
B. Start a third-generation cephalosporin
C. Start 5% albumin
D. Continue only antibiotics
E. A, B, and C

The answer is E

Diuretics should be discontinued. A third-generation cephalosporin, either cefotoxime (2 g IV Q8 H) or ceftriaxone (1 g Q12 h) should be started based on eGFR. 5% albumin at 1.5 g/kg at diagnosis and 1 g/kg on day 3 may substantially decrease the development of hepatorenal syndrome. This combination (antibiotic and albumin) therapy should be continued for a minimum of 5 days.

Suggested Reading

EASL clinical practice guidelines on the management of ascites, spontaneous bacterial peritonitis, and hepatorenal syndrome in cirrhosis. J Hepatol. 2010;53:397–417.

Pericleousa M, Sarnowskib A, Moorea A, et al. The clinical management of abdominal ascites, spontaneous bacterial peritonitis and hepatorenal syndrome: a review of current guidelines and recommendations. Eur J Gastroenterol Hepatol. 2016;28:e10–e18.

72. Despite the combination therapy and adequate volume replacement with albumin and a few boluses of normal saline, his bilirubin and creatinine increased to 10 mg/dL and 2.4 mg/dL, respectively. His urine analysis is still benign. **Which one of the following is the MOST likely diagnosis?**

A. Prerenal AKI
B. AKI with acute tubular necrosis
C. IgA nephropathy
D. Hepatorenal syndrome (HRS)
E. None of the above

The answer is D

Renal failure in cirrhosis is defined by the Acute Kidney Injury Network stages 1 to 3. In a patient with AKI, prerenal renal azotemia, acute tubular necrosis, underlying parenchymal diseases such as IgA nephropathy, and HRS should be considered. HRS is thus a diagnosis of exclusion. HRS is a functional defect with almost normal renal architecture. Benign urinalysis rules out acute tubular necrosis and IgA nephropathy. Prerenal AKI can also be safely ruled out in view of adequate hydration. It seems that the patient developed type 1 HRS, since 30% of patients with SBP develop HRS. Thus, D is correct.

In 2019, the diagnostic criteria of HRS have been revised, as shown below.

Diagnostic criteria
Cirrhosis; acute liver failure; acute-on-chronic liver failure
Increase in serum creatinine ≥0.3 mg/dL within 48 h or ≥50% from baseline value according to ICA consensus document and/or Urinary output ≤0.5 ml/kg B.W. ≥6 h[a]
No full or partial response, according to the ICA consensus document 20, after at least 2 days of diuretic withdrawal and volume expansion with albumin. The recommended dose of albumin is 1 g/kg of body weight per day to a maximum of 100 g/day
Absence of shock
No current or recent treatment with nephrotoxic drugs
Absence of parenchymal disease as indicated by proteinuria >500 mg/day, microhematuria (>50 red blood cells per high power field), urinary injury biomarkers (if available) and/or abnormal renal ultrasonography[b]
Suggestion of renal vasoconstriction with FE_{Na} of <0.2% (with levels <0.1% being highly predictive)

[a]The evaluation of this parameter requires a urinary catheter

[b]This criterion would not be included in cases of known preexisting structural chronic kidney disease (e.g., diabetic or hypertensive nephropathy). AKI, acute kidney injury; FE_{Na}, fractional excretion of sodium; HRS, hepatorenal syndrome; ICA, International Club of Ascites

Suggested Reading

Angeli P, Garcia-Tsao G, Nadim MK, et al. News in pathophysiology, definition and classification of hepatorenal syndrome: a step beyond the International Club of Ascites (ICA) consensus document. J Hepatol. 2019;71:811–22.

EASL clinical practice guidelines on the management of ascites, spontaneous bacterial peritonitis, and hepatorenal syndrome in cirrhosis European Association for the Study of the Liver. J Hepatol. 2010;53:397–417.

Pericleousa M, Sarnowskib A, Moorea A, et al. The clinical management of abdominal ascites, spontaneous bacterial peritonitis and hepatorenal syndrome: a review of current guidelines and recommendations. Eur J Gastroenterol Hepatol. 2016;28:e10–e18.

73. **Which one of the pathophysiologic mechanisms is implicated in hepatorenal syndrome (HRS)?**

A. Splanchnic vasodilation
B. Systemic inflammation
C. Activation of vasoconstrictor system and nonosmotic release of antidiuretic hormone (ADH)
D. Renal cortical vasoconstriction
E. All of the above

The answer is E

Although the exact mechanisms leading to HRS are incompletely understood, the available studies so far implicate all of the above mechanisms (A–D). Thus, E is correct. Of these mechanisms, splanchnic vasodilation is an important mechanism for HRS. In the initial stages of cirrhosis, inflammation of hepatocytes leads to hepatic stellate cells located in the perisinusoidal space to secrete collagen and deposition in the sinusoids, leading to portal vein resistance. With progression of liver disease, the increase in portal resistance/hypertension causes release of vasodilators such as nitric oxide (NO) by shear stress. Also, vasodilators such as cannabinoids and carbon monoxide are released. Increased shear stress also causes development of collaterals in mesenteric arteries, resulting in profound splanchnic vasodilation.

Splanchnic vasodilation causes a reduction in systemic vascular resistance because the splanchnic circulation is a major part of the peripheral circulation. In early cirrhosis, cardiac output increases with maintenance of arterial volume and BP. With advancing cirrhosis, this cardiac output may increase further, but not sufficient because of severe reduction in systemic vascular resistance. Effective circulating arterial blood volume also decreases. The result is a further increase in cardiac output, which is related to activation of sympathetic nervous system, renin-AII-aldosterone system, and nonosmotic release of ADH. Not only Na^+ but also water is reabsorbed, resulting in edema and ascites. Relative hypotension develops because of increased splanchnic vasodilation despite adequate salt and water retention. Thus, circulatory dysfunction occurs in cirrhosis (A and C are correct).

Another mechanism that has been proposed for HRS is systemic inflammation hypothesis. It is proposed that portal HTN increases intestinal permeability and bacterial overgrowth. Pathologic bacteria translocate from intestine to mesenteric nodes and systemic circulation. Bacteria and bacterial products called PAMPs (pathogen-associated molecular patterns) are recognized by pattern recognition receptors (PRRs) such as Toll-like receptor 4 on immune cells and trigger the release of proinflammatory cytokines (tumor necrosis factor-α and interleukin-1 and 6) and these cytokines stimulate NO production, causing splanchnic vasodilation. Norfloxacin seems to inhibit NO production and improve vasodilation. There is also evidence to suggest that bacterial translocation can cause cardiac and kidney dysfunction

Renal cortical (arcuate and interlobular) vasoconstriction in HRS has been clearly demonstrated by imaging studies, resulting in AKI. Intense renal vasoconstriction is the result of splanchnic vasodilation and activation of sympathetic nervous and renin-AII-aldosterone system. Although the vasoconstrictive effect of sympathetic nervous and renin-AII-aldosterone system is less effective in splanchnic bed because of severe vasodilation, their effect is more pronounced on renal arteries. As a result, a decrease in renal blood flow and GFR is seen in patients with HRS (D is correct). Thus, HRS is a hemodynamically mediated abnormality rather than an intrinsic kidney disease.

Suggested Reading

Angeli P, Garcia-Tsao G, Nadim MK, et al. News in pathophysiology, definition and classification of hepatorenal syndrome: a step beyond the International Club of Ascites (ICA) consensus document. J Hepatol. 2019;71:811–22.

Bernardi M, Moreau R, Angeli P, et al. Mechanisms of decompensation and organ failure in cirrhosis: from peripheral arterial vasodilation to systemic inflammation hypothesis. J Hepatol. 2015;63:1272–84.

Francoz C, Durand F, Kahn JA, et al. Hepatorenal syndrome. Clin J Am Soc Nephrol. 2019;14:774–81.

Ginès P, Schrier RW. Renal failure in cirrhosis. N Engl J Med. 2009;361:1279–90.

74. **Which one of the following treatment modalities is acceptable in the above patient?**

A. Terlipressin and albumin
B. Norepinephrine and albumin
C. Midodrine, octreotide, and albumin
D. Continuous venonenous hemodiafiltration (CVVHDF)
E. All of the above

The answer is E

All of the above treatments are acceptable (E). Pharmacologic treatment has been shown to improve the clinical course of type 1 HRS, and is the choice of therapy. The most commonly used combination is vasoconstrictors and albumin. Vasoconstrictors are used to counteract the splanchnic vasodilation, and albumin for expansion of arterial volume. Vasoconstrictors that have been tried frequently in clinical trials are vasopressin, terlipressin (an analogue of vasopressin with greater effect on V1 than V2 receptor), norepinephrine, midodrine, and dopamine.

Octreotide, a long-acting somatostatin analogue, reduces portal hypertension and causes splanchnic vasoconstriction. The combinations that have been tried most frequently in clinical trials are shown below.

1. **Combination 1 (terlipressin + albumin). Terlipressin (not yet approved in the United States). Starting dose is 0.5–1 mg IV q4–6h. Double the dose every 2 days by 2 mg q4–6 h to a maximum of 12 mg/day, if serum creatinine does not decrease by >30% from baseline. Start simultaneously albumin at 1 g/kg/day up to 100 g the first day and then 20 to 40 g/day in subsequent days. Continue treatment to a maximum of 14 days. This is the preferred combination.**
2. **Combination 2 (midodrine + octreotide + albumin). Midodrine (an α1-agonist). Start at 7.5 mg orally q8 h, and increase to 12.5 to 15 mg q8 h, as needed to increase the mean arterial pressure by 15 mm Hg. Also, start octreotide 100 μg subcutaneously q8 h to a maximum of 200 μg q8 h on day 2, if creatinine does not improve. Start also albumin at 1 g/kg/day up to 100 g the first day and then 20 to 40 g/day. Duration of treatment is 14 days. This is the preferred combination when terlipressin is not available.**
3. **Combination 3 (norepinephrine + albumin). Start norepinephrine at 0.5 mg/h IV, and increase the dose by 0.25–0.5 mg/h every 4 h to a maximum of 3 mg/h until the mean arterial pressure increases by at least 10 mm Hg. Start simultaneously albumin at 1 g/kg/day up to 100 g the first day and then 20 to 40 g/day. The maximum duration of treatment is 15 days.**

The above combination regimens have shown reversal of HRS in 25 to 83% compared to 8.7 to 12.5% with albumin alone. If HRS recurs, retreatment with one of the above combinations should be started. It is interesting to note that HRS due to acute liver disease with fulminant hepatic failure may not respond to any of the above combinations. There are several contraindications for vasoconstrictor therapy in HRS: (1) coronary artery disease; (2) cardiac arrhythmias; (3) respiratory or cardiac failure; (4) severe hypertension; (5) cerebrovascular accidents; (6) peripheral vascular disease; and (7) severe bronchospasm.

If pharmacologic therapy fails, patients with HRS may benefit from CVVHDF until the availability of liver transplant.

Suggested Reading

Angeli P, Garcia-Tsao G, Nadim MK, et al. News in pathophysiology, definition and classification of hepatorenal syndrome: A step beyond the International Club of Ascites (ICA) consensus document. J Hepatol. 2019;71:811–22.

Fagundes C, Ginès P. Hepatorenal syndrome: A severe, but treatable, cause of kidney failure in cirrhosis. Am J Kidney Dis 2012;59:874–85.

Francoz C, Durand F, Kahn JA, et al. Hepatorenal syndrome. Clin J Am Soc Nephrol 2019;14:774–81.

75. **Which one of the following conditions is associated with low fractional excretion of sodium (FE_{Na})?**

A. Hepatorenal syndrome
B. Contrast-induced nephropathy
C. Rhabdomyolysis
D. Prerenal azotemia
E. All of the above

The answer is E

Urine Na^+ excretion is influenced by a number of hormonal and other factors. Changes in water excretion by the kidney can result in changes in urine Na^+ concentration [Na^+]. For example, patients with diabetes insipidus can excrete 10 L of urine per day. Their urine [Na^+] may be inappropriately low due to dilution, suggesting the presence of volume depletion. Conversely, increased water reabsorption by the kidney can raise the urine [Na^+] and mask the presence of hypovolemia. To correct for water reabsorption, the renal handling of Nat^+ can be evaluated directly by calculating the FE_{Na}, which is defined as the ratio of urine to plasma Na^+ divided by the ratio of urine (U_{Cr}) to plasma creatinine concentration (P_{Cr}), multiplied by 100.

$$FE_{Na}(\%) = \frac{\text{Quantity of Na}^+\text{excreted}}{\text{Quantity of Na}^+\text{filtered}}$$

$$= \frac{U_{Na} \times P_{cr}}{P_{Na} \times U_{cr}} \times 100$$

The FE_{Na} is the excreted fraction of filtered Na^+. The major use of FE_{Na} is in patients with AKI. Patients with prerenal azotemia have low (<1%) FE_{Na} compared to patients with acute tubular necrosis (ATN), whose FE_{Na}

is generally high (>2%). When ATN is superimposed on decreased effective arterial blood volume due to hepatic cirrhosis or congestive heart failure, the FE_{Na} is <2% because of the intense stimulus to Na^+ reabsorption. Similarly, patients with ATN due to radiocontrast agents or rhabdomyolysis have low FE_{Na} for unknown reasons.

It was shown that FE_{Na} in children with nephrotic syndrome is helpful in the treatment of edema with diuretics. In these patients, FE_{Na} <0.2% is indicative of volume contraction, and >0.2% is suggestive of volume expansion. Therefore, patients with FE_{Na} >0.2% can be treated with diuretics to improve edema.

The FE_{Na} is substantially altered in patients on diuretics. In these patients, the FE_{Na} is usually high despite hypoperfusion of the kidneys. In such patients, the FE_{Urea} may be helpful. In euvolemic subjects, the FE_{Urea} ranges between 50 and 65%. In a hypovolemic individual, the FE_{Urea} is <35%. Thus, a low FE_{Urea} seems to identify those individuals with renal hypoperfusion despite the use of a diuretic.

Suggested Reading

Bhargava S, Jain A, Gupta V. Fractional excretion of sodium – a simple test for the differential diagnosis of acute renal failure. Clin Nephrol. 2002;58:79–80.
Espinel CH. The FENa test. Use in the differential diagnosis of acute renal failure. JAMA. 1976;236:579–81.
Steiner RW. Interpreting the fractional excretion of sodium. Am J Med. 1984;77:899–702.

76. A 48-year-old woman with type 2 diabetes is admitted to intensive care unit with sepsis due to urinary tract infection. Because of AKI, she is started on CVVHDF. However, because of shortage of nursing staff at night and for certain radiologic procedures at night, the intensivist plans to start the patient on an extended hybrid therapy during the day. **Which one of the following hybrid therapies is APPROPRIATE?**

A. Sustained low efficiency (daily) dialysis (SLEDD)
B. Sustained low efficiency (daily) diafiltration (SLEDD-f)
C. Extended daily dialysis (EDD)
D. Extended daily dialysis with filtration (EDDf)
E. All of the above

The answer is E

An alternate term for hybrid therapies is prolonged intermittent renal replacement therapy (PIRRT). PIRRT is a treatment modality that uses modified hemodialysis (HD) machine with extended period of dialysis at low blood and dialysate flow rates. Dialysis is done for 6 to 18 h. Blood flow rate is 70–350 mL/min, and dialysis flow rate is 70–300 mL/min. Fluid and solute removal are slower than the conventional intermittent HD and higher than continuous renal replacement therapies (CRRT). Solute removal is largely diffusive, but convective removal is achieved by using SLEDD-f and EDDf. Cost and anticoagulation needs are low compared to CRRT. A study comparing PIRRT with CRRT showed cardiovascular stability and a total fluid removal of 3 L over 12 h during treatment with PIRRT compared to 3.3 L over 24 h with CRRT. Thus, any one of the hybrid therapies mentioned in A–D can be used depending on the individual patient (answer E is correct).

Despite some advantages of PIRRT, a meta-analysis of randomized controlled studies (RCTs) showed no difference in mortality rates between EDD and CRRT, although observational studies showed mortality advantage with EDD. However, in both RCTs and observational studies, there were no significant differences in recovery of kidney function, fluid removal, or days spent in the intensive care unit. Serum chemistry, particularly, serum creatinine, BUN, and phosphate, was similar in both treatments.

Suggested Reading

Edrees F, Li T, Vijayan A. Prolonged intermittent renal replacement therapy. Adv Chronic Kidney Dis. 2016;23:195–202.
Zhang L, Yang J, GM Eastwood, et al. Extended daily dialysis versus continuous renal replacement therapy for acute kidney injury: a meta-analysis. Am J Kidney Dis. 2015;66:322–30

77. Cytokine surge is common in patients with severe sepsis and AKI. Continuous renal replacement therapies (CRRT) are used to remove proinflammatory cytokines with variable results and outcomes in these patients. **To achieve good outcomes, several novel membranes (techniques) have been introduced, including which one of the following?**

A. High cut-off (HCO) membranes
B. Adsorption
C. Coupled plasma filtration adsorption

D. High volume hemofiltration
E. All of the above

The answer is E

All of the above novel technologies were applied over the years to achieve cytokine balance and better survival outcomes in patients with sepsis and AKI. Thus, answer E is correct.

HCO membranes are characterized by large pores (average pore size 20 nm) compared to high-flux membrane (10 nm). The recommended dose is 25 to 40 mL/kg/h. Because of large pores, cytokines, light chain immunoglobulins, and myoglobin can be removed by convection. As a result, HCO hemodialysis can be used in patients with multiple myeloma and rhabdomyolysis. Removal of IL-6, an important mediator of severe acute pancreatitis, makes HCO membrane as potential therapeutic technique in this devastating disease. One of the problems with HCO membranes is removal of albumin up to 8 g/day with convective dose of 1 L/h, and replacement with plasma or albumin is required.

Although initial studies have shown removal of proinflammatory cytokines in patients with sepsis and AKI, the High Cut-Off Sepsis study did not show a 28-day mortality benefit, ICU length of stay, or lower requirement for vasopressors compared to conventional CRRT membranes.

Adsorption is performed with hemoperfusion, which involves passage of blood through a hemofilter where cytokines are adsorbed to the surface of the membrane or through a sorbent-containing cartridge. Target mediators for removal by adsorption or sorbents include endotoxins (produced in Gram-negative bacteremia), superantigen, and cytokines. Superantigen is a mediator in toxic shock Gram-positive bacterial infections. A variety of sorbents are available with different selectivity of target mediator removal. Some of these sorbents include the following, and the reader is referred to the Suggested Reading for details of these adsorbents:

1. **Polymixin B-immobilized fiber column**
2. **Cytosorb**
3. **Modified AN 69 (Oxiris)**
4. **HA-330**
5. **LPS adsorbers (Alteco)**

Coupled plasma filtration adsorption (CPFA) involves separation of plasma from blood cells by a filter followed by passage of plasma through a sorbent cartridge. After the sorbent cartridge, the plasma returns to the blood circuit where it combines with blood cells and then the whole blood undergoes hemofiltration or hemodialysis. In this way, both cytokines are adsorbed by the sorbent and fluid/solutes are removed by hemofiltration or hemodialysis. Although several observational studies reported hemodynamic stability and survival benefit, a large randomized controlled trial did not show either in-hospital mortality or ICU-free days during the first 30 days.

The 2015 Vicenza Nomenclature Standardization Initiative defines high volume hemofiltration (HVHF) as a continuous convective treatment with a (prescribed) target dosage greater than 35 mL/kg/h. Doses exceeding 45 mL/kg/h represents very HVHF (VHVHF). Both techniques were used for immunomodulation in sepsis and AKI. Early studies showed survival benefit and hemodynamic stability. However, large randomized studies did not show any benefit in sepsis. Thus, both HVHF and VHVHF are not recommended in ICU settings.

Suggested Reading

Ankawi G, Neri M, Zhang J, et al. Extracorporeal techniques for the treatment of critically ill patients with sepsis beyond conventional blood purification therapy: the promises and the pitfalls. Crit Care. 2018;22:262.

Hattori N, Oda S. Cytokine-adsorbing hemofilter: old but new modality for septic acute kidney injury. Ren Replace Ther. 2016;2:41.

Monard C, Rimmelé T, Ronco C. Extracorporeal blood purification therapies for sepsis. Blood Purif. 2019;47(suppl 3):2–15.

78. Extracorporeal liver support therapies (ELS) are technical options or devices that are used in patients with acute liver dysfunction as a bridge-to-transplantation or bridge-to-recovery. **Which one of the following therapies is applied in these patients?**

A. Molecular adsorbent recirculating system (MARS)
B. Fractionated plasma separation and adsorption (Prometheus)

C. Single-pass albumin dialysis
D. Plasma exchange
E. All of the above

The answer is E

There are at least three indications for ELS: (1) bridge-to-liver transplantation; (2) bridge-to-recovery; and (3) to relieve symptoms of liver failure. All of the above ELS therapy techniques have been applied to the patients with acute liver failure, acute-on-chronic liver failure and other indications. The first three devices are based on combined albumin dialysis that removes albumin-bound toxins and conventional dialysis that removes creatinine, BUN, NH_3, and bilirubin. Plasma exchange involves removal of entire plasma from the patient and replacing it with donor plasma. Thus, answer E is correct.

Of all the above techniques, MARS has been studied the most followed by promethius. It combines conventional dialysis against an albumin dialysate followed by a conventional dialysis to remove toxins from the dialysate. MARS has an albumin hemodialyzer, a conventional hemodialyzer, an activated carbon adsorber, and an anion exchanger. The treatment is based on the dialysis of blood against an albumin dialysate. Albumin-bound toxins and water-soluble low and middle molecular substances diffuse into the albumin dialysate, which is then passed through another conventional dialyzer counter-current to a standard dialysis solution where diffusive clearance of creatinine, BUN, and electrolytes occurs to provide acid-base balance. The albumin dialysate is then cleaned of its albumin-bound toxins by passing through an activated carbon adsorber and an anion exchange resin column. The albumin dialysate goes back to the albumin dialyzer to repeat the cycle.

Several observational and randomized studies have shown that MARS improves toxin clearance including bilirubin as well as NH_3 removal, hepatic encephalopathy grade, hepatorenal syndrome, and portal hemodynamic status. However, it did not show any evidence of improved survival in acute or chronic liver failure.

In Prometheus system, blood from the patient passes through a specific albumin-permeable polysulfone filter where albumin and other proteins are separated. This filtered albumin-containing plasma then passes through sequentially through an adsorption column and an anionic exchanger. Albumin-bound toxins and other ions are thus removed by these two columns. The detoxified plasma is sent to a conventional high-flux dialyzer where regular dialysis by diffusion occurs between plasma and HCO_3^- containing dialysate. The dialyzed plasma then returns to the blood side of the albumin filter.

Similar to MARS, the fractionated plasma separation and adsorption (Prometheus) system is effective in removing bilirubin, bile acids, and NH_3. However, the survival data are limited. The usefulness of both MARS and fractionated plasma separation and adsorption (Prometheus) in reversing hepatorenal syndrome is not clear at this time.

Single-pass albumin dialysis (SPAD) is the simplest form of albumin dialysis. It uses continuous venovenous hemodialysis that is impermeable to albumin. Dialysate that contains approximately 5% albumin is run countercurrent to blood, and low molecular weight toxins move from blood into dialysate by convection. These toxins bind to albumin and subsequently discarded. One randomized study comparing SPAD with MARS showed no difference in clinical and biochemical parameters. However, there was no survival benefit with SPAD as well. Compared to other albumin-based techniques, SPAD is less expensive and available in most hospitals.

In addition, several bioartificial support devices have also been introduced to replace all the functions of the liver by incorporating a bioreactor into an existing extracorporeal circuit. The bioreactor consists of hepatocytes that have been cultured in a matrix that is surrounded by a hollow-fiber capillary system for plasma perfusion. Hepatocyte function requires oxygen and glucose supply provided by an integrated generator. One example of the bioreactor support device is the extracorporeal liver assist device (ELAD). This device consists of a bioreactor which contains HepG2/C3A human hepatoblastoma cells and an integrated hemodialysis circuit. ELAD is found to be safe and seems to have a survival benefit in patients with viral hepatitis-induced acute-on-chronic liver failure.

Other bioartificial support devices include HepatAssist, the Academic Medical Centre Bio-artificial Liver, the modular extracorporeal liver system, and the spheroid reserve bioartificial liver. Although these bioartificial devices are great addition to treatment of patients with liver failure, their usefulness is greatly awaited.

Suggested Reading

Fisher C, Wendon J. Extracorporeal liver support devices. In: Ronco C, Bellomo R, Kellum JA, et al., editors. Critical care nephrology. 3rd ed. Philadelphia: Elsevier; 2019, p. 793–9.

Joseph NA, Kumar LK. Liver support devices: bridge to transplant or recovery. Indian J Respir Care. 2017;6:807–12.
José García Martínez J, Bendjelid K. Artificial liver support systems: what is new over the last decade? Ann Intensive Care. 2018;8:109
Lee KCL, Stadlbauer V, Jalan R. Extracorporeal liver support devices for listed patients. Liver Transpl. 2016;22:839–48.

79. A 38 year-old woman with alcoholic cirrhosis and ascites is admitted with altered mental status and serum [Na⁺] of 124 mEq/L. She is oliguric and edematous. She is started on CVVHDF at the effluent dose of 30 mL/kg/h to a total volume of 2.1 L/h of PrismaSate with Na⁺ content of 140 mEq/L (replacement fluid of 1.1 L/h (prefilter), dialysate flow rate of 0.8 L/h and 0.2 L post-filter). UF is set at 100 mL/h. The critical care physician wants you to correct [Na⁺] to 130 mEq/L in 24 h. **Approximately how much 5% dextrose in water (D5W) you need to infuse separately to increase serum [Na⁺] from 124 mEq/L to 130 mEq/L?**

A. 100 mL/h
B. 120 mL/h
C. 140 mL/h
D. 160 mL/h
E. 180 mL/h

The answer is C

Hyponatremia is a common electrolyte abnormality in patients with cirrhosis. Correction of serum [Na⁺] should not exceed 6 mEq/L in 24 h. In order to achieve target [Na⁺] of 130 mEq/L, you need to follow the following calculations:

$$\text{Target}\left[\text{Na}^+\right] = 130\,\text{mEq} / \text{L}$$

$$\text{Replacement}\left[\text{Na}^+\right] = 140\,\text{mEq} / \text{L}$$

$$\text{Desired clearance}\left[\text{equal to UF}(0.1\,\text{L}) + \text{dialysate}(0.8\,\text{L}) + \text{replacement fluid}(1.1\,\text{L})\right] = 2\,\text{L} / \text{h}$$

$$\text{D5W rate} = \frac{\text{Replacement fluid Na}^+ - \text{Target Na}^+}{\text{Replacement fluid Na}^+} \times \text{Desired clearance}$$

$$= \frac{140 - 130}{140} \times 2 = 0.14\,\text{L or } 140\,\text{mL} / \text{h}$$

$$\text{Rate of replacement fluid} = 1.1\,\text{L} - 0.14\,\text{L} = 0.96\,\text{L} / \text{h}$$

There are no available commercial replacement or dialysate fluids that contain <140 mEq/L of Na⁺ content in all countries. Different strategies to lower Na⁺ content in the replacement/dialysate fluids have been attempted. These include diluting commercial solutions with sterile water to desired Na⁺ content, or manually prepared fluid using a combination of NaCl, $NaHCO_3$, and D5W, or adding D5W to the post-filter. The use of D5W by peripheral route to achieve target serum [Na⁺] is simple and avoids the need for a pharmacist and other complications.

Determination of serum [Na⁺] should be checked every 2–4 h for adjustment of D5W infusion rate and make sure the correction is appropriate. Thus, answer C is correct. Similar calculations can be used to correct hypernatremia with the use of 3% NaCl.

Suggested Reading

Bender FH. Successful treatment of severe hyponatremia in a patient with renal failure using continuous venovenous hemodialysis. Am J Kidney Dis. 1998;32:829–31.
Rosner MH, Connor MJ, Jr. Management of severe hyponatremia with continuous renal replacement therapies. Clin J Am Soc Nephrol. 2018;13:787–9.
Yessayan L, Yee J, Frinak S, et al. Treatment of severe hyponatremia in patients with kidney failure: Role of continuous venovenous hemofiltration with low-sodium replacement fluid. Am J Kidney Dis. 2014;64:305–10.
Yessayan L, Yee J, Frinak S, et al. Continuous renal replacement therapy for the management of acid-base and electrolyte imbalances in acute kidney injury. Adv Chronic Kidney Dis. 2016;23:203–10.
Vassallo D, Camilleri D, Moxham V, et al. Successful management of severe hyponatraemia during continuous renal replacement therapy. Clin Kidney J. 2012;5:155–7.

80. Renal functional reserve (RFR) is an important physiologic function of the kidney. Preoperative testing of RFR can be used as a marker to predict postoperative AKI in patients undergoing cardiac procedures. **Which one of the following patients is at risk for postoperative AKI?**

A. RFR >30 mL/min
B. RFR >40 mL/min
C. RFR >50 mL/min
D. RFR >55 mL/min
E. RFR <30 mL/min

The answer is E

RFR represents the capacity of the kidney to increase GFR in response to certain physiological or pathological stimuli or conditions. Once baseline GFR is determined, RFR can be assessed after an oral protein load (1–1.2 g/kg protein in the form of red meat) or iv amino acid infusion. RFR is the difference between peak "stress" GFR induced by the test and the baseline GFR. Generally, an increase in GFR ≥30 mL/min after protein meal is considered adequate RFR. Values below 30 mL/min are considered inadequate response. If RFR is <30 mL/min preoperatively in a patient with normal GFR, this patient is at risk for AKI postoperatively.

Husain-Syed et al. evaluated RFR in 110 patients undergoing coronary artery bypass graft or valve surgery. Preoperative RFR was measured by using a high oral protein load test (1.2 g/kg red meat meal). Of 110 patients, 15 (13.6%) developed AKI postoperatively. They observed that patients with preoperative RFRs not greater than 15 mL/min were 11.8 times more likely to experience AKI (95% CI: 4.62 to 29.89 times, $p < 0.001$). The authors concluded that among elective cardiac surgical patients with normal resting GFR, preoperative RFR was highly predictive of AKI. Thus, answer E is correct.

Physiologic conditions such as exercise, intake of high protein diet, exercise, and high fluid intake, and pathologic conditions such as diabetes, hypertension, anemia, and sepsis may be associated with high RFR as a compensatory mechanism.

Normal creatinine level may not indicate the underlying kidney disease because the increase in creatinine may not be apparent until 50% of nephron function is lost. RFR may unmask the silent kidney disease. Sharma and colleagues summarize the usefulness of RFR as follows:

1. **RFR is useful to assess silent kidney disease in high-risk individuals with diabetes, HTN, polycystic kidney disease, solitary kidney disease, CKD, or in patients requiring interventional studies that lead to an increase in creatinine levels**
2. **To evaluate kidney donors and recipients that nothing will happen to their kidney function after transplantation**
3. **To assess risk of postoperative AKI in patients undergoing elective cardiac procedures, and**
4. **To evaluate the level of recovery after AKI**

Suggested Reading

Husain-Syed F, Ferrari F, Sharma A, et al. Preoperative renal functional reserve predicts risk of acute kidney injury after cardiac operation. Ann Thorac Surg. 2018;105:1094–101.
Sharma A, Mucino MJ, Ronco C. Renal functional reserve and renal recovery after acute kidney injury. Nephron Clin Pract. 2014;127:94–100.

81. A 30-year-old man is admitted with sepsis. He is started on CVVHDF for AKI and anuria. He weighs 70 kg. The effluent dose is 30 mL/kg/h He received an initial dose of renally-excreted antibiotics, which are 50% albumin-bound. **The physician wants you to suggest the dose of antibiotics that is APPROPRIATE to his eGFR?**

A. 30.5 mL/min
B. 35.5 mL/min
C. 20.5 mL/min
D. 17.5 mL/min
E. 10.5 mL/min

The answer is D

Drug dosing in CVVHDF is dependent on its clearance, which is equal to the percentage of free drug times effluent rate expressed in mL/min, as follows:

- Free drug = 50%
- Effluent rate = 30 mL/kg
- Weight = 70 kg
- = 0.5 × 30 × 70 = 1050 mL/kg/h or 1050/60 = 17.5 mL/min

Dosing of the drug should be equivalent to that given to a patient with an eGFR of 17.5 mL/min. Thus, answer D is correct.

Suggested Reading

Ferrari T, Sartori M, Milla P. Antibiotic adjustment in continuous renal replacement therapy. In: Ronco C, Bellomo R, Kellum JA, et al., editors. Critical care nephrology. 3rd ed. Philadelphia: Elsevier; 2019, p. 1051–67.

Trotman RL, Williamson JC, Shoemaker DM, et al. Antibiotic dosing in critically ill adult patients receiving continuous renal replacement therapy. Clin Infect Dis. 2005;41:1159–66.

82. **Which one of the following statements regarding restrictive versus liberal fluid administration during and 24 h following major abdominal surgery is CORRECT?**

A. No difference in disability-free survival at 1 year between two fluid regimens
B. Increased rate of AKI in restrictive group
C. Increased rate of renal replacement therapy (RRT) in restrictive group
D. Increased rate of infection at suture site in restrictive group
E. All of the above

The answer is E

Patients undergoing abdominal surgery receive at least 7 L of fluids on the day of surgery. Such liberal fluid administration can lead to tissue edema and weight gain. Studies have shown that fluid restriction can prevent these complications and promote early discharge. Myles et al. investigated the effects of fluid restriction versus liberal fluid administration during and 24 h after major abdominal surgery on several outcomes, as shown in answers A–D. There was no difference in the primary outcome, which was disability-free survival at 1 year between the two treatment groups. However, secondary outcomes such as the rate of AKI need for RRT, and surgical-site infection were higher in the restrictive group. Thus, answer E is correct. However, the need for RRT and surgical-site infection complications were not significant between the groups after adjustment for multiple testing.

Suggested Reading

Myles PS, Bellomo R, Corcoran T, et al. for the Australian and New Zealand College of Anaesthetists Clinical Trials Network and the Australian and New Zealand Intensive Care Society Clinical Trials Group Restrictive versus liberal fluid therapy for major abdominal surgery. N Engl J Med. 2018;378:2263–74.

Voldby AW, Brandstrup B. Fluid therapy in the perioperative setting-A clinical review. J Intensive Care. 2016;16:427.

83. **Which one of the following statements regarding the furosemide stress test (FST) and diseased kidney transplantation is CORRECT?**

A. FST predicts transplant rejection in 30 days
B. FST predicts 1-year mortality following kidney transplantation
C. FST predicts delayed graft function (DGF) in early post-transplant period
D. FST is applicable only to critically ill patients with AKI
E. None of the above

The answer is C

The FST is one of the tests that assesses renal tubular function to predict patients who will progress to AKI stages 2–3. McMahon and colleagues investigated the urinary response to a single 100 mg i.v. dose of intraoperative furosemide to predict the DGF in patients undergoing deceased donor kidney transplant. DGF is defined as the need for dialysis within 7 days of kidney transplantation. Nonresponders to FST were defined as those who

produced urine output <600 mL at 6 h post-furosemide administration. Patients who developed DGF had a median urine output of 73 mL 2 h post FST, as compared with the non-DGF cohort who had a median urine output of 250 mL 2 h post FST. At 6 h post FST, the median urine output in the DGF cohort was 203 mL and 952 mL in the non-DGF cohort ($p < 0.001$). Thus, FST predicts DGF in deceased donor kidney transplant recipients (answer C is correct).

Following FST, there was no difference in blood pressure or serum [K^+] between responders and nonresponders. However, the length of hospital stay was longer in nonresponders than responders. During a median follow of 1.76 years, there was no difference in graft loss between responders and nonresponders. The findings of the study have the potential to guide physicians on the timing of the initiation of dialysis for DGF in patients who received deceased donor kidney transplantation. Similar findings were reported by Udomkarnjananun and colleagues. Other answers are incorrect.

Suggested Reading

Coca A, Aller C, Sánchez JR, et al. Role of the furosemide stress test in renal injury prognosis. Int J Mol Sci. 2020;21:3086.

McMahon BA, Koyner JL, Menez S, et al. The prognostic value of the furosemide stress test in predicting delayed graft function following deceased donor kidney transplantation. Biomarkers. 2018;23:61–9.

Udomkarnjananun S, Townamchai N, Iampenkhae K, et al. Furosemide stress test as a predicting biomarker for delayed graft function in kidney transplantation. Nephron. 2019;141:1–13.

84. **Which one of the following is a risk factor for AKI?**

A. Advanced age
B. Sepsis
C. Volume depletion
D. Chronic disease
E. All of the above

The answer is E

AKI is rather common in hospitalized patients. Risk for AKI is increased by exposure to factors that cause AKI or the presence of factors that increase susceptibility to AKI. It is the interaction between the exposure and susceptibility that determines the risk and the degree of AKI. Answers A–D are important causes of AKI (E is correct). Table 5.8 **shows all the causes of AKI, as proposed by The KDIGO guideline.**

Table 5.8 Causes of nonspecific AKI

Exposures	Susceptibilities
Sepsis	Dehydration or volume depletion
Critical illness	Advanced age
Circulatory shock	Female gender
Burns	Black race
Trauma	CKD
Cardiac surgery (especially with cardiopulmonary bypass)	Chronic diseases (heart, lung, liver)
Major noncardiac surgery	Diabetes mellitus
Nephrotoxic drugs	Cancer
Radiocontrast agents	Anemia
Poisonous plants and animals	

From the above table, it is possible to identify the individual risk factor that can be modified to reduce the risk of AKI. For example, dehydration can be corrected with appropriate fluid administration just before surgery or a contrast procedure. Similarly, hyperglycemia or anemia can be treated. If a patient is on nephrotoxic drugs or on angiotensin converting enzyme inhibitors or angiotensin receptor blockers, they can be stopped before any surgical procedures. Thus, it is extremely important to identify the risk factors at the time of admission to prevent AKI. Also, it is important to follow creatinine (or AKI biomarkers, if available) and urine output to prevent progression of AKI from stage 1 to stage 3. It should be noted that some 30% of patients who recover from AKI are at increased risk for development of CKD, cardiovascular disease and death.

Suggested Reading

Kidney Disease: Improving Global Outcomes (KDIGO) Acute Kidney Injury Work Group. KDIGO clinical practice guideline for acute kidney injury. Kidney Int (Suppl). 2012;2:1–138.

Neyra JA, Leaf DE. Risk prediction models for AKI in critically ill patients: opus in progressu. Nephron. 2018;140:99–104.

Tsai TT, Patel UD, Chang TI, et al. Validated contemporary risk model of acute kidney injury in patients undergoing percutaneous coronary interventions: insights from the National Cardiovascular Data Registry Cath-PCI Registry. J Am Heart Assoc. 2014;3:e001380 https://doi.org/10.1161/JAHA.114.001380.

85. A 63-year-old man had an abdominal surgery for profuse bleeding. During the intraoperative period, he had a transient hypotension. He was transferred to surgical ICU for further care. Pre- and post-surgery creatinine was 1.2 mg/dL. **Which one of the following single urinary biomarker test that can identify patients at risk for developing AKI within the ensuing 12 h in this patient?**

A. Albuminuria
B. Urine output
C. Tissue inhibitor of metalloproteinase-2 (TIMP-2) and insulin-like growth factor–binding protein-7 (IGFBP 7)
D. Kidney injury molecule-1 (KIM-1)
E. BUN

The answer is C

Several biomarkers have been assessed to predict the development of AKI and its subsequent progression to more severe stages. However, many of these biomarkers were not standardized and validated. Only urinary TIMP-2 x IGFBP 7 assay was the only test that was approved by the FDA to use in critically ill patients at risk for AKI and the need for dialysis (answer C is correct).

TIMP-2 x IGFBP 7 induces cell cycle arrest in G1 phase, which is a consequence of AKI. When these two biomarker values are multiplied together, the resultant value has a better predictive power for assessing the development of severe AKI (stages 2–3) than either biomarker. A value of >0.3 identifies patients with a high likelihood to have moderate to severe AKI within 12 h, while a value of ≤0.3 suggests patients with a low risk to develop moderate to severe AKI within 12 h. This test is also approved in Europe. Appropriate patient population for this test include those undergoing major surgery (cardiac and noncardiac), those who are hemodynamically unstable, and those with sepsis.

Meersch and colleagues showed that urinary TIMP-2 x IGFB 7 has excellent performance in predicting cardiac surgery-associated AKI. Other studies also observed similar results with this urinary test in identifying patients at increased risk for AKI following cardiac procedures.

Other biomarkers such as albuminuria, urine output, KIM-1, and BUN are risk factors for progression rather than predicting AKI in 12 h following cardiac procedures. Thus, these tests are not appropriate for this patient.

Suggested Reading

Kashani K, Al-Khafaji A, Ardiles T, et al. Discovery and validation of cell cycle arrest biomarkers in human acute kidney injury. Crit Care. 2013;17:R25.

Meersch M, Schmidt C, Van Aken H, et al. Urinary TIMP-2 and IGFBP7 as early biomarkers of acute kidney injury and renal recovery following cardiac surgery. PLoS One. 2014;9:e93460.

Vijayan A, Faubel S, Askenazi DJ, et al. on behalf of the American Society of Nephrology Acute Kidney Injury Advisory Group.*Clinical use of the urine biomarker [TIMP-2] × [IGFBP7] for acute kidney injury risk assessment. Am J Kidney Dis. 2016;68:19–28.

86. Extracorporeal membrane oxygenation (ECMO) is a procedure used in neonates, children, and adults with severe, reversible, cardiopulmonary failure. **AKI is common occurrence with ECMO. Which one of the following mechanisms is implicated in the development of AKI?**

A. Pre-ECMO risk factors for AKI
B. Hemodynamic abnormalities
C. Coagulation and systemic inflammation
D. Kidney-lung cross talk
E. All of the above

The answer is E

ECMO is a life-saving procedure for patients with cardiopulmonary failure unresponsive to conventional management. It provides temporary extracorporeal respiratory support by the use of an artificial membrane lung to respiratory failure patients. In this way, it gives rest to lungs and allows recovery from invasiveness of mechanical ventilation. ECMO can be performed in two ways. Venovenous ECMO is done in patients with respiratory failure where the blood drawn from the vein is returned to venous circulation after oxygenation, whereas venoarterial ECMO is applied to patients with cardiac failure where the blood is returned to arterial circulation.

ECMO is not without complications. One of the complications is ECMO-induced AKI (EAKI). The incidence of AKI ranges from 70 to 85%, and the mortality in conjunction with ECMO approaches 80%. Despite this high incidence, the pathophysiology of EAKI is not completely understood. However, several mechanisms, as shown in answers A–D, have been proposed. Thus, answer E is correct.

Prior to initiation of ECMO, the patient is exposed to several risk factors for AKI such as sepsis, ischemia, vasopressors, nephrotoxic drugs, respiratory failure, and cardiac failure. Thus, patient-related factors may contribute to AKI during ECMO (A is correct).

After initiation of ECMO, certain therapeutic measures may cause AKI. These include fluid management, diuretics use to improve fluid overload, vasopressor use for hypotension, and PEEP may lead to altered hemodynamics, causing AKI. Fluid overload is rather common during ECMO and when diuretic therapy is inadequate to maintain fluid balance, hemofiltration is added to the extracorporeal circuit to achieve fluid and electrolyte balance (B is correct).

When blood is exposed to extracorporeal circuit, platelets adhere to the surface of the circuit and then become activated. Indeed, activation and consumption of platelets occur throughout the course of ECMO. Simultaneously, other systems such as coagulation system and complement activation through the alternative pathway are stimulated. This results in the derangement of coagulation system and development of systemic inflammation with release of proinflammatory cytokines (IL-1, IL-6, IL-8, and TNF-α). These cytokines may induce oxidative stress with changes in microvasculature that may result in AKI and other organ dysfunction (C is correct).

Cross talk among various organs has been clearly established. In particular, interaction between kidney and lung has been studied adequately. AKI causes lung injury, which, in turn, exacerbates AKI through mediation of hypoxia, hypercapnia, and PEEP. This leads to further decrease in renal perfusion and excretory functions of the kidney. Increased intrathoracic pressure due to high PEEP during ECMO may also contribute to reduced renal perfusion and AKI (D is correct).

Suggested Reading

Kielstein JT, Heiden AM, Beutel G, et al. Renal function and survival in 200 patients undergoing ECMO therapy. Nephrol Dial Transplant. 2013;28:86–90.

Kilburn DJ, Shekar K, Fraser JF. The complex relationship of extracorporeal membrane oxygenation and acute kidney injury: causation or association? Biomed Res Int. 2016:1094296, 14 pages.

Villa G, Katz N, Ronco C. Extracorporeal membrane oxygenation and the kidney. Cardiorenal Med. 2015;6:50–60.

Zangrillo A, Landoni G, Biondi-Zoccai G, et al. A meta-analysis of complications and mortality of extracorporeal membrane oxygenation. Crit Care Resusc. 2013;15:172–8.

87. **Which one of the following cancers is associated with high incidence of AKI?**

A. Renal cell cancer
B. Multiple myeloma
C. Liver cancer
D. Lymphoma
E. All of the above

The answer is E

According to a Danish study, the incidence of AKI, as defined by RIFLE classification, was highest in patients with renal cell cancer (44%), followed by multiple myeloma (33%), liver cancer (32%), and leukemia (28%). Those patients who developed AKI, 5.1% required dialysis within 1 year. Thus, answer E is correct.

Suggested Reading

Christiansen CF, Johansen MB, Langeberg WJ, et al. Incidence of acute kidney injury in cancer patients. A Danish population based cohort study. Eur J Intern Med. 2011;22:399–406.
Rosner MH, Perazella MA. Acute kidney injury in patients with cancer. N Engl J Med. 2017;376:1776–80.

88. Anticancer drug therapy (chemotherapy) causes both beneficial effects and adverse events. **One of complications of anticancer drug therapy is AKI. Which type of nephron segment injury by anticancer drugs precipitates AKI?**

A. Renal vasculature
B. Glomerulus
C. Renal tubules
D. Renal interstitium
E. All of the above

The answer is E

Chemotherapeutic agents affect all segments of the nephron. Thrombotic microangiopathy (TMA) is a lesion of arteriolar and capillary vessel wall thickening with intraluminal platelet thrombosis with a partial or complete obstruction of the capillary lumen. Patients present with thrombocytopenia and microangiopathic hemolytic anemia. Typical examples are thrombotic thrombocytopenic purpura and hemolytic uremic syndrome. Hypertension is also a condition of TMA. Chemotherapy agents that cause TMA are shown in Table 5.9 **(A is correct).**

Table 5.9 Anticancer drugs and AKI

Causes of AKI	Chemotherapeutic agents
TMA	Conventional agents: Cisplatin, gemcitabine, mitomycin C Anti-VEGF-Ab: Bevacizumab TKIs: Sunitinib, pazopanib, sorafenib, EGFR inhibitor: Imatinib, afatinib Anti-CTL4-Ab: Ipilimumab
Proteinuria, nephrotic syndrome, minimal change disease, FSGS	Anti-VEGF-Ab: Bevacizumab TKIs: Sunitinib, pazopanib, sorafenib, imatinib Anti-CTLA4-Ab: Ipilimumab Anti-PD-1, PDL-1: Nivolumab, pembrolizumab Interferons
Renal tubules (acute tubular injury)	Conventional agents: Cisplatin, methotrexate, pemetrexed Anti-PD-1, PDL-1: Nivolumab, pembrolizumab BRAF inhibitors: Vemurafenib, dabrafenib
Acute tubulointerstitial nephritis	Anti-PD-1, PDL-1: Nivolumab, pembrolizumab BRAF inhibitors: Vemurafenib, dabrafenib

Acute glomerular disease can occur due to podocyte, endothelial, and mesangial cell injury by various mechanisms, which results in AKI. Chemotherapeutic agents induce proteinuria, nephrotic syndrome and glomerular diseases such as minimal change disease and focal segmental glomerulosclerosis. These conditions can precipitate AKI. Drugs that cause these glomerular lesions are shown in Table 5.9 **(B is correct).**

Acute tubular necrosis/injury (ATN) is caused by several mechanisms. Both conventional and newer chemotherapeutic agents can cause ATN, as shown in Table 5.9**. Similar to ATN, acute tubulointerstitial nephritis (ATID) is also caused by many chemotherapeutic drugs. Both ATN and AIN present with AKI (C and D are correct).**

CTLA-4 cytotoxic T lymphocyte-associated protein 4, EGFR epidermal growth factor, PD-1 programmed death, PDL-1 programmed death ligand-1, VGEF vascular endothelial growth factor, TKI tyrosine kinase inhibitors, TMA thrombotic microangiopathy

Suggested Reading

Campbell GA, Hu D, Okusa MD. Acute kidney injury in the cancer patient. Adv Chronic Kidney Dis. 2014;21:64–71.
Izzedine H, Perazella MA. Anticancer drug-induced acute kidney injury. Kidney Int Rep. 2017;2:504–14.
Malyszko J, Kozlowska K, Kozlowski L, et al. Nephrotoxicity of anticancer treatment. Nephrol Dial Transplant. 2017;32:924–36.

Perazella MA. Drug-induced acute kidney injury: diverse mechanisms of tubular injury. Curr Opin Crit Care. 2019;25:550–7.
Rosner MH, Perazella MA. Acute kidney injury in patients with cancer. N Engl J Med. 2017;376:1776–80.

89. **Which one of the following is a risk factor for AKI in cancer patient?**

A. Volume depletion
B. Age >65 years
C. Malignancy-induced urinary tract obstruction
D. Intrinsic glomerular diseases
E. All of the above

The answer is E

Volume depletion is rather common in cancer patients. Vomiting, diarrhea, and mucositis cause reduced oral intake of fluids and can lead to prerenal azotemia. Sepsis and hypotension is another cause of AKI. In some patients, hypercalcemia may cause nephrogenic diabetes insipidus and volume depletion. Thus, volume depletion is an important risk factor for AKI (A is correct).

Age >65 years is a risk factor for AKI. Elderly subjects have (1) reduced GFR with aging; (2) age-related structural changes in the kidney with increased number of sclerotic glomeruli, atherosclerotic changes, and tubulointerstitial fibrosis; (3) comorbid conditions such as diabetes, hypertension, and heart disease; (4) nephrotoxins such as NSAIDs and contrast exposure; (5) poor oral intake and relative volume depletion due to diuretic use; (6) preexisting CKD; and finally, urinary tract obstruction due to prostate hypertrophy or cancer in men. All of these causes predispose elderly individuals at risk for AKI (B is correct).

In addition to patient-related risk factors, urinary tract obstruction due to malignancy is rather common. Cancers such as bladder, prostate, uterus, and cervix cause obstruction. Also, massive retroperitoneal mass due to extensive lymphadenopathy or related to radiation treatment of the abdomen may obstruct the ureters and cause anuria as well as AKI. Also, intratubular obstruction due to crystals, casts or proteins in association with decreased urine output is an important cause of obstruction. Relief of the obstruction may improve creatinine (C is correct).

Malignancy and anticancer drugs cause many glomerular diseases such as minimal change disease, focal segmental glomerulosclerosis, membranous nephropathy, membranoproliferative glomerulonephritis, and thrombotic microangiopathy. In addition, acute tubular necrosis and acute tubulointerstitial disease are also renal disorders associated with malignancy. Proteinuria, nephrotic syndrome, and hematuria are common manifestations of these glomerular diseases. Also, tumor lysis syndrome can present as AKI. Thus, intrinsic kidney diseases can precipitate AKI (D is correct).

Suggested Reading

Campbell GA, Hu D, Okusa MD. Acute kidney injury in the cancer patient. Adv Chronic Kidney Dis. 2014;21:64–71.
Izzedine H, Perazella MA. Anticancer drug-induced acute kidney injury. Kidney Int Rep. 2017;2:504–14.
Malyszko J, Kozlowska K, Kozlowski L, et al. Nephrotoxicity of anticancer treatment. Nephrol Dial Transpl. 2017;32:924–936.
Rosner MH, Perazella MA. Acute kidney injury in patients with cancer. N Engl J Med. 2017;376:1776–80.

90. **Which one of the following is a cause of AKI in patients with multiple myeloma?**

A. Light chain cast nephropathy
B. Proximal tubular injury
C. Interstitial nephritis
D. Hypercalcemia
E. All of the above

The answer is E

AKI is rather common in patients with multiple myeloma at time of diagnosis or during the work-up of the disease. Uncontrolled production of immunoglobulin light chains is the cause of both AKI and CKD. Generally, these light chains are filtered at the glomerulus, which are reabsorbed by the proximal tubule and degraded in the lysosomes. When production exceeds the reabsorption, the free light chains reach the distal nephron where

they combine with Tamm-Horsfall protein to form a cast. These casts are excreted in the urine initially when urine flow and kidney function are normal. With increased production of casts, they precipitate in the renal tubules and cause obstruction. As a result, the intratubular pressure rises which opposes the glomerular filtration pressure. This leads to a decrease in glomerular filtration rate and an increase in serum creatinine levels. Thus, light chain casts cause AKI (A is correct).

In addition, the light chains are toxic to the proximal tubule, causing injury and necrosis of the cells. This results in ATN (B is correct). Also, the uncatabolized light chains by lysosomes enter the interstitium and trigger production of proinflammatory cytokines, including transforming growth factor-β1. These cytokines through different pathways promote fibrosis in the interstitium, which causes AKI (C is correct).

Hypercalcemia is present in 15–20% of patients, which is related to the production of cytokines, chemokines and parathyroid hormone-related protein as well as bone lytic lesions. Hypercalcemia causes nephrogenic diabetes insipidus with volume depletion, resulting in AKI (D is correct). It should be noted that AKI is precipitated by volume depletion, use of diuretics, NSAIDs, and contrast material.

Suggested Reading

Irish AB. Myeloma and the kidney. In: Feehally J, Floege J, Tonelli M, et al., editors. Comprehensive clinical nephrology. 6th ed. Philadelphia: Elsevier; 2019, p. 767–75.

Katagiri D, Noiri E, Hinoshita F. Multiple myeloma and kidney disease. Sci World J. 2013:Article ID 487285, 9 pages.

Ying WZ, CE Allen, LM Curtis, et al. Mechanism and prevention of acute kidney injury from cast nephropathy in a rodent model. J Clin Invest. 2012;122:1777–85.

91. The kidney is a target for novel severe acute respiratory syndrome coronavirus 2 (SARS-CoV-2 or Covid-19) infection. Acute kidney injury (AKI) is a common manifestation besides hypoxic respiratory failure and hypotension in patients with Covid-19 infection. In ICU setting, AKI occurs in >50% of patients and mortality is extremely high. **Which one of the following pathophysiologic mechanisms contributes to AKI?**

A. Acute tubular injury
B. Collapsing glomerulopathy
C. Endothelial damage and coagulopathy
D. Hypovolemia
E. All of the above

The answer is E

The available evidence suggests that AKI occurs in >20% of hospitalized patients with Covid-19 infection. Both biopsy and autopsy studies have shown acute tubular injury and the presence of viral particles within both the tubular epithelium and podocytes on electron microscopy. Also, FSGS with collapsing variant, particularly in African American has been demonstrated.

Endothelial dysfunction, which is characterized by high D-dimer levels and microvascular damage with coagulopathy, has been described. Also, thrombotic thrombocytopenic purpura and atypical hemolytic uremic syndrome due to endothelial dysfunction may contribute to AKI.

Hypovolemia is extremely common in patients with Covid-19 infection. High temperature, diarrhea, and sepsis with increased microvascular permeability may cause intravascular fluid loss and result in hypovolemia, hypotension, and decreased blood flow to the kidney. Also, pressors to support blood pressure may eventually lead to low kidney perfusion with subsequent development of AKI. Thus, answer E is correct.

In addition to the above mechanisms, inflammation may play a significant role in AKI. "Cytokine storm" has been a well-defined mechanism in multiorgan failure, including kidney failure. Organ cross talk is also an important contributor to AKI. Patient characteristics such as body habitus and comorbidities may cause AKI superimposed on CKD. Thus, several mechanisms may be involved in the development of AKI.

Suggested Reading

Chan L, Chaudhary K, Saha A, et al.; Mount Sinai COVID Informatics Center (MSCIC). AKI in hospitalized patients with COVID-19. J Am Soc Nephrol. 2021;32:151–60.

Fisher M, Neugarten J, Bellin E, et al. AKI in hospitalized patients with and without COVID-19: a comparison study. J Am Soc Nephrol. 2020;31:2145–57.

Hanley B, Naresh KN, Roufosse C, et al. Histopathological findings and viral tropism in UK patients with severe fatal COVID-19: a post-mortem study. Lancet Microbe. 2020;1:e245–e253.

Hirsch JS, Ng JH, Ross DW, et al.; Northwell COVID-19 Research Consortium; Northwell Nephrology COVID-19 Research Consortium. Acute kidney injury in patients hospitalized with COVID-19. Kidney Int. 2020;98:209–18.

Nadim MK, Forni LG, Mehta RL, et al. COVID-19-associated acute kidney injury: consensus report of the 25th Acute Disease Quality Initiative (ADQI) Workgroup. Nature Rev Nephrol. 2020;16:747–64.

Puelles VG, Lütgehetmann M, Lindenmeyer MT, et al. Multiorgan and renal tropism of SARS-CoV-2. N Engl J Med. 2020;383:590–2.

Chapter 6
Hypertension

1. A 42-year-old Caucasian man is referred to you for evaluation of a blood pressure (BP) of 136/86 mm Hg. He has no family history of hypertension (HTN) or heart disease. He does not smoke. His creatinine and glucose are normal. His estimated risk for cardiovascular disease (CVD) in 10 years is <10%. **According to the 2017 American college of Cardiology (ACC) and American Heart Association (AHA) guideline, how would you classify his BP?**

   A. Normal
   B. Elevated BP
   C. Stage 1 hypertension
   D. Stage 2 hypertension
   E. Stage 3 hypertension

   The answer is C

   In 2017, the ACC/AHA and nine other professional associations prepared and published a new guideline on blood pressure categories in adults. According to this guideline, BP is classified into normal, elevated, stage 1 HTN, and stage 2 HTN. The following Table 6.1 **shows the classification of BP, as proposed by the above guideline.**

   Table 6.1 Classification of BP in adults

BP classification	BP (mm Hg)
Normal	<120/80
Elevated	120–129/<80
Stage 1 HTN	130–139/80–89
Stage 2 HTN	≥140/≥90

   It is evident from the table that the above individual has stage 1 HTN. However, his 10-year risk for CVD is <10%, and the guideline suggests only nonpharmacologic intervention (lifestyle modification) with follow-up BP in 3–6 mon. Stage 3 HTN has been eliminated. Thus, option C is correct.

   Suggested Reading

   Whelton PK, Carey RM, Aronow WS, et al. 2017 ACC/AHA/AAPA/ABC/ACPM/AGS/APhA/ASH/ASPC/NMA/PCNA guideline for the prevention, detection, evaluation, and management of high blood pressure in adults. A report of the American College of Cardiology/American Heart Association Task Force on Clinical Practice Guidelines. J Am Coll Cardiol. 2017, https://doi.org/10.1016/j.jacc.2017.11.006.

2. A 44-year-old woman is sent to you for evaluation of her BP. During her first visit, the BP is 144/82 mm Hg (similar BP on three measurements). She brings her home BP measurements, which range from 120–124/64–68 mm Hg. **Based on these BP values, which one of the following conditions she may have at this time?**

   A. Elevated BP
   B. White coat HTN
   C. Secondary HTN
   D. Primary HTN
   E. Stage 1 HTN

The original version of the chapter has been revised. A correction to this chapter can be found at https://doi.org/10.1007/978-3-030-85958-9_12

A. S. Reddi, *Absolute Nephrology Review*, https://doi.org/10.1007/978-3-030-85958-9_6

The answer is B

White coat HTN is defined as daytime out-of-office BP < 135/85 mm Hg and an office BP > 140/90 mm Hg. This high office BP with normal home BP is found between 15% and 30%, and most common in women and the elderly. It used to be thought that white coat HTN is a benign condition, but several studies and a meta-analysis that included 27 studies showed that untreated subjects are at increased risk for cardiovascular events and all-cause mortality. Thus, pharmacotherapy is indicated. Thus, option B is correct. Other forms of HTN are not applicable to this woman.

Suggested Reading

Bloofield DA, Park A. Decoding white coat hypertension. World J Clin Cases. 2017;5:82–92.

Cohen JB, Lotito MJ, Trivedi UK, et al. Cardiovascular events and mortality in white coat hypertension. A systematic review and meta-analysis. Ann Intern Med. 2019;170:853–62.

Franklin SS, Thijs L, Hansen TW, et al. White-coat hypertension. New insights from recent studies. Hypertension. 2013;62:982–7.

Parati G, Ochoa JE. White-coat and masked hypertension. In: Bakris GL, Sorrentino MJ, editors. Hypertension. A companion to Braunwald's heart disease. 3rd ed. Philadelphia: Elsevier; 2018. p. 104–14.

3. A 32-year-old man with a family history of HTN measures his own BP daily and keeps in his diary. He visits his primary care physician, and his BP is found to be 124/72 mm Hg, which is much lower than his home BP. He insists that his BP be measured 2 h later, which was found to be 125/73 mm Hg. **He asks you to clarify about this discrepancy between office and home BP measurements, and you would say that he has:**

A. Primary HTN
B. Elevated BP
C. White coat HTN
D. Masked HTN
E. Secondary HTN

The answer is D

In the last several years, a new form of HTN has been recognized with the use of ambulatory BP or home BP measurements. This form of HTN is called masked HTN, which is defined as low office or clinic BP and high ambulatory or home BP. The prevalence of masked HTN is varied from study to study but is more prevalent in men and elderly. Similar to white coat hypertensives, subjects with masked HTN are at risk for cardiovascular morbidity. Also, masked hypertensive subjects are at higher risk for cardiovascular disease than normotensive subjects. Thus, screening for masked HTN is important by self-monitoring his or her BP regularly. Both non-pharmacologic and pharmacologic interventions may prevent long-term complications of HTN. Some subjects with masked HTN may develop elevated or sustained HTN. Thus, the answer to your patient's question is D. Other options are incorrect.

Suggested Reading

Aronow WS. White coat hypertension. Ann Transl Med. 2017;5:456.

Franklin SS, O'Brien E, Staessen JA. Masked hypertension: understanding its complexity. Eur Heart J. 2017;38:1112–8.

Parati G, Ochoa JE. White-coat and masked hypertension. In: Bakris GL, Sorrentino MJ, editors. Hypertension. A companion to Braunwald's heart disease. 3rd ed. Philadelphia: Elsevier; 2018. p. 104–14.

4. **Which one of the following factors causes variability in BP measurement?**

A. Season
B. Time of the day
C. Eating
D. Smoking
E. All of the above

The answer is E

Many factors either in the clinic or home affect BP values. BP is high in cold season because of vasoconstriction and low in summer season because of vasodilation. The BP varies during the daytime and is usually high from

10 am to 6 pm compared to BP values at nighttime (low). Eating lowers BP because of splanchnic vasodilation, and this is particularly seen in the elderly. Smoking acutely elevates BP. Thus, option E is correct.

Suggested Reading

Bakris GL, Sorrentino MJ, editors. Hypertension. A companion to Braunwald's heart disease. 3rd ed. Philadelphia: Elsevier; 2018. p. 1–474.

Kaplan NM, Victor RG. Kaplan's clinical hypertension. 10th ed. Philadelphia: Wolters/Kluwer/Lippincott Williams & Wilkins; 2012. p. 1–469.

5. A 50-year-old woman is referred to you for evaluation of HTN, and you found that systolic BP in the right arm is 6 mm Hg higher than the left arm. Her BP is 142/89 mm Hg with a pulse rate of 72 beats/min. Femoral pulses are strong and present bilaterally. You repeated her BP 1 week later and found a similar difference in both arms. **With regard to her inter-arm difference in BP and its management, which one of the following choices is CORRECT?**

   A. Obtain a Doppler ultrasound of both arms
   B. Obtain a 24-h ambulatory BP monitoring (ABPM)
   C. Order further tests for evaluation of coarctation of aorta
   D. No further evaluation of inter-arm BP difference
   E. Start drug therapy for possible peripheral arterial disease (PVD)

   The answer is D

   It is not uncommon to see a small difference in both systolic and diastolic BPs between the right and left arm. This difference is more pronounced in patients with HTN. Usually, the BP in the right arm is slightly higher than the left arm. The difference in systolic BP between the arms is usually 10 mm Hg. Systolic BP difference >10 mm Hg suggests PVD and suggests a vascular assessment. In this patient, the inter-arm difference is only 6 mm Hg, and does not warrant further evaluation. Thus, choice D is correct. Starting antihypertensive therapy is premature. It is recommended that the arm with higher BP should be used for further BP measurements in the clinic, office, or home. Coarctation of the aorta is characterized by hypertension with weak or absent femoral pulses usually in a young patient. The above patient is a middle-aged individual with strong femoral pulses bilaterally. Thus, choice C is incorrect.

   Suggested Reading

Clark CE, Campbell JL, Evans PH, et al. Prevalence and clinical implications of the inter-arm blood pressure difference: a systematic review. J Human Hypertens. 2006;20:923–31.

Clark CE, Taylor RS, Shore AC, et al. Association of a difference in systolic blood pressure between arms with vascular disease and mortality: a systematic review and meta-analysis. Lancet. 2012;379:905–14.

6. A 72-year-old African American man with hypertension is referred to you because of dizziness despite a BP of 150/102 mm Hg. There are no sitting and standing BP changes, but a slight increase in pulse rate on standing is noticed. He is on long-acting diltiazem 180 mg daily, and not on any other medications. He has no retinopathy or proteinuria. CXR is normal. However, his brachial arteries feel hardened. **Which one of the following is the MOST likely cause of his dizziness?**

   A. Autonomic insufficiency
   B. Primary hypertension
   C. Pseudohypertension
   D. Change diltiazem to a diuretic
   E. None of the above

   The answer is C

   In elderly patients with documented high BP and without target organ damage, one needs to consider pseudohypertension as a cause of dizziness. Pseudohypertension occurs when a falsely elevated BP reading obtained with a BP cuff while an intra-arterial catheter shows a normal BP. This elevated cuff BP is due to thickened or calcified brachial arteries that are not easily compressible with the BP cuff. This phenomenon of pseudohypertension came from Osler's writing that he mistrusted the BP readings in patients with stiff arteries. The Osler's maneuver is elicited when the cuff is inflated above the systolic BP and the brachial or radial pulses, which should be

obliterated, are still palpable. When patients with pseudohypertension are treated with antihypertensive medication(s), they develop hypotensive symptoms despite high cuff BP. The above patient's dizziness is compatible with pseudohypertension. Thus, option C is correct. In autonomic insufficiency, the pulse does not increase on standing. Changing to a diuretic will not improve his symptoms. Thus, options A and D are incorrect

Suggested Reading

Spence JD. Pseudo-hypertension in the elderly: still hazy, after all these years. J Hum Hypertens. 1997;11:621–3.
Zweifler AJ, Sahab ST. Pseudohypertension. J Hypertens. 1993;11:1–6.

7. A 55-year-old man with type 2 diabetes and HTN is found to have nondipping of his BP during 11 pm to 4 am despite adequate BP control. **Which one of the following complications is associated with nondipping?**

A. Left ventricular hypertrophy (LVH)
B. Proteinuria
C. Progression of kidney disease
D. Mortality from cardiovascular disease (CVD)
E. All of the above

The answer is E

BP falls at night during sleep and also during inactivity. Although arbitrary, the nocturnal fall in both systolic and diastolic BP varies from 10% to 20%. This condition is called dipping. When nocturnal BP falls <10%, the condition is called nondipping. Studies have shown that nondipping is related to sympathetic overactivity. Nondipping is a risk factor for several conditions, including LVH, CVD, stroke, progression of proteinuria or albuminuria, and loss of kidney function. Therefore, option E is correct. Studies have suggested that inhibitors of renin-AII-aldosterone system may cause dipping in nondippers and improve the above associations of nondipping.

Suggested Reading

Birkenhãger AM, van den Meiracker AH. Causes and consequences of a non-dipping blood pressure profile. J Med. 2007;65:127–31.
Peixoto AJ, White WB. Circadian blood pressure: clinical implications based on the pathophysiology of its variability. Kidney Int. 2007;71:855–60.

8. Home BP monitoring (HBPM) by hypertensive patients is being encouraged by many primary care physicians. **Which one of the following advantages does HBPM have over office BP measurement?**

A. Elimination of white coat HTN
B. Increased number of BP readings
C. Improved adherence to antihypertensive treatment
D. Assess response to antihypertensive treatment
E. All of the above

The answer is E

HBPM is becoming popular than office BP measurement for all of the above-mentioned choices. In addition, HBPM is cost-effective (reduced cost). Several studies have reported lower BPs at home compared to either office or clinic BPs. One study reported average home BP of 123/78 mm Hg compared to office BP of 130/82 mm Hg. Thus, HBPM is better and lower than office or clinic BP recordings, making E as the correct choice.

Suggested Reading

Campbell PT, White WB. Home monitoring of blood pressure. In: Black HR, Elliott WJ, editors. Hypertension. A companion to Braunwald's heart disease. 2nd ed. Philadelphia: Elsevier/Saunders; 2013. p. 45–56.
Stergiou GS, Kollias A. Home monitoring of blood pressure. In: Bakris GL, Sorrentino MJ, editors. Hypertension. A companion to Braunwald's heart disease. 3rd ed. Philadelphia: Elsevier; 2018. p. 89–95.
Weiser B, Grune S, Burger R, et al. The Dubendorf study: a population-based investigation on normal values of blood pressure self-measurement. J Hum Hypertens. 1994;8:227–31.

9. **Ambulatory BP monitoring (ABPM) is important in which one of the following conditions?**

   A. Nocturnal BP readings
   B. Assessment of target organ damage
   C. Accuracy of BP recordings
   D. BP recordings during sleep
   E. All of the above

   The answer is E

   Accurate BP readings are necessary for diagnosis of HTN and for assessment of its therapy. In general, most of the patients have high office BP readings compared to either self-monitored (home) or 24-h BP readings. ABPM accomplishes all of the conditions mentioned from A to D. Recognition of dipping or nondipping and BP readings during sleep can be accurately obtained from ABPM. BP readings from ABPM can be used to assess the risk for target organ damage for appropriate antihypertensive therapy, and also for calculating pulse pressure. Thus, ABPM has several advantages over BP recordings taken in the office setting. Thus, option E is correct.

   Suggested Reading

Krakoff LR. Ambulatory blood pressure improves prediction of cardiovascular risk: implications for better antihypertensive management. Curr Atheroscl Rep. 2013;15:317.

O'Brien E. Ambulatory blood pressure measurement; the case for implementation in primary care. Hypertension. 2008;51:1435–41.

10. **Regarding ambulatory BP monitoring (ABPM) in chronic kidney disease (CKD) patients, which one of the following statements is CORRECT?**

   A. Nondipping is more prevalent in CKD patients than non-CKD or essential hypertensive patients
   B. The prevalence of nondipping increases with loss of kidney function
   C. Compared to non-CKD patients, CKD patients have higher nighttime SBP and lower daytime DBP with increased pulse pressure
   D. ABPM provides good assessment of CKD progression and cardiovascular (CV) risk
   E. All of the above

   The answer is E

   In normal subjects, the BP drops (dipping) by 10–20% during sleep period. This circadian rhythm is lost in CKD, resulting in higher prevalence of nondipping in CKD. A patient who shows high BP during sleep is referred to as riser. The prevalence of nondipping in CKD patients is much higher compared to non-CKD or essential hypertensive patients. Also, nondipping increases with increasing loss of kidney function (i.e., decreasing eGFR). ABPM has a good predictive value of both kidney and CV outcomes. The combination of both ABPM and eGFR has an additive effect in predicting kidney and CV outcomes. Thus, option E is correct

   Suggested Reading

Boggia J, Thijis L, Li Y, et al. International Database on Ambulatory blood pressure in relation to Cardiovascular Outcomes (DACO) Investigators: risk stratification by 24-hour ambulatory blood pressure and estimated glomerular filtration rate in 5322 subjects from 11 populations. Hypertension. 2013;61:18–26.

Cohen DL, Huan Y, Townsend RR. Ambulatory blood pressure in chronic kidney disease. Curr Hypertens Rep. 2013;15:160–6.

11. **Central aortic pressure (central BP) is found to be superior to brachial (peripheral) BP in which of the following conditions?**

   A. Central aortic pressure is the composite of SBP, DBP, and pulse wave velocity (PWV)
   B. Peripheral BP does not accurately reflect central aortic pressure
   C. Central aortic pressure is a better predictor of cardiovascular (CV) outcomes than peripheral BP
   D. CV outcomes differ between different classes of antihypertensive drugs despite similar reduction in peripheral BP
   E. All of the above

The answer is E

In the initial and routine follow-up of a patient, we measure peripheral BP using a sphygmomanometer or other automatic electron devices. Thus, SBP, DBP, and pulse pressure (pressure difference between SBP and DBP) can be obtained. However, the BP obtained by these devices does not match the central aortic pressure because central aortic pressure includes SBP, DBP, and PWV. Central aortic pressure can be measured by applanation (meaning "to flatten") tonometry (meaning "measuring of pressure"), using the radial artery rather than carotid artery for convenience and comfort of the patient (see Fig. 6.1**).**

PWV is a measure of aortic stiffness, and it can be measured between the carotid and femoral artery. Arterial stiffness causes faster PWV, whereas distensible arteries cause slow PWV. With each contraction of the left ventricle during systole, a pulse wave is generated which travels from the ascending aorta to the branching points of peripheral arteries. These peripheral arteries (arteries and arterioles) resist further propagation; therefore, the wave is reflected back to the heart. In normal arteries, the reflected wave merges with the forward traveling wave in diastole and augments coronary and cerebral perfusion. If arteries are stiff due to disease conditions such as atherosclerosis, the reflected wave returns faster and merges with the forward wave in systole. This adds more BP to the SBP, and this additional increase in SBP is called augmentation pressure (see Figure below). The net result is an increase in afterload and decreased perfusion of coronary and cerebral arteries. Another metric that has been shown to predict CV outcome is augmentation index, which is obtained by dividing augmentation pressure by central pulse pressure, and the ratio is expressed as percentage (augmentation pressure/pulse pressure × 100).

Central aortic pressure is more predictive of CV events than peripheral BP. An example of this is the CAFÉ (Conduit Artery Functional Evaluation) study, where hypertensive patients were given either atenolol or amlodipine. Central aortic pressure (applanation tonometry) and peripheral BP (electronic device) were measured. Average follow-up after first tonometry measurement was 3 years. The clinical endpoint was all CV events and development of renal impairment. Peripheral BP was similar in both groups; however, central BP was much lower with tonometry. The amlodipine group had lower central BP than atenolol group. The results showed a significant 16% reduction in the composite CV events in patients treated with amlodipine compared to atenolol group. This study shows that central aortic pressure measurements can reliably determine the clinical outcomes of antihypertensive therapies. Thus, option E is correct. Although central aortic pressure measurements are superior to peripheral BP measurements, applanation tonometry is expensive and may not be available in all clinic settings.

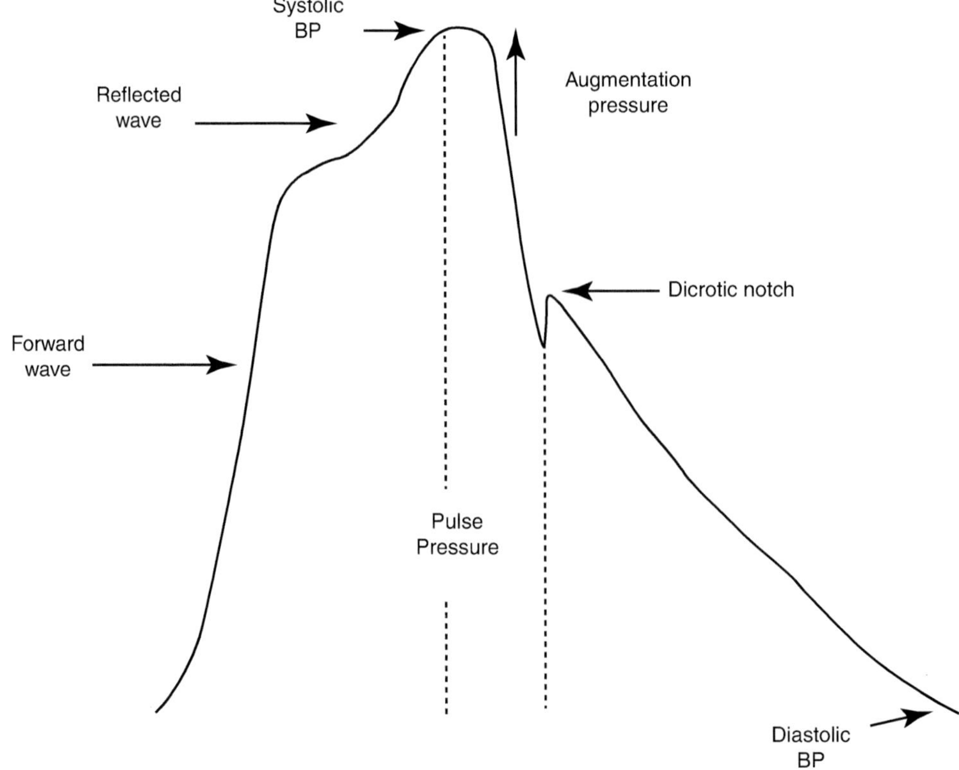

Fig. 6.1 Central aortic pressure waveform. Augmentation pressure is the pressure that is added to the forward wave by the reflected wave. Dicrotic notch represents closure of the aortic valve

Suggested Reading

Laurent S, Cockcroft J, Van Bortel L, et al. on behalf of the European Network for Non-invasive Investigation of Large Arteries. Expert consensus document on arterial stiffness: methodological issues and clinical implications. Eur Heart J. 2006;27:2588–605.

McEniery CM. Antihypertensive drugs and central blood pressure. Curr Hypertens Rep. 2009;11:253–9.

Nelson MR, Stepanek J, Cevette M, et al. Noninvasive measurement of central vascular pressures with arterial tonometry: clinical revival of the pulse pressure waveform? Mayo Clin Proc. 2010;85:460–72.

O'Rourke MF, Adji A. An updated clinical primer on large artery mechanics: implications of pulse waveform analysis and arterial tonometry. Curr opin Cardiol. 2005;20:275–81.

Williams B, Lacy PS, Thom SM, et al. Differential impact of blood pressure-lowering drugs on central aortic pressure and clinical outcomes: principal results of the Coduit Artery Function Evaluation (CAFÉ) study. Circulation. 2006;113:1213–25.

12. Aortic stiffness predicts the rate of kidney function loss, and pulse wave velocity (PWV) is one form of assessing aortic stiffness. **Which one of the following drugs does NOT improve aortic stiffness in CKD patients?**

A. Vasodilatory β-blockers
B. Angiotensin-converting enzyme-inhibitors (ACE-Is)
C. Angiotensin receptor blockers (ARBs)
D. Sevelamer carbonate
E. Statin

The answer is D

Except for sevelamer carbonate (option D), all other therapies have improved PWV and aortic stiffness in CKD and non-CKD patients.

Suggested Reading

Briet M, Boutouyrie P, Laurent S, et al. Arterial stiffness and pulse pressure in CKD and ESRD. Kidney Int. 2012; 82:388–400.

McEniery CM. Antihypertensive drugs and central blood pressure. Curr Hypertens Rep. 2009;11:253–9.

Zieman SJ, Melenovsky V, Kass DA. Mechanisms, pathophysiology, and therapy of arterial stiffness. Arterioscler Thromb Vasc Biol. 2005;25:932–43.

13. A 72-year-old man with a history of HTN and diabetes is brought to your office with complaints of dizziness, lightheadedness, reduced sweating, and occasional incontinence, particularly in morning hours. His wife, a former nurse, takes his BP twice a day. He is on hydrochlorothiazide (HCTZ) 12.5 mg per day. His morning BP on the day of his visit was 130/74 mm Hg with a heart rate of 68 beats/min (supine) and 100/64 mm Hg with a heart rate of 67 beats/min (standing). His labs: Na^+ 136 mEq/L, K^+ 3.6 mEq/L, HCO_3^- 28 mEq/L, creatinine 1.4 mg/dL, glucose 140 mg/dL, Ca^{2+} 10.2 mg/dL, and uric acid 8.4 mg/dL. **Based upon his BP, heart rate, and electrolyte pattern, which one of the following conditions is MOST likely in this patient?**

A. Diuretic (hypovolemia)-induced orthostatic hypotension
B. Orthostatic hypotension due to adrenal insufficiency
C. Neurogenic orthostatic hypotension
D. Electrolyte-induced hypotension
E. Age-related hypotension

The answer is C

The patient clearly demonstrates orthostatic hypotension, which is defined as a decrease in SBP of at least 20 mm Hg or DBP of 10 mm Hg within 3 min of standing. In patients with HTN, a decrease in SBP of 30 mm Hg is more appropriate to define orthostatic hypotension. Concomitant measurement of heart rate is extremely important, as orthostatic hypotension due to volume depletion, adrenal insufficiency, and certain medication will increase heart rate upon standing. On the other hand, neurogenic orthostatic hypotension caused by central or peripheral nervous system diseases that result in autonomic failure is not accompanied by a compensatory increase in heart rate. In this patient, the heart rate did not increase despite a fall in both SBP and DBP, suggesting the diagnosis

of neurogenic orthostatic hypotension. Thus, option C is correct. The patient's symptoms are due to his orthostatic hypotension. The electrolyte abnormalities are due to HCTZ and associated volume depletion. Adrenal insufficiency is unlikely in view of normal K^+, elevated HCO_3^-, and glucose levels.

Suggested Reading

Low PA, Singer W. Management of neurogenic orthostatic hypotension: an update. Lancet Neurol. 2008;7:451–8.

Shibao C, Lipsitz LA, Biaggioni I, et al. ASH position paper. Evaluation and treatment of orthostatic hypotension. J Am Soc Hypertens. 2013;7:317–24.

14. **Orthostatic hypotension in elderly subjects is predisposed to which one of the following conditions?**

A. Syncope and falls
B. Dementia
C. Coronary heart disease
D. Stroke
E. All of the above

The answer is E

Orthostatic hypotension, particularly in the elderly with or without HTN is associated with all of the above conditions, making E as the correct answer.

Suggested Reading

Benvenuto LJ, Krakoff LR. Morbidity and mortality of orthostatic hypotension: implications for management of cardiovascular disease. Am J Hypertens. 2011;24:135–44.

Luukinen H, Koski K, Laippala P, et al. Prognosis of diastolic and systolic hypotension in older persons. Arch Intern Med. 1999;159:273–80.

15. **Which one of the following therapeutic modalities is effective in patients with orthostatic hypotension?**

A. Adequate water and salt intake
B. Fludrocortisone
C. Midodrine
D. Pyridostigmine
E. All of the above

The answer is E

Both nonpharmacologic and pharmacologic therapies, in addition to treating the cause, have been tried to relieve symptoms of orthostatic hypotension. Nonpharmacologic interventions include fluid and salt intake to expand intravascular volume (at times 16 oz of water should be taken as a bolus), avoidance of drugs such as α1-blockers, diuretics and tricyclic antidepressants, avoidance of sudden rising and prolonged standing, use of abdominal binder or compressive waist-high stockings, and encouraging exercise such as swimming.

Pharmacologic interventions include fludrocortisones (increase volume), midodrine (α1-agonist, 5–10 mg once or twice daily), pyridostigmine (anticholine-esterase inhibitor, 30–60 mg once or twice daily), octreotide (splanchnic vasoconstrictor, 12.5–25 μg subcutaneously), and pseudoephedrine (30 mg daily) or a combination of fludrocortisone and midodrine, or midodrine, pseudoephedrine, and 16 oz of water. Thus, option E is correct.

Suggested Reading

Gupta V, Lipsitz LA. Orthostatic hypotension in the elderly: diagnosis and treatment. Am J Med. 2007;120:841–7.

Shibao C, Lipsitz LA, Biaggioni I, et al. ASH position paper. Evaluation and treatment of orthostatic hypotension. J Am Soc Hypertens. 2013;7:317–24.

16. **Which one of the following drugs does NOT cause neurogenic orthostatic hypotension?**

A. Diuretics
B. α1-blockers

C. Centrally acting drugs (clonidine)
D. Nitrates
E. Neuroleptics

The answer is C

Except for clonidine, all other drugs cause orthostatic hypotension. Clonidine reduces BP in patients with essential HTN; however, it "paradoxically" raises BP in autonomic failure or hypoadrenergic orthostatic hypotension. The mechanism seems to be arterial and/or venous constriction in patients with neurogenic orthostatic hypotension. Thus, option C is correct.

Suggested Reading

Robertson D, Goldberg MR, Hollister AS, et al. Clonidine raises blood pressure in severe idiopathic orthostatic hypotension. Am J Med. 1983;74:193–200.
Victor RG, Talman WT. Comparative effects of clonidine and dihydroergotamine on venomotor tone and orthostatic tolerance in patients with severe hypoadrenegic orthostatic hypotension. Am J Med. 2002;112:361–8.

17. A 32-year-old man is referred to you for evaluation of newly diagnosed HTN, and you made the diagnosis of essential (primary) HTN. **Which one of the following pathogenic mechanisms might be involved in the development of his HTN?**

A. Increased sympathetic activity
B. Increased renin-AII-aldosterone system (RAAS)
C. Salt sensitivity
D. Endothelial dysfunction
E. All of the above

The answer is E

The pathogenesis of essential HTN is complex and involves multiple mechanisms. Activation of sympathetic nervous system, RAAS, and increased salt intake has been involved in genesis and maintenance of HTN. Endothelial dysfunction resulting from decreased nitric oxide production and generation of endothelin may also contribute to the generation of HTN. Thus, E is correct.

In addition, hyperuricemia, metabolic syndrome, and low nephron number have been implicated. It appears that all of the mechanisms cause renal vasoconstriction and renal ischemia, finally resulting in decreased GFR and Na⁺ retention. The following figure (see Fig. 6.2**) summarizes these mechanisms.**

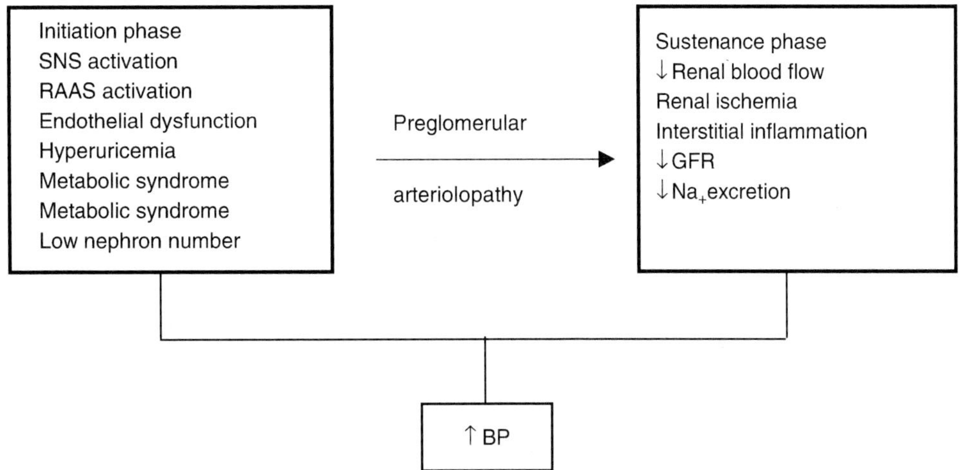

Fig. 6.2 Mechanisms that initiate and sustain blood pressure (BP) in essential hypertension. SNS = sympathetic nervous system' RAAS = renin-angiotensin-aldosterone system, GFR = glomerular filtration rate, ↓ decrease, ↑ increase

Suggested Reading

Acelajado MC, Calhoun DA, Oparil S. Pathogenesis of hypertension. In: Black HR, Elliott WJ, editors. Hypertension. A companion to Braunwald's heart disease. 2nd ed. Philadelphia: Elsevier/Saunders; 2013. p. 12–26.

Bolívar JJ. Essential hypertension: an approach to its etiology and neurogenic pathophysiology. Int J Hypertens. 2013;2013:Article ID:547809, 11 pages.

18. A 52-year-old African American woman is seen in your office for the first time for evaluation of a BP of 150/89 mm Hg with a heart rate of 64 beats per min (BPM). Phys exam is unremarkable, and serum chemistry is normal. You take a dietary history and she denies high salt intake. You order a 24-h urine Na^+ and creatinine, and the urine Na^+ is found to be 140 mEq. **According to the DASH (Dietary Approaches to Stop Hypertension), which one of the following dietary Na^+ intake you recommend, in addition to DASH combination diet (diet rich in fruits, vegetable, and low-fat dairy foods with reduced saturated fat and cholesterol) to achieve good BP control in this patient?**

A. 4000 mg
B. 3500 mg
C. 3000 mg
D. 2000 mg
E. 1500 mg

The answer is E

The DASH sodium trial tested the effects of three different Na^+ intakes separately in two diets: the DASH diet and a typical American (control) diet. From 24-h urinary Na^+ determination, the three Na^+ levels were termed low (1500 mg or 65 mEq), intermediate (2500 mg or 107 mEq), and high (3300 mg or 142 mEq). The subjects with the lowest intake of Na^+ (1500 mg/day) had the lowest BP, as compared with other Na^+ intakes. The reduction in BP occurred in both hypertensive and nonhypertensive participants. The combination of DASH diet and low Na^+ intake was more effective in lowering BP than either intervention alone. In addition to DASH study, several other studies have documented that low dietary Na^+ intake improves BP. Thus, E is correct.

Suggested Reading

Appel LJ. Diet and blood pressure. In: Black HR, Elliott WJ, editors. Hypertension. A companion to Braunwald's heart disease. 2nd ed. Philadelphia: Elsevier/Saunders; 2013. p. 151–9.

Sacks FM, Svetkey LP, Vollmer WM, et al. for the DASH-Sodium Collaborative Research Group. Effects on blood pressure of reduced dietary sodium and the dietary approaches to stop hypertension (DASH) diet. N Engl J Med. 2001;344:3–10.

19. A 50-year-old African American woman with HTN and normal kidney function follows DASH combination diet with 1500 mg Na^+ without any antihypertensive medications. **Which one of the following statements is TRUE regarding BP reduction in this woman?**

A. Her BP may not improve unless a thiazide-type diuretic is added
B. Her BP management requires a further decrease in Na^+ restriction
C. With the above diet, her BP may increase by 12/4 mm Hg
D. With the above diet, her BP may decrease by 13.2/6.1 mm Hg
E. With the above diet, the BP reduction is more in Whites than African Americans

The answer is D

The subgroup analysis of the participants from the DASH studies showed that African Americans with untreated HTN had more BP reduction than Whites (E incorrect). In hypertensive African Americans, the BP reduction was 13.2/6.1 mm Hg compared to a reduction of 6.3/4.4 mm Hg in hypertensive Whites. Among normotensive African Americans, the DASH combination diet reduced BP by 4.3/2.6 mm Hg compared to 2.0/1.2 mm Hg reduction in normotensive white participants. Thus, D is the true statement, and other statements are false. The reduction in BP in hypertensive African Americans is comparable to BP reduction in a patient on one antihypertensive drug, as shown in the following Table 6.2.

Table 6.2 BP reduction by the DASH combination diet, vegetarian diet, and other antihypertensive drugs

Treatment	BP reduction (mm Hg)
Thiazide diuretic (Hydrochlorothiazide)	11/5
β-blocker (Atenolol)	8/7
ACE-I (Captopril)	6/5
Calcium antagonist (Diltiazem)	10/9
Vegetarian diet	3–14/5–6
DASH +1500 mg sodium diet	11/6

Suggested Reading

Karanja N, Erlinger TP, Pao-Hwa L, et al. The DASH diet for high blood pressure: from clinical trial to dinner table. Clev Clin J Med. 2004;71:745–53.

Sacks FM, Svetkey LP, Vollmer WM, et al. for the DASH-Sodium Collaborative Research Group. Effects on blood pressure of reduced dietary sodium and the dietary approaches to stop hypertension (DASH) diet. N Engl J Med. 2001;344:3–10.

Svetkey LP, Simons-Mortton D, Vollmer WM, et al. for the DASH Research Group. Effects of dietary patterns on blood pressure. Subgroup analysis of the Dietary Approaches to Stop Hypertension (DASH) Randomized Clinical Trial. Arch Intern Med. 1999;159:285–93.

20. **Vegetarian diet has been shown to lower BP by which one of the following mechanisms?**

A. Weight loss
B. Increased K^+ intake
C. Lower total fat and saturated fat
D. Higher fiber intake
E. All of the above

The answer is E

A few randomized, controlled studies have shown that patients on vegetarian diets had a lower SBP (5–9 mm Hg lower) and a lower DBP (3 mm Hg lower) compared to control subjects. In one study with hypertensive patients aged 40–69 years, vegan diet for a year lowered SBP by 9 mm Hg and DBP by 5 mm Hg. Other studies have shown a BP decrease of 3–14/5–6 mm Hg. A recent meta-analysis confirmed that vegetarian diet lowers both SBP and DBP. The mechanisms by which vegetarian diet lowers BP are not fully understood; however, weight loss, high K^+, and fiber content with low total fat and low saturated fat may be responsible for lowering BP in both normotensive and hypertensive subjects.

Suggested Reading

Berkow SE, Barnard ND. Blood pressure regulation and vegetarian diets. Nutr Rev. 2005;63:1–8.

Yokoyama Y, Nishimura K, Barnard ND, et al. Vegetarian diets and blood pressure. A meta-analysis. JAMA Intern Med. 2014;174:577–87.

21. Most of the studies on Na^+ restriction and BP reduction pertain to patients with normal kidney function with normal or high BP. **A recent study in CKD 3–4 patients showed that Na^+ restriction is NOT beneficial in improving which one of the following risk factors for cardiovascular disease (CVD)?**

A. 24-h ambulatory BP
B. Proteinuria
C. Extracellular fluid (ECF) volume
D. Albuminuria
E. Pulse wave velocity (PWV)

The answer is E

Studies of Na^+ restriction on BP and other risk factors of CVD are limited in patients with CKD 3–4 and hypertension. A study by McMahon et al. showed in a double-blind, placebo-controlled, randomized, cross-over trial that CKD 3–4 patients on low Na^+ diet (mean Na^+ excretion 75 mEq with a range from 58 to 112 mEq) significantly improved BP, proteinuria, albuminuria, and ECF volume compared to high salt intake (mean Na^+ excretion 168 mEq with a range from 146 to 219 mEq). However, no effect of low salt diet was observed on PWV (option E). Although the number of patients in this study ($n = 20$) is limited, the results are extremely important that low Na^+ intake is beneficial in improving risk factors for CV and kidney disease.

Suggested Reading

McMahon EJ, Bauer JD, Hawley CM, et al. A randomized trial of dietary sodium restriction in CKD. J Am Soc Nephrol. 2013;24:2096–103.
Thijssen S, Kitzer TM, Levin NW. Salt: its role in chronic kidney disease. J Ren Nutr. 2008;18:18–26.

22. **Match the following associations between environmental exposure/agents and BP:**

Environmental exposure/agent	Influence on BP
A. Winter	1. Increase
B. Summer	2. Decrease
C. Low Vitamin D	3. No change
D. Air pollution	
E. Plant protein	
F. High K^+	
G. Alcohol >2 drinks	

Answers: A = 1; B = 2; C = 1; D = 1; E = 2; F = 2; G = 1

Temperature plays an important role in BP regulation. Many studies have recorded higher BPs during winter and lower BPs during summer seasons. These changes seem to be associated with vasoconstriction due to increased sympathetic tone during wintertime, and vasodilation probably due to increased nitric oxide production during summertime.

A few prospective cohort studies have shown that low blood levels of 25-hydroxyvitamin D are independently associated with an increased risk of HTN. Also, one study found that normotensive people who took vitamin D were less likely to develop HTN 2 decades later. Thus, low vitamin D levels were found to be associated with the development of HTN.

Air pollution is an important risk factor for the development of at least acute HTN. This has been shown in normotensive subjects, who developed acute HTN upon short-term exposure to air pollution. It seem that the particulate matter that enters the lungs can increase sympathetic tone, causing acute elevation in BP. When this particulate matter enters the systemic circulation, it increases oxidative stress and vascular inflammation.

Proteins, particularly from plant origin, have been associated with low BP. Also, supplementation of soy protein seems to lower BP in humans.

Diets rich in K^+ are found to lower BP, and BP reduction is more in African Americans compared to Whites. High K^+ causes vasodilation, thereby reducing BP.

A dose-response relationship between alcohol intake and BP showed that alcohol intake >2 drinks raises BP (1 drink is defined as 1.5 oz of 80% proof spirits, 12 oz of regular beer, and 5 oz of wine containing 12% alcohol). Binge drinkers develop severe HTN. HTN due to alcohol is related to overactivity of sympathetic nervous system. Chronic alcoholism leads to persistent HTN.

Suggested Reading

Appel LJ. Diet and blood pressure. In: Black HR, Elliott WJ, editors. Hypertension. A companion to Braunwald's heart disease. 2nd ed. Philadelphia: Elsevier/Saunders; 2013. p. 151–9.
Fares A. Winter hypertension: potential mechanisms. Internat J Health Sci. 2013;7:210–9.

23. **A scientist friend of yours asks you about garlic and BP. Regarding garlic and BP, which one of the following statements is TRUE?**

    A. Generation of hydrogen sulfide from garlic lowers BP
    B. Generation of nitric oxide from garlic lowers BP
    C. Garlic decreases oxidative stress
    D. Garlic decreases lipid peroxidation
    E. All of the above

    The answer is E

    Intake of fresh garlic or garlic powder has been shown to lower BP, improve hyperlipidemia, prevent cold and bacterial infections, and improve claudication. Garlic seems to generate hydrogen peroxide, which lowers BP by activating ATP-gated K^+ channels in vascular smooth muscle cells. Also, garlic generates nitric oxide, causing vasodilation and a decrease in BP. Garlic prevents oxidative stress and lipid peroxidation. Thus, garlic lowers BP by multiple mechanisms (E is correct).

    Suggested Reading

Gupta YK, Dahiya AK, Reeta KH. Gaso-transmitter hydrogen sulfide: potential new target in pharmacotherapy. Indian J Exp Biol. 2010;48:1069–77.

Khatua TN, Adela R, Banerjee SK. Garlic and cardioprotection: insights into the molecular mechanisms. Can J Physiol Pharmacol. 2013;91:448–58.

24. **Fructose intake in the form of sweetened beverage has been shown to raise BP by which one of the following mechanisms?**

    A. Increase in Na^+ absorption by the gut
    B. Increase in oxidative stress
    C. Increase in uric acid production
    D. Endothelial dysfunction
    E. All of the above

    The answer is E

    A close association between fructose-containing beverages and an incidental and chronic HTN has been repeatedly reported. All of the above mechanisms seem to participate in elevating BP. Na^+ absorption in the gut is due to increased Na/H exchanger and Cl/base exchanger of the apical membrane. Fructose causes preglomerular arteriolopathy, cortical vasoconstriction, and glomerular HTN, which subsequently maintain chronic HTN. During the process of fructose metabolism, ATP is consumed to generate AMP, which is converted to uric acid. In addition, fructose causes endothelial dysfunction, resulting in high BP. Thus, option E is correct.

    Suggested Reading

Brown IJ, Stampler J, van Horn L, et al. Sugar sweetened beverage, sugar intake of individuals, and their blood pressure: international study of micro/macronutrients and blood pressure. Hypertension. 2011;57:695–701.

Cohen L, Curhan G, Forman J. Association of sweetened beverage intake with accidental hypertension. J Gen Intern Med. 2012;27:1127–34.

Madero M, Perez-Pozo SE, Jalal D, et al. Dietary fructose and hypertension. Curr Hypertens Rep. 2011;13:29–35.

25. A 66-year-old African American man is referred to you for the management of HTN. Despite dietary Na^+ restriction (2 g Na^+ diet or 88 mEq) and chlorthalidone (25 mg), his BP is not well controlled. He has a strong family history of stroke. His glucose and creatinine are normal. The patient is concerned about future stroke, if his BP is not controlled. **In view of the above information, which one of the following drugs reduces stroke risk in this patient?**

    A. Angiotensin-converting enzyme-inhibitor (ACE-I)
    B. Angiotensin receptor blocker
    C. Calcium channel blocker (CCB)
    D. β-blocker
    E. Central agonist

The answer is C

Studies have shown that CCBs are better than ACE-Is for stroke outcomes in African Americans. However, ACE-Is are better than CCBs for heart failure outcomes. In both African Americans and non-African Americans, ACE-Is and CCBs are similar with respect to overall mortality and renal outcomes.

Suggested Reading

James PA, Oparil S, Canter BL, et al. 2014 Evidence-based guideline for the management of high blood pressure in adults. Report from the panel members appointed to the Eighth Joint National Committee (JNC 8). JAMA. 2014;311:507–20.

The ALLHAT Officers and Coordinators for the ALLHAT Collaborative Research Group. Major outcomes in high-risk hypertensive patients randomized to angiotensin-converting enzyme inhibitor or calcium channel blocker vs diuretic. The Antihypertensive and Lipid-Lowering Treatment to Prevent Heart Attack Trial (ALLHAT). JAMA. 2002;288:2981–97.

26. A 72-year-old man with BP of 168/94 mm Hg is treated with chlorthalidone (25 mg daily). **Lowering his BP to <150/90 mm Hg by addition of amlodipine reduces which one of the following cardiac- and cerebrovascular outcomes?**

A. Heart failure
B. Fatal stroke
C. Overall mortality
D. Coronary heart disease (CHD)
E. All of the above

The answer is E

Initiating pharmacologic therapy with antihypertensive agents to a goal BP < 150/90 mm Hg in persons 60 years or older with a SBP ≥ 160 mm Hg has been shown to reduce cerebrovascular morbidity and mortality (fatal stroke, nonfatal stroke, or both), fatal and nonfatal heart failure, overall mortality, and CHD (CHD mortality, fatal MI, nonfatal MI). Thus, E is correct.

Suggested Reading

James PA, Oparil S, Canter BL, et al. 2014 Evidence-based guideline for the management of high blood pressure in adults. Report from the panel members appointed to the Eighth Joint National Committee (JNC 8). JAMA. 2014;311(suppl):75–7.

27. **Initiating pharmacologic treatment in a 42 year-old woman with DBP of 96 mm Hg would likely reduce which one of the following cardiac- and cerebrovascular outcomes?**

A. Cerebrovascular morbidity and mortality
B. Heart failure
C. Fatal MI
D. Mortality from CHD
E. A and B

The answer is E

According to JNC 8 guideline, there is moderate to high evidence that treating DBP ≥ 90 mm Hg in adults 30 years of age or older reduces cerebrovascular morbidity and mortality (fatal stroke, nonfatal stroke, or both), and heart failure. However, there is insufficient evidence for fatal MI and mortality from CHD. Thus, E is correct.

Suggested Reading

James PA, Oparil S, Canter BL, et al. 2014 Evidence-based guideline for the management of high blood pressure in adults. Report from the panel members appointed to the Eighth Joint National Committee (JNC 8). JAMA. 2014;311(suppl):79–81.

28. **Match the following characteristics of hypertensive patients with the goal BPs, as suggested by JNC 8 (select the same BP, if applicable).**

Characteristics	Goal BP (mm Hg)
A. 60 years or older	1. <130/80
B. 18–60 years	2. <150/90
C. CKD	3. <140/80
D. Diabetes	4. <140/90

Answers: A = 2; B = 4; C = 4; D = 4

According to JNC 8 guideline, the goal BP in patients ≥60 years is <150/90 mm Hg, whereas in patients <60 years of age, it is <140/90 mm Hg. In patients with CKD and diabetes, the goal BP is <140/90 mm Hg. Other guidelines by KDIGO (Kidney Disease Improving Global Outcome, 1212) and ISHIB (International Society for Hypertension in Blacks, 2010), the goal BP in CKD patients with proteinuria and in African Americans with target organ damage is 130/80 mm Hg. The American Diabetes Association (2013) recommends a goal BP < 140/80 mm Hg for diabetic patients.

Suggested Reading

James PA, Oparil S, Canter BL, et al. 2014 Evidence-based guideline for the management of high blood pressure in adults. Report from the panel members appointed to the Eighth Joint National Committee (JNC 8). JAMA. 2014;311:507–20.

29. You are consulted on a 28-year-old man with IgA nephropathy and proteinuria of 1.2 g/day. His BP is 134/84 mm Hg with a heart rate of 70 BPM. His creatinine is 1.0 mg/dL. He has no insurance. **Which one of the following medications you recommend to improve his proteinuria?**

A. Amlodipine
B. Chlorthalidone
C. Lisinopril
D. Prednisone
E. Atenolol

The answer is C

The JNC 8 and other position statements recommend either an ACE-I or an ARB for patients with CKD and proteinuria as the drug of choice. Lisinopril costs less compared to other ACE-Is. Thus, C is correct. Amlodipine, chlorthalidone, and atenolol can be added, as needed, to control HTN. Prednisone is not indicated in this patient, as ACE-Is or ARBS can improve proteinuria and also BP.

Suggested Reading

James PA, Oparil S, Canter BL, et al. 2014 Evidence-based guideline for the management of high blood pressure in adults. Report from the panel members appointed to the Eighth Joint National Committee (JNC 8). JAMA. 2014;311:507–20.

30. You see this patient in your office 4 weeks later. Repeat labs show no change other than an increase in serum creatinine from 1.0 mg/dL to 1.2 mg/dL. His proteinuria decreased from 1.2 g to 0.9 g/day. He is euvolemic. **What is your next step in the management of this patient?**

A. Discontinue lisinopril and start losartan
B. Discontinue lisinopril and start chlorthalidone
C. Continue lisinopril and follow creatinine and other labs in 2–4 weeks
D. Discontinue lisinopril and start amlodipine
E. Add metoprolol to lisinopril

The answer is C

The patient is responding to lisinopril by improving his proteinuria. An increase in creatinine up to 30% in response to ACE-Is or ARBs is common, indicating a decrease in glomerular HTN and glomerular filtration. This is a reversible physiologic response and is not harmful. ACE-Is and ARBs also increase serum [K^+]. The best thing to do is to continue lisinopril and follow serum chemistry and proteinuria. Thus, C is correct. Other options are not appropriate for this patient at this time.

Suggested Reading

Bakris GL, Weir MR. Angiotensin-converting enzyme inhibitor-associated elevations in serum creatinine: is this a cause for concern? Arch Intern Med. 2000;160:685–93.

Hirsch S, Hirsch J, Bhatt U, et al. Tolerating increases in the serum creatinine following aggressive treatment of chronic kidney disease, hypertension and proteinuria: pre-renal success. Am J Nephrol. 2012;36:430–7.

31. A 55-year-old African American nondiabetic man is referred to you for further management of HTN. Office BP is 150/91 mm Hg with a heart rate of 70 BPM. He is on lisinopril 40 mg daily because of a strong family history of kidney disease. **Based on ALLHAT (The Antihypertensive and Lipid Lowering to prevent Heart Attack Trial), clorthalidone is more effective than lisinopril in which one of the following cardiovascular (CV) outcomes?**

A. Stroke
B. Congestive heart failure (CHF)
C. Combined CV outcomes
D. All of the above
E. No difference in outcomes between the drugs

The answer is D

The ALLHAT is the largest HTN study that was conducted in the United States, and 35% of the participants were African Americans. In the final analysis, 33,357 high-risk patients with stage 1–2 HTN aged 55 years and older and another CV risk factor was randomized to either chlorthalidone (12.5–25 mg daily), amlodipine (2.5–10 mg daily), or lisinopril (10–40 mg daily). The goal BP was <140/90 mm Hg, and the mean duration of follow-up was 4.9 years.

In African Americans, chlorthalidone was more effective in improving stroke, CHF, and combined CV outcomes, as compared with lisinopril. Therefore, a thiazide-type diuretic is recommended as the initial drug of choice in African Americans, whether they are diabetic or nondiabetic. Thus, D is correct.

Suggested Reading

James PA, Oparil S, Canter BL, et al. 2014 Evidence-based guideline for the management of high blood pressure in adults. Report from the panel members appointed to the Eighth Joint National Committee (JNC 8). JAMA. 2014;311:507–20.

The ALLHAT Officers and Coordinators for the ALLHAT Collaborative Research Group. Major outcomes in high-risk hypertensive patients randomized to angiotensin-converting enzyme inhibitor or calcium channel blocker vs diuretic. The Antihypertensive and Lipid-Lowering Treatment to Prevent Heart Attack Trial (ALLHAT). JAMA. 2002;288:2981–97.

32. The above patient refuses to change the lisinopril to chlorthalidone because he read the adverse effects of diuretics in the Internet. **Which one of the following is the appropriate next drug for this patient?**

A. Metoprolol
B. Hydralazine and metoprolol
C. Amlodipine
D. Losartan
E. Spironolactone

The answer is C

The ALLHAT also compared the health outcomes between chlorthalidone and amlodipine in African American patients. Although amlodipine was less effective than chlorthalidone in preventing CHF, there were no differences in stroke, coronary artery disease, combined CV and kidney outcomes, and overall mortality between the two

drugs. Therefore, choosing amlodipine in this patient is appropriate (choice C). Other drugs can be added, if goal BP is not achieved.

Suggested Reading

James PA, Oparil S, Canter BL, et al. 2014 Evidence-based guideline for the management of high blood pressure in adults. Report from the panel members appointed to the Eighth Joint National Committee (JNC 8). JAMA. 2014;311:507–20.

The ALLHAT Officers and Coordinators for the ALLHAT Collaborative Research Group. Major outcomes in high-risk hypertensive patients randomized to angiotensin-converting enzyme inhibitor or calcium channel blocker vs diuretic. The Antihypertensive and Lipid-Lowering Treatment to Prevent Heart Attack Trial (ALLHAT). JAMA. 2002;288:2981–97.

33. A 74-year-old man is on HCTZ 25 mg daily for his HTN for the last 5 years. His BP is 134/78 mm Hg. He denies dizziness, weakness, chest pain, or sweating. He walks 2 miles a day without any difficulty. **According to JNC 8 guideline, the goal BP in patients ≥60 years is <150/90 mm Hg. Based on JNC 8 guideline, which one of the following steps is appropriate in this patient?**

    A. Decrease the dose of HCTZ to 12.5 mg/day
    B. Increase dietary Na^+ intake to achieve SBP >140 mm Hg
    C. No change in BP medication is needed, as he is asymptomatic
    D. Add midodrine 5–10 mg/day to achieve SBP >140 mm Hg
    E. None of the above

    The answer is C

    According to the JNC 7 recommendation, the goal SBP in elderly patients is <140 mm Hg. Based on these recommendations, many of these elderly patients have SBPs lower than 140 mm Hg Yet these patients are asymptomatic. The JNC 8 developed a corollary recommendation for such asymptomatic patients with SBP < 140 mm Hg, which suggests that "it is not necessary to adjust medication to allow BP to increase." The patient is asymptomatic, and no change in BP medication (HCTZ) is needed, making C as the correct choice. It should be remembered that the JNC 8 recommends the goal BP in elderly patients to be <150/90 mm Hg, as studies have shown no benefit for a SBP < 140 mm Hg.

Suggested Reading

James PA, Oparil S, Canter BL, et al. 2014 Evidence-based guideline for the management of high blood pressure in adults. Report from the panel members appointed to the Eighth Joint National Committee (JNC 8). JAMA. 2014;311:507–20.

34. A 50-year-old man with type 2 diabetes, HTN, and coronary artery disease is referred to you for the management of HTN and proteinuria of 1.2 g/day. His BP is 148/90 mm Hg. **Adding aliskiren (renin inhibitor) is expected to cause which one of the following effects in this patient?**

    A. No effect on proteinuria
    B. Increases the risk for stroke
    C. Increases the risk for myocardial infarction (MI)
    D. Decreases the need for renal replacement therapy (RRT)
    E. Decreases death from CV and renal causes

    The answer is B

    Aliskiren is a renin inhibitor, which inhibits renin activity. In clinical studies, aliskiren lowers not only BP but also albuminuria in type 2 diabetic patients. It also improves left ventricular hypertrophy. ACE-Is and ARBS have similar effects. Therefore, the combination of aliskiren and an ACE-I or ARB should have an additive effect on CV and kidney outcomes. In a study using this combination, an increased risk for stroke (hazard ratio: 1.34; 95% CI 1.01–1.77) was observed, as compared with placebo. Because of increased stroke from the combination of aliskiren and an ACE-I or ARB, the study was prematurely terminated. Thus, choice B is correct.

    However, the study showed a decrease in proteinuria, but no change in MI, CHF, overall death, and the need for RRT.

Suggested Reading

Parving H-H, Persson F, Lewis JB, et al. for the AVOID Study Investigators. Aliskiren combined with losartan in type 2 diabetes and nephropathy. N Engl J Med. 2008;358:2433–46.

Parving H-H, Brenner BM, McMurray JJV, et al. For the ALTITUDE Investigators. Cardiorenal end points in a trial of aliskiren for type 2 diabetes. N Engl J Med. 2012;367:2204–13.

35. A 38-year-old African American woman with type 2 diabetes and HTN is brought to you by the family for the management of HTN. Her BP is 144/84 mm Hg with a heart rate of 70 BPM. Her kidney function is normal, and proteinuria is 100 mg/day. **Which one of the following antihypertensive drugs is recommended by the panel of JNC 8 as the initial drug of choice?**

A. Lisinopril
B. Clonidine
C. Chlorthalidone
D. Metaprolol
E. Hydralazine and nitrate

The answer is C

The following recommendation was made by the panel of JNC 8 for an African American with or without diabetes "In the general black population, including those with diabetes, initial antihypertensive treatment should include a thiazide-type diuretic or CCB." Thus, C is correct. This recommendation is based on the ALLHAT.

Suggested Reading

James PA, Oparil S, Canter BL, et al. 2014 Evidence-based guideline for the management of high blood pressure in adults. Report from the panel members appointed to the Eighth Joint National Committee (JNC 8). JAMA. 2014;311:507–20.

The ALLHAT Officers and Coordinators for the ALLHAT Collaborative Research Group. Major outcomes in high-risk hypertensive patients randomized to angiotensin-converting enzyme inhibitor or calcium channel blocker vs diuretic. The Antihypertensive and Lipid-Lowering Treatment to Prevent Heart Attack Trial (ALLHAT). JAMA. 2002;288:2981–97.

36. A 32-year-old African American man with CKD 3 due to HTN is seen for the first time in your office. His BP is 150/90 mm Hg with a heart rate of 72 BPM. **Which one of the following antihypertensive drugs you prescribe to this patient?**

A. A calcium channel blocker
B. An angiotensin converting enzyme-inhibitor (ACE-I)
C. A combination of ACE-I and ARB (angiotensin receptor blocker)
D. A combination of aliskiren and ARB
E. A Thiazide-type diuretic

The answer is B

Based on several studies, the JNC 8 panel recommends "In the population aged 18 years or older with CKD and hypertension, initial (or add-on) antihypertensive treatment should include an ACEI or ARB to improve kidney outcomes. This applies to all CKD patients with hypertension regardless of race or diabetes status." Thus, B is correct. It should be noted that the AASK (African American Study of Kidney Disease) trial reported beneficial effect of an ACE-I (ramipril) on kidney outcomes in African American subjects.

The AASK is a randomized, double-blind, controlled trial that randomized 1094 nondiabetic hypertensive African Americans with an eGFR between 20 and 65 mL/min, aged 18–70 years, to either amlodipine, ramipril, or metoprolol. The target mean arterial BP goals were ≤92 mm Hg or ≤102 mm Hg. Other drugs were added to achieve BP goals. The mean follow-up period was 4 years. Amlodipine arm was discontinued because ramipril had greater renoprotective effects because ramipril reduced clinical outcomes by 46%, as compared with amlodipine. Also, ramipril prevented decline in kidney function much more than metoprolol. Thus, the AASK trial provided strong evidence in support of an ACE-I for African Americans with CKD.

Suggested Reading

James PA, Oparil S, Canter BL, et al. 2014 Evidence-based guideline for the management of high blood pressure in adults. Report from the panel members appointed to the Eighth Joint National Committee (JNC 8) JAMA. 2014;311:507–20.

Wright JT Jr., Bakris G, Greene T, et al. African American Study of Kidney Disease and Hypertension Study Group. Effect of blood pressure lowering and antihypertensive drug class on progression of hypertensive kidney disease: results from the AASK trial. JAMA. 2002;288:2421–31.

37. You are asked to see a patient with an eGFR of 26 mL/min and 1+ pitting edema. Office BP is 148/92 mm Hg with a heart rate of 68 BPM. He is on HCTZ 50 mg daily, metoprolol 100 mg twice daily, and lisinopril 40 mg daily. **Which one of the following medication changes is considered appropriate for this patient?**

   A. Increase HCTZ to 100 mg daily
   B. Change lisinopril to losartan
   C. Discontinue HCTZ and start furosemide 40–80 mg daily
   D. Add spironolactone 25 mg daily
   E. No change at this time

The answer is C

The effectiveness of any diuretic is reduced in patients with CKD 3–5. Two factors control the effectiveness of thiazide diuretics. First, the filtered load of Na^+ is reduced with reduction in GFR. Second, the natriuretic response to thiazide diuretics, particularly, HCTZ, is blunted in the distal tubule. A similar blunted response occurs in proteinuric patients because HCTZ, or loop diuretics such as furosemide binds to the filtered protein, and its free drug delivery to the thick ascending limb of Henle's loop is decreased. A higher dose of furosemide is required to improve edema in patients with high proteinuria.

The patient described in the question has CKD 4. Increasing HCTZ to 100 mg may induce diuresis at the expense of severe metabolic adverse effects. Switching lisinopril to losartan may not alter the course of kidney disease or edema. Adding spironolactone may lower BP, but does not improve edema. Discontinuation of HCTZ and starting furosemide seem appropriate for this patient. Thus, C is correct.

Suggested Reading

Ellison DH, Hoorn EJ, Wilcox CS. Diuretics. In: Taal MW, Chertow GM, Marsden PA, et al., editors. Brenner & Rector's the kidney. 9th ed. Philadelphia: Elsevier Saunders; 2012. p. 1879–916.

Sica DA, Gehr TWB. Diuretic use in stage 5 chronic kidney disease (CKD) and end-stage renal disease. Curr Opin Nephrol Hypertens. 2003;2:483–90.

38. A 58-year-old nonobese man is referred to you for the management of HTN and kidney disease with an eGFR of 64 mL/min. He has a strong family history of cardiovascular disease (CVD). He is on benazepril 20 mg daily. His BP is 148/90 mm Hg. His repeat creatinine is 1.1 mg/dL with an eGFR of 62 mL/min. **In order to preserve kidney function, which one of the following add-on drugs has been shown to have a favorable effect on kidney function?**

   A. Atenolol
   B. HCTZ
   C. Amlodipine
   D. Hydralazine
   E. Losartan

The answer is C

In a randomized, double-blind trial, the investigators of the ACOMPLISH (Avoiding Cardiovascular Events through Combination Therapy in Patients Living with Systolic Hypertension) trial assigned 11,506 high-risk hypertensive patients to either benazepril and amlodipine or benazepril and HCTZ, and both CV and kidney outcomes were evaluated. As far as the renal outcomes (doubling of serum creatinine or end stage kidney disease, or need for dialysis) are concerned, the study was terminated early (mean follow-up 2.9 years) because of superior efficacy of the combination of benazepril and amlodipine, as compared with benazepril and HCTZ. In the

combination of benazepril and amlodipine, there were 2% CKD progression, as compared with 3.7% progression in the benazepril and HCTZ combination. However, peripheral edema was more in the former drug combination than the latter combination.

Based on the ACCOMPLISH results, adding amlodipine to the patient may cause less progression of his kidney disease. Therefore, C is correct. Also, the combination of benazepril and amlodipine was superior to the combination of benazepril and HCTZ in reducing the CV events in high-risk hypertensive patients.

Suggested Reading

Bakris GL, Sarafidis PA, Weir MR, et al. for the ACCOMPLISH trial investigators. Renal outcomes with different fixed-dose combination therapies in patients with hypertension at high risk for cardiovascular events (ACCOMPLISH): a prespecified secondary analysis of a randomized controlled trial. Lancet. 2010;375:1173–81.

Jamerson K, Weber MA, Bakris GL, et al. For the ACCOMPLISH trial investigators. Benazepril plus amlodipine or hydrochlorothiazide for hypertension in high-risk patients. N Engl J Med. 2008;359:2417–28.

39. You started a 32-year-old woman on HCTZ 12.5 mg daily for initial BP of 156/90 mm Hg. Four weeks later, her BP was 149/86 mm Hg despite low salt (88 mEq/day) diet. **In order to achieve goal BP < 140/90 mm Hg, which one of the following would you do next?**

A. Decrease Na^+ intake to 44 mEq/day
B. Check BP in 2 weeks
C. Increase HCTZ to 25 mg
D. Add a β-blocker
E. Discontinue HCTZ and start atenolol

The answer is C

If goal BP is not achieved within a month of treatment, the JNC 8 panelists suggest to increase the dose of the initial drug or add a second drug such as the calcium blocker, an ACE-I or ARB. In this patient, the appropriate action is to increase the dose of HCTZ to 25 mg daily. If goal BP is not reached, adding a second drug from any of the above drug classes is justified. Thus, choice C is correct.

Suggested Reading

James PA, Oparil S, Canter BL, et al. 2014 Evidence-based guideline for the management of high blood pressure in adults. Report from the panel members appointed to the Eighth Joint National Committee (JNC 8). JAMA. 2014;311:507–20.

40. A 52-year-old African American man with a strong family history of HTN comes to your office with a complaint of headache on and off. His mean BP taken three times in an hour is 164/106 mm Hg. **Which one of the following choices you select to treat his HTN?**

A. HCTZ 12.5 mg once a day
B. HCTZ 12.5 mg once a day and Na^+ (66 mEq/day) restriction
C. Start a two-drug combination
D. Start a two-drug combination after one drug failed
E. Insist only on lifestyle modification, and check BP in 2 weeks

The answer is C

This patient has stage 2 HTN. The best way to manage his HTN is to start a two-drug combination (either HCTZ 12.5 mg plus benazepril 20 mg or benazepril 20 mg plus amlodipine 5 mg) to lower BP to 150/90 mm Hg without waiting to see the effects of lifestyle modification. The dosage of the combination drugs needs to be titrated to reach goal BP. Thus, choice C is correct. Starting a two-drug combination in stage 2 hypertensive subject with other CV risk factors is also justified.

Suggested Reading

James PA, Oparil S, Canter BL, et al. 2014 Evidence-based guideline for the management of high blood pressure in adults. Report from the panel members appointed to the Eighth Joint National Committee (JNC 8). JAMA. 2014;311:507–20.

Weber MA, Schiffrin EL, White WB, et al. Clinical practice guidelines for the management of hypertension in the community. A statement of the American Society of Hypertension and the International Society of Hypertension. J Clin Hypertens. 2014;16:14–26.

41. A 65-year-old woman with HTN and a strong family history of stroke is initiated on chlorthalidone. Her office BP is 155/86 mm Hg with a heart rate of 74 BPM. **Based on clinical trials, which one of the following add-on drugs is associated with high risk for stroke?**

A. Hydralazine
B. Amlodipine
C. Losartan
D. Atenolol
E. Doxazosin

The answer is D

In general, lowering BP reduces the incidence of stroke in a hypertensive individual irrespective of the classes of antihypertensive drugs. However, calcium blockers seem to have an additional benefit in stroke prevention.

Both the ASCOT (The Anglo-Scandinavian Cardiac outcome Trial) and LIFE (Losartan Intervention For Endpoint) reduction in hypertension studies used amlodipine and atenolol (ASCOT), losartan and atenolol (LIFE) and reported that the risk for stroke is higher in atenolol than in other groups. Thus, option D is correct. Adding hydralazine or doxazosin would lower BP even further, but they are not associated with increased stroke incidence.

Suggested Reading

Dahlöf B, Devereux RB, Kjeldsen SE, Julius S, et al. for the LIFE study group: Cardiovascualr morbidity and mortality in the Losartan Intervention For Endpoint reduction in hypertension study (LIFE): a randomized trial against atenolol. Lancet. 2002;359:995–1003.

Dahlöf B, Severe PS, Poulter NR, et al. for the ASCOT Investigators. Prevention of cardiovascular events with an antihypertensive regimen of amlodipine adding perindopril as required versus atenolol adding bendroflumethiazide as required, in the Anglo-Scandinavian Cardiac Outcomes Trial-Blood Pressure Lowering Arm (ASCOT-BPLA): a multicentre randomised controlled trial. Lancet. 2005;366:895–906.

42. **Treatment of HTN with either ACE-Is or calcium blockers (CCBs) would reduce which one of the following major CV events?**

A. Stroke
B. Coronary artery disease
C. Heart failure
D. Death from any CV cause
E. All of the above

The answer is E

Meta-analyses performed on HTN treatment by the BPLTTC (the Blood Pressure Lowering Treatment Trialists' Collaboration) group demonstrated that treatment of HTN with either ACE-Is or CCBs reduced significantly all of the above listed CV events, as compared with other agents. Also, ACE-I-based regimens reduced the risk of death attributable to CV or all causes by 20% and 12%, respectively. Thus, E is correct.

Suggested Reading

Turnbull F, Neal B. Meta-analyses of hypertension trials. In: Black HR, Elliott WJ, editors. Hypertension. A companion to Braunwald's heart disease. Philadelphia: Elsevier/Saunders; 2007. p. 316–24.

43. You see a 64-year-old nondiabetic man for further management of his HTN. He is on maximum doses of chlorthalidone (25 mg), losartan (100 mg), and amlodipine (10 mg). His BP is 154/92 mm Hg. You start him on spironolactone 25 mg once daily, and in 3 weeks, his BP is 136/82 mm Hg. **Which one of the following biochemical changes you expect to see during long-term follow-up of this patient?**

A. Development of type 4 renal tubular acidosis (RTA)

B. An increase in serum [K$^+$] of 1.5 mEq/L
C. An increase in serum [K$^+$] of 0.41 mEq/L
D. A significant decrease in total and LDL cholesterol
E. C and D

The answer is E

The investigators of ASCOT-Blood Pressure Lowering Arm evaluated the effect of spironolactone (25–50 mg) as a fourth-line antihypertensive agent in 1441 participants on BP and other biochemical determinations. The median duration of spironolactone treatment was 1.3 years. Pertinent to this question, the significant findings of this study were a mean drop in BP by 21.9/9.5 mm Hg, an increase in serum [K$^+$] by 0.41 mEq/L, and a decrease in total and LDL cholesterol (0.32 and 0.36 mmol/L). No development of RTA was observed. Thus, E is correct.

Suggested Reading

Chapman N, Dobson J, Wilson S, et al., on behalf of the Anglo-Scandinavian Cardiac Outcomes Trial Investigators. Effect of spironolactone on blood pressure in subjects with resistant hypertension. Hypertension. 2007;49:839–45.

44. A 44-year-old woman with CKD 3 (eGFR 50 mL/min) due to HTN is referred to you for evaluation of proteinuria of 1.4 g/ 24 h. Her BP is 144/90 mm Hg. She is on ramipril 10 mg daily. **Which one of the following BP goals has been suggested to slow her kidney progression?**

A. <140/90 mm Hg
B. <130/80 mm Hg
C. <150/90 mm Hg
D. <120/80 mm Hg
E. None of the above

The answer is B

Older guidelines state that <130/80 mm Hg is the target BP for patients with CKD of any etiology. However, recent guidelines suggest that for patients without proteinuria (<500 mg/24 h), the goal BP is <140/90 mm Hg. At least two studies reported that patients with >500 mg proteinuria benefit from lowering BP to <130/80 mm Hg. The MDRD (Modification of Diet in Renal Disease) found that strict BP control in proteinuric patients slows the decline in GFR. According to the study, patients with proteinuria of 0.25 g to >1.0 g/24 h should have a goal BP of 130/80 mm Hg. This goal BP for proteinuric patients is confirmed by the AASK subgroup analysis study, which reported a benefit of the lower BP goal among patients with >500 mg of proteinuria. In this patient, the target BP should be <130/80 mm Hg in order to slow the progression of her kidney disease. Thus, option B is correct.

It is suggested that the BP goal for nondiabetic CKD patients without proteinuria should be <140/90 mm Hg (A). Lowering SBP to <120 mm Hg may be harmful (D), and goal BP < 150/80 is suggested for general population aged 60 years or older by the JNC 8 guideline.

It should be noted that the REIN-2 (the Ramipril Efficacy in Nephropathy 2) study did not show a benefit of tight BP control in slowing kidney progression in CKD patients with proteinuria.

Suggested Reading

Appel LJ, Wright JT Jr., Bakris GL, et al., for the AASK Collaborative Research Group. Intensive blood-pressure control in hypertensive chronic kidney disease. N Engl J Med. 2010;363:918–29.

Peterson JC, Adelr S, Burkart JM, Greene T, et al. Blood pressure control, proteinuria, and the progression of renal disease. The Modification of Diet in Renal Disease Study. Ann Intern Med. 1995;123:754–62.

Ruggenenti P, Perna A, Loriga G, et al. Blood pressure control for renoprotection in patients with non-diabetic chronic renal disease (REIN-2): a multicenter, randomized controlled trial. Lancet. 2005;365:939–46.

45. A 58-year-old type 2 diabetic man with HTN and left ventricular hypertrophy (LVH) is referred to you for control of HTN and other CV events. He is on four antihypertensive medications of different classes. His BP is 138/80 mm Hg. He has albuminuria of 280 mg/24 h. with HgbA1c of 6.8%. **Based on clinical trials and post hoc analyses, which one of the following SBPs is NOT associated with increased risk for CV outcomes in this patient?**

A. <160 mm Hg
B. <150 mm Hg
C. <140 mm Hg
D. <130 mm Hg

E. <120 mm Hg

The answer is C

Several studies tested the effect of a target SBP < 120 mm Hg on major CV events in type 2 diabetic patients with CV risk factors. One such major trial is the ACCORD (the Action to Control Cardiovascular Risk in Diabetes) BP trial. In this study, 4733 participants with type 2 diabetes were randomly assigned to either intensive SBP (<120 mm Hg) or standard SBP (<140 mm Hg) treatments. The primary composite outcome was nonfatal MI, nonfatal stroke, or death from CV causes. The patients were followed up for a mean period of 4.7 years. The achieved SBP after 1 year was 119.3 mm Hg in the intensive group and 133.5 mm Hg in the standard therapy group. The results showed that intensive therapy did not reduce any of the primary composite outcomes, as compared with the standard therapy. Also, serious adverse effects from antihypertensive treatment were higher in the intensive therapy group (3.3%), as compared with the standard therapy group (1.3%).

Also, post hoc analysis of data from the IDNT (the Irbesartan Diabetic Nephropathy Trial) showed that SBP < 120 mm Hg was associated with increased risk for CV events.

The INVEST (The International Verapamil SR-Trandolapril) trial showed that diabetic participants with SBP < 130 mm Hg had similar rates of CV outcomes but higher rates of death than those participants whose SBP was between 130 and 140 mm Hg. Thus, option C is correct.

Suggested Reading

Berl T, Hunsicker LW, Lewis, JB, et al. Impact of achieved blood pressure on cardiovascular outcomes in the Irbesartan Diabetic Nephropathy Trial. J Am Soc Nephrol. 2005;16:2170–9.

Cooper-DeHoff RM, Gong Y, Handberg EM, et al. Tight blood pressure control and cardiovascular outcomes among hypertensive patients with diabetes and coronary artery disease. JAMA. 2010;304:61–8.

Cushman W, Evans GW, Byington RP, et al. The ACCORD Study Group. Effects of intensive blood-pressure control in type 2 diabetes mellitus. N Engl J Med. 2010;362:1575–85.

46. A 42-year-old man receives a kidney transplant from a diseased donor, and presents with new-onset HTN within 2 months of transplantation. **Which one of the following mechanisms accounts for his HTN?**

A. Calcineurin inhibitors (CNIs)
B. Corticosteroids
C. Allograft dysfunction
D. Transplant renal artery stenosis (TRAS)
E. All of the above

The answer is E

The prevalence of HTN in kidney transplant patients was 50% prior to cyclosporine, which increased to 90% after its approval in 1983. Both cyclosporine and tacrolimus induce HTN by several mechanisms. Corticosteroids cause HTN mainly by salt and water retention. Allograft dysfunction may also cause volume-dependent hypertension because of salt and water retention. TRAS accounts for 1–7% of cases following kidney transplantation. Activation of renin-AII-aldosterone system is responsible for early HTN, and graft dysfunction may sustain HTN chronically. Thus, choice E is correct.

Suggested Reading

Mangray M, Vella JP. Hypertension after kidney transplant. Am J Kid Dis. 2011;57:331–41.

Thomas B, Taber DJ, Srinivas TR. Hypertension after kidney transplantation: a pathophysiologic approach. Curr Hypertens Rep. 2013;15:458–69.

Wadei HM, Textor SC. Hypertension in the kidney transplant recipient. Tansplant Rev. 2010;24:105–20.

47. **Which one of the following factors predisposes the patient to HTN after kidney transplantation?**

A. African American race
B. Donor kidney from an elderly subject
C. Pretransplant HTN
D. Obesity
E. All of the above

The answer is E

Studies have shown that 50–90% of kidney transplant recipients have either HTN or on antihypertensive medications. Patients at risk for HTN following kidney transplantation include African Americans, recipients of kidneys from elderly subjects, obese individuals, and those with pretransplant HTN. Thus, choice E is correct. In these patients, CINs and corticosteroids simply aggravate HTN.

Suggested Reading

Mangray M, Vella JP. Hypertension after kidney transplant. Am J Kid Dis. 2011;57:331–41.

Thomas B, Taber DJ, Srinivas TR. Hypertension after kidney transplantation: a pathophysiologic approach. Curr Hypertens Rep. 2013;15:458–69.

48. A 48-year-old woman with adult polycystic kidney disease develops HTN 1 month following kidney transplantation. She is on cyclosporine and steroids. Her office BP is 148/88 mm Hg with a heart rate of 72 BPM. Her serum creatinine is 1.7 mg/dL. She has proteinuria of 200 mg/24 h. There is no peripheral edema. **Which one of the following antihypertensive agents is usually recommended for this patient?**

A. A dihydropyridine calcium blocker (dCCB)
B. An ACE-I or ARB
C. A thiazide diuretic
D. A β-blocker
E. An α-blocker

The answer is A

Lowering BP to <130/80 mm Hg has been shown to improve graft survival and CV events in kidney transplant recipients. This patient is at risk for both complications, if her BP is not lowered to <130/80 mm Hg. The choice of initial antihypertensive agents depends on the individual patient's comorbidities. Also, drug interactions with CINs should be considered. In this patient, the mechanisms for her HTN seems to be cyclosporine and steroids. Based on her creatinine, a dCCB, amlodipine, or small dose of long-acting nifedipine seems appropriate because these agents counteract the renal afferent arteriolar vasoconstrictive effects of cyclosporine. Also, CCBs cause afferent arteriolar vasodilation. A meta-analysis shows that CCBs are associated with a 25% lower rate of graft loss and an increase of GFR by 2.2–6.4 mL/min, as compared with placebo or no treatment. An ACE-I or ARB use may initially raise serum creatinine, and may be confused with acute rejection. These drugs are safe to use after 2–4 months. The patient is not volume overloaded; therefore, diuretic use may not be indicated at this time. Although the other agents can be used in post-transplant hypertensive patients, their use is not indicated at this time. Thus, choice A is correct.

Suggested Reading

Cross NB, Webster AC, Masson P, et al. Antihypertensives for kidney transplant recipients: systematic review and meta-analyses of randomized controlled trials. Transplantation. 2009;88:7–18.

Kidney Disease: Improving Global Outcomes (KDIGO) Blood Pressure Work Group. KDIGO Clinical Practice Guideline for the Management of Blood Pressure in Chronic Kidney Disease. Kidney Int. 2012;(Suppl 2):337–414.

Thomas B, Taber DJ, Srinivas TR. Hypertension after kidney transplantation: a pathophysiologic approach. Curr Hypertens Rep. 2013;15:458–69.

49. An 89-year-old woman with HTN, and on four medications, including a thiazide diuretic, is admitted for headache. She is active in community service, and wants her BP to be controlled to prevent stroke. A CT of the head is normal except for age-related changes. In the Emergency Department, her headache is attributed to low glucose. Her BP is 170/78 mm Hg with a heart rate of 84 BPM. **Based on clinical trials, which one of the following goal SBPs is appropriate for this very old woman to prevent stroke?**

A. <130/80 mm Hg
B. <140/80 mm Hg
C. <150/80 mm Hg
D. >160/80 mm Hg
E. >170/80 mm Hg

The answer is C

It is well established that control of HTN (both systolic and diastolic HTN as well as isolated systolic HTN) prevents cardiovascular and renal complications. In the elderly, the reason for treating HTN is to reduce CV morbidity and mortality. However, the goal BP, particularly in the very old (>80 years of age), that is safe in reducing CV events is not well established. The investigators of all clinical studies agree that lowering SBP to <160 mm Hg (between 143 and 150) is safe and this BP goal reduces all CV events (see Table 6.3 **below). BPs <130 may not be safe in the very old people. Thus, choice C is correct.**

Table 6.3 Treatment effect of isolated systolic hypertension in the elderly

	SHEP	SYST-EUR	HYVET
No.	4736	4695	3845
Age (years)	60–80	>60	80–105
Mean entry BP (mm Hg)	170/77	174/86	173/91
BP meds	Chlorthalidone ± atenolol/reserpine	Nitrendipine ± enalapril/HCTZ	Indapamide ± perindopril
Mean follow-up (years)	4.5	2.0	1.8
Achieved BP (mm Hg)	143/64	151/79	144/78
Reduction in CV events (%)			
Stroke	33	42	30
Coronary artery disease	27	30	28
CHF	55	29	64
All CV events	32	31	34

SHEP systolic hypertension in the elderly program, *SYST-EUR* systolic hypertension in European trial, *HYVET* hypertension in the very elderly trial

Suggested Reading

Beckett NS, Peters R, Fletcher AE, et al. for the HYVET Study Group. Treatment of hypertension in patients 80 years of age or older. N Engl J Med. 2008;358:1887–98.

Lipsitz LA. A 91-year-old woman with difficult-to-control hypertension. A clinical review. JAMA. 2013;310:1274–80.

SHEP Cooperative Research Group. Prevention of stroke by antihypertensive drug treatment in older persons with isolated systolic hypertension: final results of the Systolic Hypertension in the Elderly Program. JAMA. 1991;265:3255–64.

Staessen JA, Fagard R, Thijs L, Systolic Hypertension in Europe Trial Investigators, et al. Randomised double-blind comparison of placebo and active treatment for older patients with isolated systolic hypertension. Lancet. 1997;350:757–64.

50. The granddaughter of the above patient asks you about antihypertensive treatment and cognitive function. **Which one of the following statements is CORRECT regarding her cognitive function and antihypertensive treatment?**

A. Treatment of HTN deteriorates cognitive function
B. No relationship between hypertensive treatment and cognitive function
C. Antihypertensive treatment improves cognitive function
D. All of the above
E. None of the above

The answer is C

An association between high BP and decline in cognitive function has been reported by several investigators. Although the mechanism for this association is unclear, hypertension-induced changes in the brain such as reduced cerebral blood flow, lesions in the white matter, and deposition of amyloid have been implicated. Most of the studies have shown an improvement in cognitive function following antihypertensive treatment. The investigators of the Vascular Dementia Project, SCOPE (Study on Cognition and Prognosis in the Elderly), and a meta-analysis that included HYVET-COG (Systolic Hypertension in the Very Elderly Cognition Study) showed that antihypertensive treatment decreases cognitive impairment in the elderly.

Therefore, control of systolic HTN in this patient may improve cognitive function. Thus, choice C is correct. It is of interest to note that K^+-sparing diuretics have been found to have the strongest influence on reducing the risk for dementia, possibly by K^+-induced inflammation and vasoconstriction.

Suggested Reading

Bloch MJ, Basile JN. Hypertension in older patients. In: Black HR, Elliott WJ, editors. Hypertension. A companion to Braunwald's heart disease. 2nd ed. Philadelphia: Elsevier/Saunders; 2013. p. 349–55.
Duron E, Hanon O. Hypertension, cognitive decline and dementia. Arch Cardiovasc Dis. 2008;101:181–9.
Skoog I, Gustafson D. Update on hypertension and Alzeheimer's disease. Neurol Res. 2006;28:605–11.

51. A 36-year-old obese woman body mass index of 32 kg/m^2 has BP of 149/86 mm Hg. **Regarding the pathogenesis of her HTN, which one of the following mechanisms is CORRECT?**

A. Increased Na$^+$ reabsorption by renal tubules
B. Increased sympathetic nervous system (SNS) and renin-AII-aldosterone system (RAAS) activity
C. Insulin resistance
D. Endothelial dysfunction
E. All of the above

The answer is E

A number of mechanisms have been proposed to account for the development of HTN in obesity. Na$^+$ is retained by the kidney, which is related to the activation of SNS and RAAS. Also, excess fat surrounding the kidney and kidney fat volume stimulates Na$^+$ reabsorption by intrarenal mechanisms. Pressure natriuresis is impaired in obesity. Activation of both SNS and RAAS by several factors has been described in obesity.

Hyperinsulinemia is common in obesity. Adiponectin, which sensitizes insulin, is low in obesity, causing insulin resistance. Although insulin resistance is not the major mechanism for the development of HTN, it contributes to the maintenance of HTN.

Decreased nitric oxide production and increased oxidative stress with generation of inflammatory cytokines cause endothelial dysfunction and subsequent HTN. Thus, all of the above mechanisms have been proposed to cause HTN in obesity, and choice E is correct.

Suggested Reading

DeMarco VG, Aroor AR, Sowers JR. The pathophysiology of hypertension in patients with obesity. Nature Rev Endocrinol. 2014;10:364–76.
Dorresteijn JA, Visseren FL, Spiering W. Mechanisms linking obesity to hypertension. Obes Rev. 2012;13:17–26.

52. You are consulted to see a 40-year-old obese man with a BP of 160/88 mm Hg and a heart rate of 84 BPM. **Based on clinical effectiveness and adverse effects, which one of the following antihypertensive agents is appropriate for this patient?**

A. A thiazide diuretic
B. A β-blocker
C. A central agonist
D. An ACE-I or ARB
E. A calcium blocker

The answer is D

Although all of the above drugs lower BP in this patient, they have different adverse effects. Diuretics such as chlorthalidone or HCTZ promote Na$^+$ excretion, but induce several metabolic abnormalities (see Table 6.4 **below). The heart rate may increase even further in this patient because of diuretic-induced volume contraction.**

β-blockers protect the heart, but cause metabolic abnormalities and weight gain. Calcium blockers have several advantages, but induce lower extremity edema. Centrally acting drugs such as clonidine reduce SNS activity with neutral metabolic activity, but they cause weight gain.

ACE-Is or ARBs have several advantages with minimal side effects other than cough or angioedema (ACE-Is). They also inhibit RAAS besides other beneficial effects.

Based on the above advantages and disadvantage, an ACE-I or ARB seems an appropriate initial drug for this patient, and other drugs can be added to achieve goal BP. Thus, D is correct.

Table 6.4 Pertinent advantages and disadvantages of different classes of antihypertensive drugs in obese hypertensive patient

Drug class	Advantages	Disadvantages
Diuretics	↑Na^+ excretion, ↓intravascular volume, regression of LVH	↑SNS & RAAS activity, ↑glucose, hypokalemia, hyperlipidemia, metabolic alkalosis, ankle edema with increased water intake
β-blockers	↓SNS & RAAS activity, ↓cardiac output, protection from arrhythmias	Insulin resistance, ↑glucose & triglycerides, ↓HDL-cholesterol, reduced regression of LVH, weight gain
Central agonists	↓SNS activity, ↑Na^+ excretion, neutral metabolic effects	Sedation, weight gain
ACE-Is	↓RAAS & SNS activity, ↑insulin sensitivity, ↓proteinuria, neutral lipid profile, regression of LVH	Cough, angioedema
ARBs	Same as ACE-Is	Mostly none
Calcium blockers	↑Na^+ excretion, ↓intravascular volume, regression of LVH, ↓heart rate (diltiazem, verapamil), ↓proteinuria	Edema & weight gain

Suggested Reading

Chrostowska M, Szczech R, Narkiewicz K. Antihypertensive therapy in the obese hypertensive patient. Curr Opin Nephrol Hypens. 2006;15:487–92.

Woofford MR, Smith G, Minor DB. The treatment of hypertension in obese patients. Curr Hypertens Rep. 2008;10:143–50.

53. A 32-year-old obese woman with obstructive sleep apnea (OSA) is on four antihypertensive agents, including a thiazide diuretic. Her home BP is 144/86 mm Hg. The physician adds spironolactone, but her BP remains at 140/80 mm Hg. The physician consults a pulmonologist, who orders CPAP (continuous positive airway pressure) ventilation. **Which one of the following statements is CORRECT regarding CPAP ventilation in OSA-hypertensive patient?**

A. CPAP lowers 24-h BP in combination with antihypertensive agents
B. CPAP lowers only nighttime but not daytime BP in those with medication-controlled HTN
C. CPAP is more effective in lowering BP in those with increasing severity of OSA
D. Wearing CPAP >5.8 h per night reduces BP more than those who wear less than this time
E. All of the above

The answer is E

CPAP ventilation provides an increase in pressure in airways during both inspiration and expiration. This is useful in hypertensive patients with OSA, who are at increased risk for CV events. Patients who received CPAP had reduced risk for CV events. In the above patient, all of the choices are applicable, and thus, choice E is correct.

The mechanisms underlying the BP-lowering effect of CPAP ventilation include reduction in SNS activity associated with an increase in parasympathetic activity, increased cardiac output, and decreased systemic vascular resistance. These changes are possible mediated by an increase in baroreceptor sensitivity.

Suggested Reading

Montesi SB, Edwards BA, Malhotra A, et al. The effect of continuous positive airway pressure treatment on blood pressure: a systematic review and meta-analysis of randomized controlled trials. J Clin Sleep Med. 2012;8:587–96.

Pedrosa RP, Drager LF, DePaula LK, et al. Effects of OSA treatment on BP in patients with resistant hypertension: a randomized trial. Chest. 2013;144:1487–94.

54. A 45-year-old man with a history of HTN and noncompliance to antihypertensive medications comes to the Emergency Department with a vague chest pain radiating to his back for a few hours. His BP is 220/140 mm Hg with a heart rate of 80 BPM. CXR shows widening mediastinum, and ECHO confirms acute aortic dissection. **Which one of the following drugs is appropriate to lower BP in this patient?**

A. Intravenous (IV) nitroglycerine
B. IV nicardipine
C. IV esmolol

D. IV enalapril
E. IV fenoldopam

The answer is C

Acute aortic dissection is a hypertensive emergency. It mandates lowering BP with an IV β-blocker, which reduces heart rate and shear stress on torn aorta by decreasing cardiac contractility. Short-acting β-blockers such as esmolol or labetalol should be used. Alternatively, diltiazem can be used in patients with contraindication to β-blockers. The target SBP is <120 mm Hg within 20 min. Other agents such as sodium nitroprusside can be used to achieve the target BP.

Other drugs listed above are not unreasonable, but the heart rate may not be that lowered by these drugs, as compared with a β-blocker. Thus, C is correct.

Suggested Reading

Johnson W, Nguyen M-L, Patel R. Hypertension crisis in the emergency department. Cardiol Clin. 2012;30:533–43.
Kuppasani K, Reddi AS. Emeregency or urgency? Effective management of hypertensive crises. JAAPA. 2010;23:44–9.

55. A 56-year-old man with a history of HTN is admitted for headache and a BP of 220/130 mm Hg and a heart rate of 84 BPM. A CT of the head shows acute ischemic stroke. **Which one of the following drugs is appropriate to lower BP in this patient?**

A. Nitroglycerine
B. Fenoldopam
C. Esmolol
D. Nicardipine
E. Enalapril

The answer is D

The evidence is conflicting regarding the treatment of BP in acute ischemic stroke. However, treatment is recommended in those with BP > 220/120 mm Hg, but there is no clear answer as to the use of ideal antihypertensive agent. Esmolol is an ultra-short-acting agent. It is the preferred agent in patients with acute aortic dissection. Enalapril can be used as an IV or oral agent, but its use has not been preferred in most of the studies. Nitroglycerine is the drug of choice in patients with chest pain or CHF, and it increases intracranial pressure (ICP). The American Heart Association Guidelines recommend nicardipine in patients with acute ischemic stroke whose SBP > 220 mm Hg or DBP > 120 mm Hg. IV nicardipine has been proven to be better compared to labetalol in the Emergency Department to achieve SBP target within 30 min. Of all the drugs listed above, nicardipine seems appropriate in this patient. Thus, D is correct.

Suggested Reading

Drozda J Jr., Messer JV, Spertus J, et al. ACCF/AHA/AMA-PCPI 2011 performance measures for adults with coronary artery disease and hypertension: a report of the American College of Cardiology Foundation/American Heart Association Task Force on Performance Measures and American Medical Association-Physician Consortium for Performance Improvement. J Am Coll Cardiol. 2011;58:316–36.
Peacock WF IV, Hilleman DE, Levy PD, et al. A systematic review of nicardipine vs labetalol for the management of hypertensive crises. Am J Emerg Med. 2012;30:981–93.
Ramos AP, Varon J. Current and newer agents for hypertensive emergencies. Curr Hypertens Rep. 2014;16:450.

56. **Which one of the following options is considered safe in the above patient?**

A. Do not treat BP as it falls within few days
B. Treat BP to an SBP <190 mm Hg
C. Treat BP to an SBP 140–150 mm Hg
D. Treat BP to an SBP <120 mm Hg
E. None of the above

The answer is C

Acute ischemic stroke (AIS) accounts for approximately 70% of all strokes. Most of the patients with AIS have their SBPs > 140 mm Hg at the time of presentation. The natural history of BP in AIS patients is spontaneous lowering to baseline in several days. However, in the above patient, the BP is 220/130 mm Hg. There is a U-shaped relationship between baseline SBP (within 48 h of stroke) and short-term mortality and long-term death and dependency. Both extremes of SBP (<120 and >220 mm Hg) have poor outcomes. The lowest risk seems to be between 140 and 150 mm Hg. In this patient, lowering SBP either with nicardipine or labetalol seems appropriate to prevent complications. Therefore, option C is correct.

Suggested Reading

Gorelick PB, Aiyagari V. The management of hypertension for an acute stroke: what is the blood pressure goal? Curr Cardiol Rep. 2013;15:366.

Grise EM, Adeoye O. Blood pressure control for acute ischemic and hemorrhagic stroke. Curr Opin Crit Care. 2012;18:132–8.

Manning L, Robinson TG, Anderson GS. Control of blood pressure in hypertensive neurological emergencies. Curr Hypertensive Rep. 2014;16:436.

57. A 62-year-old African American woman is admitted for severe headache. Her BP is 210/130 mm Hg. CT head showed intracerebral hemorrhage (ICH). She is started on nicardipine, and her BP is improving. Her intracranial pressure is 17 mm Hg (normal 7–15 mm Hg). **Which one of the following statements is CORRECT in this patient?**

   A. Lower SBP to <120 mm Hg
   B. Hold nicardipine drip, as her BP will spontaneously improve
   C. Lower SBP to 180 mm Hg
   D. Lower SBP to 140 mm Hg
   E. None of the above

   The answer is D

   ICH accounts for 10–15% of all strokes. Patients with ICH generally present with HTN (SBP > 140 mm Hg). Two important studies, INTERACT (Intensive Blood Pressure Reduction in Acute Cerebral Hemorrhage Trial) and ATACH (the Antihypertensive Treatment of Acute Cerebral Hemorrhage) showed that acute reduction in SBP to 140 mm Hg is safe and may improve neurological outcome. Hematoma expansion, which occurs within the first several hours after ICH, is associated with poor neurological outcome. The above two studies showed less hematoma expansion in those patients whose BP was reduced. The target BP in ICH is <140/90 mm Hg or <130/80 mm Hg in patients with diabetes or CKD. Thus, option D is correct. In patients with raised ICP, monitoring ICP and reducing SBP are usually recommended.

Suggested Reading

Gorelick PB, Aiyagari V. The management of hypertension for an acute stroke: what is the blood pressure goal? Curr Cardiol Rep. 2013;15:366.

Grise EM, Adeoye O. Blood pressure control for acute ischemic and hemorrhagic stroke. Curr Opin Crit Care. 2012;18:132–8.

Manning L, Robinson TG, Anderson GS. Control of blood pressure in hypertensive neurological emergencies. Curr Hypertensive Rep 16:436, 2014.

58. A 42-year-old woman presented to the ED with sudden onset of severe headache, nausea, vomiting, and photophobia. CT head showed ruptured aneurysm, and the diagnosis of subarachnoid hemorrhage (SAH) has been made. Her BP is 180/120 mm Hg with a heart rate of 88 BPM. **According to American Heart Association (AHA)/American Stroke Association (ASA) guidelines, which one of the following measures is important in the acute care of this patient?**

   A. Control of BP from aneurysmal rupture to aneurysmal obliteration (securing)
   B. Prevention of rebleeding after aneurysmal rupture
   C. Attainment of a reasonable SBP <160 mm Hg
   D. Management of cerebral vasospasm and delayed cerebral ischemia after aneurysmal SAH
   E. All of the above

   The answer is E

SAH accounts for 5–10% of all strokes, and it is usually due to rupture of an intracranial aneurysm. HTN is an established risk factor. In SAH, cerebral autoregulation is impaired. Therefore, lowering BP below the autoregulatory range results in cerebral ischemia. Studies have shown that rebleeding is a serious complication of SAH, and initial HTN (SBP > 160 mm Hg) is a risk factor for recurrent hemorrhage. Control of BP to <160 mm Hg is advisable.

Management of cerebral vasospasm and delayed cerebral ischemia after aneurysmal SAH is important. BP augmentation with "triple-H therapy" (hypervolemia, hypertension, and hemodilution) is indicated in those with initial low BP. In this patient, initial BP is high, and careful management with "triple-H therapy" is indicated. Thus, option E is correct.

Suggested Reading

Gorelick PB, Aiyagari V. The management of hypertension for an acute stroke: what is the blood pressure goal? Curr Cardiol Rep. 2013;15:366.

Manning L, Robinson TG, Anderson GS. Control of blood pressure in hypertensive neurological emergencies. Curr Hypertensive Rep. 2014;16:436.

59. A 38-year-old woman is referred to you for evaluation of primary aldosteronism, whose BP is not controlled despite three antihypertensive drugs (HCTZ 25 mg, lisinopril 20 mg, amlodipine 10 mg). Currently, her BP is 160/98 mm Hg. Her serum chemistry: Na^+ 145 mEq/L, K^+ 3.5 mEq/L, Cl^- 90 mEq/L, HCO_3^- 30 mEq/L, creatinine 1.5 mg/dL, glucose 120 mg/dL, aldosterone 44 ng/dL(elevated), and renin 0.2 ng/mL/h (low). **According to the Endocrine Society Guideline, which one of the following is recommended as a case detection of primary aldosteronism (PA)?**

A. Sustained BP >150/100 mm Hg on each of three measurements obtained on different days
B. Hypertension (BP >140/90 mm Hg) resistant to three conventional antihypertensive drugs (including a diuretic), or controlled BP (<140/90 mm Hg) on four or more antihypertensive drugs
C. HTN with spontaneous or diuretic-induced hypokalemia
D. HTN with adrenal incidentaloma, or HTN with a family history of early-onset HTN or cerebrovascular accident at <40 years of age
E. All of the above

The answer is E

All of the above statements are correct (E). However, it should be noted that hypokalemia is not present in all patients with PA. Studies have shown that only 9–37% of patients with PA had hypokalemia. Only 50% of the patients with aldosterone-producing adenoma and 17% of patients with idiopathic hyperaldosteronism had hypokalemia. Adrenal incidentaloma (nonfunctioning unilateral macroadenoma) is rather common in patients older than 40 years of age, and treatment for this finding is not indicated. Genetic testing is recommended for individuals <20 years of age with severe HTN and nonresponsive to antihypertensive drugs. These individuals may have glucocorticoid remediable HTN.

Suggested Reading

Funder JW, Carey RM, Montero F, et al. The management of primary aldosteronism: Case detection, diagnosis, and treatment. An Endocrine Society Clinical Practice Guideline. J Clin Endocrinol Metabol. 2016;101:1889–1916.

Harvey AM. Primary aldosteronism. Diagnosis, lateralization, and treatment. Surg Clin N Am. 2014;94:643–56.

60. **In assessing the patient with suspected primary aldosteronism (PA), which one of the following tests is appropriate to make treatment decision?**

A. Plasma aldosterone/renin ratio (ARR)
B. Confirmatory testing of ARR
C. CT/MRI of adrenal glands
D. Adrenal venous sampling (AVS)
E. All of the above

The answer is E

The ARR is the most reliable initial test available for screening PA. Several studies have indicated that ARR is superior to determinations of serum K^+, aldosterone, and renin. As with any other tests, ARR is not without false positives or false negatives. Many medications and clinical conditions affect ARR (see later question). Although there is no cut-off for abnormal value, an ARR >30 with plasma aldosterone concentration >15 ng/dL is suggestive of PA.

Increased ARR should be followed by a confirmatory test to make a positive diagnosis of PA. Four tests are available: (1) oral sodium loading test; (2) saline infusion tests; (3) fludrocortisone suppression test; and (4) captopril challenge test. The reader is referred to the Suggested Reading for details of the tests.

After confirmatory testing, the next step is adrenal imaging with CT or MRI, which provides anatomic information for surgical planning. CT is usually preferred, which may show an aldosterone-producing adenoma (APA), or normal-appearing adrenals with bilateral adrenal hyperplasia (BAH). APA requires surgery, whereas BPH requires medical management. To avoid unnecessary surgery, for example, nonfunctioning unilateral adrenal macroadenoma, lateralization of aldosterone production is done with AVS.

AVS is a difficult procedure, and therefore, an experienced interventional radiologist is needed. It is the gold standard for localizing APAs and to distinguish APA from BAH. Following both adrenal veins catheterization, baseline samples are obtained from both adrenal veins and inferior vena cava (IVC) and repeated after cosyntropin infusion. Cosyntropin is used to minimize stress-induced fluctuations in aldosterone secretion, to maximize aldosterone secretion from APA, and to confirm successful catheterization of both right and left adrenal veins. Aldosterone and cortisol levels are determined.

Interpretation of data varies among centers. First, determination of successful cannulation of both adrenal veins should be evaluated. It is done by using the cortisol levels from both adrenal veins and IVC. The adrenal vein cortisol divided by IVC cortisol ratio (vein cortisol/IVC cortisol) >10:1 assures successful catheterization. Generally, a baseline value of 3:1 or 5:1 after cosyntropin simulation is used for successful cannulation. Second, lateralization of aldosterone secretion should be assessed. It is done by calculating the ratio of aldosterone to cortisol (A/C). When A/C ratios of the affected and unaffected sides are compared, a ratio of 4:1 is used to define lateralization. At the same time, A/C values of the unaffected side and IVC should be calculated. If the A/C value of the unaffected side is less than that of IVC value, it is an evidence for suppression of the unaffected gland. Thus, a lateralization ratio >4 indicates unilateral disease, whereas a ratio <3 is suggestive of BAH. Finally, ratios between 3 and 4 represent a zone of overlap.

In a patient with PA, all of the above tests are indicated to make the decision for appropriate treatment (surgery vs medical treatment). Thus, E is correct.

Suggested Reading

Funder JW, Carey RM, Fardella C, et al. Case detection, diagnosis, and treatment of patients with primary aldosteronism: An Endocrine Society Clinical Practice Guideline. J Clin Endocrinol Metabolism. 2008;93:3266–81.

Funder JW, Carey RM, Montero F, et al. The management of primary aldosteronism: Case detection, diagnosis, and treatment. An Endocrine Society Clinical Practice Guideline. J Clin Endocrinol Metabol. 2016;101:1889–916.

Harvey AM. Primary aldosteronism. Diagnosis, lateralization, and treatment. Surg Clin N Am. 2014;94:643–56.

Sacks BA, Brook OR, Brennan IM. Adrenal venous sampling: promises and pitfalls. Curr Opin Endocrinol Diabetes Obes. 2013;20:180–5.

61. **Which one of the following drugs has the least effect on aldosterone to renin ratio (ARR)?**

A. β-blockers and central α_2 agonists
B. ACE-inhibitors and angiotensin receptor blockers (ARBs)
C. Dihydropyridine calcium blockers (DHPs)
D. K^+-sparing diuretics
E. α_1-blockers

The answer is E

Many antihypertensive drugs either increase or decrease, or have little effect on ARR, giving false-positive or false-negative results. Of all the above drugs, α_1-blockers have little effect on ARR. Thus, E is correct. The following Table 6.5 **shows the effects of various drugs and conditions on ARR.**

Table 6.5 Factors that affect ARR

Drug/condition	Aldosterone	Renin	ARR	False positive (FP)/false negative (FN)
β-blockers	↓	↓↓	↑	FP
Central α_2 agonists	↓	↓↓	↑	FP
K^+-wasting diuretics	↑	↑↑	↓	FN
ACE-Is/ARBs	↓	↑↑	↓	FN
DHPs	↓	↑	↓	FN
Non-DHPs (verapamil)	Little change (LC)	LC	LC	No effect
Na^+-loading	↓	↓↓	↑	FP
Na^+-restriction	↑	↑↑	↓	FN
Hyperkalemia	↑	↓	↑	FP
Pregnancy	↑	↑↑	↓	FN
Renal artery stenosis	↑	↑↑	↓	FN
Malignant HTN	↑	↑↑	↓	FN
CKD	LC	↓	↑	FP

↑ increase; ↓ decrease

Suggested Reading

Funder JW, Carey RM, Fardella C, et al. Case detection, diagnosis, and treatment of patients with primary aldosteronism: an Endocrine Society Clinical Practice Guideline. J Clin Endocrinol Metabolism. 2008;93:3266–81.
Harvey AM. Primary aldosteronism. Diagnosis, lateralization, and treatment. Surg Clin N Am. 2014;94:643–56.
Kumar B, Swee M. Aldosterone-renin ratio in the assessment of primary aldosteronism. JAMA. 2014;312:184–5.

62. In the patient presented in question 59, the CT of the adrenal glands is normal. The adrenal venous sampling (AVS) following cosyntropin stimulation shows the following values.

Site	Aldosterone (A)(ng/dL)	Cortisol (C) (ng/dL)	A/C ratio
Right	4002	1400	2.86
Left	3650	1310	2.79
IVC (peripheral)	50	41	1.2

Which one of the following statements is CORRECT?

A. She has aldosterone-producing adenoma (APA)
B. She has APA on the left side
C. She has CT undetectable microadenomas on the right side
D. She has bilateral adrenal hyperplasia (BAH)
E. She has hereditary primary aldosteronism (PA)

The answer is D

As stated in question 60, a lateralization ratio >4 indicates unilateral disease, whereas a ratio <3 is suggestive of BAH. In this patient, the A/C ratios of both adrenal glands are <4, suggesting the patient has BAH rather than APA. Also, aldosterone levels are high on both sides. Thus, D is correct. The age of the patient rules out possible familial form of PA.

Suggested Reading

Funder JW, Carey RM, Fardella C, et al. Case detection, diagnosis, and treatment of patients with primary aldosteronism: an Endocrine Society Clinical Practice Guideline. J Clin Endocrinol Metabolism. 2008;93:3266–81.
Sacks BA, Brook OR, Brennan IM. Adrenal venous sampling: promises and pitfalls. Curr Opin Endocrinol Diabetes Obes. 2013;20:180–5.
Young WF. Primary aldosteronism: renaissance of a syndrome. Clin Endocrinol. 2007;66:607–18.

63. (Patient in question 59). A 38-year-old woman is referred to you for evaluation of primary aldosteronism (PA), whose BP is not controlled despite three antihypertensive drugs (HCTZ 25 mg, lisinopril 20 mg, amlodipine 10 mg). PA was confirmed after appropriate tests. **Which one of the following drugs is appropriate in the initial management of her HTN?**

A. Eplerenone
B. Spironolactone
C. Amiloride
D. Losartan
E. Eplerenone and HCTZ

The answer is B

The drug of choice in this patient is spironolactone. A comparative study showed that spironolactone is superior in controlling BP compared to that of eplerenone in patients with PA. Also, a German Conn Registry showed that patients on spironolactone required less number of antihypertensive drugs than patients on eplerenone. In addition, serum [K^+] is higher and microalbuminuria is low in spironolactone group than in eplerenone group. Thus, option B is correct.

Adverse effects of spironolactone include sexual dysfunction and gynecomastia in males and mastodynia in females. These endocrine adverse effects are less with eplerenone. If the patient cannot tolerate spironolactone, eplerenone can be started. Amiloride is an alternative to both spironolactone and eplerenone, the latter is more expensive. The combination of spironolactone and HCTZ or chlorthalidone can be considered, if a single K^+-sparing drug cannot control BP. Losartan alone is not sufficient to control BP in a patient with PA.

Suggested Reading

Fourkiotis V, Vonend O, Diederich S, Mephisto Study Group, et al. Effectiveness of eplerenone or spironolactone treatment in preserving renal function in primary aldosteronism. Eur J Endocrinol. 2013;168:75–81.

Parthasarathy HK, Ménard J, White WB, et al. A double-blind, randomized study comparing the antihypertensive effect of eplerenone and spironolactone in patients with hypertension and evidence of primary aldosteronism. J Hypertens. 2011;29:980–90.

64. A 52-year-old man with primary aldosteronism has the following adrenal venous sampling (AVS) values after cosyntropin test.

Site	Aldosterone (A) (ng/dL)	Cortisol (C) (ng/dL)	A/C ratio
Right	8100	1100	7.36
Left	3100	1001	2.58
IVC (peripheral)	49	31	1.58

Which one of the following diagnoses is LIKELY in this patient?

A. Left adrenal nodule
B. Right adrenal nodule
C. Right adrenal hyperplasia
D. Left adrenal hyperplasia
E. Bilateral adrenal hyperplasia

The answer is C

In this patient, AVS did lateralize aldosterone secretion with no suppression on the left side. Therefore, the patient has right adrenal hyperplasia rather than right adrenal nodule. Thus, option C is correct.

Suggested Reading

Funder JW, Carey RM, Fardella C, et al. Case detection, diagnosis, and treatment of patients with primary aldosteronism: an Endocrine Society Clinical Practice Guideline. J Clin Endocrinol Metabolism. 2008;93:3266–81.
Sacks BA, Brook OR, Brennan IM. Adrenal venous sampling: promises and pitfalls. Curr Opin Endocrinol Diabetes Obes. 2013;20:180–5.
Young WF. Primary aldosteronism: renaissance of a syndrome. Clin Endocrinol. 2007;66:607–18.

65. A 62-year-old woman with primary aldosteronism has the following adrenal venous sampling (AVS) values after cosyntropin test.

Site	Aldosterone (A) (ng/dL)	Cortisol (C) (ng/dL)	A/C ratio
Right	310	700	0.44
Left	9460	800	11.81
IVC (peripheral)	80	36	2.2

Which one of the following diagnoses is LIKELY in this patient?

A. Left adrenal nodule
B. Right adrenal nodule
C. Right adrenal hyperplasia
D. Left adrenal hyperplasia
E. Bilateral adrenal hyperplasia

The answer is A

In this patient, AVS lateralized aldosterone secretion to the left with suppression of aldosterone secretion of the right adrenal gland. Therefore, the patient has an aldosterone-secreting nodule of left adrenal gland. Thus, A is correct. The AVS values do not support other options.

Suggested Reading

Funder JW, Carey RM, Fardella C, et al. Case detection, diagnosis, and treatment of patients with primary aldosteronism: an Endocrine Society Clinical Practice Guideline. J Clin Endocrinol Metabolism. 2008;93:3266–81.
Sacks BA, Brook OR, Brennan IM. Adrenal venous sampling: promises and pitfalls. Curr Opin Endocrinol Diabetes Obes. 2013;20:180–5.
Young WF. Primary aldosteronism: renaissance of a syndrome. Clin Endocrinol. 2007;66:607–18.

66. **Match the following histories of hypertensive patients with appropriate antihypertensive drugs:**

A. An 18-year-old man with low renin-aldosterone, hypokalemia and severe hypertension. He has mutations in the cytoplasmic COOH terminus of the β- and γ-subunits of the epithelial sodium channel (ENaC)	1. Spironolactone
B. A child with low renin-aldosterone levels, hypokalemia, severe hypertension, poor growth, short stature, and nephrocalcinosis. He has loss-of-function mutations in 11β-hydroxysteroid dehydrogenase type 2 (11β-HSD2) enzyme	2. Amiloride
C. A 16-year-old man with mild hypertension, mild hypokalemia (3.4 mEq/L), and HCO_3^- concentration of 29 mEq/L. He has a chimeric gene duplication from unequal crossover between 11β-hydroxylase and aldosterone synthase genes	3. Glucocorticoids
D. A 20-year-old pregnant woman develops severe hypertension without proteinuria during her third trimester. She was found to have a missense mutation in mineralo-corticoid receptor	4. Thiazide diuretics
E. A 22-year-old man with hypertension, hyperkalemia, metabolic acidosis, hypercalciuria, and low plasma renin but increased aldosterone levels. He has mutations in WNK 1 and WNK 4 kinases	5. No known medical treatment

Answers: A = 2; B = 2; C = 3; D = 5; E = 0.4 (see section on genetics for details). The patient described in choice A has Liddle syndrome, which is an autosomal dominant disorder. HTN responds to amiloride or triamterene, but not to spironolactone. Affected patients are at increased risk for cerebrovascular and cardiovascular disease.

The child described in choice B carries the diagnosis of the syndrome of apparent mineralocorticoid excess (AME), which is a rare autosomal recessive disorder. HTN responds to salt restriction, amiloride or triamterene but not to regular doses of spironolactone. Licorice ingestion induces a similar syndrome.

The clinical history described in choice C is consistent with the diagnosis of glucocorticoid-remediable hyperaldosteronism (GRA). Aldosterone secretion is stimulated by ACTH and not by angiotensin II. Therefore, administration of glucocorticoid suppresses excessive aldosterone secretion and improves HTN.

The possible diagnosis of the patient presented in choice D is a case of early-onset HTN with severe exacerbation during pregnancy. Pregnancy exacerbates HTN without proteinuria, edema, or neurologic changes. Aldosterone levels, which are elevated during pregnancy, are extremely low in MR gene mutation. MR antagonists such as spironolactone become agonists and increase blood pressure in patients with mutation in MR gene. Therefore, spironolactone is contraindicated in these patients. Progesterone also increases blood pressure in patients with MR gene mutation, since this hormone levels are extremely high in these patients. Hypertension improves following delivery.

The case in E represents pseudohypoaldosteronism type II (PHA II). It is called familial hyperkalemia and HTN or Gordon's syndrome. Thiazide diuretics improve HTN.

Suggested Reading

Garovic VD, Hilliard A, Turner S. Monogenic forms of low-renin hypertension. Nature Clin Pract Nephrol. 2006;2:624–30.
Williams SS. Advances in genetic hypertension. Curr Opin Pediatr. 2007;19:192–8.

67. A 72-year-old nonobese man with HTN for 2 years presents to the Emergency Department (ED) with shortness of breath. His BP is 168/102 mm Hg with a heart rate of 91 BPM. His clinic BP was 146/82 mm Hg. He is on HCTZ 25 mg, ramipril 10 mg and metoprolol succinate 100 mg (all are once daily). CXR shows pulmonary edema. His creatinine is 1.8 mg/dL (eGFR 42 mL/min), which increased from 1.2 mg/dL. **Which one of the following clinical clues is suggestive of renovascular hypertension (RVH) in this patient?**

A. BP >160/100 mm Hg (stage 2 HTN)
B. Deterioration of kidney function with treatment of HTN
C. Resistant HTN
D. Flash pulmonary edema or CHF
E. All of the above

The answer is E

There are several clues that are suggestive of RVH. Onset of HTN at age <30 years or >50 years, deterioration of kidney function despite treatment of HTN, uncontrolled HTN despite the use of three antihypertensive agents (resistant HTN), and development of flash pulmonary edema or CHF, or previous admissions for these two conditions, are some of the clinical clues to the diagnosis of RVH. This patient has all of the suggested criteria for RVH. Thus, option E is correct.

Another important clinical clue is an elderly patient with HTN who develops sudden deterioration in kidney function after the use of either an ACE-I or ARB is an indication of bilateral RVH.

Suggested Reading

Dworkin LD, Cooper CJ. Renal-artery stenosis. N Engl J Med. 2009;361:1972–8.
Textor SC. Renovascular hypertension and ischemic nephropathy. In: Taal MW, Chertow GM, Marsden PA, et al., editors. Brenner & Rector's the kidney. 9th ed. Philadelphia: Elsevier Saunders; 2012. p. 1752–91.

68. **In the above patient, which one of the following initial diagnostic tests is indicated?**

A. Captopril renography
B. CT angiography
C. Duplex Doppler ultrasonography
D. Magnetic resonance angiography (MRA)
E. Renal angiogram

The answer is C

The first four tests are noninvasive and used to diagnose RVH. However, captopril test is used to determine the renal blood flow and GFR in each kidney before and after administration of captopril. The stenotic kidney maintains GFR almost similar to the nonstenotic contralateral kidney because of high production of AII from renin. After captopril administration, GFR decreases because of suppression of AII. This indicates stenosis of the renal artery. Although it is cost-effective, the captopril test is not used widely because of several limitations. In this

patient, captopril test is not that useful, as he is already on ACE-I, and his kidney function is deteriorating. Thus, A is incorrect.

CT angiography using high-resolution multislice detector devices and contrast provides excellent images of the kidneys and vasculature. In this patient with decreased kidney function, CT angiography is not the initial choice of imaging study because of contrast use and development of AKI. Thus, B is incorrect.

MRA may require gadolinium, but it is a highly sensitive test for detecting proximal renal artery stenosis. Because of the development of nephrogenic systemic fibrosis, the use of MRA is limited, and in this patient, it is not the initial diagnostic test. Therefore, option D is incorrect.

Renal angiogram is the gold standard for defining the anatomy and vasculature of the kidney. However, it is invasive and is not the test of choice in this patient. Thus, E is incorrect.

Duplex Doppler ultrasonography provides functional and anatomic information of the kidney. With this technique, systolic flow velocity in the renal artery and aorta can be measured, and a comparative value yields the rate of stenosis. Systolic flow velocity increases in the stenotic artery, and a value >200 cm/sec represents stenosis >60%. Values >300 cm/sec represent severe stenosis. In this patient, duplex ultrasonography seems appropriate initial imaging study for detection of RVH. Thus, C is correct.

Suggested Reading

Dworkin LD, Cooper CJ. Renal-artery stenosis. N Engl J Med. 2009;361:1972–8.

Textor SC. Renovascular hypertension and ischemic nephropathy. In: Taal MW, Chertow GM, Marsden PA, et al., editors. Brenner & Rector's the kidney. 9th ed. Philadelphia: Elsevier Saunders; 2012. p. 1752–91.

69. In the above patient, duplex Doppler ultrasonography shows 50% of right renal artery stenosis. His creatinine and BP are stable. His antihypertensive medications include HCTZ 25 mg, ramipril 10 mg, and nebivolol 5 mg daily (metoprolol succinate discontinued). His pulmonary edema resolved. **The treatment of HTN in this patient with an ACE-I or ARB would result in which one of the following health outcomes?**

A. Decreased mortality
B. Decreased hospitalization for CHF
C. Delay in the initiation of chronic hemodialysis
D. Decreased incidence of stroke
E. All of the above

The answer is E

Many clinicians are reluctant to use either ACE-Is or ARBs in patients with renovascular hypertension (RVH) because of acute rise in serum creatinine and K^+. However, studies have shown that inhibition of renin-AII-aldosterone system (RAAS) is beneficial in patients with RVH. A Canadian study showed that RAAS inhibition caused lower rates of total mortality, decreased hospitalization for CHF, delayed initiation of chronic hemodialysis, and decreased incidence of stroke in elderly patients with RVH compared to patients on other antihypertensive agents. Thus, option E is correct. However, RAAS inhibition caused increased hospitalization for AKI. Despite this adverse effect, RAAS inhibition is indicated to improve CV and kidney outcomes. Additional antihypertensive drugs, such as diuretics, calcium blockers, or β-blockers, can be used to achieve goal BP.

Suggested Reading

Hackam DG, Duong-Hua ML, Mamdani M, et al. Angiotensin inhibition in renovascular disease: a population-based cohort study. Am Heart J. 2008;156:549–55.

Textor SC. Renovascular hypertension and ischemic nephropathy. In: Taal MW, Chertow GM, Marsden PA, et al., editors. Brenner & Rector's the kidney. 9th ed. Philadelphia: Elsevier Saunders; 2012. p. 1752–91.

Weber BR, Dieter RS. Renal artery stenosis: epidemiology and treatment. Int J Nephrol Renovasc Dis. 2014;13:169–81.

70. A 22-year-old woman presents to the ED with complaint of severe headache for the last 2 months, which is partially relieved by acetaminophen. Her BP is 210/110 mm Hg with a pulse rate of 82 BPM. She has no personal and family history of HTN. She is not on any medications other than occasional use of acetaminophen. Funduscopic examination shows grade 2–3 hypertensive retinopathy. Electrolytes and arterial blood gas show hypokalemic metabolic alkalosis.

Her creatinine and glucose are normal. Lipid profile is also normal. Her urine metanephrine levels are normal. Urine toxicology is negative. **Which one of the following diagnoses is MOST likely in this patient?**

A. Primary (essential) HTN
B. Pheochromocytoma
C. Atherosclerotic renovascular hypertension (aRVH)
D. Fibromuscular dysplasia
E. Drug-induced HTN

The answer is D

This patient is too young to have primary HTN with retinopathy. Also, aRVH is unlikely because of her age and normal serum creatinine and lipid levels. Pheochromocytoma is also unlikely in view of normal metanephrine and glucose levels. Drug-induced HTN will not present with retinopathy. Therefore, the most likely diagnosis is fibromuscular dysplasia, and some of the patients with this disease have the clinical presentation described in the present case.

Two most common types of RVH are fibromuscular dysplasia and atherosclerosis. Fibromuscular dysplasia is a nonatherosclerotic and noninflammatory condition with severe HTN and usually presents in childhood and child-bearing age. Most commonly the media of the vessel hypertrophies and causes stenosis, which is away from the renal artery ostium. Renal perfusion decreases with elevation in serum creatinine. However, some patients present with HTN prior to elevation in serum creatinine.

Almost all the imaging studies of RVH can be used; however, the Doppler ultrasonography is the recommended imaging technique for fibromuscular dysplasia. Renal vessels appear as "string-of-beads" on the imaging techniques.

There are no studies comparing medical treatment with revascularization in patients with fibromuscular dysplasia. Therefore, the treatment should be individualized. The goals of therapy are to control BP, to preserve renal mass and function, and to prevent CV events. Balloon angioplasty with bailout stent placement, if necessary, is chosen by many clinicians as it is safe and also reduces the number of antihypertensive agents to maintain goal BP. Surgery is indicated for patients with segmental arteries and those with microaneurysms. The cure rate of HTN with balloon angioplasty varies from 22% to 59% with no effect in 7% to 30% of patients. Thus, antihypertensive treatment is indicated in many patients even after revascularization.

Suggested Reading

Meuse MA, Turba UC, Sabri SS, et al. Treatment of renal artery fibromuscular dysplasia. Tech Vasc Intervent Radiol. 2010;13:126–33.

Slovut DP, Olin JW. Fibromuscular dysplasia. N Engl J Med. 2004;350:1862–71.

Textor SC. Renovascular hypertension and ischemic nephropathy. In: Taal MW, Chertow GM, Marsden PA, et al., editors. Brenner & Rector's the kidney. 9th ed. Philadelphia: Elsevier Saunders; 2012. p. 1752–91.

71. A 68-year-old man is found to have severe HTN and unilateral atherosclerotic renal artery stenosis. **Which one of the following criteria is an indication for revascularization (percutaneous transluminal renal angioplasty, PTRA)?**

A. Rapid elevation in BP prior to diagnosis of renal artery stenosis
B. Progression of renal dysfunction
C. Uncontrolled HTN despite the use of three or more different classes of antihypertensive agents
D. Flash pulmonary edema
E. All of the above

The answer is E

All of the above criteria warrant revascularization in a patient with unilateral renal artery stenosis (E). Surgery is indicated in those with complex anatomical lesions. PTRA with stent placement causes normalization of BP in 3–68%, improvement in BP in 5–61%, no effect on BP in 0–61%, and restenosis in 8–30% at 2 years. Thus, PTRA with stenting is beneficial in patients with unilateral stenosis who meet all of the above criteria.

Suggested Reading

Ritchie J, Green D, Chryschou C, et al. High-risk clinical presentations in atherosclerotic renovascular disease: prognosis and response to renal artery revascularization. Am J Kidney Dis. 2014;63:186–97.

Textor SC. Renal artery stenosis, renovascular hypertension, and ischemic nephropathy. In: Coffman TM, Falk RJ, Molitoris BA, et al., editors. Schrier's diseases of the kidney. 9th ed. Philadelphia: Wolters Kluwer/Lippincott Williams & Wilkins; 2013. p. 1153–96.

Textor S. Treatment of unilateral atherosclerotic renal artery stenosis. Up ToDate; 2014.

72. A 64-year-old woman with type 2 diabetes, HTN, CKD 3, and coronary heart disease is admitted for shortness of breath. CXR reveals pulmonary edema. Her BP is 164/98 mm Hg with a heart rate of 82 BPM. Her medications include furosemide 40 mg twice daily, amlodipine 10 mg daily, nebivolol 5 mg daily, and spironolactone 50 mg daily. Her HbA1c is 7.7%. She developed angioedema on ramipril, and AKI on an ARB. A captopril renogram showed decreased function in the right more than the left kidney with normal kidney size. Her serum creatinine has been increasing slowly, reaching close to stage 4 CKD. **Based on recent clinical studies of medical therapy versus revascularization, which one of the following decisions is more appropriate for this patient?**

A. Continue current management
B. Percutaneous transluminal renal angioplasty (PTRA) with stenting of the right kidney
C. PTRA with stenting of both kidneys
D. Surgery of the right kidney
E. A and B only

The answer is C

This patient's BP is high and her creatinine is increasing. Although RAAS inhibition can control her BP, it is not advisable to use angiotensin inhibitors in view of severe adverse effects, as noted previously. Flash pulmonary edema is suggestive of severe renovascular stenosis. Maintaining current management and stenting the right kidney are not appropriate decisions. Decreased function in both kidneys on captopril renogram suggests bilateral renal artery stenosis. Therefore, stenting both renal arteries is appropriate. Thus, C is correct.

A recent study showed that high-risk patients with bilateral renal artery disease and flash pulmonary edema benefit from PTRA with stenting. They also suggest that patients with both resistant HTN and declining kidney function benefit from revascularization. Therefore, this patient qualifies for bilateral stenting to improve her CV and renal outcomes.

Suggested Reading

Ritchie J, Green D, Chryschou C, et al. High-risk clinical presentations in atherosclerotic renovascular disease: prognosis and response to renal artery revascularization. Am J Kidney Dis. 2014;63:186–97.

Textor SC, Lerman LO. Reality and renovascular disease: when does renal artery stenosis warrant revascularization? Am J Kidney Dis. 2014;63:175–7.

73. **Which one of the following trials showed that renal revascularization (percutaneous renal artery angioplasty (PTRA) with stenting) is superior to medical therapy alone in improving renal and cardiovascular (CV) outcomes in patients with renal artery stenosis?**

A. DRASTIC (Dutch Renal Artery Stenosis Intervention) trial
B. ASTRAL (Angioplasty and Stent Therapy for Renal Artery Lesions) trial
C. STAR (Stent Placement in patients with Atherosclerotic Renal artery stenosis) trial
D. CORAL (Cardiovascular Outcomes in Renal Atherosclerotic Lesions) trial
E. None of the above

The answer is E

A meta-analysis of six studies excluding the CORAL trial showed that in patients with renal artery stenosis, PTRA with stenting did not show any improvement in serum creatinine or CV outcomes, as compared with medical treatment alone. Also, the CORAL trial did not show any benefit of PTRA over medical therapy alone. Thus, E is correct. The following Table 6.6 summarizes some findings of the above four studies.

Table 6.6 Characteristics of the studies that compared PTRA plus medical therapy with medical therapy alone

	DRASTIC	ASTRAL	STAR	CORAL
No. of patients	106	806	140	947
Age (mean)	60	70.5	66.5	69
Inclusion criteria	Resistant HTN	HTN/CKD	CKD	HTN/CKD
F/U (mon)	12	34 (median)	24	48 (median)
Creatinine	1.3	2.0	1.7	58 mL/min (eGFR)
BP decrease (mm Hg)				
Medical therapy alone	17/1	8/4	8/3	15.6 (SBP)
PTRA + meds	19/11	6/3	9/6	16.6 (SBP)
Outcomes between groups	No difference	No difference	No difference	No difference

Suggested Reading

Box L, Woittiez AJ, Kouwenberg HJ, et al. Stent placement in patients with atherosclerotic renal artery stenosis and impaired renal function: a randomized trial. Ann Intern Med. 2009;150:840–8.

Cooper CJ, Murphy TP, Cutlip DE, et al. For the CORAL Investigators. Stenting and medical therapy for atherosclerotic renal-artery stenosis. N Engl J Med. 2014;370:13–22.

Kumbhani DJ, Bavry AA, Harvey JE, et al. Clinical outcomes after percutaneous revascularization versus medical management in patients with significant renal artery stenosis: a meta-analysis of randomized controlled trials. Am Heart J. 2011;161:622–30.

The ASTRAL Investigators. Revascularization versus medical therapy for renal-artery stenosis. N Engl J Med. 2009;361:1953–62.

van Jaarsveld BC, Krijnen P, Pieterman H, et al. The effect of balloon angioplasty on hypertension in atherosclerotic renal-artery stenosis. Dutch Renal Artery Stenosis Intervention Cooperative Study Group. N Engl J Med. 2000;342:1007–14.

74. A 68-year-old woman with severe right atherosclerotic renal artery stenosis (>80% occlusion) receives angioplasty with stent placement. **After 3 months of the procedure, improvement in which one of the following biochemical and hemodynamic changes can occur?**

A. GFR
B. Inflammatory markers
C. Tissue hypoxia
D. Renal blood flow
E. C and D

The answer is E

In animals, microvascular changes occur distal to the renal artery stenosis. These microvascular changes lead to tissue hypoxia, rarefaction of the vessels, inflammation, and fibrogenesis. Such studies are lacking in humans. Recently, Saad et al. showed that renal artery stent placement in patients with >60% occlusion of one renal artery improves hypoxia and renal blood flow. However, there is no improvement in GFR and inflammatory mediators (TNF-α, or monocyte chemoattractant protein-1). Also, neutrophil gelatinase-associated lipocalin, a marker of tubulointerstitial disease, is not reversed by stent placement. Additional measures to improve GFR and inflammatory cytokines are needed. Thus, E is correct.

Suggested Reading

Saad A, Herrmann SMS, Crane J, et al. Stent revascularization restores cortical blood flow and reverses tissue hypoxia in atherosclerotic renal artery stenosis, but fails to reverse inflammatory pathways or glomerular filtration rate. Circ Cardiovasc Interv. 2013;6:428–35.

Textor SC, Lerman LO. Reality and renovascular disease: when does renal artery stenosis warrant revascularization? Am J Kidney Dis. 2014;63:175–7.

75. A 56-year-old non-obese man is brought to the ED for severe headache, tremor, and increased sweating. His BP is 220/140 mm Hg with a heart rate of 128 BPM. Laboratory data are normal except for glucose of 160 mg/dL. His daughter says that he lost 10–15 lbs. in the last 3 months. The patient is alert and oriented. **Which one of the following diagnoses is MOST likely in this patient?**

A. Hypertensive urgency
B. Primary aldosteronism
C. Renovascular HTN
D. Pheochromocytoma
E. Cushing's syndrome

The answer is D

The patient presents with typical manifestations of pheochromocytoma, which is a catecholamine-secreting tumor of adrenal chromaffin cells. About 10% of the pheochromocytomas occur outside the adrenal glands, and are referred to as paragangliomas. The triad of headache, sweating, and tachycardia is a common presentation of pheochromocytomas, but orthostatic hypotension and dizziness can also present in some patients. As there are no electrolyte or renal abnormalities, which commonly accompany primary aldosteronism, renovascular HTN, and Cushing's syndrome, these diagnoses can be ruled out. Hypertensive urgency does not present with above symptoms. Thus, D is the most likely diagnosis in this patient.

Suggested Reading

Adler JT, Meyer-Rochow GY, Chen H, et al. Pheochromocytoma: current approaches and future directions. Oncologist. 2008;13:779–93.

Young WF Jr. Adrenal causes of hypertension: pheochromocytoma and primary aldosteronism. Rev Endocrinol Met Disord. 2007;8:309–20.

76. The diagnosis of pheochromocytoma was made with appropriate laboratory tests and imaging studies. The tumor was removed and postoperative course was uneventful. No residual tumor activity was noticed. **Regarding long-term follow-up, which one the following tests is appropriate?**

A. Yearly CT of the abdomen
B. Yearly genetic testing
C. Yearly plasma metanephrines only
D. Yearly plasma metanephrines and CT of abdomen
E. No further follow-up

The answer is C

Successful resection of tumor does not guarantee recurrence after many years. Indeed, it has been reported the recurrence of the tumor, or the development of malignant disease years later. Therefore, yearly plasma or urine metanephrine measurements should be performed. Imaging and biochemical studies are required, if the patient presents with signs and symptoms of recurrent pheochromocytoma. Annual follow-up for life is required for patients with genetic disease, whereas an indefinite follow-up is required for sporadic cases of pheochromocytoma. Thus, option C is correct.

Many clinicians recommend measurement of plasma metanephrines as a first-line test because of its high sensitivity (99%) and specificity (85–90%). However, the routine practice is to measure plasma and 24-h urinary catecholamines (norepinephrine, epinephrine, and dopamine) and normetanephrine and metanephrine. Genetic testing is required in young patients.

Suggested Reading

Adler JT, Meyer-Rochow GY, Chen H, et al. Pheochromocytoma: current approaches and future directions. Oncologist. 2008;13:779–93.

Plouin PF, Chatellier G, Fofol I, et al. Tumor recurrence and hypertension persistence after successful pheochromocytoma operation. Hypertension. 1997;29: 1133–9.

Young WF Jr. Adrenal causes of hypertension: pheochromocytoma and primary aldosteronism. Rev Endocrinol Met Disord. 2007;8:309–20.

77. A 48-year-old African American woman is referred to you for the management of HTN. Her BP is 168/102 mm Hg with a heart rate of 74 BPM. She is on nifedipine XL 90 mg daily, labetalol 300 mg twice daily, and chlorthalidone 25 mg daily. Despite on diuretic, she started gaining weight, and she could not wear her wedding ring. She attributes her weight due to fat accumulation. Gradually, her face started to swell, and she gained 10 kg in 2 months. **Which one of the following initial tests is MOST cost-effective in this patient?**

A. Plasma catecholamines and metanephrine
B. Plasma renin and aldosterone
C. CT of abdomen
D. 24-h urine cortisol
E. Ultrasound of abdomen

The answer is D

Based on the history and uncontrolled HTN, this patient has clinical manifestations of Cushing's syndrome. Therefore, the measurement of 24-h urinary cortisol is an appropriate and cost-effective test. A 24-h urinary cortisol reflects daily circulating serum cortisol levels. Once cortisol level is high, CT of abdomen is the next appropriate study for evaluation of adrenal mass. Thus, D is correct. She has no signs and symptoms of pheochromocytoma, and the measurement of plasma catecholamines and metanephrines may not be necessary. Patients with primary aldosteronism may present with resistant hypertension, but such an increase in weight is unlikely. Ultrasound of abdomen may give nonspecific findings. Thus, choices A, B, C, and E are incorrect.

In this patient, CT of abdomen was negative, but an MRI of head revealed a pituitary microadenoma, and resection of the tumor resulted in normalization of BP. Thus, she had Cushing's disease.

Suggested Reading

Singer E, Strohm S, Göbel U, et al. Cushing's disease, hypertension, and other sequels. Hypertension. 2008;52:1001–5.
Singh Y, Kotwal N, Menon AS. Endocrine hypertension-Cushing's syndrome. Indian J Endocrinol Metab. 2011;15(suppl):S313–6.

78. A 65-year-old man with CKD 4 and resistant HTN (≥3 antihypertensive drugs, including a diuretic) had renal denervation. **Renal denervation influences which one of the following hemodynamic changes in this patient?**

A. A decrease in BP
B. Stabilization of GFR
C. A decrease in albuminuria
D. A nonsignificant increase in hemoglobin (Hgb)
E. All of the above

The answer is E

Renal denervation has been shown to improve resistant hypertension. The requirement for the number of antihypertensive medications has also decreased after renal denervation. Although most of the studies included patients with normal kidney function, a study by Schlaich's group reported their findings on 15 patients with CKD stages 3–4 (mean eGFR 31 mL/min/1.73 m^2) and resistant hypertension. Prior to bilateral denervation, their mean blood pressure was 174/91 mm Hg despite on >4 antihypertensive medications. Renal denervation reduced their blood pressure by 34/14, 25/11, 32/15, and 33/19 mm Hg at 1, 3, 6, 12 months, respectively. Also, a significant decrease in nighttime ambulatory blood pressure was observed, suggesting restoration of physiologic dipping. There was no change in eGFR during the follow-up period. In these patients, a substantial decrease in proteinuria was reported at 3 and 6 months after renal denervation. Also, a trend toward an increase in Hgb was also noticed following renal denervation. In patients with normal kidney function, a decrease in renal resistive index has been reported following renal denervation. Thus, E is correct.

Suggested Reading

Hering D, Mahfoud F, Walton AS, et al. Renal denervation in moderate to severe CKD. J Am Soc Nephrol. 2012;23:1250–7.
Xu J, Hering D, Sata Y, et al. Renal denervation: current implications and future perspectives. Clin Sci. 2014;126:41–53.

79. **Similar to renal denervation, baroreflex activation therapy (BAT) has also been shown to improve which one of the following hemodynamic changes in patients with resistant HTN and congestive heart failure (CHF)?**

A. Sustained decrease in BP of 30/17 mm Hg for 5 years
B. Sustained decrease in heart rate for 5 years
C. An increase in cardiac output in a canine model of CHF
D. No change in GFR at 1 year
E. All of the above

The answer is E

Baroreceptors are stretch receptors that respond to changes in BP via sympathetic and parasympathetic nerves. Thus, the carotid baroreflex is an important mechanism in the maintenance of short- and long-term BP. Diminished baroreflex activation is seen in patients with high and resistant HTN. Several recent trials have shown that BAT maintains sustained decrease in BP and heart rate for as long as 5 years. In a canine model of CHF, BAT increased ejection fraction, and stroke volume. However, in a study of 12 patients, BAT did not show any changes in GFR at 1 year. Thus, option E is correct.

Suggested Reading

Bakris G, Nadim M, Haller H, et al. Baroreflex activation therapy safely reduces blood pressure for at least five years in a large hypertension cohort. J Am Soc Hypertens. 2014;8:e10.
Bisognano JD, Bakris G, Nadim MK, et al. Baroreflex activation therapy lowers blood pressure in patients with resistant hypertension. Results from the double-blind, randomized, placebo-controlled Rheos pivotal trial. J Am Coll Cardiol. 2011;58:765–73.
Taylor JC, Bisognano JD. Baroreflex stimulation in antihypertensive treatment. Curr Hypertens Rep. 2010;12:176–81.

80. Many epidemiological studies have associated serum uric acid level with the development of HTN. **Which one of the following statements is CORRECT regarding the link between uric acid and HTN?**

A. Serum uric acid level >5.5 mg/dL confers a twofold rise of HTN in adolescents
B. Early HTN is reversible with reduction in uric acid
C. Early HTN is caused by increased renal renin secretion and low plasma nitrate levels
D. Chronic HTN, which is irreversible, is caused by altered vascular changes
E. All of the above

The answer is E

The link between uric acid and incident HTN has been suggested as early as 1972, and this association has been confirmed by many epidemiological studies. Possible mechanisms of this association include increased production of renin and reduced circulating levels of nitrate with resultant vasoconstriction. Later, HTN is related to altered vascular architecture caused by uric acid-induced changes in vascular smooth muscle cells and subsequent induction of cytokines. Early HTN can respond to allopurinol with improvement in BP and kidney function. Thus, E is correct.

Suggested Reading

Feig DI. Serum uric acid and the risk of hypertension and CKD. Curr Opin Rheumatol. 2014;26:176–85.
Reynolds TM. Serum uric acid new-onset hypertension: a possible therapeutic avenue. J Hum Hypertes. 2014;28:519–20.

81. Activation of renin-AII-aldosterone system (RAAS) is an important mechanism for the maintenance of chronic HTN. ACE-Is inhibit angiotensin-converting enzyme (ACE), and improve BP. A new enzyme has been identified, which is called ACE 2. **Which one of the following statements is CORRECT regarding ACE 2 of the renin-AII system?**

A. ACE 2 converts AII (octapeptide) to angiotensin 1–7 peptide
B. ACE 2 has vasodilatory properties
C. ACE 2 does not convert AI to AII
D. Compounds that enhance ACE 2 activity lower BP
E. All of the above

The answer is E

AII is formed from AI by the action of ACE, and AII exerts its vasoconstrictor effects via AT1 receptor. Recently, an endogenous antagonist of AII has been identified and is called angiotensin 1–7 peptide. This peptide is formed from AII by the enzyme ACE 2. Angiotensin 1–7 peptide is vasodilatory and opposes the pressor, proliferative, and profibrotic actions of AII. The actions of this peptide occur via Mas receptor. ACE-Is and ARBs increase the plasma levels of angiotensin 1–7 peptide. ACE 2 deficiency is associated with the development of HTN. Studies using compounds that enhance the activity of ACE 2 are found to lower BP in hypertensive rats. Xanthenone, an activator of ACE 2, caused a dose-dependent decrease in BP in spontaneously hypertensive rats with resultant remodeling of the myocardium and improvement in renal fibrosis. Thus, activators of ACE 2 appear to be novel therapeutic agents for the treatment of HTN. However, ACE 2 has no effect on ACE; therefore, it does not convert AI to AII. Thus, option E is correct.

Suggested Reading

Ferrario CM. ACE2: more of Ang-(1-7) or less AII. Curr Opin Nephrol Hypertens. 2011;20:1–6.

Tikellis C, Bernardi S, Burns WC. Angiotensin-converting enzyme 2 is a key modulator of the renin-angiotensin system in cardiovascular and renal disease. Curr Opin Nephrol Hypertens. 2011;20:62–8.

Chapter 7
Renal Pharmacology

1. A 50-year-old man with edema is given furosemide 80 mg orally to improve his edema. **In order to be familiar with pharmacokinetics of the drugs, which one of the following statements regarding volume of distribution (Vd) of a drug is CORRECT?**

   A. Protein binding
   B. Molecular weight and solubility
   C. Changes in extracellular fluid (ECF) volume status
   D. Tissue penetration and binding
   E. All of the above

   The answer is E

   Simply Vd (also called the apparent volume of distribution) refers to the distribution of a drug in body compartments, which include plasma, water, red blood cells, and tissue or organ binding. Vd is not a real but a theoretical volume. It is defined as the ratio of total amount of drug in the body to its concentration in plasma, or

$$\mathbf{Vd = \frac{Total\ amount\ of\ drug\ in\ the\ body}{Plasma\ drug\ concentration}}$$

   The following example gives an idea of Vd of a drug:
   The patient receives a bolus of 500 mg of a drug intravenously, and 1 h later the plasma concentration of the drug is 20 mg/L. The Vd of the drug is as follows:

$$\mathbf{\frac{500}{20} = 25\,L}$$

   This means that the Vd for this drug is 25 L, or the drug is distributed in 25 L (0.36 L/kg in a 70 kg subject).

   A drug that is highly protein bound (mostly to albumin) remains in plasma. Water-soluble drugs remain in the extracellular fluid space and have a small Vd. The Vd increases, if the patient has edema, ascites, or infection. In such cases, the plasma concentration of a particular drug is decreased. As a result, usual doses of a drug will result in low plasma concentrations. When total body water decreases as in volume depletion, the plasma concentration of a drug increases, but the Vd is decreased. Lipid-soluble drugs have a high Vd because the drug can penetrate the cell membrane and accumulate in adipose tissue. The increase in Vd causes low plasma concentration of the drug. Thus, an inverse relationship exists between Vd and plasma concentration. Certain drugs such as chloroquine bind to liver DNA or tetracycline to bone. Patients on these or similar drugs have tissue concentrations several times higher than blood concentrations, and improper dosing may cause severe adverse reactions. Thus, option E is correct.

A. S. Reddi, *Absolute Nephrology Review*, https://doi.org/10.1007/978-3-030-85958-9_7

Suggested Reading

Dooque MP, Polasek TM. The ABCD of clinical pharmacokinetics. Ther Adv Drug Saf. 2013;4:5–7.
Greenblatt DJ, Abourjally PN. Pharmacokinetics and pharmacodynamics for medical students: a proposed course outline. J Clin Pharmacol. 2016;56:1180–95.
Varghese JM, Roberts JA, Lipman J. Pharmacokinetics and pharmacodynamics in critically ill patients. Curr Opin Anaesthesiol. 2010;23:472–8.

2. A 46-year-old woman with hepatitis C cirrhosis and ascites is on furosemide 80 mg/day and spironolactone 200 mg/day. Her serum albumin is 2.4 g/dL. **Regarding volume of distribution (Vd) of furosemide, which one of the following choices is CORRECT?**

   A. Decreased
   B. Increased
   C. Not measurable
   D. Unchanged from normal subject without ascites
   E. None of the above

   The answer is B

   Furosemide is highly albumin bound (90–95%). In a normal individual with serum albumin concentration of 4.2 g/dL, furosemide is bound to albumin, and <5–10% of the drug is free. Therefore, the Vd of furosemide is about 3.4 L. In a hypoalbuminemic patient, the amount of free drug is extremely large, and therefore, the Vd is large or increased. Thus, choice B is correct, and other choices are inappropriate.

Suggested Reading

Brater DC. Diuretic pharmacokinetics and pharmacodynamics. In: Seldin D, Giebisch G, editors. Diuretic agents. Clinical physiology and pharmacology. San Diego: Academic Press; 1997. p. 189–208.
Hoorn EJ, Wilcox CJ, Ellison DH. Diuretics. In: Yu ASL, Chertow GM, Luyckx VA, et al., editors. Brenner & Rector's the kidney. 11th ed. Philadelphia: Elsevier Saunders; 2020. p. 1708–40.

3. **Many drugs are bound to albumin. Which one of the following statements regarding drug-albumin binding is CORRECT?**

   A. Formation of drug-albumin complex is a reversible process that is dependent on the concentration of drug and albumin
   B. Only the unbound drug is able to have a pharmacological effect
   C. Only the unbound drug is able to distribute into body tissues and determines the drug's volume of distribution (Vd)
   D. Only the unbound fraction of drug is available for elimination from the vascular compartment
   E. All of the above

   The answer is E

   All of the statements are correct regarding the drug-albumin binding. Binding of a drug to albumin is mostly a reversible process that is dependent on the concentration of drug and albumin. Pharmacologically, the drug-albumin complex has three important implications: first, it is the free (unbound) drug that has a pharmacologic effect; second, it is the only free drug that distributes into various tissues of the body and can influence drug's Vd; and finally, the bound fraction of the drug acts as a reservoir in the vascular compartment where dissociation of the drug-albumin complex provides free drug availability for further action and, subsequently, elimination from the body.

Suggested Reading

Buxton ILO, Benet LZ. Pharmacokinetics: the dynamics of drug absorption, distribution, metabolism, and elimination. In: Brunton LL, editor. Goodman and Gilman's the pharmacologic basis of therapeutics. 12th ed. New York: McGraw Hill; 2011. p. 17–37.
Ulldemolins M, Roberts J, Rello J, et al. The effects of hypoalbuminemia on optimizing antibacterial dosing in critically ill patients. Clin Pharmacokinet. 2011;50:99–110.

4. Chronic kidney disease (CKD), particularly CKD stages 4 and 5, affects pharmacokinetics of several drugs that are commonly used in patients with these stages of CKD. There is now evidence that severe CKD may lead to reductions in nonrenal clearance of many drugs. **Which one of the following alterations accounts for the reduction in nonrenal clearance of drugs?**

   A. Inhibition of hepatic cytochrome P450 enzymes
   B. A defect in intestinal transport mechanisms
   C. Altered pharmacokinetics of drugs can be reversed by kidney transplantation or temporarily by hemodialysis
   D. All of the above
   E. None of the above

   The answer is D

   The pharmacokinetic principles of drug absorption, distribution, metabolism, and excretion are influenced by the coordinated action of many different drug metabolism enzymes, including CYP 450 (CYP), and drug transporters in the intestines, liver, and kidney. CYPs are a family of enzymes located in the endoplasmic reticulum of the cell, which are responsible for the metabolism of 90% of the drugs. There are several classes of CYPs and named differently. For example, CYP3A4 refers to the root CYP family 3, subfamily A, and gene number 4. There are six classes of CYPs that are involved in pharmacokinetic processes of drugs, namely CYP1A2, CYP2C9, CYP2C19, CYP2D6, CYP3A4, and CYP3A5. A drug can be metabolized by either a single CYP enzyme or multiple CYP enzymes, and the drug is converted into more polar inactive metabolite that is readily eliminated in the bile or urine than the parent compound.

   CYP enzymes are predominantly localized in the liver, and uremic toxins are found to inhibit both the synthesis and activity of these enzymes. Thus, severe CKD alters the pharmacokinetic properties of the drugs by inhibiting the hepatic CYP enzymes so that the metabolism of the drugs is reduced. As a result, the half-life of the parent compound is prolonged (answers A is correct).

   CYPs are also present in the intestine and play an important role in orally absorbed drugs. In CKD, CYPs levels are decreased with resulting decrease in first-pass extraction. In general, bioavailability of oral drugs (i.e., the quantity of drug reaching the blood circulation) depends mostly on intestinal and hepatic metabolism and intestinal drug transport. Intestinal drug transport is mediated by several membrane transporters, such as P-glycoprotein and multidrug resistance-related protein-2. Studies have shown that uremic toxins inhibit these intestinal transporters and decrease the bioavailability of the oral drug. Thus, answer B is correct.

   Studies have shown that kidney transportation normalizes both the hepatic and intestinal abnormalities of drug metabolism. Also, hemodialysis temporarily reverses the abnormal pharmacokinetics of the drugs (answer C is correct).

   It should be noted that drug clearance is generally decreased in AKI. Data from animal and human studies suggest that nonrenal clearance of drugs is also decreased. Therefore, clinicians should consider dose adjustments of hepatically metabolized drugs in patients with AKI. Monitoring serum drug concentrations can avoid severe adverse effects in both AKI and CKD patients.

   Suggested Reading

Ladda MA, Goralski KB. The effects of CKD on cytochrome P450-mediated drug metabolism. Adv Chronic Kidney Dis. 2016;23:67–75.

Lea-Henry TN, Carland JE, Stocker SL, et al. Clinical pharmacokinetics in kidney disease. Fundamental principles. Clin J Am Soc Nephrol. 2018;13:1085–95.

Naud J, Michaud J, Boisvert C, et al. Down-regulation of Intestinal drug transporters in chronic renal failure in rats. J Pharmacol Exp Ther. 2007;320:978–85.

Robersts DM, Sevastos J, Carland JE, et al. Clinical pharmacokinetics in kidney disease. Application to rational design of dosing regimens. Clin J Am Soc Nephrol. 2018;13:1254–63.

5. A 40-year-old obese woman is being treated with vancomycin for methicillin-resistant *Staphalococcus aureus*. She has an eGFR of >60 mL/min and albumin concentration of 2.1 g/dL. **Which one of the following statements regarding vancomycin in hypoalbuminemic obese patient is FALSE?**

   A. Total body weight–based initial dosing achieves adequate therapeutic levels
   B. Vd of vancomycin increases in obese patients irrespective of albumin levels

C. Only obese patients with hypoalbuminemia demonstrate increased Vd for vancomycin
D. Clearance of vancomycin increases in obesity
E. Patients with >101 kg and/or with doses >4.5 g/day are at risk for nephrotoxicity

The answer is C

Obesity is associated with altered pharmacokinetic properties of several antibiotics, including vancomycin. Studies have shown that the Vd increases in obesity due to hydrophilic nature of vancomycin even in the presence of normal albumin levels. Thus, answer C is false. Clearance of vancomycin is increased in obesity. Also, binding of vancomycin to proteins is increased in obese patients, thus making less availability of unbound drug. Initial dose of vancomycin should be based on the total body weight (25 mg/kg initially up to 2 g and subsequent dose not to exceed 4.5 g per day) to achieve adequate therapeutic levels, and subsequent dosages are dependent on trough levels. It has been shown that obese patients >100 kg in weight and those who receive >4.5 g/day are at increased risk for vancomycin-induced nephrotoxicity. Therefore, dose adjustment and frequency are necessary in patients with renal dysfunction. Maintenance dose should also be based on total body weight.

Recently, many nomograms were developed for vancomycin dosage in obese individuals. This dose was calculated based on the area under the curve (AUC) of vancomycin dose for 24 h. Use of AUC dose avoids nephrotoxicity. The clinician needs the advice of pharmacist in the calculation of vancomycin dose for patients with normal or decreased kidney function.

Please remember the following calculations in case of calculating IDW and adjusted body weight:

$$\textbf{Total body wt}\left(\textbf{TBW}\right) = \textbf{Patient's actual body wt}$$
$$\textbf{Ideal body wt}\left(\textbf{IBW}\right) = \textbf{Male : 50 kg + 2.3 kg for each inch above 5 feet}$$
$$\textbf{Female : 45 kg + 2.3 kg for each inch above 5 feet}$$
$$\textbf{Adjusted body wt}\left(\textbf{kg}\right) = \textbf{IBW} + \textbf{0.4}\left(\textbf{TBW} - \textbf{IBW}\right)$$

Suggested Reading

Crass RL, Dunn R, Hong J, et al. Dosing vancomycin in the super obese: less is more. J Antimicrob Chemother. 2018;73:3081–86.

Grace E. Altered vancomycin pharmacokinetics in obese and morbidly obese patients: what we have learned over the past 30 years. Antimicrob Chemother. 2012;67:1305–10.

Johnson B, Thursky K. Dosing of antibiotics in obesity. Curr Opin Infect Dis. 2012;25:634–49.

6. **Regarding vancomycin adverse effects, which one of the following choices is CORRECT?**

A. Acute kidney injury (AKI)
B. Ototoxicity in combination with aminoglycosides
C. Red man syndrome (infusion reaction)
D. Thrombocytopenia
E. All of the above

The answer is E

Vancomycin-induced nephrotoxicity has been well established with both the first- and second-generation preparations of the drug. The incidence of vancomycin-induced AKI may be related to several factors, including staphylococcal epidemic, healthcare-associated pneumonia, osteomyelitis due to prosthetic hardwares, drug abuse, diabetes, etc., and the development of methicillin-resistant *staphylococcus aureus*. On kidney biopsy, acute tubulointerstitial nephritis is commonly demonstrated as a cause of AKI. Combination of vancomycin and aminoglycosides is more nephrotoxic than either drug alone.

Red man syndrome is an idiopathic infusion reaction of vancomycin. Some authors prefer to use the term "infusion-reaction" instead of Red man syndrome. Any way, it is a hypersensitivity reaction characterized by flushing, erythema, and pruritis in the upper body, neck, and face. Hypotension, muscle spasm, and chest tightness may also occur.

Vancomycin-induced thrombocytopenia is rather rare, but several cases have been reported. Thrombocytopenia is due to the development of antiplatelet antibodies, and severe bleeding can occur. Thus, choice E is correct.

Suggested Reading

Alvarez-Arango S, Ogunwole SM, Sequist TD, et al. Vancomycin infusion reaction – moving beyond "Red Man Syndrome". N Engl J Med. 2021;384:1283–6.

Bilal A, Abu-Romeh A, Rousan TA, et al. Vancomycin-induced nephrotoxicity. In: Sahay M, editor. Basic nephrology and acute kidney injury. InTech; 2012. p. 183–226.

Morales-Alvarez MC. Nephrotoxicity of antimicrobials and antibiotics. Adv Chronic Kidney Dis. 2020;27:31–7.

Sivagnanam S, Deleu D. Commentary. Red man syndrome. Crit Care. 2003;7:110–20.

von Drygalski A, Curtis BR, Bougie DW, et al. Vancomycin-induced immune thrombocytopenia. N Engl J Med. 2007;356:904–10.

7. A 46-year-old man with cirrhosis due to hepatitis C and chronic kidney disease (CKD) stage 3b is admitted for fever, elevated white blood cell (WBC) count, and bacteremia. He was admitted with similar diagnosis 3 months ago and was successfully treated with penicillin-related antibiotics. He is now started on high doses of penicillin products with improvement in fever and WBC count. While he is being planned for discharge, the nurse noticed seizure activity, which lasted for 3 min. **What is the next appropriate step in the management of his seizure activity that is CORRECT?**

   A. Request a nephrology consult for hemodialysis
   B. Request a neurology consult for EEG monitoring
   C. Reduce the dose of penicillin and related antibiotics to <6 g/day
   D. Start antiseizure medications for life
   E. Do nothing

   The answer is C

   Many antibacterial agents are water soluble with low molecular weight. They are also less protein bound. As a result, they appear in the urine unchanged. In renal failure, dosage reduction in these antibiotics is required. About 20% of the penicillin dose is also excreted in bile. Penicillins and related antibiotics reduce seizure threshold even in normal subjects. Besides seizures, other central nervous system (CNS) toxicities include myoclonus and coma. High doses of penicillin >8–12 g/day (>20 million units of penicillin G/day) predispose patients with CKD and liver failure to seizures. Also, localized CNS lesions and hyponatremia predispose patients to seizure activity with high doses of penicillins.

   In the above patient, reducing penicillin dosage to <6 g/day (option C) is appropriate. Other options are incorrect.

Suggested Reading

Petri WA Jr. Penicillins, cephalosporins, and other β-lactam antibiotics. In: Brunton LL, editor. Goodman and Gilman's the pharmacologic basis of therapeutics. 12th ed. New York: McGraw Hill; 2011. p. 1477–503.

Wallace KL. Antibiotic-induced convulsions. Crit Care Clin. 1997;13:741–62.

8. A 26-year-old woman with recurrent urinary tract infection is admitted for acute pyelonephritis. Urine culture shows *E. coli*, which is sensitive only to gentamicin. Her kidney function is normal. After a loading dose, she is maintained on therapeutic doses of gentamicin. Ten days later, she develops hypokalemia, metabolic alkalosis, hypomagnesemia, and hypocalcemia with normal blood pressure. **Which one of the following syndromes has been described with the use of gentamicin?**

   A. Gitelman syndrome
   B. Bartter syndrome type V
   C. Liddle syndrome
   D. Gordon syndrome
   E. Laboratory error

   The answer is B

   Gentamicin and other aminoglycosides have been shown to induce a Bartter-like syndrome characterized by hypokalemia, metabolic alkalosis, hypomagnesemia, hypocalcemia, normal serum creatinine levels, and normal blood pressure. Gentamicin, a polyvalent, cationic molecule, is thought to activate the extracellular calcium-sensing receptor (CaSR) in the thick ascending limb of Henle's loop. Thus, aminoglycoside treatment can lead to abnormalities that resemble those seen in patients with autosomal dominant hypocalcemia, which is caused by

mutations in the CaSR gene. This condition is also termed type V Bartter syndrome (option B). Calcimimetic agents can improve this syndrome.

Although Gitelman syndrome has also the same biochemical characteristics as Bartter syndrome, it is differentiated from Bartter syndrome by hypocalciuria. Liddle and Gordon syndromes are characterized by hypertension. Thus, option B is correct.

Suggested Reading

Chen Y-S, Fang H-C, Chou K-J, et al. Gentamicin-induced Bartter-like syndrome. Am J Kidney Dis. 2009;54:1158–61.
Singh J, Patel ML, Gupta KK, et al. Acquired Bartter syndrome following gentamicin therapy. Indian J Nephrol. 2016;26:461–3.
Zietse R, Zoutendijk R, Hoorn EJ. Fluid, electrolyte and acid–base disorders associated with antibiotic therapy. Nat Rev Nephrol. 2009;5:193–202.

9. A 60-year-old man with sepsis, requiring intubation, developed *Candida albicans* infection after a prolonged course of antibiotics. He is on amphotericin B. **Which one of the following adverse effects of amphotericin B is CORRECT?**

A. Hypokalemia
B. Inability to concentrate urine
C. Nephrogenic diabetes insipidus (NDI)
D. Distal renal tubular acidosis (dRTA)
E. All of the above

The answer is E

Amphotericin B disrupts cell membrane integrity, leading to leakage of cell contents. It causes electrolyte (hypokalemia and hypomagnesemia), acid–base (dRTA due to backleak of H^+ into the distal tubule cell), and tubular (NDI due to inhibition of vasopressin action) abnormalities. Thus, E is correct. Acute tubular necrosis is also common due to renal vasoconstriction and reduced renal blood flow. Adequate hydration of patient with normal saline may prevent acute kidney injury. Many of the electrolyte, acid–base, and tubular disorders may persist for a period of time even after amphotericin B is discontinued.

Suggested Reading

Morales-Alvarez MC. Nephrotoxicity of antimicrobials and antibiotics. Adv Chronic Kidney Dis. 2020;27:31–7.
Zietse R, Zoutendijk R, Hoorn EJ. Fluid, electrolyte and acid–base disorders associated with antibiotic therapy. Nat Rev Nephrol. 2009;5:193–202.

10. A patient is treated for vancomycin-resistant *Enterococcus faecium* with linezolid 600 mg twice a day. **Which one of the following acid accumulations is MOST likely to occur with linezolid therapy?**

A. Acetoacetic acid
B. β-hydroxybutyric acid
C. Lactic acid
D. Pyroglutamic acid
E. None of the above

The answer is C

Many case reports have documented that patients treated with linezolid can develop severe high anion gap metabolic acidosis due to lactic acid production. Although it is unclear, mitochondrial toxicity has been suggested as the underlying mechanism for lactic acid production. Thus, option C is correct.

Suggested Reading

Apodaca AA, Rakita RM. Linezolid-induced lactic acidosis. N Engl J Med. 2003;348:86–7.
Carlos J, Velez Q, Janech MG. A case of lactic acidosis induced by linezolid. Nat Rev Nephrol. 2010;6:236–42.
Morales-Alvarez MC. Nephrotoxicity of antimicrobials and antibiotics. Adv Chronic Kidney Dis. 2020;27:31–7.

11. **Food intake affects drug absorption. Which one of the following food and drug interactions is FALSE?**

   A. Food intake increases cinacalcet absorption
   B. Food intake reduces iron absorption
   C. High-fat meal increases sirolimus absorption
   D. Food intake increases tacrolimus absorption
   E. Food intake reduces tacrolimus absorption

   The answer is D

   Food intake may have several effects on drug absorption. These effects, called drug-food interactions, can be classified into five categories: (1) those causing reduced absorption; (2) those causing increased absorption; (3) those causing delayed absorption; (4) those causing accelerated absorption; and (5) those that do not have any interaction or food has no effect on drug absorption.

   Gastric emptying, fat content in food, nature of food either solids or liquids, and pH may influence drug absorption. Splanchnic circulation also influences drug absorption. A high protein meal increases splanchnic blood flow by 35%, whereas a liquid glucose meal increases by 8%. It is understandable that splanchnic vasodilation increases drug absorption to a different degree depending on the nature of the meal.

   Except for option D, other options are correct. It is well established that food intake and phosphate binders reduce iron and tacrolimus absorption, whereas absorption of cinacalcet increases with food intake. High-fat meal has been shown to increase sirolimus absorption.

   Suggested Reading

Cervelli MJ, Russ GR. Principles of drug therapy, dosing, and prescribing in chronic kidney disease and renal replacement therapy. In: Floege J, Johnson RJ, Feehally J, editors. Comprehensive clinical nephrology. 4th ed. Philadelphia: Saunders/Elsevier; 2010. p. 871–93.

Welling PG. Effects of food on drug absorption. Ann Rev Nutr. 1996;16:384–415.

12. **In many clinical trials of chronic kidney disease (CKD) and hemodialysis (HD) patients, the participation of a clinical pharmacist has some positive impact on which one of the following clinical measures?**

   A. Decrease in hospitalization rates
   B. Achieving hemoglobin (Hgb) to target levels in many CKD patients
   C. Improvement in overall quality of life in HD patients
   D. Increased medication knowledge
   E. All of the above

   The answer is E

   Only a few trials addressing the benefit and impact of clinical pharmacy services in CKD and HD patients have been published. Most of these studies have reported that involvement of a clinical pharmacist has a positive effect on decreased hospital rates, improving Hgb levels in many CKD patients, improvement in overall quality of life in HD patients, and increased medication-related knowledge. Thus, choice E is correct. It is of interest to note that none of the studies reported a negative impact of pharmacists' involvement on patient care.

   Suggested Reading

Lee H, Ryu K, Sohn Y, et al. Impact on patient outcomes of pharmacist participation in multidisciplinary critical care teams: a systematic review and meta-analysis. Crit Care Med. 2019;47:1243–50.

Pandey S, Hiller JE, Nikansah N, et al. The effect of pharmacist-provided non-dispensing services on patient outcomes, health service utilization and costs in low- and middle-income countries. Cochrane Database Syst Rev. 2013;(2).

Stemer G, Lemmens-Gruber R. Clinical pharmacy activities in chronic kidney disease and end-stage renal disease patients: a systematic literature review. BMC Nephrol. 2011;12:35.

13. A 36-year-old woman with medullary sponge kidney is admitted for urinary tract infection with *E. coli* which is sensitive to aminoglycosides only. Her eGFR is 49 mL/min. **After a loading dose of gentamicin, which one of the following dose schedules minimizes nephrotoxicity?**

    A. Three times daily
    B. Two times daily
    C. Once daily
    D. Four times daily
    E. Once every 3 days

    The answer is C

    Frequently used aminoglycosides (gentamicin, tobramycin, and amikacin) are filtered at the glomerulus and reabsorbed in the proximal tubules. They cause nephrotoxicity and ototoxicity. Because of these adverse effects, they are less commonly used. However, they are bactericidal and less expensive.

    In patients with low GFR (<60 mL/min), once daily dose has been shown to minimize nephrotoxicity compared to other dosage schedules. In this patient with CKD 4, the appropriate dose is once daily. Thus, choice C is correct.

    Suggested Reading

De Broe ME. Antibiotic- and immunosuppression-related renal failure. In: Coffman TM, Falk RJ, Molitoris BA, et al., editors. Schrier's diseases of the kidney. 9th ed. Philadelphia: Wolters Kluwer/Lippincott Williams & Wilkins; 2013. p. 901–42.

Nicolau DP, Freeman CD, Belliveau PP, et al. Experience with a once-daily aminoglycoside program administered to 2184 adult patients. Antimicrob Agents Chemother. 1995;39:650–5.

14. An 18-year-old woman with soft tissue sarcoma is consulted for a persistent electrolyte abnormality and weakness. She is on ifosfamide. **Which one of the following electrolyte abnormalities is the MOST likely cause of her weakness?**

    A. Hyponatremia
    B. Hypocalcemia
    C. Hypokalemia
    D. Hypernatremia
    E. Hypermagnesemia

    The answer is C

    Ifosfamide is an alkylating agent used for treatment of soft tissue sarcomas. It causes proximal renal tubular acidosis and Fanconi syndrome. Ifosfamide-induced hypokalemia is the most likely electrolyte abnormality, causing muscle weakness. Thus, option C is correct.

    Suggested Reading

Husband DJ, Watkins SVV. Fatal hypokalaemia associated with ifosfamide/mesna chemotherapy. Lancet. 1988;14(1):1116.

Nicolaysen A. Nephrotoxic chemotherapy agents: old and new. Adv Chronic Kidney Dis. 2020;27:38–49.

Skinner R, Pearson AD, English MW, et al. Risk factors for ifosfamide nephrotoxicity in children. Lancet. 1996;348:578–80.

15. **Which one of the following drugs is associated with proximal renal tubular acidosis (pRTA)?**

    A. Carbonic anhydrase inhibitors
    B. Aminoglycosides
    C. Valproic acid
    D. Tenofovir
    E. All of the above

    The answer is E

    All of the above drugs have been shown to cause pRTA with different mechanisms.

Suggested Reading

Kashoor I, Battle D. Proximal renal tubular acidosis with and without Fanconi syndrome. Kidney Res Clin Pract. 2019;38:267–81.
Mathew G, Knaus SJ. Acquired Fanconi's syndrome associated with tenofovir therapy. J Gen Intern Med. 2006;21:C3–5.
Rodriguez-Soriano J. Renal tubular acidosis; the clinical entity. J Am Soc Nephrol. 2002;13:2160–70.

16. An HIV patient sees his primary care physician for management of disease. His eGFR is <60 mL/min. **Which one of the following antiretroviral drug categories/agents needs dosage adjustment in patients with CKD 3–5?**

A. Integrase inhibitors (raltegravir)
B. Protease inhibitors (indinavir)
C. Nucleoside reverse transcriptase inhibitors (zidovudine)
D. Nucleotide reverse transcriptase inhibitors (tenofovir)
E. C and D

The answer is E

Except for nucleoside and nucleotide reverse transcriptase inhibitors, other categories of antiretroviral drugs do not require dosage adjustment in CKD 3–5 patients.

Suggested Reading

Cattaneo D, Gervasoni C. Novel antiretroviral drugs in patients with renal impairment: Clinical and pharmacokinetic considerations. Eur J Drug Metab Pharmacokinet. 2017;42:559–72.
Jao J, Wyatt CM. Antiretroviral medications: Adverse effects on the kidney. Adv Chronic Kidney Dis. 2010;17:72–82.
Kalayjian RC. The treatment of HIV-associated nephropathy. Adv Chronic Kidney Dis. 2010;17:59–71.

17. A 42-year-old woman with CKD 4 complaints of depression due to her kidney disease during routine follow-up. She is started on fluoxetine, one of the selective serotonin reuptake inhibitors (SSRIs). **Which one of the following adverse effects of SSRIs is expected to see in this patient?**

A. Hypertension
B. Seizures
C. Hyponatremia
D. Increased upper gastrointestinal (GI) bleeding
E. C and D

The answer is E

SSRIs cause hyponatremia due to syndrome of inappropriate antidiuretic hormone (SIADH) and increased upper GI tract bleeding. The latter effect is frequently seen with concomitant use of nonsteroidal antiinflammatory drugs (NSAIDs). The bleeding tendency is related to deficiency of platelet serotonin, resulting in decreased platelet aggregation.

Hypertension and SIADH are caused by serotonin-norepinephrine reuptake inhibitor such as duloxetine, whereas seizures are caused by norepinephrine-dopamine reuptake inhibitor (bupropion). It is advisable to avoid duloxetine in CKD patients with hypertension. Dosage reduction is needed for bupropion in patients with CKD 4–5.

Suggested Reading

Jacob S, Spinler SA. Hyponatremia associated with selective serotonin-reuptake inhibitors in older adults. Ann Pharmacother. 2006;40:1618–22.
Mort JR, Aparasu RR, Baer RK. Interaction between selective serotonin reuptake inhibitors and nonsteroidal anti-inflammatory drugs: review of the literature. Pharmacotherapy. 2006;26:1307–13.

18. **Which one of the following vaptans is available as intravenous preparation?**

A. Tolvaptan
B. Lixivaptan
C. Conivaptan

D. Satavaptan
E. Mozavaptan

The answer is C

Of the above vaptans only conivaptan is available as an intravenous preparation. Only conivaptan and tolvaptan are available in the United States. Conivaptan is a combined $V1_a$/V2 receptor antagonist. $V1_a$ receptors are present in hepatocytes and splanchnic circulation. Use of conivaptan in cirrhotic patient is expected to cause splanchnic vasodilation and cause an increase in portal pressure. Thus, option C is correct.

Suggested Reading

Lehrich RW, Ortiz-Melo DI, Patel MB, et al. Role of vaptans in the management of hyponatremia. Am J Kidney Dis. 2013;62:364–76.
Naafs MAB. The vasopressin V2 receptor antagonists: the vaptans. Glob J Endocrinol Metab. 2018;2(1): GJEM.000529.2018.
Reddi AS. Disorders of water balance: hyponatremia. In: Reddi AS, editor. Fluid, electrolyte, and acid-base disorders. Clinical evaluation and management. 2nd ed. New York: Springer; 2018. p. 107–45.

19. Lithium is used widely to treat bipolar and depressive disorders. It has a narrow therapeutic and toxic range. **Which one of the following lithium-induced nephrotoxicities is CORRECT?**

A. Polyuria
B. Inability to concentrate urine
C. Hypernatremia
D. Prerenal azotemia
E. All of the above

The answer is E

Lithium is filtered at the glomerulus and reabsorbed mostly in the proximal tubule. A fraction of lithium is reabsorbed in the distal nephron via ENaC. Lithium causes nephrogenic diabetes insipidus, resulting in urinary concentrating defect and polyuria as well as hypernatremia. Prerenal azotemia is not uncommon. Use of loop and thiazide diuretics and ACE-Is/ARBs and NSAIDs aggravate lithium toxicity. Hydration with normal saline initially improves blood pressure, volume status, and azotemia. Subsequent fluid administration depends on serum [Na^+]. Amiloride treatment blocks ENaC uptake of lithium with improvement in polyuria and urinary concentrating ability. Dialysis is indicted to improve lithium toxicity. Thus, option E is correct.

Suggested Reading

Azab AN, Shnaider A, Osher Y, et al. Lithium nephrotoxicity. Indian J Bipolar Disord. 2015;3:13.
Davis J, Desmond M, Berk M. Lithium and nephrotoxicity: a literature review of approaches to clinical management and risk stratification. BMC Nephrol. 2018;19:305.
Grüünfeld JP, Rossier BC. Lithium nephrotoxicity revisited. Nat Rev Nephrol. 2009;5:270–6.
Oliveira JP, Silva Junior GB, Abreu KL, et al. Lithium nephrotoxicity. Rev Assoc Med Bras. 2010;56:600–6.

20. A 55-year-old man with multiple myeloma is admitted for paraparesis. An MRI of the spinal cord is normal. Neurologic exam shows muscle weakness of the lower limbs with tendinous areflexia and absence of pyramidal syndrome. His medications at the time of admission include dexamethasone 4 mg Q6H and thalidomide 200 mg/day. Blood pressure and pulse rate are normal. Except for serum K^+ of 8.4 mEq/L, the other laboratory tests are normal. **What is the most likely cause of this hyperkalemia and sudden paraparesis?**

A. Hyperkalemia due to steroid use
B. Hyperkalemia due to remission of multiple myeloma
C. Hyperkalemia due to thalidomide
D. Hyperkalemia due to volume depletion
E. Pseudohyperkalemia

The answer is C

Thalidomide is being used by some investigators as the first-line treatment of multiple myeloma. In both dialysis and CKD patients, thalidomide has been shown to cause severe hyperkalemia, which may be related to either cell lysis or cellular shift. Thus, option C is correct. Both steroid use and remission of multiple myeloma are unlikely causes of hyperkalemia. Also, pseudohyperkalemia has not been reported with thalidomide. Severe volume depletion may cause hyperkalemia by limiting delivery of glomerular filtrate to the distal nephron, but this patient does not have either renal insufficiency or volume depletion.

Suggested Reading

Izzedine H, Launay-Vacher V, Deray G. Thalidomide for the nephrologist. Nephrol Dial Transplant. 2005;20:2011–2.
Lee C-C, Wu Y-H, Chung S-H, et al. Acute tumor lysis syndrome after thalidomide therapy in advanced hepatocellular carcinoma. Oncologist. 2006;11:87–8.
Wanchoo R, Abudayyeh A, Doshi M, et al. Renal toxicities of novel agents used for treatment of multiple myeloma. Clin J Am Soc Nephrol. 2017;12:176–89.

21. A 32-year-old woman with tubulointerstitial disease has serum [K^+] of 5.1 mEq/L without any EKG changes. She is on low K^+ diet. **Which one of the following is NOT associated with exacerbation of her serum [K^+]?**

A. Trimethoprim
B. Amiloride
C. Pentamidine
D. Nafamostat (a serine protease inhibitor)
E. Licorice

The answer is E

Except for licorice (causes hypokalemia), all other medications inhibit ENaC, and cause hyperkalemia. Nafamostat is a serine protease inhibitor that is used in acute pancreatitis and disseminated intravascular coagulation.

Suggested Reading

Ben Salem C, Badreddine A, Fathallah F, et al. Drug-induced hyperkalemia. Drug Saf. 2014;37:677–92.
Bhalla V, Hallows KR. Mechanisms of ENaC regulation and clinical implications. J Am Soc Nephrol. 2008;19:1845–54.

22. A 46-year-old Indian woman with type 2 diabetes for 12 years is found to have a serum [K^+] of 5.8 mEq/L, HCO_3^- 24 mEq/L, and glucose 100 mg/dL on a follow-up visit. One month ago her serum [K^+] was 4.2 mEq/L. Her eGFR is 48 mL/min, which is stable for the last 1 year. She is on glipizide (5 mg/day) and sitagliptin (50 mg/day). She denies taking any dietary supplements or NSAIDs. The only complaint is fatigue. **Which one of the following is NOT a cause of her hyperkalemia?**

A. Noni juice
B. Raw coconut juice
C. COX-2 inhibitors
D. Oral hypoglycemic agents
E. Alfaalfa

The answer is D

Except for oral hypoglycemic agents, all other food supplements cause hyperkalemia. Noni juice contains 56 mEq/L and raw coconut juice 44.3 mEq/L of K^+. COX-2 inhibitors cause hypoaldosteronism, whereas alfalfa is rich in K^+. Thus, option D is correct.

Suggested Reading

Ben Salem C, Badreddine A, Fathallah F, et al. Drug-induced hyperkalemia. Drug Saf. 2014;37:677–92.
Montford JR, Linas S. How dangerous is hyperkalemia? J Am Soc Nephrol. 2017;28:3155–65.
Reddi AS. Disorders of potassium balance: hyperkalemia. In: Reddi AS, editor. Fluid, electrolyte, and acid-base disorders. Clinical evaluation and management. 2nd ed. New York: Springer; 2018. p. 193–210.

23. **Match the following drugs that cause hyperkalemia and their mechanism of action (use all applicable answers):**

Drug	Mechanism of action
A. Digitalis intoxication	1. Transports K^+ out of cells
B. Arginine	2. Inhibits Na/K-ATPase activity
C. Amiloride, trimethoprim, and pentamidine	3. Decrease aldosterone synthesis
D. ACE-Is	4. Decrease renin/aldosterone
E. Nonsteroidal antiinflammatory drugs	5. Inhibits Na^+ channel in principal cells
F. Salt substitutes	6. Increase K^+ intake
G. Heparin	7. Decrease K^+ channel activity
H. Cyclosporine and tacrolimus	
I. Chan su, toad skin, and oleander	

Answers: A = 2; B = 1; C = 7; D = 3; E = 4; F = 6; G = 3; H = 2, 3, 7; I = 2

A large number of drugs have been shown to cause hyperkalemia by a variety of mechanisms. Na/K-ATPase transports 3 Na^+ ions out and 2 K^+ ions into the cell. Inhibition of this transport mechanism causes mild hyperkalemia in a euvolemic subject. Infusion of arginine causes shift of K^+ out of cells. Amiloride, trimethoprim, and pentamidine block Na^+ uptake by Na^+ channel (ENaC) in principal cells of the cortical collecting duct with resultant decrease in K^+ secretion via K^+ channel (ROMK). ACE-Is and heparin cause hypoaldosteronism and hyperkalemia. Nonsteroidal antiinflammatory drugs inhibit renin production, resulting in decreased aldosterone levels and hyperkalemia. Hypertensive individuals who take salt substitutes develop hyperkalemia because of K^+ overload. Cyclosporine and tacrolimus commonly cause hyperkalemia by a variety of mechanisms, including a decrease in Na/K-ATPase activity and aldosterone synthesis as well as cyclosporine-induced inhibition of K_{ATP} channel activity. Herbal medications such as chan su, toad skin, and oleander inhibit Na/K-ATPase activity and increase in serum [K^+], particularly in CKD patients.

Suggested Reading

Ben Salem C, Badreddine A, Fathallah F, et al. Drug-induced hyperkalemia. Drug Saf. 2014;37:677–92.
Montford JR, Linas S. How dangerous is hyperkalemia? J Am Soc Nephrol. 2017;28:3155–65.
Reddi AS. Disorders of potassium balance: hyperkalemia. In: Reddi AS, editor. Fluid, electrolyte, and acid-base disorders. Clinical evaluation and management. 2nd ed. New York: Springer; 2018. p. 193–210.

24. A 30-year-old man with HIV/AIDS is found to have hypercalcemia, which is thought to be medication induced. **Which one of the following drugs is NOT associated with hypercalcemia?**

A. Vitamin A
B. Omeprazole
C. Silicone
D. Lithium
E. Chloroquine

The answer is E

Except for chloroquine, all other medications have been shown to cause hypercalcemia. Vitamin A intoxication causes bone resorption and elevates serum [Ca^{2+}]. Also, vitamin A analogs, used in dermatologic and malignant conditions, cause hypercalcemia.

Omeprazole, a proton pump inhibitor (PPI), has been shown to cause acute tubulointerstitial granulomatous disease and hypercalcemia with normal PTH levels. PPIs may also cause hypocalcemia.

The use of liquid silicone for soft tissue augmentation (breast and hip) has been shown to induce granulomas and hypercalcemia. Renal stones and renal failure due to obstruction and hypercalcemia do occur in some patients. Hypercalcemia improves with steroids. TNF-α inhibitors have also been used to prevent granuloma formation, as TNF-α induces granuloma formation. Chloroquine and denosumab can be used to treat hypercalcemia.

Lithium has been known for years to cause hypercalcemia by stimulating PTH secretion. This effect occurs probably through interaction with CaSR to alter the set point for PTH secretion in relation to plasma [Ca^{2+}].

Chloroquine causes hypocalcemia by decreasing the production of $1,25(OH)_2D_3$ Thus, option E is correct.

Suggested Reading

Hariri A, Mount DB, Rastegar A. Disorders of calcium, phosphorus, and magnesium metabolism. In: Mount DB, Sayegh MH, Singh AJ, editors. Core concepts in the disorders of fluid, electrolytes and acid-base balance. New York: Springer; 2013. p. 103–46.

Hoorn EJ, Zietse R. Disorders of calcium and magnesium balance: a physiology-based approach. Pediatr Nephrol. 2013;28:1195–206. https://doi.org/10.1007/s00467-012-2350-2.

Reddi AS. Disorders of calcium: hypercalcemia. In: Reddi AS, editor. Fluid, electrolyte, and acid-base disorders. Clinical evaluation and management. 2nd ed. New York: Springer; 2018. p. 233–50.

25. **Match the following drugs that cause hyperphosphatemia with their possible mechanism of action:**

Drug	Mechanism
A. Excess vitamin D	1. Increased gastrointestinal absorption (GI) of phosphate
B. Bisphosphonates	2. Decreased phosphate excretion and cellular shift
C. Growth hormone	3. Increased proximal tubule reabsorption
D. Liposomal amphotericin B	4. Contains phosphatidyl choline and phosphatidyl serine
E. Sodium phosphate (oral)	5. GI absorption of phosphate

Answers: A = 1; B = 2; C = 3; D = 4; E = 5

Suggested Reading

Hariri A, Mount DB, Rastegar A. Disorders of calcium, phosphorus, and magnesium metabolism. In: Mount DB, Sayegh MH, Singh AJ, editors. Core concepts in the disorders of fluid, electrolytes and acid-base balance. New York: Springer; 2013. p. 103–46.

Reddi AS. Disorders of phosphate: hyperphosphatemia. In: Reddi AS, editor. Fluid, electrolyte, and acid-base disorders. Clinical evaluation and management. 2nd ed. New York: Springer; 2018. p. 273–86.

26. **Which one of the following drugs does NOT cause hypomagnesemia?**

A. Cisplatin
B. Amphotericin B (Amp B)
C. Proton pump inhibitor (PPI)
D. Alcohol
E. Vancomycin

The answer is E

Except for vancomycin, all other drugs cause hypomagnesemia. Cisplatin and Amp B cause renal wasting of Mg^{2+}. Both drugs also cause hypocalciuria. PPIs have been shown to induce hypomagnesemia by various mechanisms. Not only hypomagnesemia but also hypokalemia and hypocalcemia have been reported with PPIs. Hypokalemia is due to renal wasting of K^+. Patients with chronic alcoholism may develop hypomagnesemia by several mechanisms, including inadequate dietary intake, steatorrhea, diarrhea, phosphate deficiency, fatty acid or ATP-Mg complex formation, and alcohol-induced magnesuria. To date, vancomycin has not been shown to cause hypomagnesemia, making E as correct choice.

Suggested Reading

Lameris AL, Monnens LA, Bindels RJ, et al. Drug-induced alterations in Mg^{2+} homeostasis. Clin Sci. 2012;123:1–4.

Reddi AS. Disorders of magnesium: hypomagnesemia. In: Reddi AS, editor. Fluid, electrolyte, and acid-base disorders. Clinical evaluation and management. 2nd ed. New York: Springer; 2018. p. 293–305.

27. A 55-year-old man with chronic alcoholism presents to the emergency department with agitation, blurred vision, and eye pain. Blood pressure and pulse rate are normal. He is afebrile. He has a high AG metabolic acidosis with an osmolal gap of 26 mOsm/L. **Which one of the following toxic alcohol ingestions is the MOST likely cause of his symptoms?**

A. Ethanol
B. Ethylene glycol
C. Methanol

D. Toluene
E. Isopropyl alcohol

The answer is C

Only formic acid formed from methanol is toxic to the optic nerve, causing visual impairment, blurred vision, eye pain, and blindness. Therefore, early institution of fomepizole is recommended to inhibit alcohol dehydrogenase and conversion of methanol to formaldehyde and formic acid.

Suggested Reading

Barceloux DG, Krenzelok EP, Olson K, et al. American Academy of Clinical Toxicology practice guidelines on the treatment of methanol poisoning. J Toxicol Clin Toxicol. 2002;40:415–46.
Kraut JA, Kurtz I. Toxic alcohol ingestions: clinical features, diagnosis, and management. Clin J Am Soc Nephrol. 2008;3:208–25.

28. **Which one of the following supportive care measures you would implement at this time for the above patient?**

A. Hydration with normal saline, and glucose for hypoglycemia
B. IV $NaHCO_3$ to maintain blood pH >7.2
C. Fomepizole (4-methylpyrazole)
D. Ethanol, if fomepizole not available
E. All of the above

The answer is E

Immediate supportive care includes: (1) hydration with normal saline, and glucose for hypoglycemia; (2) IV $NaHCO_3$ to maintain blood pH > 7.2; (3) IV folinic acid (1 mg/kg) one dose, and then folate supplementation to accelerate formate metabolism to CO_2 and water by tetrahydrofolate synthetase. This may benefit some alcoholics with folate deficiency; and (4) fomepizole (4-methylpyrazole), which is the drug of choice in the United States. Ethanol is also the drug of choice, if fomepizole is not available. Thus, option E is correct.

Suggested Reading

Barceloux DG, Krenzelok EP, Olson K, et al. American Academy of Clinical Toxicology practice guidelines on the treatment of methanol poisoning. J Toxicol Clin Toxicol. 2002;40:415–46.
Kraut JA, Xing SX. Approach to the evaluation of a patient with an increased serum osmolal gap and high-anion gap metabolic acidosis. Am J Kidney Dis. 2011;58:480–4.

29. **Match the drug effects of lactic and pyroglutamic acids shown in Column A with the mechanisms of action shown in Column B:**

Column A	Column B
A. Metformin	1. Uncoupling of oxidative phosphorylation
B. Propofol	2. Inhibition of pyruvate dehydrogenase complex
C. Flucoxacillin	3. Inhibition of 5-oxoprolinase
D. Thiamine deficiency	4. Increase in NADH/NAD$^+$ ratio, inhibition of gluconeogenesis from lactate, and inhibition of mitochondrial respiration

Answers: A = 4; B = 1; C = 3; D = 2

Suggested Reading

Kraut JA, Madias NE. Lactic acidosis. N Engl J Med. 2014;371:2309–19.
Kraut JA, Madias NE. Lactic acidosis: current treatments and future directions. Am J Kidney Dis. 2016;68:473–82.
Reddi AS. Lactic acidosis. In: Acid-base disorders. Clinical evaluation and management. New York: Springer; 2020. p. 63–83.

30. A 32-year-old woman with seizure disorder and migraine is consulted for hyperchloremic metabolic acidosis with serum [HCO_3^-] of 19 mEq/L. Her urine pH is 6.4. **Which one of the following medications causes this acid–base disorder?**

A. Phenytoin
B. Topiramate
C. Levetiracetam
D. Carbamazepine
E. Gabapentin

The answer is B

Except for topiramate, all other drugs are not known to cause hyperchloremic metabolic acidosis. Topiramate is an inhibitor of carbonic anhydrase, causing HCO_3^- loss in the urine. This results in alkaline urine pH. It is a neuromodulator that is approved for use in the treatment of seizure activity and for migraine prophylaxis. Initially, it was observed that topiramate causes type II RTA and hyperchloremic metabolic acidosis in children. Since then, a number of case reports in adults have been described. Discontinuation of the drug improves serum [HCO_3^-] with resolution of RTA. Thus, option B is correct.

Suggested Reading

Mathews KD, Stark JE. Hyperchloremic, normal anion-gap, metabolic acidosis due to topiramate. Am J Health Syst Pharm. 2008;65:1430–4.
Mirza N, Marson AG, Pirmohamed M. Effect of topiramate on acid-base balance: extent, mechanism, and effects. Br J Clin Pharmacol. 2009;68:655–61.

31. A 28-year-old woman was brought to the emergency department for agitation and respiratory distress, requiring intubation. She required fentanyl and lorazepam for sedation. Kidney function was normal. Two days later she had a low serum [$HCO3^-$] of 12 mEq/L, a drop of 10 mEq/L from baseline value. An ABG shows a high anion gap metabolic acidosis. **Which one of the following acids may have contributed to her anion gap metabolic acidosis?**

A. Acetoacetate
B. Methanol
C. Ethylene glycol
D. Lactic acid
E. Hippuric acid

The answer is D

The patient received lorazepam probably at high doses for sedation. Propylene glycol (PG) is a diluent found in many intravenous and oral drugs, including lorazepam. PG is metabolized by alcohol and aldehyde dehydrogenases to lactic acid. Each milliliter of lorazepam injection contains 828 mg of PG. Thus, high doses of lorazepam administration results in high circulating levels of lactic acid. PG is water soluble and is removed by hemodialysis and also continuous venovenous hemofiltration. Thus, choice D is correct.

Suggested Reading

Zar T, Graeber C, Perazella MA. Recognition, treatment, and prevention of propylene glycol toxicity. Sem Dial. 2007;20:217–9.
Zosel A, Egelhoff E, Heard K. Severe lactic acidosis after an iatrogenic propylene glycol overdose. Pharmacotherapy. 2010;30:219.

32. **Match the following drugs that cause hypocalcemia with their possible mechanism of action:**

Drug	Mechanism (s)
A. Anticonvulsants	1. Increased metabolism of 25(OH)D_3, decreased Ca^{2+} release from bone, and decreased intestinal absorption of Ca^{2+}
B. Bisphosphonates	2. Inhibits bone resorption (↓ osteoclast activity)
C. Calcitonin	3. Inhibits bone resorption
D. Citrate	4. Chelates Ca^{2+}
E. Foscarnet and fluoride	5. Chelate Ca^{2+}
F. Antibiotics	6. Hypocalcemia (consequence of hypomagnesemia)
G. Cinacalcet	7. Inhibition of PTH secretion by activation of CaSR (calcium-sensing receptor)

Answers: A = 1; B = 2; C = 3; D = 4; E = 5; F = 6; G = 7

Suggested Reading

Hoorn EJ, Zietse R. Disorders of calcium and magnesium balance: a physiology-based approach. Pediatr Nephrol. 2013;28:1195–206. https://doi.org/10.1007/s00467-012-2350-2.

Reddi AS. Disorders of calcium: hypocalcemia. In: Reddi AS, editor. Fluid, electrolyte, and acid-base disorders. Clinical evaluation and management. 2nd ed. New York: Springer; 2018. p. 219–31.

33. **Match the following drugs that cause hypercalcemia with their possible mechanism of action:**

Drug	Mechanism (s)
A. Lithium	1. Increased PTH secretion
B. Vitamin D	2. Increased GI absorption of Ca^{2+}
C. Vitamin A	3. Increased bone resorption
D. Estrogens/antiestrogens	4. Increased bone resorption
E. Theophylline	5. Decreased sensitivity of parathyroids to Ca^{2+} and β_2-agonist mediation

Answers: A = 1; B = 2; C = 3; D = 4; E = 5

Suggested Reading

Hoorn EJ, Zietse R. Disorders of calcium and magnesium balance: a physiology-based approach. Pediatr Nephrol. 2013;28:1195–206. https://doi.org/10.1007/s00467-012-2350-2.

Reddi AS. Disorders of calcium: hypercalcemia. In: Reddi AS, editor. Fluid, electrolyte, and acid-base disorders. Clinical evaluation and management. 2nd ed. New York: Springer; 2018. p. 233–50.

34. A 52-year-old man with history of gout and hypertension is admitted for acute gouty attack. His uric acid is elevated and is on hydrochlorothiazide (HCTZ). His blood pressure is 154/88 mm Hg with a pulse rate of 90 beats/min. **Which one of the following antihypertensive agents promotes uric acid excretion?**

A. Enalapril
B. Lisinopril
C. Losartan
D. Telmisartan
E. Candesartan

The answer is C

Of all the above drugs, losartan is the only angiotensin receptor blocker (ARB) that has been shown to promote urate excretion in both normal and hypertensive subjects. HCTZ decreases urate excretion. Even in HCTZ-treated patients, losartan has shown lower serum uric acid level by promoting its renal excretion. This unique property of losartan is not shared by other ARBs or angiotensin-converting enzyme inhibitors.

Suggested Reading

Edwards RM, Trizna W, Stack EJ, et al. Interaction of nonpeptide angiotensin II receptor antagonists with the urate transporter in rat renal brush-border membranes. J Pharmacol Exp Ther. 1996;276:125–9.

Shahinfar S, Simpson RL, Carides AD, et al. Safety of losartan in hypertensive patients with thiazide-induced hyperuricemia. Kidney Int. 1999;56:1879–85.

35. A 72-year-old man with bipolar disorder and hypertension is treated with lithium (Li). His physician added enalapril 10 mg/day for improvement of his hypertension and possible congestive heart failure. Two months later, he was confused and admitted to the hospital with LI toxicity. **Which one of the following choices explains his Li toxicity?**

A. Combination of Li and an angiotensin-converting enzyme inhibitor (ACE-I) enhances Li toxicity
B. No relationship exists between Li and ACE-Is
C. Combination of an ACE-I and Li enhances estimated glomerular filtration rate (eGFR)
D. Combination of an ACE-I and Li has no effect on eGFR
E. None of the above

The answer is A

Patients on both Li and an ACE-I demonstrate drug interaction, causing Li toxicity. The mechanisms seem to be related to sodium and water depletion with resultant decrease in eGFR. Both of these mechanisms cause reduced Li clearance. A Canadian study showed that patients admitted to the hospital for Li toxicity had exposure to an ACE-I 1 month prior to their hospitalization. Other drugs that predispose to Li toxicity are diuretics and NSAIDs. Thus, choice A is correct. The combination of Li and an ACE-I reduces eGFR, and therefore, choice C is incorrect.

Suggested Reading

Hommers L, Fischer M, Reif-Leonhard C, et al. The combination of lithium and ACE inhibitors: hazardous, critical, possible? Clin Drug Invest. 2019;39:485–9.

Nagamine T. Lithium intoxication associated with angiotensin II type 1 receptor blockers in women. Clin Neuropharmacol Ther. 2013;4:23–5.

36. Interaction between antihypertensive drugs and food has been well documented. Diuretics are commonly used for many clinical conditions. **Of the following drugs, which one of the following diuretics is NOT affected by food intake?**

A. Hydrochlorothiazide (HCTZ)
B. Furosemide
C. Sustained released indapamide
D. Spironolactone
E. Acetazolamide

The answer is C

Food affects the bioavailability of many diuretics. Food intake (simultaneous intake of food and drug) increases the bioavailability of HCTZ and spironolactone by increasing their absorption, whereas the bioavailability of furosemide and bumetanide is substantially decreased. Indapamide (sustained released) absorption is not affected by food intake. The absorption of acetazolamide is not affected by food. Thus, option C is correct.

Suggested Reading

Jáuregui-Garrido B, Jáuregui-Lobera I. Interactions between antihypertensive drugs and food. Nutr Hosp. 2012;22:1866–75.

Welling PG. Effects of food on drug absorption. Ann Rev Nutr. 1996;16:384–415.

37. A 34-year-old woman with acute leukemia is admitted for tumor lysis syndrome with acute kidney injury, elevated serum [K^+], phosphate, uric acid (16 mg/dL), and creatinine levels. **Besides hydration with normal saline, which one of the following interventions is MOST appropriate for this patient?**

A. Allopurinol
B. Colchicine
C. Losartan
D. Rasburicase
E. Febuxostat

The answer is D

Allopurinol is used prophylactically with hydration prior to chemotherapy. It inhibits xanthine oxidase, which converts xanthine into uric acid. Thus, uric acid formation and serum levels of uric acid are lowered. However, allopurinol has no direct effect on uric acid conversion to more soluble allantoin. Therefore, initiation of allopurinol in this patient does not lower uric acid levels. Thus, option A is incorrect.

Colchicine reduces inflammation in gouty patients and does not reduce uric acid levels in this patient. Also, colchicine is not indicated in tumor lysis syndrome. Thus, option B is incorrect. Losartan is an angiotensin receptor blocker and has uricosuric properties. In this patient with elevated serum creatinine levels (acute kidney injury), losartan may not have any beneficial effect. Also, it is not the drug of choice in this patient. Therefore, option C is incorrect. Febuxostat is a novel nonpurine xanthine oxidase inhibitor, which is recommended for prevention of hyperuricemia and gout. So far, no clinical trial results are available for its use in tumor lysis syndrome. Thus, option E is incorrect.

Rasburicase is a recombinant urate oxidase. This enzyme converts urate into allantoin, which is excreted. Human subjects lack this enzyme. Since the patient has high uric acid levels, the use of rasburicase seems appropriate in this patient, as it converts urate into allantoin. Either a single dose (0.2 mg/kg) or daily dose for 5 days lowers uric acid levels within few hours in children, adults, and elderly. Therefore, option D is correct. Rasbubicase should be avoided in patients with glucose-6-phosphate dehydrogenase deficiency, as it may generate hydrogen peroxide and cause hemolytic anemia and methemoglobinemia.

Suggested Reading

Feng X, Dong K, Pence S, et al. Efficacy and cost of single-dose rasburicase in prevention and treatment of adult tumour lysis syndrome: a meta-analysis. J Clin Pharm Ther. 2013;38:301–8.

Howard SC, Jones DP, Pui C-H. The tumor lysis syndrome. N Engl J Med. 2011;364:1844–54.

Lopez-Olivo MA, Pratt G, Palla SL, et al. Rasburicase in tumor lysis syndrome of the adult: a systematic review and meta-analysis. Am J Kidney Dis. 2013;62:481–92.

Wilson IP, Berns JS. Onco-nephrology: tumor lysis syndrome. Clin J Am Soc Nephrol. 2012;7:1730–39.

38. A 65-year-old man is found to have a colorectal carcinoma on routine colonoscopy. He has a past medical history of hypertension and tobacco use. His blood pressure is 136/78 mm Hg on two antihypertensive medications. His oncologist decides to treat him with bevascizumab, an antivascular endothelial growth factor (VEGF), as he has seen successful results with this drug. **Which one of the following adverse effects of the drug is MOST commonly seen during the follow-up of this patient?**

A. Hypotension
B. Hypertension
C. Hypokalemia
D. Hypomagnesemia
E. Hypocalcemia

The answer is B

Antiangiogenic medications are the first-line therapies for metastatic renal cell carcinoma, and other malignancies. One of the most common adverse effects of these drugs is the new-onset hypertension or aggravation of existing hypertension. Blood pressure drops after cessation of these drugs. An increase in blood pressure can be seen in <24 h after introduction of VEGF inhibitors. Evidence implicates endothelin-1 as the causative factor for the development of hypertension. Also, decreased synthesis of nitric oxide has been proposed. Dihydropyridine calcium blockers (amlodipine and nifedipine) and renin-AII-aldosterone blockers seem to control blood pressure better than other antihypertensive agents. Nifedipine seems to induce VEGF secretion. Nondihydropyridine calcium blockers (diltiazem and verapamil) are not recommended because these drugs inhibit CYP3A4. Thus, option B is correct. Other adverse effects, as listed in the question, have not been reported consistently.

It has been reported that patients who develop hypertension on antiangiogenic medications seem to have better antitumor response than those who do not develop hypertension.

Suggested Reading

Izzedine H, Ederhy S, Goldwasser F, et al. Management of hypertension in angiogenesis inhibitor-treated patients. Ann Oncol. 2009;20:807–15.

Robinson ES, Khankin EV, Karumanchi SA, et al. Hypertension induced by vascular endothelial growth factor signaling pathway inhibition: mechanism and potential use as a biomarker. Sem Nephrol. 2010;30:591–601.

39. A 62-year-old man is referred to you for evaluation of proteinuria (2.4 g/day). He had a nonmyeloablative allogenic hematopoietic cell transplantation (HCT) for acute myelogenous leukemia 6 years ago. Blood pressure and serum complement are normal. ANCA is negative. Renal biopsy shows stage 2 membranous nephropathy. Immunofluorescence shows strong positivity for IgG1. **Regarding membranous nephropathy and HCT, which one of the following statements is TRUE?**

A. Membranous nephropathy in HCT patients is not linked to formation of antibodies to phospholipase A2 receptor
B. Membranous nephropathy is rather common in patients with nonmyeloablative allogenic HCT
C. Membranous nephropathy is a form of renal-limited graft versus host disease following HCT

D. Membranous nephropathy secondary to HCT is characterized by predominant staining for IgG1, IgG2, or IgG3 on immunofluorescence microscopy
E. All of the above

The answer is E

Nephrotic syndrome is a common complication following HCT. A study by Srinivasan et al. showed development of nephrotic syndrome in 7 of 147 patients. Of these seven patients, four had membranous nephropathy on renal biopsy. Minimal change disease is also common in HCT patients. Membranous nephropathy is secondary to HCT. In contrast to secondary membranous nephropathy, idiopathic membranous nephropathy is linked to podocyte-expressed phospholipase A2 receptor antibody. It has been reported that membranous nephropathy is a form of renal-related graft versus host disease in patients following HCT.

IgG4 is the predominant form of immunoglobulin seen on immunofluorescence microscopy in idiopathic membranous nephropathy, whereas IgG1, IgG2, or IgG3 are the predominant immunoglobulins in secondary membranous nephropathy. Thus, answer E is true regarding HCT and membranous nephropathy.

Suggested Reading

Brukamp K, Doyle AM, Bloom RD, et al. Nephrotic syndrome after hematopoietic cell transplantation: do glomerular lesions represent renal graft-versus-host disease. Clin J Am Soc Nephrol. 2006;1:685–94.

Srinivasan R, Balow JE, Sabnis S, et al. Nephrotic syndrome: An under-recognized immune-related complication of non-myeloablative allogenic hematopoietic cell transplantation. Br J Hematol. 2005;131:74–9.

40. **Match the following cancer-specific causes of hypokalemia with their mechanisms:**

Drug	Mechanism
A. Cetuximab (antiepidermal growth factor receptor (EGF) antibody)	1. Excess production of mineralocorticoid
B. Cisplatin	2. Chronic diarrhea
C. Light chains	3. Lysozyme-induced tubular injury
D. ACTH-secreting tumor	4. Fanconi syndrome
E. Villous adenoma	5. Hypomagnesemia-induced hypokalemia
F. Myelomonocytic leukemia	

Answers: A = 5; B = 5; C = 4; D = 1; E = 2; F = 3

EGF binds to its receptor on the basolateral membrane of the distal tubule epithelial cell, causing the translocation of the transient receptor potential M6 channel to facilitate Mg^{2+} transport across the apical membrane. Anti-EGF receptor antibodies inhibit Mg^{2+} reabsorption and promote its excretion. As a result, hypomagnesemia develops. Hypokalemia is due to hypomagnesemia. The option 5 is correct.

Although cisplatin causes massive magnesuria, the mechanism is different. It seems that cisplatinum accumulates in renal tubules, resulting in cell death. Magnesuria is due to cell death of renal tubules, and hypokalemia is the result of hypomagnesemia. Thus, option 5 is correct.

Excretion of light chains induces proximal tubular injury, and partial Fanconi syndrome with resultant hypokalemia. Thus, option 4 is correct.

ACTH-producing tumors generate mineralocorticoid, which promotes K^+ excretion and hypokalemia (1). Patients with villous adenoma develop chronic diarrhea, which causes hypokalemia (2).

Kidney failure with severe hypokalemia has been reported in patients with acute myelomonocytic leukemia, which is due to lysozyme-induced tubular injury. Thus, option 3 is correct.

Suggested Reading

Nicolaysen A. Nephrotoxic chemotherapy agents: old and new. Adv Chronic Kidney Dis. 2020;27:38–49.

Perazella MA. Onco-nephrology: renal toxicities of chemotherapeutic agents. Clin J Am Soc Nephrol. 2012;7:1713–21.

Sahni V, Choudhury D, Ahmed Z. Chemotherapy-associated renal dysfunction. Nat Rev Nephrol. 2009;5:450–62.

41. A 50-year-old man with renal cell carcinoma is on several new therapies, including antiangiogenic agent, bevacizumab. **Which one of the following adverse effects of bevacizumab is anticipated in this patient?**

A. Proteinuria
B. Renal thrombotic microangiopathy (TMA)
C. Acute kidney injury
D. Hematuria
E. All of the above

The answer is E

Besides severe hypertension, all of the above adverse effects can be expected in patients on antiangiogenic therapy. On kidney biopsy, characteristics of TMA such as mesangiolysis, endothelial swelling (endotheliosis), and double contours of capillary basement membrane are evident.

Suggested Reading

Eremina V, Jefferson JA, Kowalewska J, et al. VEGF inhibition and renal thrombotic microangiopathy. N Engl J Med. 2008;358:1129–36.
Nicolaysen A. Nephrotoxic chemotherapy agents: old and new. Adv Chronic Kidney Dis. 2020;27:38–49.
Perazella MA. Onco-nephrology: renal toxicities of chemotherapeutic agents. Clin J Am Soc Nephrol. 2012;7:1713–21.

42. A 51-year-old woman is admitted for severe anemia and acute kidney injury (AKI) with a serum creatinine level of 12.3 mg/dL. Despite severe renal failure, her serum [Ca^{2+}] is 10.6 mg/dL. Urine analysis was normal without proteinuria. Sulfosalicylic acid yielded a thick white precipitate. Both creatinine and Ca^{2+} did not improve despite adequate hydration. Kidney biopsy confirmed our clinical diagnosis of cast nephropathy. The patient was started on hemodialysis, plasma exchange, and chemotherapy. Serum [Ca^{2+}] remains elevated. **Regarding bisphosphonate use in this patient, which one of the following statements is TRUE?**

A. All bisphosphonates are renally excreted.
B. Case reports suggest that pamidronate use in CKD to be safe at reduced doses every 1 to 2 months.
C. Slower infusion and lower doses than those of total osteoporosis management are generally recommended in patients with severe renal impairment.
D. Zoledronate or Ibandronate might be useful in patients with renal impairment due to multiple myeloma.
E. All of the above.

The answer is E

Bisphosphonates are used to treat hypercalcemia in patients with malignancy. They inhibit osteoclast-induced bone resorption. All available bisphosphonates are renally excreted, and they are nephrotoxic. Despite their nephrotoxicity, some case reports have appeared in the literature of successful treatment of hypercalcemia with pamidronate and ibandronate in dialysis patients. Both drugs are removed by dialysis. No prospective trials of bisphosphonates use in CKD patients are available.

In clinical trials, zoledronate (zoledronic acid) was found to be superior to pamidronate. Also, zoledronate is available in most of the countries and the infusion time is shorter than pamidronate. Although not indicated in patients with creatinine clearance <30 mL/min, many clinicians prefer to use zoledronate at 3–4 mg as slow intravenous infusion (over 60 min) to treat hypercalcemia of malignancy after adequate hydration with normal saline, as an alternative therapy. This avoids procedures such as hemodialysis. If zoledronate is not available, either pamidronate (30–45 mg IV over 4 h) or ibandronate (2 mg IV over 60–90 min) seem effective in patients with eGFR <30 mL/min. Thus, option E is correct.

It should be noted that zoledronic acid is available as Zometa and Reclast in the United States. The Food and Drug Administration issued a warning that Reclast (available as Aclasta outside the United States) should not be used in patients with serum creatinine levels <35 mL/min or in patients with acute renal impairment.

It is of interest to note that denosumab, an antibody to the receptor activator of nuclear factor κB-ligand, which inhibits osteoclastic activity, can be used in patients with renal impairment because it is hepatically metabolized. However, it is expensive and not approved for use in hypercalcemic patient with renal impairment.

Suggested Reading

Asonitis N, Angelousi A, Zafeiris C, et al. Diagnosis, pathophysiology and management of hypercalcemia in malignancy: a review of the literature. Horm Metab Res. 2019;51:770778.
Lameire N. Nephrotoxicity of recent anti-cancer drugs. Clin Kidney J. 2014;7:11–22.
Sahni V, Choudhury D, Ahmed Z. Chemotherapy-associated renal dysfunction. Nat Rev Nephrol. 2009;5:450–62.
Toussaint ND, Elder GJ, Kerr PG. Bisphosphonates in chronic kidney disease; Balancing potential benefits and adverse effects on bone and soft tissue. Clin J Am Soc Nephrol. 2009;4:221–33.

43. A patient with history of stone disease asks you for cough medication that contains pseudoephedrine. You advise him to avoid pseudoephedrine because it promotes stone formation. **Besides pseudoephedrine, which one of the following drugs is associated with stone formation?**

A. Vitamin C
B. Melamine-cyanuric acid
C. Acyclovir
D. Indinavir
E. All of the above

The answer is E

A large number of agents are associated with crystal nephropathy. Chronic use of pseudoephedrine was found to be associated with urolithiasis, which is radiolucent. Vitamin C is metabolized to oxalate, and high doses of vitamin C should be avoided in patient with history of nephrolithiasis. Melanine was a contaminant in infant milk formula manufactured in China and distributed worldwide. Cyanuric acid is a derivative of melamine. Melamine-cyanuric acid precipitates in distal tubules and renal papillae, causing crystalluria. Acyclovir and indinavir are well-known causes of crystalluria and crystal nephropathy. Thus, option E is correct.

Suggested Reading

Hau AK-C, Kwan TH, Li PK-t. Melamine toxicity and the kidney. J Am Soc Nephrol. 2009;20:245–50.
Perazella MA. Crystal-induced acute renal failure. Am J Med. 1999;106:459–65.
Smith CL, Gemar SK, Lewis MJ. Pseudoephedrine urolithiasis associated wit acute renal failure. Nephrol Dial Transplant. 2004;19:263–4.

44. A 26-year-old woman with sickle cell disease with serum creatinine of 1.4 mg/dL (eGFR <30 mL/dL) is admitted for seizure disorder. She is on meperidine 50 mg BID for pain by her primary care physician. Her pain was controlled for many weeks. She does not want to change her medication. **Regarding pain management, which one of the following drugs should best be avoided in CKD 3–5 patients?**

A. Codeine
B. Fentanyl
C. Methadone
D. Meperidine
E. Hydromorphone

The answer is D

Pain is common in patients with sickle cell disease. Also, pain is a comorbid condition in dialysis patients. Hepatically metabolized drugs such as fentanyl and methadone are safe for use in nondialysis and dialysis patients. Codeine is also metabolized by the liver to codeine-6-glucuronide, norcodeine, and morphine. It can be used in renal failure patients with reduction in dosage. Hydromorphone is also metabolized by the liver, and a reduced dose is safe in CKD patients. However, meperidine should be avoided in CKD 3–4 and dialysis patients, as it is metabolized to normeperidine. This metabolite is renally excreted and accumulates in renal failure. Normeperidine causes neuroexcitation and seizures. Toxicity of normeperidine is not reversed by naloxone but is removed by hemodialysis. Thus, option D is correct.

Suggested Reading

Conway BR, Fogarty DG, Nelson WE, et al. Opiate toxicity in patients with renal failure. BMJ. 2006;332:345–6.

Dean M. Opioids in renal failure and dialysis patients. J Pain Symptom Manage. 2004;28:497–508.

45. **In a type 2 diabetic patient with eGFR <40 mL/min, which one of the following antidiabetic medications does not require dosage reduction?**

A. Insulin
B. Glyburide
C. Glipizide
D. Metformin
E. Sitagliptin

The answer is C

Diabetes management in CKD patients is rather difficult because most of the antidiabetic drugs are renally excreted. Therefore, dosage adjustment is necessary to prevent hypoglycemia. Insulin is partly metabolized by the kidney. The American College of Physicians recommends decreasing dosage of insulin by 25% for patients with eGFR between 10 and 50 mL/min, and decreasing dose by 50% for those with eGFR <10 mL/min.

Similarly, the metabolites of glyburide or glibenclamide have hypoglycemic effects, and these metabolites are renally excreted. Therefore, these drugs should be avoided in patients with eGFR <50 mL/min.

Metformin should be avoided in women with serum creatinine 1.4 mg/dL or greater, and men 1.5 mg/dL or greater.

Sitagliptin and exenatide are incretins that increase glucose-stimulated insulin secretion. Both are renally excreted. Dosage reduction is required for sitagliptin in renal failure. Normal dose is 100 mg/day, and 50 mg/day in patients with eGFR 30–50 mL/min, and 25 mg/day in those with eGFR <30 mL/min. Exenatide should be avoided in patients with eGFR <30 mL/min.

Glipizide is metabolized by the liver to inactive metabolytes. Therefore, it is the choice of oral hypoglycemic agents in patients with diabetes and renal failure (C is correct).

Suggested Reading

Barone RJ, Beresan M, Pattin M, et al. Management of type 2 diabetes in patients with chronic kidney disease. Arch Clin Nephrol. 2017;3:053–6.

Yale J-F. Oral antihyperglycemic agents and renal disease: new agents, new concepts. J Am Soc Nephrol. 2005; 16:S7–10.

Zanchi A, Lehmann R, Philippe J. Antidiabetic drugs and kidney disease. Recommendations of the Swiss Society for Endocrinology and Diabetology. Swiss Med Wkly. 2012;142: w13629.

46. Many drugs are removed by intermittent hemodialysis and continuous renal (kidney) replacement therapies. **Which one of the following physicochemical characteristics affects drug removal by these renal (kidney) replacement therapies?**

A. Molecular weight
B. Protein binding
C. Volume of distribution (Vd)
D. Membrane characteristics
E. All of the above

The answer is E

The extent to which the drug is affected by dialysis is determined by all of the above physicochemical characteristics of the drug and dialysis membranes. Molecular weight or size of the drug is an important determinant of its removal. In general, smaller molecular weight drugs pass through the membrane more easily than larger molecular weight drugs. It should be noted that molecular weight of a drug may not be that important in high-flux dialyzers, as their membranes have large pores. For example, the molecular weights of many antibiotics are lower than the membrane pore size, and therefore, these antibiotics are easily removed.

Another important factor in dialyzability is protein binding. Proteins that are bound to proteins are less dialyzable than water-soluble drugs. Similarly, Vd plays an important role in removal of the drug. Drugs with large

Vd are removed less efficiently than drugs with small Vd. As described above, the characteristics of the dialysis membranes such as pore size, surface area, and geometry are important in drug removal. In addition, blood and dialysis flow rates will have great impact on drug removal. Thus, option E is correct.

Suggested Reading

Pea F, Viale P, Pavan F, et al. Pharmacokinetic considerations for antimicrobial therapy in patients receiving renal replacement therapy. Clin Pharmacokinet. 2007;46:997–1038.

Ŝefer S, Degorïja V. About drug dialyzability. Acta Clin Croa. 2003;42:257–67.

47. Drug removal occurs by diffusion, convection, or both. **Which type of renal (kidney) replacement therapy (RRT) mostly removes the drug by both diffusion and convection?**

A. Hemodialysis (HD)
B. Continues venovenous hemofiltration (CVVH)
C. Continuous venovenous hemodiafiltration (CVVHDF)
D. All of the above
E. None of the above

The answer is C

HD removes the drugs mostly by diffusion, as the removal is dependent on concentration difference between blood and dialysate. CVVH removes the drugs preferentially by convection (solvent drag), whereas CVVHDF combines both diffusion and convection. Thus, C is correct. Table 7.1 shows some of the comparisons between HD and CVVHDF.

Table 7.1 Comparisons of drug removal by HD and CVVHDF

Characteristic	HD	CVVHDF
Drug removal	Diffusion	Convection and diffusion
Process	Passive	Active
Time to equilibrate	Long	Short
Replacement fluid	No	Yes (pre- or postdilution)
Efficiency of drug removal	Less	More

Suggested Reading

Olyaei AJ, Wahba I, Bennett WM. Prescribing drugs for dialysis patients. In: Lerma EV, Weir MR, editors. Henrich's Principles and practice of dialysis. 5th ed. Philadelphia: Wolters Kluwer/Lippincott Williams & Wilkins; 2017. p. 533–61.

Pea F, Viale P, Pavan F, et al. Pharmacokinetic considerations for antimicrobial therapy in patients receiving renal replacement therapy. Clin Pharmacokinet. 2007;46:997–1038.

48. **Which one of the following drugs does NOT need supplementation following hemodialysis (HD)?**

A. Vancomycin
B. Gentamicin
C. Piperacillin/tazobactam
D. Meropenam
E. Phenytoin

The answer is E

Except for phenytoin, all other drugs require supplementation as they are partially removed by HD. Phenytoin removal is negligible during HD, and supplementation is not required. Thus, E is correct.

Suggested Reading

Matzke GR, Keller F, Battistella M. Drug dosing considerations in patients with acute kidney injury and chronic kidney disease. In: Yu ASL, Chertow GM, Luyckx VA, et al., editors. Brenner & Rector's the kidney. 11th ed. Philadelphia: Elsevier Saunders; 2020. p. 1989–2014.e8.

Olyaei AJ, Wahba I, Bennett WM. Prescribing drugs for dialysis patients. In: Lerma EV, Weir MR, editors. Henrich's Principles and practice of dialysis. 5th ed. Philadelphia: Wolters Kluwer/Lippincott Williams & Wilkins; 2017. p. 533–61.

49. You started a 52-year-old woman with sepsis and acute kidney injury on CVVHDF. She is on pipercillin/tazobactam 3.375 g every 6 hours. **Which one of the following choices is CORRECT regarding replacement of this antibiotic during CVVHDF?**

A. Continue the same dose every 6 hours
B. Decrease the dose to 2.25 g every 12 hours
C. Increase the dose to 4.5 g every 8 hours
D. Replace pipercillin/tazobactam with another antibiotic as the drug accumulates during CVVHDF
E. None of the above

The answer is A

Pipercillin/tazobactam is removed extensively during CVVHDF. It is suggested that this drug at 3.375 g every 6 hours is expected to produce desirable trough concentrations. Therefore, continuation of the drug at the same dosage maintains trough level above the MIC level. Thus, choice A is correct. It should be noted that tazobactam may accumulate over a period of time, but the toxicity of this β-lactamase inhibitor is unknown. Other choices are not appropriate for this patient.

Suggested Reading

Pea F, Viale P, Pavan F, et al. Pharmacokinetic considerations for antimicrobial therapy in patients receiving renal replacement therapy. Clin Pharmacokinet. 2007;46:997–1038.

Trotman RL, Williamson JC, Shoemaker DM, et al. Antibiotic dosing in critically ill adult patients receiving continuous renal replacement therapy. Clin Infect Dis. 2005;41:1159–66.

50. **Regarding vancomycin supplementation during CVVHDF, which one of the following statements is CORRECT?**

A. Vancomycin is not removed by CVVHDF and no supplementation is required
B. Vancomycin is removed by CVVHDF and supplementation is require
C. A trough level >25 mg/L should be maintained during CVVHDF
D. Maintenance dose of vancomycin during CVVHD should be >2 g/day
E. None of the above

The answer is B

Vancomycin is frequently used in patients on renal replacement therapies. The half-life of vancomycin increases in renal failure patients; therefore, dose adjustment is necessary. All renal replacement therapies, such as high-flux hemodialysis, CVVH, CVVHD, and CVVHDF, effectively remove vancomycin. Therefore, supplementation is recommended. Vancomycin maintenance dosing for patients receiving CVVHD or CVVHDF varies from 1 to 1.5 g/24 h depending on the trough level. A trough level of 5–10 mg/L is adequate for skin and soft tissue infections, or uncomplicated bacteremia, whereas a trough concentration of 10–15 mg/L is indicated for infections of endocarditis, osteomyelitis, or meningitis. It is recommended that trough levels of 15–20 mg/L are necessary for treatment of healthcare-associated pneumonia. Any trough level >25 mg/L may cause toxicity, and can reach this level if vancomycin dosage exceeds >2 g/24 h in a renal failure patient. Thus, A, C, D, and E are incorrect.

Suggested Reading

Pea F, Viale P, Pavan F, et al. Pharmacokinetic considerations for antimicrobial therapy in patients receiving renal replacement therapy. Clin Pharmacokinet. 2007;46:997–1038.

Trotman RL, Williamson JC, Shoemaker DM, et al. Antibiotic dosing in critically ill adult patients receiving continuous renal replacement therapy. Clin Infect Dis. 2005;41:1159–66.

51. A 64-year-old woman with severe sepsis is seen by you for acute kidney injury. She is on vancomycin for *S. aureus*. You started the patient on CVVHDF to manage fluid status and rising creatinine. One day later, the blood culture and sensitivity report is available, which indicates the need for aminoglycoside use. **How should aminoglycosides be adjusted in CVVHDF?**

A. All frequently used aminoglycosides are removed by CVVHDF, and replacement (supplementation) is required
B. Only gentamicin is removed and not tobramycin or amikacin
C. If gentamicin is used for synergy for Gram-positive organisms, the target peak level is >10 μg/mL
D. The loading dose of tobramycin during CVVHDF is 2 mg/kg every 24–48 h
E. None of the above is applicable

The answer is A

Aminoglycosides are renally excreted. In renal failure, reduced dose and increased interval of dosing is required. The clinically useful aminoglycosides (gentamicin, tobramycin, and amikacin) to treat infection are removed by CVVHD, CVVHDF, and hemodialysis at a rate equivalent to an eGFR of 10–40 mL/min. Therefore, replacement of these drugs is indicated during renal replacement therapies. Monitoring aminoglycoside levels are important. If peak levels are high, the interval for dosing is increased. Thus, option A is correct. Among the three aminoglycosides, only gentamicin is used for synergy in patients with Gram-positive organisms, and the target peak level is 3–4 μg/mL rather than 10 μg/mL. Thus, option C is incorrect. The loading dose of tobramycin is 3 mg/kg and the maintenance dose is 2 mg/kg; therefore, option D is incorrect. Table 7.2 provides dosing recommendations for aminoglycosides in critically ill patients on CVVHDF

Table 7.2 Dosing recommendations of aminoglycosides during CVVHDF in critically ill patients

Drug	Synergy dose	Loading dose[a]	Maintenance dose[a]
Gentamicin	1 mg/kg Q24–36 h	2.5–3 mg/kg	2 mg/kg Q24–48 h
Tobramycin	Not applicable	3 mg/kg	2 mg/kg Q24–48 h
Amikacin	Not applicable	10 mg/kg	7.5 mg/kg Q24–48 h

[a]Infection with Gram-negative bacteria

Suggested Reading

Churchwell MD, Mueller BA. Drug dosing during continuous renal replacement therapy. Sem Dial. 2009;22:185–8.
Trotman RL, Williamson JC, Shoemaker DM, et al. Antibiotic dosing in critically ill adult patients receiving continuous renal replacement therapy. Clin Infect Dis. 2005;41:1159–66.

52. **Which one of the following antibiotics does not require dose adjustment during continuous renal (kidney) replacement therapies?**

A. Amphotericin
B. Ceftriaxone
C. Linezolid
D. Voriconazole
E. All of the above

The answer is E

All of the above drugs do not require any dose adjustment during continuous renal replacement therapies (answer E is correct). The other common drugs that do not require dose adjustment include micafungin, azithromycin, doxycycline, clindamycin, metronidazole, rifampin, and tigecycline.

Suggested Reading

Choi G, Gomersall CD, Tian Q, Joynt GM, Freebairn R, Lipman J. Principles of ntibacterial dosing in continuous renal replacement therapy. Crit Care Med. 2009;37:2268–82.
Heintz BH, Matzke GR, Dager WE. Antimicrobial dosing concepts and recommendations for critically ill adult patients receiving continuous renal replacement therapy or intermittent hemodialysis. Pharmacotherapy. 2009;29:562–77.

Matzke GR, Keller F, Battistella M. Drug dosing considerations in patients with acute kidney injury and chronic kidney disease. In: Yu ASL, Chertow GM, Luyckx VA, et al., editors. Brenner & Rector's the kidney. 11th ed. Philadelphia: Elsevier Saunders; 2020. p. 1989–2014.e8.

Scheetz MH, Scarsi KK, Ghossein C, et al. Adjustment of antimicrobial dosages for continuous venovenous hemofiltration based on patient-specific information. Clin Infect Dis. 2006;42:436–7.

Trotman RL, Williamson JC, Shoemaker DM, et al. Antibiotic dosing in critically ill adult patients receiving continuous renal replacement therapy. Clin Infect Dis. 2005;41:1159–66.

53. A 60-year-old woman with type 2 diabetes is started on maintenance hemodialysis 3 months ago. She has a permcath with good blood flow. She develops fever with elevated white blood cell count. Blood culture reveals Gram-positive cocci that are sensitive to vancomycin and gentamicin. The patient receives both drugs with appropriate trough levels. **Which one of the following drugs has been shown to reduce ototoxicity in dialysis patients?**

A. Mannitol
B. Carnitine
C. N-acetylcysteine (NAC)
D. 25(OH)D_3
E. Carbonic anhydrase inhibitor

The answer is C

The combination of vancomycin and gentamicin causes severe irreversible ototoxicity, particularly in dialysis patients. This combination is used to treat catheter-associated infections in hemodialysis (HD) patients and peritonitis in chronic ambulatory peritoneal dialysis (CAPD) patients. Two clinical studies, one in HD and another in CAPD patients, showed that NAC 600 mg twice daily orally reduced the incidence of ototoxicity compared to those without NAC. The mechanisms by which NAC reduces ototoxicity is not clearly understood. However, increased oxidative stress, genetic predisposition, and aminoglycoside-induced apoptosis in inner ear hair cells have been proposed. NAC seems to modify these mechanisms and reduces the incidence of ototoxicity. Thus, option C is correct. Other drugs have not been tested.

Suggested Reading

Feldman L, Efrati S, Eviatar E, et al. Gentamicin-induced ototoxicity in hemodialysis patients is ameliorated by N-acetylcysteine. Kidney Int. 2007;72:359–63.

Feldman L, Sherman RL, Weissgarten J. N-acetylcysteine use for amelioration of amioglycnoside-induced ototoxicity in dialysis patients. Sem Dial. 2012;25:491–4.

Tokgoz B, Ucar C, Kocyigit I, et al. Protective effect of N-acetylcysteine from drug-induced ototoxicity in uraemic patients with CAPD peritonitis. Nephrol Dial Transplant. 2011;26:4073–8.

54. A 64-year-old woman with end-stage kidney disease and on maintenance hemodialysis (HD) develops intradialytic hypotension during each session of treatment. **Which one of the following pharmacologic agents has been shown to improve hypotension in this patient?**

A. Clonidine
B. Midodrine
C. Hydralazine
D. Enalapril
E. Losartan

The answer is B

Intradialytic hypotension (IDH) is a vexing problem in some HD patients, including the diabetic and elderly patients. Also, patients with LVH, myocardial stunning, or ischemia are vulnerable to IDH. IDH is defined as an absolute intradialytic nadir systolic BP <90 mm Hg, which is associated with adverse cardiovascular outcomes, whereas previous definition of a drop in systolic BP ~20 mm Hg, or a drop in mean arterial BP ~10 mm Hg is not associated with adverse outcomes. It is usually associated with nausea, vomiting, dizziness, and disturbance in the stomach. Clotting of A-V access is rather frequent. Of all the above drugs, only midodrine, which is an α1-agonist, raises BP and prevents intradialytic hypotension. Other drugs lower BP. Thus, answer B is correct.

Suggested Reading

Reeves PB, Mc Causland FR. Mechanisms, clinical implications, and treatment of intradialytic hypotension. Clin J Am Soc Nephrol. 2018;13:1297–303.
Reilly RF. Attending Rounds: a patient with intradialytic hypotension. Clin J Am Soc Nephrol. 2014;9:798–803.
Sars B, van der Sande FM, Kooman JP. Intradialytic hypotension: mechanisms and outcome. Blood Purif. 2020;49:158–67.

55. A 50-year-old man on hemodialysis (HD) develops heparin-induced thrombocytopenia (HIT). **Which one of the following anticoagulants has been tried in HD patients with HIT?**

A. Enoxaparin
B. Danaparoid
C. Lepirudin
D. Citrate
E. All of the above

The answer is E

HIT is a serious condition that results from antibodies formed against platelet factor 4 and heparin. It occurs in 0–12% of HD patients. HIT is classified into type I and types II types, the latter being the most significant entity. Type II HIT is characterized by the development of thrombocytopenia in 5–10 days and development of both venous and arterial thrombosis. Discontinuation of unfractionated heparin is the first step in the treatment of HIT.

In HD patients, alternatives to heparin treatment have been developed. These include the use of low molecular weight heparins (enoxaparin), nonheparin glycosaminoglycan heparin sulfate (danaparoid), direct thrombin inhibitors (lepirudin and argatroban), and regional citrate anticoagulation. Each one of these anticoagulants causes many adverse events, including bleeding, development of antibodies, and electrolyte disturbances. Table 7.3 shows the protocol for these alternative anticoagulants.

Table 7.3 Common protocols of alternative anticoagulants during hemodialysis

Category	Drug (s)	Dose (predialysis)	Adverse events
Low-molecular-weight heparin	Enoxaparin Dalteparin Tinzaparin	100 IU/kg as a bolus 70 IU/kg as a bolus 4500 IU as a bolus with adjustment of the dose as indicated	HIT and bleeding
Heparinoid	Danaparoid	35 units/kg as a bolus	Bleeding (rare, if cautiously used)
Direct thrombin inhibitors	Lepirudin Argatroban	0.1–0.15 mg/kg as a bolus 250 μg/kg bolus with a repeat dose at midsession, or continuous infusion of 2 μg/kg/min (reduce dose in liver disease)	Bleeding and antibody production (both)
Citrate	Citrate (trisodium)	60 mL/h (62.1 mmol/L)	Hypernatremia, metabolic alkalosis, hypocalcemia, secondary hyperparathyroidism, and tetany

Suggested Reading

Dahms WJ Jr. Anticoagulation strategies during hemodialysis procedures. In: Lerma EV, Weir MR, editors. Henrich's Principles and practice of dialysis. 5th ed. Philadelphia: Wolters Kluwer/Lippincott Williams & Wilkins; 2017. p. 62–9.
Fischer K-G. Essentials of anticoagulation in hemodialysis. Hemodial Int. 2007;11:178–89.

56. A 70-year-old woman with end-stage kidney disease due to hypertension and on hemodialysis (HD) is admitted with stroke. The neurologist wants an MRI with contrast. **Which one of the following gadolinium-based contrast agents is contraindicated in this patient?**

A. Gadopentate dimeglumine (Magnevist)
B. Gadoversetamide (Optiamark)
C. Gadodiamide (Omniscan)
D. All of the above
E. A and C only

The answer is D

Currently, there are nine gadolinium-based contrast agents (GBCAs) approved for MRI imaging in the United States and the European Union. GBCAs are more nephrotoxic than iodinated contrast agents in equimolar concentrations. Because of the use of low volume for MRI and other studies, the incidence of nephrotoxicity with MRI agents is much lower than iodinated contrast agents. However, in diabetic patients, nondialysis patients with CKD stages 4–5, and dialysis patients, GBCAs induce nephrotoxicity called nephrogenic systemic fibrosis (NSF) even at standard doses.

NSF was first observed in 1997, and subsequently reported in 2000. It was originally identified as a cutaneous lesion with indurated plaques and papules on the extremities and trunk in patients on HD and failed kidney transplant patients. Thickening of the skin, resembling scleroderma, is a common feature. In 2006, a relationship between NSF and GBCAs has been suggested.

Gadolinium is extremely toxic because of its deposition in skin, lungs, lymph nodes, bone, and other organs. It may stimulate many cytokines that promote fibrosis. Joint contractures and limitations in mobility are common. Deep vein thrombosis, pulmonary embolism, atrial thrombus, and clotting of arteriovenous fistulas have been reported in patients with NSF. These patients seem to have antiphospholipid antibody syndrome. Fibrosis of several organs, including lungs, muscle, and diaphragm, may lead to morbidity and mortality. Sudden death from respiratory failure has been reported.

The above mentioned three GBCAs are contraindicated in HD patients, as they cause NSF. Thus, option D is correct.

Suggested Reading

Cohan R, Chovke P, Cohen M, et al. Nephrogenic systemic fibrosis. Am Coll Radiol Manual Contrast Media. Version 7. 2010: 49–55.

Leisman S. Radiocontrast toxicity. Adv Chronic Kidney Dis. 2020;27:50–5.

Perazella MA. Current status of gadolinium toxicity in patients with kidney disease. Clin J Am Soc Nephrol. 2009;4:461–9.

57. A 52-year-old type 2 diabetic patient with CKD 3 is referred to you for evaluation of hyperkalemia (6.9 mEq/L). He has pedal edema with occasional pain. His fasting glucose is 310 mg/dL. **Which one of the following combinations is MOST likely to cause hyperkalemia?**

    A. Angiotensin-converting enzyme inhibitor (ACE-I), furosemide and diltiazem
    B. ACE-I, furosemide and spironolactone
    C. Angiotensin receptor blocker (ARB), furosemide, and nonsteroidal antiinflammatory agent (NSAID)
    D. ACE-I, spironolactone, hyperglycemia, and NSAID
    E. ACE-I, ARB, and furosemide

The answer is D

The combination of ACE-I, spironolactone, hyperglycemia, and NSAID causes severe hyperkalemia, particularly in a diabetic subject. An ACE-I or ARB and NSAID cause hyperkalemia by lowering aldosterone levels, whereas spironolactone antagonizes the action of aldosterone. Hyperglycemia causes hyperkalemia by solvent drag. Thus, the combination in option D causes such a severe hyperkalemia. The drug combination in other options may raise serum [K^+] to the upper limit of normal range and not to this extent because of furosemide-induced kaliuresis.

Suggested Reading

Juurlink DN, Mamdani MM, Lee DS, et al. Rate of hyperglycemia after publication of the Randomized Aldactone Evaluation Study. N Engl J Med. 2004;351:543–51.

Van Buren PN. Adams-Huet B, Nguyen M, et al. Potassium handling with dual renin-angiotensin system inhibition in diabetic nephropathy. Clin J Am Soc Nephrol. 2014;9:295–301.

58. A 32-year-old woman with kidney transplant 4 years ago presents to her primary care physician with gingival hyperplasia. She is on low dose of cyclosporine and mycophenolate mofetil (MMF) (500 mg twice daily). She was initially on prednisone, tacrolimus, and sirolimus, and then switched to cyclosporine and MMF. Physical exam shows gingival

hyperplasia and thick hair growth on the trunk and lower extremities. **Which one of the following drugs is responsible for her gingival hyperplasia and hypertrichosis?**

A. MMF
B. Sirolimus
C. Tacrolimus
D. Cyclosporine
E. Prednisone

The answer is D

Of all the above drugs, cyclosporine is the most common cause of gingival hyperplasia and hirsutism. This is particularly a bothersome cosmetic problem in women. A number of case reports have been published on both gingival hyperplasia and hirsutism in patients receiving cyclosporine. Thus, option D is correct. Other agents are less likely to cause both gingival hyperplasia and hirsutism.

Suggested Reading

Boratyriska M, Radvan-Oczko M, Falkiewicz K, et al. Gingival overgrowth in kidney recipients treated with cyclosporine and its relationship with chronic graft nephropathy. Transplant Proc. 2003;35:2238–40.
Lutz G. Cyclosporin A on hair growth. Skin Pharmacol. 1994;7:1001–104.

59. A 34-year-old woman with type 2 diabetes and eGFR of 26 mL/min is admitted to the hospital for altered mental status. Her serum glucose is 42 mg/dL. She was admitted four times with similar hypoglycemic episodes in the last 3 months. She is on glyburide 5 mg, and metformin and sitagliptin combination (100 mg/1000 mg). **In order to prevent her hypoglycemic episodes, which one of the following therapeutic options you recommend at this time?**

A. Decrease the combination dose of metformin and sitagliptin to 50/500 mg daily
B. Substitute glipizide 5 mg daily with glyburide
C. Start metformin 500 mg daily
D. Start low dose of insulin
E. Increase carbohydrate intake and maintain the same oral hypoglycemic agents

The answer is D

It is not uncommon for a diabetic patient to experience hypoglycemic episodes either on insulin or oral hypoglycemic agents. However, hypoglycemic episodes are more common in patients with reduced kidney function. In this patient, the best option is to start insulin and follow glucose levels carefully and titrate dose to maintain HbA1c levels ~7.5%. Metformin should not be continued in a patient with eGFR <30 mL/min because of lactic acidosis. Increasing carbohydrate diet and switching to glipizide in this patient are of little benefit, although glipizide can be used in CKD patients without hypoglycemic episodes. Thus, option D is correct.

Suggested Reading

Reilly JB, Berns JS. Selection and dosing of medications for management of diabetes in patients with advanced kidney disease. Sem Dialysis. 2010;23:163–8.
Zanchi A, Lehmann R, Philippe J. Antidiabetic drugs and kidney disease. Recommendations of the Swiss Society for endocrinology and diabetology. Swiss Med Wkly. 2012;142: w13629.

60. **Match the following drugs with the clinical abnormalities:**

Drug	**Clinical manifestations**
A. Voriconazole	1. Hyperphosphatemia
B. Lorazepam	2. Experiencing flashing lights without eye pain
C. Propofol	3. L- and D-lactic acidosis
D. Liposomal amphotericin B (L-AMP)	4. Lactic acidosis, rhabdomyolysis, and acute kidney injury

Answers: A = 2; B = 3; C = 4; D = 1

Cyclodextrin is a solubilizing agent in voriconazole, and photopsia (seeing flashing or colored light) is an adverse event of cyclodextrin. Lorazepam contains propylene glycol as a diluent, which is metabolized to L- and D-lactic acid. Propofol is an anesthetic that causes propofol-related infusion syndrome (PRIS). This PRIS syndrome is characterized by lactic acidosis, rhabdomyolysis, acute kidney injury, hyperkalemia, and cardiovascular collapse. L-AMP is amphotericin B that is embedded in a phospholipid bilayer of unilamellar liposomes. Measurement of phosphate with a specific autoanalyzer, Synchron LX20, gives a high level of phosphate (pseudohyperphosphatemia) without any symptoms of hyperphosphatemia.

Suggested Reading

Mike LN. Propofol-related infusion syndrome. Pract Gastroenterol. 2010;16–23.

Pea F, Viale P. Hallucinations during voriconazole therapy: who is at high risk and could benefit from therapeutic drug monitoring? Ther Drug Monit. 2009;31:135–6.

61. A 50-year-old obese type 2 diabetic woman is started on canagliflozin (sodium glucose transporter-2 inhibitor, SGLT-2 inhibitor) for management of her diabetes. **Which one of the following effects of SGLT-2 inhibitor is expected in this patient?**

A. Reduction in serum glucose levels
B. Reduction in body weight
C. Reduction in BP
D. Reduction in albuminuria
E. All of the above

The answer is E

Canagliflozin inhibits glucose absorption in the proximal tubule by inhibiting Na-glucose transporter-2. As a result, the patient loses glucose in the urine. Studies on canagliflozin show that this drug lowers not only glucose but also BP. It also causes weight loss. This suggests that canagliflozin reduces cardiovascular risk in diabetic patients. Also, canagliflozin improves not only albuminuria but also GFR in type 2 diabetic patients. Thus, E is correct. Other SGLT-2 such as dapagliflozin and empagliflozin are shown to have similar beneficial effects on renal and cardiovascular outcomes.

Suggested Reading

Perkovic V, Jardine MJ, Neal B, et al. for the CREDENCE Trial Investigators. Canagliflozin and renal outcomes in type 2 diabetes and nephropathy. N Engl J Med. 2019;380:2295–306.

Schernthaner G, Gross JL, Rosenstock J, et al. Canagliflozin compared with sitagliptin for patients with type 2 diabetes who do not have adequate glycemic control with metformin plus sulfonylurea: a 52-week randomized trial. Diabetes Care. 2013;36:2508–15.

Stenlöf K, Cefalu WT, Kim KA, et al. Efficacy and safety of canagliflozin monotherapy in subjects with type 2 diabetes mellitus inadequately controlled with diet and exercise. Diabetes Obes Metab. 2013;15:372–82.

62. An 18-year-old man is referred to you for evaluation of nephrotic syndrome due to minimal change disease. His BP is 140/80 mm Hg with a heart rate of 80 beats/min. He is on steroids 40 mg daily, furosemide 80 mg twice daily, and ramipril 10 mg daily. He has 3+ pitting edema. His creatinine is 0.7 mg/dL with proteinuria of 6.5 g/24 h. He is on salt restriction of 88 mEq (2 g Na^+). Although his proteinuria reduced from 8.2 g/24 h to 6.5 g/24 h, his edema has not improved. **The patient may benefit from the addition of which one of the following drugs?**

A. Metolazone
B. Amiloride
C. Cyclophosphamide
D. Amlodipine
E. Losartan

The answer is B

The major site for Na^+ reabsorption in the kidney in patients with nephrotic syndrome is the collecting duct. According to a recent theory, Na^+ retention in patients with nephrotic syndrome occurs by overactivity of the

epithelial Na^+ channel (ENaC) in principle cells of the collecting duct. ENaC is inhibited by amiloride. It seems that ENaC activity is increased by locally generated plasmin from plasminogen. Plasminogen is filtered at the glomerulus in nephrotic syndrome. When it reaches the cortical collecting duct, it is split into plasmin by urokinase, and plasmin activates the ENaC to reabsorb Na^+, resulting in low excretion of Na^+. Thus, formation of edema is enhanced in nephrotic syndrome. Since amiloride inhibits ENaC, it is appropriate to start this patient on amiloride and follow his edema (B). Addition of any of the above drugs may not be appropriate at this time.

Suggested Reading

Svenningsen P, Bistrup C, Friis UG, et al. Plasmin in nephrotic urine activates the epithelial sodium channel. J Am Soc Nephrol. 2009;20:299–310.

RRondon-Berrios H. New insights into the pathophysiology of oedema in nephrotic syndrome. Nefrologia. 2011;31:148–54.

63. **Match the following antiretroviral drugs with their mechanisms and clinical manifestations:**

Drug	Mechanism (s)	Clinical manifestations
A. Acyclovir	1. Acute tubular injury and intratubular crystal deposition	Acute tubular necrosis (ATN) and nephrolithiasis
B. Interferon-α	2. Podocyte injury and proximal tubule injury	ATN and collapsing focal segmental glomerulosclerosis
C. Tenofovir	3. Proximal tubule injury	ATN and Fanconi syndrome
D. Foscarnet	4. Proximal tubule injury and intraglomerular crystal deposition	ATN, acute glomerulonephritis, and nephrogenic diabetes insipidus
E. Indinavir	5. Intratubular crystal deposition	Nephrolithiasis

Answers: A = 1; B = 2; C = 3; D = 4; E = 5

Suggested Reading

Coroneos E, Petrusevsk G, Varghes F, et al. Focal segmental glomerulosclerosis with acute renal failure associated with α-interferon therapy. Am J Kidney Dis. 1996;28:888–92.

Kim SY, Moon A. Drug-induced nephrotoxicity and its biomarkers. Biomol Ther (Seoul). 2012;20:268–72.

Perazella MA. Drug-induced renal failure: update on new medications and unique mechanisms of nephrotoxicity. Am J Med Sci. 2003;325:349–62.

64. **Match the following antibiotic drugs with their mechanisms and clinical manifestations:**

Drug	Mechanism(s)	Clinical manifestations
A. Aminoglycosides	1. Proximal tubule injury	Acute tubular necrosis (ATN)
B. Fluoroquinolones	2. Proximal tubule injury	ATN, acute tubulointerstitial disease, (ATID), and thrombotic microangiopathy
C. Trimethoprim/sulfamethoxazole	3. ENaC inhibition	Acute rise in serum creatinine, ATID
D. Daptomycin	4. Rhabdomyolysis	ATN

ENaC epithelial sodium channel

Answers: A = 1; B = 2; C = 3; D = 4

Suggested Reading

Abraham G, Finkelberg D, Spooner LM. Daptomycin-induced acute renal and hepatic toxicity without rhabdomyolysis. Ann Pharmacother. 2008;42:719–21.

Bird ST, Etminan M, Brophy JM, et al. Risk of acute kidney injury associated with the use of fluoroquinolones. CMAJ. 2013;185:E475–82.

Moore RD, Smith CR, Lipsky JJ, et al. Risk factors for nephrotoxicity in patients treated with aminoglycosides. Ann Intern Med. 1984;100: 352–7.

Pisoni R, Ruggenenti P, Remuzzi G. Drug-induced thrombotic microangiopathy: incidence, prevention and management. Drug Saf. 2001;24:491–501.

65. **Which one of the following angiotensin-converting enzyme inhibitors (ACE-Is) requires dose adjustment in patients with eGFR <10 mL/min?**

A. Benazepril
B. Enalapril
C. Lisinopril
D. Quinapril
E. All of the above

The answer is E

All of the above ACE-Is require dose adjustments in patients with an eGFR <10 mL/min (E is correct). Table 7.4 shows ACE-Is dosing in kidney disease.

Table 7.4 ACE-Is dosing in kidney disease

Drug	Normal dosage	Renal excretion (%)	eGFR >50 mL/min	eGFR 10–50 mL/min	eGFR <10 mL/min
Benazepril	10–80 mg QD	20	100%	75%	25–50%
Enalapril	5 mg QD–20 mg BID	45	100%	75%	50%
Lisinopril	2.5 mg QD–20 mg BID	85	100%	50–75%	25–50%
Quinapril	10 mg QD–40 mg QD	30	100%	75–100	75%

Suggested Reading

Olyaei AJ, Wahba I, Bennett WM. Prescribing drugs for dialysis patients. In: Lerma EV, Weir MR, editors. Henrich's Principles and practice of dialysis. 5th ed. Philadelphia: Wolters Kluwer/Lippincott Williams & Wilkins; 2017. p. 533–61.

66. **Which one of the following angiotensin receptor blockers (ARBs) requires dose adjustment in patients with eGFR <10 mL/min?**

A. Losartan
B. Valsartan
C. Telmisartan
D. Irbesartan
E. Candesartan

The answer is E

Only candesartan requires lower dose in patients with an eGFR <10 mL/min (E is correct). Table 7.5 provides some dose adjustment of ARBs.

Table 7.5 Dose adjustment of ARBs in renal failure

Drug	Normal dosage	Renal excretion (%)	eGFR >50 mL/min	eGFR 10–50 mL/min	eGFR <10 mL/min
Losartan	50–100 mg QD	13	100%	100%	100%
Valsartan	80–160 mg BID	7	100%	100%	100%
Telmisartan	20–80 mg QD	<5	100%	100%	100%
Irbesartan	150–300 mg QD	20	100%	100%	100%
Candesartan	16–32 mg QD	33	100%	100%	50%

Suggested Reading

Olyaei AJ, Wahba I, Bennett WM. Prescribing drugs for dialysis patients. In: Lerma EV, Weir MR, editors. Henrich's Principles and practice of dialysis. 5th ed. Philadelphia: Wolters Kluwer/Lippincott Williams & Wilkins; 2017. p. 533–61.

67. **Which one of the following drugs is NOT dialyzable by hemodialysis?**

A. Clonidine
B. Carvedilol
C. Amlodipine
D. Furosemide
E. All of the above

The answer is E

None of the above drugs is removed by hemodialysis. Therefore, dose adjustment postdialysis is not required (E is correct).

Suggested Reading

Olyaei AJ, Wahba I, Bennett WM. Prescribing drugs for dialysis patients. In: Lerma EV, Weir MR, editors. Henrich's Principles and practice of dialysis. 5th ed. Philadelphia: Wolters Kluwer/Lippincott Williams & Wilkins; 2017. p. 533–61.

68. A hemodialysis (HD) patient receives an antibiotic, which is 50% protein bound, prior to dialysis. The nurse draws blood for antibiotic level prior to starting HD, and the levels are 70 mg/L. The patient receives HD for 4 h with a blood flow rate of 400 mL/min and dialysis flow rate of 800 mL/min. Post-HD antibiotic levels are 60 mg/L. **What is the clearance of this antibiotic?**

A. 85 mL/min
B. 75 mL/min
C. 67 mL/min
D. 57 mL/min
E. 37 mL/min

The answer is D

The clearance of the drug by HD is calculated as follows:

$$\begin{aligned}&\textbf{Clearance of the drug} = \textbf{Blood flow rate} \times \textbf{Drug extraction rate, where extraction ratio is calculated as}:\\&\left(\textbf{predialysis drug concentration} - \textbf{postdialysis concentration}\right) / \textbf{predialysis concentration}\\&\qquad = \mathbf{70 - 60 / 70 \text{ or } 10 / 70 = 0.14} \ \left(\textbf{means 14\% extraction or 14\% of the drug was removed}\right)\\&\textbf{Clearance} = \textbf{Blood flow rate} \times \textbf{drug extraction ratio}\\&\qquad = \mathbf{400 \times 0.14 = 57\, mL} / \text{min}\left(\textbf{answer D is correct}\right)\end{aligned}$$

Suggested Reading

Launay-Vacher V, Izzedine H, Baumelou A, et al. F_{HD}: An index to evaluate drug elimination by hemodialysis. Am J Nephrol. 2005;25:342–51.
Lea-Henry TN, Carland JE, Stocker SL, et al. Clinical pharmacokinetics in kidney disease. Fundamental principles. Clin J Am Soc Nephrol. 2018;13:1085–95.

69. A 70 kg hemodialysis (HD) male has been receiving vancomycin for infection of his A-V fistula. His trough level is 15 μg/mL. He receives 1 g of vancomycin prior to HD. Post-HD vancomycin level is 55 μg/mL. The current dose of vancomycin is based on its published apparent volume of distribution (V_d) of 0.72 L/kg. **What is your recommendation of next dose of vancomycin?**

A. Increase
B. Decrease
C. No change
D. All of the above
E. None of the above

The answer is B

In order to implement next vancomycin dose, one needs to calculate its current V_d, which is calculated as follows:

$$\mathbf{Vd = Dose / (post - HD\,concentration - Pre - HD\,concentration)}$$
$$\mathbf{= 1{,}000 / (55 - 15) = 1{,}000 / 40 = 25\,L}$$

Since V_d is expressed as L/kg, the current V_d is 25/70 = 0.36 L/kg.

Generally, if patient's V_d is higher than the published V_d, a higher dose of vancomycin is recommended. If it is lower than the published value, a lower dose is recommended. The patient's current V_d of 0.36 L/kg is exactly half of the published V_d (0.72 L/kg); therefore, a dose reduction (i.e., 500 mg) is recommended. Thus, answer B is correct.

Suggested Reading

Estes KS, Derendorf H. Comparison of the pharmacokinetic properties of vancomycin, linezolid, tigecyclin, and daptomycin. Eur J Med Res. 2010;15:533.

Rybak MJ. The pharmacokinetic and pharmacodynamic properties of vancomycin. Clin Infect Dis. 2006;42(suppl 1): S35–9.

70. A 70-kg patient is started on CVVH for AKI and fluid overload. He receives vancomycin for suspected Gram-positive infection. The CVVH prescription is as follows:

$$\text{Effluent rate} = 1.75\,\text{L/h}\,(25\,\text{mL/kg})$$
$$\text{Prefilter fluid replacement rate}\,(Q_{rep}) = 1.5\,\text{L/h or } 25\,\text{mL/min}$$
$$\text{Postfilter fluid replacement rate} = 0.25\,\text{L/h}$$
$$\text{Blood flow rate}\,(Q_b) = 200\,\text{mL/min}$$
$$\text{Fluid removal rate}\,(Q_f) = 200\,\text{mL/h or } 3.3\,\text{mL/min}$$

What is the vancomycin clearance in this patient?

A. 20.6 mL/min
B. 20.2 mL/min
C. 24.6 mL/min
D. 26.6 mL/min
E. 28.6 mL/min

The answer is B

Solute transport across the filter occurs by convection during CVVH procedure. Simply, drug clearance by CVVH can be calculated from the ultrafiltration (UF) rate and the drug's specific sieving coefficient (SC). SC is defined as the ability of the drug to cross the membrane, which is determined by the ratio of the drug concentration in the ultrafiltrate to the concentration in the plasma. An SC of 1 indicates that the drug can cross the membrane easily, and an SC of zero (0) indicates no crossing of the membrane and no drug removal. The SC of vancomycin is 0.8, indicating that 80% of the drug is free and 20% is bound to protein.

The clearance of the drug by CVVH depends on the method of fluid replacement. Prefilter replacement fluid dilutes the drug, and its removal is less than the postfilter replacement, because the blood entering the filter is diluted by the replacement fluid. Therefore, a dilution factor must be used:

$$\textbf{Dilution factor} = (Q_b / Q_b + Q_{rep})$$

The drug clearance for prefilter replacement can then be calculated by the following formula:

$$\textbf{Rate of clearance} = \textbf{UF rate} \times \textbf{SC} \times [(Q_b / Q_b + Q_{rep})]$$

where UF rate refers to the combined amount of fluid removal rate and replacement fluid rate (mL/min); SC for vancomycin is 0.8.

$$\mathbf{UF\,rate = 25 + 3.3 = 28.3}$$
$$\mathbf{SC = 0.8}$$
$$\mathbf{\left(Q_b / Q_b + Q_{rep}\right) = \left(200 / 200 + 25\right) = 0.89}$$

By applying the above values, we obtain:

$$\mathbf{Rate\ of\ vancomycin\ clearance = 28.3 \times 0.8 \times 0.89}$$
$$\mathbf{= 20.15\,mL / \mathrm{min}\left(answer\ B\,is\ correct\right)}$$

If the same UF rate is maintained with the same amount of postfilter replacement fluid (1.5 L/h or 25 mL/min + fluid removal 200 mL/h or 3.3 mL/min), the following formula can be used to calculate the clearance of vancomycin:

$$\mathbf{Rate\ of\ clearance = UF\,rate \times SC}$$
$$\mathbf{= 28.3 \times 0.8 = 22.64\,mL / \mathrm{min}}$$

Note that postfilter clearance is higher by 2.11 mL/min than prefilter clearance.

Suggested Reading

Choi G, Gomersall CD, Tian Q, et al. Principles of antibacterial dosing in continuous renal replacement therapy. Blood Purif. 2010;30:195–212.

Pea F. Principles of pharmacodynamics and pharmacokinetics of drugs used in extracorporeal therapies. In: Ranco C, Bellomo R, Kellum JA, et al., editors. Critical care nephrology. 3rd ed. Philadelphia: Elsevier; 2019. p. 892–6.

Schetz M, Joannes-Boyau O, Bouman C. Drug removal by CRRT and drug dosing in patients on CRRT. In: Oudemans-van Straaten H, Forni L, Groeneveld A, editors. Acute nephrology for the critical care physician. Cham: Springer; 2015. p. 233–43.

71. The above patient was started on CVVHDF because of a further increase in serum creatinine and also to manage fluid balance. The CVVHDF prescription is as follows:

$$\text{Effluent fluid rate}\left(30\,\mathrm{mL/kg}\right) = 2{,}100\,\mathrm{mL/h\,or\,35\,mL/min}$$
$$\text{Pre filter fluid replacement rate}\left(Q_{rep}\right) = 1.0\,\mathrm{L/h\,or\,17\,mL/min}$$
$$\text{Dialysate fluid rate}\left(Q_d\right) = 0.9\,\mathrm{L/kg\,or\,15\,mL/min}$$
$$\text{Post filter fluid replacement rate} = 0.2\,\mathrm{L/h}$$
$$\text{Blood flow rate}\left(Q_b\right) = 200\,\mathrm{mL/min}$$
$$\text{Fluid removal rate}\left(Q_f\right) = 180\,\mathrm{mL/h\,or\,3\,mL/min}$$

What is the vancomycin clearance in this patient?

A. 24 mL/min
B. 26 mL/min
C. 28 mL/min
D. 30 mL/min
E. 32 mL/min

The answer is B

CVVHDF uses both convection and diffusion for solute transfer across the filter. Drug clearance using prefilter fluid replacement can be calculated by the following formula:

$$\textbf{Effluent rate} \times \textbf{SC} \times \left[\mathbf{Q_b} / \left(\mathbf{Q_b} + \mathbf{Q_{rep}}\right)\right]$$

Where effluent rate includes prefilter replacement fluid + dialysate fluid rate + fluid removal rate, SC is sieving coefficient and $Q_b/(Q_b + Q_{rep})$ is dilution factor.

$$\textbf{Effluent fluid}\left(\mathbf{1\,L + 0.9\,L + 0.18\,L = 2.08\,L / h}\right)\textbf{or } \mathbf{34.7\,mL} / \text{min}$$

$$\mathbf{SC = 0.8}$$

$$\textbf{Dilution factor} = \left(\mathbf{200 / 200 + 15}\right) = \mathbf{0.93}$$

By applying the above values, we obtain:

$$\mathbf{34.7 \times 0.8 \times 0.93 = 25.82\,mL} / \text{min}\left(\textbf{B is correct}\right)$$

Suggested Reading

Choi G, Gomersall CD, Tian Q, et al. Principles of antibacterial dosing in continuous renal replacement therapy. Blood Purif. 2010;30:195–212.

Pea F. Principles of pharmacodynamics and pharmacokinetics of drugs used in extracorporeal therapies. In: Ronco C, Bellomo R, Kellum JA, et al., editors. Critical care nephrology. 3rd ed. Philadelphia: Elsevier; 2019. p. 892–6.

Schetz M, Joannes-Boyau O, Bouman C. Drug removal by CRRT and drug dosing in patients on CRRT. In: Oudemans-van Straaten H, Forni L, Groeneveld A, editors. Acute nephrology for the critical care physician. Cham: Springer; 2015. p. 233–43.

72. A 70-kg woman is admitted for sepsis and is on CVVH for fluid removal. She is receiving vancomycin and meropenem. Her random vancomycin levels are 20 mg/L. Her CVVH prescription is as follows:

$$\text{Effluent rate} = 1.75\,\text{L} / \text{h}\left(25\,\text{mL} / \text{kg}\right)$$

$$\text{Prefilter fluid replacement rate}\left(Q_{rep}\right) = 1.5\,\text{L} / \text{h or } 25\,\text{mL} / \text{min}$$

$$\text{Postfilter fluid replacement rate} = 0.25\,\text{L} / \text{h}$$

$$\text{Blood flow rate}\left(Q_b\right) = 200\,\text{mL} / \text{min}$$

$$\text{Fluid removal rate}\left(Q_f\right) = 200\,\text{mL} / \text{h or } 3.3\,\text{mL} / \text{min}$$

Calculate the amount of vancomycin that is cleared per hour?

A. 20 mg/h
B. 22 mg/h
C. 24 mg/h
D. 26 mg/h
E. 28 mg/h

The answer is C

The drug clearance for prefilter replacement can be calculated, as above, with the inclusion of antibiotic concentration, by the following formula:

$$\textbf{Rate of clearance} = \textbf{UF rate} \times \textbf{Antibiotic concentration} \times \textbf{SC} \times \left[\left(\mathbf{Q_b} / \mathbf{Q_b} + \mathbf{Q_{rep}}\right)\right]$$

where UF rate refers to the combined amount of fluid removal rate and replacement fluid rate (mL/h); SC for vancomycin is 0.8.

$$\mathbf{UF\ rate = 1.5 + 0.2 = 1.7\,L/h}$$

$$\mathbf{Antibiotic\ concentration = 20\,mg/L}$$

$$\mathbf{SC = 0.8}$$

$$\mathbf{\left(Q_b / Q_b + Q_{rep}\right) = \left(200/200 + 25\right) = 0.89}$$

By applying the above values, we obtain:

$$\mathbf{Rate\ of\ vancomycin\ clearance = 1.7 \times 20 \times 0.8 \times 0.89}$$
$$\mathbf{= 24.2\,mg/h\left(answer\ C\ is\ correct\right)}$$

The drug clearance for postfilter replacement can be calculated by the following formula:

$$\mathbf{Rate\ of\ clearance = UF\ rate \times Antibiotic\ concentration \times SC}$$
$$\mathbf{= 1.7 \times 20 \times 0.8 = 27.2\,mg/h}$$

Suggested Reading

Choi G, Gomersall CD, Tian Q, et al. Principles of antibacterial dosing in continuous renal replacement therapy. Blood Purif. 2010;30:195–212.

Pea F. Principles of pharmacodynamics and pharmacokinetics of drugs used in extracorporeal therapies. In: Ronco C, Bellomo R, Kellum JA, et al., editors. Critical care nephrology. 3rd ed. Philadelphia: Elsevier; 2019. p. 892–6.

Schetz M, Joannes-Boyau O, Bouman C. Drug removal by CRRT and drug dosing in patients on CRRT. In: Oudemans-van Straaten H, Forni L, Groeneveld A, editors. Acute nephrology for the critical care physician. Cham: Springer; 2015. p. 233–43.

73. **Which one of the following statements regarding pain and narcotics is CORRECT?**

A. Morphine active metabolites accumulate in renal failure
B. Meperidine active metabolite accumulates and lowers the seizure threshold in patients with renal failure
C. Fentanyl clearance is reduced in renal failure, and is not dialyzable
D. The sensitivity to the effects of narcotics is increased in renal failure
E. All of the above

The answer is E

Opioids cause several adverse effects in patients with renal failure because of decreased elimination and accumulation of active metabolites and also parent compounds. Many of the adverse effects are related to central nervous system (CNS) and respiratory system. Also, patients with renal failure have increased sensitivity to these metabolites.

Morphine is metabolized in the liver mostly to morphine-3-glucuronide (M3G) and to a lesser account to morphine-6-glcuronide (M6G) and normorphine. Normally, all of these metabolites as well as 10% of the original compound are excreted by the kidneys. In renal failure, these compounds accumulate, if the dose of morphine is not adjusted. Adverse effects such as CNS depression and behavioral excitation.

Meperidine is metabolized in the liver to primarily normeperidine, which has a long half-life and exerts toxic effects such as a decrease in seizure threshold. Therefore, meperidine should be avoided or prescribed with great caution in patients with kidney failure.

Fentanyl is also metabolized in the liver to inactive metabolites. However, the clearance of fentanyl is decreased in renal failure. Also, it is not dialyzable because of its pharmacokinetic properties. Reduced dose of fentanyl is recommended, and patients should be followed postoperatively for signs and symptoms of respiratory distress. Thus, answer E is correct.

Suggested Reading

Davison SN. Clinical pharmacology considerations in pain management in patients with advanced kidney failure. Clin J Am Soc Nephrol. 2019;14:917–31.
Davison SN, Koncicki H, Brennan F. Pain in chronic kidney disease: a scoping review. Sem Dial. 2014;27:188–204.
Dean M. Opioids in renal failure and dialysis patients. J Pain Symptom Manage. 2004;28:497–504.

74. **Select the appropriate analgesic agent to the patient presented below.**

1. Gabapentin
2. Fentanyl patch
3. Tramadol

A. A 52-year-old woman with diabetes, hypertension, and CKD stage 3 visits her primary care physician with severe burning pain in her feet for 6 weeks, which became severe at night. She is on insulin and lisinopril. The intensity of pain is 3 out of 10

B. A 60-year-old man is on hemodialysis for 4 years, who complains of back pain for the last 6 months. He took acetaminophen without any relief. He went to his primary care physician, who prescribed tramadol 50 mg twice daily. He felt better for a month, but his pain came back. The patient asks you to recommend a stronger pain medication. You ordered a CT of the spine, which showed a lytic lesion. With additional studies, you made the diagnosis of multiple myeloma. The intensity of pain is 8 out of 10

C. A 62-year-old man with type 2 diabetes and hypertension is on maintenance hemodialysis for 6 years. He was admitted for gangrene of the left foot, which required below knee amputation. He complained of severe pain (10 out of 10 pain intensity) postoperatively

Answers: A = 1; B = 2, C = 2

Body pain is one of the most common complaints of patients with CKD stages 3-5D. Patients use different types of pain medications on their own or prescribed by a physician. Evaluation of pain requires a good social and medical history, physical examination, intensity of pain, and quality of life. Prescribing a suitable drug depends on considering the above evaluation.

The World Health Organization (WHO) introduced a stepwise approach to the management of pain in order to avoid inappropriate medications. This approach called WHO Ladder Step was originally introduced to control pain in cancer patients. This ladder step approach is found to be useful for patients with CKD. Pain is classified into three steps: mild, moderate, and severe. The intensity of pain is quantified by a subjective 10-point scoring system, where 0 denoted no pain and 10 the worst pain imaginable. The score for mild pain is 1–3, 4–6 for moderate pain, and 7–10 for severe pain. The following Fig. 7.1 shows modified WHO analgesic ladder in patients with CKD.

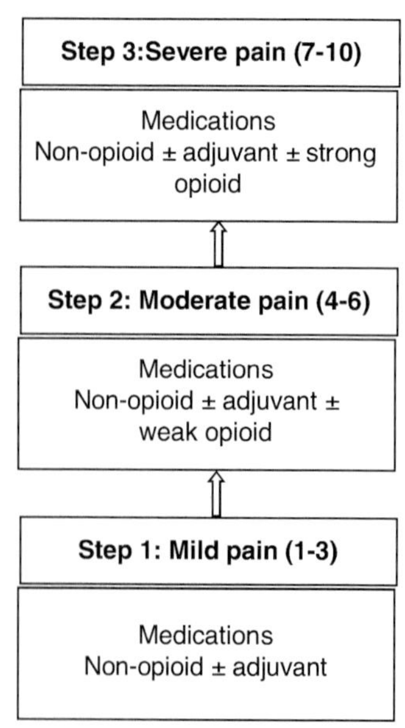

Fig. 7.1 Modified WHO analgesic ladder in patients with CKD. Nonopioids include acetaminophen; adjuvants include gabapentin, carbamazepine, pregablin, and tricyclic antidepressants; weak opioid includes tramadol; and strong opioids include oxycodone, hydromorphone, fentanyl, or fentanyl patch

The patient described in A has diabetic neuropathic pain, which requires an adjuvant medication. An adjuvant is a medication with a primary indication other than pain. Any of the adjuvant such as gabapentin, carbamazepine, pregablin, or tricyclic antidepressant is an appropriate analgesic for this patient. Nonopioid or opioid medication is inappropriate for this patient (answer 1 is correct).

The patient described in B has bone pain due to multiple myeloma. He is on dialysis, and metabolites of strong opioids such as codeine, morphine, and meperidine accumulate, resulting in severe adverse effects (seizures and respiratory depression). Fentanyl is rather safe in dialysis patients, but its dose should be reduced. Thus, the appropriate analgesic for this patient is fentanyl with 25–50% reduction in dosage preferably a patch (answer 2 is correct).

The patient described in C benefits from IV fentanyl at reduced dose and subsequently a transdermal patch until pain subsides. Other opioids are not appropriate for the reasons described in patient B (answer 2 is correct).

Tramadol is a weak opioid analgesic. It is metabolized in the liver. About 60% of tramadol metabolite, O-desmethyltramadol, and 30% of the original compound are excreted by the kidney. In renal failure, cautious use with reduction in dosage is recommended. As an inhibitor of serotonin and norepinephrine reuptake, tramadol must be used with caution in patients with selective serotonin reuptake inhibitors. Tramadol is not an appropriate analgesic for all the patients described above.

Suggested Reading

Davison SN. Clinical pharmacology considerations in pain management in patients with advanced kidney failure. Clin J Am Soc Nephrol. 2019;14:917–31.

Davison SN, Koncicki H, Brennan F. Pain in chronic kidney disease: a scoping review. Sem Dial. 2014;27:188–204.

Dean M. Opioids in renal failure and dialysis patients. J Pain Symptom Manage. 2004;28:497–504.

Gelot S, Nakhla E. Opioid dosing in renal and hepatic impairment. US Pharmacist. August 20, 2014.

75. **Which one of the following statements regarding antihypertensive drugs is CORRECT?**

A. Except for fosinopril, other angiotensin-converting enzyme inhibitors are dialyzable
B. Angiotensin receptor blockers are not dialyzable
C. Among β-blockers, labetalol and carvedilol are not dialyzable, but atenolol and metoprolol are dialyzable
D. Among calcium channel blockers, amlodipine and nifedipine XL are not dialyzable
E. All of the above

The answer is E

All of the above statements are correct. Therefore, dose adjustment for undialyzable drugs is not required (E is correct).

Suggested Reading

Olyaei AJ, Wahba I, Bennett WM. Prescribing drugs for dialysis patients. In: Lerma EV, Weir MR, editors. Henrich's Principles and practice of dialysis. 5th ed. Philadelphia: Wolters Kluwer/Lippincott Williams & Wilkins; 2017. p. 533–61.

76. **Which one of the following drugs elevates serum creatinine by interfering with creatinine assay and its secretion?**

A. Trimethoprim
B. Cephalosporins
C. Probenecid
D. Cimetidine
E. All of the above

The answer is E

As shown in Table 7.6, all of the above drugs either interfere with the creatinine assay or inhibit proximal tubular secretion of creatinine, and thus spuriously elevate its serum concentration. However, the kidney function (GFR) is not altered (answer E is correct).

Table 7.6 Drugs that increase serum creatinine levels

Factor or condition	Mechanism
Cephlosporins	Increase in chromogens
5-Flucytosine	Increase in chromogens
Trimethoprim	Decrease in proximal tubular secretion of creatinine
Cimetidine	Same as above
Triamterene	Same as above
Spironolactone	Same as above
Amiloride	Same as above
Probenecid	Same as above

Suggested Reading

Nigam PK, Chandra A. Positive and negative false estimates of serum creatinine. Interv Cardiol. 2017;9:163–7.
Samra M, Abcar AC. False estimates of elevated creatinine. Perm J. 2012;16:51–2.

77. **Match the following chemotherapy agents with their kidney injury:**

Agent	Kidney injury
A. Gemcitabine (nucleoside analog)	1. HTN, TMA/HUS, and proteinuria
B. Bortezomib (proteasome inhibitor)	2. TMA
C. Bevacizumab and sunitinib (VEGF inhibitors)	3. TMA, HTN, and proteinuria
D. Ibrutinib (Bruton's tyrosine kinase inhibitor	4. AKI, HTN, and tumor lysis syndrome (TLS)
E. Venetoclax (BCL-2 inhibitor)	5. TLS
F. Ipilimubab (immune checkpoint inhibitor, CTLA-4, and PD-1 inhibitor)	6. AKI
G. Pembrolizumab (immune checkpoint inhibitor)	7. Acute tubulointerstitial disease
H. Rivolumab (immune checkpoint inhibitor)	8. TMA, glomerulonephritis, and nephrotic syndrome

AKI acute kidney injury, *CTLA-4* cytotoxic T-lymphocyte–associated antigen 4, *PD-1* programmed cell death 1 protein, *HTN* hypertension, *TMA* thrombotic microangiopathy

Answers: A = 1; B = 2; C = 3; D = 4; E = 5; F = 6; G = 7; H = 8

Suggested Reading

Nicolaysen A. Nephrotoxic chemotherapy agents: old and new. Adv Chronic Kidney Dis. 2020;27:38–49.
Perazella MA, Shirali AC. Nephrotoxicity of cancer immunotherapies: past, present and future. J Am Soc Nephrol. 2018;29:2039–52.

78. Erythropoiesis-stimulating agents (ESAs) are used to manage anemia both in chemotherapy-treated cancer patients and patients with CKD. They raise hemoglobin (Hgb) levels and reduce the need for RBC transfusions. **Regarding ESAs and cancer-associated anemia, which one of the following statements is CORRECT**?

A. ESAs may be recommended to patients with chemotherapy-associated anemia whose cancer may not be cured and whose Hgb is <10 g/dL
B. ESAs should not be offered to those whose cancer is curative with appropriate treatment
C. ESAs should not be offered to those patients with nonchemotherapy-associated anemia
D. Hgb may be increased to the lowest concentration needed to avoid or reduce the need for RBC transfusion
E. All of the above

The answer is E

ESAs have been extensively used to treat anemia in patients with CKD because anemia is due to deficiency of erythropoietin. This management avoided RBC transfusion. Subsequently, ESAs have been used to treat chemotherapy-associated anemia in cancer patients. It was shown that tumor cells may possess receptors for

erythropoietin, and administration of ESAs may promote tumor growth. Another concern of ESAs is high-Hgb-induced venous thrombosis. Because of these concerns, The American Society of Clinical Oncology (ASCO) and the American Society of Hematology (ASH) published joint evidence-based clinical practice guidelines for the management of chemotherapy-associated anemia. The committee made ten recommendations, which include those mentioned from A to D in the question. Thus, answer E is correct.

ESA administration should be offered to cancer patients only to treat chemotherapy-associated anemia rather than anemia caused by other causes. For example, other causes such as iron deficiency, bleeding, or cancer-induced anemia should be ruled out prior to ESA use. When ESA has been started, and an increase in Hgb is not observed in 6–8 weeks, ESA should be discontinued. For other details, the reader is referred to the review quoted in Suggested Reading.

Suggested Reading

Bohlius J, Bohlke K, Castelli R, et al. Management of cancer-associated anemia with erythropoiesis-stimulating agents: ASCO/ASH clinical practice guideline update. Blood Adv. 2019;3:1197–210.

79. Prolyl hydroxylase domain inhibitors (PHDIs), which stimulate erythropoietin production through the activation of hypoxia-inducible factor (HIF), are novel therapeutic agents used for treating renal anemia. **Which one of the following drugs is NOT a PHDI?**

A. Daprodustat
B. Molidustat
C. Roxadustat
D. Vadadustat
E. Montelukast

The answer is E

Hypoxia-inducible factor (HIF) is a transcription factor that regulates several genes for cell survival during conditions of hypoxia. HIF is a heterodimer consisting of α- and β-subunits. The α-subunit exists in three isoforms: HIF-1α, HIF-2α, and HIF-3α. HIF-1α is ubiquitously expressed, whereas HIF-2α has restricted distribution. One of the important functions of HIF is production of red blood cells (erythropoiesis).

Under normoxic conditions, HIFs are inactivated by hydroxylation of prolyl residues by prolyl hydroxylase domain (PHD) enzymes. Three isoforms of PHDs have been identified: PHD1, PHD2, and PHD3. PHDs require O_2, Fe^{2+}, 2-oxyglutarate, and ascorbate for their action.

Anemia is a major problem in patients with CKD 4-5D. It is reasonable to assume that inhibition of PHDs can potentiate the action of HIFs so that endogenous erythropoiesis can be stimulated. A number of compounds have been introduced including those listed from A to D. Another PHDI is enarodustat. The pharmacologic profile of the five PHDIs is shown in Table 7.7.

Table 7.7 PHD inhibitors (summarized from several studies)

Drug	Dose in clinical trials	Dosing schedule	Half-life in healthy/CKD (h)
Daprodustat	5–25 mg (50 and 100 mg used)	Once daily by mouth	1/7
Molidustat	25–150 mg	Once daily by mouth	4–10/7–13
Enarodustat	2–6 mg	Once daily by mouth	<9/9
Roxadustat	0.7–2.5 mg/kg	Thrice weekly by mouth	12/15[a]
Vadadustat	150–600 mg	Once daily by mouth	4.7/9.1

[a]Mild hepatic impairment

Montelukast is a leukotriene receptor antagonist. It works by blocking the action of substances that cause the symptoms of asthma and allergic rhinitis (option E is correct).

Suggested Reading

Gupta N, Wish JB. Hypoxia-inducible factor prolyl hydroxylase inhibitors: a potential new treatment for anemia in patients with CKD. Am J Kidney Dis. 2017;69:815–26.

Hasegawa S, Tanaka T, Nangaku M. Hypoxia-inducible factor stabilizers for treating anemia of chronic kidney disease. Curr Opin Nephrol Hypertens. 2018;27:331–8.

Kurata Y, Tanaka T, Nangaku M. Prolyl hydroxylase domain inhibitors: a new era in the management of renal anemia. Ann Transl Med. 2019;7(suppl 8):S334.

Sanghani NS, Haase VH. Hypoxia-inducible factor activators in renal anemia: Current clinical experience. Adv Chronic Kidney Dis. 2019;26:253–66.

Wyatt CM, Drüeke TM. HIF stabilization by prolyl hydroxylase inhibitors for the treatment of anemia in chronic kidney disease. Kidney Int. 2016;90:923–5.

80. **Match the following herbal medicines with their nephrotoxicity:**

Toxic compound from the herb	Major uses	Nephrotoxicity
A. Aristolochic acid	Weight loss, liver disease, improve edema, and headache	1. Chronic tubulointerstitial disease, Fanconi syndrome, and uroepithelial carcinoma
B. Flavinoid (sciadopitysin)	Vascular disease and diabetes	2. Acute tubular necrosis and acute tubulointerstitial disease
C. Glycyrrhizic acid	Cough, arthritis, weight loss, and sore throat	3. Hypokalemia, proximal tubular injury, acute tubular necrosis, and hypertension
D. Anthraquinones and oxalic acid	Laxative	4. Tubulointerstitial fibrosis and tubular atrophy
E. Andrographolide	Diarrhea, and upper and lower respiratory infections	5. Acute tubular necrosis
F. Star fruit (carambola) juice	Weight loss and antioxidant	6. Oxalate stones

Answers: A = 1; B = 2; C = 3; D = 4; E = 5; F = 6

Suggested Reading

Charen E, Harbord N. Toxicity of herbs, vitamins, and supplements. Adv Chronic Kidney Dis. 2020;27:67–71.

Yang B, Xie Y, Guo M, et al. Nephrotoxicity and Chinese herbal medicine. Clin J Am Soc Med. 2018;13:1605–11.

Chapter 8
Genetic Diseases and Pregnancy

1. A 35-year-old man with a strong family history of polycystic kidney disease (PKD) sees his primary care physician for mild abdominal discomfort for 10 days. He is found to have a blood pressure of 144/96 mm Hg. An ultrasound of the abdomen shows bilateral large kidneys (>13.6 cm). He is subsequently referred to a nephrologist who confirms the diagnosis of autosomal dominant polycystic kidney disease (ADPKD). The patient asks about the relationship between the large kidneys (total kidney volume) and subsequent complications of ADPKD. **Which one of the following statements is FALSE regarding total kidney volume (TKV) and pathophysiologic changes?**

   A. Patients with ADPKD and hypertension (HTN) have larger kidneys, as compared with those patients who have ADPKD with normotension
   B. There is an inverse correlation between increasing TKV and decreasing glomerular filtration rate (GFR)
   C. Men have a larger TKV than women and develop end-stage kidney disease (ESKD) faster than women
   D. Patients with polycystic kidney disease 1 (PKD1) genotype have larger kidneys than patients with polycystic kidney disease 2 (PKD2) genotype
   E. The kidneys fail to enlarge in childhood, but start to increase once the patient reaches the age of 30 years

   The answer is E

   Determination of TKV with magnetic resonance imaging (MRI) has become an important prognostic factor in patients with ADPKD. It associates with the development of ESKD. It was shown initially that a fall in GFR occurred at TKV of approximately 600 mL in adult women and at 1100 mL in adult men, and the progression to ESKD is faster in men than women. Patients with HTN have larger kidneys and TKV, as compared with those patients who have normal blood pressure (BP). Also, there is an inverse correlation between increasing TKV and decreasing GFR. ADPKD is genetically determined by two genes: PKD1 and PKD2. About 85% of patients have PKD1 genotype, and the remaining 15% have PKD2 genotype. The TKV is much higher in PKD1 than PKD2 patients. The kidneys start enlarging even in childhood, but the GFR remains within normal range for 3–5 decades. Thus, option E is false.

   Suggested Reading

Chapman AB, Bost JE, Torres VE, et al. Kidney volume and functional outcomes in autosomal polycystic kidney disease. Clin J Am Soc Nephrol. 2012;7:479–86.

Grantham JJ, Chapman AB, Torres VE. Volume progression in autosomal dominant polycystic kidney disease: the major factor determining clinical outcomes. Clin J Am Soc Nephrol. 2006;1:148–57.

Grantham JJ, Torres VE, Chapman AB, et al. Volume progression in polycystic kidney disease. N Engl J Med. 2006;354:2122–30.

Schrier RW. Renal volume, renin-angiotensin-aldosterone system, hypertension, and left ventricular hypertrophy in patients with autosomal dominant polycystic kidney disease. J Am Soc Nephrol. 2009;20:1888–93.

2. **Which one of the following statements regarding height-adjusted total kidney volume (htTKV) and onset of kidney insufficiency is CORRECT?**

   A. htTKV can prospectively predict the development of CKD stage 1 in 8 years
   B. htTKV can prospectively predict the development of CKD stage 2 in 8 years
   C. htTKV can prospectively predict the development of CKD stage 3 in 8 years

A. S. Reddi, *Absolute Nephrology Review*, https://doi.org/10.1007/978-3-030-85958-9_8

D. htTKV can prospectively predict the development of CKD stage 4 in 8 years
E. htTKV can prospectively predict the development of CKD stage 5 in 8 years

The answer is C

A previous study showed that TKV is associated with decline in GFR in patients with ADPKD. In another study, htTKV was examined whether this biomarker can predict the onset of kidney insufficiency. Chapman et al. prospectively examined the association of htTKV and the onset of kidney insufficiency 241 adults with ADPKD and preserved kidney function. After a mean follow-up of 8 years, stage 3 CKD developed in 30.7% of the enrollees. Baseline htTKV of 600 mL/m most accurately defined the risk of developing stage 3 CKD within 8 years. Thus, answer C is correct.

Suggested Reading

Chapman AB, Bost JE, Torres VE, et al. Kidney volume and functional outcomes in autosomal dominant polycystic kidney disease. Clin J Am Soc Nephrol. 2012;7:479–86.

3. **Which one of the following kidney function abnormalities is reported to occur in early stages of patients with ADPKD?**

A. Impaired urinary concentrating ability, despite increased vasopressin levels
B. Preserved urine diluting ability
C. Decreased kidney blood flow
D. Proteinuria >2 g/day
E. A, B, and C

The answer is E

Studies have shown that patients with ADPKD with normal renal function demonstrate impaired urinary concentrating ability, despite increased vasopressin levels. Both urinary concentrating defect and elevated vasopressin values may contribute to cystogenesis, which results in glomerular hyperfiltration seen in children and young adults (answer A is correct). In contrast, urinary diluting capacity is preserved (answer B is correct).

Decreased renal blood flow is another early functional defect, which is caused by changes in intrarenal pressures, neurohumoral or local mediators, and/or intrinsic vascular abnormalities (answer C is correct).

In early stages of ADPKD, proteinuria >2 g/day is extremely unlikely, but proteinuria up to 1500 mg/day is seen in moderate to late stages of kidney disease and may promote kidney progression (answer D is incorrect).

Suggested Reading

Torres VE, Bankir L, Grantham JJ. A case for water in the treatment of polycystic kidney disease. Clin J Am Soc Nephrol. 2009;4:1140–50.
Torres VE, Harris PC. Cystic diseases of the kidney. In: Yu ASL, Chertow GM, Luyckx VA, et al., editors. Brenner & Rector's the kidney. 11th ed. Philadelphia: Elsevier Saunders; 2020. p. 1490–533.

4. You are following a 40-year-old patient with ADPKD, who complains of occasional abdominal pain. **Which one of the following is the LEAST likely cause of his abdominal pain?**

A. Cyst hemorrhage
B. Passage of renal stone
C. Urinary tract infection (UTI)
D. Renal cell carcinoma (RCC)
E. No cause other than the cyst itself

The answer is D

Abdominal pain occurs in approximately 60% of patients with ADPKD. At times, rupture of the cyst causing pain and hematuria is rather common. Patients with ADPKD are at risk for uric acid and calcium oxalate stone formation. Low urine pH, low citrate and NH_4^+ excretion, and urinary stasis account for predisposition to kidney stone formation. Urinary tract infection is also a common cause of abdominal pain. Some patients have chronic pain due to growth of the cyst or distension of the abdomen due to large kidneys. Renal cell carcinoma (RCC) in this young patient is very unlikely. However, in a patient older than 50 years of age, renal cell carcinoma should be considered as one of the causes of abdominal pain. Thus, option D is a very unlikely cause of pain in this patient.

Suggested Reading

Chapman AB, Rahbari-Oskoui FF. Renal cystic disorders. In: Wilcox CS, editor. Therapy in nephrology and hypertension. Philadelphia: Saunders/Elsevier; 2008. p. 539–46.

Torres VE, Harris PC. Cystic diseases of the kidney. In: Yu ASL, Chertow GM, Luyckx VA, et al., editors. Brenner & Rector's the kidney. 11th ed. Philadelphia: Elsevier Saunders; 2020. p. 1490–533.

5. **Which one of the following statements regarding hypertension (HTN) in ADPKD patients is FALSE?**

A. The median age at diagnosis of hypertension (HTN) is 32 years for men and 34 years for women
B. Left ventricular hypertrophy (LVH) and left ventricular mass index (LVMI) are increased in normotensive autosomal dominant polycystic kidney (ADPKD) subjects, compared to age-matched controls
C. Hypertensive ADPKD patients with a normal renal function have larger kidney volumes than their age-matched normotensive individuals
D. Goal blood pressure (BP) in young healthy individuals with a relatively intact kidney function is >130 mm Hg
E. Treatment of HTN with diuretics was found to be associated with faster progression to ESKD than treatment with angiotensin-converting enzyme inhibitors (ACE-Is)

The answer is D

HTN develops in the majority (60%) of patients with ADPKD, which is one of the risk factors for progression of renal disease, besides age and renal volume. It occurs at an early age in both men (median age 32 years) and women (median age 34 years), compared to the general population (answer A is correct).

Lifestyle modification is an important part of HTN management. However, many patients require pharmacologic intervention. Cardiovascular (CV) death is common in ADPKD patients. LVH and LVMI are higher, even in normotensive ADPKD patients with normal renal function than age-matched controls. Hypertensive individuals have large renal volumes than normotensive individuals (answers B and C are correct).

Treatment of HTN is highly beneficial in the prevention of renal and extrarenal complications of ADPKD. Long-term therapy with ACE-Is is found to reduce albuminuria and LVH as well as LVMI. Hemodynamic effects of ACE-Is include an increase in renal blood flow and a reduction in filtration fraction (FF), so that renal Na^+ absorption is decreased. Thus, ACE-Is or angiotensin receptor blockers seem to be the first choice for ADPKD patients with or without target organ damage. The goal blood pressure (BP) for all ADPKD patients has not been established but it has been suggested to be <130/80 mm Hg (office BP). However, in young and healthy individuals with a relatively intact kidney function, maintaining BP <110/75 mm Hg can provide cardiovascular benefit and reduce the rate of cyst growth. Thus, option D is false.

The effect of a low BP target (95/60 to 110/75 mm Hg) on annual change in total kidney volume was examined in ADPKD patients with estimated glomerular filtration rate (eGFR) >60 mL/min and compared with the standard BP target (120/70 to 130/80 mm Hg). BP-lowering agents were lisinopril plus placebo in one group and lisinopril and telmisartan in another group. The results showed that the annual percentage increase in total kidney volume was significantly lower in the low BP group than in the standard BP group without significant differences between the lisinopril-placebo and lisinopril-telmisartan groups. Although there was no overall change in eGFR, a greater decline in LVMI, and a greater reduction in urinary albumin excretion, was observed in the low BP group. Addition of telmisartan had no effect. Thus, control of BP to <110/75 mm Hg with lisinopril is beneficial in hypertensive patients with ADPKD between 15 and 49 years of age.

In another study with a similar BP regimen, monotherapy with lisinopril was associated with BP control in most patients with ADPKD and stage 3 chronic kidney disease with a similar decline in eGFR. The addition of an angiotensin receptor blocker (ARB) did not alter the decline in eGFR. This study also supports an ACE-I rather than the combination of an ACE-I and ARB.

Comparative studies in ADPKD patients have demonstrated that diuretic use was associated with faster decline in renal function, as compared with ACE-Is (answer E is correct). However, ACE-Is and β-blockers were found to have similar effects on the rate of renal disease progression. Cautious use of diuretics is recommended to control volume when lifestyle modification is inadequate.

It should be noted that a rigorous control of BP (MAP (mean arterial pressure) <93 mm Hg) than moderate control of BP (MAP 100–107 mm Hg) in the Modification of Diet in Renal Disease (MDRD) study, which enrolled a large number of ADPKD patients, demonstrated reduction in LVMI independent of the type of antihypertensive agent used.

Suggested Reading

Jafar TH, Stork PC, Schmid CH, et al. The effect of angiotensin-converting enzyme inhibitors on progression of advanced polycystic kidney disease. Kidney Int. 2005;67:265–71.
Schrier RW. Optimal care of autosomal polycystic kidney disease patients. Nephrology. 2006;11:124–30.
Schrier RW, Abebe KZ, Perrone RD, et al. for HALT-PKD. Blood pressure in early autosomal dominant polycystic kidney disease. N Engl J Med. 2014;371:2255–66.
Torres VE, Abebe KZ, Chapman AB, et al. for HALT-PKD Trial Investigators. Angiotensin blockade in late autosomal dominant polycystic kidney disease. N Engl J Med. 2014;371:2267–76.
Torres VE, Harris PC. Cystic diseases of the kidney. In: Yu ASL, Chertow GM, Luyckx VA, et al., editors. Brenner & Rector's the kidney. 11th ed. Philadelphia: Elsevier Saunders; 2020. p. 1490–533.

6. **Besides total kidney volume (TKV), which one of the following modifiable predictors is associated with deterioration in kidney function in ADPKD patients?**

A. Body surface area
B. 24-h urine osmolality
C. 24-h urine Na^+ excretion
D. Low high-density lipoprotein (HDL) cholesterol
E. All of the above

The answer is E

The National Institutes of Health sponsored a Consortium for Radiologic Imaging Studies of Polycystic Kidney Disease (CRISP) to develop imaging techniques to analyze and follow disease progression in ADPKD patients. In the CRISP I study, higher TKV and cyst volumes are associated with faster decline in GFR. The participants in this study were followed up for 3 years. The follow-up of these patients was extended up to 6 years. During this follow-up, higher body surface area, 24-h urine osmolality (a surrogate marker of vasopressin effect on kidney), 24-h Na^{2+} excretion (a surrogate marker of salt intake), and low HDL cholesterol (a possible surrogate marker of vascular disease) were found to be risk factors for decline in renal function. Correction of these abnormalities may be important in preventing the progression of renal disease in patients with ADPKD.

Suggested Reading

Grantham JJ, Torres VE, Chapman AR, et al. Volume progression in polycystic kidney disease. N Engl J Med. 2006;354:2122–30.
Torres VE, Grantham JJ, Chapman AB, et al. Potentially modifiable factors affecting the progression of autosomal dominant polycystic kidney disease. Clin J Am Soc Nephrol. 2012;6:640–7.

7. **Which one of the following drugs has been approved in 2018 by the US Food and Drug Administration (FDA) for use in patients with ADPKD?**

A. Long-acting somatostatin analog
B. Tolvaptan (vasopressin V_2-receptor antagonist)
C. Everolimus (mammalian target of rapamycin (mTOR) inhibitor)
D. Tyrosine kinase inhibitors
E. All of the above

The answer is B

The initial 3-year trial using tolvaptan was published in 2012 (Tolvaptan Efficacy and Safety in Management of Autosomal Dominant Polycystic Kidney Disease and Its Outcomes [TEMPO] 3:4). This trial showed that tolvaptan slowed the increase in total kidney volume (TKV) by 45% and the decline in renal function by 26% over 3 years in early (eGFR ≥ 60 mL/min) ADPKD patients, as compared with those on placebo. However, elevations in liver enzymes and bilirubin were higher in tolvaptan than in the placebo group. Despite these beneficial effects, tolvaptan was not approved for use in ADPKD patients by the US Food and Drug Administration in 2012.

The study was extended for another 2 years (TEMPO 4:4) and found a slower decline in GFR in tolvaptan compared to the placebo group. However, the efficacy and safety of tolvaptan in patients with lower GFRs are not known. This led the investigators of TEMPO 3:4 and 4:4 to study in patients with eGFR between 25 and 65 mL/min (Replicating Evidence of Preserved Renal Function: an Investigation of Tolvaptan Safety and Efficacy in

ADPKD [REPRISE]) trial. In this trial, 1370 patients with ADPKD who were either 18 to 55 years of age with an eGFR of 25 to 65 mL/min or 56 to 65 years of age with an eGFR of 25 to 44 mL/min were randomly assigned in a 1:1 ratio to receive tolvaptan or placebo for 12 months. Similar to the other two trials, the REPRISE trial also showed that tolvaptan caused a slower decline in eGFR by 35% in advanced ADPKD patients, as compared with placebo. Alanine aminotransferase (ALT) elevation (>3 times the upper limit of the normal range) occurred in 5.6% in the tolvaptan group and in 1.2% in the placebo group. These elevations were reversible after stopping tolvaptan. However, elevations in the bilirubin level of more than twice the upper limit of the normal range were not observed. On the basis of these studies, the FDA approved tolvaptan to slow kidney function decline in adults at risk of rapidly progressing ADPKD (answer B is correct).

Somatostatin inhibits cell proliferation and several hormones, including insulin and growth hormone. The half-life of somatostatin is approximately 3 min; therefore, more stable synthetic peptides such as octreotide, lanreotide, and pasireotide have been developed for clinical use. Half-lives in the circulation are 2 h for octreotide and lanreotide and 12 h for pasireotide.

An Italian study evaluated the efficacy of long-acting somatostatin analog (octreotide long-acting release) in 38 patients with ADPKD on TKV and compared with 37 patients on placebo. At 1 year, TKV progression was significantly less in the octreotide group compared with the placebo group. At 3 years, however, the TKV was much smaller in the octreotide group compared with that in the placebo group, but the difference was not statistically significant. The adverse effects were not different between the two groups. Thus, octreotide long-acting release seems to have a beneficial effect in reducing TKV at 1 year but not at 3 years.

The DIPAK1 (Developing Interventions to Halt Progression of ADPKD 1) randomized trial evaluated the effect of lanreotide on kidney function and TKV in advanced ADPKD patients. In this trial, patients between 18 and 60 years of age with an eGFR of 30 to 60 mL/min were treated with lanreotide (N = 153) or managed with standard care (N = 152) and their annual rate of change in eGFR and TKV followed for 2.5 years. The results showed no difference either in the annual rate of change in eGFR or in the decline in kidney function between the groups. However, the rate of growth in TKV was significantly lower in the lanreotide group than in the standard care group. Based on these results, the authors do not support the use of lanreotide for treatment of later-stage ADPKD.

Overactivation of mTOR is implicated in cell proliferation and growth. As a result, the inhibitors of mTOR have been tried in ADPKD patients. Although mTOR inhibitors have slowed the progression of TKV, the results on slowing the decline in GFR are unclear. A meta-analysis has shown no long-term benefit of mTOR use in ADPKD patients.

The tyrosine kinase inhibitor bosutinib has been studied in patients with eGFR ≥ 60 mL/min. The trial showed a reduction in the annual rate of TKV increase compared with placebo, but no difference in eGFR decline between the groups at 2 years.

From the available trial results, tolvaptan remains the only drug that can be recommended at this time for treatment of patients with ADPKD.

Suggested Reading

Cornec-Le Gall E, Alam A, Perrone RD. Autosomal dominant polycystic kidney disease. Lancet. 2019;393:919–35.

Caroli A, Perico N, Perna A, et al. for the ALADIN Study Group. Effect of long acting somatostatin analogue on kidney and cyst growth in autosomal dominant polycystic kidney disease (ALADIN): a randomised, placebo-controlled, multicentre trial. Lancet. 2013;382:1485–95.

He Q, Lin C, Ji S, et al. Efficacy and safety of mTOR inhibitor therapy in patients with early-stage autosomal polycystic kidney disease: a meta-analysis of randomized controlled studies. Am J Med Sci. 2012;344:491–7.

Tesar V, Ciechanowski K, Pei Y, et al. Bosutinib versus placebo for autosomal dominant polycystic kidney disease. J Am Soc Nephrol. 2017;28:3404–13.

Torres VE, Chapman AB, Devuyst O, et al. Tolvaptan in patients with autosomal dominant polycystic kidney disease for the TEMPO 3:4 Trial Investigators. N Engl J Med. 2012;367:2407–18.

Torres VE, Chapman AB, Devuyst O, et al. Multicenter, open-label, extension trial to evaluate the long-term efficacy and safety of early versus delayed treatment with tolvaptan in autosomal dominant polycystic kidney disease: the TEMPO 4:4 trial. Nephrol Dial Transplant. 2017;33:477–89.

Torres VE, Chapman AB, Devuyst O, et al. Tolvaptan in later-stage autosomal dominant polycystic kidney disease. N Engl J Med. 2017;77:1930–42.

8. **Which one of the following statements regarding ADPKD is CORRECT?**

   A. Genetic testing should be considered to confirm the diagnosis of ADPKD in an individual with negative family history and only a few cysts are present
   B. Patients with mutations in PKD2 have a more favorable renal prognosis than patients with mutations in PKD1.
   C. PKD1 patients with truncated mutations ($PKD1^T$) have worse renal prognosis than those with nontruncated mutations ($PKD1^{NT}$)
   D. The Predicting Renal Outcomes in Polycystic Kidney Disease (PROPKD) score can provide an accurate stratification of the risks of decline in eGFR and progression to end-stage kidney disease (ESKD)
   E. All of the above

   The answer is E

   The clinical course of ADPKD is variable, as some patients reach ESKD at an early age and some other patients do not reach ESKD. This variability was clarified by several elegant genotype-phenotype correlation studies. These studies have demonstrated that the gene and the type of mutation are important factors that could explain much of this clinical variability. Studies have shown that genetic testing should be done in those individuals with no documented family history and have only few cysts to confirm the diagnosis of ADPKD (answer A is correct).

   ADPKD patients with mutations in PKD1 gene are at higher risk for kidney disease progression than those with mutations in PKD2 gene (answer B is correct). Also, patients with PKD1 gene mutations have larger TKV and larger cysts at any given age than patients with PKD2 gene mutations.

   It was also reported that truncated PKD1 gene mutation carries worse kidney prognosis than nontruncated PKD 1 gene mutation (answer C is correct).

   Based on genetic and clinical data, Cornec-Le Gall et al. introduced a prognostic model that can predict kidney outcomes in patients with ADPKD. This model (PROPKD) included a point system from 0 to 9 by combining genetic and clinical factors such as $PKD1^T$, $PKD1^{NT}$, PKD2, sex, HTN before 35 years of age, age at first event of macroscopic hematuria, or flank pain related to cyst or cyst infection. From this point system, three risk categories were identified as low risk (0–3 points), intermediate risk (4–6 points), and high risk (7–9 points). The median ages for onset of ESKD were 70.6, 56.9, and 49 years, respectively, for low-, intermediate-, and high-risk categories. In the TEMPO 3:4 study, the patients who were in the high-risk PROPKD category had higher htTKV, htTKV growth, and faster eGFR decline, as compared with patients in the intermediate- and low-risk categories. Thus, PROPKD score can predict the development of ESKD in patients with ADPKD (answer D is correct).

   Suggested Reading

   Chebib FT, Perrone RD, Chapman AB, et al. A practical guide for treatment of rapidly progressive ADPKD with tolvaptan. J Am Soc Nephrol. 2018;29:2458–70.

   Cornec-Le Gall E, Audrezet MP, Chen JM, et al. Type of PKD1 mutation influences renal outcome in ADPKD. J Am Soc Nephrol. 2013;24:1006–13.

   Cornec-Le Gall E, Audrezet MP, Rousseau A, et al. The PROPKD score: a new algorithm to predict renal survival in autosomal dominant polycystic kidney disease. J Am Soc Nephrol. 2016;27:942–51.

   Hwang YH, Conklin J, Chan W, et al. Refining genotype-phenotype correlation in autosomal dominant polycystic kidney disease. J Am Soc Nephrol. 2016;27:1861–8.

   Magistroni R, He N, Wang K, et al. Genotype-renal function correlation in type 2 autosomal dominant polycystic kidney disease. J Am Soc Nephrol. 2003;14:1164–74.

9. **Match the following case histories of ADPKD patients with the kidney prognosis using Mayo Imaging Classification:**

   A. A 31-year-old man with height-adjusted total kidney volume (htTKV) of 250 mL, an eGFR of 100 mL/min, and nontruncating mutation in PKD1
   B. A 32-year-old man with htKTV of 460 mL, an eGFR of 110 mL/min, and truncating mutation in PKD1
   C. A 33-year-old man with htTKV of 1350 mL, an eGFR of 116 mL/min, and truncating mutation in PKD1

   1. Class 1A
   2. Class 1C
   3. Class 1E

   Answers: A = 1; B = 2, C = 3.

The Mayo imaging classification uses htTKV and age to identify ADPKD patients who are at greater risk for progression independent of kidney function. Approximately 95% of patients have a typical disease with diffuse and symmetric distribution of cysts throughout the kidney. These patients are classified as class 1. This class is further stratified into five subclasses (A to E) on the basis of annual htTKV growth rates of 1A 1.5%, 1B 1.5–3%, 1C 3–4.5%, ID 4.5–6%, and 1E >6%.

The remaining 5% of patients have asymmetric focal cyst distribution, substantial fibrosis, or solitary kidneys, and these patients are classified as class 2. This class does not predict eGFR decline.

Patient A has small htTKV and nontruncating mutation in the PKD1 gene. He is at low risk for progression of kidney disease (decline in eGFR), and he is classified as 1A.

Patient B has truncating mutation in the PKD1 gene, and he is classified as 1C. He is at intermediate risk for decline in eGFR, despite low htTKV.

Patient C is at high risk for progression of kidney disease, as he has high htTKV and truncating mutation in PKD1. His cyst growth rate is >6% and belongs to the Mayo imaging classification of 1E. This patient may benefit from the use of tolvaptan, if his eGFR starts to decline.

Suggested Reading

Chebib FT, Perrone RD, Chapman AB, et al. A practical guide for treatment of rapidly progressive ADPKD with tolvaptan. J Am Soc Nephrol. 2018;29:2458–70.

Cornec-Le Gall E, Alam A, Perrone RD. Autosomal dominant polycystic kidney disease. Lancet. 2019;393:919–35.

Irazabal MV, Rangel LJ, Bergstralh EJ, et al. CRISP Investigators. Imaging classification of autosomal dominant polycystic kidney disease: a simple model for selecting patients for clinical trials. J Am Soc Nephrol. 2015;26:160–72.

10. A 34-year-old woman with autosomal polycystic kidney disease (ADPKD) is referred to a nephrologist for the evaluation and management of HTN. She asks you whether she needs a computed tomography (CT) of head for possible aneurysms. **Regarding screening for the presence of intracranial aneurysms (ICA) in patients with ADPKD, which one of the following choices is FALSE?**

A. Patients with a strong family history of ICA
B. Airline pilots and scuba drivers
C. Magnetic resonance angiography (MRA) rather than CT angiography (CTA) is the most sensitive technique for the detection of aneurysms
D. For patients where knowledge of either a positive or negative test would improve their quality of life
E. All patients deserve at least one screening test after diagnosis of ADPKD

The answer is E

ADPKD patients carrying PKD1 and PKD2 genes are at higher risk for developing ICA than the general population. The prevalence of unruptured ICA in these patients is 10–11.5% (five times higher than in the general population), but this prevalence increases to 21% in those with a family history of ICA or subarachnoid hemorrhage. The most sensitive imaging technique for detection of these aneurysms is MRA than CT angiography which requires iodinated contrast with potential for acute kidney injury (AKI). Screening for ICA should be considered in those (1) with a strong family history of ICA or subarachnoid hemorrhage; (2) who are at high-risk occupations (airline pilots or scuba divers); (3) prior to major elective surgeries; and (4) patients who request screening for the purpose of reassurance. Therefore, routine screening for ICA in patients after diagnosis of ADPKD is not warranted. Except for E, the other choices apply to patients with ADPKD.

Another concern regarding ICA is the risk of rupture of asymptomatic ICA and its management. It has been suggested that the risk of growth or rupture of aneurysms <7 mm in diameter is small. For those patients with aneurysms ≥10 mm in diameter or aneurysms in the posterior circulation, endovascular management may be the treatment of choice in patients over 50 years of age. Control of HTN and hyperlipidemia as well as smoking cessation is recommended to reduce the risk of aneurysmal rupture.

When aneurysms do rupture, the combined morbidity and mortality rate is 35–55%. Complications include subarachnoid hemorrhage, vasospasm, and cerebral ischemia. Rupture occurs a decade earlier in patients with ADPKD, compared with patients with sporadic intracranial aneurysm.

Based on the Markov decision-analytic model, Malhotra et al. suggest MRA screening every 5 years with annual MRA follow-up in asymptomatic ADPKD patients. Despite various recommendations, there is currently no standardized screening protocol for ICA in patients at the initial diagnosis of ADPKD.

Suggested Reading

Cagnazzo F, Gambacciani C, Morganti R, et al. Intracranial aneurysms in patients with autosomal dominant polycystic kidney disease: prevalence, risk of rupture, and management-a systematic review. Acta Neurochir (Wien). 2017;159:811–21.

Malhotra A, Wu X, Matouk CC, et al. MR angiography screening and surveillance for intracranial aneurysms in autosomal dominant polycystic kidney disease: a cost-effectiveness analysis. Radiology. 2019;291:400–8.

Torres VE, Harris PC. Cystic diseases of the kidney. In: Yu ASL, Chertow GM, Luyckx VA, et al., editors. Brenner & Rector's the kidney. 11th ed. Philadelphia: Elsevier Saunders; 2020. p. 1490–533.

11. **Which one of the following statements regarding ADPKD is CORRECT?**

A. Patients with mutations in PKD1 have worse kidney prognosis than patients with mutations in PKD2
B. Patients with truncating mutation in PKD1 show progressive kidney enlargement and reduction in eGFR, leading to ESKD at a median age of 55 years
C. Height-adjusted total kidney volume (htTKV) is a predictor of future GFR decline
D. The Mayo imaging classification uses htTKV and age to identify patients at the highest risk for kidney disease progression, independent of renal function
E. All of the above

The answer is E

The importance of each one of the above statements is explained in previous questions with regard to ADPKD. Thus, all of the statements are correct.

Suggested Reading

Chebib FT, Perrone RD, Chapman AB, et al. A practical guide for treatment of rapidly progressive ADPKD with tolvaptan. J Am Soc Nephrol. 2018;29:2458–70.

Cornec-Le Gall E, Alam A, Perrone, RD. Autosomal dominant polycystic kidney disease. Lancet. 2019;393:919–35.

Irazabal MV, Rangel LJ, Bergstralh EJ, et al. CRISP Investigators. Imaging classification of autosomal dominant polycystic kidney disease: a simple model for selecting patients for clinical trials. J Am Soc Nephrol. 2015;26:160–72.

12. A 50-year-old man on maintenance hemodialysis (HD) for over 10 years is found to have gross hematuria, fever, flank pain, and rising hematocrit level. Physical examination shows bilateral flank pain and palpable masses. A tentative diagnosis of the acquired cystic kinetic disease (ACKD) is made. **Which one of the following statements is FALSE in patients with ACKD?**

A. ACKD develops not only in hemodialysis (HD) patients but also in peritoneal dialysis (PD) and nondialysis patients
B. ACKD patients are at high risk for development of renal cell carcinoma (RCC)
C. ACKD may not regress after a successful kidney transplantation
D. CT scan with or without contrast is the preferred diagnostic technique for the detection of ACKD
E. Nephrectomy is recommended in those with retroperitoneal hemorrhage and renal cell carcinoma cannot be ruled out

The answer is C

ACKD develops in the remnant kidneys in >90% of patients who are maintained on HD for more than 8 years. ACKD is a clinically recognized complication of long-term HD and PD therapy. The incidence approximates >90% after 8 years of HD. ACKD occurs even in CKD patients without dialysis. Clinical manifestations include gross hematuria, flank pain, fever, palpable renal mass, and rising hematocrit.

An important complication of ACKD is the development of renal cell carcinoma, which is due to the pronounced epithelial hyperplasia lining the cyst. A CT scan with or without contrast is the preferred technique in suspect patients with renal cell carcinoma. This CT can distinguish simple cysts from multiple acquired cysts. An ultrasound or MRI can be used in CKD patients to prevent contrast-induced further deterioration in renal function.

Persistent hemorrhage may require nephrectomy. Also, retroperitoneal hemorrhage may underlie undetected renal cell carcinoma. Nephrectomy is recommended in those patients where carcinoma cannot be ruled out.

ACKD has been shown to regress after successful kidney transplantation. Therefore, option C is false.

Suggested Reading

Chen K, Huang HH, Aydin H, et al. Renal cell carcinoma in patients with end-stage renal disease is associated with more favourable histological features and prognosis. Scand J Urol. 2015;49:200–4.

Scandling JD. Acquired cystic kidney disease and renal cell cancer after transplantation: time to rethink screening? Clin J Am Soc Nephrol. 2007;2:621–2.

Torres VE, Harris PC. Cystic diseases of the kidney. In: Yu ASL, Chertow GM, Luyckx VA, et al., editors. Brenner & Rector's the kidney. 11th ed. Philadelphia: Elsevier Saunders; 2020. p. 1490–533.

13. An 18-year-old African American female student comes to the Emergency Department with complaints of weakness, dizziness, and poor appetite. On physical examination, she is a thin female with normal growth, but tachypnic. History reveals nocturia and polydipsia. Her BP is 100/60 mm Hg with a pulse rate of 102 (supine) and 80/40 mm Hg with a pulse rate of 120 (standing). She weighs 52 kg. The rest of the physical examination is unremarkable, except for a pericardial friction rub. Initial labs:

Na^+ = 132 mEq/L
K^+ = 5.8 mEq/L
Cl^- = 100 mEq/L
HCO_3^- = 10 mEq/L
Creatinine = 9.6 mg/dL
BUN = 110 mg/dL
Glucose = 90 mg/dL
Uric acid = 10.2 mg/dL
Hgb = 8 g/dL
Urinalysis = no hematuria or proteinuria
FE_{Na} = 15%

Which one of the following is the MOST likely diagnosis?

A. Autosomal dominant polycystic kidney disease (ADPKD)
B. Juvenile nephronophthisis(NPHP)
C. Autosomal dominant medullary cystic kidney disease (MCKD)
D. Medullar sponge kidney (MSK)
E. Percutaneous renal biopsy is needed to make the diagnosis

The answer is C

The clinical history and laboratory data are consistent with the diagnosis of autosomal dominant MCKD, which is now called autosomal dominant interstitial kidney disease (ADIKD). MCKD is of two types: type 1 and type 2. Type 1 MCKD is due to mutation in MUC1 gene, which encodes mucoprotein mucin 1. This protein is expressed on the surface of epithelial cells. Clinically, it presents with a slow decline in kidney function with a median age of ESKD of 50 years. The urine is bland with no hematuria. Uric acid is elevated with ESKD.

Type 2 MCKD is a progressive disease with onset of ESKD usually in the 2nd and 3rd decades of life. It is due to mutations in UMOD gene, which encodes uromodulin (Tamm-Horsfall protein). Despite kidney failure, patients develop relative hypotension due to renal salt wasting and volume depletion. The inability to concentrate urine is also an early finding. Gout is an early manifestation of type 2 MCKD. The kidneys tend to be small and an open renal biopsy is needed to make the definitive diagnosis in patients with MCKD (answer E is incorrect). Both kidneys are involved. The kidney surface has a granular appearance, and the cysts are located preferentially at the corticomedullary junction. Cysts are not present in organs other than the kidney. Histologically, interstitial fibrosis rather than glomerular disease is prominent. This patient has type 2 rather than MCKD type 1 disease (answer C is correct).

Flank pain, hematuria, nephrolithiasis, and HTN are uncommon and distinguish type 2 MCKD disease from ADPKD and medullary sponge kidney (answers A and D are incorrect).

NPHP is an autosomal recessive disorder and is grouped under ciliopathies. It is characterized by the inability to concentrate urine, polyuria, and polydipsia. At least mutations in 20 genes have been described. Three clinical forms of NPHP have been described by age of onset of ESKD: (1) infantile; (2) juvenile; and (3) adolescent. The median age for the development of ESKD for these three forms is 1 year, 13 years, and 15 years, respectively. Generally, NPHP is associated with retinal degeneration, optic atrophy, and retinitis pigmentosa. For this reason, NPHP is also termed renal-retinal dysplasia.

Previously, NPHP and MCKD were grouped together because of clinical and pathologic similarities. However, MCKD is distinct from NPHP because of the following conditions: (1) as explained above, MCKD is an autosomal dominant disease; (2) ESKD occurs during the 2nd and 3rd decades of life; and (3) there is no extrarenal involvement other than hyperuricemia and gout in MCKD. Thus, answer B is incorrect.

Suggested Reading

Benzing T, Walz G. Pathogenesis of nephronophthisis and medullary cystic kidney disease. In: Mount DB, Pollack MR, editors. Molecular and genetic basis of renal disease. Philadelphia: Saunders; 2008. p. 131–40.
Bleyer AJ. Improving the recognition of hereditary interstitial kidney disease. J Am Soc Nephrol. 2009;20:11–3.
Hildebrandt F, Benzing T, Katsanis N. Ciliopathies. N Engl J Med. 2011;364:1533–43.
Sayer JA. Nephronophthisis and medullary cystic kidney disease: overview. In: Turner N, Lameire N, Goldsmith DJ, et al., editors. Oxford textbook of clinical nephrology. 4th ed. Oxford: Oxford University Press; 2016. p. 2674–6.
Torres VE, Harris PC. Cystic diseases of the kidney. In: Yu ASL, Chertow GM, Luyckx VA, et al., editors. Brenner & Rector's the kidney. 11th ed. Philadelphia: Elsevier Saunders; 2020. p. 1490–533.

14. A 35-year-old woman is referred to a nephrologist for frequent urinary tract infections (UTIs), hematuria, and a renal stone. There is no weight loss. Physical examination is otherwise unremarkable. Labs are as follows:

Na^+ = 138 mEq/L
K^+ = 3.4 mEq/L
Cl^- = 112 mEq/L
HCO_3^- = 18 mEq/L
Creatinine = 1.1 mg/dL
BUN = 16 mg/dL
Glucose = 100 mg/dL
Hgb = 13.6%
Urine pH = 7.1

An intravenous pyelography (IVP) showed pronounced tubular ectasia of all papillae. **Which one of the following statements characterizes the patient's condition?**

A. Progression to ESKD is rare
B. Nephrolithiasis due to recurrent UTIs
C. Renal tuberculosis (TB)
D. Primary hyperparathyroidism
E. Medullary sponge kidney and routine preventive measures for UTI are not warranted

The answer is E

Based upon the history and the excretory urographic findings, the most likely diagnosis is the medullary sponge kidney (MSK). The diagnosis of MSK is usually made by excretory urography, which shows the presence of radial striations or cystic collection of contrast medium in the affected papillae. Sonography and CT of abdomen are generally not required, but CT is helpful to distinguish MSK from renal tumors, renal abscesses, papillary necrosis, or polycystic kidney disease.

A variety of terms have been used to describe the radiologic findings, including "streaking" or "brush-like" pattern of affected papillae, or "bouquets of flowers" or "bunches of grapes" for ectatic lesions that appear as spherical or cystic images filled with contrast medium.

MSK is a benign condition and progression to ESKD is uncommon. In this condition, only tubular dilatation of the collecting ducts and formation of multiple cysts are found in the medullary pyramids.

Clinically, patients with MSK present with microscopic or gross hematuria alone or in association with UTIs, nephrolithiasis or nephrocalcinosis. Both UTI and nephrolithiasis are frequent complications of MSK. Sterile pyuria is occasionally observed in patients with MSK without UTI. The incidence of UTI is higher in women than in men.

Renal stones are mostly composed of calcium oxalate and calcium phosphate. Renal colic is a frequent clinical manifestation. The risk factors for stone formation include urine stasis in ectatic tubules, absorptive hypercalciuria, hypocitraturia, and defective urinary acidification (alkaline urine pH) due to distal form of renal tubular acidosis (RTA). Therefore, recurrent UTIs are not responsible for renal stone formation.

Renal tubular ectasia, resulting in abnormal precalyceal opacification, is also seen in renal TB, renal papillary necrosis, and medullary nephrocalcinosis in primary hyperparathyroidism. These diseases should be included in the differential diagnosis of MSK and can be excluded based upon the associated clinical signs and etiologic conditions.

Suggested Reading

Fabris A, Anglani F, Lupo A, et al. Medullary sponge kidney: state of the art. Nephrol Dial Transplant. 2013;28:1111–9.

Torres VE, Harris PC. Cystic diseases of the kidney. In: Yu ASL, Chertow GM, Luyckx VA, et al., editors. Brenner & Rector's the kidney. 11th ed. Philadelphia: Elsevier Saunders; 2020. p. 1490–533.

15. **Match the following clinical histories of patients with the molecular defects:**

A. An 18-year-old man with low renin-aldosterone, hypokalemia, and severe HTN, who responds to amiloride but is unresponsive to spironolactone
B. A child with low renin-aldosterone, hypokalemia, severe HTN, poor growth, short stature, and nephrocalcinosis
C. A 16-year-old male with mild HTN, serum [K^+] of 3.4 mEq/L, and [HCO_3^-] of 29 mEq/L. His HTN is unresponsive to angiotensin-converting enzyme inhibitors (ACE-Is) and β-blockers, but responsive to glucocorticoids
D. A 20-year-old pregnant woman develops severe HTN without proteinuria during her 3rd trimester. Her 17-year-old brother is also hypertensive, whose BP rises on spironolactone
E. A child with hypotension, hyponatremia, hyperkalemia, and metabolic acidosis with elevated plasma renin and aldosterone levels
F. A 22-year-old man with HTN, hyperkalemia, metabolic acidosis, hypercalciuria, and low plasma renin but increased aldosterone levels

1. Mutations in the cytoplasmic COOH-terminus of the β- and γ-subunits of the epithelial sodium channel (ENaC)
2. Loss-of-function mutations in 11β-hydroxysteroid dehydrogenase type 2 (11β-HSD2) enzyme gene
3. A chimeric gene duplication from unequal crossover between 11β-hydroxylase (CYP11B1) and aldosterone synthase (CYP11B2) genes
4. A missense mutation in mineralocorticoid receptor (MR)
5. Inactivating mutations in either α-, β-, or γ-subunits of the ENaC
6. Mutations in lysine-deficient protein kinase 1 (WNK1) and lysine-deficient protein kinase 4 (WNK4)

Answers: A = 1; B = 2; C = 3; D = 4; E = 5; F = 6.

The patient described in choice A has Liddle syndrome, which is an autosomal dominant disorder. It is caused by mutations in the cytoplasmic COOH-terminus of the β- and γ-subunits of the ENaC. Activation of this channel results in increased Na^+ reabsorption with blunted Na^+ excretion, hypokalemia, and low-renin-aldosterone HTN. However, HTN responds to triamterene or amiloride, but not to spironolactone. Affected patients are at increased risk for cerebrovascular and cardiovascular diseases.

The child described in choice B carries the diagnosis of the syndrome of apparent mineralocorticoid excess (AME), which is a rare autosomal recessive disorder. It is due to a loss-of-function mutation in the gene encoding the enzyme 11β-hydroxysteroid dehydrogenase type 2 (11β-HSD2). This enzyme converts cortisol to the inactive cortisone. As a consequence of the mutation, the 11β-HSD2 enzyme activity is decreased with resultant accumulation of cortisol. Cortisol acts like a mineralocorticoid by occupying its receptor, causing Na^+ reabsorption, hypokalemic metabolic alkalosis, and low-renin-aldosterone HTN. Suppression of renin and aldosterone is due to volume excess caused by Na^+ and water retention. Children with AME demonstrate low birth weight and nephrocalcinosis, the latter due to hypokalemic nephropathy. HTN responds to salt restriction, amiloride or triamterene, but not to regular doses of spironolactone. Licorice ingestion induces a similar syndrome. Complications include cardiac events, including stroke and renal failure.

The clinical history described in choice C is consistent with the diagnosis of glucocorticoid-remediable aldosteronism (GRA). This disorder, also called familial hyperaldosteronism type 1, is caused by a chimeric gene duplication from unequal crossover between 11β-hydroxylase and aldosterone synthase. Some patients with GRA may have severe HTN, hypokalemia, and metabolic alkalosis. Some other patients may have mild HTN, normal to low serum [K^+], and a mild increase in serum [HCO_3^-]. Plasma renin is suppressed, but aldosterone levels are increased. Aldosterone secretion is stimulated by adrenocorticotropic hormone (ACTH) and not by angiotensin II. Therefore, administration of glucocorticoid suppresses excessive aldosterone secretion and improves HTN.

The possible diagnosis of the patient presented in choice D is a case of early-onset HTN with severe exacerbation during pregnancy. This disorder is caused by an activating heterozygous missense mutation in the mineralocorticoid receptor (MR) gene called S810L mutation. Clinically, the patient presents with HTN before the age of 20 years with low plasma K^+, renin, and aldosterone levels. Pregnancy exacerbates HTN without proteinuria, edema, or neurologic changes. Aldosterone levels, which are elevated during pregnancy, are extremely low in MR gene mutation. MR antagonists such as spironolactone become agonists and increase BP in patients with mutation in MR gene. Therefore, spironolactone is contraindicated in these patients. Progesterone also increases BP in patients with MR gene mutation, since these hormone levels are extremely high in these patients. It should be remembered that heterozygous loss-of-function mutations in the MR gene (locus symbol NR3C2) result in pseudohypoaldosteronism type I (PHA I), an autosomal dominant disorder that causes salt wasting and hypotension. This disease remits with age.

The clinical history present in choice E is similar to PHA I, but it is an autosomal recessive disorder. It is caused by mutations in any of the three (α, β, γ) subunits of the ENaC. This autosomal recessive disorder can manifest in the neonate as failure to thrive or in childhood which is a rare disease. It is characterized by salt wasting, hypotension, hyperkalemia, and metabolic acidosis. Other biochemical abnormalities include hyponatremia, high plasma and urine aldosterone levels despite hyperkalemia, and high plasma renin activity. Treatment includes lifelong high salt supplementation (at least 50 mEq/kg/day) and K^+ restriction as well as cation exchange resin (kayexalate).

The case in choice F represents pseudohypoaldosteronism type II (PHA II). It is called familial hyperkalemia with HTN or Gordon syndrome. The disease is caused by mutations in the genes that encode WNK (with-no-lysine (K)) family of serine-threonine kinases, WNK1 and WNK4. Both mutated kinases are present in the distal nephron and promote transcellular or paracellular Cl^- conductance. As a result, more salt is absorbed, causing an increase in intravascular volume. This expansion in intravascular volume suppresses renin activity, but increases BP. At the same time, both K^+ and H^+ secretions are reduced, resulting in hyperkalemia and metabolic acidosis. Aldosterone levels vary from low to high concentrations depending on the severity of hyperkalemia. Thus, patients with PHA II disorder, which may present in the neonate or adult, are characterized by hyperkalemia, metabolic acidosis, low-renin and low- to high aldosterone levels, and volume-dependent HTN. Thiazide diuretics correct both metabolic abnormalities and HTN.

Suggested Reading

Bonnardeaux A, Bichet DG. Inherited disorders of the renal tubule. In: Yu ASL, Chertow GM, Luyckx VA, et al., editors. Brenner & Rector's the kidney. 11th ed. Philadelphia: Elsevier Saunders; 2020. p. 1450–89.

Seidel E, Scholl UI. Genetic mechanisms of human hypertension and their implications for blood pressure physiology. Physiol Genomics. 2017;49:630–52.

Williams SS. Advances in genetic hypertension. Curr Opin Pediatr. 2007;19:192–8.

16. **Match the following disease conditions with the molecular defects:**

A. Cystinosis
B. Type A cystinuria
C. Dent disease
D. Primary hyperoxaluria (type 1)
E. Familial hypomagnesemia with hypercalciuria and nephrocalcinosis
F. X-linked hypophosphatemic rickets

1. Mutation in the SLC3A1 (solute carrier family 3, member 1) gene, which encodes the proximal tubule and intestinal dibasic amino acid transporter
2. Inactivating mutations in CTNS encoding the protein called cystinosin that is responsible for cystine export from lysosomes
3. Inactivating mutations in CLCN5 encoding a renal-specific chloride channel
4. Absolute or functional deficiency of AGTX (alanine-glycoxylate aminotransferase) gene
5. Mutations in PHEX (phosphate-regulating endopeptidase homolog, X-linked) gene
6. Mutations in paracellin-1

A = 2; B = 1; C = 3; D = 4; E = 6; F = 5

Cystinosin is an important cause of Fanconi syndrome in children. It is caused by inactivating mutations in CTNS which encodes a lysosomal membrane protein called cystinosin. It is a membrane transporter that is responsible for cystine export from lysosomes. Because of this mutation, the transport of cystine is impaired, with resultant accumulation of cystine in renal tubules and other organs. Nephropathic cystinosis manifests in the first year of life with failure to thrive, increased thirst, polyuria, and hypophosphatemic rickets. Increased urinary loss of Na^+, Ca^{2+}, and Mg^{2+} occurs in cystinosis. ESKD occurs by 10 years of age and cystinosis does not recur in a transplanted kidney.

Cystinuria is an autosomal recessive disorder with a defective transport of cystine and the dibasic amino acids (lysine, ornithine, and arginine) in the renal tubules and gastrointestinal (GI) tract. Three types of cystinuria have been described: type A, type B, and type AB. All three types are classified based on cystine excretion. Type A cystinuria is due to mutations in the SLC3A1 gene, which encodes the proximal tubule S3 segment and intestinal dibasic amino acid transporter. Cystinuria presents as nephrolithiasis usually during the 1st and 3rd decades of life but may occur in infants. Urinalysis shows cystine (hexagonal) crystals in the sediment. Type B cystinuria is secondary to mutations in the SLC7A9 (solute carrier family 7, member 9) gene, whereas type AB cystinuria is caused by mutations in both SLC3A (solute carrier family, member 3A) and SLC7A9 genes.

Dent disease is an X-linked recessive disease with associated Fanconi syndrome. It is caused by inactivating mutations in the CLCN5 (chloride voltage-gated channel) gene, which encodes a renal chloride channel, CLC-5. The disease is characterized by varying degrees of low-molecular-weight proteinuria, hypercalciuria, nephrolithiasis, hyperphosphaturia, and rickets. Renal failure gradually develops in patients with Dent disease. Renal biopsy shows chronic tubulointerstitial disease with calcium deposits. Glomeruli are normal. Treatment of Dent disease is largely supportive.

Primary hyperoxaluria type 1, the most common and severe form of the primary hyperoxalurias, is due to absolute or functional deficiency of the AGTX gene. This gene encodes the liver-specific AGT (alanine-glyoxylate aminotransferase) enzyme. AGT is a pyridoxal-PO_4-dependent enzyme, which catalyzes the conversion of glyoxalate to glycine which is deposited in the kidney and other organs. Excess production of oxalate presents as calcium oxalate nephrolithiasis and progressive renal failure. ESKD may occur in 80% of patients by 30 years of age. In the absence of this enzyme, the result is high levels of glycolic and oxalic acids, which readily convert to oxalate.

Familial hypomagnesemia with hypercalciuria and nephrocalcinosis is an autosomal recessive disease caused by mutations in paracellin-1, a protein that is present in tight junctions of the thick ascending limb of Henle's loop. The disease is characterized by renal Mg^{2+} wasting and hypomagnesemia. Hypercalciuria is also present, resulting in bilateral nephrocalcinosis and progressive renal failure. Serum parathyroid hormone (PTH) levels are abnormally increased with normal serum concentrations of Ca^{2+}, phosphate, and K^+. Hypomagnesemia is unresponsive to oral or intravenous (IV) magnesium administration. Kidney transplantation normalizes renal tubular handling of Mg^{2+} and Ca^{2+}.

X-linked hypophosphatemic rickets, a dominant disorder, are caused by a mutation in the PHEX gene. This gene encodes a protein that has similarities with neutral endopeptidases. Patients with this disease are characterized by short stature, femoral or tibial bowing, and evidence of rickets and osteomalacia. Biochemically, these patients have hypophosphatemia, phosphaturia, normal plasma Ca^{2+} and PTH, and increased alkaline phosphatase levels. The most important serum abnormality is inappropriately normal $1,25(OH)_2D_3$ (1,25-dihydroxyvitamin D3) levels in the presence of hypophosphatemia (<2.5 mg/dL). Males are affected more severely than females. Treatment includes calcitriol and phosphate therapy.

Suggested Reading

Bonnardeaux A, Bichet DG. Inherited disorders of the renal tubule. In: Yu ASL, Chertow GM, Luyckx VA, et al., editors. Brenner & Rector's the kidney. 11th ed. Philadelphia: Elsevier Saunders; 2020. p. 1450–89.

Monico CG, Rumbsy G, Milliner DS. The primary hyperoxalurias: molecular and clinical insights. In: Mount DB, Pollack MR, editors. Molecular and genetic basis of renal disease. Philadelphia: Saunders; 2008. p. 179–93.

17. **Which one of the following observations is LEAST likely in patients with Fabry's disease?**

A. Mutations resulting in deficient activity of serum or leukocyte α-galactosidase A, resulting in accumulation of globotriaosylceramide (ceramidetrihexoside)
B. Angiokeratomas of the skin, palmar erythema, peripheral and autonomic neuropathy, corneal opacities, hypertrophic cardiomyopathy, and early onset of stroke are commonly seen in male hemizygotes
C. Hematuria, nephrotic-range proteinuria, and progressive renal failure occur in males

D. Electron microscopy (EM) findings on renal biopsy include "myelin figures" or "zebra bodies" within the cytoplasm of the podocytes
E. Nephrotic-range proteinuria is due to deficient nephrin and podocin proteins in slit diaphragms rather than glycosphingolipid accumulation in podocytes

The answer is E

Fabry's disease is an X-linked disorder of abnormal glycosphingolipid metabolism. It is caused by deficient activity of lysosomal α-galactosidase A, resulting in accumulation of globotriaosylceramide in various organs, including the kidney, skin, brain, and vascular tissue. Male hemizygotes are affected more severely than female heterozygotes whose clinical manifestations vary from asymptomatic to severe disease.

In male hemizygotes, the clinical manifestations may begin in childhood with pain in extremities and acroparesthesias. LVH and coronary artery disease and stroke may occur at a younger age. Accumulation of globotriaosylceramide in podocytes rather than deficient nephrin and podocin causes proteinuria and renal failure. Therefore, statement E is false.

The diagnosis of Fabry's disease is usually made by measuring plasma or leukocyte levels of α-galactosidase activity in affected males. Prenatal diagnosis can also be made by measuring the enzyme activity in amniotic fluid.

Treatment of the disease includes replacement of recombinant human α-galactosidase (agalsidase α, agalsidase β). Enzyme replacement therapy slows or prevents irreversible damage in the cardiac and renal complications if started at an earlier stage, but it has lower efficacy in advanced stages. Both these enzymes require iv administration. Another drug for Fabry's disease is migalastat, sold under the brand name galafold, is an oral compound, which has advantage over the iv forms.

Suggested Reading

del Pino M, Andres A, Bernabeu AA, et al. Fabry nephropathy: an evidence-based narrative review. Kidney Blood Press Res. 2018;43:406–21.

Ortiz A, Germain DP, Desnick RJ, et al. Fabry disease revisited: management and treatment recommendations for adult patients. Mol Genet Metab. 2018;123:416–27.

18. A 30-year-old woman is referred to a nephrologist for proteinuria, hematuria, and elevation in serum creatinine level. She complained of eye pain and limping. She has a family history of glaucoma and proteinuria, but none on dialysis. Her serum creatinine is 3.6 mg/dl and serum antinuclear antibody (ANA) is negative. Her serum complement levels are normal. A 24-h urine collection reveals 3.6 g of proteinuria. The renal biopsy findings are as follows:

LM (light microscopy): mild increase in mesangial matrix

IF (immunofluorescence): unremarkable

EM (electron microscopy): thickened basement membranes (BMs) with irregular lucent areas and moth-eaten appearance

Based upon the above information, which one of the following is the MOST likely diagnosis?

A. Minimal change disease
B. Membranous nephropathy
C. Nail-patella syndrome
D. Fabry's disease
E. Lupus nephritis

The answer is C

This patient has clinical and morphologic evidence of nail-patella syndrome, which is characterized by hypoplastic or absent patellae, dystrophic finger and toenails, and other skeletal abnormalities. Heterochromia of the iris and glaucoma are associated eye findings. Nail-patella syndrome is inherited as an autosomal dominant disorder, which is caused by mutations in the LMXIB gene on human chromosome 9q34. This transcription factor regulates the expression of COL4A3 (collagen type IV alpha 3) and COL4A4 (collagen type IV alpha 4) chains in the glomerular basement membrane (GBM) and podocin and CD2AP (CD2-associated protein) in the podocyte.

Affected members demonstrate micro- and macroalbuminuria. Some patients develop nephrotic syndrome and HTN. Progressive renal failure occurs in 5 to 10% of the patients. LM findings are usually nonspecific. However, the GBM on electron microscopy shows characteristic moth-eaten appearance. Based upon these

findings, minimal change disease, membranous nephropathy, and Fabry's disease can be ruled out. Lupus nephritis is also unlikely based upon normal complement levels as well as negative ANA. Also, the renal pathology is not consistent with lupus nephritis.

Suggested Reading

Ghoumid J, Petit F, Holder-Espinasse M, et al. Nail-Patella Syndrome: clinical and molecular data in 55 families raising the hypothesis of a genetic heterogeneity. Eur J Hum Genet. 2016;24:44–50.

Heiget L, Gubler MC. Nail patella syndrome. In: Turner N, Lameire N, Goldsmith DJ, et al., editors. Oxford textbook of clinical nephrology. 4th ed. Oxford: Oxford University Press; 2016. p. 2711–3.

Sweeney E, Fryer A, Mountford R, et al. Nail patella syndrome: a review of the phenotype aided by developmental biology. J Med Genet. 2003;40:153–62.

Witzgall R. Nail-patella syndrome. In: Mount DB, Pollack MR, editors. Molecular and genetic basis of renal disease. Philadelphia: Saunders; 2008. p. 173–8.

19. A 40-year-old man is referred to you for evaluation of HTN and hematuria. There is no history of seizure disorder. Physical examination reveals retinal hemangiomas. An MRI of the kidney shows numerous cysts with possible tumor growth in some cysts. There were no renal angiomyolipomas. **Based upon the above information, which one of the following choices is the MOST likely diagnosis?**

A. Tuberous sclerosis complex (TSC)
B. Von Hippel-Lindau (VHL) disease
C. ADPKD
D. Hereditary renal cell papillary carcinoma
E. Papillary cystadenoma

The answer is B

The clinical history of the patient is consistent with the diagnosis of VHL disease, which is an autosomal dominant disease. It is characterized by retinal and cerebellar hemangiomas, clear cell renal cell carcinoma, pheochromocytoma, pancreatic tumors, and epididymal cystadenoma. Genetic analysis showed mutations in the VHL gene, which is linked to an oncogene locus that is possibly involved in spontaneous development of renal cell carcinoma. HTN is usually due to pheochromocytoma, and hematuria is attributed to cysts and the development of tumors. Because of the presence of numerous and large cysts, VHL disease may simulate ADPKD, and this disease should be included in the differential diagnosis.

Tuberous sclerosis complex is also an autosomal dominant disorder, which is characterized by hamartomas in the skin, retina, brain, bone, kidney, liver, and lung. Affected individuals develop seizures and mental retardation. Typical facial lesions and adenoma sebacium are characteristic features. The combination of renal angiomyolipomas and cysts is pathognomonic of tuberous sclerosis complex. This disorder is caused by mutations in one of the two genes: TSC1 (tuberous sclerosis protein 1) and TSC2 (tuberous sclerosis protein 2). TSC1 encodes a protein called hamartin, whereas TSC2 encodes tuberin. Normally, both proteins interact together and function as tumor suppressor genes. Abnormal function of these proteins may lead to tumors in the kidney.

Hereditary papillary renal cell carcinoma (HPRCC) is caused by activating mutations of the gene c-Met encoding tyrosine kinase receptor for hepatocyte growth factor/scatter factor. Hepatocyte growth factor/Met signaling leads to many cellular events, including growth, invasion, tumor metastasis, tissue regeneration, and wound healing. Patients with this tumor bear trisomy in chromosomes 7 and 17. Physical findings presented in the case are not found in patients with HPRCC.

Papillary cystadenoma, also called benign cystic nephroma, arises from metanephric blastema. When examined microscopically, the nephroma or mass consists of many cysts. These masses are benign and require no specific therapy. At times, however, the mass may contain sarcoma or renal cell carcinoma, which may require partial nephrectomy.

Suggested Reading

Maher ER, Neumann HP, Richard S. Von Hippel-Lindau disease: a clinical and scientific review. Eur J Hum Genet. 2011;19:617–23.

Torres VE, Harris PC. Cystic diseases of the kidney. In: Yu ASL, Chertow GM, Luyckx VA, et al., editors. Brenner & Rector's the kidney. 11th ed. Philadelphia: Elsevier Saunders; 2020. p. 1490–533.

20. **Regarding the heritability of idiopathic nephrolithiasis, which one of the following statements is FALSE?**

A. Pedigree studies of severe forms of absorptive hyperoxaluria have been mapped to a gene on chromosome 1
B. Transmembrane erythrocyte oxalate flux is much higher in patients with idiopathic calcium nephrolithiasis than controls
C. First-degree relatives of stone formers are 3 times at higher risk of developing renal stones than the general population
D. Most of the studies suggest that the mode of inheritance of stone disease is complex and polygenic
E. Studies suggest that the prevalence of monogenic kidney stone disease in patients attending kidney stone clinics is 35%

The answer is E

The genetic basis for idiopathic nephrolithiasis was explored as early as in 1894 when familial aggregations of urinary calculi were recorded. Furthermore, it was shown that the first-degree relatives of stone formers have 3 times the risk of developing nephrolithiasis, as compared with the general population. A number of other studies addressed this problem and suggested the mode of inheritance to be either monogenic, autosomal dominant, or polygenic. However, a strong evidence exists only for the polygenic mode of inheritance, as a trimodal distribution of calciuria, oxaluria, and citraturia was attributed to three genes with codominant alleles.

Although there is some evidence for a monogenic basis for idiopathic hyperoxaluria, the evidence is not as strong as for polygenic mode of inheritance. The prevalence of monogenic kidney stone disease is ~15%. Thus, choice E is not correct.

Sequence variations in a gene on chromosome 1 may be responsible for the absorptive hypercalciuria found in some patients with idiopathic stone disease.

Studies using erythrocytes have shown increased transmembrane oxalate flux in patients with idiopathic calcium nephrolithiasis than controls, and this defect is correctable with diuretics.

Suggested Reading

Coe FL, Worcester EM, Evan AP. Idiopathic hypercalciuria and formation of calcium renal stones. Nat Rev Nephrol. 2016;12:519–33.
Goldfarb DS, Avery AR, Beara-Lasic L, et al. A twin study of genetic influences on nephrolithiasis in women and men. Kidney Int Rep. 2019;4:535–40.
Halbritter J, Baum M, Hynes AM, et al. Fourteen monogenic genes account for 15% of nephrolithiasis/nephrocalcinosis. J Am Soc Nephrol. 2015;2:543–51.
Howles SA, Thakker RV. Genetics of kidney stone disease. Nat Rev Urol. 2020;17:407–21.

21. **Match the glomerular diseases with the implicated genes shown below:**

A. Focal segmental glomerulosclerosis (FSGS)
B. Lupus nephritis
C. Sickle cell nephropathy
D. C1q nephropathy
E. Autosomal dominant FSGS

1. Apolipoprotein L1 gene (APOL1)
2. Formin gene (inverted formin 2 gene (INF2))
3. MYH9 gene (myosin heavy chain 9)

Answers: A = 1; B = 1; C = 1; D = 3; E = 2

The development of techniques, such as single nucleotide polymorphisms (SNPs), admixture linkage disequilibrium (MALD), and genome-wide association studies (GWAS), made it possible to scan the entire genome to detect CKD and glomerular diseases. Initial studies have shown that nonmuscle myosin heavy chain 9 gene (MYH9) accounts for about 43% of ESKD in African Americans and is also responsible for the development of idiopathic

FSGS, collapsing variant of FSGS in HIV (human immunodeficiency virus) patients, and focal global sclerosis (formerly labeled "hypertensive ESKD"). However, recent MALD studies have identified an APOL1 gene close to the MYH9 gene. Two variants of the APOL1 gene, G1 and G2, have been found to be strongly associated with multiple different types of kidney diseases previously thought to represent distinct entities. Currently, they are considered to be caused by G1 and G2 variants of the APOL1 gene. The diseases that are associated with G1 and G2 variants include idiopathic FSGS, HIV-associated collapsing variant of FSGS, solidified (global) glomerulosclerosis (GS), severe lupus nephritis, sickle cell nephropathy, and HTN-attributed nephropathy in African Americans. It seems that the G1 and G2 forms of APOL1 confer protection against the trypanosomes that cause African sleeping sickness in African Americans.

Reeves-Daniel et al. reported two non-HIV African American patients with collapsing C1q nephropathy and a rapid loss of kidney function to have SNPs in the MYH9 gene. This suggests that C1q nephropathy in African Americans appears to reside in the MYH9 gene or probably APOL1-associated glomerular diseases.

Brown et al. presented evidence in 11 unrelated families that missense mutations in formin gene (INF2) cause autosomal dominant adult FSGS. Formins are a group of proteins that accelerate actin filament assembly and are localized in the podocytes. This activity is different from the activity of Actin4 gene protein on podocyte cytoskeleton. A number of mutations have now been identified in the INF2 gene and they all cluster in the same domain of the gene called the diaphanous inhibitory domain. Thus, the mutations in the above families were confined to the diaphanous inhibitory domain of the INF2 gene. It has been estimated that INF2 gene mutations account for up to 17% of autosomal dominant familial FSGS cases and 1% of sporadic cases.

Suggested Reading

Brown EJ, Schlöndorff JS, Becker DJ, et al. Mutations in the forming gene INF2 cause focal segmental glomerulosclerosis. Nat Genet. 2010;42:72–6.

Freedman BI, Limou S, Ma L, et al. APOL1-associated nephropathy: a key contributor to racial disparities in CKD. Am J Kidney Dis. 2018;72(Suppl 1):S8–16.

Friedman DJ, Pollack MR. APOL1 nephropathy: from genetics to clinical applications. Clin J Am Soc Nephrol. 2021;16:294–303.

Labat-de-Hoz L, Alonso MA. The formin INF2 in disease: progress from 10 years of research. Cell Mol Life Sci. 2020;77:4581–4600.

Lepori N, Zand L, Sethi S, et al. Clinical and pathological phenotype of genetic causes of focal segmental glomerulosclerosis in adults. Clin Kidney J. 2018;11:179–90.

Reeves-Daniel AM, Iskandar SS, Bowden DW, et al. Is collapsing C1q nephropathy another MYH9-associated kidney disease? A case report. Am J Kidney Dis. 2010;55:e21–4.

22. **Match the appropriate gene mutations with the following glomerular diseases:**

A. NPHS1
B. NPHS2
C. CD2AP
D. TRPC6
E. Actin4
F. LMX1B
G. WT1

1. Childhood FSGS, congenital nephrotic syndrome of the Finnish type
2. Early childhood, adolescent, or adult FSGS
3. Childhood or adulthood FSGS
4. Adult FSGS
5. Familial FSGS
6. Childhood or adolescent FSGS

Answers: A = 1; B = 2; C = 3; D = 4; E = 5; F = 6.

The following table shows genes, their proteins, mode of inheritance, and age of onset of nephrotic syndrome and FSGS.

Gene	Protein	Mode of inheritance	Age of onset	Comment
NPHS1	Nephrin	AR	Childhood congenital nephrotic syndrome of the Finnish type. Disease occurs 1 in 10,000 children	Nephrin is a component of slit diaphragm (SD)
NPHS2	Podocin	AR	Early childhood, adolescent, or adults	Podocin is a component of SD and causes steroid-resistant nephrotic syndrome
CD2AP	CD2-associated protein (CD2AP)	AD, rarely AR	Childhood or adulthood FSGS	CD2AP is a SD scaffolding molecule involved in actin cytoskeleton regulation. Its absence causes nephrotic syndrome. A case of apparent recessive CD2AP-associated FSGS has been reported in a 10-month-old child
TRPC6	TRP cation channel 6	AD	Adulthood and rarely childhood	TRPC6 is expressed in SD and reported to interact with nephrin and podocin, with both affecting the TRPC6 function
ACTIN4	α-Actinin4	AD	Adulthood	α-Actinin4 is a podocyte cytoskeleton protein. Mutations in the ACTIN4 gene alter the interaction of α-actinin4 with actin filaments
LMX1B	LIM homeobox transcription factor 1β	AD	Adulthood	LMX1B is a transcription factor. It plays a crucial role in the transcriptional regulation of essential podocyte genes
WT1	Wilms tumor 1	AD	Child and adulthood	Mutations in the WT1 gene cause a spectrum of urogenital disorders that include FSGS as a prominent feature

Suggested Reading

De Vriese AS, Sethi S, Nath KA, et al. Differentiating primary, genetic, and secondary FSGS in adults: a clinicopathologic approach. J Am Soc Nephrol. 2018;29:759–74.

Lepori N, Zand L, Sethi S, et al. Clinical and pathological phenotype of genetic causes of focal segmental glomerulosclerosis in adults. Clin Kidney J. 2018;11:179–90.

Li AS, Ingham JF, Lennon R. Genetic disorders of the glomerular filtration barrier. Clin J Am Soc Nephrol. 2020;15:1818–28.

Schlöndorff J, Pollack MR. Inherited disorders of the glomerulus. In: Yu ASL, Chertow GM, Luyckx VA, et al., editors. Brenner & Rector's the kidney. 11th ed. Philadelphia: Elsevier Saunders; 2020. p. 1434–49.

23. **Which one of the following statements regarding genetics of diabetic kidney disease (DKD) is TRUE?**

A. Familial clustering of DKD, independent of risk factors such as hyperglycemia and hypertension, has been reported by several studies
B. Heritability of DKD and its phenotypes such as albuminuria and glomerular filtration rate has been estimated >0.3 (30%) by most of the studies
C. Initial studies on insertion/deletion (I/D) polymorphism of the ACE gene showed that the DD phenotype carries a higher risk for development of ESKD than other genotypes
D. The SUMMIT Consortium report from >5000 individuals with Type 1 diabetes suggested an association of AFF3 (AF4/FMR2 family, member 3), CNTNAP2 (contactin associated protein 2), NRG3 (neuregulin 3), and PTPN13 (tyrosine-protein phosphatase nonreceptor type 13) genes with DKD
E. All of the above

The answer is E

The pathogenesis of DKD remains incompletely understood, although metabolic, genetic, and epigenetic mechanisms have been implicated. The genetic basis of DKD was initially suggested by the study of Seaquist and associates in 1989. In this study, two sets of families consisting of both probands and siblings with type 1 diabetes were evaluated. In one set, the probands had no evidence of DKD, while the other set of probands had kidney transplantation because of DKD. During follow-up, 83% of siblings without history of DKD had a normal renal function and only 17% had albuminuria (>45 mg of albumin/24-h). None of the patients had ESKD. On the other hand, 41% of siblings with a history of DKD had albuminuria, 41% ESKD, and 17% normal renal function. This disparity of renal dysfunction between siblings with and without history of DKD suggested the involvement of

genetic predisposition to DKD. Following this study, many other investigators have confirmed the familial aggregation of DKD in patients with both Type 1 and Type 2 diabetes (answer A is correct).

In addition to familial clustering of DKD, heritability (h^2) of DKD phenotypes such as creatinine, glomerular filtration rates, albuminuria, and hypertension have been reported in Type 2 and Type 1 diabetes with h^2 0.3 to 0.75 or 30 to 75%. Thus, answer B is correct.

Among the genes of renin-angiotensin system, polymorphism of the ACE gene has been studied the most. The ACE gene polymorphism is characterized by the insertion (I) or deletion (D) of 287 base-pair segments in intron 16. Each person carries two copies (II, DD or ID) of the gene. Studies have shown that patients with DD genotype have increased risk for progression to ESKD and experience higher mortality, once the dialysis is initiated. Also, patients with DD genotype showed a faster decline in glomerular filtration rate and less reduction in albumin excretion rate than those with II or ID genotypes following treatment with an ACE-inhibitor (answer C is correct).

Various genetic studies have identified more than 150 genes, but only 30 genes were found to be associated with DKD. However, most of these studies lack adequate power and confirmation. In addition, the effect of associated obesity, hypertension, or hyperlipidemia on DKD in Type 2 diabetics has not been adequately studied. Thus, the association of a specific gene with DKD in both types of diabetics is lacking. These issues were addressed by the SUMMIT Consortium. In this Consortium, 2563 Type 1 patients with DKD and 2593 controls (Type 1 patients with a normal kidney function) from four international studies were reevaluated for genetic variants that were associated with DKD. Despite sophisticated genetic analysis and power, the study could not identify any single variant that can influence the risk of DKD. However, the investigators found suggestive variant signals in or near AFF3, CNTNAP, and PTPN13 genes, but additional studies are suggested to confirm these signals (answer D is correct). The Consortium also found the heritability of DKD in 35% of the cases.

Suggested Reading

Bain SC, Chowdhury TA. Genetics of diabetic nephropathy and microalbuminuria. J R Soc Med. 2000;93:62–6.

Gu HF. Genetic and epigenetic studies in diabetic kidney disease. Front Genet. 2019;10:507.

Mooyaart AL, Valk EJJ, va Es LA, et al. Genetic associations in diabetic nephropathy: a meta-analysis. Diabetologia. 2011;54:544–53.

Parving H-H, Tarnow L, Rossing P. Genetics of diabetic nephropathy. J Am Soc Nephrol. 1996;7:2509–17.

Sandholm N, van Zuydam N, Ahlqvist E, et al. on behalf of the SUMMIT Consortium. The genetic landscape of renal complications in type 1 diabetes. J Am Soc Nephrol. 2017;28:557–74.

Seaquist ER, Goetz FE, Rich S, et al. Familial clustering of diabetic kidney disease, evidence for genetic susceptibility to diabetic nephropathy. N Engl J Med. 1989;120:1161–5.

Wei L, Xiao Y, Li L, et al. The susceptibility genes in diabetic nephropathy. Kidney Dis. 2018;4:226–37.

24. **A 16-year-old male student is diagnosed with Alport syndrome. Which one of the following statements regarding this syndrome is FALSE?**

    A. Antisera or monoclonal antibodies to type IV collagen chains reveal the loss of immunoreactivity for the α5 and α3 chains from the glomerular basement membrane (GBM) of males with X-linked disease
    B. Proteinuria and hypertension increase with age and occur much more probably in affected males than females in the X-linked disease
    C. X-linked male patients with deletions in the α5 chain of type IV collagen progress to ESKD during the 2nd or 3rd decade of life with deafness
    D. Male patients with autosomal dominant disease with heterozygous mutations in α3 or α4 subunits of type IV collagen will have gross hematuria and rapid progression to ESKD
    E. Autosomal recessive disease has no expression or immunostaining for α3 or α4 chain of type IV collagen in the GBM

The answer is D

Alport syndrome is a progressive hereditary disorder in children or young adults with characteristic ultrastructural changes of the glomerular basement membrane (GBM) associated with sensorineural hearing loss and eye abnormalities. There are three forms of the disease that are caused by mutations in type IV collagen. Type IV collagen is found in all GBMs, Bowman's capsule, distal tubular basement membranes, epidermal basement membrane, lens capsule, and cochlea.

Type IV collagen consists of six α-chains, designated α1 to α6. Each α chain is encoded by one gene. For example, α1 chain, usually designated α1 (IV), is encoded by the COL4A1 (collagen type IV alpha 1 chain) gene.

Thus, there are six genes that are located in three different chromosomes and encode all six chains. Pertinent to Alport syndrome, the COLA4A3 and COLA4A4 genes reside on chromosome 2 and COL4A5 (collagen type IV alpha 5 chain) gene on X chromosome. Each α-chain has a collagenous and a noncollagenous domain. Three α-chains fold at the collagen domain to form a triple helix, and only three sets of triple helical molecules can be formed from all six chains and are called promoters. These promoters have the composition of 1.1.2, 3.4.5, and 5.5.6. chains. The promoters, in turn, interact to form three types of collagen networks: 1.1.2/1.1.2 in all basement membranes, 3.4.5/3.4.5 in GBMs, tubular basement membranes, eye, and cochlea, and 1.1.2/5.5.6 in skin and Bowman's capsule. In general, mutations in the collagen IV α345 molecule cause all forms of Alport syndrome. The following discussion is a brief summary of the new classification of Alport syndrome, as proposed by Kashtan et al. In this new classification, three genetic forms of the Alport syndrome have been described: (1) X-linked; (2) autosomal (either recessive or dominant); and (3) digenic.

X-linked Alport syndrome is due to mutations in COL4A5, the gene encoding the α5 chain of type IV collagen. Over 200 mutations have been reported in this form of Alport syndrome. Hemizygous males are at 100% risk for progression to ESKD. Heterozygous females have lower frequency (25%) lifetime risk of progression to ESKD. In these females, the risk factors for progression to ESKD include a history of gross hematuria in childhood, sensorineural deafness, proteinuria, and extensive GBM thickening and lamellation. It should be noted that the females, once considered carriers and exhibit benign course, seem to have some form of Alport system and require a timely and appropriate treatment to prevent ESKD.

Patients with hematuria, thin GBMs, and heterozygous mutations in COL4A3 or COL4A4 genes are included into autosomal Alport syndrome. Thus, the new classification eliminates thin basement membrane nephropathy as a separate diagnostic entity. Autosomal Alport syndrome results from biallelic (homozygous or compound heterozygous) or heterozygous mutations in the COL4A3 or COL4A4 gene. Biallelic mutations demonstrate a recessive inheritance pattern and patients are at 100% risk for development of ESKD. As in X-linked disease, patients with autosomal recessive disease have sensorineural deafness and eye lesions in association with renal disease.

Heterozygous mutations in COL4A3 or AOL4A4 are inherited in an autosomal dominant fashion. The clinical symptoms may be asymptomatic or symptomatic. In symptomatic patients, the risk for ESKD may reach up to 20% in later life. Risk factors for ESKD include proteinuria, family history of ESKD, sensorineural deafness, focal segmental glomerulosclerosis, or GBM thickness or lamellation. Prognosis is generally good, if hematuria is absent. The reason for redefining thin basement membrane nephropathy as a form of autosomal dominant Alport syndrome is to avoid inadequate monitoring and therapy, thereby preventing the development of ESKD.

Digenic Alport syndrome refers to patients and families with mutations in two of the COL4A3, COL4A4, or COL4A5 genes. This is a new form of non-Mendelian inheritance. However, some patients with mutations in *trans* behave like autosomal recessive and some with mutations in *cis* behave like autosomal dominant mode of inheritance.

The association of X-linked Alport syndrome (XLAS) with leiomyomatosis of the esophagus or tracheobronchial tree is due to large deletions that span the adjacent 5' ends of the COL4A5 and COL4A6 genes.

The diagnosis of Alport syndrome is suspected based upon the identification of characteristic symptoms, a thorough history, and clinical evaluation. Also, the family history of Alport syndrome, kidney failure without known cause, early deafness, or hematuria aid in the diagnosis of Alport syndrome. However, a definitive diagnosis requires either kidney or skin biopsy in addition to genetic testing. On renal biopsy, immunofluorescence staining of various chains of type IV collagen has become a routine procedure to establish the diagnosis of Alport syndrome. Patients with X-linked Alport syndrome have absent or negative staining for α5 chain, which is accompanied by the loss of α3 chain in the kidney. In the autosomal form, staining for α3 and α4 chains is absent in the kidney.

Microscopic hematuria is the cardinal feature of Alport syndrome. Proteinuria may be absent in early phase of the disease. However, proteinuria and hypertension develop with aging much more commonly in males than females in the X-linked disease. The clinical course in X-linked males is largely dependent on the type of mutation in the COL4A5 gene. Large deletions in the gene confer a 90% probability of ESKD before the age of 30 years, with 50% reaching ESKD by age 20. Deafness is not congenital but occurs during adolescence or early in about 55% of males and 45% of females. Ocular defects (anterior lenticonus) are restricted to patients who progress to ESKD. Autosomal recessive disease is diagnosed with similar clinical manifestations as X-linked disease, and both sexes may reach ESKD before the age of 30. Autosomal dominant disease is a much milder form compared to other forms of the disease, and patients with this disease do not progress rapidly to ESKD. However, ESKD occurs after 50 years of age. Therefore, option D is incorrect.

Suggested Reading

Hudson BG, Tryggvason K, Sundaramoorthy M, Neilson EG. Alport's syndrome, Goodpasture's syndrome, and type IV collagen. N Engl J Med. 2003;348:2543–56.

Kashtan CE. Familial hematuria. Pediatr Nephrol. 2009;24:1951–8.

Kashtan CE, Ding J, Garosi G, et al. Alport syndrome: a unified classification of genetic disorders of collagen IV α345: a position paper of the Alport syndrome Classification Working Group. Kidney Int. 2018;93:1045–51.

Mencarelli MA, Heidet L, Storey H, et al. Evidence of digenic inheritance in Alport syndrome. J Med Genet. 2015;52:163–74.

25. **Match the following urinary findings with the appropriate management and treatment of Alport syndrome:**

A. Hematuria with normal albuminuria
B. Hematuria and albuminuria of 30–300 mg/24-h
C. Hematuria and albuminuria >300 mg/24-h
D. Progressive proteinuria, despite adequate ACE-inhibitor therapy

1. Monitor BP, creatinine, and albuminuria annually
2. Follow above evaluations every 6 months, consider the ACE-inhibitor in patients with mutations (deletion, frameshift, nonsense, splicing), deafness, and family history of ESKD before the age of 30 years
3. Start ACE-inhibitor or an angiotensin receptor blocker (ARB) and titrate as tolerated
4. Control BP to <130/80 mm Hg by adding any class of antihypertensive drugs, including aldosterone antagonists, statin for hyperlipidemia, and management of mineral bone disorder

Answers: A = 1; B = 2; C = 3; D = 4

Management of children with Alport syndrome includes early screening for hematuria in suspected cases, determination of urinary protein (albumin) excretion rate, and initiation of renin-angiotensin system inhibitors (RASIs) in patients with albuminuria >300 mg/24-h. If 24-h urine collection is not possible, the determination of protein:creatinine ratio in a single voided specimen should be done.

The initial antihypertensive drug of choice is RASI, either an ACE-inhibitor or an ARB. Generally, ACE-inhibitors are cheaper than ARBs and are available worldwide. A recent trial, EARLY PRO-TECT (Prospective Therapy European Community Trial), in children with Alport syndrome showed that early treatment with ramipril (an ACE-inhibitor) was effective in slowing renal disease. In this study, 66 children with a mean age of 8.8 ± 4.2 yr, normal glomerular filtration rate, and either isolated microscopic hematuria or albuminuria ranging from 19.1 to 82.9 mg/g creatinine were included. Of these 66 children, 20 were randomized to either ramipril or placebo, and 42 treated with ramipril only (open-ramipril treatment arm) completed the treatment. The data from the open-ramipril treatment arm were compared with the data from 28 untreated children. The patients were followed up for up to 6 yr. Overall, the data showed a nonsignificant decrease in the risk of disease progression, diminished the slope of albuminuria progression, and the decline in glomerular filtration rate. Thus, early treatment of patients with an ACE-inhibitor in children with Alport syndrome delays the onset of ESKD by several years. Also, control of hypertension, hyperlipidemia, and proteinuria may delay ESKD.

Suggested Reading

Gross O, Tönshoff B, Weber LT, et al. for the German Pediatric Nephrology (GPN) Study Group and EARLY PRO-TECT Alport Investigators. A multicenter, randomized, placebo-controlled, double-blind phase 3 trial with open-arm comparison indicates safety and efficacy of nephroprotective therapy with ramipril in children with Alport's syndrome. Kidney Int. 2020;97:1275–86.

Kashtan CE, Ding J, Garosi G, et al. Alport syndrome: a unified classification of genetic disorders of collagen IV α345: a position paper of the Alport syndrome Classification Working Group. Kidney Int. 2018;93:1045–51.

Rheault MN, Smoyer WE. Long-term ACE inhibition in Alport syndrome: are the benefits worth the risks? Kidney Int. 2020;97:1104–6.

26. A 30-year-old man with X-linked Alport syndrome (XLAS), deafness and anterior lenticonus and a functioning renal allograft from a living-related donor 9 months ago is concerned about his long-term function and survival of transplanted kidney. His creatinine is 1.2 mg/dL. **Which one of the following diseases can occur and cause acute allograft loss in this patient?**

A. Focal segmental glomerulosclerosis (FSGS)

B. Recurrence of Alport syndrome
C. Minimal change disease
D. Anti-GBM antibody disease
E. Membranous nephropathy

The answer is D

Kidney transplantation, besides dialysis, is the only long-term treatment modality available for patients with XLAS. The survival rate of renal allograft in an XLAS patient is similar to those of patients with other diseases. Recurrence of Alport syndrome does not occur in the transplant because the donor GBM is normal; however, 3% and 5% of patients develop de novo anti-GBM antibody disease. Usually, anti-GBM antibody disease occurs within a year of transplantation, but occurrence after several years has been described. As stated in the previous question, the antibodies are usually directed against the α-5 chain of type IV collagen. Affected patients have high titers of these antibodies and are at high risk for crescentic glomerulonephritis (GN) and loss of graft function. Treatment with plasmapheresis and cyclophosphamide is of limited benefit, and retransplantation is associated with a high recurrence rate of anti-GBM antibody disease. The occurrence of FSGS, minimal change disease, and membranous nephropathy has not been reported. Thus, option D is correct.

Suggested Reading

Byrne MC, Budisavljevic MN, Fan Z, et al. Renal transplant in patients with Alport's syndrome. Am J Kidney Dis. 2002;39:769–75.

Gumber MR, Kute EB, Gopalani KR, et al. Outcome of renal transplantation in Alport's syndrome: a single-center experience. Transplant Proc. 2012;44:261–3.

Kashtan CE. Renal transplantation in patients with Alport syndrome. Pediatr Transplant. 2006;10:651–7.

27. A 35-year-old Caucasian man is referred to a nephrologist for episodic hematuria. More specifically, hematuria occurs following an upper respiratory tract infection. There is no history of extrarenal manifestations. Serum creatinine is normal (eGFR=100 mL/min). Urinalysis shows microscopic hematuria and proteinuria. A spot urine protein-to-creatinine ratio is 0.4. A kidney biopsy shows no specific lesion on light microscopy (LM). Also, immunofluorescent microscopy (IF) studies are negative. **Based on the following electron microscopy (EM) photomicrograph** (Fig. 8.1), **which one of the following is the MOST likely diagnosis?**

A. IgA (immunoglobulin A) nephropathy
B. X-linked Alport syndrome
C. Autosomal recessive Alport syndrome
D. Thin basement membrane nephropathy (Autosomal dominant Alport syndrome)
E. Minimal change disease

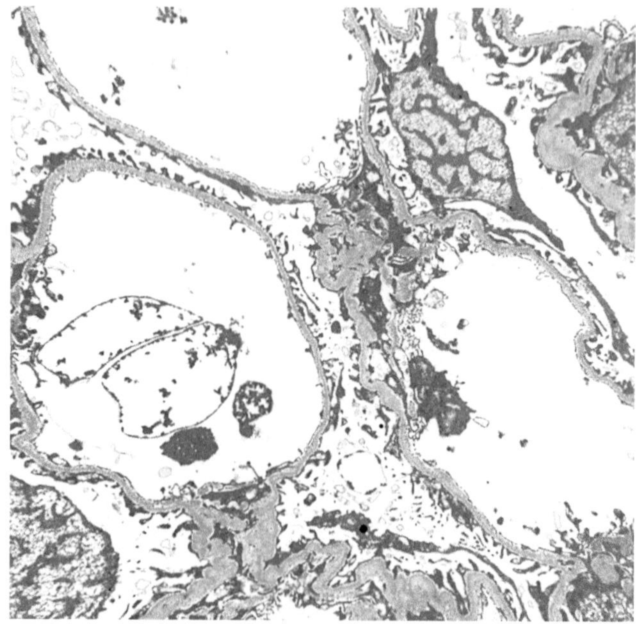

Fig. 8.1 EM micrograph of the above patient

The answer is D

Except for minimal change disease, all other disease conditions initially present with hematuria. The clue for diagnosis is the finding on EM, which shows a uniformly thin basement membrane. Thin basement membranes are also found in the Alport syndrome and IgA nephropathy; however, these two diseases can be distinguished from thin basement membrane nephropathy by LM and IF findings and clinically. In the Alport syndrome, the cardinal ultrastructural abnormality is the variable thickening, thinning, basket weaving, and lamellation of the glomerular basement membrane. According to one study, the normal range for basement membrane width in adult males is 373 ± 42 nm, and in females 326 ± 45 nm. In thin basement membrane nephropathy, the glomerular basement membrane width is <200 nm (for comparison, the normal GBM is shown in the right of Fig. 8.2 **below). At present, 40% of thin basement membrane nephropathy is caused by mutations in COL4A3 and COL4A4 genes that encode α3 and α4 chains of type IV collagen.**

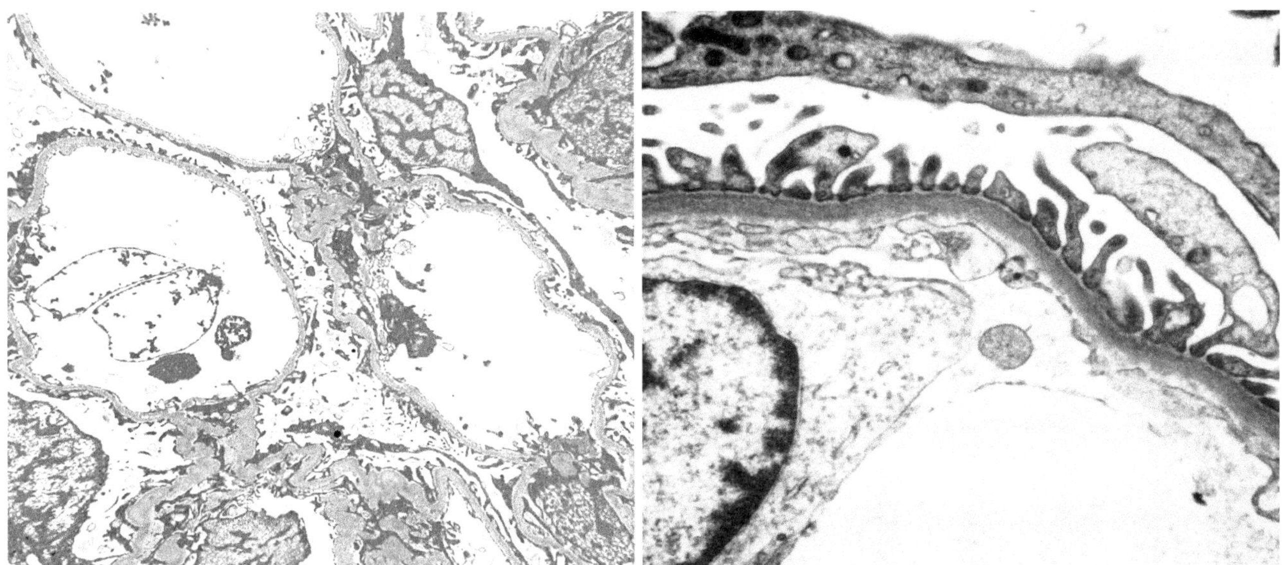

Fig. 8.2 EM micrograph showing thin basement membrane width (left) and normal basement membrane width (right)

In children, the diagnosis of thin basement membrane is rather difficult, unless each laboratory establishes its own age-related normal glomerular basement membrane width. In one study, the range varied from 146 to 273 nm in a male child at 1 year of age to 230–430 nm at age 9 or older.

It should be noted that the term thin basement membrane disease is eliminated in the new classification of the Alport syndrome and is now included under the classification of autosomal dominant Alport syndrome.

Suggested Reading

Hashimoto H, Ohashi N, Tsuji N, et al. A case report of thin basement membrane nephropathy accompanied by sporadic glomerulocystic kidney disease. BMC Nephrol. 2019;20:248.

Kashtan CE, Ding J, Garosi G, et al. Alport syndrome: a unified classification of genetic disorders of collagen IV α345: a position paper of the Alport syndrome Classification Working Group. Kidney Int. 2018;93:1045–51.

Savige J, Rana K, Tonna S, et al. Thin basement membrane nephropathy. Kidney Int. 2003;64:1169–78.

Savige J, Gregory M, Gross O, et al. Expert guidelines for the management of Alport syndrome and thin basement membrane nephropathy. J Am Soc Nephrol. 2013;24:364–75.

Tryggvason K, Patrakka J. Thin basement membrane nephropathy. J Am Soc Nephrol. 2006;17:813–22.

28. A pregnant woman in her 3rd trimester first noticed frequent urination (polyuria) associated with thirst and polydipsia. Her urine osmolality is 100 mOsm but failed to sustain the maximum osmolality, despite highly frequent administration of vasopressin. Her serum [Na^+] is 142 mEq/L. **Which one of the following treatments is APPROPRIATE for this woman?**

    A. Increase vasopressin dose to 50 U once daily

B. Limit fluid intake to improve polyuria
C. Match intake and output to maintain fluid status
D. Administer dDAVP (desmopressin) to improve polyuria
E. Do nothing until delivery

The answer is D

Infrequently, pregnant women in their late gestation develop polyuria, thirst, and polydipsia. The urine is dilute, and vasopressin administration transiently increases the osmolality; however, vasopressin levels decrease within 30 min due to degradation by the enzyme, vasopressinase. This enzyme is produced by the placenta, and women with polyuria have high circulating levels of vasopressinase. Polyuria, which is called transient diabetes insipidus of pregnancy, disappears after delivery. Vasopressinase degrades vasopressin, but not its synthetic analog dDAVP (desmopressin). Therefore, women with transient diabetes insipidus of pregnancy respond to treatment with dDAVP. Thus, option D is correct. Other options are inappropriate for this woman.

Suggested Reading

Ananthakrishnan S. Gestational diabetes insipidus: diagnosis and management. Best Pract Res Clin Endocrinol Metab. 2020;34:101384.
Durr A, Hoggard JG, Hunt JM, Schrier RW. Diabetes insipidus in pregnancy associated with abnormally high circulating vasopressinase activity. N Engl J Med. 1987;316:1070–4.
Marques P, Gunawardana K, Grossman A. Transient diabetes insipidus in pregnancy. Endocrinol Diabetes Metab Case Rep. 2015;2015:150078.

29. **Which one of the following laboratory findings is a major CONCERN during midpregnancy in a woman with no history of kidney disease and hypertension?**

A. Na^+ = 130 mEq/L
B. Hematocrit = 33 g/L
C. Uric acid = 6.5 mg/dL
D. GFR 134 = mL/min
E. Filtration fraction (FF) <20%

The answer is C

Except for uric acid, all other laboratory findings are normal in an uncomplicated pregnant woman. Both the excretion and clearance are increased in early and midpregnancy. As a result, serum uric acid levels are decreased by 25%. Serum uric acid levels range from 2.5 to 4.9 mg/dL in early and midpregnancy, and the values approach near normal at term. Serum uric acid levels vary among ethnic groups, and also exhibit a diurnal variation, being highest in the morning and lowest in the evening. Pregnant women with multiple fetuses usually have high uric acid levels.

It is thought that serum uric acid level in the high normal range is considered abnormal in a pregnant woman with normal renal function and BP levels. This high normal value may be a risk factor for impending preeclampsia and also a better predictor of fetal risk than BP, although some studies suggest no prognostic implication of uric acid. Roberts et al. examined the fetal risk in 972 pregnancies by the presence of or absence of combinations of gestational hypertension, proteinuria, and hyperuricemia. In women with hypertension, hyperuricemia was associated with shorter gestations, small-for-gestational-age infants, and increased risk for preterm birth. Hyperuricemia increased the risk of these complications in the absence or presence of proteinuria. Thus, hyperuricemia should be considered a risk factor for poor fetal outcomes.

FF is that fraction of plasma that is filtered at the glomerulus. It is calculated as follows:

$$FF = \frac{GFR}{RPF} \times 100$$

For example, if GFR is 120 mL/min and the renal plasma flow (RPF) is 600 mL/min; then FF is:

$$\frac{120}{600} \times 100 = 20\%$$

This calculation reveals that only 20% of the plasma entering the glomerulus is filtered. The remaining 80% of the plasma leaves the glomerular capillaries via the efferent arteriole into the peritubular capillaries and

subsequently into the systemic circulation. The FF may be a useful indicator in following renal function changes in certain physiologic and pathologic conditions. When FF increases, there is an increase in filtration of plasma (>20%) at the glomerulus. As a result, the protein concentration in the plasma leaving the efferent arteriole is increased. Consequently, the oncotic pressure in the peritubular capillaries is increased more than normal. Because of this increase in oncotic pressure, reabsorption of solutes is increased in the proximal tubule.

In early pregnancy, the increase in GFR is less than the increase in RPF, resulting in low FF. In late pregnancy, however, the RPF decreases slightly relative to GFR, causing FF to rise. The following Table 8.1 **shows some important laboratory values in a normal pregnant woman.**

Table 8.1 Some important laboratory values in pregnancy

Labs	Pregnancy	Reference values (nonpregnant)
Serum		
Na^+ (mEq/L)	130–135	140
K^+(mEq/L)	3.0–4.0	4.5
HCO_3^- (mEq/L)	18–22	24
BUN (mg/dL)	7–10	12
Creatinine (mg/dL)	0.4–0.6	0.8–1.2
Albumin (g/dL)	3.0–4.0	3.5–4.5
Uric acid (mg/dL)	2.5–4.9 (early-midpregnancy)	4.5
Hct (g/dL)	30–33	40
Urine		
Glucose	High	Absent
Amino acids	High	Normal
Protein	Normal	Normal (<150 mg/day)
Calcium	High	Normal
Others		
ABG	pH = 7.43; pCO_2 = 31; HCO_3^- = 19	pH = 7.40; pCO_2 = 40; HCO_3^- = 24
BP	105/60 mm Hg	115/70 mm Hg

Suggested Reading

Abbassi-Ghanavati M, Greer LG, Cunningham FG. Pregnancy and laboratory studies. A reference table for clinicians. Obstet Gynecol. 2009;114:1326–31.

Morton A, Teasdale S. Review article: Investigations and the pregnant woman in the emergency department – part 1: Laboratory investigations. Emerg Med Australas. 2018;30:600–9.

Roberts JM, Bodner LM, Lain KY, et al. Uric acid is as important as proteinuria in identifying fetal risk in women with gestational hypertension. Hypertension. 2005;46:1263–9.

30. A 24-year-old woman with type 1 diabetes and serum creatinine level of 1.8 mg/dL is contemplating pregnancy. She has proteinuria of 2.5 g per day. **Which one of the following advices is INAPPROPRIATE?**

A. Adverse maternal and fetal outcomes are common during pregnancy
B. Pregestational microalbuminuria predisposes to preeclampsia
C. Preterm delivery is rather common
D. Progression of kidney disease is uncommon following delivery
E. Postpone pregnancy until successful kidney transplantation

The answer is D

Women with pregestational diabetes experience higher maternal and fetal outcomes during pregnancy, as compared with nondiabetic women. Also, diabetic women are at increased risk for preeclampsia than nondiabetic women. In addition, the presence of microalbuminuria before pregnancy is an added risk for preeclampsia and preterm delivery. Also, the study by Klemetti et al. showed high rates of preeclampsia and preterm delivery in type 1 diabetic patients with diabetic nephropathy. Therefore, it is better for a diabetic woman with nephropathy to postpone pregnancy until successful kidney transplantation.

Purdy et al. studied 11 type 1 diabetic women with proteinuria and serum creatinine levels >1.4 mg/dL before pregnancy and found that seven patients progressed to dialysis in 6–57 months following delivery. In five of these

seven patients, acceleration of renal disease during pregnancy accounted for dialysis dependency. Renal function was stable only in 27%. Proteinuria increased in 79%, and exacerbation of hypertension or preeclampsia occurred in 73%. During pregnancy, mean creatinine rose from 1.8 mg/dL to 2.5 mg/dL in the 3rd trimester. Thus, pregnancy in type 1 diabetic patients with nephropathy causes progression of renal disease (answer D is incorrect).

Suggested Reading

Hladunewich MA, Melam N, Bramham K. Pregnancy across the spectrum of chronic kidney disease. Kidney Int. 2016;89:995–1007.

Ekbom P, Damm P, Feldt-Rasmussen B, et al. Pregnancy outcome in type 1 diabetic women with microalbuminuria. Diabetes Care. 2001;24:1739–44.

Klemetti MM, Laivuori H, Tikkanen M, et al. Obstetric and perinatal outcome in type 1 diabetes patients with diabetic nephropathy during 1988–2011. Diabetologia. 2015;58:678–86.

Purdy LS, Hantsch CE, Molitch ME, et al. Effect of pregnancy on renal function in patients with moderate-to-severe diabetic renal insufficiency. Diabetes Care. 1996;19:1067–74.

31. **In a patient with primary glomerulonephritis (GN) and serum creatinine <1.4 mg/dL, which one of the following statements is FALSE during pregnancy?**

   A. An increase in serum creatinine is seen in some patients
   B. Occurrence of de novo hypertension is common in some patients
   C. Increase in proteinuria is common
   D. Decline in renal function postpartum is much faster than in nonpregnant women with a similar primary glomerular disease
   E. Maternal and fetal complications are higher in women with serum creatinine >1.4 mg/dL than women with serum creatinine <1.4 mg/dL

The answer is D

There is a relationship between the degree of renal impairment prior to conception and pregnancy outcomes. Based on serum creatinine levels, the women with CKD are divided arbitrarily into three categories: mild (creatinine <1.4 mg/dL); moderate (creatinine 1.5–2.0 mg/dL); and severe (creatinine >2.4 mg/dL). There is little or no decline in renal function during pregnancy, if creatinine is <1.4 mg/dL. In women with moderate renal impairment, there is a 40% decline in renal function but most of the patients return their renal function to baseline after delivery. However, in women with severe renal dysfunction there is >50% decline in renal function with requirement for renal replacement therapy after delivery.

In 1980, Katz et al. analyzed the outcomes of 121 pregnancies and the effect of pregnancy on the underlying disease in 89 women with various renal diseases and creatinine levels <1.4 mg/dL. They observed an increase in serum creatinine in 16%, exacerbation or de novo occurrence of hypertension in 28%, and an increase in protein excretion in 50% of pregnancies. Proteinuria exceeded 3.0 g in 68% (39 of 57 pregnancies). All of the above changes resolved after delivery. Long-term follow-up of these patients showed that the decline in renal function was similar to that expected for the underlying disorder. This study shows that most of the women with normal or near-normal renal function and primary glomerular disease are not at higher risk for progression of the underlying disease following delivery than nonpregnant women with a similar primary renal disease. Thus, option D is false. Preterm delivery (<37 wk) was 20%, as compared with 11% in the general population.

The pregnancy outcomes are different, if serum creatinine is >1.4 mg/dL. Hou et al. gathered data on 25 pregnancies in 23 women with serum creatinine levels of 1.4 mg/dL or greater prior to or at the onset of pregnancy. Twelve women had primary renal disorders. In five women with serum creatinine between 1.7 and 2.7 mg/dL, pregnancy caused a rapid decline in renal function which is thought to be greater than expected from the natural history of the disease. In 14 women, the renal function remained stable or declined similar to the natural history of the disease. In 14 pregnancies, hypertension became worse, and 9 of them required premature delivery. Twenty-three of 25 pregnancies had live births, and 14 of 23 were premature. Two of 23 babies died, indicating a high fetal survival. Thus, in women with moderate renal insufficiency, pregnancy is associated with a decline in renal function. Similar complications were reported by Jones and Hayslett in patients with moderate or severe renal insufficiency. Also, increase in adverse outcomes (new-onset hypertension, new-onset or doubling of proteinuria, CKD stage shift, or renal replacement therapy) with increase in CKD stages were also observed by Piccoli et al.

Suggested Reading

Hou SH, Gossman SD, Madias NE. Pregnancy in women with renal disease and moderate renal insufficiency. Am J Med. 1985;78:185–94.

Hayslett JP. Renal disease in pregnancy. In: Burrow GN, Duffy TP, Copel JA, editors. Medical complications during pregnancy. 6th ed. Philadelphia: Elsevier Saunders; 2004. p. 247–58.

Jones DC, Hayslett JP. Outcome of pregnancy in women with moderate or severe renal insufficiency. N Engl J Med. 1996;335:226–32.

Katz AI, Davison JM, Hayslett JP, et al. Pregnancy in women with kidney disease. Kidney Int. 1980;8:192–206.

Piccoli GB, Cabiddu G, Attini R, et al. Risk of adverse pregnancy outcomes in women with CKD. J Am Soc Nephrol. 2015;26:2011–22.

32. An 18-year-old African American woman has recently been diagnosed with systemic lupus erythematosus (SLE) and is on prednisone 10 mg/day. On renal biopsy, she has class II lupus nephritis and proteinuria of 750 mg. Her disease is currently in remission, and she has no antiphospholipid antibodies. She contemplates pregnancy and seeks your advice. **Which one of the following statements is INCORRECT?**

A. Exacerbation of lupus is a possible complication during pregnancy
B. A renal biopsy may be necessary, if urine sediment shows red cell casts
C. Fetal survival rate is >90% with inactive disease prior to pregnancy
D. Proteinuria may increase during pregnancy
E. Prophylactic use of high doses of prednisone may be required to prevent flares of lupus and preeclampsia

The answer is E

It is not uncommon for a woman with established SLE to seek counseling with regard to her successful pregnancy. The physician should discuss before the pregnancy about the impact of pregnancy on SLE and of SLE on the safety of the mother and fetus. Exacerbation of lupus has been reported in most of the series, and serology and urinalysis are extremely helpful in distinguishing preeclamsia from flare of the underlying renal disease. If urine shows red blood cells (RBCs) and red cell casts, a renal biopsy is required before 30 weeks' gestation. If flare occurs after 32 weeks' gestation, a meticulous follow-up is required until delivery. Prophylactic use of steroids does not seem to prevent a lupus flare during pregnancy. Thus, option E is incorrect. With good prenatal care, fetal survival is >90%. Proteinuria may increase due to hyperfiltration, but this increase should not be ignored in the presence of new onset of hypertension and before 20th week because of preeclampsia.

A study by Gladman et al. showed that lupus patients with kidney disease had a high degree of pregnancy-induced hypertension and flares of lupus, as compared with those lupus patients without kidney disease. Predictors of poor pregnancy outcome include baseline creatinine >0.9 mg/dL, proteinuria >0.5 g/24-h, antiphospholipid syndrome, hypertension, non-White ethnicity, and maternal disease flare. Women with anti-Ro and anti-La antibodies should be counseled regarding the risk for fetal heart block and neonatal cutaneous lupus, respectively.

Suggested Reading

Buyon JP, Kim MY, Guerra MM, et al. Predictors of pregnancy outcomes in patients with lupus: a cohort study. Ann Intern Med. 2015;163:153–63.

Buyon JP, Kim MY, Guerra MM, et al. Kidney outcomes and risk factors for nephritis (flare/de novo) in a multiethnic cohort of pregnant patients with lupus. Clin J Am Soc Nephrol. 2017;12:940–6.

Do SC, Druzin ML. Systemic lupus erythematosus in pregnancy: high risk, high reward. Curr Opin Obstet Gynecol. 2019;31:120–6.

Eudy AM, Siega-Riz AM, Engel SM, et al. Effect of pregnancy on disease flares in patients with systemic lupus erythematosus. Ann Rheum Dis. 2018;77:855–60.

Gladman DD, Tandon A, Ibañez D, Urowitz MB. The effect of lupus nephritis on pregnancy outcome and fetal and maternal complications. J Rheumatol. 2010;37:754–8.

Knight CL, Nelson-Piercy C. Management of systemic lupus erythematosus during pregnancy: challenges and solutions. Open Access Rheumatol. 2017;9:37–53.

Lateef A, Petri M. Systemic lupus erythematosus and pregnancy. Rheum Dis Clin North Am. 2017;43:215–26.

Wei S, Lai K, Yang Z, Zeng K. Systemic lupus erythematosus and risk of preterm birth: a systematic review and meta-analysis of observational studies. Lupus. 2017;26:563–71.

33. A 28-year-old woman with lupus nephritis is found to have anti-Ro and anti-La antibodies. Her lupus is quiescent for 1 year. She wants to conceive. **Which one of the following statements about her pregnancy is CORRECT?**

A. She should not have any concerns about her pregnancy
B. Treatment with prednisone during pregnancy will result in normal baby
C. She should be counseled regarding the risk for fetal heart block and neonatal cutaneous lupus
D. Hydroxychloroquine may reduce the risk for recurrent fetal heart block in women with a previously affected infant, and this should be encouraged
E. C and D

The answer is E

Women with anti-Ro and anti-La antibodies should be informed of the potential risk of development of fetal heart block due to placental transfer of immunoglobulin (Ig) leading to endocardial fibroelastosis. In one study of 186 pregnancies, 5% of offspring were affected only in women with titers >50 U/mL. Similarly, neonatal cutaneous lupus was reported to be more common in women with high-titer anti-La antibody (>100 U/mL), occurring in 57% of infants. Initially, it was shown that Toll-like receptor (TLR) signaling participates in the pathogenesis of neonatal lupus and hydroxychloroquine inhibits TLR signaling, and this drug was shown to reduce the cardiac effects of neonatal lupus. A subsequent study showed that hydroxychloroquine was effective in reducing the risk for recurrent fetal heart block in women with a previously affected infant. Thus, answer E is correct. Other options are incorrect.

Suggested Reading

Blom K, Odutayo A, Bramham K, et al. Pregnancy and glomerular disease. A systematic review of the literature with management guidelines. Clin J Am Soc Nephrol. 2017;12:1862–72.

Izmirly PM, Kim MY, Llanos C, et al. Evaluation of the risk of anti-SSA/Ro-SSB/La antibody-associated cardiac manifestations of neonatal lupus in fetuses of mothers with systemic lupus erythematosus exposed to hydroxychloroquine. Ann Rheum Dis. 2010;69:1827–30.

Izmirly PM, Costedoat-Chalumeau N, Pisoni CN, et al. Maternal use of hydroxychloroquine is associated with a reduced risk of recurrent anti-SSA/Ro-antibody-associated cardiac manifestations of neonatal lupus. Circulation. 2012;126:76–82.

34. **With regard to pregnancy in the kidney transplant patient, which one of the following statements is INCORRECT?**

A. Pregnancy can be considered in a year of posttransplant, if the woman is stable with normal renal function, on low-dose immunosuppressive drugs and had no previous episodes of rejection
B. Approximately 22% of pregnancies end in the 1st trimester
C. Low birth weight and preterm delivery are common
D. No effect of pregnancy on renal dysfunction in a woman with moderate renal insufficiency (creatinine >1.5 mg/dL) prior to conception
E. Urinary tract infection (UTI) rates are much higher than nontransplant individual

The answer is D

Successful kidney transplantation restores fertility in 6 months in about 90% of women with child-bearing age. Current consensus opinion is that pregnancy can be considered by 1 year after transplant, if the woman is receiving low doses of immunosuppressive drugs, allograft function is adequate (creatinine <1.5 mg/dL), proteinuria <500 mg/day, and had no previous rejections. In Europe, waiting for 2 years after transplantation is recommended. Approximately, 22% of pregnancies end before the 1st trimester. Also, there is a high risk for low birth weight babies and preterm delivery. Hypertension and preeclampsia are the two main reasons for the high rate of preterm babies in kidney transplant recipients. Because of immunosuppression, the rates of UTI are much higher compared to a woman without kidney transplantation. According to the UK experience, serum creatinine level in excess of 2.3 mg/dL prior to conception should be regarded as a contraindication to pregnancy because all pregnant women with the above creatinine levels had progression of their renal dysfunction, requiring renal replacement therapy within 2 years of delivery. Thus, option D is incorrect.

Suggested Reading

McKay DB, Josephson MA. Pregnancy in recipients of solid organs-effects on mother and child. N Engl J Med. 2006;354:1281–93.

Vidaeff AC, Yeomans ER, Ramin SM. Pregnancy in women with renal disease. Part I: General principles. Am J Perinatol. 2008;25:385–98.

35. **Which one of the prepregnancy factors is associated with graft loss or decline in kidney function during pregnancy?**

A. Serum creatinine >1.4 mg/dL
B. Proteinuria >500 mg/24-h
C. Hypertension (BP > 140/90 mm Hg)
D. All of the above
E. C only

The answer is D

Transplant Registry Data show that pregnancy itself has no impact on graft function in the absence of the above three risk factors. Best pregnancy outcomes have been reported if prepregnancy serum creatinine is <1 mg/dL, proteinuria <500 mg/24-h, and treated or untreated BP < 140/90 mm Hg. Thus, answer D is correct.

Suggested Reading

Chittka D, Hutchinson JA. Pregnancy after renal transplantation. Transplantation. 2017;101:675–8.

Cotovio P. The challenge of pregnancy after kidney transplantation. Port J Nephrol Hypert. 2018;32(2):117–22.

Ong SC, Kumar V. Pregnancy in a kidney transplant patient. Clin J Am Soc Nephrol. 2020;15:120–2.

36. **Which one of the following immunosuppressive drugs is contraindicated in pregnancy?**

A. Prednisone
B. Cyclosporine
C. Tacrolimus
D. Azathioprine
E. Sirolimus and mycophenolate mofetil

The answer is E

Immunosuppression needs to be continued during the entire pregnancy. As a result, the fetus is exposed to potential teratogenic and fetotoxic drugs throughout development. The following Table 8.2 **summarizes the drugs and their safety during pregnancy in a transplant recipient.**

Table 8.2 Immunosuppressive medications that are commonly used in transplantation

Drug	FDA category[a]	FDA safety profile
Prednisone	B	Safe at low doses (5–10 mg/day)
Cyclosporine	C	Safe at low-to-moderate doses
Tacrolimus	C	Safe at low-to-moderate doses
Azathioprine[b]	D	Safe at dosages <2 mg/kg/day
Sirolimus	C	Contraindicated; teratogenic in animals
Mycophenolate mofetil	C	Contraindicated; teratogenic in animals and humans
OKT-3	C	Safe, but limited data
Antithymocyte globulin	C	No data
Basiliximab	B	No data

[a]FDA categories: A (no human risk); B (risk in animal studies, but no evidence of human risk); C (human risk not ruled out); D (evidence of human risk); and X (absolutely contraindicated).

[b]Higher doses cause congenital anomalies and growth retardation. If possible azathioprine should be avoided.

Suggested Reading

Chittka D, Hutchinson JA. Pregnancy after renal transplantation. Transplantation. 2017;101:675–8.
McKay DB, Josephson MA. Pregnancy in recipients of solid organs-effects on mother and child. N Engl J Med. 2006;354:1281–93.
McKay DB, Josephson MA. Pregnancy after kidney transplantation. Clin J Am Soc Nephrol. 2008; 3(Suppl 2):S117–25.
Ong SC, Kumar V. Pregnancy in a kidney transplant patient. Clin J Am Soc Nephrol. 2020;15:120–2.

37. The obstetrician consults you to see a 32-year-old woman with nephrotic syndrome due to membranous nephropathy in 1st trimester and wants to know the impact of preconception nephrotic syndrome on maternal and fetal complications. Her creatinine is <1.4 mg/dL and has mild edema. **Which one of the following statements is INCORRECT?**

A. The mother is at risk for thromboembolism
B. Routine use of diuretics to treat edema
C. Low birth weight is common
D. Preterm delivery is common
E. Nephrotic syndrome due to primary renal disease carries better prognosis than nephrotic syndrome caused by preeclampsia

The answer is B

It used to be thought that nephrotic syndrome has benign course on the mother and fetus, except for low birth weight. However, several studies have shown that nephrotic syndrome prior to conception may cause maternal thromboembolism, fetal growth retardation, and premature delivery. Nephrotic syndrome and hypertension that develop after 20th week of gestation imply that preeclampsia has poor prognosis on the mother and fetus.

Edema, a common symptom of normal pregnancy and preeclampsia, does not require treatment with diuretics routinely because of intravascular volume depletion, hypotension, low blood flow to the fetus, AKI, and tendency toward maternal thromboembolism. Thus, option B is incorrect.

It is interesting to note that nephrotic syndrome caused by membranoproliferative GN carries poor maternal and fetal prognosis than nephrotic syndrome caused by membranous nephropathy. A case report of de novo development of nephrotic syndrome during pregnancy (17th wk) resulted in fetal growth retardation and death, despite steroid treatment. Renal biopsy at the onset of nephrotic syndrome showed focal segmental glomerulosclerosis.

Suggested Reading

Basgul A, Kavak ZN, Sezen D, et al. A rare case of early onset nephrotic syndrome in pregnancy. Clin Exp Obstet Gynecol. 2006;33:127–8.
Bramham K, Brown MA. Pregnancy with pre-existing kidney disease. In: Feehally J, Floege J, Tonelli M, et al., editors. Comprehensive clinical nephrology. 6th ed. Philadelphia: Elsevier; 2019. p. 522–31.

38. A 28-year-old woman is on maintenance hemodialysis for 4 years and found to be pregnant. She has a urine output of approximately 100 mL/day. Her BP is well controlled with antihypertensive medications other than ACE-I or ARB. **Of the following factors, which one leads to poor fetal outcome?**

A. Urine output >50 mL/day
B. Maintenance of hypovolemia to control pregnancy-induced volume expansion
C. Daily hemodialysis of at least 4-h duration with low blood flow
D. Weekly dialysis >36 hours
E. Maintenance of predialysis BUN <50 mg/dL

The answer is B

The reported incidence of pregnancy in women on dialysis was <1% in the 1980s, but recent incidence is 1–7% because of improved dialysis and anemia. However, premature delivery, intrauterine growth retardation, and maternal hypertension still remain as important complications of pregnant women on dialysis. Because of these complications, the rate of surviving infants remains around 50%.

There are some factors that can improve fetal outcome. Nakabayashi et al. reported that women who were on dialysis for <6 years and who had a urine output >50 mL/day had surviving infants, as compared with those who

were on hemodialysis for >9 years and no residual renal function had no surviving infants. Daily dialysis of at least 4-h duration with low blood flow to avoid hypotension or weekly dialysis of >20 h carries better prognosis than <20 h a week. A recent study showed that hemodialysis >36 h/week had a high birth rate (85%) compared to a birth rate of 48% for hemodialysis ≤20 h/week. Also, maintenance of prediadialysis blood urea nitrogen (BUN) <50 mg/dL avoids intrauterine uremic environment and improves fetal survival. The maintenance of low blood urea nitrogen (BUN) is probably facilitated by daily and long dialysis sessions. Also, daily dialysis allows the pregnant women to have a high protein intake of at least 1.8 g/kg/day, in addition to maintenance of intradialytic weight gain of ~1 kg.

Avoidance of hypovolemia and hypotension helps in maintaining normal blood flow to the fetus, so that fetal hypoxia and growth retardation can be minimized. Thus, option B is incorrect. The following Table 8.3 **summarizes the recommendations for dialysis management in a pregnant woman.**

Table 8.3 Hemodialysis management in a pregnant woman

Treatment factor	**Recommendation**
Dialyzer	Biocompatible small surface area dialyzer to avoid excess ultrafiltration
Duration & frequency	Daily or 6 times/wk, >4 h or >20-h/ wk of treatment (also a recent study suggested >36-h/wk has better outcome compared to ≤20-h/wk)
Heparin	Judicious use to avoid bleeding
Dialysate composition	HCO_3^- 25 mEq/l; K^+ 3–4 mEq/L. Adjust according to serum chemistry. Blood pH ~ 7.40
Predialysis BUN	<50 mg/dL
Hgb	10–11 g/dL with the use of erythropoietin and IV iron. Note that the erythropoietin requirements may increase during pregnancy
Diet	Protein 1–1.8 g/kg/day. Folate 5 mg/day. Continue water-soluble vitamins
Interdialytic weight gain	~1 kg
Ultrafiltration	Avoid hypotension
Maternal BP Consider aspirin 80 mg	Diastolic 80–90 mm Hg To prevent preeclampsia
Fetal monitoring by an obstetrician	Frequent

Suggested Reading

Bramham K, Brown MA. Pregnancy with pre-existing kidney disease. In: Feehally J, Floege J, Tonelli M, et al., editors. Comprehensive clinical nephrology. 6th ed. Philadelphia: Elsevier; 2019. p. 522–31.

Hladunewich MA, Hou S, Odutayo A, et al. Intensive hemodialysis associates with improved pregnancy outcomes: a Canadian and United States cohort comparison. J Am Soc Nephrol. 2014;25:1103–9.

Manisco G, Poti M, Maggiulli G, et al. Pregnancy in end-stage renal disease patients on dialysis: how to achieve a successful delivery. Clin Kidney J. 2015;8:293–9.

Tangren J, Nadela M, Hladunewich MA. Pregnancy and end-stage renal disease. Blood Purif. 2018;45:194–200.

39. You are called to consult on a 24-year-old African American woman, gravida 2. para 1, at 14 weeks of gestation for a BP of 142/98 mm Hg. There are no orthostatic changes. She has no previous follow-up by a physician for a year. She has no history of HTN. She is not on any medications. She denies nausea and vomiting. The only positive medical history is that she had preeclampsia during her previous pregnancy. However, she had an uneventful delivery. Physical examination is unremarkable, except for A-V nicking and narrowing on funduscopic examination. Her labs:

    Na^+ = 135 mEq/L
    K^+ = 4.2 mEq/L
    Cl^- = 92 mEq/L
    HCO_3^- = 20 mEq/L
    Creatinine = 0.9 mg/dL
    BUN = 16 mg/dL
    Glucose = 80 mg/dL
    Uric acid = 5.2 mg/dL
    Albumin = 3.1 g/dL
    AST/ALT = 20/15 U/L

Urinalysis: pH 5.8; SG 1012; RBC 2; WBC (white blood cell) 2; protein 1+; glucose trace; few granular casts. A 24-h urine protein 259 mg

Which one of the following is the MOST likely diagnosis?

A. Preeclampsia
B. Gestational hypertension
C. Acute kidney injury (AKI) due to volume depletion
D. Chronic kidney disease (CKD)
E. None of the above

The answer is D

Preeclampsia is a very likely possibility; however, it occurs most commonly after the 20th week. In women with preexisting renal disease, preeclampsia can occur before 20th week; however, normal proteinuria can exclude this possibility. Proteinuria up to 300 mg is normal in a pregnant woman. Gestational hypertension occurs after 20th week and eye examination is normal. AKI due to volume depletion is also unlikely because urinalysis and BP do not suggest any evidence of volume depletion.

A-V (arteriovenous) nicking and narrowing suggests that the patient has hypertension for at least 5 years. Although her creatinine is 0.9 mg/dL, it is high for a pregnant woman. Also, uric acid of 5.2 mg/dL is high for this patient. The most likely diagnosis appears to be CKD due to hypertension. Thus, option D is correct.

Suggested Reading

Bateman BT, Bansil P, Hernandez-Diaz S, et al. Prevalence, trends, and outcomes of chronic hypertension: a nationwide sample of delivery admissions. Am J Obstet Gynecol. 2012;206:e131–8.

Maynard SE, Ananth Karumanchi S, Thadani R. Pregnancy and kidney disease. In: Yu ASL, Chertow GM, Luyckx VA, et al., editors. Brenner & Rector's the kidney. 11th ed. Philadelphia: Elsevier Saunders; 2020. p. 1622–52.

40. The patient described above had induction of labor at 36 weeks because of severe hypertension, requiring several antihypertensive medications. Follow-up serum creatinine rose to 1.2 mg/dL 4 weeks postpartum. At 6 months of follow-up, her creatinine stabilized at 1.6 mg/dL. One year later, she and her husband discuss that they contemplate another pregnancy. **How do you counsel the couple?**

A. Preeclampsia is likely
B. Hypertensive emergency is likely
C. Preterm delivery can be contemplated
D. Renal function may deteriorate further
E. All of the above

The answer is E

The patient had complications during her two previous pregnancies. She has CKD and nephrosclerosis. She may develop all of the above complications. Also, the kidney function may deteriorate postpartum, requiring a renal replacement therapy. The following Table 8.4 **shows maternal and fetal complications that follow pregnancy in a CKD patient.**

Table 8.4 Adverse effects of pregnancy in CKD patients

Maternal complications	Fetal complications
Deterioration in kidney function	Preterm births
Preeclampsia (HELLP syndrome)	Still births
Preterm delivery	Small for gestational age infants
Adverse effects from medications	Low birth weight
Flare from underlying disease (e.g., SLE)	Fetal deaths
Miscarriages	

Suggested Reading

Bateman BT, Bansil P, Hernandez-Diaz S, et al. Prevalence, trends, and outcomes of chronic hypertension: a nationwide sample of delivery admissions. Am J Obstet Gynecol. 2012;206:134.e1–8.

Piccoli GB, Alrukhaimi M, Liu ZH, et al. World Kidney Day Steering Committee. What we do and do not know about women and kidney diseases; questions unanswered and answers unquestioned: reflection on World Kidney Day and International Woman's Day. BMC Nephrol. 2018;19(1):66.

Zhang JJ, Ma XX, Hao L, et al. A systematic review and meta-analysis of outcomes of pregnancy in CKD and CKD outcomes in pregnancy. Clin J Am Soc Nephrol. 2015;10:1964–78.

41. A 34-year-old African American woman with 34 weeks of gestation was admitted for nausea and vomiting for 3 days. Her creatinine was 1.1 mg/dL with regular follow-up by renal and obstetrics and gynecology services. Her blood pressure (BP) was 120/80 mm Hg prior to conception. In the Emergency Department, her BP was 164/100 mm Hg with a pulse rate of 102 beats/min. She did not have any seizure activity. She was started on magnesium sulfate, labetalol, and hydralazine, and BP was lowered to 136/82 mm Hg with a pulse rate of 90 beats/min. Significant labs: creatinine 2.1 mg/dL; Hgb 10.1 g/dL; and platelets 82,000/μL (platelets before pregnancy were 210,000/μL). Urinalysis showed no proteinuria. A diagnosis of preeclampsia was made. **Which one of the following findings CONFIRMS the diagnosis of preeclampsia?**

A. BP ≥ 140/90 mm Hg measured 4 h apart
B. Acute increase in serum creatinine
C. Thrombocytopenia
D. Presence or absence of proteinuria
E. All of the above

The answer is E

In 2013, the American College of Obstetricians and Gynecologists (ACOG) published new diagnostic criteria for preeclampsia. These criteria are shown in Table 8.5.

Table 8.5 Diagnostic criteria for preeclampsia

Hypertension (HTN)	Systolic BP ≥ 140 mmHg or diastolic BP ≥ 90 mmHg after 20 wks of gestation on two occasions at least 4 h apart in a woman with a previously normal BP or With systolic BP ≥ 160 mmHg or diastolic BP ≥ 105 mmHg. HTN can be confirmed within a short interval (minutes) to facilitate timely antihypertensive therapy
And Proteinuria	≥300 mg/24-h or Protein-to-creatinine ratio ≥0.3 mg protein/mg creatinine or Dipstick 2+ (when quantitative methods not available)
OR If no proteinuria is present, new onset of any one of the following:	
Thrombocytopenia	<100,000/μL
Creatinine	>1.1 mg/dL or doubling of serum creatinine concentration in the absence of other renal disease
Transaminases	Twice upper limits of normal levels
Pulmonary edema Cerebral or visual symptoms (headache, blurred vision, or flashing lights)	
Preeclampsia with severe features	
HTN	Systolic BP 160 mmHg or more, or diastolic BP 110 mmHg or more on two occasions at least 4 h apart (unless antihypertensive therapy is initiated before this time)
Thrombocytopenia	<100,000/μL
Creatinine	>1.1 mg/dL or doubling of serum creatinine concentration in the absence of other renal disease
Transaminases	Twice upper limits of normal levels
Pulmonary edema New-onset headache unresponsive to medication and not accounted for by alternative diagnoses Visual disturbances	or severe persistent right upper quadrant or epigastric pain unresponsive to medications

It is evident from the above table that proteinuria is not necessary to make the diagnosis of preeclampsia. In the absence of proteinuria, either new onset of HTN, thrombocytosis, creatinine >1.1 mg/dL, pulmonary edema, or brain or visual symptoms may be enough to make the diagnosis of preeclampsia. Thus, answer E is correct.

Suggested Reading

Gestational hypertension and preeclampsia. ACOG Practice Bulletin No. 222. American College of Obstetricians and Gynecologists. Obstet Gynecol. 2020;135:e237–60.

Hypertension in pregnancy. Report of the American College of Obstetricians and Gynecologists' Task Force on Hypertension in Pregnancy. Obstet Gynecol. 2013;122:1122–31.

42. A 24-year-old primiparous woman in her 34 weeks of gestation is admitted because of nausea, vomiting, and epigastric pain. Physical examination shows BP 150/110 mm Hg, peripheral edema, and segmental arteriolar narrowing of the fundus. The remaining examination is normal. Labs:

    Hct 40%
    Platelets 70,000/μL
    Creatinine 1.7 mg/dL
    BUN 15 mg/dL
    Bilirubin. 2.4 mg/dL
    AST 500 U/L
    ALT 300 U/L
    LDH 500 U/L
    Glucose: 100 mg/dL
    PT: normal
    Antithrombin III: Low
    Urinalysis: 1+ protein; no red cells or white cells
    Peripheral smear: schistocytes and helmet cells

    What is the MOST likely diagnosis?

    A. Hypertensive emergency
    B. Acute fatty liver of pregnancy
    C. Thrombotic thrombocytopenic purpura (TTP)
    D. Atypical hemolytic uremic syndrome (aHUS)
    E. Preeclampsia

    The answer is E

    The physical examination and the degree of BP do not support the diagnosis of hypertensive emergency. Furthermore, hypertensive emergency occurs in a patient with chronic hypertension and noncompliance or inappropriate antihypertensive medications (A is incorrect).

    Acute fatty liver of pregnancy (AFLP) is a possibility, but the extent of liver failure does not support this diagnosis. AFLP is a rare, life-threatening condition that is characterized by microvesicular fatty infiltration of the liver leading to hepatic failure. It is usually identified at 36th week. Risk factors include twin pregnancies and low body mass index (BMI). Early recognition, prompt delivery, and supportive care are important to optimize maternal and fetal health. In particular, total bilirubin is extremely elevated in AFLP. Hypoglycemia, prolonged PT, and low antithrombin III levels are common in AFLP. Generally, patients with AFLP are encephalopathic, and our patient is alert and oriented, making this diagnosis unlikely (B is correct).

    TTP can occur at any time of pregnancy, but rather common during the 3rd trimester of pregnancy. The findings on peripheral smear and low platelet count are consistent with TTP, but these findings are also present in hemolytic uremic syndrome (HUS) and preeclampsia because of hemolysis. More importantly, antithrombin III levels are normal in TTP. HUS occurs usually within a week to 3–6 months postpartum. Again, antithrombin III levels are normal in HUS. Furthermore, the liver function tests are slightly abnormal or normal in both TTP and HUS. Thus, options C and D are incorrect.

    Preeclampsia occurs after 20th week in an otherwise normal woman with no preexisting renal disease or hypertension. Symptoms such as nausea, vomiting, and epigastric pain are usually present in a woman with preeclampsia. Epigastric pain or right upper quadrant pain may be due to hepatic ischemia or even liver rupture. Segmental arteriolar narrowing is also seen in preeclampsia. The laboratory findings and abnormal liver

function tests are consistent with preeclampsia. High hematocrit is related to volume contraction. Hematocrit may be low if there is massive hemolysis. Thus, option E is correct. HEELP syndrome (hemolysis, elevated liver enzymes, low platelets) is a variant of severe preeclampsia, and is characterized predominantly by liver and platelet abnormalities. HELLP affects a minority of pregnancies but complicates up to 20% of cases of severe preeclampsia/eclampsia. Normal glucose levels and relatively normal PT distinguish HEELP syndrome from AFLP. The patient seems to have preeclampsia complicated by HEELP syndrome. The following Table 8.6 **shows the clinical and laboratory findings of preeclampsia, acute fatty liver of pregnancy, TTP, and HUS.**

Table 8.6 Clinical and laboratory characteristics of complications of pregnancy

Clinical/Labs	Preeclampsia (HEELP)	Acute fatty liver of pregnancy	TTP	aHUS
Onset	3rd trimester	3rd trimester	Any time	Postpartum
HTN	Yes (3+)	Yes (2+)	No/Yes	Yes/No
Creatinine	Increased (+)	Increased (2+)	Increased (3+)	Increased (3+)
Proteinuria	Yes/No (1–2+)	Variable (1+)	Variable (1+)	Yes/Variable (1+)
CNS symptoms	Yes/No	Yes	Yes	Yes/No
Anemia	Yes	Yes/No	Yes	Yes
Platelet count	Low (2+)	Low (1+)	Low (3+)	Low (3+)
NH_3	Normal	High	Normal	Normal
Liver enzymes	High (2+)	Very high (3+)	Normal	Normal
Bilirubin LCHAD[a]	High Normal	Very high Deficient	Normal Normal	Normal Normal
PT Glucose	Normal/High Normal	Very high Low	Normal Normal	Normal Normal
Antithrombin III	Low	Low	Normal	Normal
ADMITS 13 ADMITS 13-antibody	Normal Negative	Normal Negative	Low Positive	Normal Negative
Effect of delivery	Recovery	Recovery	No effect	No effect
Treatment	Supportive care/delivery	Supportive care/delivery	Plasma exchange	Plasma exchange/ Eculizumab

[a]LCHAD: Long-chain 3-hydroxyacyl-CoA dehydrogenase (fatty acid oxidation)

Suggested Reading

Brown MA, Magee LA, Kenny LC, et al. on behalf of the International Society for the Study of Hypertension in Pregnancy (ISSHP). Hypertensive disorders of pregnancy. ISSHP classification, diagnosis, and management recommendations for international practice. Hypertension. 2018;72:24–43.

Gestational hypertension and preeclampsia. ACOG Practice Bulletin No. 222. American College of Obstetricians and Gynecologists. Obstet Gynecol. 2020;135:e237–60.

Hypertension in pregnancy. Report of the American College of Obstetricians and Gynecologists' Task Force on Hypertension in Pregnancy. Obstet Gynecol. 2013;122:1122–31.

Rana S, Lemoine E, Granger JP, et al. Preeclampsia: pathophysiology, challenges, and perspectives. Circ Res. 2019;124:1094–112.

Scully M, Thomas M, Underwood M, et al. Thrombotic thrombocytopenic purpura and pregnancy: presentation, management, and subsequent pregnancy outcomes. Blood. 2014;124:211–9.

Tran TT, Ahn J, Reau NS. ACG clinical guideline: liver disease and pregnancy. Am J Gastroenterol. 2016;111:176–94.

43. The above patient is treated with fluids and labetalol and her BP is 130/88 mm Hg. However, her liver function tests are worsening and her platelet count decreased to 50,000/μL. She is alert and oriented to place, time, and name but she complains of mild headache and epigastric pain. **What is the next step in her management?**

    A. Follow her until 37th week and then prepare for delivery
    B. Lower BP to 120/70 mm Hg
    C. Prepare her for delivery
    D. High-dose steroid therapy
    E. Assume that her headache is related to her low BP

The answer is C

Although the BP is adequate, the patient continues to have liver abnormalities and becoming symptomatic. Of all the options, delivery may be the best choice for this patient. This would prevent both maternal and fetal complications. Some indications for delivery are:

- **progressive maternal organ dysfunction, such as kidney failure, hepatic failure, worsening thrombocytopenia, or onset of neurologic signs or symptoms**
- **inadequate fetal growth**
- **inadequate BP control**
- **epigastric pain**

The consensus statement of the American College of Obstetricians and Gynecologists recommends that women with HEELP syndrome should be delivered, regardless of their gestational age. In the USA, preeclampsia/eclampsia account for 20% of all pregnancy-related maternal deaths. The risk of death is high in African American women, women with no prenatal care, women over 35 years of age, and early-onset preeclampsia. Steroid use has been advocated for HEELP syndrome for fetal lung maturity as well as to improve other maternal and fetal complications; however, recent studies have shown uncertain clinical value of steroids.

Suggested Reading

Brown MA, Magee LA, Kenny LC, et al. on behalf of the International Society for the Study of Hypertension in Pregnancy (ISSHP). Hypertensive disorders of pregnancy. ISSHP classification, diagnosis, and management recommendations for international practice. Hypertension. 2018;72:24–43.

Gestational hypertension and preeclampsia. ACOG Practice Bulletin No. 222. American College of Obstetricians and Gynecologists. Obstet Gynecol. 2020;135:e237–60.

Hypertension in pregnancy. Report of the American College of Obstetricians and Gynecologists' Task Force on Hypertension in Pregnancy. Obstet Gynecol. 2013;122:1122–31.

Report of the National High Blood Pressure Education Program Working Group on high blood pressure in pregnancy. Am J Obstet Gynecol. 2000;183:S1–22.

Vernier N, Brown MA, Reynolds M, et al. Indications for delivery in pre-eclampsia. Pregnancy Hypertens. 2018;11:12–7.

44. Women with preeclampsia with severe features (see Table 8.5) are at increased risk for acute and long-term complications for the mother and the newborn. **Which one of the following maternal complications is CORRECT?**

A. Myocardial infarction
B. Stroke
C. Pulmonary edema
D. Kidney failure
E. All of the above

The answer is E

Maternal complications include, in addition to the above, acute respiratory distress syndrome, coagulopathy, and retinal injury. These complications are more likely to occur in the presence of preexisting medical conditions. The clinical course of preeclampsia with severe features is characterized by progressive deterioration of maternal and fetal condition. Therefore, delivery is recommended when gestational HTN or preeclampsia with severe features is diagnosed at or beyond 34 weeks of gestation, after the patient is stabilized. Thus, answer E is correct.

Suggested Reading

Gestational hypertension and preeclampsia. ACOG Practice Bulletin No. 222. American College of Obstetricians and Gynecologists. Obstet Gynecol. 2020;135:e237–60.

Piccoli GB, Alrukhaimi M, Liu ZH, et al. World Kidney Day Steering Committee. What we do and do not know about women and kidney diseases; questions unanswered and answers unquestioned: reflection on World Kidney Day and International Woman's Day. BMC Nephrol. 2018;19(1):66.

Phillips EA, Thadani R, Benzing T, et al. Pre-eclampsia: pathogenesis, novel diagnostics and therapies. Nat Rev Nephrol. 2019;15:275–89.

Rana S, Lemoine E, Granger JP, et al. Preeclampsia: pathophysiology, challenges, and perspectives. Circ Res. 2019;124:1094–112.

45. A 20-year-old African American pregnant woman at her 16th week of gestation is found to have proteinuria >500 mg/24-h. She has no previous follow-up by a physician. Her BP is 118/80 mm Hg. **Which one of the following is LIKELY to suggest the diagnosis of preeclampsia superimposed on chronic HTN?**

   A. Nonoliguria
   B. Hematuria
   C. Sudden increase in HTN and proteinuria
   D. Normal liver enzymes
   E. None of the above

   The answer is C

   Many young black women are not aware of preexisting HTN prior to pregnancy, which becomes more pronounced before the 20th week of gestation. Because of vasodilation, their BP in the early weeks of pregnancy is normal. The following features either alone or in combination suggest superimposed preeclampsia on chronic HTN prior to 20 weeks of pregnancy: (1) sudden increase in HTN; (2) sudden increase in proteinuria; (3) abnormal aminotransferases; and (4) thrombocytopenia. Thus, option C is correct.

   Oliguria is usually present in preeclampsia; however, nonoliguria may be present at onset of pregnancy. Hematuria is common in normal pregnancy; but it has to be followed with microscopic examination of the urine by an experienced physician to exclude the possibility of an underlying primary renal disease. Slight elevation in liver enzymes is usually seen in preeclampsia.

   Suggested Reading

   Gestational hypertension and preeclampsia. ACOG Practice Bulletin No. 222. American College of Obstetricians and Gynecologists. Obstet Gynecol. 2020;135:e237–60.

   Hypertension in pregnancy. Report of the American College of Obstetricians and Gynecologists' Task Force on Hypertension in Pregnancy. Obstet Gynecol. 2013;122:1122–31.

46. The BP in the above patient rose to 170/110 mm Hg on repeated measurements. The patient is asymptomatic. **Which one of the following intravenous (IV) medications is recommended for the patient?**

   A. Nitroprusside
   B. Hydralazine
   C. Labetalol
   D. Furosemide
   E. Magnesium sulfate

   The answer is C

   When BP is severe (160/100 mm Hg), antihypertensive treatment is indicated to prevent maternal cardiovascular complications, including stroke. Although several antihypertensive medications are available, only IV labetalol and nicardipine are recommended for severe hypertension (HTN). Good safety data are available for these two drugs. Intravenous (IV) hydrazine is also recommended as a first-line drug for HTN during preeclampsia; however, a meta-analysis of 21 trials comparing IV hydralazine with IV labetalol or oral nifedipine for acute management of HTN showed that hydralazine caused maternal hypotension, maternal oliguria, low Apgar score, and placental abruption. Thus, hydralazine is not recommended as a first-line drug for acute management of HTN.

   Sodium nitroprusside is a good drug for lowering BP; however, its use should be avoided because of fetal cyanide poisoning if used for >4-h. Furosemide or any other diuretic should be used cautiously because of volume contraction in preeclampsia. If the patient has pulmonary edema, IV furosemide is recommended. Magnesium sulfate is used routinely to prevent seizures (to prevent preeclampsia to eclampsia); however, it also lowers BP. In a patient with severe HTN, magnesium sulfate alone is not adequate. Thus, options A, B, D, and E are incorrect. The following Table 8.7 **shows the choice of antihypertensive agents in pregnant women.**

Table 8.7 Choice of antihypertensive drugs in pregnancy

Drug	Dosage	Comment
Oral: first line		
Methyldopa	1–4 g/day in divided doses	Extensive safety data
Labetalol	100 mg BID (2400 mg maximum)	Safe
Long-acting nifedipine	30–120 mg/day	Safe
IV: first-line		
Labetalol	20 mg initially, then 40 mg 10 min later. Then 80 mg every 10 min for 3 doses (300 mg/day maximum)	Safe
Nicardipine	5 mg/h and titrate to 15 mg/h, if needed	Safe
To be avoided		
Diuretics		Volume depletion
Atenolol		Low birth weight
Nitroprusside		Fetal cyanide poisoning
Contraindicated		
ACE-Is & ARBs		Fetal anomalies

Suggested Reading

Gestational hypertension and preeclampsia. ACOG Practice Bulletin No. 222. American College of Obstetricians and Gynecologists. Obstet Gynecol. 2020;135:e237–60.

Hypertension in pregnancy. Report of the American College of Obstetricians and Gynecologists' Task Force on Hypertension in Pregnancy. Obstet Gynecol. 2013;122:1122–31.

Magee LA, Cham C, Waterman EJ, et al. Hydralazine for treatment of severe hypertension in pregnancy: meta-analysis. BMJ. 2003;327:955–60.

47. A 36-year-old African American woman gravida 4, para 3 with history of chronic hypertension was admitted at 30 weeks of gestation for management of headache and blurred vision for 3 days. Admission BP was 160/112 mm Hg with a pulse rate of 94 beats/min. Her previous pregnancy was complicated by preeclampsia. She was started on magnesium sulfate and labetalol, and BP gradually improved to 138/84 mm Hg and pulse rate of 86 beats/min. Three days later, her BP decreased to 130/80 mm Hg with a pulse rate of 58 beats/min, but she became lethargic. Both magnesium sulfate and labetalol were discontinued. Physical examination was significant for decreased deep tendon reflexes. Pertinent serum chemistry showed creatinine of 3.2 mg/dL (admission creatinine was 1.2 mg/dL), Mg^{2+} 14.2 mg/dL, and Ca^{2+} 7.8 mg/dL. Urine output was 10 mL/h and urinalysis showed 1+ proteinuria. **In addition to IV calcium gluconate, which one of the following therapeutic decisions is APPROPRIATE to improve her clinical manifestations?**

A. Continue calcium gluconate until the symptoms improve
B. Use loop diuretics to promote magnesium excretion
C. Start hemodialysis
D. Start peritoneal dialysis (PD)
E. Prepare for delivery

The answer is C

This woman has Mg^{2+} toxicity, which is related to its serum levels. The following Table 8.8 **shows the serum levels of Mg^{2+} and related clinical manifestations.**

Table 8.8 Clinical manifestations of hypermagnesemia

Serum [Mg^{2+}] (mg/dl)	Signs/symptoms
3.6–6.0	Nausea and vomiting
4.8–8.4	Sedation, hyporeflexia, muscle weakness
6.0–12.0	Bradycardia, hypotension
12.0–18.0	Absent reflexes, respiratory paralysis, coma
>18.0	Cardiac arrest

$MgSO_4$ has been widely used for the management and prevention of preeclampsia/eclampsia for decades to prevent seizure activity and also lower BP. The US Food and Drug Administration issued a warning label due to adverse fetal bone effects with long-term (>5–7 days) use. Despite this warning, short-term (<48 h) IV $MgSO_4$ is recommended by the American College of Obstetricians and Gynecologists for the prevention and treatment of seizures in women with preeclampsia and eclampsia. Frequent monitoring of Mg^{2+} levels is necessary to maintain therapeutic range (5 to 9 mg/dL) and to avoid toxicity. Since Mg^{2+} is excreted by the kidneys, the toxic levels reach much earlier in patients with decreased kidney function and low urine output.

The above patient developed acute kidney injury superimposed on CKD (creatinine of 1.2 mg/dL is high in a pregnant woman). Also, her urine output is low. Loop diuretics with saline administration would promote Mg^{2+} excretion in an individual with normal kidney function; however, in this patient the loop diuretics may not lower Mg^{2+} levels sufficient to improve her symptoms. Therefore, HD seems to be a preferred option to improve her symptoms (answer C is correct). PD may not be an appropriate choice and also preparing for delivery is not a good approach (answers D and E are incorrect). Continuing calcium gluconate may improve symptoms transiently but does not decrease serum Mg^{2+} levels (answer A is incorrect). HD was done with improvement in both the symptoms and serum levels.

Suggested Reading

Gestational hypertension and preeclampsia. ACOG Practice Bulletin No. 222. American College of Obstetricians and Gynecologists. Obstet Gynecol. 2020;135:e237–60.

Okusanya B, Oladapo O, Long Q, et al. Clinical pharmacokinetic properties of magnesium sulphate in women with preeclampsia and eclampsia. BJOG. 2016;123:356–66.

48. **Which one of the following statements regarding gestational hypertension is CORRECT?**

A. Gestational hypertension is defined as a systolic BP > 140 mm Hg or a diastolic BP > 90 mm Hg or both, on two occasions at least 4 h apart after 20 weeks of gestation in a woman with a previously normal BP in the absence of features of preeclampsia. BP returns to normal in the postpartum period
B. The above definition suggests that gestational hypertension is not a benign condition, and at least 25% of such cases may progress to develop preeclampsia
C. Treatment of gestational hypertension includes control of BP 110–140/85 mm Hg, monitoring preeclampsia development, monitoring fetal growth particularly in women with elevated uric acid and delay delivery beyond 36 weeks, if BP is controlled
D. There is no specific test to project which woman with gestational hypertension will develop preeclampsia, although the risk is highest among those who present with gestational hypertension before 34 weeks
E. All of the above

The answer is E

In addition to the above correct statements, gestational hypertension seems to have several underlying etiologies. For example, a subset of women with gestational hypertension may have previously undiagnosed primary hypertension, which becomes manifest during pregnancy. It is likely that these women with undiagnosed preexisting hypertension progress to preeclampsia. Eye examination may help in making the diagnosis of chronic hypertension in such women. Although women with gestational hypertension normalize their BP after delivery, they are at risk for development of chronic hypertension and cardiovascular complications.

Suggested Reading

Brown MA, Magee LA, Kenny LC, et al. on behalf of the International Society for the Study of Hypertension in Pregnancy (ISSHP). Hypertensive disorders of pregnancy. ISSHP classification, diagnosis, and management recommendations for international practice. Hypertension. 2018;72:24–43.

Davis GK, Mackenzie C, Brown MA, et al. Predicting transformation from gestational hypertension to preeclampsia in clinical practice: a possible role for 24 hour ambulatory blood pressure monitoring. Hypertens Pregnancy. 2007;26:77–87.

Gestational hypertension and preeclampsia. ACOG Practice Bulletin No. 222. American College of Obstetricians and Gynecologists. Obstet Gynecol. 2020;135:e237–60.

49. A 32-year-old woman 1 week postpartum is seen for anuria, HTN, and creatinine of 5.5 mg/dL. She is gravida 3 and para 2. The first pregnancy resulted in spontaneous abortion, and her second pregnancy was complicated by preeclampsia, but had a vaginal delivery at 36th week. She had a normal third pregnancy course, except for gestational hypertension. She denies diarrhea. Physical examination shows a BP of 150/100 mm Hg with no orthostatic BP and pulse changes, normal chest, cardiovascular and neurologic exam. There is no peripheral edema. One of her cousins had postpartum acute kidney injury (AKI), requiring hemodialysis. Pertinent labs:

Na^+ = 138 mEq/L
K^+ = 4.2 mEq/L
Cl^- = 90 mEq/L
HCO_3^- = 18 mEq/L
Creatinine = 5.5 mg/dL
BUN = 60 mg/dL
Glucose = 100 mg/dL
Uric acid = 6.0 mg/dL
Bilirubin = 1.8 mg/dL
AST/ALT = 20/18 U/L
Hct = 30 g%
Platelets = 100,000/μL
ADAMTS 13 = normal
ADAMTS antibody titer = negative
PT/PTT = normal
C3 = slightly low
Peripheral smear = schistocytes
Urinalysis = trace blood, 1–2 RBCs, no RBC casts
Renal ultrasound = slightly enlarged kidneys with echogenicity

Which one of the following is the MOST likely etiology of her AKI?

A. Prerenal azotemia
B. Diarrhea-associated hemolytic uremic syndrome (D+HUS)
C. Thrombotic thrombocytopenic purpura (TTP)
D. Atypical HUS (aHUS)
E. Disseminated intravascular coagulation (DIC)

The answer is D

This patient has a typical clinical picture of either TTP or HUS. TTP and D+HUS are ruled out based upon normal ADAMTS 13 (a disintegrin and metalloproteinase with a thrombospondin type 1 motif, member 13) levels as well as negative antibody titers to ADAMITS 13 and absence of diarrhea, respectively. Subsequent laboratory test showed that shiga toxin was absent, confirming that she does not have D+HUS. DIC can be ruled out based upon normal PT/PTT (prothrombin time/partial thromboplastin time) levels. Prerenal azotemia is a possibility, but the history and physical examination do not suggest AKI due to volume depletion. Thus, options A, B, C, and E are incorrect. This woman developed aHUS, which typically occurs during postpartum period (option D is correct).

aHUS is a well-recognized thrombotic microangiopathy both in pediatric and adult populations. Pregnancy-associated aHUS has been well recognized. It occurs anywhere from few days to few months postpartum. Both sporadic and familial forms have been described. Like TTP or D+HUS, aHUS presents with nonimmune hemolytic anemia, thrombocytopenia, and renal failure. Unlike D+HUS, aHUS carries a poor prognosis, either with development of ESKD or death in 50 to 80%.

Pregnancy-associated aHUS occurs 1 in 25,000 pregnancies. It seems that pregnancy triggers this complication. The underlying pathogenesis is the activation of an alternative complement system, which is caused by mutations in complement factor H (CFH), complement factor I (CFI), C3, and membrane cofactor protein (MCP). This activation leads to the loss of endothelial cell function, resulting in the stimulation of procoagulation pathways and development of thrombotic microangiopathy. Low C3 may be due to consumption or mutation or a combination of both.

It should be noted that in a normal individual, the complement system is tightly regulated by plasma proteins, including factor H and factor I and MCP. Impaired regulation can lead to pathology and complement-mediated aHUS.

More than 80 mutations in CFH have been described. Also, 6 to 10% of patients with aHUS are found to have autoantibodies to CFH. Overall, 40–50% of mutations in CFH, 10–20% in CFI, 14% in C3, and 10% in MCP affect patients with aHUS.

The study of Fakhouri et al. showed that 21 women out of 100 pregnant women developed pregnancy-associated aHUS. Of these 21 women, 18 had mutations in complement factors: 45% in CFH, 9% in CFI, and 4% in MCP. Fourteen percent had mutations in more than one complement factor. aHUS occurred in 79% during the postpartum period. Treatment consisted mostly of plasma exchange, and in some only plasma infusion. About 76% of patients developed ESKD, requiring either hemodialysis or kidney transplantation during the follow-up period of 6 years or longer.

Recurrence of aHUS in a patient with history of aHUS responds well to treatment with eculizumab. The patient described above had a cousin with postpartum AKI. Thus, the patient requires genetic studies of her complement.

Suggested Reading

Brocklebank V, Wood KM, Kavanagh D. Thrombotic microangiopathy and the kidney. Clin J Am Soc Nephrol. 2018;13:300–17.

Fang CJ, Richards A, Liszewski MK, et al. Advances in understanding of pathogenesis of aHUS and HEELP. Br J Hematol. 2008;143:336–48.

Fakhouri F, Roumenina L, Provôt F, et al. Pregnancy-associated hemolytic-uremic syndrome revisited in the era of complement gene mutations. J Am Soc Nephrol. 2010;21:859–67.

Fakhouri F, Scully M, Provôt F, et al. and the International Working Group on Pregnancy-Related Thrombotic Microangiopathies. Management of thrombotic microangiopathy in pregnancy and postpartum: report from an international working group. Blood. 2020;136:2103–17.

Kavanagh D, Sheerin N. Thrombotic microangiopathies. In: Yu ASL, Chertow GM, Luyckx VA, et al., editors. Brenner & Rector's the kidney. 11th ed. Philadelphia: Elsevier Saunders; 2020. p. 1178–95.

Noris M, Remuzzi G. Atypical hemolytic-uremic syndrome. N Engl J Med. 2009;361:1676–87.

50. **Regarding atypical HUS (aHUS) and treatment, which one of the following statements is FALSE?**

A. Plasma exchange should be started within 24 h after diagnosis with 1.5 times the plasma volume in patients with CFH and CFI mutations. Also, in patients with CFH mutations, long-term plasma infusion alone is not enough to induce disease remission

B. In patients with documented mutations only in MCP, plasma exchange or plasma infusion is as effective as in patients with CFH and CFI mutations

C. The duration of plasma exchange is dependent on the basis of individual response as well as full recovery of hematological abnormalities. Platelet count and serum lactate dehydrogenase (LDH) are the most sensitive markers of responsiveness to plasma exchange

D. Eculizumab (a human anti-C5 monoclonal antibody) is the drug of choice to treat aHUS and to induce remission of aHUS refractory or dependent on plasma exchange therapy

E. Living-related donor transplantation is contraindicated in patients with aHUS because of high recurrence of the disease

The answer is B

Except for B, all other statements are true. According to the guidelines of treatment of atypical HUS, plasma exchange should be started within 24-h after the diagnosis is made with 1–2 times the plasma volume. Fresh frozen plasma (FFP) provides the defective CFH and CFI, but plasma exchange not only removes autoantibodies to CFH but also removes dysfunctional CFH, which FFP alone cannot achieve. Furthermore, FFP alone is not enough to replace CFH after long-term therapy. Thus, plasma exchange is superior to infusion of FFP in patients with CFH mutations. For patients with known MCP mutations and no mutations in other complements, spontaneous remission occurs in 80 to 90% of patients without plasma exchange or FFP therapy. Thus, statement B is false.

Eculizumab is a monoclonal humanized immunoglobulin G (IgG) that inhibits the cleavage of C5 and thus, prevents the generation of C5a, a powerful anaphylatoxin, and C5b, which initiates the formation of the membrane attack complex. Thus, eculizumab blocks the common terminal activation step of all three complement pathways. Thus, eculizumab has been shown to remit aHUS and related complications, such as improvement in kidney function.

In a retrospective study of 22 patients with pregnancy-associated aHUS, Huerta et al. reported that 17 patients underwent plasma treatments with a positive renal response in only three cases. In contrast, 10 patients received

eculizumab for a mean period of 9.8 months with an excellent hematologic and renal response in all, independent of carrying or not inherited complement abnormalities. Thus, eculizumab seems to help patients with aHUS.

Kidney transplantation has been done in some patients with aHUS. Recurrence of the disease is variable, depending on the nature of the mutation, but seen in around 50% of the patients, and graft failure occurs in 80–90% of those with recurrent disease. Living-related donor kidney transplantation is contraindicated because of the high risk of recurrent disease. Also, donors who carry a mutation may be at risk for the disease in the single kidney. A case report shows such a recurrence of the disease in the father who donated one of the kidneys to his child. Thus, genetic evaluation of complement genes is warranted in individuals seeking living-related donor kidney.

Suggested Reading

Brocklebank V, Wood KM, Kavanagh D. Thrombotic microangiopathy and the kidney. Clin J Am Soc Nephrol. 2018;13:300–17.

Fakhouri F, Vercel C, Frémeaux-Bacchi V. Obstetric nephrology: AKI and thrombotic microangiopathies in pregnancy. Clin J Am Soc Nephrol. 2012;7:2100–6.

Fakhouri F, Scully M, Provôt F, et al. and the International Working Group on Pregnancy-Related Thrombotic Microangiopathies. Management of thrombotic microangiopathy in pregnancy and postpartum: report from an international working group. Blood. 2020;136:2103–17.

Huerta A, Arjona E, Portoles J, et al. A retrospective study of pregnancy-associated atypical hemolytic uremic syndrome. Kidney Int. 2018;93:450–9.

Kavanagh D, Sheerin N. Thrombotic microangiopathies. In: Yu ASL, Chertow GM, Luyckx VA, et al., editors. Brenner & Rector's the kidney. 11th ed. Philadelphia: Elsevier Saunders; 2020. p. 1178–95.

51. **Which one of the following statements regarding counseling a woman with history of atypical HUS (aHUS) who contemplates pregnancy is CORRECT?**

A. Pregnancy is not a contraindication in a woman with history of aHUS
B. Approximately 12 months of aHUS remission and stable kidney function are necessary prior to pregnancy anticipation
C. Relapse of aHUS occurs more frequently during pregnancy than after delivery in women with previous aHUS
D. Women with previous history of aHUS should be considered a high-risk pregnancy
E. All of the above

The answer is E

Counseling women with a history of aHUS about pregnancy includes all of the above statements (answer E is correct). Currently, pregnancy is not contraindicated in a woman with history of aHUS. This is related to the introduction of anticomplement therapy during pregnancy and after delivery in reversing acute kidney injury. Despite this treatment, a close supervision clinically and biochemically from conception to 3–4 months after delivery is extremely important because the relapse of aHUS triggered by pregnancy is difficult to predict. Prophylaxis of anticomplement therapy is not recommended, and CKD may be a limiting factor to pregnancy.

Suggested Reading

Fakhouri F, Scully M, Provôt F, et al. and the International Working Group on Pregnancy-Related Thrombotic Microangiopathies. Management of thrombotic microangiopathy in pregnancy and postpartum: report from an international working group. Blood. 2020;136:2103–17.

52. The occurrence of chronic HTN in pregnancy is rather common. However, the onset of preeclampsia is difficult to distinguish from chronic HTN. **Which one of the following is FALSE regarding chronic HTN in pregnancy?**

A. Onset of HTN before 20th week
B. Proteinuria <300 mg/day
C. Drop in systolic BP > 10 mm Hg by 13–20 weeks
D. Drop in diastolic BP > 10 mm Hg by 13–20 weeks
E. Increase in BP to prepregnancy level during 3rd trimester

The answer is C

Chronic HTN can be diagnosed easily in a pregnant woman when BP is ≥140/90 mm Hg before 20 weeks of gestation and proteinuria <300 mg/day. Normally, BP falls in early pregnancy; however, systolic BP changes very little.

In contrast, diastolic BP falls by >10 mm Hg during 10 to 20 weeks of gestation, with a nadir (lowest) at 24 weeks, and then rises to prepregnancy level during 28 to 40 weeks (3rd trimester). This physiological fall may be more exaggerated in women with chronic HTN. This exaggerated fall in BP may pose a diagnostic problem when chronic hypertensive woman is seen for the first time during the 2nd trimester and erroneously label her as normotensive. When BP returns to prepregnancy level during the 3rd trimester, this woman may be labeled as having gestational HTN or new onset of preeclampsia. It is important, therefore, to follow the dip in diastolic than systolic BP during 13–20 weeks of gestation. Thus, option C is false.

In women with chronic HTN and proteinuria >300 mg/day before 20 weeks of gestation, the diagnosis of preeclampsia can be made. Also, preeclampsia can be considered if proteinuria or BP increases and evidence of HEELP syndrome is present.

Suggested Reading

Malha L, Padymon T, August P. Hypertension in pregnancy. In: Bakris GL, Sorrentino MJ, editors. Hypertension: a companion to Braunwald's heart disease. 3rd ed. Philadelphia: Elsevier; 2018. p. 361–73.

Seely EM, Ecker J. Chronic hypertension in pregnancy. N Engl J Med. 2011;365:439–46.

53. Hypertension during pregnancy is rather common, but BP targets were not clearly defined until the Control of Hypertension in Pregnancy Study (CHIPS). The CHIPS examined the effects of tight control (diastolic BP 85–105 mm Hg) versus less-tight control (diastolic BP 90–105 mm Hg) on clinical outcomes in women who had nonproteinuric preexisting or gestational hypertension from 14 weeks 00 days to 33 weeks 6 days of pregnancy. **Which one of the following observations is CORRECT between the two BP targets?**

    A. No difference in the pregnancy loss
    B. No difference in high-level neonatal care
    C. No difference in overall maternal complications
    D. Higher frequency of severe maternal hypertension in the less-tight control group
    E. All of the above

    The answer is E

    CHIPS was an open, international, multicenter trial that included 987 women from 95 sites in 16 countries. Of these 987 women, 490 were assigned to tight control and 497 to less-tight control. About 75% had preexisting hypertension. Baseline BP was similar in both groups (140/92 mm Hg). During follow-up, the diastolic BP was higher by 4.6 mm Hg in the less-tight control group. The composite primary outcome was pregnancy loss and high-level neonatal care for more than 48 h during the first 28 postnatal days. The secondary outcome was serious maternal complications. The study showed no difference in primary outcome between the groups. Also, no difference in maternal complications was observed, except for severe hypertension (>160/110 mm Hg) that developed in 27.5% of the women in the tight control group compared to 40.6% of the women in the less-tight control group ($p < 0.001$). Thus, answer E is correct.

    Suggested Reading

Magee LA, von Dadelzen P, Rey E, et al. Less-tight versus tight control of hypertension in pregnancy. N Engl J Med. 2015;372:407–17.

54. A number of agents have been used to prevent preeclampsia. **Which one of the following agents has been shown to have a preventive effect on preeclampsia?**

    A. ACE-Is
    B. Vitamin C and E
    C. Aspirin
    D. Calcium
    E. Sodium

    The answer is C

    Since preeclampsia causes both maternal and fetal complications, prevention of its onset is clearly warranted. Preventive measures need to start early in pregnancy, around 12 to 14 weeks of gestation. ACE-Is or ARBs are contraindicated in pregnancy because of fetal anomalies (renal dysgenesis, fetal oliguria, pulmonary hypoplasia, fetal growth retardation, and neonatal AKI).

Oxidative stress has been implicated in preeclampsia, therefore, vitamin C and E have been used. Although a few studies have shown some benefit, other large studies showed no benefit. Thus, routine use of vitamin C and E is not recommended. In the study of VIP (The Vitamins in Pre-eclampsia), it was observed that vitamin C and E supplementation was associated with more severe and earlier onset preeclampsia, HTN, lower birth weight and increased neonatal morbidity. Also, a study published in the New England Journal of Medicine showed that vitamin C and E supplementation to 10,154 low-risk nulliparous women in the 9th to 16th week of gestation did not reduce the rate of adverse maternal or perinatal outcomes related to pregnancy-associated HTN.

Pregnancy induces hypercalciuria. In preeclampsia, calcium excretion is reduced, therefore, calcium supplementation is recommended to prevent preeclampsia; however, randomized studies have failed to show the benefit of calcium supplementation. However, calcium supplementation is recommended only in women with a daily intake of calcium <600/mg/day. Sodium restriction, once thought to be helpful, is not effective in reducing either gestational HTN or preeclampsia.

Platelet activation, their consumption and aggregation commonly occur in preeclampsia, due to increased thromboxane activity. To prevent thromboxane activity, antiplatelet agents such as aspirin are routinely recommended during pregnancy. The American College of Obstetricians and Gynecologists and the Society for Maternal-Fetal Medicine recommend "Low-dose aspirin (81 mg/day) prophylaxis is recommended in women at high risk of preeclampsia and should be initiated between 12 weeks and 28 weeks of gestation (optimally before 16 weeks) and continued daily until delivery." Thus, option C is correct.

Suggested Reading

Low-dose aspirin use during pregnancy. ACOG Committee Opinion No. 743. American College of Obstetricians and Gynecologists. Obstet Gynecol. 2018;132:e44–52.

Roberts JM, Myatt L, Spong CY, et al. Vitamin C and E to prevent complications of pregnancy-associated hypertension. N Engl J Med. 2010;362:1282–91.

Rolnik DL, Wright D, Poon LC, et al. Aspirin versus placebo in pregnancies at high risk for preterm preeclampsia. N Engl J Med. 2017;377:613–22.

55. Angiogenic imbalance has been proposed as one of the major contributing mechanisms for the development of preeclampsia. **Which one of the following is an antiangiogenic factor?**

A. Soluble fms-like tyrosine kinase-1 (sFlt-1)
B. Soluble endoglin
C. Placental growth factor (PlGF)
D. Vascular endothelial growth factor (VEGF)
E. A and B only

The answer is E

It has been proposed that an imbalance between the angiogenic and antiangiogenic factors plays an important role in the pathogenesis of preeclampsia. Angiogenic factors are VEGF and PlGF. Both VEGF and PlGF induce the synthesis of nitric oxide (NO) and prostaglandins in endothelial cells, causing vasodilatation. The antiangiogenic factors are sFlt-1, soluble endoglin, and hypoxia-inducible factor-1.

sFlt-1 is synthesized by the placenta, and its circulating levels are increased in preeclampsia. It is a splice variant of the VEGF receptor Flt-1 and lacks the transmembrane cytoplasmic domain of the membrane-bound receptor. Thus, sFlt-1 antagonizes the angiogenic potential of VEGF and PlGF, resulting in vasoconstriction, HTN, hypoxia, and proteinuria. Indeed, administration of sFlt-1 to pregnant and nonpregnant rats produces HTN, proteinuria, and glomerular endotheliosis that are seen in human preeclampsia.

Soluble endoglin, a truncated form of endoglin, is a cell surface coreceptor for TGF-β (transforming growth factor beta). It binds and antagonizes TGF-β in the extracellular milieu. It is also produced by the placenta. It appears that soluble endoglin may act in concert with sFlt-1 in causing severe preeclampsia and HEELP syndrome.

To support the roles of antiangiogenic factors in the pathogenesis of preeclampsia, the circulating levels of both sFlt-1 and soluble endoglin were measured and found to be elevated before the onset of preeclampsia. In particular, the levels of sFlt-1 are 2–4 times higher in clinically severe preeclampsia. Thus, these two antiangiogenic factors may be used as serum markers for detection of preeclampsia. Thus, option E is correct. It is of interest to note that sFlt-1 levels are decreased in women with smoking, which has been shown to have a protective effect on preeclampsia.

Suggested Reading

Karumanchi SA. Angiogenic factors in preeclampsia: from diagnosis to therapy. Hypertension. 2016;67:1072–9.

Karumanchi SA, Maynard SE, Stillman IE, et al. Preeclampsia: a renal perspective. Kidney Int. 2005;67:2101–13.

Levine RJ, Maynard SE, Qian C, et al. Circulating angiogenic factors and the risk of preeclampsia. N Engl J Med. 2004;350:672–83.

Phipps EA, Thadhani R, Benzing T, et al. Pre-eclampsia: pathogenesis, novel diagnostics and therapies. Nat Rev Nephrol. 2019;15:275–89.

Steinberg G, Khankin EV, Karumanch SA. Angiogenic factors and preeclampsia. Thromb Res. 2009;123(suppl 2): S93–9.

Verlohren S, Dröge LA. The diagnostic value of angiogenic and antiangiogenic factors in differential diagnosis of preeclampsia. Am J Obstet Gynecol. 2020 Sept 28:S0002-9378(20)31169–8. https://doi.org/10.1016/j.ajog.2020.09.046. Epub ahead of print. PMID: 33002498.

56. Screening for preeclampsia was based on history, physical examination, and laboratory values. In addition to these traditional criteria, the inclusion of antiangiogenic and proangiogenic factors (biomarkers) made the diagnosis of preeclampsia much easier than before. **Which one of the following statements regarding biomarkers of preeclampsia is CORRECT?**

    A. Plasma sFlt-1 levels rise and PlGF (placental growth factor) levels decrease and the ratio of sFlt-1/PlGF seems to be an ideal biomarker for the detection of preeclampsia
    B. Plasma sFlt-1/PlGF ratio on presentation predicts adverse maternal and perinatal outcomes (occurring within 2 weeks) in the preterm setting
    C. Plasma sFlt-1/PlGF ratio alone performs better than the standard battery of clinical diagnostic measures such as BP, proteinuria, uric acid, and other laboratory assays
    D. Measurement of plasma sFlt-1 and PlGF levels can be used to differentiate preeclampsia from other diseases that mimic preeclampsia, such as CKD, chronic hypertension, gestational hypertension, and gestational thrombocytopenia
    E. All of the above

    The answer is E

    It is well established that an imbalance in circulating antiangiogenic (sFlt-1) and proangiogenic (PlGF) protein levels is involved in the development of preeclampsia (see the above question). Increased plasma levels of sFlt-1 and low levels of PlGF have been reported in women with preeclampsia by several studies. In addition, prospective studies have shown that the ratio of sFlt-1/PlGF is a better biomarker to predict the onset of preeclampsia and the pregnancy outcomes. Cut-off values for this ratio have been published in women with singleton pregnancies in whom preeclampsia was suspected between 24 and 36 weeks and 6 days of gestation. A value <38 rules out short-term preeclampsia and this number was found to have a negative predictive value of 99.3% with 80% sensitivity and 78.3% specificity. This suggests that these women can be followed in an outpatient setting. The positive predictive value for a value >38 for diagnosis of preeclampsia within 4 weeks was 36.7% with 66.2% sensitivity and 83.1% specificity. It was also shown that a value ≥85 correlates with diagnosis of preeclampsia and predicts adverse outcomes and delivery within 2 weeks presenting <34 weeks of gestation. These women need hospitalization with close follow-up. Thus, the ratio of sFlt-1/PlGF is a better biomarker in diagnosing preeclampsia in suspected women than BP or other traditional laboratory parameters (answers A-C are correct). The following Table 8.9 **illustrates management of pregnancy using sFlt-1:PlGF ratios at different gestation periods.**

Table 8.9 sFlt-1/PlGF ratios and the risk-stratification (adapted from Suresh and Rana)

Risk	Ratio at <34 wk	Ratio at >34 wk	Comment
Low-risk ratio	<38	<38	Follow traditional criteria
Intermediate-risk ratio	38–85	38–110	Follow traditional criteria, clinical evaluation, and ratios every week and manage individually
High-risk ratio	>85	>110	No further testing, admission preferred, follow maternal and fetal well-being

In a study of Dröge et al., risk-stratification of the cut-off values into high (>85), intermediate (38–85), and low (<38) showed a significantly shorter time to delivery in high-risk (4 days), intermediate-risk (8 days), and low-risk (29 days) in women with suspected preeclampsia. This study showed that combining sFlt-1/PlGF ratio with BP and proteinuria increased detection of adverse outcomes in women with preeclampsia than the ratio alone.

A few studies have shown that the ratio of sFlt-1/PlGF can differentiate preeclampsia from CKD. In one study, this ratio was 436 (individual values expressed in pg/mL) compared to 4 in CKD and 9 in normal (control) individuals. Another study reported elevated sFlt-1/PlGF ratios in chronic hypertensive woman with superimposed preeclampsia, compared to those chronic hypertensive women without preeclampsia.

Similarly, higher levels of antiangiogenic factors and lower angiogenic PlGF levels were found in patients with HELLP thrombocytopenia than patients with non-HELLP syndrome. Angiogenic factor abnormalities in patients with preeclampsia were similar to patients with HELLP syndrome, suggesting a common pathogenesis. Patients with non-HELLP thrombocytopenia had angiogenic profiles similar to normotensive controls.

Patients with active SLE have higher levels of VEGF, PlGF, and sFlt-1 than controls. sFlt-1 was also higher in patients with active SLE than patients with inactive SLE. Furthermore, sFlt-1/PlGF ratios were higher in preeclamptic lupus, primary antiphospholipid, and secondary antiphospholipid women than women without preeclampsia (D is correct).

Suggested Reading

Dröge LA, Holger F, Natalia P, et al. Prediction of preeclampsia-related adverse outcomes with sFlt1/PlGF (soluble fms-like tyrosine kinase 1)/PlGF (placental growth factor)-ratio in the clinical routine. A real-world study. Hypertension. 2021;77:461–71.

Karumanchi SA. Angiogenic factors in preeclampsia: from diagnosis to therapy. Hypertension. 2016;67:1072–9.

Kim MY, Buyon JP, Guerra MM, et al. Angiogenic factor imbalance early in pregnancy predicts adverse outcomes in patients with lupus and antiphospholipid antibodies: results of the PROMISSE study. Am J Obstet Gynecol. 2016;214:108.e1–14.

Phipps EA, Thadhani R, Benzing T, et al. Pre-eclampsia: pathogenesis, novel diagnostics and therapies. Nat Rev Nephrol. 2019;15:275–89.

Suresh SC, Rana S. Real-world use of biomarkers in management of hypertension during pregnancy. Hypertension. 2021;77:472–4.

Verlohren S, Dröge LA. The diagnostic value of angiogenic and antiangiogenic factors in differential diagnosis of preeclampsia. Am J Obstet Gynecol. 2020 Sept 28:S0002-9378(20)31169–8. https://doi.org/10.1016/j.ajog.2020.09.046. Epub ahead of print. PMID: 33002498.

Zeisler H, Llurba E, Chantraine F, Predictive value of the sFlt-1:PlGF ratio in women with suspected preeclampsia. N Engl J Med. 2016;374:13–22.

57. A 28-year-old woman with preeclampsia during her 1st pregnancy 2 years ago is found to have HTN and proteinuria of 750 mg/24-h at 30 weeks of pregnancy. Her soluble fms-like tyrosine kinase-1 (sFlt-1) levels were found to be elevated. **Which one of the following treatments has been found to be beneficial in the removal of sFlt-1?**

A. Hemodialysis (HD)
B. Continuous venovenous hemofiltration (CVVH)
C. Plasma exchange
D. Dextran sulfate cellulose apheresis
E. None of the above

The answer is D

As stated in the previous question, sFlt-1 is an antiangiogenic factor and causes preeclampsia. Its levels are elevated in this condition. It is, therefore, of interest to observe whether lowering sFlt-1 levels are beneficial to patients who are diagnosed to have preeclampsia. Thadhani et al. observed initially in a pilot study that removal of sFlt-1 by dextran sulfate cellulose extracorporeal apheresis can prolong pregnancy with reduction in proteinuria and stabilization of BP in preeclamptic women. This procedure was found to be safe to the mother and fetus and was well tolerated by all patients. These beneficial effects were subsequently confirmed in another study with an increased number of preeclamptic patients (D is correct). So far, neither HD nor CVVH, or plasma exchange has been tried.

Suggested Reading

Thadhani R, Kisner T, Hagmann H, et al. Pilot study of extracorporeal removal of soluble fms-like tyrosine kinase 1 in preeclampsia. Circulation. 2011;124:940–50.

Thadhani R, Hagmann H, Schaarschmidt W. et al. Removal of soluble fms-like tyrosine kinase-1 by dextran sulfate apheresis in preeclampsia. J Am Soc Nephrol. 2016;27:903–13.

58. A 30-year-old woman had preeclampsia during her pregnancy. Her HTN and proteinuria were resolved postpartum. Despite this improvement, she may be at risk for long-term cardiovascular (CV) and renal complications. **Which one of the following is NOT a long-term complication in a woman with history of preeclampsia?**

    A. Hypertension (HTN)
    B. Stroke
    C. Microalbuminuria
    D. Chronic kidney disease (CKD)
    E. Dementia

    The answer is E

    Women with a history of preeclampsia/eclampsia are at increased risk for CV and cerebrovascular complications later in life. One meta-analysis showed that the odds ratios (OR) with 95% confidence interval (CI) were for HTN 3.1 (CI 2.51–3.89), CV disease 2.28 (CI 1.87–2.78), and cerebrovascular disease 1.77 (CI 1.43–2.21), as compared with or without preeclampsia/eclampsia. Another meta-analysis on renal disease and preeclampsia showed that 31% of women with a history of preeclampsia had microalbuminuria, compared to 7% of women without a history of preeclampsia (4-fold increase). However, this study did not show any difference either in serum creatinine levels or eGFR between preeclamptic and normal pregnant women. A study by Vikse et al. reported a relative risk of ESKD of 4.7 (CI 3.6–6.1) in women who had one or two pregnancies but preeclampsia during the 1st pregnancy. However, the absolute risk for ESKD was low. This study shows that women with a history of preeclampsia are at increased risk for CKD and ESKD. Dementia may be attributed to cerebrovascular disease, but a direct causal relationship between a history of preeclampsia and dementia has not been reported. Thus, E is unlikely.

    Suggested Reading

Brown MC, Best KE, Pearce MS, et al. Cardiovascular disease risk in women with pre-eclampsia: systematic review and meta-analysis. Eur J Epidemiol. 2013;28:1–9.

McDonald SD, Han Z, Walsh MW, et al. Kidney disease after preeclampsia: a systematic review and meta-analysis. Am J Kidney Dis. 2010;55:1026–39.

Rana S, Lemoine E, Granger JP, et al. Preeclampsia: pathophysiology, challenges, and perspectives. Circ Res. 2019;124:1094–112.

Vikse BE, Irgens LM, Leivestad T, et al. Preeclampsia and the risk of end-stage renal disease. N Engl J Med. 2008;359:800–9.

59. A 29-year-old primigravida is seen at 34 weeks' gestation for severe headache, palpitations associated with diaphoresis. Her BP is 180/110 mm Hg with a pulse rate of 120 beats per min. Other than basilar crackles, the physical examination is normal. BP did not respond to either methyldopa or hydralazine. However, labetalol initially lowered the heart rate with a slight improvement in BP. Pertinent labs: Serum creatinine is 0.7 mg/dL; K^+ level is 4.4 mg/dL; HCO_3^- level is 23 mg/dL; and glucose is 120 mg/dL. Urinalysis shows trace proteinuria. At night, the BP became normal (130/84 mm Hg with a pulse rate of 92 beats per min) without treatment and headache improved. **Which one of the following laboratory tests you order next?**

    A. Plasma renin and aldosterone levels
    B. Plasma insulin
    C. Plasma and urine catecholamines
    D. Plasma T_3, T_4, and TSH
    E. Plasma PTH levels

    The answer is C

    Although HTN and proteinuria are suggestive of preeclampsia, the classic triad of headache, palpitations, and diaphoresis is suggestive of pheochromocytoma (Pheo). This triad is due to excess release of catecholamines (norepinephrine, epinephrine, and to some extent dopamine). The incidence of Pheo in pregnancy is <0.2% per 10,000 pregnancies. Despite this rarity, the mortality for untreated Pheo is as high as 58% for both the mother and fetus. The paroxysmal attacks begin abruptly and last for minutes to hours and then subside. BP is normal in between surges. Patients with Pheo demonstrate orthostatic hypotension. Plasma and urine catecholamines, and most importantly, 24-h urine metanephrines are appropriate laboratory tests to diagnose Pheo. The patient has a typical presentation of Pheo and warrants determinations of catecholamines and their metabolites, particularly urine metanephrines. Thus, option C is the appropriate next step in this patient.

Clinical clues such as labile hypertension and failure to respond to conventional antihypertensive medications should prompt physicians to include the diagnosis of Pheo in their differential diagnosis. Also, several factors that trigger Pheo should be considered, including increases in abdominal pressure, uterine contractions, and fetal movements. Surgery and anesthesia can precipitate Pheo. Phenoxybenzamine is the drug of choice, and surgery is the definitive treatment for Pheo. Metabolically, patients with Pheo develop insulin resistance and hyperglycemia. Because of insulin resistance, the insulin levels might be high; however, they have no diagnostic significance.

Renovascular HTN and primary aldosteronism are associated with hypokalemia and metabolic alkalosis. The patient's K^+ and HCO_3^- levels are normal. Thus, determination of renin and aldosterone will not be that helpful.

Hyperthyroidism is a consideration; however, high diastolic BP excludes this diagnosis. MEN type 2A (multiple endocrine neoplasia type 2A) is characterized by Pheo, medullary thyroid cancer, and hyperparathyroidism. Determination of PTH is thus warranted but the patient has no clinical manifestations of MEN 2A syndrome.

Suggested Reading

Desai AS, Chutkow WA, Edelman E, et al. A crisis in late pregnancy. N Engl J Med. 2009;361:2271–7.

Oliva R, Angelos P, Kaplan E, et al. Pheochromocytoma in pregnancy. A case series and review. Hypertension. 2010;55:600–6.

Rao F, Friese R, Weu G, et al. Catecholamines, pheochromocytoma and hypertension: genomic insights. In: Lip GYH, Hall JE, editors. Comprehensive hypertension. Philadelphia: Mosby; 2007. p. 895–911.

Yulia A, Seetho IW, Ramineni A, et al. Pheochromocytoma in pregnancy: a review of the literature. Obstet Gynecol Cases Rev. 2016;3:096.

60. **Which one of the following kidney function changes returns to preconception level following delivery in a nonhypertensive woman?**

A. Glomerular filtration rate (GFR)
B. Renal plasma flow (RPF)
C. Filtration fraction (FF)
D. All of the above
E. B only

The answer is B

Pregnancy is characterized by structural and physiologic functions of the kidney. Both kidney length and volume are enlarged early in pregnancy with resultant increase in cardiac output, GFR, and RPF. Changes in FF (GFR/RPF) also occur. The following Table 8.10 **shows renal function changes at different points during gestation in a normal pregnant woman.**

Table 8.10 Changes in GFR, RPF, and FF (adapted from Odutayo and Hladunewich)

Gestation period (wk)	GFR (% change)	RPF (% change)	FF (% change)
1–20	37	41	−1.9
21–30	38	29	11
31–40	39	10	29
Postpartum (1 wk)	31	-2	18

It is evident from the above table that GFR remains elevated during pregnancy and 1 week postpartum and RPF decreases, as pregnancy progresses and reaches prepregnancy level following delivery. Thus, answer B is correct. FF decreases early in pregnancy but remains elevated until delivery.

Suggested Reading

Odutayo A, Hladunewich M. Obstetric nephrology: renal hemodynamic and metabolic physiology in normal pregnancy. Clin J Am Soc Nephrol. 2012;7:2073–80.

Chapter 9
Hemodialysis

1. A 62-year-old man with CKD 5 (eGFR 11 mL/min) due to HTN comes to the clinic for routine follow-up with no complaints of nausea, vomiting, fatigue, or poor appetite. An arteriovenous fistula (AVF) was placed 1 year ago when his eGFR was 12 mL/min and the fistula is ready for use. His BP is 134/80 mm Hg. He walks 2 miles everyday without shortness of breath, chest pain, or fatigue. Pertinent labs include Na^+ 139 mEq/L, K^+ 4.4 mEq/L, HCO_3^- 22 mEq/L, BUN 68 mg/dL, Ca^{2+} 8.8 mg/dL, phosphate 4.2 mg/dL, and albumin 4.1 g/dL. He expresses hemodialysis (HD) as his choice of renal replacement therapy (RRT). **According to the KDIGO guideline, which one of the following is the MOST appropriate management in this patient?**

   A. Start HD in 2 weeks at the outpatient dialysis unit
   B. Start peritoneal dialysis (PD) in 4 weeks
   C. Convince for preemptive kidney transplantation
   D. Start HD when signs and symptoms of kidney failure are present
   E. Suggest no RRT at any time, as he may do well with conservative management

   The answer is D

   Of all the choice, choice D is appropriate. According to the KIDIGO guideline, dialysis should be considered when signs and symptoms of kidney failure such as serositis, acid-base or electrolytes abnormalities, and pruritus are present. In addition, dialysis should be initiated when volume status and BP cannot be controlled. Thus, D is correct. The patient wants HD when appropriate. Convincing him at this time for preemptive kidney transplantation is unwise. The patient wishes to have HD rather than PD. Starting PD and suggesting conservative management are not appropriate at this time.

   According to KDIGO "initiation of dialysis is usually considered when one or more of the following are present: symptoms or signs attributable to kidney failure (e.g., neurological signs and symptoms attributable to uremia, pericarditis, anorexia, medically resistant acid-base or electrolyte abnormalities, reduced energy level, weight loss with no other potential explanation, intractable pruritus, or bleeding); inability to control volume status or blood pressure; and a progressive deterioration in nutritional status refractory to interventions. Depending on the patient's preferences and circumstances, an aggressive trial of medical nondialytic management of advanced CKD symptoms may be warranted before initiating maintenance dialysis."

   Suggested Reading

Chan CT, Blankestijn PJ, Dember LM, et al. Dialysis initiation, modality choice, access, and prescription: conclusions from a Kidney Disease: Improving Global Outcomes (KDIGO) controversies conference. Kidney Int. 2019;96:37–47.

Kidney Disease Improving Global Outcomes. KIDIGO 2012 clinical practice guideline for the evaluation and management of chronic kidney disease. Kidney Int. 2013;(Suppl 3):1–150.

Rivara MB, Mehrotra R. Timing of dialysis initiation- What has changed since IDEAL?. Sem Nephrol. 2017;37:181–93.

2. **Which one of the following statements in CKD 5 patients regarding early (eGFR 10–14 mL/min) versus late (eGFR 5–7 mL/min) initiation of HD is CORRECT?**

   A. Early initiation of HD improves mortality and morbidity of patients
   B. Late initiation of HD improves mortality and morbidity of patients

A. S. Reddi, *Absolute Nephrology Review*, https://doi.org/10.1007/978-3-030-85958-9_9

C. No difference between early and late initiation of HD either in survival or other outcomes such as hospitalizations or quality of life
D. Compared to early initiation, late initiation is better in controlling mortality only
E. None of the above

The answer is C

Initial small observational studies reported beneficial effects of early initiation of dialysis (hemo- or peritoneal dialysis). However, there are no large studies that evaluated the outcomes of early versus late initiation of HD. The large study by Cooper et al. randomized 828 adults (mean age 60.4 years) in 32 centers in Australia and New Zealand to begin early or late HD treatment. During the median follow-up of 3.59 years, 37% in the early-start group and 36.6% in the late-start group died. Also, there was no difference between the groups in cardiovascular events, infections, or complications of dialysis. The median time to initiation of dialysis was 1.8 months in the early-start groups compared to 7.4 months in the late-start group. Therefore, the correct answer is C.

It should be remembered that this study cannot be extrapolated to all ethnic group because the majority of the study patients were under the care of a nephrologist (approximately 32.5 months for the early group and 29.4 months for the late group), and such a follow-up may not be available to most other patients. Also, 70–73% of the patients were white. Therefore, initiation of RRT should be individualized.

A meta-analysis of 15 cohort studies and the above large study concluded that higher GFR at the initiation of dialysis therapy is associated with higher mortality risk. It also showed that a 1-mL/min GFR increment was associated with a 4% higher adjusted hazard for all-cause mortality.

Suggested Reading

Cooper BA, Branley P, Bulfone L, et al. for the IDEAL Study. A randomized, controlled trial of early versus late initiation of dialysis. N Engl J Med. 2010;363: 609–19.
Rivara MB, Mehrotra R. Is early initiation of dialysis harmful?. Sem Dial. 2014;27:250–2.
Rivara MB, Mehrotra R. Timing of dialysis initiation- What has changed since IDEAL?. Sem Nephrol. 2017;37:181–93.

3. **Which one of the following decisions is important for conservative management of patients with ESKD is CORRECT?**

A. Patient's choice
B. Presence of severe comorbidities
C. Functional status of the patient
D. Severe vascular dementia
E. All of the above

The answer is E

For some patients with ESKD, offering conservative (palliative) care may be a satisfactory alternative to renal replacement therapy (RRT). In a survey of nephrologists from 11 European countries, a decision was made to offer conservative care for 15% (10% by nephrologists, and 5% by patients) of patients in 2009. Patients' preference (93%), severe clinical conditions (93%), vascular dementia (84%), and low physiological functional status (75%) were considered important in the decision-making of not to start RRT.

In another study from Australia, about 14% of patients with CKD 5 preferred conservative care when presented as a treatment option. The median age of these patients was 80 years. Of interest is that those patients with private health insurance did not prefer conservative care. Therefore, the option of conservative care should be presented to certain patients who do not benefit from dialysis.

RRT is not without adverse effects, particularly in the elderly. A study by Brown et al. described a cohort of 467 older patients with advanced CKD. Of these 467 patients, 122 (26%) chose to forego dialysis. Mean age of these patients was 82 years, who had many comorbid conditions, including dementia. The median survival time of patients who chose conservative management was 16 months, with a 53% 1-year survival rate.

Suggested Reading

Brown MA, Collett GK, Josland EA, et al. CKD in elderly patients managed without dialysis; survival, symptoms, and quality of life. 2015;Clin J Am Soc Nephrol. 10:260–9.

Morton RL, Turner RM, Howard K, et al. Patients who plan for conservative care rather than dialysis: A national observational study in Australia. Am J Kidney Dis. 2012;59:419–27.

Murtagh FE, Burns A, Moranne O, et al. Supportive Care: Comprehensive conservative care in end-stage kidney disease. Clin J Am Soc Nephrol. 2016;11:1909–14.

van de Luijtgaarden MW, Noordzi M, van Biesen W, et al. Conservative care in Europe-nephrologists' experience with the decision not to start renal replacement therapy. Nephrol Dial Transpl. 2013;28:2604–12.

4. A 56-year-old woman is started on hemodialysis (HD) using a fistula that was created 1 year ago. She is diabetic with HTN. **Which one of the following dialysis prescriptions is appropriate to improve dialysis outcomes?**

A. Dialysis should be delivered at least 3 times per week, and the total duration should be at least 12-h/week, unless supported by significant kidney function
B. In anuric patient treated 3 times per week, the prescribed target eKt/V should be at least 1.2. Higher eKt/V up to 1.4 should be considered in women and in patients with comorbidity
C. Delivered dialysis dose should be measured monthly
D. Dialysis treatment time and/or frequency should be increased in patients who remain hypertensive despite maximum possible fluid removal
E. All of the above

The answer is E

The current European Best Practice Guideline recommendations for dialysis strategies include all of the above dialysis prescriptions to improve dialysis outcomes (E is correct).

In addition, the guideline recommends the use of synthetic high-flux membranes to delay or reduce long-term complications of HD therapy, such as dialysis-related amyloidosis, to improve hyperphosphatemia, to reduce cardiovascular risk, and to improve anemia.

Suggested Reading

Kuhlmann MK, Kotanko P, Levine NW. Hemodialysis: Dialysis prescription and adequacy. In: Feehally J, Floege J, Tonelli M, et al., editors. Comprehensive clinical nephrology. 6th ed. Philadelphia: Elsevier; 2019. p. 1082–9.

Tattersall J, Martin-Malo A, Pedrini L, et al. EBPG guideline on dialysis strategies. Nephrol Dial Transpl. 2007;22(suppl 2): ii5–ii21m.

5. You started a 50-year-old man with eGFR 7 mL/min on hemodialysis (HD) 3 times per week because of poor appetite. He has a functional AVF created 9 months ago. The patient wants more frequent in-center HD sessions in preparation for home HD in the future, and he wants to know the benefits and risks associated with frequent HD. **Which one of the following choices regarding the risks and benefits of frequent HD is CORRECT?**

A. Improved death outcome
B. Improved LV mass index
C. Improved HTN and phosphate
D. More vascular access complications
E. All of the above

The answer is E

Several small studies have shown better outcomes in patients who received frequent HD treatments. Compared to these small studies, a larger study with 245 patients on frequent in-center HD was published in 2010. In this study, called Frequent Hemodialysis Network (FHN) trial, 125 patients were allocated to conventional HD (3 times per week) and 120 patients to 6 times per week schedule. The study duration was 12 months. Table 9.1 **shows the study design, characteristics, achieved time, fluid removal (ultrafiltration, UF), and Kt/v of the two cohorts of patients.**

Table 9.1 FHN trial results

Mode of dialysis	No.	Hr/week	UF/week	Kt/v/week
Conventional (3×/week)	125	10.4	8.99 L	2.49
Frequent (6×/week)	120	12.7	10.58 L	3.54

The following improved outcomes were observed in the frequent HD patients:

1. **Coprimary outcomes: Death and decrease in LV mass index**
2. **HTN with less number of antihypertensives**
3. **Phosphate**
4. **Physical-health composite score**

In both groups, there were few deaths and the authors of FHN trial concluded that the study was not sufficiently powered to allow for a survival conclusion.

Adverse events

1. **More AV access thromboses and other complications, most likely related to frequent cannulations**

No changes were observed in

1. **Cognitive function**
2. **Anemia and ESA use**
3. **Albumin**

In a subsequent study, the long-term follow-up of the above two cohorts (245 patients) was reported. After the initial 12-month intervention, all patients returned to the conventional HD (3×/week) schedule. The patients were followed for a median of 3.6 years (range 1.5–5.3 years) to observe the long-term outcomes of the 12-month frequent in-center HD intervention. During the follow-up, 16% (20 of 125 patients) in the frequent HD cohort and 28% (34 of 120 patients) in the conventional HD cohort died. The difference between the cohorts was significant, suggesting that frequent HD has survival advantage over conventional HD. Thus, option E is correct.

However, the FHN Nocturnal Trial, which included only 87 patients (45 conventional HD, and 42 nocturnal HD), did not find any difference in any one of the above observations.

Suggested Reading

Chertow GM, Levin NW, Beck GJ, et al. In-center hemodialysis six times per week versus three times per week. FHN Trial Group. N Engl J Med. 2010;363:2287–300.

Chertow GM, Levin NM, Beck GJ, et al. Frequent Hemodialysis Network (FHN) Trials Group. Long-term effects of frequent in-center hemodialysis. J Am Soc Nephrol. 2016;27:1830–6.

Diaz-Buxo JA, White SA, Himmele R. Frequent hemodialysis: a critical review. Sem Dial. 2013;26:578–89.

Morfin JA, Fluck RJ, Weinhandl ED, et al. Intensive hemodialysis and treatment complications and tolerability. Am J Kidney Dis. 2016;68(suppl 1):S43–S50.

Rocco MV, Lockridge RS, Beck GJ, et al. The effects of frequent nocturnal home hemodialysis: the Frequent Hemodialysis Network Nocturnal trial. Kidney Int. 2011;80:1080–91.

6. Six months later, the above patient showed interest in home HD. **Which one of the following regarding home HD compared to in-center HD is CORRECT?**

   A. Home HD is the best modality for patients with uncontrolled seizures
   B. Patients with hypoglycemia should be recommended to have home HD
   C. Improved patient survival has been reported with home HD
   D. In-center HD < 4 h is better to improve extracellular fluid volume than home HD
   E. In-center HD is the best approach to improve cardiovascular complications than home HD

The answer is C

There are no specific guidelines to address the selection of RRT for patients with ESKD; many nephrologists offer several options to patients with ESKD, including preemptive transplantation, conservative care, and other dialysis modalities. If the patient's preference is dialysis, either peritoneal dialysis or home HD is recommended. Although there are more patients on in-center HD, the preference for home HD is increasing. The prevalence rate of home HD varies from 5 to 15%. The most important prerequisite for home HD is the patient's willingness or partner who is able to perform dialysis safely. The suitability of home environment for HD will then be assessed.

Uncontrolled seizures, recurrent hypoglycemia, noncompliance to medical care and volume status, and frequent nursing interventions are relative contraindications for home HD. Thus, all choices except C are incorrect.

Weinhandl and colleagues reviewed the evidence for survival rate between daily home HD and matched thrice-weekly in-center HD patients and concluded that risk of death in the former treatment group was 13% and 18% lower in intention-to-treat and as-treated analyses, respectively. They attributed this lower risk of death in daily

home HD patients to reduced cardiovascular and other unknown causes. Also, another study by Stack and colleagues showed that home HD patients are 26% less likely to die compared to in-center HD patients. Thus, these reports suggest survival benefit in patients who are on home HD (C is correct).

Other investigators in their reviews of home HD also demonstrated improved clinical outcomes such as improved survival, cardiovascular, nutritional, and quality of life. Although home HD may not be preferred by all patients, the nephrologist should offer it as a modality choice for renal replacement therapy.

Suggested Reading

Miller BW, Himmele R, Sawin D-A, et al. Choosing home hemodialysis: a critical review of patient outcomes. Blood Purif. 2018;45:224–9.

Nesrallah GE, Suri RS, Lindsay RM, et al. Home and intensive hemodialysis. In: Daugirdas JT, Blake PG, Ing TS, editors. Handbook of dialysis. 5th ed. Philadelphia: Wolters Kluwer; 2015. p. 305–20.

Stack AG, Mohammed W, Elsayled M, et al. Survival difference between home dialysis therapies and in-center haemodialysis: a national cohort study. J Am Soc Nephrol. 2014;SA-PO957.

Walker RC, Howard K, Morton RL. Home hemodialysis: a comprehensive review of patient-centered and economic considerations. Clinicoecon Outcomes Res. 2017;9:149–61.

Weinhandl ED, Liu J, Gilbertson DT, et al. Survival in daily home dialysis and matched thrice-weekly in-center hemodialysis patients. J Am Soc Nephrol. 2012;23:895–904.

7. A 60-year-old thin small woman on a 4-h session HD 3 times per week asks you to reduce her time to 3 and ½ h, as her eKt/V is 1.4. Her postdialysis BP is 150/86 mm Hg, and her interdialytic weight gain is 3 kg. **Which one of the following choices regarding short in-center HD is CORRECT?**

   A. Short HD is associated with an increase in systolic BP (SBP)
   B. Short HD is associated with inadequate solute removal
   C. Short HD causes intradialytic hypotension
   D. Similar to skipped dialysis treatments, short HD is associated with increased mortality
   E. All of the above

   The answer is E

   Studies have shown that shorter delivered HD treatments were associated with high SBP, inadequate solute removal, intradialytic hypotension, as well as high mortality. Thus, E is correct. Similar to shortening dialysis, skipped dialyses are associated with high all-cause mortality. It was found that each skipped HD session was associated with a 10% increase in mortality rate. However, shortening of three or more sessions in a month was associated with 20% mortality.

   In this thin and small person, a longer session time and maintenance of Kt/V of 1.4 is recommended by the HEMO study.

   Suggested Reading

Hakim RM, Saha S. Dialysis frequency versus dialysis time, that is the question. Kidney Int. 2014;85:1024–9.

Tandon T, Sinha AD, Agarwal R. Shorter delivered dialysis times associated with a higher and more difficult to treat blood pressure. Nephrol Dial Transpl. 2013;28:1562–8.

8. Fluid gain during interdialytic HD treatments is a risk factor for all-cause and cardiovascular (CV) mortality. Your patient with congestive heart failure (CHF) who weighs 80 kg gained 5 kg between 2 successive treatments. **Which one of the following is the desired and recommended ultrafiltration (UF) rate in this patient?**

   A. Remove all 5 kg in 4 h
   B. Remove 25 mL/h/kg
   C. Remove 10 mL/h/kg
   D. Remove 10–13 mL/h/kg
   E. Remove 5 mL/h/kg

   The answer is C

   Interdialytic fluid gain is rather common in many HD patients. Patients who have excess fluid gain are at increased risk for HTN, LVH, CHF, and CV-associated mortality. At the start of HD, each patient has prescribed an estimated dry weight (EDW), which is defined as "the lowest tolerated postdialysis weight achieved with minimal

signs or symptoms of hypo- or hypervolemia." Although this definition is incomplete, most of the nephrologists try to achieve EDW in their patients. This requires frequent adjustment of EDW because of weight gain due to fluid intake, Na⁺ intake, or improvement in nutritional status.

Despite adequate education, some patients have excess interdialytic weight gain of >2.5 L. In such patients, data from the Hemodialysis (HEMO) study showed that UF rate >13 mL/h/kg was associated with increased all-cause or CV mortality. UF rates between 10 and 13 mL/h/kg were not associated with all-cause or CV mortality, but they were significantly higher in patients with CHF. Cubic spine analysis showed a steep rise in the risk for all-cause and CV mortalities at UF rates >10 mL/h/kg. Thus, UF rate of 10 mL/h/kg seems appropriate (C is correct), and other UF rates or removal of the entire gained volume are inappropriate in this patient. Additional treatments or longer treatment sessions may be appropriate to achieve EDW in this patient.

Suggested Reading

Flythe JE, Kimmel SE, Brunelli SM. Rapid fluid removal during dialysis is associated with cardiovascular morbidity and mortality. Kidney Int. 2011;79:250–7.

Huand S-H S, Filler G, Lindsay R, et al. Euvolemia in hemodialysis patients: a potentially dangerous goal?. Sem Dial. 2015;28:1–5.

9. The above patient received several additional sessions of HD with an UF rate of 10 mL/h/kg. His eKt/v is 1.3, and serum albumin is 4.1 g/dL. His interdialytic weight gain is 1.6 kg with fluid and sodium restriction. His BP at time of dialysis initiation is 144/82 mm Hg. During one of his sessions, he started developing hypotension without any UF. His hypotension improves with administration of 500 mL of normal saline. During the next HD session, the patient develops intradialytic hypotension. **Which one of the following approaches seems reasonable to improve his hypotension?**

   A. Lower his antihypertensive medications
   B. Prescribe Na^+ modeling
   C. Continue saline infusion during each session
   D. Evaluate estimated dry weight (EDW)
   E. Midodrine 10 mg 1 h before HD

   The answer is D

   The appropriate choice to improve his interdialytic hypotension is reevaluation of his EDW (D is correct). Lowering EDW may prevent the development of hypotension. Lowering his antihypertensive medication may increase his predialysis BP, and Na^+ modeling will raise his serum Na^+ as well as thirst. Without addressing his dry weight, saline infusion should not be continued, and midodrine is inappropriate in this patient as his predialysis BP is adequate.

   Suggested Reading

Hecking M, Karaboyas A, Antlanger M, Significance of interdialytic weight gain versus chronic volume overload: consensus opinion. Am J Nephrol. 2013;38:78–90.

Huand S-H S, Filler G, Lindsay R, et al. Euvolemia in hemodialysis patients: a potentially dangerous goal?. Sem Dial. 2015;28:1–5.

10. A 52-year-old man is being dialyzed 3 times per week using high-flux dialyzer for removal of fluid at 10 mL/h/kg for an interdialytic weight gain of 4 kg. Despite adequate education from the dietician, physician, and additional dialysis session, his interdialytic weight gain did not improve. He says he is depressed because of family troubles, and he does not want to take any antidepressants. **Besides Na^+ restriction in diet, which one of the following therapeutic modalities will improve his interdialytic weight gain?**

   A. Restrict his fluid intake to 600 mL /day
   B. Increase ultrafiltration rate to 15 mL/h/kg
   C. Provide chairside cognitive behavioral therapy
   D. Switch him to peritoneal dialysis (PD)
   E. Switch him to home HD

   The answer is C

   Depression is common in patients on dialysis. About 20 to 44% of ESKD patients have depression. The American Psychiatric Association guidelines suggest that psychotherapy, particularly cognitive behavioral therapy, and

selective serotonin reuptake inhibitors (SSRIs; fluoxetine, sertraline) will help those patients with nonpsychotic major depression. The use of SSRIs in ESKD and PD patients improved depressive scores.

Cukor et al. evaluated the efficacy of individual chairside cognitive behavioral therapy in 33 HD depressive patients and 26 waitlist control groups on depression, quality of life, and fluid adherence for 3 months. The effect was assessed at 3 and 6 months. Depression was measured in three different ways. Overall, the study showed that individual cognitive behavioral therapy is effective in improving depression scores, fluid adherence, and quality of life (C is correct). However, this positive effect did not last after 6 months, suggesting the requirements for persistent cognitive behavioral therapy.

Other choices such as fluid restriction, switching him to PD or home dialysis, are not appropriate for this patient. It is known that UF >15 mL/h/kg is associated with increased cardiovascular morbidity and should not be applied for any fluid overloaded patient.

Suggested Reading

Cukor D, Ver Halen N, Asher DR, et al. Psychosocial intervention improves depression, quality of life, and fluid adherence in hemodialysis. J Am Soc Nephrol. 2014;25:196–206.

Kimmel PL. Psychosocial factors in dialysis patients. Kidney Int. 2001;59: 1599–613.

11. Hemodiafiltration (HDF) combines both diffusion and convection. **Which one of the following clinical benefits of HDF is FALSE?**

A. HDF removes middle molecules more efficiently than high-efficiency or high-flux dialysis
B. Phosphate removal is much higher than high-efficiency or high-flux dialysis
C. Removal of inflammatory cytokines is better or higher with HDF than high-efficiency or high-flux dialysis
D. Preservation of residual kidney function is much better with HDF than high-efficiency or high-flux dialysis
E. Improvement in albumin and other markers of nutrition is better with HDF than high-efficiency or high-flux dialysis

The answer is E

HDF is a modality that combines both diffusion and convection. This technique requires large ultrapure volumes of replacement fluid. This fluid can be infused pre-, post-, or mixed dilution modes. Because of convection, many uremic toxins that have a molecular weight of up to 40,000 daltons can be removed. As a result, many biochemical abnormalities associated with ESKD or uremia can be improved. Removal of middle molecules such as β_2-microglobulin is 30–40% higher with HDF compared to high-flux dialysis. Similarly, removal of phosphate mass with HDF is 15–20% higher than other HD modalities. It has been shown that cytokine removal is much higher with HDF, and preservation of residual kidney function is prolonged with HDF. However, most studies did not find any significant benefit of HDF in improving nutritional, as measured by either albumin or prealbumin concentrations. Thus, E is false.

HDF has been shown to improve β_2-microglobulin-associated amyloidosis and carpal tunnel syndrome. Also, some studies have shown reduced incidence of intradialytic hypotensive episodes. However, most studies showed no effect of HDF on the usage of erythropoietic-stimulating agents and anemia.

Suggested Reading

Canaud B, Bowry S, Stuard S. Hemodiafiltration. In: Daugirdas JT, Blake PG, Ing TS, editors. Handbook of dialysis. 5th ed. Philadelphia: Wolters Kluwer; 2015. p. 321–32.

Ronco C. Hemodiafiltration: technical and clinical issues. Blood Purif. 2015;40(suppl 1):2–11.

Susantitaphong P, Siribamrungwong M, Jaber BL. Convective therapies versus low-flux hemodialysis for chronic kidney failure: a meta-analysis of randomized controlled trials. Nephrol Dial Transpl. 2013;28:2859–74.

Tattersall JE, Ward RA, on behalf of the EUDIAL group. Online hemodiafiltration: definition, dose quantification and safety revisited. Nephrol Dial Transpl. 2013;28:542–0.

12. **Regarding survival benefit of hemodiafiltration (HDF), which one of the following choices is CORRECT?**

A. The study of Grooteman et al. found no survival benefit compared to low-flux hemodialysis (HD)
B. The study of Ok et al. also found no survival benefit compared to low-flux HD
C. Post hoc analyses of the above two studies found a survival benefit of HDF
D. The ESHOL study of Moduell et al. found that replacement (convection) volume >23 L/session reduces all-cause mortality by 40%
E. All of the above

The answer is E

There are few large trials that evaluated the effect of HDF on all-cause mortality, cardiovascular mortality, and hospitalizations in HD patients. The initial study was that of Grooteman et al., called CONTRAST (CONvective TRAnsport Study) and another Turkish OL-HDF study by Ok et al. showed no difference either in all-cause mortality or death from cardiovascular or nonfatal adverse events, or hospitalizations. However, post hoc analyses of these studies showed a trend toward survival benefit among patients who received high-volume HDF.

The study by Maduell et al. from Spain showed that HDF with postdilution infusion of convection volume between 23 and 25 L/session and >25 L/session caused a 40 and 45% mortality risk reduction, respectively. Also, other outcomes such as cardiovascular mortality, hospitalization, and intradialytic hypotensions were much lower in those patients who received HDF. This study confirmed the post hoc analyses of the above two studies, suggesting that HDF with convections volumes >23 L/session can improve patient survival and other adverse events.

Another study by See and colleagues included 26,961 patients from Australia and New Zealand (HDF = 4110; HD = 22,851) and followed-up for a median of 5.31 (interquartile range 2.87–8.36) years. Compared with standard HD, HDF was associated with a significantly lower risk of all-cause mortality. In Australian patients, there was also an association between HDF and reduced cardiovascular mortality. Thus, HDF seems to have better survival and also lower CV mortality compared to HD (E is correct).

Suggested Reading

Grooteman MPC, van den Dorpel MA, Bots ML, et al. Effect of online hemodiafiltration on all-cause mortality and cardiovascular outcomes. J Am Soc Nephrol. 2012;23:1087–96.

Maduell F, Moreso F, Pons M, et al. High-efficiency postdilution online hemodiafiltration reduces all-cause mortality in hemodialysis patients. J Am Soc Nephrol. 2013;24:487–97.

Mostovaya IM, Blankestijn PJ, Bots ML, et al. Clinical evidence on hemodiafiltration: a systematic review and a meta-analysis. Sem Dial. 2014;27:119–27.

Ok E, Asci G, Toz H, et al. Mortality and cardiovascular events in online haemodiafiltration (OL-HDF) compared with hig-flux dialysis: results from the Turkish OL-HDF Study. Nephrol Dial Transpl. 2013;28:192–202.

See EJ, Hedley J, Agar JWM, et al. Patient survival on haemodiafiltration and haemodialysis: a cohort study using the Australia and New Zealand Dialysis and Transplant Registry. Nephrol Dial Transpl. 2019;34:326–38.

13. In hemodiafiltration, ultrapure dialysate and nonpyrogenic substitution fluid are generally used. Some of the complications observed in hemodialysis patients have been attributed to contaminants such as bacteria and endotoxins in ultrapure dialysate. **Which one of the following choices regarding ultrapure dialysate is FALSE?**

    A. Ultrapure dialysate is defined as the fluid that contains viable bacteria of <0.1 colony-forming units (CFU)/mL and endotoxin <0.03 endotoxin units (EU)/mL
    B. By definition, the standard dialysate contains <200 CFU/mL and endotoxin <2 EU/mL
    C. Cuprophane and polyacrylonitrile dialysis membranes are more permeable to endotoxins and promote inflammatory cytokine production than polysulfone and polyamide dialysis membranes
    D. There is substantial evidence that ultrapure dialysate is superior to standard dialysate in reducing the inflammatory cytokine production
    E. The production of inflammatory cytokines in blood of dialysis patients depends on the endotoxin levels and type of dialysis membranes than ultrapure dialysate

The answer is D

Except for choice D, all other choices are correct. The Association for the Advancement of Medical Instrumentation reduced the target limits of viable bacteria and endotoxin to <0.1 CFU/mL and 0.03 EU/mL, respectively, for ultrapure dialysate and to <200 CFU/mL and 2 EU/mL, respectively, for standard dialysate. Thus, choices A and B are correct. Cuprophane and polyacrylonitrile dialysis membranes are more permeable to endotoxins and promote inflammatory cytokine production than polysulfone and polyamide dialysis membranes (C is correct). Because of this high permeability of certain membranes, inflammatory cytokine levels are high in the serum of dialysis patients. Also, the levels of these cytokines are dependent on the level of endotoxin that enters the blood via the permeable membranes (E is correct). However, there are no randomized trials to confirm that ultrapure dialysate is superior to standard dialysate in reducing the cytokine levels and associated complications. Thus, D is false.

However, the use of ultrapure dialysate has been reported to improve anemia, dialysis-related amyloidosis, and nutritional status. Also, reduction in mortality was reported by some studies.

Suggested Reading

Bommer J, Jaber BL. Ultrapure dialysate: facts and myths. Sem Dial. 2006;19:115–9.

Glorieux G, Neirynck N, Veys N, et al. Dialysis water and fluid purity: more than endotoxin. Nephrol Dial Transpl. 2012;27:4010–21.

14. A 51-year-old woman with multiple myeloma (biopsy-proven cast nephropathy) is admitted with a serum creatinine of 10.6 mg/dL and [Ca^{2+}] of 11.8 mg/dL. She is started on thalidomide and bortezomib, and hemodialysis (HD). She responded initially to chemotherapy but became resistant to the second cycle of chemotherapy. She is continued on HD. She asks you about high cut-off HD (HCO-HD). **Which one of the following statements regarding HCO-HD is CORRECT?**

A. HCO-HD is a better modality in removing monoclonal free light chains (FLC) than conventional HD
B. Removal of FLC by plasmapheresis is more efficient than HCO-HD
C. Several early nonrandomized clinical trials have shown dialysis independence in more than 50% of patients with HCO-HD who responded to chemotherapy
D. Clinical trials done so far with HCO-HD did not include any controls to evaluate the efficacy of this procedure
E. Recent randomized clinical trials showed no long-term dialysis independence

The answer is E

The most common cause of acute kidney injury in patients with multiple myeloma is cast nephropathy. The casts are composed of monoclonal FLC and Tamm-Horsfall protein that are formed in the distal and collecting ducts, and cause tubular obstruction and atrophy with the release of inflammatory cytokines. The net result is interstitial damage and fibrosis.

Light chains are of two types: k-chains and λ-chains with molecular weights of 22,500 and 45,000 daltons (or 22.5 and 45 kDa), respectively. These FLCs are freely filtered at the glomerulus and reabsorbed by the proximal tubules. The proximal tubule cannot handle the excess production of these FLC in multiple myeloma, resulting in cast formation and tubular obstruction. Therefore, extracorporeal therapies have been used in addition to chemotherapy to remove the excess FLC. Rapid reduction of FLC has been shown to improve kidney function. It was shown that HCO-HD is a better mode of monoclonal free light chain (FLC) removal than conventional HD.

Plasmapheresis removes FLCs because these are confined to the extracellular space. A 2-h treatment is able to remove only 25% of these FLCs, and rebound of these FLCs is substantial following discontinuation of plasmapheresis. Probably this is one of the reasons for the lack of effect of plasmapheresis on the recovery of kidney function in one of the larger studies involving 104 patients with AKI. Similarly, high-flux HD cannot remove these FLCs unless hemodiafiltration is applied.

In order to achieve a better removal of FLCs, the HCO-HD was introduced. In this technique, the hemofilters with large pores that can remove proteins with 45,000 to 65,000 daltons and large surface area 1.1 to 2.1 m² have been developed. Using one of these filters, a few clinical trials, involving 5, 19, and 67 patients, showed that >50% of patients improved their kidney function without dialysis. However, this improvement was seen in those patients who responded to chemotherapy. Non-responders did not improve their kidney function. One of the major problems with these clinical trials is lack of appropriate controls. Therefore, the renal recovery in >50% of patients cannot be attributed to HCO-HD alone.

Two randomized clinical trials have reported their results on the efficacy of HCO-HD in patients with cast nephropathy. The first trial, called the MYRE study, randomized 46 patients to HCO-HD (8 5-h sessions over 10 days) and 48 patients to a conventional high-flux dialyzer. All patients received the same chemotherapy regimen of bortezomib and dexamethasone. The primary end point was HD independence at 3 months, and secondary end points were HD independence rates at 6 and 12 months as well as HD and chemotherapy-related adverse effects. At 3 months, there was no difference in dialysis independence between the two treatment modalities. However, at 6 and 12 months, more patients in the HCO-HD patients achieved dialysis independence compared to the high-flux HD patients. Despite these beneficial effects, the overall survival was not different between the two groups of patients. Thus, the study did not show any benefit of HCO-HD on survival in patients with cast nephropathy and acute kidney injury. Also, there were more adverse effects with HCO-HD modality.

The second randomized trial, EuLITE trial, randomized 43 patients to HCO-HD and 47 patients to high-flux HD. After 3 months, 24 (56%) patients in the HCO-HD group and 24 (51%) patients in the high-flux-HD group were independent of dialysis. This difference was not statistically different. Adverse events were more in the HCO-HD than in the high-flux-HD group at 3 months and also at 2-year follow-up. Similar to the first trial, this trial also did not observe any benefit of HCO-HD in patients with cast nephropathy and acute kidney injury (answer E is correct).

The answer to the patient's question is that the HCO-HD may not be that helpful to her in terms of dialysis independence, survival, and adverse events.

Suggested Reading

Bridoux F, Carron P-L, Pegourie B, et al. for the MYRE Study Group. Effect of high-cutoff hemodialysis vs conventional hemodialysis on hemodialysis independence among patients with myeloma cast nephropathy a randomized clinical trial. JAMA. 2017;318:2099–110.

Cockwell P, Cook M. The rationale and evidence base for the direct removal of serum-free light chains in the management of myeloma kidney. Adv Chronic Kidney Dis. 2012;19:324–32.

Curti A, Schwarz A, Trachsler J, et al. Therapeutic efficacy and cost effectiveness of high cut-off dialyzers compared to conventional dialysis in patients with cast nephropathy. PLos One. 2016. https://doi.org/10.1371/journal.pone.0159942.

Finkel KW. Is high cut-off hemodialysis effective in myeloma kidney?. Sem Dial. 2014;27:234–6.

Hutchison CA, Cockwell P, Moroz V, et al. High cutoff versus high-flux haemodialysis for myeloma cast nephropathy in patients receiving bortezomib-based chemotherapy (EuLITE): a phase 2 randomised controlled trial. Lancet Haematol. 2019;6:e217–228.

15. You are following a patient with CKD 4 (eGFR 22 mL/min) and you plan to place a native arteriovenous (AV) fistula. **Which one of the following is the MOST preferred fistula for your patient?**

   A. Radiocephalic fistula
   B. Brachiocephalic fistula
   C. Brachiobasilic transposition fistula
   D. AV graft
   E. Any one of the above

   The answer is A

   Currently, there are several options for creation of vascular accesses at different anatomical locations of the body. In general, the preferred initial site is the wrist in a nondominant arm. Therefore, the radiocephalic access is the preferred AV fistula for any patient (A is correct). Once distal sites are exhausted, creation of a fistula in the upper arm should be considered, and brachiocephalic or brachiobasilic fistulas are placed. The AV graft has less survival compared to the fistula, and is not the preferred access in most of the patients. The concept of FISTULA FIRST is introduced because of superior outcomes with a fistula compared to a graft.

   Suggested Reading

Agarwal AK. Vascular access for hemodialysis: types, characteristics, and epidemiology. In: Asif A, Agarwal AK, Yevzlin AS, Wu S, Beathard G, editors. Interventional nephrology. New York: McGraw Hill; 2012, p. 101–20.

Fistula First: National Vascular Access Improvement Initiative. Available at http://www.fistulafirst.org.

Lok CE, Huber TS, Lee T, et al. KDOQI Vascular Access Guideline Work Group. KDOQI clinical practice guideline for vascular access: 2019 update. Am J Kidney Dis. 2020;75(4)(suppl 2):S1–S164.

Santoro D, Benedetto F, Mondello P, et al. Vascular access for hemodialysis: current perspectives. Int J Nephrol Renovasc Dis. 2014;7:281–94.

16. The above patient has radiocephalic fistula, and he comes to your office 4 weeks after fistula creation. **Which one of the following measurements suggests that the fistula is functioning properly and will be ready in 3 months for cannulation?**

   A. Vein diameter 2 mm and access flow rate 300 mL/min
   B. Vein diameter 3 mm and access flow rate 400 mL/min

C. Vein diameter 4 mm and access flow rate 450 mL/min
D. Vein diameter 6 mm and access flow rate 600 mL/min
E. Vein diameter 2.8 mm and access flow rate 350 mL/min

The answer is D

Generally, 28–53% of AV accesses never mature adequately to be usable for dialysis. When mature, the median time for maturity is 98 days. The KDOQI guidelines defined the "rule of 6s" as the criteria for maturation of the fistula, which include (1) vein diameter of 6 mm, (2) access flow rate of 600 mL/min, and (3) access depth of 6 mm below the skin. According to the study of Robbin et al., the vein diameter >4 mm and access flow rate >500 mL/min are highly predictive of fistula maturation and adequate for cannulation. Based on these criteria, choice D is correct, suggesting that the fistula is maturing properly. Other choices are incorrect.

Suggested Reading

Huber TS. Hemodialysis access: general considerations. In: Cronenwett JL, editor. Rutherford's vascular surgery. 8th ed. Philadelphia: Elsevier Saunders; 2012. p. 1082–98.

Robbin ML, Chamberlain NE, Lockhart ME, et al. Hemodialysis arteriovenous fistula maturity. US evaluation. Radiology. 2002;225:59–64.

17. A radiocephalic arteriovenous fistula (AVF) was created in your 60-year-old African American diabetic woman 4 weeks ago and is currently not maturing. **Which one of the following variables is associated with failure of fistula maturation (primary failure) is CORRECT?**

A. Age ≥65 years
B. Coronary artery disease (CAD)
C. Peripheral vascular disease (PVD)
D. Hyperlipidemia
E. All of the above

The answer is E

Primary failure of an AVF is defined as the fistula that has never been usable for dialysis or that fails within 3 months of use. A Canadian study by Lok et al. showed that all of the above variables are associated with primary failure of the native fistula by univariate analysis (E is correct). Although diabetes was found to be associated with primary failure of the fistula by univariate analysis, it was not significant by multivariate analysis. However, other studies found that diabetes is a risk factor for maturation of the fistula. In the study of Lok et al., male gender and white race were found to decrease the risk for maturation.

By using age, CAD and PVD, and other variables, Lok et al. developed a predictive risk score system to assess the most appropriate choice of access for an individual patient. They classified the risk categories into low risk (score <2 points), moderate risk (2–3 points), high risk (3.1–7.9 points), and very high risk (≥8 points). Accordingly, low-risk patients will have a failure rate of 24%, moderate risk 34%, high risk 50%, and very high risk 69%. Therefore, patients with very high risk should have a graft rather than a native fistula because of poor maturity. However, one study concluded that Lok model is not predictive of primary failure. It is clear from Lok model that creation of a fistula should be based on patient preference, comorbidities, and other relevant factors.

Bosanquet et al. proposed a different prediction score for radiocephalic fistula patency or survival. Five significant factors were identified: (1) ipsilateral central venous access; (2) age >73 years; (3) anastomosed Vein <2.2 mm; (4) previous lower limb angioplasty; and (5) absent intraoperative thrill (1 point for first three variables, 2 points for the latter two). The CAVeA2 T2 score (maximum 7 points) significantly predicted reduced fistula patency and a reduced rate of successful dialysis. Fistulae with CAVeA2 T2 scores ≥2 had 6-week and 1-year patency rates significantly below pooled published rates. Thus, the above two prediction scores can be used for their patency and use for dialysis before creating a radiocephalic fistula.

Factors that promote AV access maturation include male sex, younger age, nondiabetic status, lower body mass index, and lack of peripheral vascular and coronary artery disease. The reader is referred to the publications of the hemodialysis fistula maturation study for details of the anatomic, physiologic, and functional factors that influence maturation of AVF.

Suggested Reading

Bosanquet DC, Rubasingham J, Imam M, et al. Predicting outcomes in native AV forearm radio-cephalic fistulae; the CAVeA2 T2 scoring system. J Vasc Access. 2015;16:19–25.

Dember LM, Imrey PB, Beck GJ, et al. on behalf of the Hemodialysis Fistula Maturation Study Group. Objectives and design of the Hemodialysis Fistula Maturation Study. Am J Kidney Dis. 2013;63:104–12.

Lok CE, Allon M, Moist L, et al. Risk equation determining unsuccessful cannulation events and failure to maturation in arteriovenous fistula (REDUCE FTM I). J Am Soc Nephrol. 2006;17:3204–12.

Smith GE, Gohil R, Chetter IC. Factors affecting the patency of arteriovenous fistulas for dialysis access. J Vasc Surg. 2012;55:849–55.

Zangan SM, Falk A. Optimizing arteriovenous fistula maturation. Sem Intervent Radiol. 2009;26:144–150.

18. About 20–60% of AV fistulas (AVFs) that are created fail to mature successfully for dialysis use. Pharmacologic intervention has been used to promote postoperative maturation of AVF. **Which one of the following pharmacologic adjuvant therapies as suggested by the 2019 National Kidney Foundation's Kidney Disease Outcomes Quality Initiative (KDOQI) clinical practice guideline for vascular access maturation is CORRECT?**

A. Heparin
B. Clopidogrel
C. Glyceryl-trinitrate
D. Cholecalciferol
E. None of the above

The answer is E

The 2019 KDOQI clinical practice guideline for vascular access does not recommend any one of the above pharmacologic agents as an adjuvant therapy in the perioperative period to improve AVF maturation and reduce the likelihood of primary failure. Thus, answer E is correct. Also, KDOQI does not make a recommendation on the use of clopidogrel-prostacyclin for AVF patency or usability because of inadequate evidence.

Suggested Reading

Lok CE, Huber TS, Lee T, et al. KDOQI Vascular Access Guideline Work Group. KDOQI clinical practice guideline for vascular access: 2019 update. Am J Kidney.Dis. 2020;75(4)(suppl 2):S1–S164.

19. On dialysis rounds, your 58-year-old woman diabetic patient with brachiocephalic fistula complains of hand pain, coldness, and diminished sensation for the past 2 weeks. The fistula was created 6 months ago. You confirm his complaints on your physical examination of the hand and think that the patient has hand ischemia due to steal syndrome. **Which one of the following risk factors predisposes to AV access steal?**

A. Brachiocephalic AV fistula
B. Diabetes
C. Peripheral vascular disease
D. Female sex
E. All of the above

The answer is E

The hemodynamic changes following creation of HD accesses such as an AVF or AVG in the upper extremity can lead to hand ischemia. This phenomenon, termed the "steal syndrome," can lead to significant disability. Steal syndrome can occur within few days (1 week) or several weeks after construction of these accesses. According to the hemodialysis fistula maturation study, 7% of their patients experienced hand ischemia. Terms such as "steal," "arterial steal syndrome," hand "ischemia," "dialysis access-associated syndrome" (DAAS), or "distal hypoperfusion ischemic syndrome" describe the same entity.

An AV access is created by connecting an artery to a vein. Blood flows from the artery to the vein, causing a high-flow low resistance circuit. As a result, distal perfusion pressure decreases because of increased arterial flow into the vein. Also, retrograde flow from the distal artery into the access occurs during each cardiac cycle. Both these processes cause a decrease in distal pressure in the forearm and hand. This phenomenon is called "physiologic steal," which is common in any AV fistula or graft. With time, patients overcome this physiologic steal by

developing inflow arteries, collaterals, and augmenting cardiac output. These hemodynamic changes provide adequate distal pressure to the forearm and hand. Hand ischemia occurs when these adaptive hemodynamic changes fail to compensate for distal hypoperfusion. In addition to the above risk factors (A to D), advanced age (>60 years), large outflow conduits, multiple prior access surgeries of the same arm, and history of hand ischemic episodes may precipitate hand ischemia. The incidence of DASS is much higher with brachiocephalic than with radiocephalic fistula and also higher with AVF than with graft. Thus, answer D is correct.

A patient with DASS has a cool and pale extremity. Tropic changes of the skin and nails may occur. Muscle atrophy and weakness may develop. Some patients may complain of tingling, cramps, numbness, and decreased motor function. Hand pain at rest or on exertion may occur. Some patients may complain of extreme hand pain while receiving hemodialysis. In severe cases, muscle and nerve paralysis, ischemic ulcers, absence of pulses, dry gangrene of the digits, and tissue loss may develop. These signs and symptoms can be categorized into various stages for proper management (Table 9.2)**.**

Table 9.2 Stages of DASS

Stage	Signs and symptoms
1	Pale and cool hand without pain. No or slight cyanosis of nail beds, mild coldness of skin
2	Disturbing coldness in hand or fingers, hand pain on excursion, or during dialysis, cramps, numbness
3	Rest pain, motor dysfunction of hand or fingers
4	Gangrene of digits, ulcers, or tissue loss

Suggested Reading

Beathard GA, Spergel LM. Hand ischemia associated with dialysis vascular access: an individualized access flow-based approach to therapy. Sem Dial. 2013;26:287–314.

Iwuchukwu CO, Costanza MJ. Access Complications. In: Gahtan V, Costanza MJ, editors. Essentials of vascular surgery for the general surgeon. New York: Springer; 2015. p. 267–84.

Huber TS, Larive B, Imrey PB, et al. for the HFM Study Group. Access related hand ischemia and the hemodialysis fistula maturation study. J Vasc Surg. 2016;64:1050–8.

Lok CE, Huber TS, Lee T, et al. KDOQI Vascular Access Guideline Work Group. KDOQI clinical practice guideline for vascular access: 2019 update. Am J Kidney Dis. 2020;75(4)(suppl 2):S1–S164.

Salman L, Asif A. New horizons in dialysis access: approach to hand ischemia. Adv Chronic Kidney Dis. 2020;27:208–13.

20. **Which one of the following treatment options is available for a patient with dialysis access-associated syndrome (DASS)?**

A. Percutaneous balloon angioplasty (PBA)
B. Insertion of intravascular stent
C. Banding
D. Proximalization of arterial inflow (PAI)
E. All of the above

The answer is E

The goal of DASS treatment is to improve hand ischemia and preserve AV access. Treatment of DASS depends on the severity of signs and symptoms. As shown in Table 9.1**, treatment for stages 1 and 2 is conservative management and following the patient for progression of the disease. Vasodilating drugs such as calcium channel blockers may relieve some pain. At times, endovascular interventions such as PBA or insertion of intravascular stent may be required for stage 2 symptoms (A and B are correct). Urgent surgical procedures such as banding, access ligation, PAI, DRIL, and RUDI are required for stages 3 and 4 (C and D are correct). Advantages and disadvantages of these interventions are presented in** Table 9.3**.**

Table 9.3 Some surgical treatment options for dialysis access-related syndrome (adapted from Iwuchukwu and Costanza)

Procedure	Advantages	Disadvantages
Banding	Technically easy Saves (preserves) access	Risk of access thrombosis
Access ligation	Technically easy Improves hand perfusion	Loss of access
Proximalization of arterial inflow (PAI)	Saves access	Less effective in accesses with high flow or tissue loss Needs prosthetic conduit
Distal revascularization-interval ligation (DRIL)	Saves access	Technically demanding Brachial artery ligated
Revision using distal inflow (RUDI)	Saves access with shorter bypass conduit Brachial artery remains in continuity	High failure rate

Suggested Reading

Beathard GA, Spergel LM. Hand ischemia associated with dialysis vascular access: an individualized access flow-based approach to therapy. Sem Dial. 2013;26:287–314.

Iwuchukwu CO, Costanza MJ. Access complications. In: Gahtan V, Costanza MJ, editors. Essentials of vascular surgery for the general surgeon. New York: Springer; 2015. p. 267–84.

Lok CE, Huber TS, Lee T, et al. KDOQI Vascular Access Guideline Work Group. KDOQI clinical practice guideline for vascular access: 2019 update. Am J Kidney Dis. 2020;75(4)(suppl 2):S1–S164.

Salman L, Asif A. New horizons in dialysis access: approach to hand ischemia. Adv Chronic Kidney Dis. 2020;27:208–13.

21. You have been dialyzing a patient with a graft with a blood flow of 400–500 mL/min for 6 months without any complications. One day you get a call from your nurse that the venous pressure is high and she needs to reduce blood flow to 300 mL/min, and the nurse suspects thrombosis of the graft. **Which one of the following methods of vascular access clinical monitoring would have prevented the access flow dysfunction of the graft?**

    A. Measurement of monthly access flow
    B. Measurement of monthly static venous dialysis pressures
    C. Monthly duplex ultrasound
    D. Physical examination by a qualified health practitioner
    E. None of the above

    The answer is D

    Access flow dysfunction is due to stenosis or thrombus rather than the presence of aneurysms. Clinical monitoring of AV access flow dysfunction includes physical examination (inspection, palpation, and auscultation) to check the vascular access by a knowledgeable and qualified health practitioner to detect signs that suggest the presence of pathology. Of all the above choices, physical examination and clinical assessment are the keys to access maintenance. Although the most common screening tests are access flow and dialysis venous pressure measurements, a review of vascular access monitoring suggests that the physical examination and clinical assessment are the initial assessment strategies than hemodynamic studies. Also, the recent KOQI guideline does not suggest routine AVG surveillance by measuring access blood flow, pressure monitoring, or imaging for stenosis, other than clinical monitoring to improve AVG patency. Thus, D is correct. Follow-ups of other measures have not consistently shown any improvements in outcomes of graft function.

Suggested Reading

Koirala N, Anvari E, McLennan G. Monitoring and surveillance of hemodialysis access. Sem Intervent Radiol. 2016;33:25–30.

Lok CE, Huber TS, Lee T, et al. KDOQI Vascular Access Guideline Work Group. KDOQI clinical practice guideline for vascular access: 2019 update. Am J Kidney Dis. 2020;75(4)(suppl 2):S1–S164.

22. You found no bruit or thrill during physical examination of the newly created radiocephalic fistula and suspected access flow dysfunction. Decreased blood flow in the circuit was also noticed. **Which one of the following choices regarding angioplasty is CORRECT?**

A. Angioplasty should be performed if >20% stenosis is present
B. Angioplasty should be performed if >30% stenosis is present
C. Angioplasty should be performed if >40% stenosis is present
D. Angioplasty should be performed if >50% stenosis is present
E. Angioplasty should be performed if >60% stenosis is present

The answer is D

In 2006, a collaborative group that consisted of nephrologists, vascular surgeons, transplant surgeons, and interventional radiologists created and published the KDOQI guidelines and the Fistula First program for the management of dialysis patients. These guidelines recommended that fistulas and grafts should be evaluated routinely for such complications as stenosis, thrombus, and low blood flows. According to these guidelines, angioplasty should be performed if >50% stenosis is present in either the arterial or venous limbs. Successfully treated lesions should have <30% residual stenosis. Thus, option D is correct.

Suggested Reading

Bountouris J, Kritikou G, Degermetzoglou N, et al. A review of percutaneous transluminal angioplasty in hemodialysis fistula. Int J Vasc Med. 2018;Article ID 1420136, 5 pages.
KDOQI: Clinical practice guidelines for vascular access. Am J Kidney Dis. 2006;48(suppl 1):S176–S247.
Navuluri R, Regalado S. The KDOQI 2006 vascular access update and fistula first program synopsis. Sem Intervent Radiol. 2009;26:122–4.

23. Pharmacologic treatment is an important preventive measure of AV access flow dysfunction. **As per KDOQI 2019 guideline, which one of the following pharmacologic recommendations regarding prevention of AV access flow dysfunction is CORRECT?**

A. Routine use of fish oil or aspirin is not recommended to prevent AVF flow dysfunction
B. Oral fish oil supplementation is recommended to patients with newly created AV grafts to reduce frequency of thrombosis
C. There is inadequate evidence for oral fish oil supplementation to prolong AV graft cumulative patency
D. There is inadequate evidence for simvastatin and ezetimibe to reduce AV graft thrombosis
E. All of the above

The answer is E

Several randomized clinical studies have evaluated the effect of pharmacologic agents such as warfarin, aspirin, dipyridamole, clopidogrel, prostacyclin, simvastatin, ezetimibe alone, or in combination on the prevention of AV access flow dysfunction (stenosis and thrombosis). The results are variable when compared to placebo.

Irish et al. in a randomized clinical study evaluated the effect of fish oil/aspirin or placebo in patients with new AV fistulas and found no benefit in improving primary failures, thrombosis, hospitalizations/emergency department visits, or mortality between fish oil and placebo after 1-year follow-up.

Two studies evaluated the effect of fish oil versus placebo on patency of AV graft. Lok et al. followed patients for 1 year and Bowden et al. for 8 months. In Lok et al. study, primary patency was better at 1 year with fish oil compared to placebo ($P = 0.045$) and no difference at 6 months in Bowden et al. study. However, Bowden et al. reported that the proportion of AVG with thrombosis or required angioplasty was 50% with fish oil versus 40% with placebo. Overall, fish oil has low-risk profile; risks and benefits can be considered within the patient's ESKD Life-Plan. For answers C and D, there was not enough evidence to suggest either oral fish oil to prolong AV graft cumulative patency or simvastatin and ezetimibe to reduce AV graft thrombosis (E is correct).

Suggested Reading

Bowden RG, Wilson RL, Gentile M, et al. Effects of omega-3 fatty acid supplementation on vascular access thrombosis in polytetrafluorethylene grafts. J Renal Nutr. 2007;17:126–31.

Irish AB, Viecelli AK, Hawley CM, et al. for the Omega-3 Fatty Acids (Fish Oils) and Aspirin in Vascular Access Outcomes in Renal Disease (FAVOURED) Study Collaborative Group Effect of fish oil supplementation and aspirin use on arteriovenous fistula failure in patients requiring hemodialysis. A randomized clinical trial. JAMA Intern Med. 2017;177:184–94

Lok CE, Moist L, Hemmelgarn BR, et al. for the Fish Oil Inhibition of Stenosis in Hemodialysis Grafts (FISH) Study Group. Effect of fish oil supplementation on graft patency and cardiovascular events among patients with new synthetic arteriovenous hemodialysis grafts. A randomized controlled trial. JAMA. 2012;307:1809–16.

Lok CE, Huber TS, Lee T, et al. KDOQI Vascular Access Guideline Work Group. KDOQI clinical practice guideline for vascular access: 2019 update. Am J Kidney Dis. 2020;75(4)(suppl 2):S1–S164.

24. A 70-year-old woman is receiving hemodialysis (HD) with an AVF 3 times a week. She is trained to feel pulsation and thrill over the fistula. Twelve hours after completing her HD, she found no pulsation or thrill over the fistula. She calls her HD nurse and told that her fistula is not working. The nurse asked her to come to the dialysis facility for check-up of the fistula. Upon physical examination, the nurse confirms that the fistula is thrombosed. **Which one of the following statements regarding the management of thrombosis is CORRECT?**

    A. Wait until the next HD session for aspiration of the thrombus
    B. Perform ultrasound for access blood follow
    C. Refer patient immediately to an interventionalist for endovascular thrombectomy within 24–48 h
    D. Call a surgeon for an appointment
    E. Arrange for a central venous catheter for next dialysis treatment

    The answer is C

    Thrombosis is a common complication of both AV fistula and graft, the rate is lower in former than the latter. AV graft thrombosis can account for up to 80% of the graft failures due to an underlying stenosis at the venous anastomosis. Therefore, monitoring of either AV fistula or graft is important during each HD treatment by the trained personnel. Once the diagnosis of thrombus is confirmed by physical examination, immediate referral to an interventionalist is mandatory for endovascular thrombectomy. The optimal timing between discovery of thrombus and thrombectomy is not well defined until Hsieh and associates reported that thrombectomy within 24 h of diagnosis confers a higher rate of access patency. In this study, the authors introduced a before- and after-quality initiative thrombectomy policy, and compared data of 165 cases who had thrombectomies 1 year before (control group) and 164 cases who had thrombectomies after the initiation of early intervention thrombectomy policy (intervention group). In the early intervention group, endovascular thrombectomies were performed within 24 to 48 hours of thrombosis diagnosis. At 3 months, the intervention group had a higher primary patency rate than the control group, although this did not reach statistical significance. However, after stratification into AV fistula and graft groups, a significantly higher rate of patency was observed in the fistula and not in the graft group at 3 and 6 months. Thus, the study suggests that a timely thrombectomy approach, in which salvage is attempted within 24 h of thrombosis diagnosis, improves postintervention primary patency of fistula but not graft accesses for dialysis (C is correct). Other options are incorrect.

    Suggested Reading

Hsieh M-Y, Timely thrombectomy can improve patency of hemodialysis arteriovenous fistulas. J Vasc Surg. 2018;67:1217–26.

Lok CE, Huber TS, Lee T, et al. KDOQI Vascular Access Guideline Work Group. KDOQI clinical practice guideline for vascular access: 2019 update. Am J Kidney Dis. 2020;75(4)(suppl 2):S1–S164.

25. **Which one of the following considerations regarding surgical intervention for a failing AV access is CORRECT?**

    A. Endovascular treatment failures
    B. Clinically significant lesions not amenable to endovascular treatment
    C. Situations in which the surgical outcomes are deemed markedly better
    D. All of the above
    E. A and B are only

    The answer is D

    The 2019 KDOQI guideline considers all of the above options for a failing AV access in situations where surgical outcomes are anticipated to be better than alternative options. Thus, answer D is correct.

Suggested Reading

Lok CE, Huber TS, Lee T, et al. KDOQI Vascular Access Guideline Work Group. KDOQI clinical practice guideline for vascular access: 2019 update. Am J Kidney Dis. 2020;75(4)(suppl 2):S1–S164.

26. **Which one of the following statements regarding hemodialysis access type and clinical outcomes is FALSE?**

A. Patients with central venous catheters (CVCs) had increased risk of all-cause mortality, infection rate, major cardiovascular (CV) events, and hospitalization compared to patients with fistulas
B. Patients with CVCs had increased risk of all-cause mortality, nonfatal infection rate, major CV events, and hospitalization compared to patients with grafts
C. Patients with fistulas had increased risk of all-cause mortality, nonfatal infection rate and hospitalization compared to patients with grafts
D. Patients with grafts had increased risk of all-cause mortality, nonfatal infection rate, major CV events, and hospitalization compared to patients with fistulas
E. Patients with native fistulas have decreased all-cause mortality. Decreased infection rate, and decreased hospitalization compared to patients with either CVCs or grafts

The answer is C

Except for choice C, all other choices are correct. A review by Ravani et al. showed that patients with fistulas had lower all-cause mortality, infection rate, and hospitalization compared to patients with either a graft or CVCs. Also, the conclusion of this review was that patients with CVCs have the highest risk for death, infections, and CV events compared to patients with other vascular access types. Of interest is the observation that there was no difference in CV events between patients with fistulas and those with grafts.

It has been reported by the National Healthcare Safety Network that CVCs for HD are more likely to cause central line-associated bloodstream infections (CLABSI) than are AV fistulas and AV grafts by factors of 8.4 and 4.7, respectively. Each CLABSI event is estimated to cost about $45,000. Thus, CVCs for HD cause high morbidity than AV fistulas or grafts.

Suggested Reading

Klevens RM, Edwards JR, Andrus ML, et al. NHSN Participants in Outpatient Dialysis Surveillance: dialysis surveillance report: National Healthcare Safety Network (NHSN)-data summary for 2006. Sem Dial. 2008;21:24–8.
Ravani P, Palmer SC, Oliver MJ, et al. Associations between hemodialysis access type and clinical outcomes: a systematic review. J Am Soc Nephrol. 2013;24:465–73.
Rupp ME, Karnatak R. Intravascular catheter-related bloodstream infections. Infect Dis Clin North Am. 2018;32:765–87.

27. **A tunneled central venous catheter (CVC) for short-term hemodialysis (HD) is considered in which one of the following situations?**

A. AV fistula or AV graft created but not ready for use and dialysis is required
B. Acute transplant rejection or other complications requiring dialysis
C. Peritoneal dialysis patient with complications that require time-limited peritoneal rest or resolution of complication (e.g., pleural leak)
D. Patient has a living donor transplant confirmed with an operation date in the near future (<90 days) but requires dialysis
E. All of the above

The answer is E

The 2019 KDOQI guideline considers all of the above situations for placement of a tunneled CVC for urgent dialysis. Also, tunneled CVC can be used when AV fistula or AV graft complication such as major infiltration injury or cellulitis that results in temporary nonuse until problem is resolved. Thus, option E is correct.

Suggested Reading

Lok CE, Huber TS, Lee T, et al. KDOQI Vascular Access Guideline Work Group. KDOQI clinical practice guideline for vascular access: 2019 update. Am J Kidney Dis. 2020;75(4)(suppl 2):S1–S164.

28. Your patient has a central venous catheter for hemodialysis, and the infection rate is much higher than an AV graft. **Which one of the following sources for infection of the catheter is CORRECT?**

A. Catheter connectors
B. Catheter lumen during dialysis
C. Infused solutions
D. Migration of patient's skin flora into the cannulation site
E. All of the above

The answer is E

Venous catheters can be infected from several sources, including the above despite following the best practice guidelines proposed by the Centers for Disease Control and KDOQI. Also, catheters can colonize infective organisms from recently treated bacteremia (E is correct).

Suggested Reading

Almasri J, Alsawas M, Mainou M, et al. Outcomes of vascular access for hemodialysis: a systematic review and meta-analysis. J Vasc Surg. 2016;64:236–43.
KDOQI: Clinical practice guidelines for vascular access. Am J Kidney Dis. 2006;48(suppl 1): S176–247.
Landry D. Editorial. Central venous catheters and central line-associated bloodstream infections: The best prevention is elimination. NephSAP. 2019;18(3):119–24.
Salman L, Asif A, Allon M. Venous catheter infections and other complications. In: Daugirdas JT, Blake PG, Ing TS, editors. Handbook of dialysis. 5th ed. Philadelphia: Wolters Kluwer; 2015. p. 155–71.

29. On a routine examination, you found erythema, discharge, and tenderness at the exit site of the venous catheter. There is no tunnel tenderness or purulence. **Which one of the following steps in the management of the catheter is CORRECT?**

A. Meticulous care of the exit site
B. Apply antibiotic to the exit site and start oral antibiotics to cover Gram-positive organisms
C. Nasal swab for colonization of Staphylococcal (Staph) organisms
D. Remove catheter once the blood cultures are positive, or the patient has fever and leukocytosis
E. All of the above

The answer is E

All of the above choices are correct in the management of exit site or systemic infections (E is correct). Meticulous cleaning of the exit site is always helpful. Generally, infection with coagulase-negative Staph species is common. Application of mupirocin cream or ointment at the exit site and oral antibiotics such as clindamycin (300–600 mg BID) and trimethoprim-sulfamethoxazole (800/150 mg once daily) for 7–10 days may be sufficient for superficial infection. However, some patients may require parenteral therapy, if no improvement in erythema or tenderness. Nasal swab culture is required in some patients to diagnose nasal carriage of Staph aureus and treatment with mupirocin (half tube into each nostril twice a day for 5 days). For systemic infection, removal of catheter and IV antibiotics (vancomycin alone or in combination with aminoglycoside or a third-generation cephalosporin, linezolid for methicillin-resistant Staph aureus, or daptomycin) is indicated.

It should be noted that exchange of the catheter over a guidewire 48–72 h after antibiotic treatment and improvement in fever was found to be more effective than antibiotics alone. This type of treatment is equal to the removal of catheter. However, there are no randomized studies to confirm this observation.

Suggested Reading

Kumbar L, Yee J. Current concepts in hemodialysis vascular access infections. Adv Chronic Kidney Dis. 2016;26:16–22.
Langer JM, Cohen RM, Berns JS, et al. Staphylococcus-infected tunneled dialysis catheters: Is over-the-wire exchange an appropriate management option?. Cardiovasc Intervent Cardiol. 2011;34:1230–4.
Salman L, Asif A, Allon M. Venous catheter infections and other complications. In: Daugirdas JT, Blake PG, Ing TS, editors. Handbook of dialysis. 5th ed. Philadelphia: Wolters Kluwer; 2015, p. 155–71.

30. One of the ways to prevent or treat catheter-associated infection in addition to systemic antibiotics is the antibiotic lock. **Which one of the following organisms is MOST susceptible to the antibiotic lock?**

    A. Staph aureus
    B. Staph epidermidis
    C. Gram-negative organisms
    D. Enterococcus
    E. All of the above organisms

    The answer is C

    The antibiotic lock is indicated as an adjunctive therapy to systemic antibiotics to treat catheter-related blood-borne infections. Therefore, it should not be used alone. The lock consists of very high concentrations of antibiotics, which are instilled into the lumen of the catheter. The antibiotic is usually mixed with either heparin (1000–5000 U/mL) or 4% sodium citrate. This lock sterilizes the catheter biofilm in two-thirds of the patients without removal of the catheter. In the remaining one-third of patients, removal of catheter is necessary because of persistence of infection.

    The antibiotic lock is effective with the following cure rate of the organisms:

    - **Gram-negative bacteria: 87–100%**
    - **Staph epidermidis: 75–84%**
    - **Enterococcus: 61%**
    - **Staph aureus: 40–55%**

    Thus, choice C is correct. It is obvious that the lock is not indicated for Staph aureus infections.

    It is of interest to note that sodium citrate, as a locking solution, is found to lower catheter failure rates and use of thrombolytics compared to heparin (5000 U) locking solution. Also, sodium citrate use was found to be cost-effective compared to heparin.

    Suggested Reading

Allon M. Treatment guidelines for dialysis catheter-related bacteremia: an update. Am J Kidney Dis. 2009;54:13–7.
Arechabala M, Catoni M, Claro JC, et al. Antimicrobial lock solutions for preventing catheter-related infections in haemodialysis. Cochrane Database of 2018, Issue 4. Art. No.: CD010597.
Salman L, Asif A, Allon M. Venous catheter infections and other complications. In: Daugirdas JT, Blake PG, Ing TS, editors. Handbook of dialysis. 5th ed. Philadelphia: Wolters Kluwer; 2015. p. 155–71.
Tapia G, Yee J. Biofilm: its relevance in kidney disease. Adv Chronic Kidney Dis. 2006;13:215–24.

31. **Which one of the following physical examination findings differentiates AV aneurysm/pseudoaneurysm urgent from nonurgent intervention?**

    A. Size of the aneurysm/pseudoaneurysm
    B. Overlying skin depigmentation and thinness
    C. Erosion on aneurysm/pseudoaneurysm
    D. Bleeding from cannulation sites
    E. All of the above

    The answer is E

    After creation of an AV access, particularly AV fistula, several hemodynamic changes occur in both the artery and the vein. These changes lead to an increase in vessel diameter, blood volume, and its flow in the circuit. Although these are physiologic changes, they can become problematic if the vein continues to dilate and becomes aneurysmal. A true aneurysm is a pathologic dilatation of the blood vessel involving all layers of the vessel wall. On the other hand, a pseudoaneurysm is an extraluminal bulging anatomical defect that is common in AV grafts. These aneurysms can cause serious problems, including thrombosis, and life-threatening hemorrhage. Therefore, close monitoring and surveillance of these aneurysms are important.

Aneurysms should be monitored by physical examination during each dialysis treatment for changes in size, the overlying skin for depigmentation, tightness, thinning, ulcerations, and spontaneous bleeding. If the skin is very thin, it is not possible to pinch between the index finger and thumb. This indicates an ominous sign of rupture.

If the size of the aneurysm is enlarging rapidly, the overlying skin depigmented and thin, erosion and ulceration on the skin, and spontaneous bleeding from cannulation sites, urgent intervention is required to save the AV access. There are certain nonurgent interventions that should be recognized to avoid unnecessary treatments. The options presented in the question can differentiate urgent from nonurgent intervention (E is correct, see Table 9.4**).**

Suggested Reading

Inston N, Mistry H, Gilbert J, et al. Aneurysms in vascular access: state of the art and future developments. J Vasc Access. 2017;18:464–72.

Lok CE, Huber TS, Lee T, et al. KDOQI Vascular Access Guideline Work Group. KDOQI clinical practice guideline for vascular access: 2019 update. Am J Kidney Dis. 2020;75(4)(suppl 2):S1–S164.

Valenti D, Mistry H, Stephenson M. A novel classification system for autogenous arteriovenous fistula aneurysms in renal access patients. Vasc Endovasc Surg. 2014;48:491–6.

32. One of your long-standing hemodialysis (HD) patients returns from a 4-week vacation for his regular treatments. He has a brachiocephalic fistula with a large aneurysm. On physical examination, the overlying skin of the aneurysm is depigmented, shiny, and thin. There was some clotted blood, and the patient did not notice it because it was covered with gauge. The dialysis nurse calls you and describes the findings. **Which one of your responses is APPROPRIATE regarding further management is CORRECT?**

A. Clean the blood clot and cannulate in the area next to the aneurysm
B. Refer the patient to his office for examination
C. Ask the nurse to refer the patient to a vascular surgeon immediately
D. Reschedule the dialysis treatment and send the patient home
E. Refer the patient for Doppler ultrasound

The answer is C

From Table 9.4**, one can understand that the patient needs urgent intervention of his fistula and aneurysm. The appropriate next step in the management is a referral to the vascular surgeon for repair of the aneurysm because the physical examination findings are suggestive of impending aneurysmal rupture. Thus, answer C is correct. Other answers are inappropriate.**

Table 9.4 Urgent and nonurgent intervention of aneurysm/pseudoaneurysm by physical examination (adapted from 2019 KDOQI guideline)

Finding	Urgent	Nonurgent
Size	Enlarging	Not enlarging, pseudoaneurysm
Overlying skin appearance	Shiny, thin, depigmented	Mobile skin, supple
Erosions of skin	Ulcers, scabs	None
Arm elevation	No aneurysmal collapse	Aneurysmal collapses
Bleeding from cannulation site	Prolonged	None

Suggested Reading

Balaz P, BjörckM. True aneurysm in autologous hemodialysis fistulae: definitions, classification and indications for treatment. J Vasc Access. 2015;16:446–53.

Inston N, Mistry H, Gilbert J, et al. Aneurysms in vascular access: state of the art and future developments. J Vasc Access. 2017;18:464–72.

33. A 44-year-old woman with diabetes and hypertension is started on hemodialysis (HD) with a central venous catheter (CVC) because of uremia. She was noncompliant with follow-up appointments and medications. She is scheduled for an AV fistula, which will mature in 4–6 months. **What changes in certain laboratory parameters such as hemoglobin**

(Hgb), white blood cell count (WBC), serum albumin, and erythropoietin (ESA) use are expected to observe after switching from CVC to AV fistula or graft for HD?

A. A decrease in WBC
B. An increase in Hgb
C. An increase in albumin
D. A decrease in ESA use
E. All of the above

The answer is E

The study of Wystrychowski et al. reported a change in several laboratory parameters in HD patients after changing their dialysis accesses. Some patients in their cohort required changes from CVCs to AV fistulas or grafts (*N* = 271) and some required switching from AV accesses to CVCs (*N* = 69). The data were compared between these two groups and a group who had only accesses (control; *N* = 1846). They showed that a change from a catheter to an AV fistula or graft was associated with a significant rise in Hgb (0.41 g/dL) and serum albumin (0.12 g/dL), and a decrease in WBC (370 μL). Thus, answer E is correct. Conversely, switching from an AV fistula to a catheter was followed by a significant fall in albumin and a rise in ESA dosage as compared with controls. This study reiterates that a change from CVCs to AV accesses is associated with an improvement in nutrition, anemia, and inflammation, which may account for high survival in HD patients.

Suggested Reading

Wystrychowski G, Kitzler TM, Thijssen S, et al. Impact of switch of vascular access type on key clinical and laboratory parameters in chronic haemodialysis patients. Nephrol Dial Transpl. 2009;24:2194–200.

34. You started a male patient with an AV fistula on hemodialysis, and he wants you to order buttonhole (constant site) cannulation. **Which one of the following complications of buttonhole cannulation compared to the traditional rope-ladder technique or rotating cannulation sites is CORRECT?**

A. Increases hematoma formation
B. Improves patency rate
C. Increases infection rate
D. Increases pain
E. Increases needle sticks

The answer is C

Buttonhole cannulation or technique is a good approach for patients with new fistulas or limited cannulation sites. This technique causes not only few infiltrations and hematoma formation but also causes less pain (one study showed no difference in pain score with buttonhole needling) and fewer needle sticks. However, buttonhole technique causes more infectious complications than the traditional techniques. Thus, C is correct. One study showed that buttonhole technique is not superior to rope-ladder technique in improving primary patency rate (B is incorrect). Increase in hematoma formation is common with rope-ladder technique.

Suggested Reading

Ball LK. The buttonhole technique for arteriovenous fistula cannulation. Nephrol Nurs J. 2006;33:299–305.
Chan MR, Shobande O, Vats H, et al. The effect of buttonhole cannulation vs. rope-ladder technique on hemodialysis access patency. Sem Dial. 2014;27:210–6.
Di Nicolò P, Marina Cornacchiari M, Mereghetti M, et al. Buttonhole cannulation of the AV fistula: a critical analysis of the technique. Sem Dial. 2017;30:32–8.
MacRae JM, Ahmed SB, Atkar R, et al. A randomized trial comparing buttonhole with rope ladder needling in conventional hemodialysis patients. Clin J Am Soc Nephrol. 2012;7:1632–8.

35. A 52-year-old woman with CKD stages 4–5 due to hypertension asks you about her future renal replacement therapies. After discussion of all available modalities, she expresses interest in hemodialysis (HD) and wants to know about AV access in detail from you and your healthcare associates. **A multidisciplinary educational intervention regarding early placement of an AV access is associated with which one of the following favorable outcomes?**

   A. Lower catheter usage at initiation of HD
   B. Delayed initiation of HD
   C. Increases home HD therapy
   D. Lower cost of care, particularly in the first 6 months of HD
   E. All of the above

   The answer is E

   Predialysis educational intervention is an integral part of the management of a patient with stages 4–5. This intervention provides choices from conservative management to modalities of renal replacement therapies, including preemptive kidney transplantation. Once the patient prefers HD, the multidisciplinary team (nephrologist, vascular surgeon, nurse practitioner, dietician, social worker, and a psychiatrist or psychologist) should plan for an AV access placement. Studies have shown that early placement of an AV access for HD therapy is associated with all of the above outcomes. Thus, answer E is correct.

   Suggested Reading

Devins GM, Mendelssohn DC, Barre PE, et al. Predialysis psychoeducational intervention and coping styles influence time to dialysis in chronic kidney disease. Am J Kidney Dis. 2003;42:693–703.
Goldstein M, Yassa T, Dacouris N, et al. Multidisciplinary predialysis care and morbidity and mortality of patients on dialysis. Am J Kidney Dis. 2004;44:706–14.
Lacson E Jr., Wang W, DeVries C, et al. Effects of a nationwide predialysis educational program on modality choice, vascular access, and patient outcomes. Am J Kidney Dis. 2011;58: 235–42.
Wilson SM, Robertson JA, Chen G, et al. The IMPACT (Incident Management of Patients, Actions Centered on Treatment) program: a quality improvement approach for caring for patients initiating long-term hemodialysis. Am J Kidney Dis. 2012;60:435–43.
Yu YJ, Wu IW, Huang CY, et al. Multidisciplinary predialysis education reduced the inpatient and total medical costs of the first 6 months of dialysis in incident hemodialysis patients. PLoS One. 2014;9:e112820.
Zukmin K, Ahmad I, Wynn AK, Lim YY, Naing L, Chong VH, et al. A comparative study to evaluate factors that influence survival in multidisciplinary predialysis educated patients and "Crashlanders". Saudi J Kidney Dis Transpl. 2017;28:743–50.

36. Serum Ca^{2+} plays a significant role in several biologic functions, but it also causes calcification. Dialysate Ca^{2+} concentration varies from ≤2 mEq/L to ≥3 mEq/L in dialysis centers of the world. **From recent clinical studies, which one of the following appears to be the ideal dialysate Ca^{2+} concentration?**

   A. 1.75–2.1 mEq/L
   B. 2.2–2.5 mEq/L
   C. 2.5–2.75 mEq/L
   D. 3.0–3.2 mEq/L
   E. 3.3–3.6 mEq/L

   The answer is C

   Low dialysate Ca^{2+} concentration (<2.5 mEq/L) causes intradialytic hypotension, cardiac arrhythmias, sudden cardiac arrest, and increased PTH secretion. On the other hand, high dialysate Ca^{2+} concentration (>3 mEq/L) causes calcification in a maintenance HD patient. Therefore, prescribing an ideal Ca^{2+} dialysate bath is difficult, and the practice is variable. Studies of Basile et al. and others suggest that the ideal dialysate Ca^{2+} concentration is between 2.5 and 2.75 mEq/L. Also, Ok et al. evaluated the effect of low dialysate Ca^{2+} (2.5 mEq/L) versus high dialysate Ca^{2+} (3.5 mEq/L) bath on coronary artery calcification (CAC) and low bone-turnover disease for 24 months in HD patients. The results showed that progressions of both CAC and low bone-turnover were much less with low dialysate than with high dialysate Ca^{2+} bath (C is correct).

Suggested Reading

Basile C, Libutti P, Di Turo AL, et al. Effect of dialysate calcium concentrations on parathyroid hormone and calcium balance during a single dialysis session during bicarbonate hemodialysis: a crossover clinical trial. Am J Kidney Dis. 2012;59:92–101.

Langote A, MD, Ahearn M, Zimmerman D. Dialysate calcium concentration, mineral metabolism disorders, and cardiovascular disease: deciding the hemodialysis bath. Am J Kidney Dis. 2015;66:348–58.

McGill RI, Weiner DE. Dialysis composition for hemodialysis: changes and changing risk. Sem Dial. 2017;30: 112–20.

Ok E, Asci G, Bayraktaroglu S, et al. Reduction of dialysate calcium level reduces progression of coronary artery calcification and improves low bone turnover in patients on hemodialysis. J Am Soc Nephrol. 2016;27:2475–86.

Pun PH, Horton JR, Middleton JP. Dialysate calcium concentration and the risk of sudden cardiac arrest in hemodialysis patients. Clin J Am Soc Nephrol. 2013;8:797–803.

Rhee CM, Chou JA, Kalantar-Zadeh K. Dialysis prescription and sudden death. Sem Nephrol. 2018;38:570–81.

37. **Which one of the following statements regarding calciprotein particles (CPPs) and vascular calcification (VC) is correct?**

A. Serum CPPs are colloidal nanoparticles that have a prominent role in the initiation and progression of VC
B. The T_{50} test measures the conversion of primary to secondary CPPs, indicating the tendency of serum to calcify in both CKD 4-5 and hemodialysis (HD) patients
C. A higher T_{50} indicates a higher potency of the serum to inhibit calcification, whereas a lower T_{50} suggests progression of VC
D. Higher dialysate Mg^{2+} concentration (>1 mEq/L) increases T_{50} in HD patients
E. All of the above

The answer is E

Serum CPPs are colloidal nanoparticles consisting of proteins such as fetuin-A (major component) albumin and Gla-rich protein and calcium phosphate. These protein-calcium complexes, called calciprotein monomers, undergo further aggregation and maturation to form primary CPP I, which is subsequently converted into secondary CPP II. CPPII has been shown to cause vascular smooth muscle cell calcification, and a simple laboratory test is needed to assess the extent of VC in CKD and dialysis patients. T_{50} test, also called serum calcification propensity test, may fulfill this requirement to follow VC in these patients.

The conversion from CPP I to CPP II is called "ripening" that occurs naturally in serum. The time that takes for this conversion can be measured by nephelometry, and T_{50} represents one-half maximal conversion time of primary to secondary CPPs. A higher T_{50} is beneficial since serum with a higher T_{50} is less prone to calcify tissues compared to serum that has a lower T_{50}. Thus, higher T_{50} is associated with lower risk of VC, cardiovascular events, and death in CKD 4-5 and dialysis patients. Conversely, lower T_{50} represents higher calcification propensity and is associated with higher risk of cardiovascular events and death in these patients.

Bressendorff et al. compared the effect of higher dialysate Mg^{2+} (1 to 2 mEq/L) with that of standard dialysate Mg^{2+} (1 mEq/L) concentration for 28 days on T_{50} in HD patients. The primary end point was the value of T_{50} at the end of the intervention. This study showed that increasing dialysate Mg^{2+} from 1 to 2 mEq/L increased T_{50}, suggesting that higher dialysate Mg^{2+} concentration can decrease calcification propensity and eventually a decrease in cardiovascular events in subjects undergoing maintenance HD. Thus, answers A to D are correct.

Suggested Reading

Bressendorff I, Hansen D, Schou M, et al. The effect of increasing dialysate magnesium on serum calcification propensity in subjects with end-stage kidney disease: a randomized controlled clinical trial. Clin J Am Soc Nephrol. 2018;13:1373–80.

Pasch A. Novel assessments of systemic calcification propensity. Curr Opin Nephrol Hypertens. 2016;25:278–84.

Pasch A, Block GA, Bachtler M, et al. Blood calcification propensity, cardiovascular events, and survival in patients receiving hemodialysis in the EVOLVE Trial. Clin J Am Soc Nephrol. 2017;12:315–22.

Silaghi CN, Ilyés T. Van Ballegooijen AJ, et al. Calciprotein particles and serum calcification propensity: hallmarks of vascular calcifications in patients with chronic kidney disease. J Clin Med. 2020;9:1287. https://doi.org/10.3390/jcm9051287.

38. **Which one of the following statements regarding dialysate Na^+ concentration is CORRECT?**

A. Dialysate Na^+ concentration that is higher than patient's Na^+ concentration reduces symptoms of disequilibrium and intradialytic hypotension
B. Low dialysate Na^+ concentration (5 mEq below serum Na^+) was found to be associated with lower systolic BP and ameliorated intradialytic hypertension compared to high dialysate Na^+ concentration (5 mEq above serum Na^+)
C. The DOPPS (The Dialysis Outcomes and Practice Patterns Study) showed lowest mortality in patients with serum Na^+ concentration <137 mEq/L who were dialyzed with a dialysate Na^+ concentration >142 mEq/L
D. High dialysate Na^+ concentration is associated with high mortality only in those with high predialysis serum Na^+ concentration
E. All of the above

The answer is E

The usual dialysate Na^+ concentration varies between 135 and 145 mEq/L. However, the ideal dialysate Na^+ concentration remains unclear. Low predialysis serum Na^+ level (<135 mEq/L) is associated with low BP and cramps, whereas serum Na^+ level >138 mEq/ L causes increased thirst, weight gain, and high BP. It is known that dialysate Na^+ concentration that is higher than patient's Na^+ concentration reduces symptoms of disequilibrium and intradialytic hypotension (A is correct). A recent study by Inrig et al. showed that low dialysate Na^+ concentration (5 mEq below serum Na^+) is associated with significantly low systolic BP with amelioration of intradialytic hypertension compared to high dialysate Na^+ concentration (5 mEq above serum Na^+). Thus, option B is correct.

The DOPPS showed that the mortality is lower in patients with predialysis serum Na^+ concentration <137 mEq/L when dialyzed against dialysate Na^+ concentration >142 mEq/L (C is correct). This study, therefore, suggests that the risk associated with low serum Na^+ is ameliorated by a higher dialysate Na^+ concentration. However, dialysis of a patient with high predialysis Na^+ concentration against a dialysate that contains high Na^+ concentration can cause several adverse events, including death (D is correct). Therefore, following predialysis serum Na^+, predialysis weight gain, and BP is extremely important in the management of a dialysis patient.

It should be noted that dialysis patients may have individualized "set point" for Na^+, and that low predialysis serum Na^+ concentration does not always reflect over hydration or fluid overload. If a patient's serum Na^+ concentration is low because of low "set point," dialysis with low dialysate Na^+ concentration is advisable.

It should be noted that predialysis serum Na^+ levels are associated with mortality risk. Rhee et al. observed a U-shaped association between predialysis Na^+ level and mortality such that sodium levels <138 mEq/L and ≥144 mEq/L were associated with high mortality risk compared to levels between 138 and 144 mEq/l.

Suggested Reading

Causland FR, Waikar SS. Optimal dialysate sodium-What is the evidence. Sem Dial. 2014;27:128–34.

Hecking M, Karaboyas A, Saran R, et al. Predialysis serum sodium level, dialysate sodium, and mortality in maintenance hemodialysis patients: The Dialysis Outcomes and Practice Patterns Study (DOPPS). Am J Kidney Dis. 2012;59:238–48.

Inrig JK, Molina C, D'silva K, et al. Effect of low versus high dialysate sodium concentration on blood pressure and endothelial-derived vasoregulators during hemodialysis: a randomized crossover study. Am J Kidney Dis. 2015;65:464–73.

Mendoza JM, Arramreddy R, Schiller B. Dialysis sodium: choosing the optimal hemodialysis bath. Am J Kidney Dis. 2015;66:710–20.

Rhee CM, Ravel VA, Ayus JC et al. Pre-dialysis serum sodium and mortality in a national incident hemodialysis cohort. Nephrol Dial Transpl. 2016;31:992–1001.

Rhee CM, Ayus JC, Kalantar-Zadeh K. Hyponatremia in the dialysis population. Kidney Int Rep. 2019;4:769–80.

39. **Which one of the following statements regarding serum potassium (K^+) levels in hemodialysis (HD) patients is CORRECT?**

A. In a study of 2134 patients on HD, a predialysis serum K^+ level of 5.1 mEq/L was associated with the lowest risk of peridialytic sudden cardiac arrest, whereas K^+ levels above and below 5.1 mEq/L were associated with increased risk
B. In another study of 81,013 patients on HD, predialysis serum K^+ levels between 4.6 and 5.3 mEq/L were associated with the lowest incidence of all-cause mortality, and K^+ levels ≥5.6 mEq/L were associated with significantly higher rates of mortality

C. The decrease in serum K^+ levels is much higher with higher dialysate bicarbonate (35 mEq/L) and <2 mEq/L K^+ bath than with lower dialysate bicarbonate (30 mEq/L) and 2 mEq/L K^+ bath during a single HD treatment
D. Consider the use of dialysate K^+ profiling (i.e., start with dialysate concentration of 4 mEq/L and gradually reduce it during the treatment to 2 mEq/L) when predialysis K^+ levels ≥6.5 mEq/L or higher
E. All of the above

The answer is E

About 98% of total body K^+ is present in the intracellular fluid compartment, and only 2% is present in the extracellular fluid compartment. In a patient on HD, dietary K^+ intake is limited to 60 mEq/day. Any additional intake will increase serum K^+ level in an anuric HD patient, and K^+ balance is mostly positive in these patients. Therefore, the function of HD is to remove excess K and to maintain normokalemia. A typical HD treatment of 4 h will remove 70–100 mEq of K^+, and 3 times per week treatments will remove 210–300 mEq. Also, >10% of K^+ is removed from the stool. If intake of K^+ exceeds the removal from these two sources, the patient is in a positive K^+ balance and is prone to develop hyperkalemia. During HD, K^+ removal occurs by diffusion (85%) from the extracellular fluid compartment and by convection (15%) from the intracellular fluid compartment. Rebound of K^+ during postdialysis period is mostly from the intracellular fluid compartment.

All of the above statements are correct with regard to K^+ levels in HD patients. Predialysis hyperkalemia is rather common in HD patients despite adequate dietary and other management efforts. Both hyperkalemia and hypokalemia predispose HD patients to arrhythmias. However, hyperkalemia is more common than hypokalemia in HD patients. Depending on the laboratory, the serum K^+ ranges from 3.5 to 5 mEq/L in the general population. Above 5 mEq/L is generally considered hyperkalemia and may cause adverse effects in this population. Although this definition applies even to HD patients, the adverse effects of hyperkalemia are not that common at this level of K^+. For example, in the study of Pun and associates involving 2134 HD patients, a predialysis serum K^+ level of 5.1 mEq/L was associated with the lowest risk of peridialytic sudden cardiac arrest, whereas K^+ levels above and below 5.1 mEq/L were associated with increased risk (A is correct).

In another study by Kovesdy et al. involving 81,013 patients on HD, predialysis serum K^+ levels between 4.6 and 5.3 mEq/L were associated with the lowest incidence of all-cause mortality, and K^+ levels ≥5.6 mEq/L were associated with significantly higher rates of mortality (B is correct). Another multinational study (DOPPS: Dialysis Outcomes and Practice Patterns Study) also confirmed that predialysis serum K^+ levels between 4 and 5.5 mEq/K were associated with lowest risk and predialysis serum K^+ levels ≥5.6 mEq/L with increased risk of death and arrhythmias. Thus, the definition of hyperkalemia that causes complications varies from study to study.

Generally, bicarbonate lowers K^+ levels in dialysis patients. Using high-flux dialyzers and high dialysate bicarbonate bath, a substantial decrease in serum K^+ was found during a 4-h dialysis treatment compared to a low dialysate bicarbonate bath (Table 9.5). **Also, postdialysis rebound of K^+ was much higher with high dialysate bicarbonate than with low bicarbonate bath. Similarly, dialysate <2 mEq/L K^+ bath lowers serum K^+ level much more than dialysate 2 mEq/L K^+ bath. Thus, adjustment of dialysate bicarbonate and K^+ is necessary to prevent hypokalemia when hyperkalemia is managed during HD treatment (C is correct). It should be noted that removal of K^+ during HD is dependent on serum-dialysate gradient. The following table shows the effect of low and high dialysate bicarbonate levels on serum K^+ level during different times of HD treatment.**

Table 9.5 Effect of dialysate bicarbonate on serum K^+ level (adapted from Heguilén et al.)

Dialysate bicarbonate (mEq/L)	Baseline K^+ level (mEq/L)	15 min	30 min	60 min	240 min
27	5.40	4.96	4.90	4.68	4.24
35	5.38	5.01	4.70	4.30	3.80
39	5.45	4.79	4.48	3.86	3.34

Similar to bicarbonate, dialysate K^+ profiling is also important in managing severe hyperkalemia. It is reasonable to use a 4 mEq/L K^+ initially in patients with predialysis K^+ levels 6.5 or higher to avoid sudden drop in serum K^+ to hypokalemic level by using 1 mEq K^+ bath to avoid any arrhythmia. Then gradual decrease in dialysate K^+ to 2–3 mEq/L is appropriate (D is correct). Postdialysis determination of plasma K^+ level in such hyperkalemic patients is suggested, as the prognosis of postdialysis hypokalemia is not known. In this context, it is important to note that arrhythmias are rather common in patients during and also immediately after the treatment of HD, as reported by Wan and colleagues.

Suggested Reading

Bansal S, Pergola PE. Current management of hyperkalemia in patients on dialysis. Kidney Int Rep. 2020;5:779–89.
Heguilén RM, Sciurano C, Bellusci AD, et al. The faster potassium-lowering effect of high dialysate bicarbonate concentrations in chronic haemodialysis patients. Nephrol Dial Transpl. 2005;20:591–7.
Hung AM, Hakim RM. Dialysate and serum potassium in hemodialysis. Am J Kidney Dis. 2015;66:125–32.
Karaboyas A, Zee J, Brunelli SM, et al. Dialysate potassium, serum potassium, mortality, and arrhythmia events in hemodialysis: Results from the Dialysis Outcomes and Practice Patterns Study (DOPPS). Am J Kidney Dis. 2017;69:266–77.
Kovesdy CP, Regidor DL, Mehrotra R, et al. Serum and dialysate potassium concentrations and survival in hemodialysis patients. Clin J Am Soc Nephrol. 2007;2:999–1007.
Pun PH, Lehrich RW, Honeycutt EF, et al. Modifiable risk factors associated with sudden cardiac arrest within hemodialysis clinics. Kidney Int. 2011;79:218–27.
Pun PH, Middleton JP. Dialysate potassium, dialysate magnesium, and hemodialysis risk. J Am Soc Nephrol. 2017;28:3441–51.
Wan C, Herzog CA, Zareba W, et al. Sudden cardiac arrest in hemodialysis patients with wearable cardioverter defibrillator. Ann Noninvasive Electrocardiol. 2014;19:247–57.

40. **Which one of the following electrolyte abnormalities in hemodialysis (HD) patients is ASSOCIATED with frequent Emergency Department (ED) visits:**

A. Hypercalcemia
B. Hypermagnesemia
C. Hyperphosphatemia
D. Hyperkalemia
E. Hypernatremia

The answer is D

Brunelli and associates investigated an independent association between serum K^+ level and short-term hospitalization risk, mortality risk, and risk for ED visits among 52,734 in-center HD patients, who were treated 3 times a week. Hyperkalemia (serum K^+ between 5.5 and 6 mEq/L) was more common on Friday or Tuesday before long interdialytic interval (about 72 h) than Monday or Wednesday with short interdialytic interval (about 48 h). Higher hospitalization rate was observed when hyperkalemia occurred during long interdialytic interval compared to those whose serum K^+ level was between 4 and 4.5 mEq/L. Also, death and ED visits were significantly higher in those with serum K^+ level >6 mEq/L (answer D is correct). In comparison to hyperkalemia, ED visits for other electrolyte abnormalities are rare, and their abnormalities are detected only when HD patients are admitted for a different cause.

Suggested Reading

Brunelli SM, Du Mond C, Oestreicher N, et al. Serum potassium and short-term clinical outcomes among hemodialysis patients: impact of the long interdialytic interval. Am J Kidney Dis. 2016;70:21–9.
Rhee CM, Chou JA, Kalantar-Zadeh K. Dialysis prescription and sudden death. Sem Nephrol. 2018;38:570–81.

41. **Which one of the following statements regarding magnesium (Mg^{2+}) level and complications in hemodialysis (HD) patients is CORRECT?**

A. Hypomagnesemia is common in HD patients who are malnourished, dialyzed on low dialysate Mg^{2+} (<1 mEq/L) bath, and those receiving proton pump inhibitors (PPIs)
B. Hypomagnesemia is associated with intradialytic hypotension, impaired endothelial function, insulin resistance, and inflammation in HD patients
C. Hypomagnesemia is associated with cardiovascular (CV) and non-CV mortality in HD patients
D. A J-shaped relationship between serum Mg^{2+} level and all-cause mortality was reported in HD patients
E. All of the above

The answer is E

In recent years, Mg^{2+} is receiving great attention with regard to its serum levels and outcomes in HD patients. It plays an important role in cellular activities. Normal levels of serum (plasma) Mg^{2+} range from 1.7 to 2.7 mg/dL

(1.4–2.3 mEq/L). Any deviation from these levels causes serious adverse effects on health and disease. Hypermagnesemia is more common in CKD stages 4–5, and hypomagnesemia is commonly seen in HD patients because of low dialysate Mg^{2+} bath, malnutrition, diarrhea, and PPI use (A is correct).

Hypomagnesemia has been shown to cause intradialytic hypotension, impaired endothelial dysfunction, elevated glucose levels by causing metabolic syndrome, inflammation, and pruritus in HD patients (B is correct).

Observational studies in HD patients have shown that hypomagnesemia causes increased CV mortality (e.g., mitral annular calcification, peripheral arterial calcification, and increased carotid intima-media thickness).

Sakaguchi et al. showed in 142,555 Japanese in-center HD patients a J-shaped relationship between serum Mg^{2+} levels and mortality risk such that Mg^{2+} levels <2.3 mg/dL and levels >3.8 mg/dL were associated with higher mortality, with an optimal level of approximately 2.8 mg/dL. These authors also reported excess non-CV mortality (related infections) in patients with hypomagnesemia. In another study of 27,544 HD patients, Lacson et al. reported that serum levels <1.3 mEq/L were associated with higher rates of death compared to serum levels of >2.1 mEq/L. Another study by Li et al. also showed that serum Mg^{2+} levels <2.0 mg/dL were associated with higher mortality in 9359 HD patients (C and D are correct).

It is of interest to note that very few studies have examined the relationship between dialysate Mg^{2+} concentration and clinical outcomes in HD patients. In a secondary analysis of the study by Lacson et al., no mortality risk was found between dialysate Mg^{2+} concentrations of 0.75 to 1.5 mEq/L and mortality risk. However, a small German study found that HD patients with dialysate Mg^{2+} concentration of 1.5 mEq/L had a better survival rate than patients who received 1.0 mEq/L dialysate bath. More prospective studies are needed to recommend the appropriate dialysate Mg^{2+} concentration for maintenance HD patients.

Suggested Reading

Alhosaini M, Leehey DJ. Magnesium and dialysis: the neglected cation. Am J Kidney Dis. 2015;66:523–31.

Lacson E Jr, Wang W, Ma L, et al. Serum magnesium and mortality in hemodialysis patients in the United States: a cohort study. Am J Kidney Dis. 2015;66:1056–66.

Li L, Streja E, Rhee CM, et al. Hypomagnesemia and mortality in incident hemodialysis patients. Am J Kidney Dis. 2015;66:1047–55.

McGill RI, Weiner DE. Dialysis composition for hemodialysis: changes and changing risk. Sem Dial. 2017;30:112–20.

Pun PH, Middleton JP. Dialysate potassium, dialysate magnesium, and hemodialysis risk. J Am Soc Nephrol. 2017;28:3441–51.

Rhee CM, Chou JA, Kalantar-Zadeh K. Dialysis prescription and sudden death. Sem Nephrol. 2018;38:570–81.

Sakaguchi Y, Fujii N, Shoji T, et al. Hypomagnesemia is a significant predictor of cardiovascular and non-cardiovascular mortality in patients undergoing hemodialysis. Kidney Int. 2014;85:174–81.

Schmaderer C, Braunisch MC, Suttmann Y, et al. Reduced mortality in maintenance haemodialysis patients on high versus low dialysate magnesium: a pilot study. Nutrients. 2017;9(9).

42. Metabolic acidosis is rather common in hemodialysis (HD) patients. Whenever Na^+ modeling is applied, the delivery of HCO_3^- is also altered and acid-base balance is affected. Low serum HCO_3^- concentration is associated with high mortality. **Which one of the following statements regarding serum HCO_3^- concentration in dialysis patients is FALSE?**

A. Serum HCO_3^- concentration <22 mEq/L is associated with higher all-cause mortality in both HD and peritoneal dialysis (PD) patients compared to reference group HCO_3^- concentration (24–25 mEq/L)
B. PD patients were found to have higher serum HCO_3^- concentration compared to HD patients
C. In DOPPS (Dialysis Outcomes and Practice Patterns Study) registry, the dialysate HCO_3^- concentration was positively associated with mortality rate
D. In prevalent PD patients, the mortality rate is higher than prevalent HD patients with time-averaged serum HCO_3^- concentration <19 mEq/L
E. Survival data suggest maintenance of serum HCO_3^- concentration >22 mEq/L in both HD and PD patients

The answer is D

Both metabolic acidosis and metabolic alkalosis are associated with high mortality rate in HD and PD patients. Therefore, maintenance of serum HCO_3^- concentration between 24 and 25 mEq/L is appropriate, but in clinical practice, it is difficult to maintain these reference values in all patients. Several studies have suggested that serum HCO_3^- concentration, 22 mEq/L, is associated with high all-cause mortality (A is correct) in both HD and PD patients. However, PD patients seem to maintain high serum HCO_3^- levels than HD patients at the same dialysate HCO_3^- concentration (B is correct).

Data from the DOPPS registry showed that dialysate HCO_3^- concentration was positively associated with mortality with an adjusted hazard ratio (HR) of 1.08 per 4 mEq/L higher, and this HR was similar (1.07) when dialysate HCO_3^- concentrations between ≥38 and 33–37 mEq/L were compared. Thus, C is correct.

The study of Vashistha et al. suggests a survival advantage for both HD and PD patients who maintain their serum HCO_3^- concentration >22 mEq/L (E is correct). In the same study, the authors reported that the time-averaged serum HCO_3^- concentration <19 mEq/L was associated with 18% risk for all-cause and CV mortality in PD patients compared to 25% risk in HD patients. Thus, statement D is False.

Suggested Reading

Basile C, Rossi L, Lomonte C. The choice of dialysate bicarbonate: do different concentrations make a difference?. Kidney Int. 2016;89:1008–15.

Dobre M, Rahman M, Hostetter TH. Current status of bicarbonate in CKD. J Am Soc Nephrol. 2015;26:515–23.

Kraut JA, Madias NE. Metabolic acidosis of CKD: an update. Am J Kidney Dis. 2016;67:507–17.

Tentori F, Karaboyas A, Robinson BM, et al. Association of dialysis bicarbonate concentration with mortality in the Dialysis Outcomes and Practice Patterns Study (DOPPS). Am J Kidney Dis. 2013;62:738–46.

Vasistha T, Kalantar-Zadeh K, Molnar MZ, et al. Dialysis modality and correction of uremic metabolic acidosis: relationship with all-cause and cause-specific mortality. Clin J Am Soc Nephrol. 2013;8:254–64.

Wu, DY, Shinaberger CS, Regidor DL, et al. Association between serum bicarbonate and death in hemodialysis patients: is it better to be acidotic or alkalotic?. Clin J Am Soc Nephrol. 2006;1:70–8.

43. In prevalent hemodialysis (HD) patients, 25–33% of all deaths are due to sudden cardiac arrest (SCD) or cardiac arrhythmias. **Which of the following predictors is associated with SCD in HD patients?**

A. Age >60 years
B. Diabetes
C. Ischemic heart disease (ISH)
D. Peripheral vascular disease (PVD)
E. All of the above

The answer is E

Cardiovascular disease is the major cause of morbidity and mortality in HD patients, and the single most cause of this mortality is the SCD or arrhythmias. Shastri and associates analyzed the predictors of SCD in 1745 HEMO participants during a median of 2.5-year follow-up, and reported that increasing age, diabetes, ISH, and PVD as predictors of SCD (E is correct). In addition, low serum creatinine and elevated alkaline phosphatase levels were found to be independently associated with SCD. Most of these risk factors are similar to those previously reported by other investigators. It should also be noted that dialyzing patients against low K^+ (<2 mEq/L) and low Ca^{2+} (<2.5 mEq/L) are associated with SCD.

Of interest is that traditional risk factors such as smoking and cholesterol were not associated with SCD. It should be noted that the HD procedure is itself a risk factor for SCD.

In the DOPPS study, the reported rate of SCD was 33.4% in the United States and 6.8% in Sweden, and higher rates of death were associated with shorter dialysis time, low Kt/V, large volumes of ultrafiltration, low dialysate K^+, and use of amiodarone.

Suggested Reading

Bleyer AJ, Hartman J, Brannon PC, et al. Characteristics of sudden death in hemodialysis patients. Kidney Int. 2006;69:2268–73.

Jadoul M, Thumma J, Fuller DS, et al. Modifiable practices associated with sudden death among hemodialysis patients in the Dialysis Outcomes and Practice Patterns Study. Clin J Am Soc Nephrol. 2012;7:765–74.

Makar MS, Pun PH. Sudden cardiac death among hemodialysis patients. Am J Kidney Dis. 2017;69:684–95.

Parekh RS, Meoni LA, Jaar BG, et al. Rationale and design for the Predictors of Arrhythmic and Cardiovascular Risk in End Stage Renal Disease (PACE) study. BMC Nephrology. 2015;16:63.

Pun PH, Middleton JP. Sudden cardiac death in hemodialysis patients: a comprehensive care approach to reduce risk. Blood Purif. 2012;33:183–9.

Rhee CM, Chou JA, Kalantar-Zadeh K. Dialysis prescription and sudden death. Sem Nephrol. 2018;38:570–81.
Shastri S, Tangri N, Tighiourt H, et al. Predictors of sudden cardiac death: a competing risk approach in the hemodialysis study. Clin J Am Soc Nephrol. 2012;7:123–30.

44. **Which one of the following mechanisms is an important cause of sudden cardiac death (SCD) in hemodialysis (HD) patients?**

A. Bradyarrhythmia
B. Ventricular tachycardia
C. High dialysate bicarbonate concentration
D. Left ventricular hypertrophy (LVH) and heart failure with reduced ejection fraction (HFrEF)
E. All of the above

The answer is E

SCD is defined as "an unexpected death due to cardiac causes in a person with known or unknown cardiac disease, within 1 h of symptom onset (witnessed SCD) or within 24 h of the last proof of life (unwitnessed SCD)" (Genovesi et al. 2019). It is the most common cause of death in HD population. The incidence of death is rather difficult to establish because SCD is usually combined that occurred during postdialysis period with sudden cardiac arrest (SCA) occurring during treatment of HD session. For this reason, the European Dialysis Working Group of ERA-EDTA classifies SCD into two separate extradialysis SCD and intradialysis SCA.

It was shown that both bradyarrhythmia and ventricular tachycardia, particularly ventricular fibrillation, may underlie SCD in HD patients. Recent data suggest that the former may be most frequently responsible for the fatal event in HD patients. Some studies also reported asystole for SCD. A relationship between the timing of SCDs and the dialysis session in HD patients was reported by two studies. These studies showed two frequency peaks: one at the end of the longer interdialytic interval and the second immediately after the first dialysis session (Monday or Tuesday) of the week (A and B are correct). It is of interest to note that diabetic patients seem to be particularly vulnerable to SCD, even in the presence of a normal LV ejection fraction and should therefore be monitored more carefully.

Bradyarrhythmias in HD patients seems to be related to β-blockers, predialysis hyperkalemia, cardiac valvular calcification, and obstructive sleep apnea.

A study published in 2008 reported 110 intradialysis SCA cases in HD facilities during a period of 14 years. The initial EKG rhythm was ventricular fibrillation (VF) in 70 (65%) cases, ventricular tachycardia in 2 (2%), pulseless electrical activity in 25 (23%) cases, and asystole in 11 (10%) cases. Thus, VF seems to be the initial arrhythmia for SCA. Of 110 SCAs, 72 (71%) occurred during dialysis treatment, 10 (9.8%) occurred before dialysis, 20 (19.6%) occurred after dialysis, and data for the remaining 8 patients could not be obtained. Installation of automated external defibrillators (AEDs) in dialysis facilities with trained dialysis nurses and timely application of these AEDs prior to the arrival of Emergency Medical service support has been shown to prevent SCAs.

The incidence of intradialysis SCA seems to occur frequently during the first dialysis session of the week. This is attributed to predialysis hyperkalemia and metabolic acidosis. Use of high dialysate bicarbonate concentration and <2 mEq/L dialysate K^+ bath may contribute to SCA. A high dialysate bicarbonate bath can increase CO_2 production and metabolic alkalosis. Also, metabolic acidosis can lower ionized Ca^{2+}. Dialysis can lower K^+ by its removal and also by transporting it into intracellular compartment as metabolic acidosis is corrected by bicarbonate. Thus, bicarbonate can cause hypocalcemia and hypokalemia, which prolong QT interval and predispose to arrhythmias (C is correct).

It has been shown that LVH alone or HFrEF (<35%) alone is a risk factor for arrhythmias and SCD in HD patients. Patients on HD have both concentric and eccentric hypertrophies; the latter is related to fluid overload. Left ventricular mass index seems to be the strongest predictor of ventricular arrhythmias. There is a cumulative effect on SCD if both LVH and HFrEF are combined. The following mechanisms (Table 9.6) **have been attributed to arrhythmogenesis in general population and may apply to CKD patients as well (adapted from Stevens et al.). Thus, answer D is correct.**

Table 9.6 Arrhythmogenic mechanisms in patients with LVH and HFrEF

LVH	HFrEF
↑Subendocardial ischemia ↑Early after depolarizations ↑Sensitivity to pro-arrhythmias due to wall stress Genetic predisposition to LVH and ion channelopathies Diffuse myocardial fibrosis causing conduction and repolarization changes Atrial stretch/dilatation due to fluid overload	Prolonged action potential duration ↑Sympathetic tone ↑Renin-AII-aldosterone axis ↑Interstitial and myocardial fibrosis Scars from previous myocardial infarctions Stunned myocardium (decreased myocardial perfusion) during HD

Suggested Reading

Charytan DM, Foley R, McCullough PA, et al. on behalf of the MiD Investigators and Committees. Arrhythmia and sudden death in hemodialysis patients: protocol and baseline characteristics of the monitoring in dialysis study. Clin J Am Soc Nephrol. 2016;11:721–34.

Canaud B, Kooman JP, Selby NM, et al. Dialysis-induced cardiovascular and multiorgan morbidity. Kidney Int Rep. 2020;5:1856–69.

Genovesi S, Boriani G, Covic A, et al. on behalf of the EUDIAL Working Group of ERA-EDTA. Sudden cardiac death in dialysis patients: different causes and management strategies. Nephrol Dial Transplant. 2019;1–10. https://doi.org/10.1093/ndt/gfz182.

Makar MS, Pun PH. Sudden cardiac death among hemodialysis patients. Am J Kidney Dis. 2017;69:684–95.

Poulikakos D, Hnatkova K, Skampardoni S, et al. Sudden cardiac death in dialysis: arrhythmic mechanisms and the value of non-invasive electrophysiology. Front Physiol. 2019. https://doi.org/10.3389/fphys.2019.00144.

Rhee CM, Chou JA, Kalantar-Zadeh K. Dialysis prescription and sudden death. Sem Nephrol. 2018;38:570–81.

Saravanan P, Davidson NC. Risk assessment for sudden cardiac death in dialysis patients. Circulation: Arrhythm Electrophysiol. 2010;3:553–9.

Stevens SM, Reinier K, Chugh SS. Increased left ventricular mass as a predictor of sudden cardiac death: is it time to put it to the test?. Circ Arrhythm Electrophysiol. 2013;6:212–7.

Wong MC, Kalman JM, Pedagogos E, et al. Bradycardia and asystole is the predominant mechanism of sudden cardiac death in patients with chronic kidney disease. J Am Coll Cardiol. 2015;65:1263–5.

45. Blood pressure (BP) management is rather difficult in hemodialysis (HD) patients. **Despite the availability of several classes of antihypertensive medications, are available, the first-line pharmacologic agent for management of hypertension (HTN) is still debated. Based on the available evidence, which one of the following antihypertensive drugs has been shown to have improved cardiovascular (CV) and other outcomes in dialysis patients?**

A. β-blockers
B. Angiotensin-converting enzyme inhibitors (ACE-Is)/ angiotensin receptor blockers (ARBs)
C. Calcium channel blockers (CCBs)
D. Mineralocorticoid receptor antagonists (MRAs)
E. All of the above

The answer is E

Two meta-analyses reported that lowering of blood pressure (BP) in hypertensive HD patients reduced CV events and all-cause mortality irrespective of drug class (E is correct). Diuretics are less effective in anuric HD patients, but they may be of some use in patients with residual kidney function in improving fluid status. Therefore, clinical trials have been conducted mostly with drugs other than diuretics. All the trials showed reduced CV events and all-cause mortality in dialysis patients. The results of these studies are summarized in Table 9.7.

Table 9.7 Effect of antihypertensive agents on cardiovascular and all-cause mortality in HD patients

Antihypertensive Agents	Results	References
β-blockers	Carvedilol reduced mortality (prolonged survival by 2 years) compared to placebo (standard therapy) in HD patients with dilated cardiomyopathy. Also, hospitalizations were reduced in carvedilol group	Cice et al.
	Atenolol 3×/week reduced CV events and hospitalizations for heart failure compared to 3×/week lisinopril in HD patients with HTN and LVH	Agarwal et al.
ACE-Is/ARBs	Fosinopril did not reduce CV events and mortality compared to placebo in HD patients with LVH	Zannad et al.
	ACE-I/ARB-containing regimens were associated with a lower risk of death compared with β-blockers-containing regimens, but there was no association with CV hospitalizations in HD patients	Shafi et al.
	Losartan/valsartan/candesartan reduced CV events and mortality compared to treatment that did not include ACE-Is or ARBs in HD patients	Takahashi et al.
	Olmesartan did not reduce CV events or all-cause mortality compared to treatment that did not include ACE-Is or ARBs in HD patients with HTN	Suzuki et al.
CCB	Amlodipine reduced CV events compared to placebo in HD patients with HTN	Tepel et al.
MRAs	Spironolactone may reduce cardiocerebral events and mortality compared to placebo in HD patients	Matsumoto et al.
	Spironolactone reduced cardiocerebral events and mortality in HD and PD patients compared to placebo	Lin et al.

Although β-blockers have been suggested as first-line therapy for management of HTN in dialysis patients (Shaman et al.), the study of Shafi et al. suggested that β-blockers are associated with higher CV risks than renin-angiotensin blockers in two large cohorts of patients. Therefore, choosing one of these as first-line or second-line therapy agents depends on the comorbidities of the patients. CCBs, particularly dihydropyridines, as second- or third-line therapy agents may control BP in most of the patients. However, some patients may have resistant HTN and require MRAs to control their BP. Other drugs such as clonidine are also frequently used.

Suggested Reading

Agarwal A, Cheung AK. Mineralocorticoid receptor antagonists in ESKD. Clin J Am Soc Nephrol. 2020;15:1047–9.

Agarwal R, Sinha AD, Pappas MK, et al. Hypertension in hemodialysis patients treated with atenolol or lisinopril: a randomized controlled trial. Nephrol Dial Transpl. 2014;29:672–81. 189.

Cice G, Ferrara L, D'Andrea A, et al. Carvedilol increases two-year survival in dialysis patients with dilated cardiomyopathy: a prospective, placebo-controlled trial. J Am Coll Cardiol. 2003;41:1438–44.

Fravel MA, Bald E, Mony F. Antihypertensive agents in the dialysis patient. Curr Hypertens Rep. 2019;21:5 https://doi.org/10.1007/s11906-019-0909-z.

Iseki K, Arima H, Kohagura K, et al. Effects of angiotensin receptor blockade (ARB) on mortality and cardiovascular outcomes in patients with long-term haemodialysis: a randomized controlled trial. Nephrol Dial Transpl. 2013;28:1579–89.

Lin C, Zhang Q, Zhang H, et al. Long-term effects of low-dose spironolactone on chronic dialysis patients: a randomized placebo-controlled study. J Clin Hypertens (Greenwich). 2016;18:121–8.

Matsumoto Y, Mori Y, Kageyama S, et al. Spironolactone reduces cardiovascular and cerebrovascular morbidity and mortality in hemodialysis patients. J Am Coll Cardiol. 2014;63:528–36.

Sarafidis PA, Persu A, Agarwal R, et al. Hypertension in dialysis patients: a consensus document by the European Renal and Cardiovascular Medicine (EURECA-m) working group of the European Renal Association- European Dialysis and Transplant Association (ERA-EDTA) and the Hypertension and the Kidney working group of the European Society of Hypertension (ESH). J Hypertens. 2017;35:657–76.

Shafi T, Sozio SM, Luly J, et al. For The DEcIDE Network Patient Outcomes in End Stage Renal Disease Study Investigators. Antihypertensive medications and risk of death and hospitalizations in US hemodialysis patients. Evidence from a cohort study to inform hypertension treatment practices. Medicine. 2017;96:5(e5924).

Shafi T, Miskulin DC. Drug selection for treating hypertension in dialysis patients. More to consider than bp-lowering potency. Clin J Am Soc Nephrol. 2020;15:1084–6.

Shaman AM, Smyth B, Arnott C, et al. Comparative efficacy and safety of BP-lowering pharmacotherapy in patients undergoing maintenance dialysis. A network meta-analysis of randomized, controlled trials. Clin J Am Soc Nephrol. 2020;15:1129–38.

Suzuki H, Kanno Y, Sugahara S, et al. Effect of angiotensin receptor blockers on cardiovascular events in patients undergoing hemodialysis: an open-label randomized controlled trial. Am J Kidney Dis. 2008;52:501–6.

Takahashi A, Takase H, Toriyama T, et al. Candesartan, an angiotensin II type-1 receptor blocker, reduces cardiovascular events in patients on chronic haemodialysis- a randomized study. Nephrol Dial Transpl. 2006;21:2507–12.

Tepel M, Hopfenmueller W, Scholze A, et al. Effect of amlodipine on cardiovascular events in hypertensive haemodialysis patients. Nephrol Dial Transpl. 2008;23:3605–12.

Zannad F, Kessler M, Lehert P, et al. Prevention of cardiovascular events in end-stage renal disease: results of a randomized trial of fosinopril and implications for future studies. Kidney Int. 2006;70:1318–24.

46. Your dialysis nurse calls you and reports that BP in one of your patients is high compared to starting (predialysis) BP 2 h after ultrafiltration. She also says that the intradialytic hypertension has been observed during the last six HD sessions. **Which one of the following pathophysiologic mechanisms regarding intradialytic hypertension is CORRECT?**

A. Volume overload
B. Activation of renin-AII-aldosterone system
C. Increased cardiac output and systemic vascular resistance
D. Removal of antihypertensive agents
E. All of the above

The answer is E

All of the above mechanisms have been implicated in the development of intradialytic hypertension (E is correct). Although there are no prospective studies to define intradialytic hypertension, the suggestion of an increase in mean arterial pressure (MAP) of 15 mm Hg above starting MAP is considered intradialytic hypertension. When intradialytic hypertension is defined as systolic BP >10 mm Hg, from pre- to postdialysis, its prevalence varied from 12.2 to 22.3%.

In addition to the above mechanisms, inability to achieve the estimated dry eight, hypokalemia, high dialysate Na^+ and Ca^{2+} composition, endothelial dysfunction, high hematocrit, and erythropoietin use also play a role in increasing BP during dialysis. Figure 9.1 **illustrates the pathogenesis of intradialytic hypertension.**

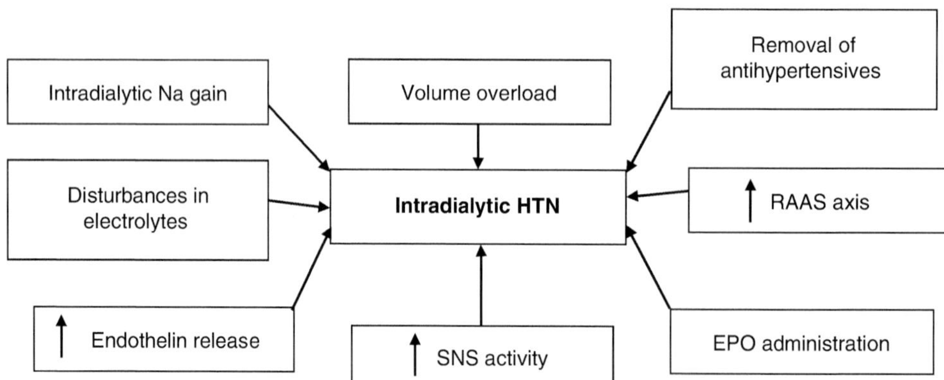

Fig. 9.1 Pathogenesis of intradialytic hypertension

Most frequently, intradialytic hypertension is seen in patients with increased interdialytic weight gain and vigorous ultrafiltration. Also, dialysis against high dialysate Na^+ concentration leads to diffusion of Na^+ from dialysate into plasma with resultant hypertension.

Intradialytic hypertension has been shown to be independently associated with increased all-cause mortality, adverse CV outcomes, and hospitalization.

Table 9.8 **shows the dialyzability of antihypertensive drugs.**

Table 9.8 Dialyzability of commonly used antihypertensive drugs

Drug class	Extensively removed	Partially removed
β-blockers	Metoprolol, atenolol. Nadolol	Carvedilol, pindolol, propranolol,
α, β-blockers		Labetalol, prazosin, terazosin
Sympatholitics	Methyldopa	Clonidine, guanabenz
ACE inhibitors	Captopril, enalapril, lisinopril, ramipril, perindopril	Fosinopril
Angiotensin receptor blockers		None
Ca blockers	None	Amlodipine, nifedipine, isradipine, felodipine, diltiazem, verapamil
Vasodilators		Hydralazine, minoxidil (partial)

Suggested Reading

Chen J, Gul, A Sarnak MJ. Management of intradialytic hypertension: the ongoing challange. Sem Dial. 2006;19:141–5.

Fravel MA, Bald E, Mony F. Antihypertensive agents in the dialysis patient. Curr Hypertens Rep. 2019;21:5 https://doi.org/10.1007/s11906-019-0909-z.

Georgianos PI, Sarafidis PA, Zoccali C. Intradialysis hypertension in end-stage renal disease patients. Hypertension. 2015;66:456–63.

Inrig JK. Antihypertensive agents in hemodialysis patients: a current perspective. Sem Dial. 2010;23:290–7.

Santos SF, Peixoto AJ, Perazella MA. How should we manage adverse intradialytic blood pressure changes?. Adv Chronic Kidney Dis. 2012;19:158–65.

van Buren PN. Pathophysiology and implications of intradialytic hypertension. Curr Opin Nephrol Hypertens. 2017;26:303–10.

47. **Which one of the following measures you would take in the management of intradialytic hypertension in the above patient?**

A. Adjust the dry weight
B. Avoid high dialysate Na^{+} and Ca^{2+} concentration
C. Avoid fluid overload
D. Consider carvedilol to treat hypertension
E. All of the above

The answer is E

All of the above measures are necessary to improve intradialytic hypertension (E is correct). A study by Inrig et al. showed that carvedilol, up to 50 mg twice daily, improved posthemodialysis, intradialytic, and 44-h ambulatory BP in hemodialysis patients. Also, the frequency of intradialytic hypertensive episodes was reduced. These changes were related to carvedilol-induced improvement in endothelial dysfunction and vasodilation.

Suggested Reading

Georgianos PI, Sarafidis PA, Zoccali C. Intradialysis hypertension in end-stage renal disease patients. Hypertension. 2015;66:456–63.

InrigJK, Van Buren P, Kim C, et al. Probing the mechanisms of intradialytic hypertension: a pilot study targeting endothelial dysfunction. Clin J Am Soc Nephrol. 2012;7: 1300–9.

Santos SF, Peixoto AJ, Perazella MA. How should we manage adverse intradialytic blood pressure changes?. Adv Chronic Kidney Dis. 2012;19:158–65.

48. Your HD patient has persistent interdialytic weight gain of 5 kg with BP of 194/102 mmMg. He weighs 100 kg. You order ultrafiltration rate at 10 mL/h/kg. His BP drops with removal of fluid. His postdialysis BP after a 5-h dialysis session was 144/90 mm Hg. Epidemiologic studies have shown U-shaped association between BP during hemodialysis (HD) and mortality. Also, post-HD change in systolic BP has prognostic significance. **Based on the available evidence,**

which one of the following post-HD changes in systolic BP (post-HD minus pre-HD) has the greatest survival advantage in HD patients?

A. 0 50 mm Hg drop
B. 0–40 mm Hg drop
C. 0–35 mm Hg drop
D. 0–14 mm Hg drop
E. 20 mm Hg increase

The answer is D

The optimal BP range in HD patients is unclear. However, a U-shaped curve was observed between systolic BP and mortality. Predialysis systolic BP values <130 mm Hg and >150 mm Hg were found to be associated with high mortality rate. However, another large retrospective study in 113, 255 HD patients concluded that a modest decrease in systolic BP during dialysis (−30 to 0 mm Hg) was associated with the best survival. The greatest survival was associated with a change in systolic BP -14 mm Hg (D is correct). Similarly, a change in diastolic BP -6 mm Hg was associated with greatest survival. A U-shaped curve was observed at −40–50 and +10–30 mm Hg. Thus, the study suggests that changes in systolic BP rather than predialysis BP are important to monitor in HD patients.

Zhang et al. reported that a high prehemodialysis systolic BP (pre-HD SBP) combined with a high peridialytic SBP rise was associated with higher mortality. In contrast, when concurrent with low pre-HD SBP, a peridialytic SBP rise was associated with better survival. This study suggests that both pre-HD SBP and peridialytic SBP should be taken into consideration in the evaluation of mortality in HD patients.

Suggested Reading

Inrig JK. Peri-dialytic hypertension and hypotension: another U-shaped BP-outcome association. Kidney Int. 2013;84:641–4.

Park J, Rhee CM, Sim JJ, et al. Comparative effectiveness research study of the change in blood pressure during hemodialysis treatment and survival. Kidney Int. 2013;84:795–802.

Port FK, Robinson BM, McCullough KP et al. Predialysis blood pressure on survival in hemodialysis patients. Kidney Int. 2017;91:755–6.

Robers MA, Pilmore HL, Tonkin AM, et al. on behalf of the Beta-Blocker to Lower Cardiovascular Dialysis Events (BLOCADE) Feasibility Trial Management Committee. Challenges in blood pressure management in patients treated with maintenance hemodialysis. Am J Kidney Dis. 2012;60:463–72.

Zhang H, Preciado P, Wang Y, et al. Association of all-cause mortality with pre-dialysis systolic blood pressure and its peridialytic change in chronic hemodialysis patients. Nephrol Dial Transplant. 2020;35:1602–8.

49. A 64-year-old woman with end-stage kidney disease and on maintenance hemodialysis (HD) develops intradialytic hypotension during each session of treatment. **Which one of the following interventions is appropriate for this patient to improve hypotension?**

A. Carnitine
B. Midodrine
C. Cool dialysate
D. Avoidance of food intake during dialysis
E. All of the above

The answer is E

Intradialytic hypotension (IDH) is a vexing problem in some HD patients. IDH is defined as an absolute intradialytic nadir systolic BP < 90 mm Hg, which is associated with poor cardiovascular outcomes, whereas previous definitions of a drop in systolic BP ~ 20 mm Hg, or a drop in mean arterial BP ~ 10 mm Hg, are not associated with poor outcomes. It is usually associated with nausea, vomiting, dizziness, muscle cramps, and disturbance in the stomach. Clotting of AV access is rather frequent. All of the above interventions have been shown to improve IDH. Thus, option E is correct.

Suggested Reading

Chou JA, Streja E, Nguyen DV, et al. Intradialytic hypotension, blood pressure changes and mortality risk in incident hemodialysis patients. Nephrol Dial Transpl. 2018;33:149–59.

Reeves PB, Mc Causland FR. Mechanisms, clinical implications, and treatment of intradialytic hypotension. Clin J Am Soc Nephrol. 2018;13:1297–303.

Reilly RF. Attending rounds: a patient with intradialytic hypotension. Clin J Am Soc Nephrol. 2014;9:798–803.

Sars B, van der Sande FM, Kooman JP. Intradialytic hypotension: mechanisms and outcome. Blood Purif. 2020;49:158–67.

50. **Which one of the following risk factors for development of intradialytic hypotension (IDH) is CORRECT?**

A. Systolic and diastolic heart failure
B. Poor nutritional status, including hypoalbuminemia
C. Low body mass index
D. Autonomic dysfunction
E. All of the above

The answer is E

In addition to the above risk factors, female sex, diabetes, increased interdialytic weight, and vascular calcification predispose patients to IDH (E is correct).

Suggested Reading

Kanbay M, Ertuglu LA, Afsar B, et al. An update review of intradialytic hypotension: concept, risk factors, clinical implications and management. Clin Kidney J. 2020;1–13.

Reeves PB, Mc Causland FR. Mechanisms, clinical implications, and treatment of intradialytic hypotension. Clin J Am Soc Nephrol. 2018;13:1297–303.

Reilly RF. Attending rounds: a patient with intradialytic hypotension. Clin J Am Soc Nephrol. 2014;9:798–803.

Sars B, van der Sande FM, Kooman JP. Intradialytic hypotension: mechanisms and outcome. Blood Purif. 2020;49:158–167.

51. Intradialytic hypotension (IDH) is a serious complication of chronic hemodialysis (HD), which is linked to adverse cardiovascular and all-cause mortality. **Which one of the following pathophysiologic mechanisms is involved in IDH?**

A. Decreased intravascular or blood volume
B. Impaired compensatory responses to low blood volume
C. Decreased myocardial perfusion (myocardial stunning)
D. Plasma osmolality changes
E. All of the above

The answer is E

Interdialytic weight gain is common in the majority of HD patients, as they are anuric and have more than recommended water intake. This excess water is removed by ultrafiltration (UF) to achieve the estimated dry weight. This UF results in decreased intravascular volume, which causes a decline in cardiac output and subsequently hypotension. The drop in BP is more pronounced in patients with cardiac disease who do not have either an increase in myocardial contractility or heart rate. In healthy individuals, low BP is accompanied by compensatory mechanisms such as activation of sympathetic nervous system and renin-angiotensin-aldosterone axis, which restore BP by vascular constriction and increased peripheral vascular resistance. Such compensatory mechanisms are impaired in HD patients. Many HD patients have left ventricular hypertrophy, which demand more O_2 supply, and this increased oxygen demand may make the cardiac tissue more vulnerable to a decline in BP. Thus, answers A and B are correct.

It has been reported that dialysis procedure itself can cause decreased myocardial perfusion and ischemia. Myocardial stunning refers to a transient myocardial hypoperfusion during HD. It has been shown that hemodiafiltration with high ultrafiltration rates induced a decline in myocardial hypoperfusion more than conventional HD, as shown by cardiac MRI. These changes lead to decreased cardiac output and low BP. In turn, low BP causes further decrease in myocardial perfusion and precipitates IDH (answer C is correct).

During dialysis, plasma osmolality changes occur due to removal of BUN and other osmotically active solutes. Studies have shown that plasma osmolality decreases by up to 33 mOsm/kg during HD treatment. Although urea is considered an ineffective osmole, its rapid removal creates an osmotic gradient for water to move from extracellular to intracellular compartment, resulting in a decrease in intravascular volume and a decline in BP. It has been shown that infusion of mannitol or hypertonic saline attenuates the decline in plasma osmolality and BP (answer D is correct).

Suggested Reading

Buchanan C, Mohammed A, Cox E, et al. Intradialytic cardiac magnetic resonance imaging to assess cardiovascular responses in a short-term trial of hemodialfiltration and hemodialysis. J Am Soc Nephrol. 2017;28:1268–77.

Chou JA, Streja E, Nguyen DV, et al. Intradialytic hypotension, blood pressure changes and mortality risk in incident hemodialysis patients. Nephrol Dial Transpl. 2018;33:149–59.

Kanbay M, Ertuglu LA, Afsar B, et al. An update review of intradialytic hypotension: concept, risk factors, clinical implications and management. Clin Kidney J. 2020;1–13.

Reeves PB, McCausland FR. Mechanisms, clinical implications, and treatment of intradialytic hypotension. Clin J Am Soc Nephrol. 2018;13:1297–303.

Singh AT, Mc Causland FR. Osmolality and blood pressure stability during hemodialysis. Sem Dial. 2017;30:509–17.

Sars B, van der Sande FM, Kooman JP. Intradialytic hypotension: mechanisms and outcome. Blood Purif. 2020;49:158–67.

52. A 50-year-old woman on hemodialysis (HD) due to hypertensive nephrosclerosis frequently develops intradialytic hypotension (IDH) despite use of midodrine 10 mg 1 h before the treatment. Her interdialytic weight gain is 1 kg, and her predialysis BP is 110/70 mm Hg. BP drops to 88/68 mm Hg after 90 min of dialysis treatment with an increase in heart rate. Her estimated dry weight has been appropriately adjusted. Measurement of her intravascular volume shows evidence of depletion, but BP failed to improve with normal saline up to 1L. **Which one of the following is the most important cause of her IDH?**

A. Subclinical infection
B. Myocardial ischemia
C. Needs to have large interdialytic weight gain
D. Cold dialysate
E. Dialysate Na^+ concentration greater than plasma Na^+ concentration

The answer is B

IDH is rather common (10–30%) in patients whose predialysis BP is low. Generally, <90 systolic BP is considered IDH. Frank sepsis rather than subclinical infection may cause IDH (A is incorrect). Volume-related causes such as excess fluid removal because of large interdialytic weight gain results in IDH (C is incorrect).

Dialysate temperature generally maintains patient's arterial blood temperature. When dialysate temperature is high, blood temperature is also high, which causes cutaneous vasodilation with resultant hypotension. Cold dialysate improves IDH (D is incorrect).

When dialysate Na^+ concentration is less than patient's Na^+ concentration, the blood returning from the dialyzer is hypotonic to the surrounding tissues. This causes movement of water from blood to other compartments, which results in relative hypovolemia and hypotension (E is incorrect).

HD induces cardiac stress and causes HD-associated cardiomyopathy and ischemia. Repeated ischemic episodes result in myocardial stunning and hibernation, leading to myocardial remodeling and scarring and irreversible contractile function. This patient's low predialysis BP is an indirect measure of abnormal contractility, and midodrine failed to improve her BP during HD. Thus, B appears to be the best possible answer for her IHD.

HD-associated myocardial ischemia, which, in the absence of coronary artery disease, may be due to coronary microvascular dysfunction. Myocardial stunning may be important in the development of heart failure in long-term HD patients.

During intravascular volume depletion, cardiac output decreases despite an increase in heart rate. Venous pooling of blood probably increases during HD, and addition of midodrine may not have any effect in increasing cardiac output other than increasing heart rate. Furthermore, midodrine may enhance cardiac ischemia. Thus, switching the patient from HD to peritoneal dialysis may prevent IHD.

Suggested Reading

Canaud B, Kooman JP, Selby NM, et al. Dialysis-induced cardiovascular and multiorgan morbidity. Kidney Int Rep. 2020;5:1856–69.

Kott J, Reichek N, Butler J, et al. Cardiac imaging in dialysis patients. Kidney Med. 2020;2:629–38.

McIntyre CW, Odudu A. Hemodialysis-associated cardiomyopathy: a new defined disease entity. Sem Dial. 2014;27:87–97.

53. A 64-year-old woman with ESKD due to diabetes and on hemodialysis (HD) is admitted for new-onset tachycardia of 130 beats/min. A 12-lead EKG shows atrial fibrillation (AF). Her BP is well controlled. **Which one of the following statements regarding anticoagulation with warfarin in this patient is Correct?**

A. Warfarin use does not have any effect on the incidence of ischemic stroke
B. Warfarin use increases hemorrhagic stroke
C. Warfarin use is not a risk for major bleeding and does not have an effect on overall mortality
D. Warfarin is associated with significantly higher bleeding risk compared with apixaban or no anticoagulation
E. All of the above

The answer is E

AF is a risk factor for thromboembolism in both patients with normal and reduced kidney function. Regarding anticoagulation in HD patients with AF, there is no general conclusion on whether to use or not to use anticoagulation because of lack of prospective randomized controlled studies. However, there are several meta-analyses that included only observational studies and reported conflicting results. Two such meta-analyses were published in 2020 with large number of studies and patients. The meta-analysis of Randhawa et al. concluded that "warfarin use is not associated with any benefit in the prevention of ischemic stroke. Instead, it is associated with a significant increase in the risk of hemorrhagic stroke, no significant difference in the risk of major bleeding, and no association with overall mortality" (options A to C are correct).

The meta-analysis of Kuno et al. concluded that "Warfarin, dabigatran, and rivaroxaban were associated with significantly higher bleeding risk compared with apixaban and no anticoagulant" (option D is correct). This meta-analysis also showed that the above oral anticoagulants did not show any reduced risk of thromboembolism in HD patients with AF. However, apixaban 5 mg twice daily had a significantly lower risk of mortality than apixaban 2.5 mg twice daily compared to either warfarin or no anticoagulation.

It should be noted that warfarin causes valvular calcification and calciphylaxis. Therefore, warfarin therapy should be individualized, if indicated.

Suggested Reading

Belley-Cote EM, Eikelboom JW. Anticoagulation for stroke prevention in patients with atrial fibrillation and end-stage renal disease- First, do no harm. JAMA Network Open. 2020;3:e202237.

Kuno T, Takagi H, Ando T, et al. Oral anticoagulation for patients with atrial fibrillation on long-term hemodialysis. J Am Coll Cardiol. 2020;75:273–85.

Randhawa MS, Vishwanath R, Rai MP, et al. Association between use of warfarin for atrial fibrillation and outcomes among patients with end-stage renal disease: a systematic review and meta-analysis. JAMA Network Open. 2020;3:e202175.

54. Mineral and bone disorders (Ca^{2+}, phosphate, and PTH), called CKD-MBD, are implicated in cardiovascular (CV) morbidity and mortality in hemodialysis (HD) patients because of tissue calcification. **Which one of the following statements regarding CKD-MBD and CV hospitalizations in HD patients is TRUE?**

A. Patients with normal PTH (range 150–600 pg/mL), normal Ca^{2+} (range 8.4–10.2 mg/dL), and normal phosphate (range 3.5–5.5 mg/dL) are at risk for CV hospitalizations
B. Patients with normal PTH, normal Ca^{2+}, and high phosphate are at risk for CV hospitalizations
C. Patients with PTH >300 pg/mL, high Ca^{2+}, and normal phosphate are at risk for CV hospitalizations
D. Patients with normal PTH, high Ca^{2+}, and high phosphate are at risk for CV hospitalizations
E. Patients with normal PTH, high Ca^{2+}, and high phosphate are at risk for CV hospitalizations

The answer is C

Several studies have analyzed individual components of CKD-MBD on CV outcomes. Such analyses may introduce bias in the interpretation of the results. To overcome these barriers, Block et al. analyzed data from USRDS and Davita centers to evaluate the effect of CKD-MBD on CV hospitalizations or death in 26,221 HD patients. They combined serum Ca^{2+}, phosphate, and PTH as a single composite variable, and compared this variable as target reference group to different phenotypes (patients divided into various categories based on PTH, Ca^{2+}, and phosphate levels) with each phenotype consisting of at least 100 patients. Based on their analysis, patients with high PTH (>300 pg/mL), high Ca^{2+}, and normal to high phosphate had a higher risk of death or the composite end point of death or CV hospitalization. Thus, C is a true statement. It is of interest to note that patients with high PTH with high phosphate and normal Ca^{2+} were also at risk for CV hospitalization. Thus, PTH plays a significant role in CKD-MBD and CV disease.

Suggested Reading

Block GA, Kilpatrick RD, Lowe KA, et al. CKD-mineral and bone disorder and risk of death and cardiovascular hospitalization in patients on hemodialysis. Clin J Am Soc Nephrol. 2013;8:2132–40.

Palmer SC, Hayen A, Macaskill P, et al. Serum levels of phosphorus, parathyroid hormone, and calcium and risk of death and cardiovascular disease in individuals with chronic kidney disease: a systematic review and meta-analysis. JAMA. 2011;305:1119–27.

55. An ESKD patient with serum PTH levels of 1, 900 pg/mL is started on cinacalcet 30 with increasing doses to 120 mg with food intake. However, the patient complains of nausea, vomiting, and stomach upset. The physician ordered 5 mg of IV etelcalcetide, a calcimimetic drug, thrice weekly. Compared to oral cinacalcet, **which one of the following complications is frequently observed with etelcalcetide?**

A. Hypomagnesemia
B. Hyperphosphatemia
C. Hypocalcemia
D. Hyponatremia
E. All of the above

The answer is C

Etelcalcetide is an octapeptide type 2 calcimimetic that interacts with the calcium-sensing receptor at a site distinct from cinacalcet. It is an IV form of calcimimetic and is an alternative to suppress PTH secretion in patients who cannot tolerate oral cinacalcet. In a randomized, double-blind, double-dummy active clinical trial, etelcalcitide was compared with daily oral cinacalcet in 683 adult hemodialysis (HD) patients on PTH (>500 pg/mL), Ca^{2+}, phosphate, and fibroblast growth factor-23. The study was conducted for 27 weeks. The results show that 68.2% of patients randomized to receive etelcalcetide versus 57.7% randomized to receive cinacalcet experienced more than a 30% reduction in mean PTH concentrations over 27 weeks, a significant difference. Although phosphate concentration was found to be lower in etelcalcitide group, the most common adverse effect was decreased blood calcium (68.9% vs. 59.8%). Thus, answer C is correct. In a second trial, etelcalcitide also lowered PTH levels in HD patients compared to placebo.

Suggested Reading

Block GA, Bushinsky DA, Cheng S, et al. Effect of etelcalcetide vs cinacalcet on serum parathyroid hormone in patients receiving hemodialysis with secondary hyperparathyroidism. A randomized clinical trial. JAMA. 2017;317:156–64.

Block GA, Bushinsky DA, Cunningham J, et al. Effect of etelcalcetide vs placebo on serum parathyroid hormone in patients receiving hemodialysis with secondary hyperparathyroidism. Two randomized clinical trials. JAMA. 2017;317:146–55.

56. A 58-year-old woman on hemodialysis (HD) for 4 years is found to have hyperphosphatemia (serum phosphate level of 6.4 mg/dL) despite several different types of nonCa-phosphate binders. Her major problems happen to be pill burden and some adverse effects such as constipation. She heard of tenapanor and she wants to try it. **Which one of the following mechanisms by which tenapanor lowers serum phosphate level?**

A. It binds to phosphate in the gut
B. It inhibits Na/H exchanger isoform 3 (NHE3) in the intestine

C. It promotes fecal excretion of phosphate by unknown mechanism
D. It inhibits paracellular phosphate absorption
E. B, C, and D

The answer is E

Hyperphosphatemia causes secondary hyperparathyroidism, cardiovascular disease, including vascular calcification, fractures, progression of kidney disease, and death. Therefore, control of hyperphosphatemia is extremely important in HD patients. Dietary restriction of phosphate, education, and phosphate binders are extensively used in HD patients to control hyperphosphatemia. However, most of the patients do not adhere to this kind of management.

Recently, a new and simple treatment of hyperphosphatemia was introduced by Block and associates. These investigators studied the effect of tenapanor, which is a minimally absorbed small-molecule inhibitor of NHE3 transporter in the small intestine. This transporter promotes Na^+ reabsorption and secretes H^+ into the lumen. Tenapanor inhibits Na^+ absorption and eliminates it into the stool. At the same time, this agent also prevents absorption of phosphate with excretion into the stool (options B and C are correct).

Block et al. used six different dosages (3 or 30 mg once daily or 1, 3, 10, or 30 mg twice daily) or placebo in 162 HD patients for 4 weeks and found a dose-related decrease in serum phosphate levels (least squares mean change: tenapanor = 0.47–1.98 mg/dL; placebo = 0.54 mg/dL; $P = 0.01$). Patients tolerated the drug well; however, diarrhea seems to be the most common adverse effect in these patients.

It seems that tenapanor reduces intestinal phosphate absorption by two mechanisms: (1) by reducing paracellular phosphate absorption (D is correct) and (2) by preventing active transcellular phosphate absorption via decreasing the expression of NaPi2b, the major active intestinal phosphate transporter. These two mechanisms promote excess removal of phosphate in the stool and decreased excretion in the urine. Also, Na^+ and water excretion are promoted in the stool as well. The net result of these effects is a reduction in serum phosphate level, as reported by Block and associates in HD patients.

Suggested Reading

Block GA, Rosenbaum DP, Leonsson-Zachrisson M, et al. Effect of tenapanor on serum phosphate in patients receiving hemodialysis. J Am Soc Nephrol. 2017;28:1933–42.

King AJ, Siegel M, He Y, et al. Inhibition of sodium/hydrogen exchanger 3 in the gastrointestinal tract by tenapanor reduces paracellular phosphate permeability. Sci Transl Med. 2018;10(456). https://doi.org/10.1126/scitranslmed.aam6474.

57. Serum phosphate is usually elevated above 5.5 mg/dL in hemodialysis (HD) patients. High-flux dialyzers remove phosphate. **Which one of the following statements regarding intradialytic phosphate kinetics is CORRECT?**

A. Phosphate is removed throughout the dialysis session with higher rates at the end of dialysis
B. Pre- and post-HD phosphate levels are similar
C. Phosphate levels decrease during the first 90–120 min, and then stabilize
D. No change in phosphate level in some patients because they eat before HD session
E. Phosphate level decreases in those who take sevelamer compared to those who take calcium acetate

The answer is C

Phosphate is removed during dialysis like urea, but less than creatinine. Its kinetics during dialysis was studied in HD patients by several investigators. It was found that during the first 90 to 120 min into dialysis, serum phosphate levels decrease substantially by elimination into the dialysate and then stabilize (C is correct). The study of Eliasa et al. showed that the fall in serum phosphate is approximately 44% during the first hour of HD using the high-flux membrane dialyzer, if serum phosphate is <5.5 mg/dL. The percentage removal was 49%, if serum phosphate level is >5.5 mg/dL. At the end of the 4-h session, the removal was similar to 1-h removal.

Stabilization occurs due to mobilization of phosphate from other compartments at a rate similar to its removal so that the plasma concentration of phosphate remains at predialysis level (B is incorrect). This suggests that phosphate kinetics involves two or more compartment modeling. Phosphate kinetics is not altered by food intake or phosphate binders (D and E are incorrect).

Suggested Reading

Eliasa RM, Alvaresa VRC, Moysés RMA. Phosphate removal during conventional hemodialysis: a decades-old misconception. Kidney Blood Press Res. 2018;43:110–4.
Koolenga L. Phosphorus balance with daily dialysis. Sem Dial. 2007;20:342–5.
Laursen SH, Vestergaard P, Hejlesen OK. Phosphate kinetic models in hemodialysis: a systematic review. Am J Kidney Dis. 2017;71:75–90.

58. Iron deficiency is rather common in hemodialysis (HD) patients. **Which one of the following mechanisms accounts for iron deficiency in these patients?**

A. HD patients lose 2–3 g of iron annually
B. HD patients absorb oral iron poorly
C. Consumption of iron by erythropoiesis-stimulating agents (ESAs)
D. Poor dietary intake due to inadequate dialysis adequacy
E. All of the above

The answer is E

Total iron amounts to approximately 3000–4000 mg in a 70 kg adult (35–50 mg/kg). Females have less iron compared to males. Most of this iron is distributed in erythrocytes as Hgb and as a stored iron in the form of ferritin and hemosiderin in reticuloendothelial system. Iron deficiency is rather common in HD patients (A is correct). Several mechanisms have been proposed. First, HD patients lose 2 to 3 g of iron every year. This is mostly due to loss of blood in dialysis tubing, bleeding from AV accesses, frequent phlebotomies in and out of hospital setting, and subclinical loss of blood in the GI tract due to telangiectasia. Second, HD patients absorb iron poorly by mouth. This was shown by ferrokinetic studies (B is correct). HD patients receive ESA for anemia treatment, and new RBCs are formed with high content of iron. Loss of these RBCs in the tubing and other sites of body may result in iron loss (C is correct).

A typical American diet contains 10–20 mg of iron; however, all of this iron is not absorbed. Approximately, 1–2 mg of this iron is absorbed daily in an adult. This amount is enough to replace iron loss mostly in the stool. The loss is contributed by sloughed off cells from the gastrointestinal (GI) tract and skin. In order to maintain iron-requiring functions of the body, dietary absorption of 1–2 mg of iron alone is not adequate. To maintain iron homeostasis, at least 20 mg of iron is required daily for production of Hgb for generation of new erythrocytes. Therefore, most functional iron is derived from recycling of iron already present in the body.

In HD patients, nausea and vomiting, loss of appetite, and early satiety due to inadequate dialysis therapy may account for poor oral intake. Intake of foods that contain phytates, oxalates, and phosphate complex with iron prevents its absorption. Also, achlorhydria impairs iron absorption. Thus, option D is correct.

The single most regulator of systemic iron homeostasis is a peptide hormone called hepcidin. It is predominantly synthesized by hepatocytes. It is excreted by the kidneys. Hepcidin inhibits GI absorption and also blocks the release of stored iron from hepatocytes and macrophages, leading to low plasma levels of iron.

Suggested Reading

Camaschella C, Nai A, Silvestri L. Iron metabolism and iron disorders revisited in the hepcidin era. Haematologica. 2020;105:260–72.
Eschbach JW, Cook JD, Scribner BH et al. Iron balance in hemodialysis patients. Ann Intern Med. 1977;87:710–3.
Nissenson AR, Strobos J. Iron deficiency in patients with renal failure. Kidney Int. 1999;55(suppl 69):S-18-S21.
Yu MK, Chertow GM. Testing two (of several) intravenous iron dosing strategies in hemodialysis. Ann Transl Med. 2019;7(Suppl 3):S129.
Wish JB, Aronoff GR Bacon BR, et al. Positive iron balance in chronic Kidney disease: how much is too much and how to tell?. Am J Nephrol. 2018;47:72–83.

59. In managing anemia in hemodialysis (HD) patients, intravenous (IV) iron therapy is used to maintain target hemoglobin (Hgb) level. Two general regimens are used for iron therapy: high dose and low dose. When iron sucrose is used, high dose includes 100 mg given in 5 to 10 consecutive HD sessions (500–1000 mg/month), whereas low dose includes 25–50 mg weekly (100–200 mg/month). **Which one of the following effects of iron therapy in HD patients is CORRECT?**

A. Low-dose iron therapy is associated with low infection rate
B. Serum ferritin levels are almost equal with low- and high-dose iron administration
C. Both high- and low-dose iron therapies are associated with increased risk of infection and infection-related hospitalization compared to low-dose therapy
D. High-dose iron therapy lowers erythropoiesis-stimulating agent (ESA) dose as compared with low-dose iron therapy
E. There is no relationship between iron and infection

The answer is D

Intravenous iron therapy is usually initiated prior to ESA therapy and subsequently both in HD patients for management of anemia, whose transferrin saturation (TSAT) is <20% and ferritin levels are <200 ng/mL. This combination treatment is continued until TSAT reaches 30–50% or serum ferritin up to 800 ng/mL (threshold levels for ferritin vary among centers and countries). As IV iron is continued, the dose of ESA is reduced to prevent high ESA-induced adverse cardiovascular (CV) events.

It is well known that iron promotes bacterial growth, and iron is held when a dialysis patient is suspected to have infection. In some studies, high-dose iron was associated with adverse CV events and increased hospitalizations. Other studies did not observe such adverse effects. For a summary of all these studies, the reader is referred to a review by Macdougall (2017). Also, a recent study by the same investigator and his colleagues addressed the safety and adverse effects of high-dose versus low-dose IV iron therapy in HD patients, as described below.

In a prospective randomized multicenter, open-label trial, Macdougall and colleagues assigned adult patients <12 months on HD to receive either high-dose IV iron sucrose ($N = 1093$), in a proactive fashion (400 mg monthly, unless the ferritin level was >700 μg/L or the TSAT was ≥40%), or low-dose iron sucrose ($N = 1048$) in a reactive fashion (0 to 400 mg monthly, with a ferritin level <200 μg/L or the TSAT was <20%), and were followed for a median of 2.1 years. The dose of ESAs was selected by the clinician in order to maintain a target Hgb concentration of 10–12 g/dL. The primary outcome was the composite of nonfatal myocardial infarction, nonfatal stroke, hospitalization for heart failure, or death. The secondary outcome was death, infection rate, and dose of ESA.

The data revealed that the high-dose group received a median monthly iron dose of 264 mg as compared with 145 mg in the low-dose group. The median monthly dose of ESA was 29,757 IU in the high-dose group and 38,805 IU in the low-dose group (median difference of −7539 IU). The primary outcome occurred in 29.3 (320 patients) in the high-dose group compared to 32.3% (338 patients) in the low-dose group ($p < 0.001$). The infection rate was the same in both groups. Thus, a high-dose IV iron regimen administered proactively was safe and superior to a low-dose iron regimen administered reactively in preventing nonfatal myocardial infarction, nonfatal stroke, hospitalization for heart failure, or death without any effect on infection rate. Furthermore, patients on high-dose IV iron therapy required lower doses of ESA (option D is correct). Other options are incorrect.

A meta-analysis that included 7 randomized, controlled trials and 15 observational studies also reported that higher dose IV iron is not associated with higher risk of mortality, infection, CV events, or hospitalizations in adult HD patients.

Suggested Reading

Brookhart MA, Freburger JK, Ellis AR, et al. Infection risk with bolus versus maintenance iron supplementation in hemodialysis patients. J Am Soc Nephrol. 2013;24:1151–8.
Hougen I, Collister D, Bourrier M, et al. Safety of intravenous iron in dialysis a systematic review and meta-analysis. Clin J Am Soc Nephrol. 2018;13:457–67, 2018.
Macdougall IC. Intravenous iron therapy in patients with chronic kidney disease: recent evidence and future directions. Clin Kidney J. 2017;10:(suppl 1):i16–i24.
Macdougall IC, White C, Anker SD, et al. for the PIVOTAL Investigators and Committees. Intravenous iron in patients undergoing maintenance hemodialysis. N Engl J Med. 2019;380:447–58.
Rhee CM, Kalantar-Zadeh K. Is iron maintenance therapy better than load and hold?. J Am Soc Nephrol. 2013;24:1028–31.
Yu MK, Chertow GM. Testing two (of several) intravenous iron dosing strategies in hemodialysis. Ann Transl Med. 2019;7(suppl 3):S129.

60. Hypoxia-inducible factor (HIF) prolyl hydroxylase domain inhibitors (PHDIs) are novel therapeutic agents used for treating renal anemia. **Which one of the following beneficial effects of renal anemia has been observed with PHDIs?**

A. Increase in endogenous erythropoietin (epo) secretion
B. Increase in total iron-binding capacity (TIBC)
C. Decrease in serum ferritin

D. Decrease in serum hepcidin level
E. All of the above

The answer is E

All PHDIs reported that an increase in epo levels with an increase in Hgb concentration and TIBC and a decrease in serum ferritin and hepcidin were reported in nondialysis and dialysis CKD patients. Thus, answer E is correct. Also, a decrease in total cholesterol and low-density lipoprotein levels has also been found to be decreased in these patients.

Suggested Reading

Akizawa T, Nangaku M, Yonekawa T, et al. Efficacy and safety of daprodustat compared with darbepoetin alfa in Japanese hemodialysis patients with anemia. A randomized, double-blind, phase 3 trial. Clin J Am Soc Nephrol. 2020;15:1155–65.
Chen N, Hao C, Liu B-C, et al. Roxadustat treatment for anemia in patients undergoing long-term dialysis. N Engl J Med. 2019;381:1011–22.
Gupta N, Wish JB. Hypoxia-inducible factor prolyl hydroxylase inhibitors: a potential new treatment for anemia in patients with CKD. Am J Kidney Dis. 2017;69:815–26.
Hasegawa S, Tanaka T, Nangaku M. Hypoxia-inducible factor stabilizers for treating anemia of chronic kidney disease. Curr Opin Nephrol Hypertens. 2018;27:331–8.
Kurata Y, Tanaka T, Nangaku M. Prolyl hydroxylase domain inhibitors: a new era in the management of renal anemia. Ann Transl Med. 2019;7(suppl 8):S334.
Sanghani NS, Haase VH. Hypoxia-inducible factor activators in renal anemia: current clinical experience. Adv Chronic Kidney Dis. 2019;26:253–66.
Wyatt CM, Drüeke TM. HIF stabilization by prolyl hydroxylase inhibitors for the treatment of anemia in chronic kidney disease. Kidney Int. 2016;90:923–5.

61. A 60-year-old diabetic man is on hemodialysis (HD) for 2 years, and his Hgb is 9.2 g/dL despite erythropoietin α 30,000 U weekly. His ferritin is 515 μg/L. He was started on roxadustat 100 mg orally thrice weekly. **Which one of the following electrolyte abnormalities is expected with roxadustat?**

A. Hyponatremia
B. Hypomagnesemia
C. Hypokalemia
D. Hyperkalemia
E. Hypocalcemia

The answer is D

Studies in dialysis and nondialysis CKD patients have shown that hyperkalemia (7.4% in HD patients) and metabolic acidosis were more frequent in the roxadustat group than in the placebo group (D is correct).

The mechanism for hyperkalemia is not known. It is proposed that metabolic acidosis may have promoted K^+ entry from extracellular to intracellular compartment. For metabolic acidosis, it is postulated that HIF during hypoxic conditions stimulates glycolysis and lactate production, which may account for PHDIs-induced metabolic acidosis. It should be remembered that lactic acidosis does not cause hyperkalemia; therefore, the mechanism for hyperkalemia needs further investigation.

Suggested Reading

Chen N, Hao C, Peng X, et al. Roxadustat for anemia in patients with kidney disease not receiving dialysis. N Engl J Med. 2019;381:1001–10.
Chen N, Hao C, Liu B-C, et al. Roxadustat treatment for anemia in patients undergoing long-term dialysis. N Engl J Med. 2019;381:1011–22.
Kurata Y, Tanaka T, Nangaku M. Prolyl hydroxylase domain inhibitors: a new era in the management of renal anemia. Ann Transl Med. 2019;7(suppl 8):S334.

62. One of your diabetic hemodialysis (HD) patients with peripheral neuropathy complains of unpleasant or uncomfortable sensation in lower extremities during periods of rest, and relief by movement. You made the diagnosis of restless leg syndrome (RLS). **Besides peripheral neuropathy, which one of the following pathophysiologic mechanisms is implicated in RLS?**

A. Anemia with iron depletion
B. Dysfunction of the dopaminergic system
C. Activation of sympathetic nervous system
D. Disturbed mineral metabolism
E. All of the above

The answer is E

The prevalence of RLS in HD patients varies from 7 to 45%. All of the above mechanisms have been implicated in the pathogenesis of RLS. Also, hyperhomocysteinemia has been implicated. Many pharmacologic agents, including dopaminergic agents (ropinirole, pramipexole, rotigotine, pergolide, cabergoline) and gabapentin, have been used with 60–75% relief of symptoms. Of all these drugs, the non-ergot dopaminergic agonists ropinirole and pramipexole are the drugs of choice for RLS.

Nonpharmacologic therapies such as cooling of the dialysate solution from 37⁰ C to 36⁰ C seem to reduce the motor and sensory symptoms of uremic RLS and are considered safe. Aerobic exercise is also helpful.

Suggested Reading

Gade K, Blaschke S, Rodenbeck A, et al. Uremic rest leg syndrome (RLS) and sleep quality in patients with end-stage renal disease on hemodialysis: potential role of homocystein and parathyroid hormone. Kidney Blood Press Res. 2013;37:458–63.

Giannaki CD, Hadjigeorgiou GM, Karatzaferi C, et al. Epidemiology, impact, and treatment options of rest leg syndrome in end-stage renal disease patients; An evidence-based review. Kidney Int. 2014;85:1275–82.

Kambampati S, Wasim S, Kukkar V, et al. Restless leg syndrome in the setting of patients with end-stage renal disease on hemodialysis: a literature review. Cureus. 2020;12(8):e9965.

Schere JS, Combs SA, Brennan F. Sleep disorders, restless legs syndrome, and uremic pruritus: diagnosis and treatment of common symptoms in dialysis patients. Am J Kidney Dis. 2017;69:117–28.

63. A 56-year-old man on hemodialysis (HD) complains of pruritus despite adequate control of Ca^{2+}, phosphate, PTH, and application of lotions. His eKt/V is 1.2. **Which one of the following is helpful in improving his pruritus?**

A. Nalfurafine
B. Gabapentin
C. Pregabalin
D. Antihistamines
E. All of the above

The answer is E

Although the pathophysiology of pruritus is poorly understood, involvement of immunologic and opioidergic mechanisms has been suggested.

According to immunohypothesis, systemic inflammation rather than local skin inflammation is responsible for uremic pruritus. Accordingly, immunomodulating therapies such as thalidomide, calcineurin inhibitors, and ultraviolet B phototherapy have been shown to improve pruritus.

The opioid hypothesis proposes that an imbalance between μ and κ-opioid receptors causes pruritus. Activation of μ receptors increases pruritus that is common in both HD and PD patients. The DOPPS reported that 42% of the study patients experienced pruritus. The prevalence is similar in PD patients, whereas κ receptor stimulation decreases pruritus. Therefore, use of nalfurafine, a κ receptor agonist, for 2 weeks was effective in improving pruritus. Similarly, gabapentin, pregabalin, and antihistamines were found to be effective in improving uremic pruritus (E is correct). In addition, increasing the dialysis dose to achieve eKt/V around 1.4–1.5 may improve pruritus.

In a prospective, multicenter, randomized, double-blind, placebo-controlled trial, Mathur et al. studied the effectiveness of nalbuphine, a μ-opioid antagonist and κ-opioid agonist, in HD patients and found that

extended-release (ER) tablet 120 mg improved itching intensity compared to placebo. Thus, nalbuphine ER 120 mg seems to help pruritus in HD patients.

Interestingly, a review of 44 randomized control trials examined 39 different treatments, including gabapentin, pregabalin, mast cell stabilizers, phototherapy, HD modifications, and multiple other systemic and topical treatments and found that gabapentin was effective in the treatment of pruritus.

Suggested Reading

Mathur VS, Kumar J, Crawford PW, et al. for the TR02 Study Investigators. A multicenter, randomized, double-blind, placebo-controlled trial of nalbuphine ER tablets for uremic pruritus. Am J Nephrol. 2017;46:450–8.

Mettang T, Kremer AE. Uremic pruritus. Kidney Int. 2015;87:685–91.

Patel TS, Freedman BI, Yosipovitch G. An update on pruritus associated with CKD. Am J Kidney Dis. 2007;50:11–20.

Rayner HC, Larkina M, Wang M, et al. International comparisons of prevalence, awareness, and treatment of pruritus in people on hemodialysis. Clin J Am Soc Nephrol. 2017;12:2000–7.

Simonsen E, Komenda P, Lerner B, et al. Treatment of uremic pruritus: a systematic review. Am J Kidney Dis. 2017;70:638–55.

64. You are called by your dialysis nurse that the patient has severe cramps 2 h after starting hemodialysis (HD). **Which one of the following factors is predisposed to muscle cramp in HD patients?**

A. Low estimated body weight (EDW) and hypovolemia
B. Hypotension
C. Increased ultrafiltration rate and fluid removal
D. Low dialysate Na^+ concentration
E. All of the above

The answer is E

All of the above factors predispose the patient to develop muscle cramps by causing vasoconstriction and decreased blood flow to muscle (E is correct). The management includes replacement of volume with normal saline in hypovolemic and hypotensive patients. However, giving large volumes of normal saline is not appropriate all the time; therefore, hypertonic solutions such as saline (1.5–3%), glucose (10 or 50%), or mannitol (12.5–25 g) can cause muscle vasodilation and improve blood flow.

Other agents such as biotin (1 mg), carnitine (330 mg twice or 3 times daily), oxazepam, and vitamin E (400 IU) have been shown to improve muscle cramps. Quinine, once used to treat cramps, is no longer used because of its predisposition to TTP/HUS.

Suggested Reading

Flythe JE, Hilliard T, Lumby E, et al. for the Kidney Health Initiative Prioritizing Symptoms of ESRD Patients for Developing Therapeutic Interventions Stakeholder Meeting Participants. Fostering innovation in symptom management among hemodialysis patients paths forward for insomnia, muscle cramps, and fatigue. Clin J Am Soc Nephrol. 2019;14:150–60.

Sherman RA, Daugirdas JT, Ing TS. Complications during hemodialysis. In: Daugirdas JT, Blake PG, Ing TS, editors. Handbook of dialysis. 5th ed. Philadelphia: Wolters Kluwer; 2015. p. 215–36.

65. As medical director of a dialysis facility, you noticed that one of your colleague's patients has consistently low eKt/V of 1.1 despite a 4-h session 3 times a week on a high-flux dialyzer and a functioning AV fistula. **Which one of the following factors can affect delivered Kt/V?**

A. AV access recirculation
B. Delivered blood and dialysate flow rates
C. Treatment time
D. Dialyzer KoA (mass transfer area coefficient)
E. All of the above

The answer is E

All of the above factors can affect Kt/V (E). Whenever goal Kt/V is not met, the function of AV access should be evaluated initially by physical examination and then by radiologic procedure. Also, recirculation can lower Kt/V. Blood and dialysate flow rates should be checked. If blood flow is 350 mL/min and dialysate flow is 500 mL/min, increasing dialysate flow to 800 mL/min can increase Kt/V by 10–15%. Also, blood flow rate of 400–450 may increase Kt/V.

Increasing treatment time without any cutting in time can increase Kt/V. This approach has been proven to be very effective in improving HD-associated outcomes.

KoA represents the efficiency of the dialyzer, which is the equivalent of glomerular filtration coefficient (surface area x porosity) of the native glomerular capillary. The higher the value of KoA, the more is the solute clearance. Thus, using a filter with high KoA will occasionally improve Kt/V. However, it should be remembered that little benefit occurs when extremely large area dialyzer is used.

Suggested Reading

Ahmad S, Misra M, Hoenich N, Daugirdas JT. Hemodialysis apparatus. In: Daugirdas JT, Blake PG, Ing TS, editors. Handbook of dialysis. 5th ed. Philadelphia: Wolters Kluwer; 2015. p. 66–88.

Daugirdas JT. Physiologic principles and urea kinetic modeling. In: Daugirdas JT, Blake PG, Ing TS, editors. Handbook of dialysis. 5th ed. Philadelphia: Wolters Kluwer; 2015, p. 34–65.

66. Patients on either hemodialysis (HD) or peritoneal dialysis (PD) experience several benefits if they have some residual kidney function (RKF). RKF of even 2–3 mL/min will improve volume control, uremic toxicity, and LV hypertrophy. Also, malnutrition in PD patients is attributed to loss of RKF. Therefore, clinicians should try to preserve RKF in their patients on dialysis. **Which one of the following factors contributes to loss of RKF?**

A. Intradialytic hypotension
B. Radiocontrast agents
C. Aminoglycoside use
D. Congestive heart failure
E. All of the above

The answer is E

RKF is extremely important in dialysis patients. Early studies have shown that RKF is associated with increased survival rate in both HD and PD patients. It was estimated that every 1 mL/min increase in GFR was associated with a 40% reduced risk of death in dialysis patients. Of interest is the observation that the risk of death was much lower in PD than in HD patients. It was subsequently shown that PD preserves RKF better than HD because of hemodynamic stability and less oxidative stress.

Another study also showed that a decline in RKF, both renal clearance of urea and urine volume separately, showed a graded association with higher mortality among incident HD patients.

All of the above factors have been shown to contribute to loss of RKF (E is correct). In addition, ACE-Is and NSAIDs use is found to decrease RKF.

Strategies to preserve RKF include maintenance of hemodynamic stability, avoidance of nephrotoxins, and prevention of peritonitis in PD patients.

Suggested Reading

Brener ZZ, Kotanko P, Thijssen S, et al. Clinical benefit of preserving residual renal function in dialysis patients: an update for clinicians. Am J Med Sci. 2010;339:453–6.

Liu X, Dai C. Advances in understanding and management of residual renal function in patients with chronic kidney disease. Kidney Dis. 2016;2:187–96.

Obi Y, Rhee CM, Mathew, AT, et al. Residual kidney function decline and mortality in incident hemodialysis patients. J Am Soc Nephrol. 2016;27:3758–68.

Wang A-M, Lai K-N. The importance of residual renal function in dialysis patients. Kidney Int. 2006;69:1726–32.

67. A 48-year-old woman was just restarted on hemodialysis (HD) after failed transplant kidney. She had a deceased donor kidney transplant 2 years ago. Her maintenance immunosuppressive drugs are tacrolimus, mycophenolate mofetil, and prednisone. Her allograft biopsy showed antibody-mediated rejection. Her BP is well controlled, and she looks healthy.

Her eGFR is 10 mL/min. Her appetite and exercise tolerance are good. **Regarding reinitiation of her dialysis after allograft failure, which one of the following statements is CORRECT?**

A. Initiation of HD at higher eGFR >10 mL/min is better than early initiation (<10 mL/min) to improve mortality
B. Her infection-related hospitalization after initiation of HD is greatly reduced compared to those patients on maintenance HD who are waiting for kidney transplant
C. She will have a survival advantage with allograft nephrectomy than without nephrectomy
D. Abrupt discontinuation of immunotherapy will prevent infection-related hospitalization
E. She may not have a survival benefit with retransplantation compared to those on maintenance HD

The answer is C

In recent years, the number of patients starting dialysis after a failed transplant kidney has increased substantially (the number increased from 2463 in 1988 to 5588 in 2010). In the United States, the failed kidney transplant patients comprise 5% of all incident dialysis patients. Reinitiation of dialysis at an eGFR >10 mL/min was associated with a higher mortality compared to those patients whose dialysis was started at an eGFR <10 mL/min (A is incorrect). It is estimated that each 1 mL/min higher eGFR at reinitiation of dialysis was associated with 1–6% higher risk of death. Thus, reinitiation of dialysis at lower eGFR has survival advantage.

The DOPPS showed that patients with a failed kidney transplant had a 17% higher risk of hospitalization and 32% higher risk of death compared to patients on dialysis who are eligible for a transplant. The hazard ratio for infection-related hospitalization was 1.4 (RI 1.12–1.76). Thus, option B is incorrect.

Abrupt discontinuation of immunotherapy was found to be associated with high risk of infection rate, as withdrawal of immunosuppressive drugs may precipitate chronic inflammatory state and also anemia due to erythropoietin resistance. Therefore, gradual tapering of immunosuppressive drugs is suggested (D is incorrect).

It has been shown that retransplantation for the second time has a survival benefit compared to those on HD. Thus, E is incorrect.

Nephrectomy is usually performed when the allograft is inflamed with clinical presentation of abdominal pain, fever, hematuria, or anemia resistant to erythropoietin. Also, nephrectomy is performed due to surgical complications, thrombosis, and acute rejection. The USRDS data showed that nephrectomy was associated with a 13% increased risk of death in those whose transplant kidneys failed within 12 months of transplantation. On the other hand, an 11% lower risk of death was observed when nephrectomy was performed >12 months after transplantation. Another study showed that nephrectomy was associated with a 32% reduction in death rate over an average of 2.9-year follow-up. Thus, nephrectomy has a survival advantage in patients who are on dialysis with a failed kidney transplant (C is correct).

It should be noted that starting PD in failed kidney transplant patients has similar outcomes as HD, and PD should be considered an alternative modality of renal replacement therapy in these patients.

Suggested Reading

Gómez-Dos-Santos V, Lorca-Álvaro J, Hevia-Palacios V, et al. The failing kidney transplant allograft. transplant nephrectomy: current state-of-the-art. Curr Urol Rep. 2020;21(1):4.
Molnar MZ, Ichii H, Lineen J, et al. Timing of return to dialysis in patients with failing kidney transplants. Sem Dial. 2013;26:667–74. Curr Urol Rep. 2020;21:4.
Perl J, Hasan O, Bargman JM, et al. Impact of dialysis modality on survival after kidney transplant failure. Clin J Am Soc Nephrol. 2011;6:582–90.
Perl J, Zhang J, Gillespie B, et al. Reduced survival and quality of life following return to dialysis after transplant failure: the dialysis outcomes and practice patterns. Nephrol Dial Transpl. 2012;27:4464–72.
Pham P-T, Everly M, Faravardeh A, et al. Management of patients with a failed kidney transplant: dialysis reinitiation, immunosuppression weaning, and transplantectomy. World J Nephrol. 2015;4:148–59.

68. Malnutrition is rather common in some dialysis patients. Serum albumin is considered a marker of nutritional status in dialysis patients. Efforts to improve albumin status have been undertaken with the use of oral nutritional supplementation to patients whose serum albumin levels are either ≤3.5 g/dL or <3.8 g/dL during each visit of hemodialysis (HD) session. **Which one of the following statements regarding oral protein supplementation is CORRECT?**

A. Oral protein supplementation improves albumin to >4.5 g/dL
B. Oral protein supplementation improves survival rate by 50%

C. Oral protein supplementation lowers hospitalization rate at 1 year
D. Oral protein supplementation improves handgrip strength in all patients
E. Oral protein supplementation improves cognitive function

The answer is C

The Fresenius Medical Care of North America introduced an elective program of oral nutrition supplementation (ONS) in HD patients treated in their facilities, and two publications came out of this program. One is a retrospective study involving patients with serum albumin level ≤3.5 g/dL, and ONS was continued for a year until serum albumin reached 4 g/d (A is incorrect). This study found lower mortality rate at 2 years and increased survival rate in patients on ONS compared to controls. The increase in survival rate ranged from 9 to 34%, depending on the statistical evaluation. Thus, option B is incorrect. NeproCarb Steady, ProStat RC, ZonePerfect, and VitalProteinRxin were used in the first study. The protein content varied from 10 to 20 g per serving.

The second study included 470 patients. Of these, 276 patients received ONS, and 194 did not receive ONS (controls). Ensure Plus (nondiabetics) and Glucerna (diabetics) were used. Protein content ranged from 10 to 13 g. Baseline albumin level was <3.8 g/dL. ONS was continued until albumin reached ≥3.8 g/dL. ONS increased albumin by 0.058 g/dL, but this increase disappeared at 12 months of study. The analyses showed that ONS reduced the hospitalization rate at 1 year (68.4% in ONS group and 88.7% in controls; $p < 0.01$). Thus, option C is correct. However, unlike the first study, this study did not show any survival benefit of ONS. The above studies did not evaluate either handgrip strength or cognitive function (D and E are incorrect).

A small study showed that anabolic steroid (oxymetholone) use for 24 weeks showed an improvement in handgrip strength, physical function, and fat-free muscle mass.

Suggested Reading

Cheu C, Pearson J, Dahlerus C, et al. Association between oral nutritional supplementation and clinical outcomes among patients with ESRD. Clin J Am Soc Nephrol. 2013;8:100–7.
Lacson E Jr., Wang W, Zebrowski B, et al. Outcomes associated with intradialytic oral nutritional supplements in patients undergoing maintenance hemodialysis: a quality improvement report. Am J Kidney Dis. 2012;60:591–60.
Supasyndh O, Satirapoj B, Aramwit P, et al. Effect of oral anabolic steroid on muscle strength in hemodialysis patients. Clin J Am Soc Nephrol. 2013;8:271–9.

69. Normalized protein nitrogen appearance (nPNA) is a calculated number that represents the daily protein intake in a dialysis patient. In a stable patient, nPNA 1.0–1.2 g/kg/day suggests adequate protein intake. **Which one of the following conditions alters nPNA that may reflect either adequate or inadequate daily protein intake?**

A. Protein anabolic condition
B. Protein catabolic condition
C. Residual kidney function (RKF)
D. A, B, and C
E. None of the above

The answer is D

As stated above, nPNA is a calculated number from generation rate of urea nitrogen from protein. nPNA 1.0–1.2 g/kg/day is normal, and <1.0 g/kg/day suggests low protein intake. It should be noted that low number does not always represent inadequate protein intake. For example, a patient with adequate Kt/V and hemodynamically stable eats 1.0–1.2 g/kg/day protein and generates very little urea nitrogen (estimated as BUN) because most of this urea nitrogen is utilized for generation of protein. In such a case, nPNA is <1.0/g/kg/day (A is correct).

On the other hand, if the patient is highly catabolic due to intercurrent illness, more BUN is generated and the nPNA will be >1.0 g/kg/day (B is correct). Therefore, clinical examination and serum albumin levels will help the clinician in the evaluation of nPNA.

A patient with RKF may lose urea nitrogen in the urine but otherwise stable can have low nPNA. Therefore, RKF should be taken into consideration in the evaluation of nPNA (C is correct).

Based on the above discussion, it cannot be stated that nPNA is one of the best markers of clinical outcome. However, studies have shown that serum albumin and nPNA are associated with both mortality and hospitalization outcomes.

Suggested Reading

Daugirdas JT. Physiologic principles and urea kinetic modeling. In: Daugirdas JT, Blake PG, Ing TS, editors. Handbook of dialysis. 5th ed. Philadelphia: Wolters Kluwer; 2015. p. 34–65.

Kalantar-Zadeh K, Supasyndh O, Lehn RS, et al. Normalized protein nitrogen appearance is correlated with hospitalization and mortality in hemodialysis patients with Kt/V greater than 1.20. J Renal Nutr. 2003;13:13–25.

70. A 62-year-old diabetic woman is on hemodialysis (HD) for 4 years. She complains of occasional chest pain during HD only. ECHO for evaluation of heart function shows LV hypertrophy with an ejection fraction of 62%. She refuses coronary angiogram. The cardiologist believes that she has asymptomatic coronary artery disease (CAD). **Which one of the following screening tests for CAD is recommended in this patient?**

A. Routine measurements of cardiac troponins
B. Quantification of coronary Ca^{2+} score
C. CT coronary angiography
D. Cardiac MRI
E. Myocardial perfusion scintigraphy (MPS) with dipyridamole

The answer is E

Asymptomatic CAD is rather common in HD patients. In patients with diabetes, the prevalence of asymptomatic CAD is very high (about 83%) compared to nondiabetic (54%) HD patients. In one study, 75% of diabetic patients on HD with confirmed coronary artery stenosis had no symptoms. Thus, asymptomatic CAD is common in HD patients irrespective of their causative disease.

There are several screening tests to document asymptomatic CAD. Elevated troponins T and I are sensitive markers of myocardial damage. However, elevated troponin T levels are frequently seen without acute coronary syndrome and are attributed to LV hypertrophy, LV remodeling, silent myocardial ischemia, and congestive heart failure. Therefore, cardiac troponins alone may not indicate asymptomatic CAD (A is incorrect).

Multislice computed tomography and electron-beam computed tomography are sensitive methods to document and quantify the presence of Ca^{2+} in coronary arteries. Since coronary Ca^{2+} scores predict mortality in dialysis patients, no correlation between these scores and luminal stenosis has been established (B is incorrect).

CT coronary angiogram is used when there is intermediate probability of CAD. However, it is not routinely used in dialysis patients because of contrast material, decrease in residual kidney function, and interference with coronary calcification (C is incorrect).

Cardiac MRI is usually not recommended in dialysis patients because of exposure to gadolinium and fear of nephrogenic systemic sclerosis (D is incorrect).

The correct answer is E. Although MPS has low sensitivity compared to coronary angiogram, it is the recommended test with dipyridamole as the cardiac stressor of choice in dialysis patients. MPS-dipyridamole test measures only coronary blood flow, whereas coronary angiogram provides anatomical information, such as stenosis. Studies have shown that abnormal MPS and diabetes were found to be independent predictors of death. Also, in patients assessed for kidney transplantation, MPS was superior to coronary angiography in predicting all-cause mortality. Thus, MPS with dipyridamole appears to be the screening test for asymptomatic CAD patients on dialysis.

Suggested Reading

De Vriese AS, Vandecasteele SJ, Van Den Berg B, et al. Should we screen for coronary artery disease in asymptomatic chronic dialysis patients?. Kidney Int. 2012;81:143–51.

Raggi P, Alexopoulous N. Cardiac imaging in chronic kidney disease patients. Sem Dial. 2017;30:353–60.

Venkataraman R, Hage FG, Dorfman T, et al. Role of myocardial perfusion imaging in patients with end-stage renal disease undergoing coronary angiography. Am J Cardiol. 2008;102:1451–6.

71. Cardiovascular disease is the major cause of morbidity and mortality in patients on hemodialysis (HD). In recent years, several imaging techniques have been developed for analysis of cardiac structural changes in asymptomatic patients. **Match the following cardiac imaging techniques with their evaluation (use), advantages, and limitations in these patients:**

Imaging technique	Evaluation	Advantage	Limitations
A. ECHO	1. Myocardial structure and function Coronary artery flow Valvular and interstitial structure	Gold standard of cardiac imaging, better imaging quality than ECHO	Expensive and limited availability. Risk for nephrogenic systemic fibrosis
B. CMRI	2. Structure and function Assessment of cardiac valves LV mass, volume, and EF	Less expensive and noninvasive, assessment of LV function, EF, and left atrial volume	High interobserver variability on various measurements than other imaging procedures
C. PET	3. Myocardial perfusion Microvascular and macrovasculature LV function	Reliably detect ischemia and microvascular changes	Variable radiotracer uptake by myocardium in HD patients

ECHO echocardiography, *MRI* cardiac magnetic resonance imaging, *PET* positron emission tomography, *EF* ejection fraction

Answers. A = 2; B = 1; C = 3

Suggested Reading

Kott J, Reicheck N, Butler J, et al. Cardiac imaging in dialysis patients. Kidney Med. 2020;2:629–38.

Loutradis C, Sarafidis PA, Papadopoulos CE, et al. The ebb and flow of echocardiographic cardiac function parameters in relationship to hemodialysis treatment in patients with ESRD. J Am Soc Nephrol. 2018;29:1372–81.

Raggi P, Alexopoulous N. Cardiac imaging in chronic kidney disease patients. Sem Dial. 2017;30:353–60.

72. Hospitalization for dialysis patients is rather common that involves not only monetary burden on taxpayers but also morbidity on these patients. Also, rehospitalization after discharge within 30 days is high. **Which one of the following strategies can improve rehospitalization?**

A. Frequent face-to-face visits by the physician or healthcare worker
B. Frequent phone conversation with the patient
C. Long visit time once a month by the physician
D. Counseling about health issues
E. Care by the patient himself/herself can prevent rehospitalization

The answer is A

One of the goals of healthcare reform is to prevent or reduce the rate of 30-day rehospitalization. In 2004, the Medicare cost for unplanned rehospitalization was $17.4 billion. With regard to ESKD patients, 30-day rehospitalization is rather common. An observational study has shown that checking hemoglobin within a week of discharge followed by modification of erythropoietin dose significantly reduced the rehospitalization. Also, administration of vitamin D within a week was found to be associated with reduced rehospitalization.

A more recent study showed that frequent physician visits following hospital discharge were found to reduce rehospitalizations in HD patients (A is correct). Other options are incorrect.

Suggested Reading

Chan KE, Lazarus JM, Wingard RL, et al. Association between repeat hospitalization and early intervention in dialysis patients following hospital discharge. Kidney Int. 2009;76:331–41.

Erickson KF, Winkelmayer WC, Chertow GM, et al. Physician visits and 30-day hospital readmission in patients receiving hemodialysis. J Am Soc Nephrol. 2014;25:2079–87.

73. A 54-year-old African American woman with type 2 diabetes was started on hemodialysis (HD) with a functioning AV fistula. Her medications are insulin, amlodipine, lisinopril, and atorvastatin (20 mg/day), which were continued from predialysis care. Her cholesterol is 132 mg/dL, and LDL cholesterol is 89 mg/mL. **Regarding statin use in HD patients, which one of the following statements is CORRECT?**

A. Decrease the dose to 10 mg, as she may be at increased risk for rhabdomyolysis
B. Start coenzyme Q 10 to prevent rhabdomyolysis

C. Continue statin to decrease cardiovascular (CV) death
D. Continue statin at 20 mg/day, as she has been on the drug for long time
E. All the studies on statin use showed CV benefit in HD patients

The answer is D

Statins have shown a beneficial effect on all-cause and CV-related mortality in individuals with normal kidney function. However, their effect in HD patients is controversial. Initial studies have shown no CV benefit in HD patients. The 4D study (Deutsche Diabetes Dialyse Study) in 1255 HD patients with type 2 diabetes showed no benefit of atorvastatin (20 mg) during a mean follow-up of 4 years on any CV events. Although LDL cholesterol levels were reduced, atorvastatin was associated with increased risk for stroke. Similarly, the AURORA (A Study to Evaluate the Use of Rosuvastatin in Subjects on Regular Dialysis) on 2.776 dialysis patients did not show any CV benefit during a 3.8-year follow-up. In the SHARP (Study of Heart and Renal Protection), simvastatin (20 mg) and ezetimibe (10 mg) use for 4.9 years in 2527 HD and 496 PD patients did not have any effect CV events. The KDIGO guideline does not recommend the use of LDL cholesterol to assess the coronary risk in CKD patients.

Based on the above large studies, initiation of statin therapy is not routinely recommended to prevent CV events in dialysis patients. However, if the patient is already on a statin, it should be continued without adding coenzyme Q 10, if no myopathy is present. Thus, D is correct.

It should be noted that one meta-analysis of 31 studies showed a benefit of 28% reduction in CV events in CKD patients.

Suggested Reading

Baigent C, Landray MJ, Reith C, et al. SHARP Investigators. The effects of lowering LDL cholesterol with simvastatin plus ezetimibe in patients with chronic kidney disease (Study of Heart and Renal Protection): a randomized controlled placebo trial. Lancet. 2011;377:2181–92.

Fellström BC, Jardine AG, Schmieder RE, et al. AURORA Study Group. Rosuvastatin and cardiovascular events in patients undergoing hemodialysis. N Engl J Med. 2009;360:1395–407.

Hou W, Lv J, Perkovic V, et al. Effect of statin therapy on cardiovascular and renal outcomes in patients with chronic kidney disease: a systematic review and meta-analysis. Eur Heart J. 2013;34:1807–17.

Wanner C, Krane V, März W, et al. German Diabetes and Dialysis Study Investigators. Atorvastatin in patients with type 2 diabetes mellitus undergoing hemodialysis. N Engl J Med. 2005;353:238–48.

Wanner C, Tonelli M. KDIGO Clinical Practice Guideline for Lipid Management in CKD: summary of recommendation statements and clinical approach to the patient. Kidney Int. 2014;85:1303–9.

74. A 74-year-old woman, on hemodialysis (HD) for 5 years, develops ascites which is found to be an exudate. She complains of poor appetite. Tuberculosis (TB) is strongly suspected. **Which one of the following tests for TB detection is appropriate in dialysis patients?**

A. Tuberculin skin test (TST)
B. Chest X-ray
C. QuantiFERON test
D. Physical examination will detect TB most of the time
E. None of the above

The answer is C

There are no specific and uniformly accepted guidelines for TB testing in dialysis patients. Since HD-dependent patients are immunocompromised, TST may be negative to detect latent TB (A is incorrect). However, a TST is an acceptable alternative, especially in situations where an interferon γ release assay is not available, too costly, or too burdensome.

Chest X-ray findings may not always be present in TB patients; therefore, detection of TB is delayed (B is incorrect). Physical examination may give a clue to the diagnosis of TB, but it is not always reliable (D is incorrect). Interferon γ release assays such as quantiFERON test and T-SPOT.TB test (enzyme-linked immunosorbent spot) can detect latent TB, and therefore, C is correct. A meta-analysis by Rogerson et al. suggests that quantiFERON test and T-SPOT.TB tests determined by ELISA are strongly associated with radiologic evidence of past TB and prior contact with acute TB.

Suggested Reading

Lewinsohn DM, Leonard MK, LoBue PA, et al. Official American Thoracic Society/Infectious Diseases Society of America/Centers for Disease Control and prevention clinical practice guidelines: diagnosis of tuberculosis in adults and children. Clin Infect Dis. 2017;64:111–5.

Rogerson TE, Chen S, Kok J, et al. Tests for latent tuberculosis in people with ESRD: a systematic review. Am J Kidney Dis. 2013;61:33–43.

Chapter 10
Peritoneal Dialysis

1. Peritoneal dialysis (PD) offers several advantages over hemodialysis (HD), at least during the first 2–3 years of treatment. **Which one of the following statements regarding PD is FALSE?**

   A. PD maintains hemodynamic stability better than HD
   B. Peritoneal membrane is more biocompatible than HD membrane
   C. Preservation of residual kidney function is better with PD than with HD
   D. The incidence and severity of delayed graft function is greatly reduced in PD patients after kidney transplantation compared to patients on HD
   E. Small solute clearance (Na^+, K^+, creatinine, urea) is similar in both PD and HD during short dialysis sessions

   The answer is E

   Except for E, all other statements are correct. In addition, PD allows the patient independency to travel and have flexible schedules for dialysis. PD treatment also allows more fluid and dietary intake. However, small solute clearance is far less in PD than in HD patients in short dialysis sessions. For this reason, adequacy of PD is calculated on a weekly basis.

   PD has been shown to have a better survival than HD during the first 2 years of dialysis treatment. The cost of PD is much less than HD. Also, the rate of infection-related complications has been declining over the last decade in patients on PD than patients on HD. Thus, many nephrologists offer PD as the first choice of renal (kidney) replacement therapy.

   Suggested Reading

   Chaudhary K, Sangha H, Khanna R. Peritoneal dialysis first: rationale. Clin J Am Soc Nephrol. 2012;6:447–56.
   Javaid MM, Khan BA, Subramanian S. Peritoneal dialysis as initial dialysis modality: a viable option for late presenting end stage renal disease. J Nephrol. 2019;32:51–6
   Tang SCW, Lai KN. Peritoneal dialysis: the ideal bridge from conservative therapy to kidney transplant. J Nephrol. 2020;33:1189–94.

2. One of your 52-year-old female patients with an eGFR of 12 mL/min comes to your office with complaints of fatigue and poor appetite due to metallic taste in the mouth for the last 2 years. She has no chest pain or hyperkalemia. Her BP is 130/80 mm Hg. Her serum [HCO_3^-] is 20 mEq/L. During her previous visit (3 months ago), you discussed about the choice of her future renal replacement therapies, including transplantation. After prolonged discussion, she feels that PD is a reasonable choice in view of her daily work in the school. **Based on her clinical history, which one of the following choices is MOST appropriate regarding the management of her symptoms and selection of dialysis modality is CORRECT?**

   A. Admit to hospital and start HD with a central vein catheter (CVC), and then start PD
   B. Tell her that she would receive in-center HD once acute HD treatment is over
   C. Admit to hospital and place a PD catheter, and then train her for continuous ambulatory PD with small volume exchanges initially

The original version of the chapter has been revised. A correction to this chapter can be found at https://doi.org/10.1007/978-3-030-85958-9_12

A. S. Reddi, *Absolute Nephrology Review*, https://doi.org/10.1007/978-3-030-85958-9_10

D. Change her diet and increase her $NaHCO_3$ to 1350 mg every 8 hours
E. Tell her that she may not need any renal (kidney) replacement therapy (either HD or PD) until her eGFR falls to 7 mL/min

The answer is C

This patient has either no PD catheter or an arteriovenous fistula or graft; therefore, HD using a CVC or femoral catheter is a default modality for dialysis initiation. This is usually the practice in unplanned mode of treatment for acute dialysis. However, this patient expressed PD as her choice of dialysis. If she agrees to PD, a PD catheter can be inserted and acute PD can be started to improve her symptoms. Then she can be trained for CAPD. Thus, choice C is correct. Option A is the choice of many nephrologists, however, this patient prefers PD. Moreover, PD catheters have low infection rates than CVCs. A study by Koch et al. showed that initiation of PD within 12 h after PD catheter insertion for unplanned dialysis had a lower rate of infection compared to HD catheters. A study from the United States also showed that PD for unplanned dialysis is safe, efficacious, and feasible alternative to unplanned initiation of HD. Therefore, choice A is incorrect. Other choices are also not appropriate.

Suggested Reading

Ghaffari A. Urgent-start peritoneal dialysis: a quality improvement report. Am J Kidney Dis. 2012;59:400–08.
Koch M, Kohnle M, Trapp R, et al. Comparable outcome of acute unplanned peritoneal dialysis and hemodialysis. Nephrol Dial Transplant. 2012;27:375–80.

3. A 65-year-old woman with diabetic kidney disease preferred PD, and her granddaughter is trained to do automated peritoneal dialysis (APD) with four exchanges at night without daytime dwell ("dry day"). The patient is brought to the emergency department with complaints of fever and chills. Her admission labs: Na^+ 130 mEq/L, K^+ 4.1 mEq/L, HCO_3^- 17 mEq/L, creatinine 12.6 mg/dL, BUN 72 mg/dL, and glucose 172 mg/dL. **Which one of the following factors can maximize PD clearance of a solute?**

A. No dry time
B. More frequent exchanges
C. Larger dwell volumes
D. Maximum fluid removal
E. All of the above

The answer is E

The solute and fluid clearance occurs by three processes in PD: diffusion, convection, and fluid reabsorption. The best accepted model of peritoneal transport is the three-pore model. In this model, the peritoneal capillary, which is the only barrier to the peritoneal transport, consists of three pores of different sizes. The smallest pores (<0.5 nm) represent aquaporin-1 channels that allow only water to pass through them, and solute transport is inhibited. The following figure shows three-pore model of capillary transport and water and solute movement from capillary lumen to the interstitium and then into the dialysate.

All of the above factors are involved to increase the peritoneal clearance of small solutes during APD. Increasing dialysate dwelling time (no dry time) with frequent exchanges which increases the concentration gradient will increase solute clearance.

In addition, larger dwell volumes increase the peritoneal surface area and maximum fluid removal by increasing the osmotic gradient with 4.25% dextrose can improve fluid removal and solute clearance. Thus, E is correct.

Suggested Reading

Devuyst O, Rippe B. Water transport across the peritoneal membrane. Kidney Int. 2014;85:750–58.
Flessner MF. Peritoneal transport physiology: insights from basic research. J Am Soc Nephrol. 1991;2:122–35.
Rippe B. A three-pore model of peritoneal transport. Perit Dial Int. 1993;13 Suppl 2:S35–8.

4. One of your 50-year-old male patients with CKD 5 is considering PD as one of his choices for renal (kidney) replacement therapy. He asks you about indications and contraindications about PD. **Which one of the following choices is a contraindication for PD?**

A. Abdominal hernia not amenable to surgery
B. Adhesions from previous surgery

C. Severe inflammatory bowel disease
D. Diaphragmatic fluid leak
E. All of the above

The answer is E

All of the above choices are contraindications to PD (E is correct). The contraindications can be absolute or relative. Table 10.1 summarizes these contraindications for PD.

Table 10.1 Contraindications for PD

Absolute contraindications	Relative contraindications
1. Abdominal adhesions, fibrosis, or malignancy 2. Uncorrectable abdominal hernias 3. Loss of peritoneal function 4. Ostomies (colostomy, ileostomy, etc.) 5. Third trimester pregnancy 6. Severe active psychiatric disorder 7. Lack of suitable assistance to do PD at home 8. Pleuroperitoneal fistulas not corrected by surgery	1. Recent abdominal surgery with aortic prostheses (may cause infection of prostheses) 2. Severe malnutrition 3. Abdominal wall cellulitis (may cause peritonitis) 4. Severe respiratory failure 5. Morbid obesity 6. Severe diabetic gastroparesis 7. Presence of ventriculoperitoneal shunt 8. Severe nephrotic syndrome

It should be noted that some of the absolute contraindications can be considered relative contraindications by some nephrologists.

There are some indications for PD, which are shown in Table 10.2.

Table 10.2 Indications for PD

Indication	Strong indication for PD	Preference for PD
Age	0–5 years	6–16 years
Medical issues	1. Patient choice 2. Independency 3. Severe vascular disease and difficulty in creating vascular access 4. Severe congestive heart failure refractory to medical management 5. Frequent hypotensive episodes and intolerability to hemodialysis 6. Long distance to in-center hemodialysis unit	1. Bleeding disorders 2. Seeking kidney transplantation 3. Transfusion reactions 4. Cardiovascular instability 5. Persistent volume-related hypertension 6. No in-center hemodialysis for patients with positive hepatitis B antigenemia
Psychosocial		1. Flexible diet 2. Frequent travel 3. Variable schedule

Suggested Reading

Khosla N. Patient selection for peritoneal dialysis. In: Haggerty S, editor. Surgical aspects of peritoneal dialysis. China: Springer; 1917. p. 17–21.

Reynar HC, Imai E, Kher V. Approach to renal replacement therapy. In: Feehally J, Floege J, Tonelli M, et al., editors. Comprehensive clinical nephrology. 6th ed. Philadelphia: Elsevier; 2019. p. 1036–49.

Shahab T, Khanna R, Nolph KD. Peritoneal dialysis or hemodialysis? A dilemma for the nephrologist. Adv Perit Dial. 2006;22:180–5.

5. A 50-year-old diabetic woman is on PD for 1 year. Her ultrafiltrate Na^+ concentration is 128 mEq/L 1 h after instillation of 2 L of 4.25% dextrose into the peritoneum. Simultaneous determination of plasma Na^+ concentration is 144 mEq/L. **Which one of the following statements regarding the difference in Na^+ concentration between plasma and ultrafiltrate is CORRECT?**

A. Sieving of Na^+
B. Dialysis to plasma ratio (D/P) of Na^+ <1 during the first hour and then reaches unity after several hours of dwell
C. The difference between plasma and ultrafiltrate Na^+ level (Na^+ dip) indicates adequate aquaporin-1 function

D. The Na^+ dip does not occur with icodextrin
E. All of the above

The answer is E

All of the above statements are correct (E). During the first-hour dwell of hypertonic (hyperosmolar) dialysis solutions, such as 2.5% and 4.5% dextrose solutions, the osmotic pressure in the peritoneum is higher than in the peritoneal capillaries. This osmotic gradient causes water movement from blood into the peritoneum and dilutes Na^+ concentration. This water movement is a process of diffusion via aquaporin-1 channels. These channels are stimulated by dialysate osmolality. Na^+ does not move with aquaporin-stimulated water movement. Therefore, Na^+ concentration in blood increases due to water movement into the dialysate. This process is called sieving of Na^+ (A is correct).

Because of an increase in plasma Na^+ and a decrease in dialysate Na^+, the D/P ratio decreases during the first hour of dwell. If the dwell time increases to 4 or more hours, there is an equilibration, and water movement decreases across the transcellular pores (see Fig. 10.1 in question 3) and convection increases through other pores. As a result, Na^+ and other solutes as well as water move into the peritoneal cavity, and the D/P ratio of Na^+ reaches unity (B is correct).

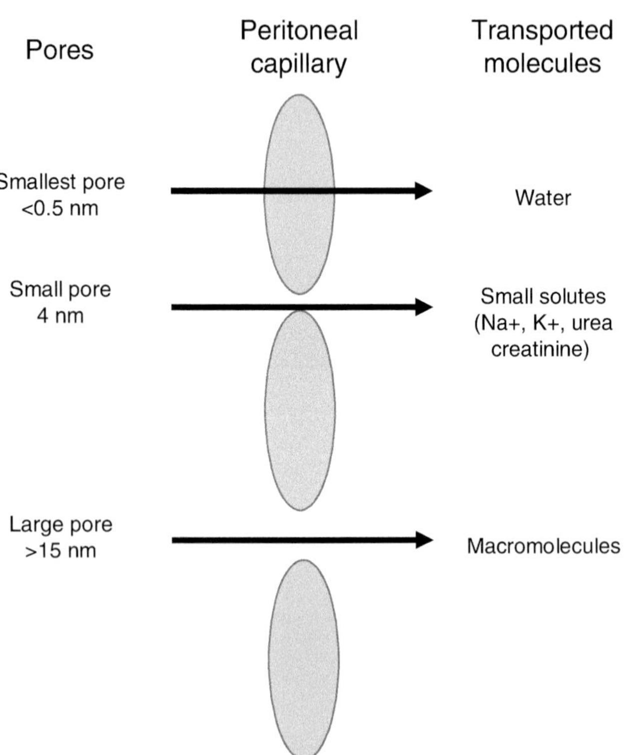

Fig. 10.1 Three-pore model of peritoneal transport

When sieving of Na^+ occurs (Na^+ dip), it is an indication of adequate aquaporin function. On the other hand, failure to decrease Na^+ concentration in the dialysis solution during the first hour of dwell is an indication of aquaporin deficiency. This suggests ultrafiltration failure.

Icodextrin is a glucose polymer derived from starch and is iso-osmotic. Unlike dextrose, icodextrin does not stimulate aquaporin channels in the three-pore model of transport. Therefore, sieving of Na^+ does not occur. Icodextrin creates a colloidal osmotic pressure (similar to albumin) with resultant water and solute movement across the small and large pores. Here, the D/P ratio of Na^+ does not alter, and Na^+ dip does not occur (D is correct).

It should be noted that Na^+ sieving causes hypernatremia, thirst, and hypertension, which are seen with hyperosmolar dialysis solutions.

The osmotic agents that are commonly used in clinical practice are glucose-containing solutions, usually referred to as dextrose solutions. It is, therefore, important for the nephrologists to be familiar with the concentrations, osmolarities, and the expected rate of ultrafiltration with these different glucose solutions (see Table 10.3).

Table 10.3 Various concentrations of glucose solutions

Dextrose (g/dL)[a]	Glucose (g/dL)	Osmolarity (mOsm/L)	Ultrafiltrate (mL)/2 L exchange/60 min dwell
1.5	1.36	346	40–150
2.5	2.27	396	100–300
4.25	3.86	486	300–400

[a]Glucose monohydrate that is 10% higher in weight than anhydrous glucose

Suggested Reading

Devuyst O, Goffin E. Water and solute transport in peritoneal dialysis: models and clinical applications. Nephrol Dial Transplant. 2008;23:2120–23.

Rusthoven E, Krediet RT, Willems HL, et al. Sodium sieving in children. Perit Dial Int. 2005;25 Suppl 3:S141–42.

6. A 54-year-old man is started on continuous ambulatory peritoneal dialysis (CAPD) 6 weeks ago. You ask your PD nurse to perform a test to evaluate the peritoneal membrane transport characteristics to prescribe appropriate PD therapy for the patient. **Which one of the following is MOSTLY used tests in this incident patient?**

A. Traditional peritoneal equilibration test (PET)
B. Fast PET
C. Modified PET
D. Dialysis adequacy and transport test (DATT)
E. All of the above

The answer is A

There is insufficient evidence to suggest that one test is superior to another test to evaluate peritoneal membrane characteristics. However, the traditional (original) test, which was introduced by Twardowski et al. in 1987, is the most widely used test in clinical practice. This test uses 2 L of 2.5% dextrose solution, and a sample of dialysate is taken immediately after completion of instillation and then at 2 and 4 h. The samples are sent for determination of urea, creatinine, glucose, and Na^+. A blood sample is taken at 2 h and sent for urea, creatinine, glucose, and Na^+ determination. At the end of 4 h, the dialysate is drained and its volume is recorded. Blood for creatinine is also collected. Dialysate to plasma (D/P) ratios are calculated. Glucose samples are drawn immediately after instillation (0 time) and then at 2 and 4 h to calculate D/D_0 ratio.

Based on 4 h D/P ratios of creatinine and glucose, the patients are classified into four groups of transporters, as shown in Table 10.4. Other ratios are also used to evaluate the membrane characteristics.

Table 10.4 Types of transporters

Type of transporter	$D/P_{Creatinine}$	$D/D_{0(glucose)}$
High (fast)	0.82–1.03	0.092–0.25
High average	0.66–0.81	0.26–0.37
Low average	0.50–0.65	0.39–0.48
Low (slow)	0.34–0.49	0.49–0.61

The above traditional test does not quantify ultrafiltration rate, because it does not involve Na^+ sieving. Therefore, use of 4.25% dextrose is recommended. With this test, ultrafiltration (UF) can be calculated. The PET is done 4–6 weeks following initiation of PD.

The fast PET is a simplified test of the traditional PET. In this test, only 4-h dialysate and blood creatinine and dialysate glucose are measured after instillation of 2.5% dextrose. The volume of drained dialysate is measured. Typical values for fast PET are shown in Table 10.5. The fast PET is criticized for not having internal controls, and also difficult to interpret data in diabetic subjects.

Table 10.5 Results of fast PET[a]

Type of transporter	$D/P_{Creatinine}$	Dialysate glucose (mg)	UF (mL)
High (fast)	0.82–1.03	230–501	1580–2084
High average	0.66–0.81	502–722	2085–2367
Low average	0.50–0.65	724–944	2369–2650
Low (slow)	0.34–0.49	945–1214	2651–3326

[a]Twardowski (1990)

A modified PET is introduced in some patients who have UF failure. In this test, 2 L of 4.25% dextrose is used. After 4-h dwell, the volume is drained. UF failure is defined as an UF volume <400 mL. This suggests that the peritoneal membrane has lost its UF capacity, and a decision can be made to switch to HD for volume control. This incident patient has not shown any UF failure yet.

DATT is used by some centers to evaluate membrane permeability. This test requires 24-h drainage in a CAPD patient and blood sample on the day of drainage for creatinine to calculate $D/P_{Creatinine}$ ratio. Studies have shown reasonable correlation between TET and DATT.

Of all the above tests, the traditional PET is preferred in incident PD patients; therefore, the appropriate answer is A.

Suggested Reading

Tawardowski ZJ. The fast peritoneal equilibration test. Sem Dial. 1990;3:141–2.
Twardowski ZJ, Nolph KD, Khanna R, et al. Peritoneal equilibration test. Perit Dial Bull. 1987;7:138–47.
van Biesen W, Heimburger O, Krediet R, et al. Evaluation of peritoneal membrane characteristics: a clinical advice for prescription management by the ERBP working group. Nephrol Dial Transplant. 2010;25:2052–62.

7. The above patient is on CAPD with 2 L of 2.5% dextrose with a dwell time of 4 h. She had a traditional PET 5 weeks after initiation of PD, and the following values were obtained:

- $D/P_{Creatinine}$ 0.91 and $D/D_{0(glucose)}$ 0.2.

Which one of the following PD prescriptions is APPROPRIATE for him?

A. CAPD with 2 L of 1.5% dextrose solution and a dwell time of 4 h
B. CAPD with 2 L of 2.5% dextrose solution and a dwell time of 4 h
C. APD with 2 L of 4.25% dextrose and a dwell time of 1.5 h
D. APD with 2 L of 2.5% dextrose and a dwell time of 1.5 h
E. Continue her current regimen of PD prescription

The answer is D

Based on the above ratios, the patient is a fast (high) transporter. Approximately 15% of patients will be fast transporters at the initiation of PD. Rapid transporters have high rates of diffusive transport for small solutes like urea, creatinine, and glucose. As a result, these patients reabsorb glucose at a rapid rate, leading to dissolution of the osmotic gradient between the dialysate and blood. This causes slow diffusion and convection of water and solutes. The net result is less ultrafiltration (UF) and resultant fluid accumulation. Also, these patients develop volume-dependent HTN and LV hypertrophy. This cardiac stress leads to high mortality. It was estimated that for every 0.1 increase in D/P ratios of creatinine, there was an increase in the relative risk of death of 1.15 (CI 1.07–1.23). In low transporters, this risk is less.

This patient who is a rapid transporter will benefit from APD with shorter dwell times (1.5 h or less). Thus, D is correct.

CAPD with longer dwell times is not indicated for fast transporters because of dissipation of osmotic gradient and low UF. For low transporters, CAPD with longer dwell time or continuous cycling PD with less overnight exchanges may be appropriate. Thus, choices other than D are not appropriate for this patient.

It should be noted that PET does not provide information on adequacy of dialysis, which is obtained from Kt/V_{Urea}. This requires appropriate adjustments in the number of exchanges.

Suggested Reading

Burkart JM. Rapid transporters on maintenance peritoneal dialysis. UpToDate; 2020.

Chung SH, Heimbürger O, Lindholm B. Poor outcomes for fast transporters on PD: the rise and fall of a clinical concern. Sem Dial. 2008;21:7–10.

8. One of your patient's choices for renal (kidney) replacement therapy is PD. He read CAPD and APD from the Internet, but he could not understand completely the survival advantage between these two modalities. **Which one of the following statements you would make regarding the risk of survival between CAPD and APD?**

   A. The risk of survival is reduced in patients on CAPD compared to APD
   B. The risk of survival is reduced in patients on APD compared to CAPD
   C. The risk of survival is similar in both CAPD and APD
   D. There are no comparative studies on survival among different modalities of PD
   E. There are several comparative randomized studies, but the data are inconclusive

   The answer is C

   Most of the studies on mortality in CAPD and APD patients are observational. These studies showed no difference immortality between these two modalities. Also, a small, randomized study did not find any difference in mortality, indicating that survival is similar between CAPD and APD patients. Thus, choice C is correct. Similarly, no difference in peritonitis, volume management, and technical failure were observed between these two modalities. Larger randomized studies are needed to confirm the results of observational studies.

   Suggested Reading

Bieber SD, Burkart J, Gilper TA, et al. Comparative outcomes between continuous ambulatory and automated peritoneal dialysis: a narrative summary. Am J Kidney Dis. 2014;63:1027–37.

Mizuno M, Suzuki Y, Sakata F, et al. Which clinical conditions are most suitable for induction of automated peritoneal dialysis? Renal Replacement Ther. 2016;2:46.

9. **In selecting the modality of PD, which one of the following major considerations is important?**

   A. Patient preference
   B. Lifestyle and social activities
   C. Employment and home environment
   D. Cost
   E. All of the above

   The answer is E

   Selection of either CAPD or APD is dependent mostly on the patient preference. These preferences may include lifestyle, time for social activities, employment, ability to perform PD with or without support, unwillingness to sleep with cycler, and freedom from cycler. Although peritoneal membrane characteristics are an important consideration in the selection of PD, emphasis is placed on patient preferences. Finally, cost is an important consideration. CAPD is cheaper than APD, and frequently the patient has to bear the additional cost. Thus, all of the above choices are correct.

   Suggested Reading

Blake PG, Daugirdas JT. Adequacy of peritoneal dialysis and chronic peritoneal dialysis prescription. In: Daugirdas JT, Blake PG, Ing TS, editors. Handbook of dialysis. 5th ed. Philadelphia: Wolters Kluwer; 2015. p. 464–82.

Roumeliotis A, Roumeliotis S, Leivaditis K, et al. APD or CAPD: one glove does not fit all. Int Urol Nephrol. 2020. https://doi.org/10.1007/s11255-020-02678-6.

10. PD adequacy is expressed as Kt/V_{Urea}, which is the clearance of urea (K) per unit time (t) in relation to its volume of distribution or total body water (V). **Which one of the following choices regarding Kt/V is CORRECT?**

    A. Previous target Kt/V was 2
    B. Current target Kt/V is 1.7

C. Kt/V of 1.7 reflects weekly and not daily urea clearance
D. The V in Kt/V is calculated by Watson formula, using the actual body weight
E. All of the above

The answer is E

Clearance in PD can be calculated as Kt/V_{Urea} and also measured by creatinine clearance. The Kt/V includes peritoneal and residual kidney function components. Previous guidelines suggested a weekly Kt/V of 2 and above; however, recent studies have suggested that Kt/V of 1.7 is adequate to improve long-term outcomes. Daily Kt/V values are not adequate; therefore, daily values are multiplied by 7 to express the adequacy of PD. The V (volume of distribution of urea) is calculated by Watson formula, where age, height, and weight are included in the calculation, as follows:

- Men: V = 2.447 - 0.09516 Age (years) + 0.1704 Height (cm) + 0.3362 Weight (kg)
- Women: V = 2.097 + 0.1069 Height (cm) + 0.2466 Weight (kg)

Thus, all of the above choices are correct.

Suggested Reading

Blake PG, Bargman JM, Brimble SN, the Canadian Society of Nephrology Work Group on Adequacy of Peritoneal Dialysis, et al. Clinical practice guidelines and recommendations on peritoneal dialysis adequacy 2011. Perit Dial Int. 2011;31:218–39.

Burkart JM. Adequacy of peritoneal dialysis. In: Lerma EV, Weir MR, editors. Henrich's principles and practice of dialysis. 5th ed. Philadelphia: Wolters Kluwer/Lippincott Williams & Wilkins; 2017. p. 169–93.

Lo W-K, Bargman JM, Krediet RT, for the ISPD Adequacy of Peritoneal Dialysis Working Group, et al. Guideline on targets for solute and fluid removal in adult patients on chronic peritoneal dialysis. Peri Dial Int. 2006;26:520–22.

Woodrow G, Fan SL, Reid C, et al. Renal Association Clinical Practice Guideline on peritoneal dialysis in adults and children. BMC Nephrol. 2017;18:333.

11. **Which one of the following statements regarding total Kt/V (residual kidney clearance and peritoneal clearance) is FALSE?**

A. Both residual kidney clearance and peritoneal clearance have different effects on patient survival
B. Achieving total Kt/V above 2 by increasing dialysis therapy has no beneficial effect on survival
C. Total Kt/V <1.7 is associated with greater need for erythropoietin therapy
D. Several studies have established the lower limit of Kt/V (1.4) that is associated with mortality
E. Small solute clearance is dependent on the frequency and volume of dialysate, whereas middle molecule clearance is dependent on duration of dialysate dwell

The answer is D

PD adequacy is determined by total Kt/V or creatinine clearance. Both include residual and peritoneal clearances. Once the patient is anuric, only peritoneal clearance is calculated. The importance of residual kidney function (RKF) on CAPD patients was popularized by the initial Canada-USA (CANUSA) study, where patients with RKF had better survival with Kt/V of 2 to 2.25. A reanalysis of the original data showed that for every 5 mL/min of residual GFR, there was a 12% decrease in the risk of death. Also, for every 250 mL of urine output, the relative risk of death decreased by 36%. Thus, RKF is associated with improved survival compared to those without RKF (A is correct).

Two prospective randomized studies (Adequacy of PD in Mexico, ADMEX, and Lo et al.) showed no survival benefit of increasing Kt/V above 2. Also, HEMO study did not show any benefit of survival in patients assigned a higher Kt/V (B is correct).

In the study of Lo et al., patients with Kt/V of 1.5 and below (1.0) had greater clinical problems and required more erythropoietin dosage compared to patients whose Kt/V was 1.7–2 (C is correct). However, there are no prospective randomized studies that explored the lower limit of target clearance (Kt/V) in relation to mortality (D is false).

A significant discrepancy between small solute clearance and middle molecule clearance exists. For better clearance of small solutes such as urea and creatinine, increasing the number of exchanges per day and larger dwell volumes are recommended. For middle molecules such as β_2 microglobulin, longer dwell times are recommended (E is correct).

Suggested Reading

Blake PG, Bargman JM, Brimble SN, the Canadian Society of Nephrology Work Group on Adequacy of Peritoneal Dialysis, et al. Clinical practice guidelines and recommendations on peritoneal dialysis adequacy 2011. Perit Dial Int. 2011;31:218–39.

Kim DJ, Do JH, Huh W, et al. Dissociation between clearances of small and middle molecules in incremental peritoneal dialysis. Peri Dial Int. 2001;21:462–66.

Lo W-K, Bargman JM, Krediet RT, for the ISPD Adequacy of Peritoneal Dialysis Working Group, et al. Guideline on targets for solute and fluid removal in adult patients on chronic peritoneal dialysis. Peri Dial Int. 2006;26:520–22.

Woodrow G, Fan SL, Reid C, et al. Renal Association Clinical Practice Guideline on peritoneal dialysis in adults and children. BMC Nephrol. 2017;18:333.

12. A 70-kg anuric male is started on CAPD and you want to calculate weekly Kt/V for evaluation of adequacy of dialysis. The following values were obtained:

- 24-h drained dialysate = 8.8 L
- Dialysate urea = 90 mg/dL
- Plasma urea = 90 mg/dL
- Total body water = 42 L

Which one of the following Kt/V values is CORRECT?

A. 1.80
B. 1.70
C. 1.47
D. 1.60
E. 1.54

The answer is C

This patient is anuric and his kidney clearance is zero. One needs to calculate only peritoneal clearance. To calculate peritoneal clearance, one needs to have K, which is urea clearance, t is time of dialysis in days, and V is volume of distribution of urea in the body which is equal to total body water (60% of total body weight in kg). Also, one needs dialysate and plasma urea concentrations for calculation of urea equilibration (D/P_{Urea}). This patient has all of the above items for calculation of weekly Kt/V, which is shown as follows:

- K = 8.8 L × D/P_{Urea} = 1 or K = 8.8 L
- t = 24 h (1 day)
- V = 70 kg × 0.6 = 42 L
- Daily Kt/V = 8.8/42 = 0.21
- Weekly Kt/V = 0.21 × 7 = 1.47

Thus, answer C is correct.

Suggested Reading

Burkart JM. Measurement of solute clearance in continuous peritoneal dialysis: Kt/V and creatinine clearance. UpToDate; 2020.

Lee MJ, Ryu D-R. Peritoneal dialysis prescription. In: Kim Y-L, Kawanishi H, editors. The essentials of clinical dialysis. Singapore: Springer; 2018. p. 191–213.

Tzamaloukas AH, Murata GH, Piraino B, et al. Peritoneal urea and creatinine clearances in continuous peritoneal dialysis patients with different types of peritoneal solute transport. Kidney Int. 1998;53:1405–11.

13. A 72-year-old woman, weighing 72 kg, is started recently on CAPD and you want to calculate weekly Kt/V for evaluation of adequacy of dialysis. She has a daily urine output of 0.6 L. The following values were obtained.

Peritoneal clearance	Kidney clearance
24-h drained dialysate = 8.8 L	Urine output 0.6 L/d
Dialysate urea = 80 mg/dL	Urine urea 200 mg/dL
Plasma urea = 90 mg/dL	Plasma BUN 80 mg/dL
Total body water = 36 L	Total body water = 36 L

Which one of the following Kt/V values is CORRECT?

A. 1.53
B. 1.63
C. 1.73
D. 1.83
E. 1.93

The answer is D

In this patient who has urine output of 0.6 L, one needs to calculate both peritoneal and renal clearance for both daily and weekly urea clearance. The calculations are as follows:
Peritoneal clearance

- K = 8.8 L × D_{Urea}/P_{Urea} = 80/90 = 0.89 or 8.8 × 0.89 = 7.82 L
- t = 24 h (1 day)
- V = 72 kg × 0.5 = 36 L
- Daily Kt/V = 7.82/36 = 0.22
- Weekly Kt/V = 0.22 × 7 = 1.54

Kidney clearance

- Kt = urine urea/plasma urea × urine volume
- 200/80 × 0.6 = 1.5 L
- Daily Kt/V = 1.5/36 = 0.04
- Weekly Kt/V 0.07 × 7 = 0.29

Total clearance = peritoneal clearance + kidney clearance

- 1.54 + 0.29 = 1.83

Thus, answer D is correct.

Suggested Reading

Burkart JM. Measurement of solute clearance in continuous peritoneal dialysis: Kt/V and creatinine clearance. UpToDate; 2020.
Lee MJ, Ryu D-R. Peritoneal dialysis prescription. In: Kim Y-L, Kawanishi H, editors. The essentials of clinical dialysis. Singapore: Springer; 2018. p. 191–213.
Tzamaloukas AH, Murata GH, Piraino B, et al. Peritoneal urea and creatinine clearances in continuous peritoneal dialysis patients with different types of peritoneal solute transport. Kidney Int. 1998;53:1405–11.

14. A 48-year-old nondiabetic man is started on CAPD 6 weeks ago, and his total Kt/V is 1.4. He is on 4 × 2 L (2.5% dextrose) exchanges. He weighs 72 kg and a urine volume of 100 mL/day. Repeat Kt/V 1 week later is 1.42. **Which one of the following strategies is recommended to improve his Kt/V?**

A. Increase the frequency of daily exchanges
B. Increase the dwell volumes from 2 to 2.5 L
C. Change dialysis solution to 4.25% dextrose until target Kt/V is achieved
D. Change 2.5% dextrose to icodextrin
E. A, B, and C

The answer is E

Patients on CAPD who do not achieve target Kt/V of 1.7 may require adjustment in their prescription. Various strategies can be used, including increasing the frequency of daily exchanges from 4 to 5, increasing the dwell volumes from 2 to 2.5 L, which increases peritoneal surface area, and changing the tonicity of dialysis solution. Thus, E is correct.

Changing 2.5% dextrose to icodextrin is not appropriate in this nondiabetic patient without knowing the transporter status. Also, icodextrin is expensive. Its use may be justified once strategies given in choices A, B, and C fail, and the patient insists on continuing CAPD (D is incorrect).

Increasing the frequency of daily exchanges from 4 to 5 with a dwell time of at least 4 h may increase small solute clearances. However, noncompliance develops to frequent exchanges.

Increasing the dwell volumes may improve Kt/V. Increasing volume of dialysis solution from 2 to 2.5 L is shown to increase Kt/V by 20%. Also, increase in dwell time may increase Kt/V. In anuric patients who are >75 kg in weight can benefit from 2.5 L dwell volumes to achieve adequacy. Back pain, abdominal distention, and shortness of breath may be some of the complications of large volume dialysis solutions.

Increasing glucose concentration may achieve ultrafiltration and adequacy. However, metabolic complications such as hyperglycemia, hyperlipidemia, and obesity may occur. Also, use of long-term higher tonicity solutions may damage peritoneal membrane integrity.

Thus, each one of the above choices except D can be implemented to increase Kt/V in this patient. However, increasing dwell volume seems appropriate in this patient.

Suggested Reading

Blake PG, Daugirdas JT. Adequacy of peritoneal dialysis and chronic peritoneal dialysis prescription. In: Daugirdas JT, Blake PG, Ing TS, editors. Handbook of dialysis. 5th ed. Philadelphia: Wolters Kluwer; 2015. p. 464–82.

Burkart JM. Adequacy of peritoneal dialysis. In: Lerma EV, Weir MR, editors. Henrich's principles and practice of dialysis. 5th ed. Philadelphia: Wolters Kluwer/Lippincott Williams & Wilkins; 2017. p. 169–93.

Lee MJ, Ryu D-R. Peritoneal dialysis prescription. In: Kim Y-L, Kawanishi H, editors. The essentials of clinical dialysis. Singapore: Springer; 2018. p. 191–213.

15. Despite adequate prescription, the above patient did not reach adequacy. **Which one of the following conditions may contribute to underdialysis in this patient?**

    A. Noncompliance to prescription
    B. Errors in estimating total body water
    C. Technical problems
    D. Leakage of dialysate into tissues adjacent to peritoneal cavity
    E. All of the above

The answer is E

All of the above conditions can cause underdialysis in PD patients. Noncompliance to prescriptions such as failure to perform additional exchange, failure to instill the recommended volume, and shortening the dwell time may lead to underdialysis (A is correct).

Inaccuracies in estimating total body water in conditions such as overhydration or dehydration may not represent adequate V, and several liters of V may be missed or added. These errors are usually caused by anthropometric formulas. For example, these formulas (B is correct).

Technical problems can lead to inadequate drainage, and leakage of dialysate into tissues adjacent to the peritoneal cavity may cause underdialysis (C and D are correct).

In addition, absorption of glucose into the body may cause fluid overload and decreased peritoneal solute clearances. This may be the evidence for fast transporter.

In this patient, any one of the above problems may be responsible for his underdialysis, and proper evaluation is clearly warranted.

Suggested Reading

Lee MJ, Ryu D-R. Peritoneal dialysis prescription. In: Kim Y-L, Kawanishi H, editors. The essentials of clinical dialysis. Singapore: Springer; 2018. p. 191–213.

Lobbedez T, Boissinot L, Ficheux M, et al. How to avoid technique failure in peritoneal dialysis patients? Contrib Nephrol. 2012;178:53–7.

Tzamaloukas AH, Raj DSC, Onime A, et al. The prescription of peritoneal dialysis. Sem Dial. 2008;21:250–57.

16. A 52-year-old type 2 diabetic woman on APD for 4 years has been stable with weekly Kt/V of 1.7 and serum albumin of 4.1 g/dL. Her HbA1c is 7.4%. She has no residual kidney function and anuric. For the last 3 months, she has been gaining weight with an increase in systolic BP. On your monthly examination, you noticed 1+ pitting edema, and you

recommended 6 g (102 mEq) daily salt intake. She comes in 4 weeks for follow-up visit, and at this time she gained 1.5 kg, and edema is still present. **Which one of the following factors you need to consider for fluid overload in this patient?**

A. Noncompliance to salt and water intake
B. Noncompliance to PD prescription
C. Inappropriate prescription
D. Fast transporter with ultrafiltration (UF) failure
E. All of the above

The answer is E

All of the above factors need to be considered in this patient (E is correct). Noncompliance to salt and water intake in anuric patient can cause fluid overload. Also, noncompliance to prescription and inappropriate prescription without knowledge of her transport characteristics can lead to fluid overload. If the patient has been compliant to diet and adherent to her prescription with adequate glucose control, one needs to consider UF failure due to fast transport or inadequate aquaporin function. Therefore, PET with 4.25% dextrose needs to be performed.

Slow transporter with UF failure occurs infrequently due to low peritoneal surface area caused by adhesions and scarring, Also, increased lymphatic absorption of peritoneal fluid can cause UF failure. Abdominal leaks of fluid can easily be diagnosed on physical examination. If patients develop congestive heart failure, it may lead to fluid overload. Physical examination and ECHO can help the nature of heart failure.

Suggested Reading

Burkart JM. Management of hypervolemia in peritoneal dialysis patients. UpToDate; 2020.
Kim Y-L, Van Biesen W. Fluid overload in peritoneal dialysis patients. Sem Nephrol. 2017;37:43–53.
Trinh E, Perl J. The patient receiving automated peritoneal dialysis with volume overload. Clin J Am Soc Nephrol. 2018;13:1732–34.

17. The above patient had a PET with 4.25% dextrose. The following D/P ratios for creatinine, Na^+, and glucose (D/D_0) at 1 and 4 h were obtained:

Time	Creatinine	Na^+	Glucose
1	0.36	0.93	0.36
4	0.82	0.92	0.22

Which one of the following mechanisms is responsible for UF failure in this patient?

A. Slow transporter with UF failure
B. Aquaporin deficiency
C. Fast transporter with UF failure
D. A and B
E. B and C

The answer is E

The striking ratio is D/P_{Na} of 0.93 at 1 h. One of the properties of the peritoneal membrane is Na^+ sieving. During the first hour of dialysate dwelling, aquaporin-1 channels are stimulated by high osmolality of 4.25% dextrose and water moves via ultra small pores into the dialysate (see question 3). As a result, the dialysate [Na^+] decreases by 5–10 mEq with a small increase in plasma [Na^+]. When peritoneal membrane aquaporins are intact, the D/P ratio should be around 0.89 (assuming dialysate Na^+ drops from 132 to 124 mEq/L and serum Na^+ increases from 138 to 140 mEq/L, the D/P ratio is 0.89). This Na^+ dip in the first hour of dialysis dwell is called Na^+ sieving (see question 5). At 4 h, there is equilibration and [Na^+] in both the dialysate and plasma return to their basal levels. In this patient, D/P_{Na} in the first hour is 0.93 and remains the same at 4 h, suggesting aquaporin deficiency.

D/P creatinine and D/D_0 glucose values suggest that this patient is a fast transporter. Thus, both aquaporin deficiency and fast transporter status are responsible for UF failure (E is correct). This is an indication for a switch from PD to HD.

Suggested Reading

Devuyst O, Goffin E. Water and solute transport in peritoneal dialysis: models and clinical applications. Nephrol Dial Transplant. 2008;23:2120–23.
Devuyst O, Rippe B. Water transport across the peritoneal membrane. Kidney Int. 2014;85:750–8.
Krediet RT. Ultrafiltration failure is a reflection of peritoneal alterations in patients treated with peritoneal dialysis. Front Physiol. 2018;9:1815. https://doi.org/10.3389/fphys.2018.01815.
Rippe B, Venturoli D, Simonsen O, et al. Fluid and electrolyte transport across the peritoneal membrane during CAPD according to the three-pore model. Perit Dial Int. 2004;24:10–27.

18. A 42-year-old woman on CAPD for 6 months complains of lower extremity weakness on routine monthly examination. Physical examination confirms her complaint, and the only electrolyte abnormality is [K^+] of 3.2 mEq/L. KCl supplementation improves her weakness. **Which one of the following statements about serum [K^+] in PD patients is CORRECT?**

A. Compared to HD patients, hypokalemia (<3.5 mEq/L) in PD patients does not have any cardiovascular (CV) risk
B. Time-averaged serum [K^+] of 4.5 to <5.0 mEq/L in PD patients carries a high CV mortality
C. Time-averaged serum [K^+] <3.5 or ≥5.5 mEq/L in PD patients carries a high CV mortality
D. Time-averaged serum [K^+] 4.5 to <5.0 mEq/L in PD patients is not associated with a high CV mortality
E. C and D

The answer is E

In a retrospective analysis of 10,468 PD patients, Torlén et al. reported that there was a U-shaped relationship between time-averaged serum [K^+] and CV and all-cause mortality. Time-averaged serum [K^+] <3.5 or ≥5.5 mEq/L in PD patients was associated with a high CV and all-cause mortality. On the other hand, time-averaged serum [K^+] 4.5 to <5.0 mEq/L was not associated with either CV or all-cause mortality. Thus, E is correct.

This study points out that PD patients similar to HD patients are at risk for CV or all-cause mortality, if the serum [K^+] is <3.5 or >5.5 mEq/L. Thus, maintenance of serum [K^+] between 4.5 and 5.0 mEq/L seems appropriate in PD patients.

It is of interest to note that the study of Lee et al. did not observe a U-shaped relationship between serum K^+ levels and mortality in PD patients, but observed in HD patients. However, these investigators found higher mortality with serum K^+ levels <4.5 mEq/L in PD patients.

Suggested Reading

Lee S, Kang E, Yoo KD, Choi Y, et al. Lower serum potassium associated with increased mortality in dialysis patients: a nationwide prospective observational cohort study in Korea. PLoS One. 2017;12(3): e0171842.
Torlén K, Kalantar-Zadeh K, Molnar MZ, et al. Serum potassium and cause-specific mortality in a large peritoneal dialysis cohort. Clin J Am Soc Nephrol. 2012;7:1272–84.

19. Both hemodialysis and PD remove K^+ from the body at different rates. In PD, clearance of K^+ occurs in response to hypertonic dextrose solutions. The following data were obtained during a study of K^+ clearance in an incident (<3 months of PD initiation) patient on CAPD with 2.5% dextrose solution with 2 L exchanges every 6 h for four exchanges.

- Net removal (24 h) = 42 mEq
- Drainage volume (24 h) = 8.8 L
- Plasma [K^+] = 4.0 mEq/L

Which one of the following K^+ clearance (C_K) values is CORRECT?

A. 5.18 mL/min
B. 6.18 mL/min
C. 7.18 mL/min
D. 8.18 mL/min
E. 9.18 mL/min

The answer is C

It is customary to express clearance of a solute, including creatinine in mL/min, using the formula UV/P, where U is urine concentration of a solute, V is total volume of urine, and P is plasma concentration of a solute. In the above patient, the net removal of K^+ was calculated as follows:

- *Net removal for 24 h = ([concentration in drained dialysate × drainage volume] - [concentration in instilled solution × instilled volume])*
- *C_K (mL/min) was calculated as:*
- *([net removal/plasma K^+/1440 min])*

Please note that numbers must be expressed in the same units. By using the patient's data, we obtain:

- U = 42 mEq/8800 mL = 0.0047 mEq/mL
- V = 8800 mL/1440 min = 6.11 mL/min
- P = 4 mEq/L/100 = 0.004 mEq/mL

When the above values are included into the clearance formula UV/P, we obtain:

- 0.0047 mEq/mL × 6.11 mL/min = 7.18 mL/min

Note that mEq in the numerator and denominator cancel each other. Thus, answer C is correct.

20. One of your CAPD patients who has a urine output of 250 mL/day heard about biocompatible dialysis solutions, and the patient wants to know more about these solutions. **Which one of the following statements regarding biocompatible versus standard dextrose-based solutions is CORRECT?**

A. The time to the development of anuria is prolonged with biocompatible solutions
B. The incidence of peritonitis is lower with biocompatible solutions
C. Initially there is a higher rate of peritoneal membrane transport, which remained stable over a period of 2 years of the study with biocompatible solutions
D. Studies are mixed (benefit or no benefit) regarding preservation of residual kidney function (RKF) or urine output with biocompatible solutions
E. All of the above

The answer is E

Standard dextrose-based solutions generate glucose degradation products (GDPs) during heat sterilization. These GDPs have systemic and membrane toxic effects via generation of advanced glycation end products. Therefore, solutions containing low GDPs and neutral pH (7.40) compared to pH 5.5 in standard dextrose-based solutions have been developed. These new solutions are called biocompatible solutions. There are several studies using these biocompatible solutions. A recent review by Cho et al. who evaluated 24 studies that used lactate/bicarbonate buffered neutral pH and low GDP solutions provided greater urine output and higher RRF after 12 months of use. They concluded that "the use of these biocompatible PD solutions resulted in clinically relevant benefits without added risks of harm." This conclusion is inclusive of 12 studies that used icodextrin.

However, the balANZ trial of Johnson et al. showed no benefit in preserving RRF, but it showed that the biocompatible solution "Balance" prolonged the onset of anuria and decreased incidence of peritonitis. However, the data on peritonitis are conflicting. The balANZ trial also showed that the patients who were treated with "Balance" solution initially had a higher rate of peritoneal membrane transport which remained stable over the 2-year observation. On the other hand, patients who were treated with standard PD solution had a progressive increase in peritoneal membrane transport. Based on all of the studies, statement E is correct.

As pointed out by Blake et al., more evidence is needed by large studies on incident PD patients, which are not feasible. Therefore, the wide use of biocompatible PD solutions in the United States is questionable.

Suggested Reading

Blake PG, Jain AK, Yohanna S. Biocompatible PD solutions: many questions but few answers. Kidney Int. 2013;84:864–66.

Cho Y, Johnson DW, Craiq JC, et al. Biocompatible dialysis fluids for peritoneal dialysis. Cochrane Database Syst Rev. 2014;3:CD007554.

Johnson DW, Brown FG, Clark M, et al. balANZ Trial Investigators: effects of biocompatible versus standard fluid in peritoneal dialysis outcomes. J Am Soc Nephrol. 2012;23:1097–107.

Johnson DW, Brown FG, Clark M, et al. balANZ Trial Investigators: the effect of low glucose degradation product, neutral pH versus standard peritoneal dialysis solutions on peritoneal membrane function. The balANZ trial. Nephrol Dial Transplant. 2013;27:4445–53.

21. **Which one of the following statements regarding icodextrin is FALSE?**

A. Icodextrin is a glucose polymer derived from starch and is iso-osmolar and induces ultrafiltration (UF) by its oncotic rather than crystalloid effect
B. It is generally used as a single exchange in patients on CAPD and APD who have UF failure
C. Icodextrin has been shown to improve glycemic control and lipid abnormalities without lowering BP
D. Adverse effects include hyperglycemia, skin rash, hyponatremia, and sterile peritonitis episodes
E. It is recommended in all diabetic patients because of its low cost

The answer is E

Icodextrin is derived from corn starch with many glucose molecules bonded together. In the peritoneal cavity, icodextrin is broken down into smaller units and are retained for long periods of time. These smaller units are not absorbed by the peritoneum. It is an iso-osmolar solution and provides colloid oncotic pressure similar to albumin. Sustained UF occurs because of long dwell via small pores. Transport of water does not occur via aquaporins because these channels are not stimulated by iso-osmolarity. Icodextrin is particularly useful in fast transporters in causing UF. In CAPD patients, icodextrin can be used during nighttime and in APD patients during daytime to achieve adequate fluid removal.

All of the above statements except E are correct. Regarding hyperglycemia, icodextrin is metabolized to maltose, and maltose is read as glucose with nonglucose oxidase-containing strips. This spurious hyperglycemia may lead to unnecessary use of insulin and oral hypoglycemic agents.

Some patients (10%) may develop macular popular rash on the trunk and extremities due to starch-induced hypersensitivity reaction. Hyponatremia is due to translocation of fluids from tissues into the intravascular compartment, leading to hyponatremia. Some patients may develop sterile peritonitis as well.

The disadvantage of icodextrin for its use in diabetics is its cost. It is more expensive than standard dextrose-containing solutions. Therefore, E is false.

Icodextrin has been shown to have favorable effects on glycemia and lipids. Also, there is some evidence that icodextrin can have a sustained preservation of peritoneal membrane function.

Suggested Reading

Cho J, Johnson DW, Badve S, et al. Impact of icodextrin on clinical outcomes in peritoneal dialysis: a systematic review of randomized controlled trials. Nephrol Dial Transplant. 2013;28:1899–907.

Cho Y, Johnson DW, Craig JC, et al. Biocompatible dialysis fluids for peritoneal dialysis. Cochrane Database Syst Rev. 2014;3:CD007554.

Heimbürger O, Blake PG. Apparatus for peritoneal dialysis. In: Daugirdas JT, Blake PG, Ing TS, editors. Handbook of dialysis. 5th ed. Philadelphia: Wolters Kluwer; 2015. p. 408–24.

22. A 31-year-old woman was started on HD due to hypertensive nephrosclerosis. After 1 year, she decides to have PD because of convenience. She received PD training and learnt about advanced laparoscopic insertion of PD catheter. **Which one of the following statements regarding advanced laparoscopic insertion of PD catheter is CORRECT?**

A. The advanced laparoscopic technique includes rectus sheath tunneling and adjunctive procedures such as omentopexy, adhesiolysis, excision of appendix epiploica (epiploectomy), salpingectomy, and colopexy
B. The advanced laparoscopic technique facilitates visualization of the peritoneal cavity for adhesions and hernias
C. The incidence of catheter obstruction, migration, pericannular leak, and hernias is significantly lower, and catheter survival at 1 and 2 years is better following advanced laparoscopy as compared with open surgery
D. The advanced laparoscopic technique produces a better outcome compared with conventional open and basic laparoscopic insertion techniques
E. All of the above

The answer is E

Chronic PD catheter placement requires expertise and experience. Methods of catheter insertion include open surgery, laparoscopic, and percutaneous techniques. Although open surgery is the best method, it requires general anesthesia and possible hospital stay. Laparoscopic insertion also requires general anesthesia; however, percutaneous insertion requires local anesthesia only and can be done under fluoroscopy. Of these procedures, laparoscopy is rather popular. It creates the ability to insert the catheter under direct vision, which ensures correct position of the catheter.

The laparoscopic insertion technique may be either basic or advanced. The basic laparoscopic technique is used to verify the position of the catheter. The advanced technique includes rectus sheath tunneling and adjunctive procedures such as omentopexy, adhesiolysis, excision of appendix epiploica (epiploectomy), salpingectomy, and colopexy (A is correct). It also facilitates visualization of the peritoneal cavity for adhesions and hernias (B is correct). A meta-analysis involving seven cohort studies (1045 patients) reported less catheter obstruction, catheter migration, pericannular leak, and pericannular and incisional hernias as well as better 1- and 2-year catheter survival with advanced laparoscopy as compared with open insertion (C is correct). Similarly, catheter obstruction and migration were significantly lower in the advanced laparoscopy method as compared with basic laparoscopy, whereas catheter survival was similar in both techniques (D is correct). Thus, advanced laparoscopic insertion of PD catheter has lowest mechanical complications.

Suggested Reading

Crabtree JH, Fishman A. A laparoscopic method for optimal peritoneal dialysis access. Am Surg. 2005;71:135–43.

Crabtree JH, Shrestha BM, Chow K-M, et al. Creating and managing optimal peritoneal dialysis access in the adult patient: 2019 update. Perit Dial Int. 2019;39:414–36.

Di Cocco P, Brown EA, Papalois VE, et al. Overview of catheter choices and implantation techniques. In: Haggerty S, editor. Surgical aspects of peritoneal dialysis. Springer International Publishing AG; 2017. p. 47–69.

Shrestha BM, Shrestha D, Kumar A, et al. Advanced laparoscopic peritoneal dialysis catheter insertion: systematic review and meta-analysis. Peri Dial Int. 2018;38:163–78.

23. The PD catheters are made in different shapes and sizes. However, the outcomes and longevity of these catheters is poorly understood. **Which one of the following statements regarding the types and the number of cuffs in PD catheters is CORRECT?**

A. No difference in exit-site or peritoneal infections were observed between straight and coiled catheters
B. No difference in exit-site or peritoneal infections were observed between straight and swan-neck catheters
C. No difference in exit-site or peritoneal infections were observed between single and double cuff catheters
D. Survival of straight catheter at 1 and 2 years was superior compared to coiled catheter
E. All of the above

The answer is E

Peritoneal catheter dysfunction or failure is an important reason in switching from PD to HD. This failure may be related to catheter type. However, there is no conclusive evidence that one type of catheter is superior in function to another catheter. In order to clarify this question, Hagen et al. performed a review of 682 identified studies and a meta-analysis of 11 randomized controlled studies. The outcomes of interest were exit-site infections, peritonitis, catheter survival, drainage dysfunction, migration, leakage, and catheter removal. All catheters were surgically inserted. The results show no difference in any outcome between straight and swan neck catheters and between single and double-cuffed catheters. Similarly, no differences except for survival were found between straight and coiled-tip catheters. The survival at 1 and 2 years was significantly better with straight catheters (E is correct). Thus, the meta-analysis identifies straight with double-cuff catheters as better catheters for PD patients.

Suggested Reading

Crabtree JH, Shrestha BM, Chow K-M, et al. Creating and managing optimal peritoneal dialysis access in the adult patient: 2019 update. Perit Dial Int. 2019;39:414–36.

Di Cocco P, Brown EA, Papalois VE, et al. Overview of catheter choices and implantation techniques. In: Haggerty S, editor. Surgical aspects of peritoneal dialysis. Springer International Publishing AG; 2017. p. 47–69.

Hagen SM, Lafranca JA, Ijermans JNM, et al. A systematic review and meta-analysis of the influence of peritoneal dialysis catheter type on complication rate and catheter survival. Kidney Int. 2014;85:920–32.

Stylianou KG, Daphnis EK. Selecting the optimal peritoneal dialysis catheter. Kidney Int. 2014;85:741–43.

24. **Which one of the following statements regarding antibiotic prophylaxis during the preparation (perioperatively) of a PD catheter placement is FALSE?**

A. Perioperative intravenous (IV) antibiotic administration reduces subsequent development of peritonitis
B. A single dose of a first- or second-generation cephalosporin is recommended perioperatively to prevent exit-site infection
C. Routine prophylaxis with one dose of vancomycin is not usually recommended because of vancomycin-resistant enterococci (VRE)
D. The choice of specific antibiotic use for perioperative prophylaxis use should take center-specific susceptibility patterns and community-based susceptibility
E. Vancomycin prophylaxis should be considered perioperatively in all patients

The answer is E

Administration of an antibiotic just before PD catheter placement has been shown to prevent wound infection, catheter-related infections, including peritonitis. Therefore, IV antibiotic administration within 60 min before PD catheter insertion is recommended. Although the choice of antibiotics has not been established, generally either the first- or second-generation cephalosporin is recommended. Also, the decision of antibiotic use is dependent on the center-specific susceptibility patterns because the susceptibility of the same organism may vary among centers and communities.

Although single-dose vancomycin was found to be superior to single-dose cephalosporin, vancomycin is not recommended for prophylaxis because of subsequent colonization of VRE in all pediatric and adult patients. Thus, E is false.

Suggested Reading

Li PK-T, Szeto CC, Piraino B, et al. ISPD peritonitis recommendations: 2016 update on prevention and treatment. Perit Dial Int. 2016;36:481–508.
Wallace EL, Fissell RB, Golper TA, et al. Catheter insertion and perioperative practices within the ISPD North American Research Consortium. Perit Dial Int. 2016;36:382–86.
Warady BA, Bakkaloglu S, Newaland J, et al. Consensus guidelines for the prevention and treatment of catheter-related infections and peritonitis in pediatric patients receiving peritoneal dialysis:2012 update. Perit Dial Int. 2012; 32:S29–86.

25. You started 2 years ago, a 60-year-old type 2 diabetic woman on APD, and on monthly examination you noticed for the first time erythema around the exit site which is 10 mm in diameter. She has no complaint of pain or fever. Also, there is pain or redness over the subcutaneous tunnel catheter. You are not convinced that it is exit-site infection (ESI), but you wanted to prevent future ESI. **Based on the above findings, which one of the following measures is appropriate to prevent ESI?**

A. Oral cephalexin 500 mg BID (twice daily)
B. 2% Mupirocin ointment and gentamicin cream each daily
C. Gentamicin cream twice daily
D. Polysporin ointment twice daily
E. 2% Mupirocin ointment twice daily

The answer is E

ESI is an important risk factor for peritonitis. One study showed that patients who had an ESI developed peritonitis within 30 days even after ESI was appropriately treated. Thus, prevention of ESI is an important aspect of PD management.

The most common causative organisms of ESI are *Staphylococcus aureus* and *Pseudomonas aeruginosa*. ESI is usually diagnosed when there is erythema (>13 mm in diameter), purulent discharge, edema, or pain around the exit site. Erythema <13 mm may or may not represent infection. However, in this diabetic patient, one needs to prevent ESI.

Oral cephalexin is not indicated in this patient, as ESI has not been established (A is incorrect). Mupirocin ointment, gentamicin cream, and polysporin ointment have all been used prophylactically to prevent ESI and subsequent peritonitis. The use of gentamicin cream can cover Gram-negative organisms as well. However, routine use of gentamicin cream has caused resistance, as reported by many investigators (C is incorrect). The use of

polysporin is associated with increased rate of fungal infections, and polysporin use is not recommended (D is incorrect). The best prophylactic agent is mupirocin in the prevention of *S. aureus* ESI and peritonitis, as suggested by Xu et al. in a systematic review (E is correct). It was shown that alternating mupirocin/gentamicin is associated with increased risk of fungal peritonitis compared with gentamicin alone. The combination of mupirocin and gentamicin is not appropriate without good evidence (B is incorrect).

Suggested Reading

Li PK-T, Szeto CC, Piraino B, et al. ISPD peritonitis recommendations: 2016 update on prevention and treatment. Perit Dial Int. 2016;36:481–508.

Szeto CC, Li PK-T, Johnson DW, et al. ISPD catheter-related infection recommendations:2017 update. Perit Dial Int. 2017;37:141–54.

26. The above patient was prescribed mupirocin ointment and asked to come in 2 weeks for an examination of the exit site. However, she showed up 6 weeks later because of travel and she ran out of mupirocin. On examination, there was erythema of >16 mm in diameter, small purulent discharge, and pain on palpation. There is no pain or erythema over the tunnel catheter. She has urine output of 175 mL. **Which one of the following therapeutic strategies regarding exit-site infection (ESI) is CORRECT?**

A. Continue mupirocin ointment
B. Clean area with saline and hydrogen peroxide
C. Oral cephalexin
D. Intraperitoneal (IP) gentamicin
E. IP Fluconazole

The answer is C

This patient has ESI because of erythema >13 mm in diameter and purulent discharge. The ESI should not be considered failure of mupirocin treatment, as the patient did not continue the treatment. Since this is her first episode of ESI, an empiric treatment with oral cephalexin 500 mg twice daily may be reasonable to cover Gram-positive organisms until the culture and sensitivity results of the purulent material are available. If the culture results show *S. aureus*, the treatment should be continued for 2 weeks until the exit site looks normal. Thus, C is correct. Continuing mupirocin and cleaning the area with hydrogen peroxide may eventually lead to tunnel infection and then peritonitis in this diabetic patient. Therefore, A and B are incorrect.

This patient has residual kidney function. IP gentamicin can decrease residual kidney function (and also ototoxicity), choice D is not correct. Fungal infections are unlikely; therefore, E is incorrect.

If the response to cephalexin is slow, rifampin 600 mg/day should be considered. Vancomycin should be reserved for MRSA, though clindamycin and doxycycline can cover community-acquired MRSA.

If *Pseudomonas* is cultured, it requires two drugs: oral fluoroquinolones (are drugs of choice) and other antipseudomonal drugs, such as IP ceftazidime, cefepime, piperacillin, or meropenem. Resistance to oral fluoroquinolones develops rapidly without second antipseudomonal drug. The treatment should be continued for 3 weeks.

Suggested Reading

Li PK-T, Szeto CC, Piraino B, et al. ISPD peritonitis recommendations: 2016 update on prevention and treatment. Perit Dial Int. 2016;36:481–508.

Szeto C-C, Li PK-T, Leehey DJ. Peritonitis and exit-site infection. In: Daugirdas JT, Blake PG, Ing TS, editors. Handbook of dialysis. 5th ed. Philadelphia: Wolters Kluwer; 2015. p. 490–512.

27. Your PD patient comes to your clinic with purulent discharge and pain at the exit site. However, you are not sure about the tunnel infection because of pain on and off over the tunnel catheter. There is no discharge on milking the catheter. **What would you do next?**

A. Order an ultrasound of the exit site and tunnel catheter
B. Order a PET scan
C. Order a WBC scan
D. A only
E. C only

The answer is D

Physical examination of the exit site and tunnel catheter may not detect occult or unsuspected infection. Ultrasonography is useful in detecting not only the catheter infection, but also the extent of infection. A large number of studies have initially evaluated the tunnel infections by ultrasonography. A sonolucent zone around the catheter and external cuff is suggestive of infection. Some have performed WBC and PET scans to evaluate catheter infections. The cost of the latter scans is high compared to ultrasonography. Sequential ultrasonographic evaluations can be used to follow the effectiveness of therapy, further antibiotic use, and catheter removal. These sequential evaluations are not possible with other scans because of cost and procedural time. Thus, D is correct.

It is suggested that a sonolucent zone around the external cuff >1-mm thick following a course of antibiotic treatment and the involvement of the proximal cuff are associated with poor clinical outcome. In *Pseudomonas aeruginosa* infections, the clinical outcome is uniformly poor irrespective of ultrasound findings.

Suggested Reading

Karahan OI, Taskapan H, Yikilmaz A, et al. Ultrasound evaluation of peritoneal catheter tunnel in catheter related infections in CAPD. Int J Urol Nephrol. 2005;37:363–66.

Kwan T-H, Tong M K-H, Sue Y-P, et al. Ultrasonography in the management of exit site infections in peritoneal dialysis patients. Nephrology. 2004;9:348–52.

Li PK-T, Szeto CC, Piraino B, et al. ISPD peritonitis recommendations: 2016 update on prevention and treatment. Perit Dial Int. 2016;36:481–508.

28. A 60-year-old diabetic woman on automated PD (APD) presented to the clinic with mild abdominal pain overnight. She denied fever. The nurse drained some peritoneal fluid from the catheter, which looked cloudy. The physician makes the diagnosis of peritonitis. **Which one of following statements regarding peritonitis is CORRECT?**

A. White blood cell (WBC) count >100/μL with >50% polymorphonuclear (PMN) cells >50% is indicative of peritonitis
B. In APD patients because of short dwells, PMN count >50% suggests peritonitis despite the WBC count is <100/μL
C. Empiric antibiotic therapy is indicated once peritonitis is suspected
D. Patients with peritonitis may likely benefit from addition of heparin (500 units/L) to the dialysate to prevent occlusion of the catheter by fibrin
E. All of the above

The answer is E

Patients with peritonitis usually present with mild-to-severe abdominal pain with cloudy effluent. The degree of abdominal pain is organism specific. Patients with coagulase-negative organisms may present with less pain compared to those whose pain may be severe due to Gram-negative rods, *S. aureus*, or *Streptococcus* organisms.

All of the above statements are correct (E). Once peritonitis is suspected, effluent should be sent for cell count, Gram stain, and culture. Generally peritoneal fluid does not contain WBCs. If WBC count is >100/μL and PMNs account for >50%, the patient is considered to have peritonitis. On the other hand, if the cell count is >100/μL and all of them are monocytes, it is difficult to make the diagnosis of peritonitis.

In APD patients, who have fluid during the daytime may have cell count similar to those of CAPD patients and does not pose any difficulty in interpreting the results. However, in those APD patients who do not have daytime dwells (dry day), 1 L of dialysate is infused and drained 1–2 h later, and the effluent is sent for cell count. In these patients, the percentage of PMNs is more important than the WBC count.

It is suggested that empiric antibiotic therapy should be started once peritonitis is suspected because of serious consequences such as catheter removal, relapse, switching to HD, or death that are associated with untreated peritonitis.

It has been shown that addition of heparin to the dialysate can prevent catheter occlusion by fibrin threads that can avoid catheter malfunction.

Gram stain is helpful even in the absence of bacteria because it may detect fungus. Cultures of effluent are generally positive in 70–90% of the time, and results are dependent on culture technique. Culture-negative peritonitis should not be >20 episodes.

Suggested Reading

Li PK-T, Szeto CC, Piraino B, et al. ISPD peritonitis recommendations: 2016 update on prevention and treatment. Perit Dial Int. 2016;36:481–508.

Szeto C-C, Li PK-T, Leehey DJ. Peritonitis and exit-site infection. In: Daugirdas JT, Blake PG, Ing TS, editors. Handbook of dialysis. 5th ed. Philadelphia: Wolters Kluwer; 2015. p. 490–512.

29. The nephrologist wants to start empiric antibiotics in the above patient. **Which one of the following statements regarding peritonitis treatment is CORRECT?**

A. Empiric treatment should cover both Gram-positive and Gram-negative organisms
B. A center-specific selection of antibiotics should be chosen
C. For Gram-negative organisms, first-generation cephalosporins such as cefazolin are preferred to vancomycin unless MRSA is cultured
D. For Gram-negative organisms, a third-generation cephalosporin (ceftazidime) or an aminoglycoside (if patient is anuric) is the drug of choice
E. All of the above

The answer is E

All of the above statements are correct (E). Intraperitoneal (IP) administration of antibiotics is usually preferred to IV and oral for treatment of peritonitis. IV antibiotics are indicated for severely ill patients. A loading dose is usually given IP for both CAPD and APD patients. In the above patient, the dwell time should be at least 4–6 h, and IP administration is considered. In her, the loading dose can also be given IV. Intermittent or continuous dosing of antibiotics is equally efficacious.

Suggested Reading

Li PK-T, Szeto CC, Piraino B, et al. ISPD peritonitis recommendations: 2016 update on prevention and treatment. Perit Dial Int. 2016;36:481–508.

Salzer W. Peritoneal dialysis-related infections. In: Lerma EV, Weir MR, editors. Henrich's principles and practice of Dialysis. 5th ed. Philadelphia: Wolters Kluwer; 2017. p. 220–34.

30. **Which one of the following infection-related indications for catheter removal is CORRECT?**

A. Refractory peritonitis
B. Relapsing peritonitis
C. Fungal peritonitis
D. Refractory exit-site and tunnel infections
E. All of the above

The answer is E

Generally, most patients with peritonitis show clinical improvement within 48 h of antibiotic therapy. However, there are several conditions that warrant catheter removal in order to preserve the peritoneum for future PD treatment. All of the above conditions require removal of the catheter (E is correct).

Refractory peritonitis episodes are defined as failure of the effluent to clear after 5 days of appropriate antibiotics. Prolonged treatment of refractory peritonitis may cause peritoneal membrane damage, opportunistic fungal infections, antibiotic-induced adverse effects, prolonged hospital stay, and even death. Catheter removal should be done immediately. After catheter removal, systemic antibiotics should be continued for at least 2 weeks.

Relapsing peritonitis is defined as the occurrence of an episode of peritonitis within 4 weeks with the same organism after completion of a prior episode or a sterile peritonitis. Catheter should be removed immediately.

Fungal infections are common after prolonged antibiotic use. Catheter removal is indicated immediately after diagnosing fungal peritonitis.

Exit-site and tunnel infections refractory to antibiotics and other maneuvers warrant catheter removal.

Other indications that can be considered for removal of catheter include repeat peritonitis and peritonitis caused by multiple enteric and mycobacterial organisms.

Suggested Reading

Li PK-T, Szeto CC, Piriano B, et al. Peritoneal dialysis-related infections recommendations: 2010 update. Perit Dial Int. 2010;30:393–423.

Li PK-T, Szeto CC, Piraino B, et al. ISPD peritonitis recommendations: 2016 update on prevention and treatment. Perit Dial Int. 2016;36:481–508.

Szeto C-C, Li PK-T, Leehey DJ. Peritonitis and exit-site infection. In: Daugirdas JT, Blake PG, Ing TS, editors. Handbook of dialysis. 5th ed. Philadelphia: Wolters Kluwer; 2015. p. 490–512.

31. **Which one of the following disease states causes a high risk for the development of hernia in patients undergoing PD?**

A. Hypertension
B. Diabetes
C. Membranous nephropathy
D. Adult dominant polycystic kidney disease (ADPKD)
E. Focal segmental glomerulosclerosis

The answer is D

Hernias are one of the noninfectious complications of long-term PD. Of all the above disease conditions, ADPKD is a risk factor for the development of hernias while receiving PD (D is correct). Hernias are formed due to increased abdominal pressure caused by large dialysate volumes, sitting position, and several other conditions. Because of the cyst and dialysate burden, the abdominal wall may become thin, causing hernia. For ADPKD patients, APD with dry day or small daytime dwell volumes may be suitable to prevent hernia formation. Other diseases may not contribute to hernia formation.

Suggested Reading

Dunsmore S, Bargman JM. Peritoneal dialysis: non-infectious complications. In: Turner N, Lameire N, Goldsmith DJ, editors. Oxford textbook of clinical nephrology. 4th ed. Oxford: Oxford University Press; 2016. p. 2281–89.

Guest S. Non-infectious complications. In: Guest S, editor. Handbook of peritoneal dialysis. 2012. p. 119–41.

Kumar S, Fan SL-S, Raftery MJ, et al. Long-term outcome of patients with adult dominant polycystic kidney diseases receiving peritoneal dialysis. Kidney Int. 2008;74:746–51.

32. A 44-year-old woman on CAPD with 2.5% dextrose 2 L exchanges presented to your clinic with new-onset shortness of breath and pain on breathing. Chest X-ray showed right pleural effusion. A diagnostic tap is done. **Which one of the following tests is suggestive of peritoneal–pleural leak in this patient?**

A. Higher LDH levels in the pleural fluid compared to serum levels
B. Higher protein levels in the pleural fluid compared to serum levels
C. Higher glucose levels in the pleural fluid compared to serum levels
D. No difference in glucose levels between pleural fluid and serum
E. Pleural fluid is typically an exudate

The answer is D

Hydrothorax, particularly on the right side, is a complication of PD. The causes may be congenital or acquired. With congenital diaphragmatic defect, hydrothorax occurs immediately after one or two dialyses, whereas acquired defect causes a late complication. The pleural fluid is typically a transudate rather than an exudate.

The pleural fluid glucose is high compared to serum glucose, and this is the most diagnostic feature suggestive of peritoneal–pleural fistula or leak (D is correct). Other tests mentioned above are not diagnostic of hydrothorax due to PD treatment.

Suggested Reading

Ambarsari CG, Bermanshah EK, Putra MA, et al. Effective management of peritoneal dialysis-associated hydrothorax in a child: a case report. Case Rep Nephrol Dial. 2020;10:18–25.

Bargman JM. Hernias, leaks, and encapsulating peritoneal sclerosis. In: Daugirdas JT, Blake PG, Ing TS, editors. Handbook of dialysis. 5th ed. Philadelphia: Wolters Kluwer; 2015. p. 513–20.

Dunsmore S, Bargman JM. Peritoneal dialysis: non-infectious complications. In: Turner N, Lameire N, Goldsmith DJ, editors. Oxford textbook of clinical nephrology. 4th ed. Oxford: Oxford University Press; 2016. p. 2281–89.

Guest S. Non-infectious complications. In: Guest S, editor. Handbook of peritoneal dialysis. 2012. p. 119–41.

33. A 56-year-old man with diabetes is evaluated for nausea, vomiting, abdominal pain, abdominal distention, anorexia, and weight loss. He has been on CAPD for 12 years and was doing well until recently. His Hb is 11.1 g/dL, and there is no history of hematochezia or diarrhea. Although anorexia has been present for some time, the other complaints started 2 weeks ago. He is on daily KCl 20 mEq orally for persistent hypokalemia. Other medications include insulin, lisinopril, lactulose, and calcium acetate. A plain abdominal film shows distended bowl with possible obstruction, and a surgery consult is requested. The surgeon ordered CT of abdomen with contrast. The patient had three episodes of peritonitis. His ultrafiltration has been decreasing slowly. **Based on the history, which one of the following is the MOST likely diagnosis?**

   A. Diabetic gastroparesis
   B. Colon cancer with obstruction
   C. Ileus
   D. Encapsulating peritoneal sclerosis (EPS)
   E. Constipation

   The answer is D

   Diabetic gastroparesis is a possibility, but he is not on any motility drugs. Also, the patient has been well until recently (A is incorrect).

   Colon cancer with obstruction can explain some of the signs and symptoms, the absence of diarrhea or hematochezia can rule out this diagnosis (B is incorrect).

   Hypokalemia can cause ileus, but the extent of symptoms does not support this diagnosis (C is incorrect). It should be noted that hypokalemia is rather common because the dialysate does not contain K^+, and losses through dialysate. In this patient, hypokalemia is related not only to dialysis losses, but also insulin-induced transcellular shift.

   Constipation, although common in PD patients, is also unlikely because he is on lactulose and he did not complain of constipation (E is incorrect).

   Based on his history, duration of PD time, slow loss of ultrafiltration, and episodes of peritonitis, the most likely diagnosis is EPS. EPS is a rare but life-threatening long-term complication in patients on PD. The most reliable risk factor is duration of time on PD. Peritonitis is an added risk for EPS. Ultrafiltration failure suggests fast transport status, which accompanies EPS. The pathogenesis involves chronic exposure of the peritoneum to high glucose followed by gradual development of inflammation. Diagnosis is made by abdominal CT scan, which is the choice of imaging techniques.

   The clinical manifestations of EPS have been divided into several stages, as shown in Table 10.6.

   EPS needs to be considered in patients who switched from PD to HD and those who received kidney transplantation and present signs and symptoms similar to the present patient.

Table 10.6 Stages of EPS[a]

Stage	Clinical classification	Clinical manifestations
1	Pre-EPS period	UF failure, fast transport, ↓ protein level, ascites, hemoperitoneum, peritoneal calcification
2	Inflammatory period	Fever, ascites, weight loss, high levels of C-reactive protein
3	Progressive or encapsulating period	Nausea, vomiting, abdominal pain, constipation, abdominal mass
4	Obstructive period	Anorexia, weight loss, malnutrition, abdominal mass

[a]Adapted from suggested reading 2

Suggested Reading

Alston H, Fan S, Nakayama M. Encapsulating peritoneal sclerosis. Sem Nephrol. 2017;37:93–102.

Danford CJ, Lin SC, Smith MP, et al. Encapsulating peritoneal sclerosis. World J Gastroenterol. 2018;24:3101–11.

de Sousa E, del Peso-Gilsanz G, Baso-Rubio MA, et al. Encapsulating peritoneal sclerosis in peritoneal dialysis. A review and European initiative for approaching a serious and rare disease. Nefrologia. 2012;32:707–14.

Jagirdar RM, Bozikas A, Zarogiannis SG, et al. Encapsulating peritoneal sclerosis: Pathophysiology and current treatment options. Int J Mol Sci. 2019;20:5765.

Korte MR, Sampimon DE, Beties MG, et al. Encapsulating peritoneal sclerosis: State of affairs. Nat Rev Nephrol. 2011;7:528–38.

34. The results of CT of abdomen are available. **Which one of the following radiologic findings is suggestive of EPS?**

    A. Thickening of parietal and visceral peritoneal membrane
    B. Peritoneal calcification
    C. Bowl loop dilations and loculated ascites
    D. Thickening of the intestinal wall and intestinal encapsulation
    E. All of the above

The answer is E

All of the above observations on CT of abdomen have been described in patients with EPS. Thus, E is correct. It has been shown that these findings provide a sensitivity of 100% and specificity of 94%.

CT scan of abdomen may not detect any abnormalities in asymptomatic patient. There are no sufficient data of biomarkers to detect EPS in asymptomatic patient. With time, radiologic findings become evident. When the small intestinal loops are encapsulated by the thickened visceral peritoneum, a cocoon-like appearance is observed.

Suggested Reading

Danford CJ, Lin SC, Smith MP, et al. Encapsulating peritoneal sclerosis. World J Gastroenterol. 2018;24:3101–11.

de Sousa E, del Peso-Gilsanz G, Baso-Rubio MA, et al. Encapsulating peritoneal sclerosis in peritoneal dialysis. A review and European initiative for approaching a serious and rare disease. Nefrologia. 2012;32:707–14.

Jagirdar RM, Bozikas A, Zarogiannis SG, et al. Encapsulating peritoneal sclerosis: pathophysiology and current treatment options. Int J Mol Sci. 2019;20:5765.

Korte MR, Sampimon DE, Beties MG, et al. Encapsulating peritoneal sclerosis: State of affairs. Nat Rev Nephrol. 2011;7:528–38.

Singhal M, Krishna S, Lal A, et al. Encapsulating peritoneal sclerosis: the abdominal cocoon. RadioGraphics. 2019;39:62–77.

35. **Which one of the following strategies regarding treatment of EPS has been tried with some success?**

    A. Nutritional support
    B. Tamoxifen
    C. Corticosteroids
    D. Surgery
    E. All of the above

The answer is E

All of the above strategies have been tried with variable success. Either enteric or total parenteral nutrition (TPN) support should be started once the diagnosis is established. Adequate food supply is needed to improve malnutrition and albumin for all patients. TPN predisposes to infection; therefore, careful monitoring of vital signs is important. Usually, enteral nutrition when indicated is better than TPN, if patients can tolerate small feeds.

Tamoxifen is a selective inhibitor of estrogen receptors. It has a potential for antifibrotic effects, possibly by inhibiting the production of TGF-β. The use of tamoxifen alone or in combination with steroids has produced satisfactory results, but the experience is limited to case reports and small case series. It is of interest to note that the use of tamoxifen in long-term PD patients and those with fast transport characteristics produced promising results. Randomized studies are needed to confirm prophylactic use of tamoxifen in these patients.

The adverse effects of tamoxifen should be considered. These include thromboembolic events and risk of endometrial cancer.

Like tamoxifen, corticosteroids have been used alone or in combination with tamoxifen with variable success.

Surgery seems to be the most successful intervention in the management of advanced EPS. The mortality is greatly reduced in the hands of an experienced surgeon, and the cure rate is 70–80%. The surgical procedure involves lysis of adhesions and excision of the peritoneum while avoiding enterotomy.

It should be noted that EPS is a serious complication, and early clinical suspicion and possible diagnosis are necessary to prevent the progression of the disease.

Suggested Reading

de Sousa E, del Peso-Gilsanz G, Baso-Rubio MA, et al. Encapsulating peritoneal sclerosis in peritoneal dialysis. A review and European initiative for approaching a serious and rare disease. Nefrologia. 2012;32:707–14.

Jagirdar RM, Bozikas A, Zarogiannis SG, et al. Encapsulating peritoneal sclerosis: Pathophysiology and current treatment options. Int J Mol Sci. 2019;20:5765.

Korte MR, Sampimon DE, Beties MG, et al. Encapsulating peritoneal sclerosis: state of affairs. Nat Rev Nephrol. 2011;7:528–38.

36. During long-term PD, the peritoneal membrane undergoes structural and functional alterations that predispose to ultrafiltration failure. **Which one of the following factors contribute to these peritoneal membrane changes?**

A. Incompatible PD solutions
B. Repeated peritonitis
C. Interleukin-1β
D. Interleukin-17A
E. All of the above

The answer is E

Structurally, the peritoneal membrane consists of a layer of mesothelial cells and submesothelium (interstitium) that contains collagen, blood capillaries, and lymphatics. Fluid and solute transport is related to the number of blood capillaries rather than total peritoneal surface area. Long-term PD causes both structural and functional changes in the peritoneal membrane, leading to fibrosis, angiogenesis, mesothelial to mesenchymal transition, vasculopathy, and ultrafiltration failure.

Bioincompatible dialysis solutions contain high glucose and increased glucose degradation products (GDPs), which stimulate the production of transforming growth factor-β (TGF-β) and vascular endothelial growth factor (VEGF) by mesothelial and other cells. These growth factors promote fibrosis and angiogenesis, respectively. Also, increased GDPs stimulate inflammatory cytokines (A is correct).

Peritonitis stimulates inflammatory cytokines. Recent studies have demonstrated activation of NLRP3 (the nucleotide-binding oligomerization domain-like receptors or NOD-like receptors, also known as nucleotide-binding leucine-rich repeat receptors) inflammasome. Inflammasome is a molecular platform that is activated upon cellular infection or stress. The NLRP3 inflammasome is a multiprotein complex expressed in the cytosol of macrophages and neutrophils, which generates interleukin 1β (IL-1β). This cytokine stimulates the release of growth factors, such as TGF-β and VEGF, which promote peritoneal fibrosis and angiogenesis, resulting in structural and functional changes of the peritoneal membrane (answers B and C are correct). Elevated levels of IL-1β were found in PD fluid. Genetic and pharmacologic blockade of the NLRP3/IL-1b axis prevented morphologic alterations and transport defects during acute peritonitis, suggesting a novel therapeutic regimen for this severe complication of PD.

Another novel cytokine that has been implicated in peritoneal pathology is IL-17A. This cytokine has been shown to participate in immune-mediated glomerulonephritis. Immunostaining of IL-17A was found in inflamed but absent in healthy peritoneal membrane biopsy specimens. In animal, chronic infusion of IL-17A caused submesothelial fibrosis. Experimental studies demonstrated that IL-17A blockade ameliorated peritoneal damage caused by exposure to PD fluids (D is correct). Thus, exposure to bioincompatible PD fluids can trigger peritoneal inflammation with subsequent production of inflammatory cytokines leading to peritoneal membrane fibrosis and impaired solute and fluid transport.

Suggested Reading

Hautem N, Morelle J, Sow A, et al. The NLRP3 inflammasome has a critical role in peritoneal dialysis-related peritonitis. J Am Soc Nephrol. 2017;28:2038–52.

Marchant V, Tejera-Muñoz A, Marquez-Expósito L, et al. IL-17A as a potential therapeutic target for patients on peritoneal dialysis. Biomolecules. 2020;10(10):1361.

Rodrigues-Diaz R, Aroeira LS, Orejudo M, et al. IL-17A is a novel player in dialysis-induced peritoneal damage. Kidney Int. 2014;86:303–15.
Zhou Q, Bajo M-A, del Peso G, et al. Preventing peritoneal membrane fibrosis in peritoneal dialysis patients. Kidney Int. 2016;90:515–24.

37. A 42-year-old woman with cirrhosis due to hepatitis C is referred to you from hepatology clinic for evaluation of creatinine of 4.5 mg/dL with an eGFR of 18 mL/min. She relocated recently, and she was informed of kidney problem by her previous nephrologist. Blood pressure is 100/62 mm Hg with a pulse rate of 90 beats/min. Pertinent physical findings are ascites and 2+ pitting edema in lower extremities. She asks you about modalities of dialysis and survival, and she prefers home therapy. She has urine output of 600 mL/day. **Which one of the following maintenance dialysis modalities you recommend her based on the available evidence of survival?**

A. Hemodialysis (HD)
B. Peritoneal dialysis (PD)
C. Hemodialysis alternating with plasmapheresis
D. Molecular adsorbent recirculating system (MARS)
E. Prolonged intermittent renal (kidney) replacement therapy (PIRRT)

The answer is B

The patients with cirrhosis and ascites provide significant challenges to their physicians, especially in the management of their end-stage kidney disease due to their hemodynamic status and risk of bleeding. HD appears to be less attractive than PD in such patients. However, most of these patients receive HD support because of availability and easy accessibility. Although PD is a suitable renal (kidney) replacement therapy for cirrhotic patients with ascites, survival rates between these two renal replacement modalities have not been studied adequately.

Chou and colleagues compared the survival of cirrhotic patients on PD with the propensity score matched cirrhotic patients on HD. The study showed that patients on PD had lower mortality rates than those on HD. This lower mortality was independent of patients' comorbidity, severity of liver cirrhosis, and serum albumin levels.

The appropriate maintenance renal (kidney) replacement therapy for this patient, when needed, is PD. Thus, answer B is correct. If this patient develops untreatable infectious and noninfectious complications, the other choice is HD. The other choices are not appropriate for maintenance therapies as an outpatient (A, C, D, and E are incorrect).

Suggested Reading

Chaudhary K, Khanna R. Renal replacement therapy in end-stage renal disease patients with chronic liver disease and ascites: role of peritoneal dialysis. Perit Dial Int. 2008;28:113–17.
Chou C-Y, Wang S-M, Liang C-C, et al. Peritoneal dialysis is associated with a better survival in cirrhotic patients with chronic kidney disease. Medicine (Baltimore). 2016;95:e2465.
Guest S. Peritoneal dialysis in patients with cirrhosis and ascites. Adv Perit Dial. 2010;26:82–7.

38. The above patient comes to your clinic every 2 months and compliant with your prescription. Based on your prevision discussion with her about dialysis modalities, she agrees to have peritoneal dialysis (PD), and a PD catheter was placed. **Which one of the following noninfectious complications is expected to occur within 6 months of urgent-start PD?**

A. Hernia
B. Hydrothorax
C. Pericatheter fluid leak
D. Subcutaneous fluid leak
E. All of the above

The answer is E

Urgent start is defined in the literature as initiation of dialysis within few days (usually 7–14) days after placement of a PD catheter, and is gaining popularity for unplanned initiation of dialysis. Abdominal wall and catheter-related complications are rather common in patients with urgent-start dialysis. All of the above complications listed from A to D are expected to occur at different degrees (answer E is correct). In one study of Chinese patients, 4.8% (44/922 patients) developed complications. These include inguinal hernias (41%), umbilical hernias (14%), hydrothorax (25%), subcutaneous leaks (4%), and pericatheter leak (2%) in a median follow-up of

5.2 months. Hydrocele occurred in 14% of their patients. During the first month of PD therapy, two hernias, three hydrothoraxes, two hydroceles, one subcutaneous leak, and one pericatheter leak occurred in a total of 44 patients.

All patients were started with an initial dialysate volume of 0.5–0.8 L during the first 2 days with gradual titration to 2 L within a month or the maximum tolerable volume. Male sex and prior abdominal wall surgery were found to be risk factors for abdominal wall complications.

Regarding urgent start of PD, another 10-year retrospective study of Chinese cohort reported functional catheter malfunction in 4.1% of patients, and abdominal wall complications (including hernia, hydrothorax, hydrocele, and leakage) in 1.7% of patients within 1 month of PD catheter placement. Thus, both studies suggest that urgent-start PD is safe and feasible in CKD 5 patients who require long-term dialysis support.

Suggested Reading

Xu D, Liu T, Dong J. Urgent-start peritoneal dialysis complications: prevalence and risk factors. Am J Kidney Dis. 2017;70:102–10.

Ye H, Yang X, Yi C, et al. Urgent-start peritoneal dialysis for patients with end stage renal disease: a 10-year retrospective study. BMC Nephrol. 2019;20:238.

39. **Which one of the following statements regarding incremental peritoneal dialysis (PD) is CORRECT?**

A. Incremental PD is done with the intention of increasing peritoneal prescription when residual kidney function (RKF) declines
B. Use of PD solution and cost of PD are less compared to standard (full dose) PD
C. Renal outcomes with incremental PD are at least as good as standard PD in a patient with RKF
D. Incremental PD allows patients more time for life participation, less treatment burden, and better quality of life
E. All of the above

The answer is E

Incremental PD is a strategy by which less than standard (regular) PD is prescribed in patients initiating PD. It is done with the intention of increasing the peritoneal prescription if and when RKF declines. Use of incremental PD involves less PD solution and cost compared to standard PD treatment. Also, kidney outcomes are at least as good as standard PD prescription in those patients with preserved RKF. All of these interventions allow patients more time for life participation, less treatment burden, and better quality of life. Thus, answer E is correct.

Suggested Reading

Brown EA, Blake PG, Boudville N, et al. International Society for Peritoneal Dialysis practice recommendations: prescribing high-quality goal-directed peritoneal dialysis. Perit Dial Int. 2020;40:244–53.

40. **Which one of the following statements regarding recent observations by a multicenter international prospective cohort study of adult peritoneal dialysis (PD) patients on PD modality, PD prescription, and practice patterns in Australia/New Zealand, Canada, Japan, Thailand, the United Kingdom, and the United States is CORRECT?**

A. Thailand is unique in that it has a "PD first" policy and most patients received continuous ambulatory PD (CAPD)
B. Patients in Australia/New Zealand, Canada, the United Kingdom, and the United States predominantly received automated PD (APD)
C. Patients in the United Kingdom and Japan received ≤3 CAPD exchanges
D. Neutral pH low GDP PD solutions were prescribed more often in Japan, Australia/New Zealand, and the United Kingdom than in Canada, Thailand, and the United States
E. All of the above

The answer is E

Wang and colleagues recently updated the guideline on patterns of PD prescription among Peritoneal Dialysis Outcomes and Practice Patterns Study (PDOPPS) participants on CAPD and APD (N = 4657) from Australia/New Zealand, Canada, Japan, Thailand, the United Kingdom, and the United States and found variable PD prescription among these six countries.

In Thailand, "PD first" policy was introduced for all ESKD patients. About 90% of them are on CAPD for whom there is universal health coverage. The remaining patients have their medical expenses fully reimbursed under the Civil Servant Medical Benefit Scheme for their management. In Japan only 3% of patients were on

CAPD. In contrast to Thailand, patients in Australia/New Zealand, Canada, the United Kingdom, and the United States predominantly received APD because of their preference.

Although patients in all six countries achieved weekly Kt/V above 1.7, their CAPD and APD prescription and delivered volumes showed marked variations. Patients in the United Kingdom and Japan received ≤3 CAPD exchanges because of lower body size of patients in these countries.

Selection of PD solutions varied among countries as well. In general, neutral pH low GDP (glucose degradation product) PD solutions were prescribed more often in Japan, Australia/New Zealand, and the United Kingdom than in Canada, Thailand, and the United States. This type of PD solution has been shown to preserve RKF and delay the onset of anuria. The frequent use of neutral pH low GDP in Japan, Australia/New Zealand, and the United Kingdom is probably related to availability, reimbursement policies, or commercial costs of these solutions to providers. In the United States, the mostly used PD solutions were 2.5% (>50% of the time) and 4.25% (>40% of the time) dextrose solutions. Icodextrin is expensive and also restriction to its use in some centers make nephrologists to select high-glucose PD solutions in the United States, and probably in Canada and Thailand as well. Thus, answer E is correct.

Suggested Reading

Wang A Y-M, Zhao J, Bieber B, PDOPPS Dialysis Prescription and Fluid Management Working Group, et al. International comparison of peritoneal dialysis prescriptions from the Peritoneal Dialysis Outcomes and Practice Patterns Study (PDOPPS). Perit Dial Int. 2020;40:310–19.

Chapter 11
Transplantation

1. A 26-year-old man with ethylene glycol poisoning develops irreversible brain damage and acute kidney injury. He is on continuous venovenous hemodiafiltration for a week with no improvement in brain function. The family decides to donate his organs, and he is pronounced brain dead. **Which one of the following immunologic events is expected to occur within the donor kidney at the time of donor harvest?**

   A. Spillage of damage-activated molecular patterns (DAMPs) into the tissue milieu
   B. Activation of interstitial resident dendritic cells by DAMPs
   C. Brain death in the deceased donor causes swings in blood pressure (BP) with resultant ischemia/anoxia to the kidney
   D. Brain death is accompanied by massive release of cytokines that activate immune cells and endothelial and tubular epithelial cells of the kidney
   E. All of the above

   The answer is E

   The donor kidney consists of not only glomeruli, mesangium, tubular cells, and endothelium but also immune cells such as dendritic cells from the interstitium, which are phagocytic. These cells are usually dormant and are activated by low blood flow to the kidney following brain death. As a result of ischemia, cells in the donor kidney die and release such molecules as DAMPs. Examples of DAMPs include uric acid, ATP, heat-shock proteins, DNA, RNA, and glycosaminoglycans. DAMPs activate dendritic cells by binding to their receptors located on the epithelial, endothelial, and mesenchymal cells within the donor kidney. These receptors include toll-like receptors and nucleotide-binding oligomerization domain-like receptors. The interaction between DAMPS and their receptors triggers inflammatory cytokines which attract recipient inflammatory cells. Thus, the donor kidney is immunologically activated even before it is transplanted into the recipient.

   One of the ways that resident dendritic cells become activated is through renal ischemia/anoxia caused by low blood flow to the donor kidneys. Brain death causes initially high BP followed by low BP. These swings in BP result finally in ischemia, which starts immunologic events in the donor kidney. Thus, E is correct.

   Suggested Reading

   John R, Nelson PJ. Dendritic cells in the kidney. J Am Soc Nephrol. 2007;8:2628–35.
   Kurts C, Ginhoux F, Panzer U. Kidney dendritic cells: fundamental biology and functional roles in health and disease. Nat Rev Nephrol. 2020;16:391–407.
   Reis e Sousa C. Activation of dendritic cells: translating innate into adaptive immunity. Curr Opin Immunol. 2004;16:21–5.
   Womer KL. Immunologic principles in kidney transplantation. In: Feehally J, Floege J, Tonelli M, et al., editors. Comprehensive clinical nephrology. 6th ed. Philadelphia: Elsevier; 2019. p. 1141–53.

2. In transplant immunobiology, the human major histocompatibility complex (MHC) plays an important role in both innate (natural) and adaptive immune systems. **Regarding MHC and kidney transplantation, which one of the following statements is CORRECT?**

   A. MHC comprises a set of genes that is located on the short arm of chromosome 6
   B. MHC genes are highly polymorphic (diverse), and each individual inherits one set of genes from each parent

A. S. Reddi, *Absolute Nephrology Review*, https://doi.org/10.1007/978-3-030-85958-9_11

C. In humans, both MHC and major human leukocyte antigens (HLAs) are used interchangeably because MHC was first discovered in leukocytes
D. Among three classes of HLA genes, only class I and class II HLA genes are important for kidney transplantation
E. All of the above

The answer is E

All of the statements are correct and also self-explanatory. Successful organ transplantation depends on the donor and recipient HLAs that are encoded by HLA (MHC) genes. These antigens are called alloantigens (a cell or tissue antigens that are present in some members of species but not in others) and are recognized as foreign antigens. The genes for these alloantigens (proteins) are clustered in MHC on the short arm of chromosome 6. Because MHC genes, also called HLA genes, are polymorphic, the products of these genes are also polymorphic. A new World Health Organization classification has been introduced in 2010 to include all HLA genes and their products.

HLA genes are classified into three classes: HLA class I, HLA class II, and HLA class III. HLA class I genes include HLA-A, HLA-B, and HLA-C genes, and are present on cell surfaces of all nucleated cells. HLA class II genes include HLA-DP, HLA-DQ, and HLA-DR; the proteins of these genes are present in antigen-presenting cells such as dendritic cells, macrophages, B cells, endothelial cells, and some epithelial cells. Only HLA class I and HLA class II genes and their antigens participate in kidney transplants.

HLA class III genes encode complement proteins, heat-shock proteins, and tissue necrosis factors, and do not play a significant role in kidney transplantation.

In transplant immunobiology, the effector cells for rejection are T cells, although B cells are also important. The ability of T cells to recognize antigens is dependent on association of these antigens with either class I or class II HLA proteins. For example, T helper (CD4) cells respond to antigens in association with class II proteins, whereas cytotoxic T (CD8) cells respond to class I proteins. Thus, either the rejection or acceptance of a transplant is dependent on either class I or class II HLA proteins on donor cells. Generally, class II proteins play a major role in these processes. Matching class I and class II antigens between the donor and recipient is important for successful kidney transplantation. It should, however, be noted that many transplants are done successfully with six antigen mismatches as well.

Suggested Reading

Alelign T, Ahmed MM, Bobosha K, et al. Kidney transplantation: the challenge of human leukocyte antigen and its therapeutic strategies. J Immunol Res. 2018;2018:5986740.

Castro-Dopico T, Clatworthy MR. The immunology of transplantation. In: Knechtle SJ, Marson LP, Morris PJ, editors. Kidney transplantation: principles and practice. 8th ed. Philadelphia: Elsevier; 2020. p. 9–35.

3. **Which one of the following immunologic barriers should be considered for any successful kidney transplantation?**

A. Blood group incompatibility
B. Mismatched HLA (human leukocyte antigen) antigens
C. Anti-donor HLA antibodies in the recipient
D. Rhesus (Rh) factor positivity
E. A, B, and C

The answer is E

Prior to kidney transplantation, both donor and recipient undergo certain tests to prevent rejection. These tests include blood type matching, HLA antigen matching, and anti-HLA antibody test. The first barrier to successful transplantation is blood group mismatch (A is correct). There are four types of blood groups: A, B, AB, and O. The most frequently found blood groups in the United States are A and O (42–44%). The A and B groups are glycosylated, whereas group O lacks glycosylation. Individuals with A or B blood types produce natural antibodies to the opposite type, and individuals with group O produce antibodies to both A and B. Because group O lacks glycosylated moiety, both A and B fail to produce antibodies to group O. Thus, group O grafts can be transplanted into patients with blood types A, B, and AB. However, it is not a common practice for ethical reasons in order to prevent depletion of available transplants for type O recipients, who must receive an O transplant. When ABO-incompatible kidney is transplanted, it is immediately rejected because of preformed anti-A and/or anti-B antibodies. Table 11.1 **shows the blood compatibility between donor and recipient blood groups.**

Table 11.1 Blood type compatibility

Recipient blood type	Donor blood type compatible with recipient
A	A, O
B	B, O
AB	A, B, AB, O
O	O (A[a])

[a]Some centers accept transplantation from donors with blood type A to recipients with blood type O

The second barrier is mismatched HLA antigens. Despite many advances, HLA matching continues to be a major determinant of graft survival. The survival of grafts with no mismatches is much greater than those with one mismatch. However, concerns were raised about the HLA antigen mismatch, as no benefit in survival of grafts was observed with HLA matching in African Americans. A recent review concludes that HLA matching should continue because it allows the use of lower dosages of immunosuppressive agents. This conclusion was based on (1) HLA matching overrides the impact of cold ischemia time (as longer time has negative impact on graft survival) on graft survival; (2) HLA mismatched patients were frequently hospitalized for malignancies due to high dosages of immunosuppressive agents; finally, HLA mismatches at class II level (HLA-DR) appears to be associated with de novo development of donor-specific antibody 4.6 years after transplantation. Thus, HLA matching is important (B is correct).

The third barrier is the presence of anti-donor HLA antibodies. If not desensitized, these donor-specific antibodies cause hyperacute rejection and also limit the survival of the allograft. Prior to transplantation, crossmatch testing is done for the presence or absence of these antibodies (C is correct).

The final barrier is the presence of minor HLAs, which are not well studied. The requirement of reduced immunosuppression in recipients of HLA identical siblings suggests the presence of such minor HLAs.

The rhesus (Rh) factor either negative or positive is not an issue in kidney transplantation, as the kidney does not express this blood group. Thus, D is incorrect

Suggested Reading

Santos RD, Langewisch ED, Norman DJ. Immunological assessment of the transplant patient. In: Weir MR, Lerma EV, editors. Kidney transplantation. Practical guide to management. New York: Springer; 2014. p. 23–34.

Süsal C, Opelz G. Current role of human leukocyte antigen matching in kidney transplantation. Curr Opin Transplant. 2013;18:438–44.

4. In addition to the above tests, crossmatch testing is necessary prior to surgical transplantation to detect anti-HLA antibodies in the recipient. **Which one of the following tests is NOT used to detect anti-HLA antibodies in the recipient?**

A. Complement-dependent cytotoxicity (NIH-CDC) test
B. Anti-human globulin (AHG-CDC) enhanced test
C. T and B cell flow cytometric test
D. Solid-phase bead or ELISA assay
E. Panel-reactive antibody (PRA) test

The answer is E

Crossmatching test was introduced in transplant technology to identify the antibodies in the serum of recipients that can cause hyperacute rejection or early graft failure. The oldest test is the NIH-CDC with very low sensitivity; however, the sensitivity of this test has subsequently been increased by the addition of AHG. Further sensitivity is increased by flow cytometric crossmatch testing, and the highest sensitive test is the solid-phase bead or ELISA assay (A-D are correct). The PRA test is a screening test that is used for patients who are on the nationwide deceased donor list. Thus, option E is incorrect.

Table 11.2 **gives a list of various assays for detection of alloantibodies in the recipient.**

Table 11.2 Various alloantibody detection assays

Assays	Sensitivity
Screening tests Panel reactive antibody (T cell only) Donor-specific alloantibody detection Solid-phase beads or ELISA	
Class I HLA antibody tests	
T cell cytotoxicity (NIH-CDC)	Very low
T cell AHG-CDC	Low
T cell flow cytometric test	High
Solid-phase bead or ELISA	Very high (highest)
Both class I and class II HLA antibodies tests	
B cell cytotoxicity (NIH-CDC)	Low
B cell flow cytometric test	High
Solid-phase bead or ELISA	Very high (highest)

The reader is referred to the following suggested reading for technical aspects of these tests.

Suggested Reading

Fuggle SV, Taylor CJ. Histocompatibility in renal transplantation. In: Knechtle SJ, Marson LP, Morris PJ, editors. Kidney transplantation: principles and practice. 8th ed. Philadelphia: Elsevier; 2020. p. 139–56.

Mulley WR, Kanellis J. Understanding crossmatch testing in organ transplantation: a case-based guide for the general nephrologist. Nephrology. 2011;16:125–33.

Pham P-TT, Zhang QJ, Hickey MJ. Transplant immunobiology. In: Pham P-TT, Pham P-CT, editors. Guide to kidney transplantation. From initial evaluation to long-term post-transplant care. Philadelphia: Wolters Kluwer; 2020. p. 1–13.

Santos RD, Langewisch ED, Norman DJ. Immunological assessment of the transplant patient. In: Weir MR, Lerma EV, editors. Kidney transplantation. Practical guide to management. New York: Springer; 2014. p. 23–34.

Tambur AR, Campbell P, Claas FH, et al. Sensitization in transplantation: assessment of Risk (STAR) 2017 Working Group Meeting Report. Am J Transplant. 2018;18:1604–14.

5. Patients awaiting cadaveric kidneys have their serum screened for antibodies. **Which one of the following antibody testing is MOST important in screening these patients?**

   A. Blood group B antibody
   B. Blood group A antibody
   C. Blood group AB antibody
   D. Panel-reactive antibody (PRA)
   E. A, B, and C

   The answer is D

   The most important screening test in the recipient awaiting nationwide deceased donor kidney is the PRA test, which is expressed from 0% to 100% (D is correct). This test is done by testing the recipient serum with lymphocytes from individuals who are considered representatives of the general population. Most laboratories perform the test by using the lymphocytes from 30 to 50 subjects. A 0% of PRA indicates no antibodies against the general population. On the other hand, if the recipient has a PRA of 30, it tells that 30% of the population is not a suitable donor of the kidney. The higher the percentage, the longer is the waiting time and less likely to have a kidney transplant. This screening test should not be confused with crossmatch testing. Tests from A to C are not screening tests.

Suggested Reading

Althaf MM, El Kossi M, Jin JK, et al. Human leukocyte antigen typing and crossmatch: a comprehensive review. World J Transplant. 2017;7:339–48.

Milfrod EL, Guleria I. What is histocompatibility testing and how is it done? In: McKay DB, Steinberg SM, editors. Kidney transplantation. A guide to the care of kidney transplant recipients. New York: Springer; 2010. p. 41–55.

Murphey CL, Forsthuber TG. Trends in HLA antibody screening and identification and their role in transplantation. Expert Rev Clin Immunol. 2008;4:391–99.

Schinstock A, Stegall M. Transplantation in the sensitized recipient and across ABO blood groups. In: Knechtle SJ, Marson LP, Morris PJ, editors. Kidney transplantation: principles and practice. 8th ed. Philadelphia: Elsevier; 2020. p. 355–66.

6. The new deceased donor kidney allocation system has been revised and implemented on December 4, 2014. **Which one of the following variables is included in designing estimated posttransplant survival (EPTS)?**

   A. Age of the patient
   B. Time on dialysis
   C. Diabetes status
   D. Prior organ transplant
   E. All of the above

The answer is E

The new kidney allocation system (KAS) has been developed with the participation of transplant professionals and people who have personal experience with donation and transplantation. This KAS is designed to increase the lifespan and allograft survival in transplant recipients and to improve transplant to patients who are socially or immunologically disadvantaged by shortfalls of the previous KAS that prioritized longer wait times.

The new system was built on two designs to improve the allocation of the kidney: EPTS and KDPI (Kidney Donor Profile Index). EPTS is a tool to estimate the anticipated posttransplant survival in the recipient. It is based on four variables: age of the patient, time on dialysis in years, diabetes status, and the number of prior solid organ transplants (E is correct). A score is calculated, which is expressed as percentage from 0% to 100%. The transplanted kidney is expected to last longer in a patient with a score <20% compared to a patient with a score >20%.

KDPI incorporates 10 donor factors which provide the relative risk of posttransplant kidney graft failure. Thus, KDPI measures donor quality. KDPI is applicable to only deceased donors and not living donors. Lower KDPI scores indicate high donor quality, whereas higher KDPI scores are associated with lower donor quality.

Table 11.3 Donor factors for KDPI

1. Age
2. Height
3. Weight
4. Ethnicity
5. History of hypertension
6. History of diabetes
7. Cause of death
8. Serum creatinine
9. Hepatitis C virus status
10. Donation after circulatory death status (brain or cardiovascular death)

Table 11.3 **shows the 10 donor factors (variables).**

EPTS scores are used to divide patients on the waiting list into the top 20% and remaining 80%. The top 20% will receive the kidney with the longest estimated posttransplant survival. Based on EPTS and KDPI, the kidneys are allocated in four sequences:

Sequence A: **Top 20% KDPI kidneys to 20% EPTS candidates. The projected waiting time for these candidates is less than those of the remaining 80%**

Sequence B: KDPI between 20% and 35%. Pediatric candidates will receive priority with this score

Sequence C: KDPI from 20% to 85%. EPTS is not a factor in allocation, and kidneys are allocated based on points given for waiting time, HLA-DR matching, and calculated PRA

Sequence D: KDPI >85%. Older candidates are opted based on the time on the waiting list

Thus, this new KAS may fulfill the principles of utility and equity (justice).

Suggested Reading

Chopra B, Suresh Kumar KK. Changing organ allocation policy for kidney transplantation in the United States. World J Transplant. 2015;24:38–43.

Friedenwald JJ, Samana CJ, Kasiske BL, et al. The kidney allocation system. Surg Clin N Am. 2013;93:1395–406.

Israni AK, Salkowski N, Gustafson S, et al. New national allocation policy for deceased donor kidneys in the United States and possible effect on patient outcomes. J Am Soc Nephrol. 2014;25:1842–48.

Lee D, Kanellish J, Mulley WR. Allocation of deceased donor kidneys: a review of international practices. Nephrology. 2019;24:591–98.

7. **Since implementation of the new Kidney Allocation System (KAS), which one of the following statements is CORRECT?**

A. An increase in deceased donor kidney transplants among black candidates
B. An increase in deceased donor kidney transplants among those with calculated panel-reactive antibodies (cPRA) of 98–100%
C. A decrease in deceased donor kidney transplants among those aged 65 years or older
D. A positive trend in graft and patient survival for both deceased and living donor kidney transplants
E. All of the above

The answer is E

All of the above statements are true regarding the effects of new KAS implementation since December 2014 (E is correct). The above data were derived from the 2015 Annual Data Report. In addition, the total number of patients on the waiting list decreased for the first time in a decade, which was due to a combination of (1) a decrease in the number of candidates added to the list; (2) an increase in the number of candidates removed from the list due to deteriorating medical condition; and (3) an increase in total transplants. However, deaths on the waiting list remained flat. Candidates with cPRA of 80–97% were likely to receive a deceased donor kidney as opposed to patients with cPRA of 98–100%. Thus, the new KAS seems to have a great impact on transplant candidates.

Suggested Reading

Hart A, Smith JM, Skeans MA, et al. OPTN/SRTR 2015 annual data report: kidney. Am J Transplant. 2017;17:21–116.

8. **Which one of the following statements regarding the presence of antibodies and rejection of transplanted kidney is CORRECT?**

A. IgG antibodies against HLA-A and B antigens result in acute rejection
B. IgM antibodies against HLA-A and B antigens in the current rather than past serum is highly predictive of rejection
C. Autoimmune disease (such as lupus)-induced antibodies do not play an important role in rejection
D. Medication (hydralazine, quinidine)-induced antibodies have significant role in rejection
E. A, B, and C

The answer is E

All of the above statements except D are correct (E). Lupus or medication-induced antibodies are of IgM isotype and are not important in kidney transplantation as they do not mediate rejection (D is incorrect). However, IgM antibodies can cause a positive crossmatch.

Suggested Reading

McKay DB, Park K, Perkins. What is transplant immunology and why are allografts rejected? In: McKay DB, Steinberg SM, editors. Kidney transplantation. A guide to the care of kidney transplant recipients. New York: Springer; 2010. p. 25–39.

Milfrod EL, Guleria I. What is histocompatibility testing and how is it done? In: McKay DB, Steinberg SM, editors. Kidney transplantation. A guide to the care of kidney transplant recipients. New York: Springer; 2010. p. 41–55.

Schinstock A, Stegall M. Transplantation in the sensitized recipient and across ABO blood groups. In: Knechtle SJ, Marson LP, Morris PJ, editors. Kidney transplantation: principles and practice. 8th ed. Philadelphia: Elsevier; 2020. p. 355–66.

9. A 38-year-old Caucasian woman donates her kidney to her son with Alport syndrome. At the time of donation, her eGFR was 96 mL/min, BP 128/74 mm Hg, and normal glucose and urinalysis. Currently, she is being followed by a nephrologist for health-related issues. **Which one of the following statements regarding posttransplant medical conditions is CORRECT?**

A. Her eGFR may decrease to <30 mL/min is 0.2% in the first decade of postdonation
B. The overall prevalence of ESKD is 0.5% in the 6 months to 5 years and 1.1% in the 10 years after postdonation
C. She may develop albuminuria/proteinuria (proteinuria >500 mg/day) which is higher than controls

D. She is at risk for hypertension during her lifetime and also for gestational hypertension or preeclampsia during pregnancy
E. All of the above

The answer is E

Posttransplant development of complications in live donors is rather common. Studies have shown that during the first decade of postdonation, 40% of donors have a GFR between 60 and 80 mL/min, 12% of donors have a GFR between 30 and 59 mL/min, and 0.2% of donors have a GFR <30 mL/min (A is correct). The maintenance of the above GFRs is related to the hyperfiltration of the remaining kidney with hypertrophied nephrons.

ESKD was typically defined as donors undergoing dialysis or kidney transplantation. A meta-analysis of 12 studies involving 108,900 living kidney donors reported that the overall prevalence of ESKD is 0.5% in the 6 months to 5 years and 1.1% in the 10 years after that postdonation (answer B is correct). A report from Japan showed that follow-up of 12 live donors maintained their GFR for a median of 16 years but developed ESKD following an inciting event such as infection, hypertension, and proteinuria. Also, another study showed a 7.4-fold increase in the development of ESKD after 7.8-year postdonation, as compared with controls. Several other studies also have shown the development of ESKD with older age for whites and younger age for blacks, and male sex as risk factors. Thus, the progression to ESKD in live donors depends on several factors.

Studies have shown that follow-up of live donors for albuminuria/proteinuria showed that approximately 12% develop albuminuria/proteinuria after 7–12 years (C is correct). Development of hypertension is common and reported to occur in approximately 30% of donors. A retrospective cohort study of living kidney donors showed that gestational hypertension or preeclampsia was more common among living kidney donors than among non-donor pregnant women (D is correct).

Suggested Reading

Garg AX, Nevis IF, McArthur E, et al. For the DONOR Network. Gestational hypertension and preeclampsia in living kidney donors. N Engl J Med. 2015;372:124–33.
Ibrahim HN, Foley R, Tan L, et al. Long-term consequences of kidney donation. N Engl J Med. 2009;360:459–69.
Lentine KL, Kasiske BL, Levey AS, et al. KDIGO Clinical Practice guideline on the evaluation and care of living kidney donors. Transplantation. 2017;101(8S):S1–109.
Li SS, Huang YM, Wang M, et al. A meta-analysis of renal outcomes in living kidney donors. Medicine (Baltimore). 2016;95:e3847.
Maggiore U, Budde K, Heemann U, et al. for the ERA-EDTA DESCARTES working group. Long-term risks of kidney living donation: review and position paper by the ERA-EDTA DESCARTES working group. Nephrol Dial Transplant. 2017;32:216–23.
Matas AJ, Berglund DM, Vock DM, et al. Causes and timing of end-stage renal disease after living kidney donation. Am J Transplant. 2018;18:1140–50.
Wainright JL, Robinson AM, Wilk AR, et al. Risk of ESRD in prior living kidney donors. Am J Transplant. 2018;18:1129–39.

10. A 40-year-old woman is willing to donate her kidney to her daughter with type 2 diabetes. Her BMI is 38 kg/m^2, BP 142/92 mm Hg, and 24-h proteinuria of 310 mg. She has a history of recurrent calcium oxalate stones. **Which one of the following statements regarding her kidney donation is CORRECT?**

A. Her excess weight excludes her from donation
B. Her uncontrolled BP may exclude from donation
C. Her proteinuria indicates underlying glomerular disease
D. She is not at risk for surgical complications compared to lean donors
E. All of the above

The answer is E

All of the above statements are correct (E). A BMI >35 kg/m^2 is considered a relative contraindication for donation at many transplant centers. The obese individuals are advised to lose weight to <25 kg/m^2 before donation, as obesity >25 kg/m^2 is associated with ESKD. Uncontrolled hypertension (ambulatory BP >140/90 mm Hg) is also a relative contraindication for donation. However, the kidney donation is accepted provided the donors are >50 years of age, eGFR ≥80 mL/min, and normal urinalysis.

Proteinuria of 310 mg/day generally indicates an underlying glomerular disease. Since proteinuria is a risk factor for progression of kidney and cardiovascular disease, donor kidney is not accepted from those with proteinuria >300 mg/day with or without hypertension. Indeed, it was shown that the risk for ESKD 20 years after

donation was 93.9/10,000 for obese compared to 39.7/10,000 for nonobese live kidney donors. Generally, the obese subjects experience more surgical complications during nephrectomy than lean subjects; however, some studies reported no surgical risk at all. Recurrence of kidney stones is a contraindication for kidney donation. Weight loss may improve many of the conditions of metabolic syndrome and make the obese subjects suitable for kidney donation. The donor has many health-related issues that make her unsuitable for kidney donation.

Suggested Reading

Lentine KL, Kasiske BL, Levey AS, et al. KDIGO clinical practice guideline on the evaluation and care of living kidney donors. Transplantation. 2017;101(8S):S1–109.

Locke JE, Reed RD, Massie A, et al. Obesity increases the risk of end-stage renal disease among living kidney donors. Kidney Int. 2017;91:699–703.

Srinivas TR, Meier-Kriesche H-U. Obesity and kidney transplantation. Sem Nephrol. 2013;33:34–43.

11. A 50-year-old woman, mother of three children, develops ESKD and on hemodialysis for 2 years. Prior to transplantation, she was found to have higher titers of anti-HLA antibodies on crossmatching. **Which one of the following exposures associated with the development of antibodies is CORRECT?**

A. Pregnancy
B. Blood transfusion
C. Prior transplantation
D. Autoimmune disease
E. A, B, and C

The answer is E

Unlike anti-ABO antibodies, anti-HLA antibodies do not occur naturally. The exposure of HLA antigens and subsequent development of anti-HLA antibodies is seen in three conditions: pregnancy, blood transfusion, and prior transplantation (E is correct). Blood transfusion should be avoided in patients awaiting a kidney transplant unless the benefit outweighs the risk. Autoimmune-induced antibodies (IgM isotype) do not participate in kidney transplantation. Thus, option D is incorrect.

Suggested Reading

Pratschke J, Dragun D, Hauser IA, et al. Immunological risk assessment: the key to individualized immunosuppression after kidney transplantation. Transplant Rev. 2016;30:77–84.

Santos RD, Langewisch ED, Norman DJ. Immunological assessment of the transplant patient. In: Weir MR, Lerma EV, editors. Kidney transplantation. Practical guide to management. New York: Springer; 2014. p. 23–34.

Zhang R. Donor-specific antibodies in kidney transplant recipients. Clin J Am Soc Nephrol. 2018;13:182–92.

12. Because of the presence of anti-HLA antibodies, the above recipient is highly sensitized. **Which one of the following interventions is helpful in desensitizing (removal of antibodies) the patient?**

A. Plasmapheresis
B. Intravenous (IV) IgG
C. Immunoadsorption
D. Rituximab
E. All of the above

The answer is E

All of the above intervention modalities have been tried alone or in combination to desensitize the patient, and mixed results were obtained (E is correct). However, patients with very high titers still retain some antibodies despite the use of these techniques. Acute and chronic rejections of allografts are expected in patients with elevated titers of antibodies. However, some patients maintain graft survival and kidney function for several years after transplantation despite the presence of some ant-HLA antibodies. Splenectomy, eculizumab (inhibitor of C5 that prevents the formation of the terminal complement complex C5b-9), and proteasome inhibitor (bortezomib) have also been used as desensitization procedures.

Jordan et al. used an IgG endopeptidase derived from Streptococcus pyogenes to desensitize patients with donor-specific antibodies (DSAs) to an incompatible deceased donor kidney at the time of transplantation. This

IgG endopeptidase degrades the antibody and destroys it. This treatment seems to be an important advance for deceased donor kidney transplantation because this agent can be given at the time of surgery with complete elimination of all DSAs and permits HLA-incompatible transplantation. The elimination occurred in 24 of 25 patients. If this treatment is established, avoidance of plasmapheresis, IV IgG, rituximab, and immunoadsorbent procedures can be avoided.

Suggested Reading

Abu Jawdeh BG, Cuffy MC, Alloway RR, et al. Desensitization in kidney transplantation: review and future perspectives. Clin Transplant. 2014;28:494–507.

Formica RN, Kulkarni S. Being thoughtful about desensitization. Clin J Am Soc Nephrol. 2017;12:1878–80.

Jordan SC, Lorant T, Choi J, et al. IgG endopeptidase in highly sensitized patients undergoing transplantation. N Engl J Med. 2017;377:442–53.

Keith DS, Vranic GM. Approach to the highly sensitized kidney transplant candidate. Clin J Am Soc Nephrol. 2016;7:684–93.

Marfo K, Lu A, Ling M, et al. Desensitization protocols and their outcome. Clin J Am Soc Nephrol. 2011;6:922–36.

Sethi S, Choi J, Toyoda M, et al. Desensitization: overcoming the immunologic barriers to transplantation. J Immunol Res. 2017;2017:6804678.

13. **Which one of the following effects is expected to occur after desensitization?**

   A. Increase in fungal infections
   B. Increase in acute antibody-mediated rejection (AMR)
   C. Increase in chronic allograft nephropathy
   D. Increase in patient survival
   E. All of the above

The answer is E

Desensitization procedures are expensive, and these procedures have been associated with increased fungal infections, increased rate of AMR, and higher subclinical and chronic antibody-mediated rejection compared to non-sensitized or placebo groups. A study from Johns Hopkins reported increased patient survival following plasmapheresis/IVIG treatment, as compared with those patients on dialysis. Thus, option E is correct.

Suggested Reading

Han DJ. Complications from desensitization. In: Han DJ, editor. Kidney transplantation in sensitized patients. Singapore: Springer; 2020. p. 63–89.

Marfo K, Lu A, Ling M, et al. Desensitization protocols and their outcome. Clin J Am Soc Nephrol. 2011;6:922–36.

Montgomery RA, Lonze BE, King KE, et al. Desensitization in HLA-incompatible kidney recipients and survival. N Engl J Med. 2011;365:318–26.

14. A 72-year-old nonobese woman wants to donate her kidney to her only daughter of 50 years old with hypertensive nephrosclerosis and eGFR <15 mL/min. She approached several transplant centers, and one center decides to perform preemptive transplantation. **Which one of the following statements regarding graft and recipient survival from older donors is CORRECT?**

   A. Graft survival is similar between older and younger donors
   B. Mortality rate is not higher in kidney recipients from older donors compared to younger donors
   C. Kidneys from older donors (>70 years) should not be accepted for transplantation
   D. Transplantation of kidneys from donors >70 years of age is associated with less graft survival and increased mortality
   E. Crossmatch is not necessary when transplantation is done between mother and daughter

The answer is D

Several studies have shown that kidney donation from older individuals had increased rejection rate, lower graft function, and poor graft survival when compared to younger donors (A is false). However, other studies have shown no difference in graft survival between older and younger donors. As far as recipient death is concerned, donor age is a risk factor for recipient death, which is attributed to age-related decrease in kidney function (or increase in serum creatinine) and associated cardiovascular disease (B is false). Recently, some centers accept

kidney donation from subjects >70 years of age (C is false). Crossmatch is mandatory even between living-related individuals to evaluate donor-specific antibodies (E is false).

A study by Berger et al. showed that the graft survival from live donors aged 70 years or older was much lower than the graft survival from donors aged 50–59 years after 1, 5, and 10 years of transplantation. Similarly, patient survival was much lower in those who received kidneys from older (>70 years) compared to the recipient survival who received kidneys from younger group (50–59 years). The actual data are shown in Table 11.4.

Table 11.4 Renal data

Years	Graft failure (%) older/younger	Recipient survival (%) older/younger
1	7.4/5.0	93.1/96.4
5	14.9/12.0	74.5/83.3
10	33.3/21.6	56.2/64.2

Thus, graft failure was higher and patient survival was lower in recipients who received kidneys from donors aged >70 years compared to those who received kidneys from younger donors (D is correct). Interestingly, there was no difference in survival between donors compared to the survival of age-matched general population.

Suggested Reading

Berger JC, Muzaale AD, James N, et al. Living kidney donors ages 70 and older: recipient and donor outcomes. Clin J Am Soc Nephrol. 2011;6:2887–93.

Reule S, Matas A, Ibrahim HN. Live donor transplantation. In: Weir MR, Lerma EV, editors. Kidney transplantation. Practical guide to management. New York: Springer; 2014. p. 75–84.

Veroux M, Grosso G, Coron D, et al. Age is an important predictor of kidney transplantation outcome. Nephrol Dial Transplant. 2012;27:1663–71.

15. A 40-year-old woman is evaluated for kidney donation. All the pertinent tests are negative except for microscopic hematuria. She had menstrual cycle 15 days ago. Urine sediment shows six dysmorphic RBCs on phase-contrast microscopy. **Which one of the following tests do you recommend for this donor?**

A. Ultrasound of the kidneys
B. CT of the kidneys
C. Kidney biopsy
D. Malignancy workup
E. Workup for renal stones

The answer is C

There are no prospective studies that evaluated the issue of hematuria in live donors, although case reports suggest that donor kidneys with glomerular abnormalities had good short-term outcomes in both the donors and recipients.

In general, isolated hematuria with 3–5 isomorphic RBCs/HPF is not a contraindication for kidney donation. On the other hand, dysmorphic RBCs indicate glomerular origin and disease. In donors with dysmorphic RBCs, a renal biopsy is indicated for evaluation of IgA nephropathy, X-linked Alport syndrome, or autosomal dominant Alport syndrome (previously called thin basement membrane disease). Thus, C is correct. If the donor has IgA nephropathy, she is prohibited from donation. If the donor is a carrier for Alport syndrome and the kidney function is normal without proteinuria, or hypertension, she may donate the kidney even in the presence of microscopic hematuria. On the other hand, if the biopsy shows pathology of Alport syndrome, the donor should not be accepted because the recipient may develop anti-GBM-antibody disease. All the other tests in this donor may not provide adequate information.

Suggested Reading

Ierino F, Kanellis J. Donors at risk: haematuria. Nephrology. 2010;15:S111–13.

Lentine KL, Kasiske BL, Levey AS, et al. KDIGO clinical practice guideline on the evaluation and care of living kidney donors. Transplantation. 2017;101(8S):S1–S109.

Yachnin T, Iaina A, Schwartz D, et al. The mother of an Alport's syndrome: a safe kidney donor? Nephrol Dial Transplant. 2002;17:683.

16. **Which one of the following conditions is a contraindication for live donor kidney donation?**

A. Reduced kidney function (eGFR <60 mL/min)
B. Diagnosis of IgA nephropathy or Alport syndrome
C. Bilateral or recurrent nephrolithiasis
D. Proteinuria >300 mg/day
E. All of the above

The answer is E

According to the 2017 KDIGO clinical practice guideline, all of the above conditions are contraindications for kidney donation (E is correct). The reader is referred to the following Suggested Reading for other contraindications as well as relative contraindications.

Suggested Reading

Kidney disease: improving global outcomes (KDIGO) kidney transplant candidate work Group. KDIGO clinical practice guideline on the evaluation and management of candidates for kidney transplantation. Transplantation. 2020;104:S1–103.

Lentine KL, Kasiske BL, Levey AS, et al. KDIGO clinical practice guideline on the evaluation and care of living kidney donors. Transplantation. 2017;101(8S):S1–109.

17. **Immunosuppressive drugs act on several steps of the T cell activation. Match the signal and cell proliferation inhibitors with the appropriate immunosuppressive agents.**

Signal	Immunosuppressive agents
A. Signal 1	1. OKT3, alefacept, cyclosporine, tacrolimus
B. Signal 2	2. Belatacept
C. Signal 3	3. Basiliximab, sirolimus, everolimus
D. Cell proliferation	4. Mycophenolate mofetil, azathioprine

Answers: A = 1; B = 2; C = 3; D = 4

Immunosuppressive drugs prevent allograft rejection. The mechanisms by which these drugs prevent rejection, it is essential to understand T cell activation in the recipient. As soon as the donor kidney is transplanted, several important reactions occur, as discussed in question 1. Initially, the recipient is exposed to DAMPs (damage-activated molecular patterns) released from the donor kidney and activate dendritic cells. The activated dendritic cells enter the lymph nodes of the recipient where they encounter naïve T cells and activate them. To understand the mechanism of T cell activation, a three-signal hypothesis was introduced. The initial interaction between the antigen-presenting cell (APC) and a specific T cell receptor (TCR), the complex of TCR-CD3, represents the first signal (*signal 1*) of T cell activation.

The next required component of T cell activation is called *signal 2*, which is the costimulation signaling, and it occurs when the CD80 and CD86 molecules on the APC bind to the CD28 molecule on the T cell. In order for full T cell activation to occur, both signal 1 and signal 2 are required. Both signals subsequently trigger a cascade of signaling pathways in the cytoplasm and nucleus of the T cell for its maturation. These pathways for maturation of the T cell include (1) calcineurin pathway, (2) mitogen-activated protein kinase pathway, and (3) JAK/STAT (Janus kinase/Signal Transducers and Activators of Transcription) pathway. The first two pathways cause the production of IL-2, which binds to its receptor (IL-2R) on T cells. This binding leads to the activation of the mammalian target of rapamycin (mTOR), which allows the T cells to undergo cell division and cell proliferation. The binding of IL-2 with its receptor and activation of mTOR represents *signal 3*.

The rejection of donor kidney is prevented by several immunosuppressive agents at several signals of T cell activation. The following are the drugs that block the three signals.

Signal 1 blockers: OKT3 and rabbit-derived antithymocyte globulin (rATG) (anti-CD3 molecules that block the T cell receptor complex) and cyclosporine and tacrolimus (calcineurin inhibitors). Figure 11.1 **shows the sites of blockage by these drugs**

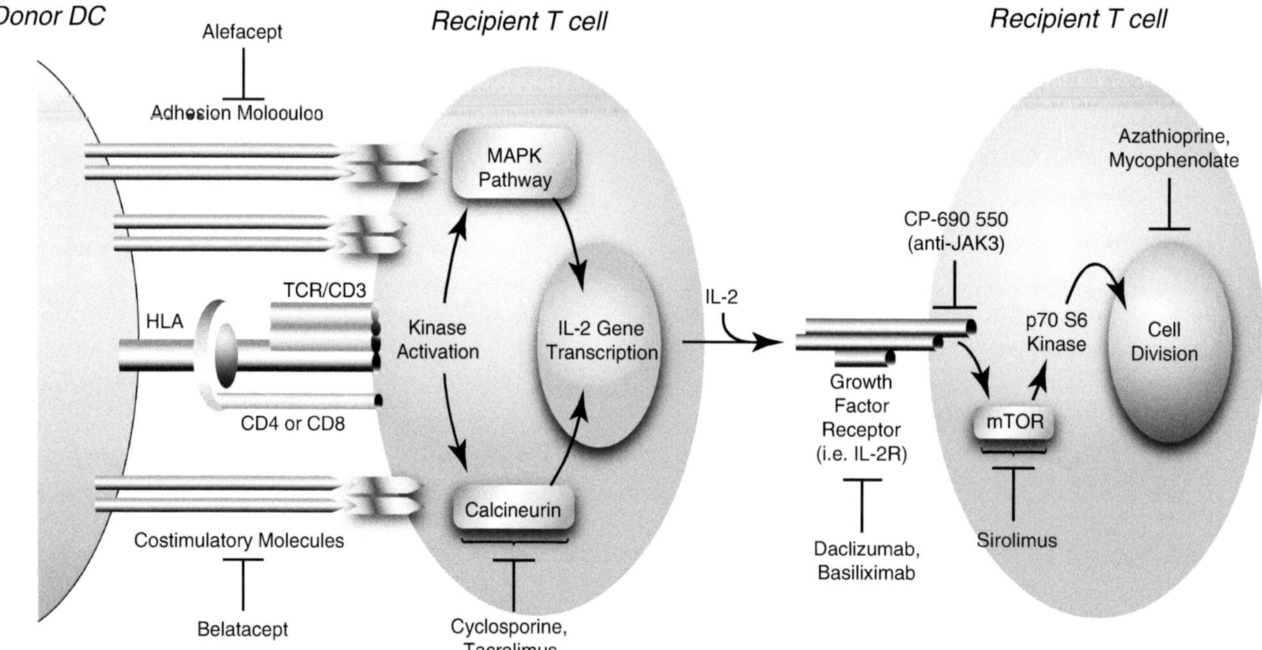

Fig. 11.1 T cell activation by the donor dendritic cell (DC) and the inhibitory sites by various immunosuppressive agents (adapted with permission from McKay DB, Steinberg SM)

Signal 2 blockers: Belatacept, which competitively binds the costimulatory molecule CD28 preventing it from binding CD80/CD86. The site of blockage is shown in Fig. 11.1

Signal 3 blockers: Basiliximab is an anti-CD25 antibody that competitively binds the IL-2R, and sirolimus and everolimus are mTOR inhibitors

In addition, mycophenolate mofetil and azathioprine inhibit cell proliferation. More specifically, mycophenolate mofetil inhibits inosine monophosphate dehydrogenase, and this enzyme controls the synthesis of RNA. Azathioprine is a purine synthesis inhibitor, and purines are involved in the synthesis of RNA, DNA, ATP, etc. JAK3 inhibitors (tofacitinib) inhibit JAK/STAT pathway. Figure 11.1 **shows T cell activation by the donor dendritic cell and the inhibitory sites by various immunosuppressive agents.**

Suggested Reading

Claes E, Vermeire K. Immunosuppressive drugs in organ transplantation to prevent allograft rejection: mode of action and side effects. J Immunological Sci. 2019;3:14–21.

McKay DB, Park K, Perkins. What is transplant immunology and why are allografts rejected? In: McKay DB, Steinberg SM, editors. Kidney transplantation. A guide to the care of kidney transplant recipients. New York: Springer; p. 25–39.

Weltz A, Scalea J, Popescu M, et al. Mechanisms of immunosuppressive drugs. In: Weir MR, Lerma EV, editors. Kidney transplantation. Practical guide to management. New York: Springer; 2014. p. 127–41.

Wiseman AC. Immunosuppressive medications. Clin J Am Soc Nephrol. 2016;5:332–43.

18. **Which one of the following drugs does NOT increase blood levels of calcineurin inhibitors (CNIs)?**

A. Ketoconazole
B. Erythromycin
C. Diltiazem
D. Atorvastatin
E. Caspofungin

The answer is E

CNIs include cyclosporine and tacrolimus and are the most commonly used immunosuppressive agents. Both agents are metabolized by cytochrome P-450 (CYP450) enzyme system, and drugs that either induce or inhibit

CYP450 may influence the levels of CNIs. Also, the levels of CNIs are influenced by a protein called P-glycoprotein. Except for caspofungin, all other drugs inhibit CYP450 and increase CNIs levels. Thus, option E is correct. Table 11.5 **shows all the drugs that either increase or decrease blood CNIs levels.**

Table 11.5 Effects of drugs on CNIs levels

Drugs that increase blood levels of CNIs by inhibition of CYP450 and/or P-glycoprotein	Drugs that decrease blood levels of CNIs by induction of CYP450 and/or P-glycoprotein
Calcium channel blockers	*Antituberculous drugs*
Diltiazem	Rifampin
Verapamil	Rifabutin
Amlodipine	Isoniazid
Nicardipine	*Anticonvulsants*
Antifungal agents	Barbiturates
Ketoconazole	Phenytoin
Fluconazole	Carbamazepine
Itraconazole	*Antidepressive herbals*
Voriconazole	St. John's wort
Antibiotics	*Antibiotics*
Erythromycin	Nafcillin
Macrolides	Imipenem
Drugs/food	Cephalosporins
Metoclopramide	
Grapefruit juice	
Statins	
Protease inhibitors	

Suggested Reading

Chang PC-W, Hricik DE. What are immunosuppressive medications? How do they work? What are their side effects? In: McKay DB, Steinberg SM, editors. Kidney transplantation: a guide to the care of kidney transplant recipients, New York: Springer; 2010; p. 119–35.

Claes E, Vermeire K. Immunosuppressive drugs in organ transplantation to prevent allograft rejection: mode of action and side effects. J Immunological Sci. 2019;3:14–21.

Sievers TM, Lum EL, Danovitch GM. Immunosuppressive medications and protocols for kidney transplantation. In: Danovitch GM, editor. Handbook of kidney transplantation. 7th ed. Philadelphia: Lippincott Williams & Wilkins; 2017. p. 101–63.

Wiseman AC. Immunosuppressive medications. Clin J Am Soc Nephrol. 2016;5:332–43.

19. Nephrotoxicity is a well-known complication of calcineurin inhibitors (CNIs). **Which one of the following renal-related complications due to CNIs is CORRECT?**

A. Hypertension
B. Hyperkalemia
C. Chronic kidney disease (CKD)
D. Hypomagnesemia, hypophosphatemia, type 4 renal tubular acidosis (RTA)
E. All of the above

The answer is E

Both cyclosporine and tacrolimus cause nephrotoxicity. Hypertension is common in posttransplant patients receiving one of these drugs. The mechanisms of hypertension include endothelial dysfunction, decreased production of nitric oxide, and other vasodilators with an increase in endothelin levels. These changes lead to renal and systemic vasoconstriction with resultant hypertension. Hyperkalemia is due mainly to inhibition of K^+ channel in the distal tubule, and decreased renin-AII-aldosterone activity. Type 4 RTA has also been reported, which is due to a decrease in NH_4^+ synthesis by hyperkalemia. Hypomagnesemia and hypophosphatemia are due to renal loss of these electrolytes. Interestingly, long-term use of cyclosporine in patients with liver and heart transplantation can lead to CKD and progression to end-stage kidney disease. Chronic tubulointerstitial disease, cytokine production (TGF-β1), and renal vasoconstriction seem to be responsible for CKD. Thus, option E is correct.

In addition to above changes, CNIs cause endothelial damage as well as renal vasoconstriction, resulting in thrombotic microangiopathy and renal ischemia.

Suggested Reading

Bennett WM, DeMattos A, Meyer MM, et al. Chronic cyclosporine nephropathy: the Achilles' heel of immunosuppressive therapy. Kidney Int. 1996;50:1089–100.

Lee CH, Kim G-H. Electrolyte and acid-base disturbances induced by calcineurin inhibitors. Electrolyte Blood Press. 2007;5:126–30.

Sievers TM, Lum EL, Danovitch GM. Immunosuppressive medications and protocols for kidney transplantation. In: Danovitch GM, editor. Handbook of kidney transplantation. 7th ed. Philadelphia: Lippincott Williams & Wilkins; 2017. p. 101–63.

20. Many drugs exacerbate calcineurin inhibitor (CNI) nephrotoxicity. **Which one of the following agents does NOT potentiate nephrotoxicity of CINs?**

    A. Amphotericin
    B. Nonsteroidal anti-inflammatory drugs (NSAIDs)
    C. Aminoglycosides
    D. Sirolimus
    E. Prostacyclin E (P_GE)

    The answer is E

    It is very important to recognize certain drugs that potentiate CNIs nephrotoxicity. These include amphotericin, NSAIDs, inappropriately high doses of aminoglycosides, and sirolimus. Also, concomitant use of ACE-Is or ARBs with CNIs requires close monitoring for hyperkalemia and acute kidney injury. P_GE is a vasodilator, which has least interaction with CNIs. Thus, option E is correct.

Suggested Reading

Chang PC-W, Hricik DE. What are immunosuppressive medications? How do they work? What are their side effects? In: McKay DB, Steinberg SM, editors. Kidney transplantation: a guide to the care of kidney transplant recipients. New York: Springer; 2010. p. 119–35.

Manitpisitkul W, Wilson NS, Lee S, et al. Drug interactions in solid organ transplant recipients. In: Weir MR, Lerma EV, editors. Kidney transplantation. Practical guide to management. New York: Springer; 2014. p. 411–25.

Sievers TM, Lum EL, Danovitch GM. Immunosuppressive medications and protocols for kidney transplantation. In: Danovitch GM, editor. Handbook of kidney transplantation. 7th ed. Philadelphia: Lippincott Williams & Wilkins; 2017. p. 101–63.

21. **Which one of the following reasons accounts for the preferred use of tacrolimus over cyclosporine?**

    A. Tacrolimus-treated patients had lower rate of acute rejection compared to cyclosporine at 1-year posttransplantation
    B. African American transplant patients treated with tacrolimus experienced less acute rejection compared to those on cyclosporine
    C. Tacrolimus causes less hirsutism and gingival hyperplasia but more alopecia than cyclosporine
    D. Requirement of antihypertensive treatment is much lower in tacrolimus-treated than cyclosporine-treated patients
    E. All of the above

    The answer is E

    In a comparison of tacrolimus and cyclosporine for immunosuppression after cadaveric kidney transplantation, a randomized, open-label study showed that 30.7% of tacrolimus-treated group experienced acute rejection compared with 46.4% of cyclosporine-treated group. Also, the degree of severity of rejection was 10.8% in the tacrolimus versus 26.5% in the cyclosporine-treated group (A is correct).

    There is also racial difference between tacrolimus and cyclosporine with regard to acute rejection. African Americans had 23.2% of acute rejection with tacrolimus compared to 47.9% with cyclosporine. When patients on cyclosporine were switched to tacrolimus (crossover) because acute rejection was counted as graft failure, there was a significant increase in 5-year survival of the graft (65.4%) in the tacrolimus group compared to 42.6%

survival in the cyclosporine group (B is correct). Crossover analysis also revealed that tacrolimus resulted in a significant increase in graft survival among African American patients at 5 years compared to those on cyclosporine (65.4% vs. 42.6%; *P* = 0.013).

Cyclosporine has been shown to cause hirsutism and gingival hyperplasia compared to tacrolimus, whereas tacrolimus causes alopecia than cyclosporine (C is correct). Interestingly, tacrolimus was found to lower mean levels of serum cholesterol, triglyceride, and low-density lipoprotein after 12 months of treatment compared to cyclosporine.

New-onset hypertension was much higher, requiring pharmacologic treatment in cyclosporine-treated group compared to tacrolimus-treated group of heart transplant and liver transplant patients. Similar results were noted in kidney transplant patients as well (D is correct). Thus, tacrolimus treatment causes less acute rejection, increased graft survival at 1 and 5 years, less lipid abnormality, and low incidence of hypertension than cyclosporine treatment for kidney transplant recipients.

Suggested Reading

Canzanello VJ, Textor SC,Taler SJ, et al. Late hypertension after liver transplantation: a comparison of cyclosporine and tacrolimus (FK 506). Liver Transplant Surg. 1998;4:328–34.

Jensik SC. Tacrolimus (FK 506) in kidney transplantation: three-year survival results of the us multicenter, randomized, comparative trial. Transplant Proc. 1998;30:1216–18.

Neylan JF. Racial differences in renal transplantation after immunosuppression with tacrolimus versus cyclosporine. Transplantation. 1998;65:515–23.

Pirsch JD, Miller J, Deierhoi MH, et al. A comparison of tacrolimus (FK506) and cyclosporine for immunosuppression after cadaveric renal transplantation. Transplantation. 1997;63:977–83.

Vincenti F, Jensik SC, Filo RS, et al. A long-term comparison of tacrolimus (FK506) and cyclosporine in kidney transplantation: evidence for improved allograft survival at five years. Transplantation. 2002;73:775–82.

Waid T. Prograf as secondary intervention versus continuation of cyclosporine in patients at risk for chronic renal allograft failure (CRAF) results in improved renal function, decreased CV risk, and no increased risk for diabetes. Am J Transplant. 2003;3 Suppl 1:436.

22. A kidney transplant patient is on cyclosporine and mycophenolate mofetil (MMF) for maintenance therapy. **Which one of the following statements is FALSE regarding the use of MMF in this patient?**

A. MMF converts into active mycophenolic acid in the stomach
B. MMF is a reversible inhibitor of inosine monophosphate dehydrogenase
C. MMF is preferred to azathioprine as the drug of choice in the maintenance of immunosuppression in renal transplant patients
D. Cyclosporine and tacrolimus equally lower MMF levels
E. MMF is associated with increased teratogenicity in pregnancy

The answer is D

MMF and enteric-coated MMF are potentially useful antiproliferative immunosuppressive drugs with wide popularity. Both drugs are metabolized to mycophenolic acid. MMF requires acid environment for absorption, whereas enteric-coated MMF requires alkaline pH for absorption. Thus, MMF is absorbed in the stomach and enteric-coated MMF in the intestine. Both drugs are potent reversible inhibitors of inosine monophosphate dehydrogenase, which is the rate-limiting enzyme in the synthesis of guanosine monophosphate. Thus, these drugs inhibit the de novo synthesis of purines. Because of few side effects, well tolerability, and documented efficacy, MMF largely replaced azathioprine as the drug of choice in the maintenance phase of immunosuppression. Both animal and human studies have shown teratogenicity with MMF during pregnancy, and azathioprine is usually recommended until pregnancy is completed. Cyclosporine but not tacrolimus lowers serum levels of MMF. Thus, option D is false.

Suggested Reading

Chang PC-W, Hricik DE. What are immunosuppressive medications? How do they work? What are their side effects? In: McKay DB, Steinberg SM, editors. Kidney transplantation: a guide to the care of kidney transplant recipients. New York: Springer; 2010. p. 119–35.

Sievers TM, Lum EL, Danovitch GM. Immunosuppressive medications and protocols for kidney transplantation. In: Danovitch GM, editor. Handbook of kidney transplantation. 7th ed. Philadelphia: Lippincott Williams & Wilkins; 2017. p. 101–63.

23. Drug-drug interactions are clinically significant. **Which one of the following drugs lowers plasma levels of sirolimus?**

A. Cyclosporine
B. Diltiazem
C. Fluconazole
D. Erythromycin
E. Rifabutin

The answer is E

Sirolimus is an antiproliferative agent, which is an mTOR (mammalian target of rapamycin) inhibitor. Another mTOR inhibitor is everolimus. Both of them are metabolized by P450 enzyme system. Thus, an interaction occurs when two P450 metabolizable drugs are used simultaneously. Because of this interaction, the primary drug's levels may be either low or elevated. Except for rifabutin, all other drugs increase plasma levels of sirolimus by decreasing its metabolism. Rifabutin lowers sirolimus levels by increasing its (sirolimus) metabolism. When cyclosporine and sirolimus are used as immunosuppressive drugs, it is preferable to administer sirolimus 4 h after cyclosporine. Adverse effects of sirolimus include hyperlipidemia, anemia, and neutropenia.

Suggested Reading

Chang PC-W, Hricik DE. What are immunosuppressive medications? How do they work? What are their side effects? In: McKay DB, Steinberg SM, editors. Kidney transplantation: a guide to the care of kidney transplant recipients. New York: Springer; 2010. p. 119–35.
Sievers TM, Lum EL, Danovitch GM. Immunosuppressive medications and protocols for kidney transplantation. In: Danovitch GM, editor. Handbook of kidney transplantation. 7th ed. Philadelphia: Lippincott Williams & Wilkins; 2017. p. 101–63.

24. **Which one of the following biologic immunosuppressive drugs does NOT deplete lymphocytes?**

A. Thymoglobulin
B. Atgam
C. Muromonab CD3 (OKT3)
D. Basiliximab
E. Alemtuzumab

The answer is D

Thymoglobulin and Atgam are polyclonal antibodies that are prepared by immunization of rabbit (Thymoglobulin) or horse (Atgam) against human lymphocytes. Atgam is largely replaced by Thymoglobulin. OKT3 is a monoclonal antibody against CD3 antigen associated with the T cell receptor. The use of OKT3 results in early activation of T cells with resultant release of cytokines followed by blocking T cell function. Alemtuzumab (Campath) is a monoclonal antibody against CD52, which was developed to treat chronic lymphocytic leukemia. Thus, thymoglobulin, atgam, OKT3, and alemtuzumab deplete both T and B lymphocytes, and thus are useful for induction of immunosuppression.

Basiliximab is a monoclonal CD25 antibody that binds to the α-chain of the IL-2 receptor-activated cells. It is an IgG1 antibody and blocks the proliferative signal without depleting lymphocytes. Thus, option D is correct.

Suggested Reading

Chang PC-W, Hricik DE. What are immunosuppressive medications? How do they work? What are their side effects? In: McKay DB, Steinberg SM, editors. Kidney transplantation: a guide to the care of kidney transplant recipients. New York: Springer; 2010. p. 119–35.
Sievers TM, Lum EL, Danovitch GM. Immunosuppressive medications and protocols for kidney transplantation. In: Danovitch GM, editor. Handbook of kidney transplantation. 7th ed. Philadelphia: Lippincott Williams & Wilkins; 2017. p. 101–63.

25. **Match the following drugs with their mechanism of action in kidney transplantation.**

Drug	Mechanism
A. Alemtuzumab	1. Anti-CD20 antibody
B. Rituximab	2. Anti-CD52 antibody
C. Intravenous immunoglobulin (IVIG)	3. Proteasome inhibitor
D. Bortezomib	4. Anti-complement 5 antibody
E. Eculizumab	5. Reduction of alloantigen antibody titers

Answers: A = 2; B = 1; C = 5; D = 3; E = 4

Alemtuzumab is a humanized IgG1 monoclonal antibody against CD52, which is present on cell surface of T and B lymphocytes, macrophages, monocytes, and granulocytes. It is approved for the treatment of B cell chronic lymphocytic leukemia. However, alemtuzumab is used in induction therapy of organ transplantation, which depletes peripheral and central lymphoid cells.

Rituximab is a monoclonal antibody that is directed against CD20 and IgG1 constant region. CD20 mediates B cell proliferation and differentiation, and rituximab inhibits these processes. B cells act as antigen-presenting cells and activate T cells, and rituximab inhibits this T cell activation.

The function of IVIG in transplantation is to deplete alloantibody titers by inhibiting their production and increasing their catabolism.

Bortezomib is a proteasome inhibitor, causing cell cycle arrest and apoptosis. It causes thrombocytopenia and peripheral neuropathy. It is also used in desensitizing patient.

Eculizumab is a humanized monoclonal antibody directed against complement factor C5 and prevents its conversion into C5a and C5b. It is used in paroxysmal nocturnal hemoglobinuria and atypical HUS. Eculizumab is used for prevention of antibody-mediated rejection. Meningococcal infection is a serious complication of eculizumab treatment.

Suggested Reading

Alquadan KF, Worner KL, Casey MJ. Immunosuppressive medications in kidney transplantation. In: Feehally J, Floege J, Tonelli M, et al., editors. Comprehensive clinical nephrology. 6th ed. Philadelphia: Elsevier; 2019. p. 1154–62.

Chang PC-W, Hricik DE. What are immunosuppressive medications? How do they work? What are their side effects? In: McKay DB, Steinberg SM, editors. Kidney transplantation: a guide to the care of kidney transplant recipients. New York: Springer; 2010. p. 119–35.

Sievers TM, Lum EL, Danovitch GM. Immunosuppressive medications and protocols for kidney transplantation. In: Danovitch GM, editor. Handbook of kidney transplantation. 7th ed. Philadelphia: Lippincott Williams & Wilkins; 2017. p. 101–63.

26. **Which one of the following statements regarding belatacept is FALSE?**

A. Belatacept inhibits T cell costimulation
B. Belatacept maintains long-term kidney function compared to cyclosporine in transplant recipients
C. Belatacept increases cardiovascular and metabolic complications compared to cyclosporine treatment
D. Belatacept is contraindicated in EBV-seronegative patients
E. Belatacept is used in combination with basiliximab for induction and in combination with MMF and steroids for maintenance therapy

The answer is C

All of the above statements except C are correct. Indeed, patients treated with belatacept had improved cardiovascular and metabolic profile, as compared with cyclosporine-treated patients. Thus, C is false. Also, belatacept has been shown to improve kidney function at 1 year and also subsequent years in kidney transplant patients, as compared to those treated with cyclosporine. However, belatacept has been shown to cause posttransplant lymphoproliferative disorders, and EBV-seronegative patients are at higher risk for these disorders. Therefore, belatacept is contraindicated in EBV-seronegative patients.

Suggested Reading

Alquadan KF, Worner KL, Casey MJ. Immunosuppressive medications in kidney transplantation. In: Feehally J, Floege J, Tonelli M, et al., editors. Comprehensive clinical nephrology. 6th ed. Philadelphia: Elsevier; 2019. p. 1154–62.

Sayed BA, Kirk AD, Pearson TC, et al. Belatacept. In: Morris PJ, Knechtle SJ, editors. Kidney transplantation-principles and practice. 7th ed. Philadelphia: Elsevier Saunders; 2013. p. 314–19.

27. A 33-year-old African American male receives a deceased donor kidney transplant and had antibody induction therapy. **Which one of the following statements regarding induction therapy is CORRECT?**

A. African American race is a risk factor for acute rejection
B. Rabbit antithymocyte globulin (rATG) is the most commonly used agent in induction therapy
C. OKT3 is off label since 2009 in the United States
D. T-cell-depleting agents are associated with future development of lymphoma compared to nondepleting agents
E. All of the above

The answer is E

It has become a common practice to use a brief course of immunosuppressive agents to prevent acute rejection in both high- and low-risk patients at the time of transplant. This strategy is called induction therapy. According to one source, 83% of kidney transplant recipients received induction therapy in the United States in 2011. There are several risk factors for acute rejection. One of them that is still considered is the African American ethnicity, although a French study found no difference in rejection rates between European Africans and European Caucasians (A is correct).

Among polyclonal antibody preparations, rATG (thymoglobulin) is the most commonly used agent for induction therapy (B is correct). OKT3 is a monoclonal antibody that is directed against CD3 complex. It causes a "cytokine storm" that is potentially dangerous. Because of this profound cytokine release, OKT3 is withdrawn from market in 2009 (C is correct).

Induction agents are classified as T-cell-depleting or nondepleting agents (see question 21). It has been shown that T-cell-depleting agents may predispose patients to the development of lymphomas compared to either nondepleting agents or no induction therapy (D is correct). Table 11.6 summarizes the drugs that are used for induction therapy.

Table 11.6 Drugs for induction therapy

Drug	Action/Effect	Dose	Comment
Methylprednisolone	Inhibition of numerous cytokine production	250–500 mg intravenously. Followed by taper over 1–5 days	Gradual tapering of steroids is important
Thymoglobulin (rATG)	Lymphocyte-depleting agent	1–1.5 mg/kg IV for 4–14 days for a total dose of 6 mg/kg	Generally used in high-risk patients. About 75% of patients received in 2016
Alemtuzumab	Anti-CD52 antibody. Lymphocyte-depleting agent	30–60 mg 1 or 2 doses on days 0 and 4 (a single 30 mg intraoperative dose is commonly used in clinical practice)	Used in a small number of US centers
Basiliximab	Inhibition of IL-2 receptor activity (non-lymphocyte-depleting agent)	20 mg IV on 0 and 4 days	Preferred in low-risk patients

Suggested Reading

Cooper JE, Stites E, Wiseman AC. Prophylaxis and treatment of kidney transplant rejection. In: Feehally J, Floege J, Tonelli M, et al., editors. Comprehensive clinical nephrology. 6th ed. Philadelphia; Elsevier: 2019. p. 1186–97.

Hanaway MJ, Woodle ES, Mulgoankar S, et al. For the INTAC Study Group. Alemtuzumab induction in renal transplantation. N Engl J Med. 2011;364:1909–19.

Hardinger KL, Brennan DC, Schnitzler MA. Rabbit antithymocyte globulin is more beneficial in standard kidney than in extended donor recipients. Transplantation. 2009;87:1372–76.

28. **Which one of the following statements regarding antibody induction therapy and outcomes is CORRECT?**
   A. Compared with rabbit antithymocyte globulin (rATG) recipients, alemtuzumab (AT) recipients had higher risk of death and death or allograft failure
   B. Compared with rATG recipients, basiliximab (BM) recipients had a nonsignificant higher risk of death and death or lymphoma
   C. One-year resource utilization was slightly lower among AT recipients than among rATG recipients
   D. Overall, rATG induction therapy is associated with lower risk of the above-listed complications compared to either AT or BM induction therapy
   E. All of the above

   The answer is E

   Less is known about long-term outcomes of induction therapy on death, allograft survival, and other complications. After linking organ procurement and transplantation network data with Medicare claims, Koyawala et al. compared three induction therapies for 18–90-year-old kidney recipients. Of 21,168 rATG-treated recipients, 5330 matched with 5330 AT-treated and 9378 with 9378 BM-treated recipients. Other medications used were tacrolimus in 75%, prednisone 87% in BM, 66% in rATG, and 29% in AT recipients. The primary outcomes were death or death and allograft failure, and the secondary outcomes were death or sepsis, death or lymphoma, death or melanoma, and healthcare resource utilization within 1 year. Compared with rATG recipients, AT recipients had higher risk of death and death or allograft failure. Except for death or sepsis, the hazard ratios (HRs) for other primary or secondary outcomes were >1.0 (A is correct). Similarly, BM recipients had higher HRs (>1.0) for both primary and secondary outcomes compared to rATG recipients (B is correct). After 1 year, the healthcare cost for AT recipients was lower by $3083 compared to that for rATG recipients with no difference between BM and rATG groups (C is correct). Overall, rATG recipients had longer survival and generally similar or better outcome compared with either AT or BM recipients (D is correct). This analysis should help the clinicians select appropriate induction therapy to avoid long-term complications.

   Suggested Reading

   Koyawala N, Silber JH, Rosenbaum PR, et al. Comparing outcomes between antibody induction therapies in kidney transplantation. J Am Soc Nephrol. 2017;28:2188–200.

29. A 52-year-old woman on hemodialysis is called for kidney transplantation from a 60-year-old deceased donor. She has explained the medical history of hypertension, smoking, alcoholism, and prostatism of the donor. She is curious about transmission of infection and malignancy from the donor. **Which one of the following statements regarding transmission of malignancy from the donor history of smoking and alcoholism and transmission of infection from prostatism is CORRECT?**
   A. Renal cell carcinoma accounts for most of the donor-derived malignancy
   B. Donor transmission rate of renal carcinoma is 0.1%
   C. Donor-derived transmission rate of infection is <1%
   D. Predonor testing for HIV, hepatitis B, and hepatitis C may be negative during "window" period
   E. All of the above

   The answer is E

   A survey from 1994 to 2001 identified a total of 21 donor-related malignancies from 14 cadaveric and 3 living donors were identified. Fifteen tumors were donor-transmitted (malignancies that were present in the donor at time of transplantation) and six were donor-derived (de novo tumors that developed after transplantation). The cadaveric donor-related tumor rate was 0.04%.

   Between 2005 and 2009, a total of 146 cases of donor-derived malignancies were reported in the United States. Of these, 64 cases (43.8%) were renal cell carcinomas, and only 7 of 64 (0.1%) were related to donor transmission cancers (A and B are correct). Also, donor-derived transmission of infection rate was <1% during 2005–2009 years (C is correct).

   Donors are routinely screened for HIV, hepatitis B, and hepatitis C. However, these tests may be negative during the "window period," a period between infection and detection by routine tests. Thus, transmission of these viruses may be missing at time of donation or removal of the kidney from a deceased donor (D is correct).

Suggested Reading

Baudoux TER, Gastaldello K, Rorive S, et al. Donor cancer transmission in kidney transplantation. Kidney Int Rep. 2017;2:134–7.

Chiang RS, Connor AA, Inman BB, et al. Metastatic urothelial carcinoma from transplanted kidney with complete response to an immune checkpoint inhibitor. Case Rep Urol. 2020;2020:8881841.

Desai R, Collett D, Watson CJ, et al. Cancer transmission in solid organ donors-an unavoidable but low risk. Transplantation. 2012;94:1200–07.

Ison MG, Nalesnik MA. An update on donor-derived disease transmission in organ transplantation. Am J Transplant. 2011;11:1123–30.

Xiao D, Craig JC, Chapman JR, et al. Donor cancer transmission in kidney transplantation: a systematic review. Am J Transplant. 2013;13:2645–52.

30. **Which one of the following statements regarding the epidemiology of malignancy in kidney transplant recipients is CORRECT?**

A. Skin cancers are the most common de novo cancers in the adult transplant patients that occurs 20–30 years earlier in immunosuppressive patients as compared with general population
B. Posttransplant lymphoproliferative disorders (PTLDs) are the most common nonskin malignant disorders in kidney recipients
C. In patients with a history of preexisting malignant neoplasms, close monitoring for recurrence is highly recommended
D. Among malignancies, recurrence rates of multiple myeloma are much higher than those of nonmelanoma skin and other cancers
E. All of the above

The answer is E

All of the statements are correct (E). In 2004, Kasiske et al. reported the rates of malignancies in a large number of first-time recipients of either deceased or living donor kidney transplants between 1995 and 2001 using Medicare billing claims. A twofold higher rate for cancers such as colon, lung, prostate, stomach, esophagus, pancreas, ovary and breast, and cancer rates was reported after kidney transplantation as compared with the general population. A fivefold higher rate for melanoma, leukemia, hepatobiliary tumors, cervical and vulvovaginal tumors, a threefold higher rate for testicular and bladder cancers, a 15-fold higher rate for kidney cancers, and >20-fold for Kaposi's sarcoma, non-Hodgkin's lymphomas, and nonmelanoma skin cancers. They concluded that the rates for most malignancies are higher after kidney transplantation as compared to the general population.

Among all cancers, skin cancers are the most common de novo posttransplant cancers in adults and their occurrence increases with time. Among nonskin malignant cancers, PTLDs are the most common type of tumors. Cancers such as Kaposi sarcoma, PTLDs, testicular cancer, cancer of the small intestine, and thyroid occur before 800 days after transplantation

In patients with a history of preexisting malignant neoplasms, close monitoring for recurrences after kidney transplantation is highly recommended. Among malignancies, the recurrence rate for multiple myeloma is 67% followed by 53% for nonmelanoma skin cancers, 29% for bladder cancers, 29% for sarcomas, 27% for symptomatic renal cell carcinomas, and 23% for breast carcinomas. The recurrence of prostate cancer is dependent on the stage of the disease, with highest rate for stage III disease. Thus, cancer screening is mandatory for recurrent disease after kidney transplantation.

Suggested Reading

Au E, Wong G, Chapman JR. Cancer in kidney transplant recipients. Nat Rev Nephrol. 2018;14:508–20.

Kasiske BL, Snyder JJ, Gilbertson DT, et al. Cancer after kidney transplantation in the United States. Am J Transplant. 2004;4:905–13.

Katabathina VS, Menias CO, Tammisetti VS, et al. Malignancy after solid organ transplantation: comprehensive imaging review. RadioGraphics. 2016;36:1390–407.

Penn I. Evaluation of transplant candidates with pre-existing malignancies. Ann Transplant. 1997;2:4–17.

Sampaio MS, Cho YW, Qazi Y, et al. Posttransplant malignancies in solid organ recipients: an analysis of the U.S. National Transplant database. Transplantation. 2012;94:990–8.

Tessari G, Nadi L, Boschiero L, et al. Incidence of primary and second cancers in renal transplant recipients: a multicenter cohort study. Am J Transplant. 2013;13:214–21.

31. De novo development of malignancy is common in recipients of solid organ transplantation. **Which one of the following choices regarding the mechanisms of malignancy after transplantation is CORRECT?**

A. Immunosuppression
B. Antigenic stimulation in the presence of immunosuppression
C. Neoplastic activity of immunosuppressive drugs
D. Increased susceptibility to oncogenic viral infection
E. All of the above

The answer is E

All of the above choices are correct (E). Immunosuppressive drugs may alter the tumor surveillance by affecting both innate and adaptive immunities. This causes potentially malignant cells to be seeded in the host and escape usual killing by the immune system. Also, the foreign HLA antigens in the allograft may stimulate its own lymphoreticular system in the development of lymphomas. In addition, immunosuppressive drugs themselves may deplete T cells and promote the development of posttransplant lymphoproliferative disorders (PTLDs) following induction therapy. Both cyclosporine and tacrolimus have been shown to cause higher rates of malignancy by stimulating transforming growth factor-β. Belatacept, an inhibitor of costimulatory signals, is associated with higher incidence of PTLDs, particularly in EBV-seronegative recipients who received kidneys from EBV-seropositive donors. Similarly, azathioprine, an antimetabolite, may sensitize skin to UV light and promote skin cancer. Finally, immunosuppressive therapy may activate latent oncogenic viruses (EBV, herpes virus, papillomavirus, hepatitis B, and C viruses), which promote the development of malignancy. In addition, preexisting cancers that were undetectable at time of transplantation may be activated by any one of the above mechanisms. Thus, E is correct.

Suggested Reading

Au E, Wong G, Chapman JR. Cancer in kidney transplant recipients. Nat Rev Nephrol. 2018;14:508–20.
Kamal AI, Mannon RB. Malignancies after transplantation and posttransplant lymphoproliferative disorder. In: Weir MR, Lerma EV, editors. Kidney transplantation. Practical guide to management. New York: Springer; 2014. p. 269–80.
Mucha K, Forencewicz B, Ziarkiewich B, et al. Post-transplant lymphoproliferative disorder in view of the new WHO classification: a more rational approach to a protean disease? Nephrol Dial Transplant. 2010;25:2089–98.
Webster AC, Rosales BM, Thompson JF Cancer in dialysis and kidney transplant patients. In: Knechtle SJ, Marson LP, Morris PJ, editors. Kidney transplantation: principles and practice. 8th ed. Philadelphia: Elsevier; 2020. p. 591–607.

32. **Match the following infections with their associated cancers in the transplant recipients.**

Infectious agent	Type of malignancy
A. Epstein Barr virus (EBV)	1. Hodgkin and non-Hodgkin lymphoma
B. Hepatitis B and hepatitis C virus	2. Kaposi sarcoma
C. Human herpes virus-8 (HHV-8)	3. Hepatocellular carcinoma
D. Human papillomavirus (HPV)	4. Cervix, vulva, vagina, penis, anus, oral cavity, pharynx
E. *H. pylori*	5. Gastric cancer

Answers: A = 1; B = 3; C = 2; D = 4; E = 5

The association between infectious agents and cancer in immunocompromised patients has been well documented. In both solid organ transplant and HIV/AIDS patients, this causal relationship has been established. EBV has been conclusively linked to certain forms of Hodgkin and non-Hodgkin lymphomas, and to nasopharyngeal carcinoma. Hepatitis B and C viruses are linked to the development of liver cancer. HHV-8 is recognized as an important cause of Kaposi sarcoma. HPV infection is associated with cancer of cervix, vulva, vagina, penis, anus, oral cavity, and pharynx. *H. pylori* accounts for approximately 60% of all stomach cancers.

Suggested Reading

Au E, Wong G, Chapman JR. Cancer in kidney transplant recipients. Nat Rev Nephrol. 2018;14:508–20.

Grulich AE, van Leeuwen MT, Falster MO. Incidence of cancers in people with HIV/AIDS compared with immunosuppressed transplant recipients: a meta-analysis. Lancet. 2007;370:59–67.

Unal E, Topcu A, Demirpolat M T, et al. Viral infections after kidney transplantation: an updated review. Int J Virol AIDS. 2018;5:40. https://doi.org/10.23937/2469-567X/1510040.

33. A 60-year-old Caucasian man with history of skin cancer received a cadaveric kidney transplant 10 years ago. His creatinine remains at 1.2 mg/dL. He is on tacrolimus and mycophenolate mofetil (MMF) 500 mg twice a day. **In view of his history of skin cancer, which one of the following immunosuppressive agents is found to lower the incidence of skin cancer?**

A. Cyclosporine
B. Prednisone
C. Sirolimus
D. Belatacept
E. Eculizumab

The answer is C

Of all the drugs listed above, only sirolimus has been found to have antineoplastic activity (C is correct). Skin cancers occur in light skin color individuals and are seen after several years; it is better for the patient to start on sirolimus and discontinue tacrolimus. Both cyclosporine and tacrolimus are found to enhance tumor development. Besides light skin color, other risk factors for skin cancer in immunosuppressed patients are sun and UV light exposure, genetic predisposition, history, or current use of azathioprine and duration of follow-up after transplantation.

Suggested Reading

Euvrard S, Morelon E, Rostaing L, et al. Sirolimus and secondary skin-cancer prevention in kidney transplantation. N Engl J Med. 2012;367:329–39.

Pham P-TT, Schaenman J, Pham P-CT. Medical management of the kidney transplant recipient: infections and malignancies. In: Feehally J, Floege J, Tonelli M, et al., editors. Comprehensive clinical nephrology. 6th ed. Philadelphia: Elsevier; 2019. p. 1198–212.

34. The above patient presents to his transplant nephrologist a few years later with a wound-like growth on his shin, which he attributes to trauma that occurred a few months ago. He was referred to a dermatologist, who did a biopsy of the lesion and found it to be skin cancer. **Of the following cutaneous malignancies, which one of the following is the MOST likely found malignancy after kidney transplantation?**

A. Basal cell cancer
B. Squamous cell cancer
C. Melanoma
D. Kaposi sarcoma
E. Lymphoma

The answer is B

Basal cell carcinoma is the most common skin cancer in the general population. However, in immunosuppressed kidney recipient patients, squamous cell cancer is twice as common as basal cell carcinoma. Thus, B is correct. At times, both basal cell and squamous cell carcinoma may occur at the same time. The other mentioned tumors also occur in kidney transplant recipients with lesser frequency.

Suggested Reading

Euvrard S, Morelon E, Rostaing L, et al. Sirolimus and secondary skin-cancer prevention in kidney transplantation. N Engl J Med. 2012;367:329–39.

Pham P-TT, Schaenman J, Pham P-CT. Medical management of the kidney transplant recipient: infections and malignancies. In: Feehally J, Floege J, Tonelli M, et al., editors. Comprehensive clinical nephrology. 6th ed. Philadelphia: Elsevier; 2019. p. 1198–212.

35. **Which one of the following malignancies requires no waiting time prior to kidney transplantation?**

A. Breast cancer
B. Renal cell cancer
C. Colon cancer
D. Basal cell skin cancer
E. Malignant melanoma (in situ)

The answer is D

Appropriate screening for malignancy in transplant donors is common, and each malignancy has a specific waiting time before listing for transplantation. Generally, for many tumors, pretransplant waiting time is 2 years, but certain tumors require 5 years (breast cancer, stage 2 or greater colon cancer, large, high-grade renal cell cancer, malignant melanoma in situ, and noninvasive bladder cancer) of waiting time. Basal cell carcinoma requires no waiting time (D is correct). Also, low-grade cancers such as carcinoma in situ, incidental renal cell carcinoma that is located within the capsule, and very low-grade bladder cancer require no waiting time.

Suggested Reading

Kamal AI, Mannon RB. Malignancies after transplantation and posttranplant lymphopriliferative disorder. In: Weir MR, Lerma EV, editors. Kidney transplantation. Practical guide to management. New York: Springer; 2014. p. 269–80.
Webster AC, Rosales BM, Thompson JF Cancer in dialysis and kidney transplant patients. In: Knechtle SJ, Marson LP, Morris PJ, editors. Kidney transplantation: principles and practice. 8th ed. Philadelphia: Elsevier; 2020. p. 591–607.

36. **Which one of the following statements regarding posttransplant lymphoproliferative disorders (PTLDs) is CORRECT?**

A. The incidence of PTLDs is lowest in kidney transplant recipients compared to intestinal transplant recipients
B. Kidney transplant patients are at 20–50 times higher risk for lymphomas than the general population
C. Most of the PTLDs are of B cell type (large non-Hodgkin lymphomas) with lesser frequency of T and NK cell types
D. A bimodal occurrence of PTLDs is common initially at 1–2 years and later at 4–5 years
E. All of the above

The answer is E

PTLDs are heterogenous group of disorders that carry high morbidity and mortality after solid organs transplantation. The incidence of PTLDs differs according to the transplanted organ with 1–2% in kidney transplant recipients (lowest) compared to 19–30% in intestinal, heart, lung, and multi-organ transplant recipients (highest). Higher incidence of PTLD in heart, lung, intestinal, and multi-organ transplants has been attributed to greater immunosuppression in these patients. Thus, A is correct. The incidence of PTLDs is much higher (20–50 times) in immunosuppressive patients than in the general population (B is correct). More than 85% of PTLDs are derived from B cells, about 14% from T cells, and 1% from NK cells (C is correct). PTLDs occur predominantly in the early posttransplant period (1–2 years) with another peak later at 4–5 years. Thus, the occurrence of PTLDs is bimodal (D is correct).

Because of pathologic diversity, PTLDs are histologically classified (WHO classification) into (1) early lesions, (2) polymorphic PTLD, (3) monomorphic PTLD (B and T cell neoplasms), and (4) classical Hodgkin lymphoma PTLD. Of all PTLDs, 90% are of host origin, and the remaining are donor-derived which are confined to the allograft.

Generally, PTLDs are linked to EBV infection. However, the percent association with above different classes of PTLDs varies. For example, patients with early lesions are 100% positive, polymorphic PTLD patients are >90% positive, monomorphic PTLD patients are either positive or negative, and Hodgkin lymphoma PTLD patients are >90% positive.

Suggested Reading

Dierickx D, Habermann TM. Post-transplantation lymphoproliferative disorders in adults. N Engl J Med. 2018;378:549–62.
Mucha K, Forencewicz B, Ziarkiewich B, et al. Post-transplant lymphoproliferative disorder in view of the new WHO classification: a more rational approach to a protean disease? Nephrol Dial Transplant. 2010;25:2089–98.

Swerdlow SH, Campo E, Harris NL, Jaffe ES, Pileri SA, Stein H, Thiele J, editors. WHO classification of tumours of haematopoietic and lymphoid tissues. 4th ed. Lyon: IARC; 2017.

Swerdlow SH, Campo E, Pileri SA, et al. The 2016 revision of the World Health Organization classification of lymphoid neoplasms. Blood. 2016;127:2375–90.

37. A 50-year-old man with a transplant from deceased donor 2 years ago presents to the clinic with fever, weight loss, and lymphadenopathy. Pertinent chemistry shows abnormal liver function tests and elevated LDH. Serum creatinine is 1.3 mg/dL. EBV PCR titers are high, which were normal 3 months ago. A clinical diagnosis of posttransplant lymphoproliferative disorder (PTLD) is made. He is on tacrolimus and mycophenolate mofetil 750 mg twice daily. **Which one of the following available choices regarding management of PTLD is CORRECT?**

    A. Reduce the dose of immunosuppressive
    B. Rituximab
    C. Cyclophosphamide, doxorubicin, vincristine, prednisolone (CHOP)
    D. Combination of rituximab and CHOP (R-CHOP)
    E. All of the above

    The answer is E

    All of the above choices are correct (E). There is no general agreement on the therapeutic strategies regarding treatment of PTLD. However, the recognition of T lymphocyte depletion by immunosuppressive drugs mandates a reduction in the dosage of these drugs (A is correct). Rituximab therapy alone has been found to be beneficial in patients with PTLD who are on low doses of immunosuppressive drugs (B is correct). CHOP treatment is the most frequently used therapy with a 5-year disease-free survival >60% (C is correct). If the treatment choices A-C have suboptimal response, the combination of R-CHOP is indicated for an aggressive disease (D is correct).

    CNS disease carries high mortality. The treatment is local radiotherapy and methotrexate, as this drug crosses the blood-brain barrier. If EBV titers are high, antiviral treatment is indicated. In certain cases, tumor resection and graft removal are suggested.

    Future therapies include

    1. **Ibrutinib (Bruton's tyrosine inhibitor)**
    2. **Idelalisib (phosphoinositide 3-kinase)**
    3. **Sirolimus (rapamycin) and everolimus (mTOR inhibitors)**
    4. **Bortezomib (proteasome inhibitor)**
    5. **Pembrolizumab, nivolumab (checkpoint inhibitors)**
    6. **Brentuximab vedotin (Anti-CD30 therapy)**
    7. **Radioimmunotherapy**

    Suggested Reading

Dierickx D, Habermann TM. Post-transplantation lymphoproliferative disorders in adults. N Engl J Med. 2018;378:549–62.

Mucha K, Forencewicz B, Ziarkiewich B, et al. Post-transplant lymphoproliferative disorder in view of the new WHO classification: a more rational approach to a protean disease? Nephrol Dial Transplant. 2010;25:2089–98.

Swerdlow SH, Campo E, Harris NL, Jaffe ES, Pileri SA, Stein H, Thiele J, editors. WHO classification of tumours of haematopoietic and lymphoid tissues. 4th ed. Lyon: IARC; 2017.

Swerdlow SH, Campo E, Pileri SA, et al. The 2016 revision of the World Health Organization classification of lymphoid neoplasms. Blood. 2016;127:2375–90.

38. A 50-year-old man on hemodialysis due to hypertension is being evaluated for kidney transplantation. **Which one of the following statements regarding immunization in transplant patients before and after transplantation is FALSE?**

    A. Vaccination should be administered 4–6 months before transplantation
    B. If no contraindications, influenza A vaccine should be given to all transplant candidates
    C. Live virus or live organism vaccine should be given to all transplant recipients
    D. Vaccines with inactivated or killed microorganisms, or recombinant vaccines are safe for kidney recipients
    E. Except for influenza vaccination, all other vaccinations should be avoided in the first 6 months after kidney transplantation

The answer is C

The risk of vaccination in kidney transplant patients is minimal, and there is no evidence that vaccination causes any rejection. Immunization is recommended 4–6 months before kidney transplantation (A is correct). As influenza infection causes increased morbidity and mortality in kidney transplant recipients, influenza vaccination is recommended in all transplant donors and recipients (B is correct). There are sufficient data to indicate that the risk of vaccination with inactivated vaccines is minimal (D is correct). On the other hand, live viral vaccines may cause infections in kidney recipients; therefore, they are contraindicated in these patients (C is false). Immunosuppression is highest in the first few months of transplantation. If there is no acute rejection, the immunosuppressive medication dose is substantially reduced in 6–12 months, and this is the best time for vaccination (E is correct). However, annual influenza vaccination is recommended after 1 month of transplantation for both the recipients and their household. Table 11.7 **shows pertinent vaccination before and after kidney transplantation.**

Table 11.7 Vaccination in transplant candidates

Vaccine	Before	After
Influenza	Yes	Yes
Pneumococcal	Yes	Yes
Meningococcal	Yes	Yes
Hepatitis A	Yes	Yes
Hepatitis B	Yes	Yes
Measles (except during outbreaks), mumps, rubella	No	No
Bacillus Calmette-Quérin	No	No
Smallpox	No	No
Live oral typhoid	No	No
Intranasal influenza	No	No
Oral polio	No	No
Yellow fever	No	No
Live Japanese B encephalitis vaccination	No	No

Suggested Reading

Arora S, Kipp G, Bhanot N, et al. Vaccinations in kidney transplant recipients: clearing the muddy waters. World J Transplant. 2019;9:1–13.

Danziger-Isakov L, Kumar D. AST Infectious diseases community of practice. Vaccination in solid organ transplantation. Am J Transplant. 2019;13 Suppl 4:311–17.

Kasiske BL, Zeier MG, Chapman JR, et al. KDIGO clinical practice guideline for the care of kidney transplant recipients: a summary. Kidney Int. 2010;77:299–311.

Pilmore H, Manley P. Vaccination. KHA-CARI adaptation of KDIGO clinical practice guideline for the care of kidney transplant recipients. Nephrology. 2012:84–9.

39. A 32-year-old type 1 diabetic woman presents to the clinic with fever, cough, sore throat, and chest pain on deep breathing 3 weeks following a living-related kidney transplant. She denies burning on urination, dysuria, or flank pain. Medications include tacrolimus, mycophenolate mofetil, and prednisone 10 mg. She is on oral nystatin. Her serum creatinine is 1.1 mg/dL. **Which one of the following infections occurs MOST commonly during the first month of transplantation?**

    A. Urinary tract infections (UTIs)
    B. Bacterial pneumonia
    C. Oral candidiasis
    D. Cryptococcosis
    E. A, B, and C

The answer is E

Generally, posttransplant infections have been classified based on the length of time from transplantation into 0–1 month, 2–6 months, and >6 months. Table 11.8 **shows this timetable for infectious agents.**

Table 11.8 Timetable showing occurrence of various infections after kidney transplantation

0–1 month	2–6 months	>6 months
Bacterial	*Opportunistic infections*	*Community acquired infections*
Pneumonia	Pneumocystis jirovecii	Bacterial pneumonias
Urinary tract infections (UTIs)	Nocardia	UTIs
Surgical (wound) infections	Aspergillus	Upper respiratory tract viral infections, including influenza
Bacteremia	Candida	Acute gastroenteritis
Viral	Mycobacteria	CMV retinitis
Herpes simplex 1 and 2	Toxoplasma gondii	Late-onset BK virus nephropathy
Fungal	Strongyloidosis	Cryptococcosis
Oral and esophageal candidiasis	*Viral*	
	Herpes (varicella zoster, EBV, CMV)	
	Other (HBV, HBC reactivation, early-onset BK virus)	
	Other infections	
	Listeria	
	Cryptococcosis	
	Other endemic mycoses	

As shown in the above table, UTIs, bacterial pneumonia, surgical wound infections, oral and esophageal candidiasis, and herpes simplex 1 and 2 infections are common in the first month of transplantation. Thus, E is correct. The patient presents with signs and symptoms of pneumonia and most likely related to bacterial infection. Oral or esophageal candidiasis is unlikely because she is on prophylactic oral nystatin, which is not absorbed. Cryptococcosis is a late infection (D is incorrect).

Suggested Reading

Fishman JA, Costa SF, Alexander BD. Infections in kidney transplant recipients. In: Knechtle SJ, Marson LP, Morris PJ, editors. Kidney transplantation: principles and practice. 8th ed. Philadelphia: Elsevier; 2020. p. 517–38.

Fishman JA. Infection in organ transplantation. Am J Transplant. 2017;17:856–79.

Karuthu S, Blumberg EA. Common infections in kidney transplant recipients. Clin J Am Soc Nephrol. 2012;7:2058–70.

40. Infections are common in the first month of kidney transplantation. **Which one of the following infections is MOST likely to occur after transplantation?**

A. Wound infections
B. Herpes simplex 1 and 2
C. Urinary tract infections (UTIs)
D. CMV infections
E. BK viremia

The answer is C

UTIs are the most common bacterial infections that occur after transplantation. The incidence rate of UTIs ranges from 35% to 79% (C is correct). Also, UTI is the most common source of bacteremia followed by the lung and surgical wounds. Prophylactic use of antibiotics (trimethoprim-sulfamethoxazole) prevents not only bacteremia but also pyelonephritis in the allograft.

Aspiration pneumonia is also a common second complication in posttransplant period. Gram-positive organisms are the most likely causative agents of pneumonia, and perioperative antibiotic use prevents this complication.

There is a decline in surgical wound infection because of perioperative antibiotics, intraoperative bladder irrigation, and improvement in surgical techniques. Reactivation of herpes simplex 1 and 2 occurs following immunosuppression, but these infections are not as common as UTIs and pneumonias. Similarly, CMV and BK virus infections occur after 1 month of transplantation.

Suggested Reading

Fishman JA, Costa SF, Alexander BD. Infections in kidney transplant recipients. In: Knechtle SJ, Marson LP, Morris PJ, editors. Kidney transplantation: principles and practice. 8th ed. Philadelphia: Elsevier; 2020. p. 517–38.

Fishman JA. Infection in organ transplantation. Am J Transplant. 2017;17:856–79.

Karuthu S, Blumberg EA. Common infections in kidney transplant recipients. Clin J Am Soc Nephrol. 2012;7:2058–70.

Pilmore H, Manley P. Urinary tract infections. KHA-CARI adaptation of KDIGO clinical practice guideline for the care of kidney transplant recipients. Am J Transplant. 2012;2012:127–9.

41. A 58-year-old man with a deceased donor kidney transplant 1 year ago is admitted to the hospital for an increase in serum creatinine from 1.2 mg/dL to 1.9 mg/dL in 2 weeks. Urinalysis shows only three red blood cells with trace proteinuria. Total proteinuria is 154 mg/24 h. He is on tacrolimus, mycophenolate mofetil, and 5 mg prednisone. Valganciclovir was recently discontinued. He denies fever, pain at the donor kidney site, weight gain, or decrease in urine output. His blood pressure remains stable at 136/80 mm Hg. The patient was adequately hydrated, but his creatinine did not improve. **Which one of the following tests is APPROPRIATE in the evaluation of acute kidney injury (AKI)?**

   A. Urinalysis for decoy cells
   B. BK viruria (virus load in urine)
   C. BK viremia (virus load in serum)
   D. CMV viremia
   E. All of the above

The answer is E

All of the choices are correct (E). It is not unreasonable to order the above-listed tests after excluding the diagnosis of prerenal AKI, acute tubular necrosis (ATN), and calcineurin nephrotoxicity in this patient. Prerenal AKI is unlikely because his creatinine did not improve with adequate hydration. Urinalysis is benign, ruling out the possibility of ATN. Tacrolimus causes nephrotoxicity, which can present as acute tubulopathy, chronic nephrotoxicity, and thrombotic microangiopathy. Kidney biopsy is necessary to evaluate calcineurin nephrotoxicity.

In this patient, CMV nephropathy is a possibility because valganciclovir was discontinued. Therefore, determination of CMV viremia is necessary to rule out CMV nephrotoxicity. BK virus resides in the kidney, and reactivation of this virus can come from the donor or recipient. Following immunosuppressive therapy, 10–60% of recipients have reactivation with shedding of the virus in the urine. The clinical course of reactivation follows viruria, viremia, and nephropathy.

In BK virus reactivation, the urine sediment contains decoy cells, which are epithelial cells with intranuclear BK virus bodies. The decoy cells can be easily seen under phase-contrast microscopy. BK viremia is a better indicator of BK nephropathy than viruria. The gold standard for the diagnosis of BK nephropathy is the biopsy of the allograft.

Suggested Reading

Bohl DL, Brennan DC. BK virus nephropathy and kidney transplantation. Clin J Am Soc Nephrol. 2007;2:S36–46.

Cohen-Bucay A, Ramirez-Andrade SE, Gordon CE, et al. Advances in BK virus complications in organ transplantation and beyond. Kidney Med. 2020;2:771–86.

Hirsch HH, Randhawa P, AST Infectious Diseases Community of Practice. BK polyomavirus in solid organ transplantation. Am J Transplant. 2013;13 Suppl 4:179–88.

Jamboti J. BK virus nephropathy in renal transplant recipients. Nephrology. 2016;21:647–54.

Pilmore H, Manley P. KHA-CARI adaptation of KDIGO clinical practice guideline for the care of kidney transplant recipients. Nephrology. 2012;2012:90–5.

42. **Which one of the following histopathological characteristics is seen in BK polyomavirus nephropathy?**

   A. Early nephropathy with minimal injury to tubular epithelium
   B. Interstitial nephritis with infiltration of mononuclear cells
   C. Enlarged tubular epithelial cells with recognition of viral nuclear inclusions
   D. The presence of simian virus (SV) 40 T antigen by immunohistochemistry
   E. All of the above

The answer is E

BK virus nephropathy occurs mostly in the first 2 years, and only 5% between 2 and 5 years after transplantation. On allograft biopsy, the leading lesion is interstitial nephritis; however, in the early stages of nephropathy the tubules appear normal without any inflammation in the interstitium. In moderate nephropathy, the tubules are enlarged with large nuclei due to the presence of viral inclusions. The BK virus infection is confirmed by the presence of SV 40 T antigen by immunohistochemistry. Positive SV 40 T antigen staining is 100% sensitive for BK virus nephropathy. Thus, E is correct.

In addition, viral DNA has been detected in BK virus nephropathy. Electron microscopy (EM) reveals the presence of intranuclear viral particles of 30–40 nm in diameter in tubular epithelium. Also, urine sediment by negative-staining EM shows cast-like aggregates called "Haufen," which are defined as aggregates of a minimum of six polyomaviruses of 40–45 nm in diameter. It is suggested that detection of "Haufen" in urine may serve as a noninvasive test for BK virus nephropathy.

Suggested Reading

Jamboti J. BK virus nephropathy in renal transplant recipients. Nephrology. 2016;21:647–54.

Nickeleit V, Singh HK, Randhawa P, et al. on behalf of the Banff Working Group on Polyomavirus Nephropathy. The Banff Working Group classification of definitive polyomavirus nephropathy: morphologic definitions and clinical correlations. J Am Soc Nephrol. 2018;29:680–93

Sawinski D, Trofe-Clark J. BK virus nephropathy. Clin J Am Soc Nephrol. 2018;13:1893–96.

Singh HK, Andreoni KA, Papadimitiou JC et al. Presence of urinary Haufen accurately predicts polyomavirus nephropathy. J Am Soc Nephrol. 2009;20:416–27.

43. **Which one of the following definitions of Banff morphologic classifications of polyomavirus nephropathy (PVN) is CORRECT?**

A. Class 1 characterizes pvl (polyomavirus replication/load level) 1 and cortex interstitial fibrosis (ci) score ≤1
B. Class 2 characterizes pvl 1 and ci score ≥2 or pvl 2 and ci score 0–3 or pvl 3 ci score ≤1
C. Class 3 characterizes pvl 3 and ci score ≥2
D. All of the above
E. Only glomerular fibrosis

The answer is D

PVN (BK nephropathy) is a common infection of renal allografts with 5% incidence. The histologic classification of definitive as opposed to presumptive PVN has been attempted by the Banff working group in 2017. Presumptive PVN is defined as high viremia without histologic evidence of kidney disease. On the other hand, definitive PVN has been introduced for patients with biopsy-proven viral nephropathy.

The Banff working group retrospectively evaluated 192 patients with biopsy-proven PVN for potential predictors of allograft function and graft failure over a period of 24 months. After evaluation of several variables for allograft function and failure over 24 months, the combination of pvl and ci formed the basis for the histologic classification of PVN. Accordingly, the PVN was classified into three classes, as shown in answers 1–3 (D is correct). Table 11.9 **defines these three classes of PVN.**

Table 11.9 Classification of PVN

Class 1		Class 2		Class 3	
pvl[1]	ci[2]	pvl	ci	pvl	ci
1	0–1	1	2–3	–	–
–	–	2	0–3	–	–
–	–	3	0–1	3	2–3

[1]Polyomavirus replication/load level
[2]Banff score is divided into zero or 1 versus 2 or 3

It should be noted that baseline serum creatinine levels (median) 4 months before kidney biopsy were 1.4 mg/dL in class 1, 1.5 mg/dL in class 2, and 1.8 mg/dL in class 3 PVN. Class 1 was diagnosed with a median of 18 weeks after allograft placement, and creatinine increased by 0.3 mg/dL from baseline during this period. In contrast, classes 2 and 3 were diagnosed at a median of 30 and 54 weeks after grafting, respectively. During these periods, the median increases in serum creatinine levels in these 2 classes were 0.6 and 0.8 mg/ dL, respectively.

Over a period of 24-month follow-up, serum creatinine levels (median) increased by 0.4 mg/dL in class 1, 1.0 mg/dL in class 2, and 4.8 mg/dL in class 3 PVN patients. Similar increases were observed in graft failure rate during these 24 months following kidney biopsy. Graft failure rates were 16%, 31%, and 50% in class 1, class 2, and class 3, respectively. Thus, Banff histologic classification of PVN is helpful not only in patient care but also following the natural course of allograft transplant.

Suggested Reading

Nickeleit V, Singh HK, Randhawa P, et al. on behalf of the Banff Working Group on Polyomavirus Nephropathy. The Banff Working group classification of definitive polyomavirus nephropathy: morphologic definitions and clinical correlations. J Am Soc Nephrol. 2018;29:680–93.

Roufosse C, Simmonds N, Clahsen-van Groningen M, et al. A 2018 reference guide to the Banff classification of renal allograft pathology. Transplantation. 2018;102:1795–814.

44. **Which one of the following MOST common infectious complications of BK virus in kidney transplant recipient is CORRECT?**

A. Urinary tract infection (UTI)
B. Proteinuria >2 g/day
C. Ureteral stenosis
D. Atypical pneumonia
E. Tuberculosis (TB)

The answer is C

The most common association between BK virus and ureteral stenosis was first described in 1971 (Gardner et al. The Lancet 1:1253–1257) when the virus was isolated in a kidney recipient and named after the initials of the patient (C is correct). The incidence of ureteral stenosis in kidney transplant patients is approximately 3%. UTIs, atypical pneumonia, and TB are common from bacterial and other infections, and are not specifically related to BK virus alone (A, D, E are incorrect). Proteinuria is also a complication of BK virus, but it is usually <1 g/day (B is incorrect).

Suggested Reading

Cohen-Bucay A, Ramirez-Andrade SE, Gordon CE, et al. Advances in BK virus complications in organ transplantation and beyond. Kidney Med. 2020;2:771–86.

Mylonakis E, Goes N, Rubin RH, et al. BK virus in solid organ transplant recipients: an emerging syndrome. Transplantation. 2001;72:1587–92.

Sanoff SL. Infectious disease in kidney transplantation. In: Lerma EV, Rosner M, editors. Clinical decisions in nephrology, hypertension and kidney transplantation. New York: Springer; 2013. p. 427–57.

45. **Which one of the following treatment strategies is MOST effective in polyomavirus nephropathy (PVN)?**

A. Reduction in immunosuppression
B. Leflunomide
C. Ciprofloxacin
D. Cidofovir
E. Intravenous immunoglobulin G (IVIG)

The answer is A

There is currently no specific antiviral therapy to treat BK nephropathy. Early detection of polyoma viremia and viruria and reducing the dose of immunosuppressive drugs remain the most effective treatment strategies for BK virus nephropathy. Thus, A is correct. Dosage reduction should be based individually and implemented when plasma titers are >10,000 copies/mL. A strategy of immunosuppressive reduction is withdrawal of antimetabolites (mycophenolate mofetil, azathioprine) and reduction in calcineurin inhibitors by 50%. The major concern of reduced immunosuppression is the fear of rejection. For this reason, gradual switching to other immunosuppressive agents has been proposed. It has been shown that polyoma viremia and nephropathy were found to be more common with tacrolimus than cyclosporine. Therefore, switching tacrolimus to cyclosporine seems effective in clearing polyoma viremia and improving allograft function. Thus, choice A is the most accepted way of treating PVN.

In addition to reducing immunosuppressive agents, adjunctive therapies are implemented by some centers. These therapies include leflunomide (an immunomodulator), cidofovir, and IVIG. In addition to immunomodulatory effect, leflunomide has antiviral effect. However, convincing efficacy of these adjunctive agents alone has not been demonstrated. A clinical trial in patients with polyoma viremia showed that a 30-day treatment of levofloxacin did not significantly improve allograft function or polyomaviral load reduction. Therefore, fluoroquinolones are not recommended for BK viremia treatment.

Solis et al. have reported that BK virus genotype-specific neutralizing antibody (NAb) titers may be a predictable marker for BK virus replication before and after kidney transplantation. They found that patients with high titers of NAb against the replicating strain had a lower risk of developing polyoma viremia, and the risk decreased with increasing titers of NAb. Thus, the NAb seems protective against developing polyoma viremia and PVN.

Suggested Reading

Cohen-Bucay A, Ramirez-Andrade SE, Gordon CE, et al. Advances in BK virus complications in organ transplantation and beyond. Kidney Med. 2020;2:771–86.

Jamboti J. BK virus nephropathy in renal transplant recipients. Nephrology. 2016;21:647–54.

Pilmore H, Manley P. BKV polyoma virus. KHA-CARI adaptation of KDIGO clinical practice guideline for the care of kidney transplant recipients. Nephrology. 2012;2012:90–5.

Solis M, Velay A, Porcher R, et al. Neutralizing antibody-mediated response and risk of BK virus-associated nephropathy. J Am Soc Nephrol. 2018;29:326–34.

46. Cytomegalovirus (CMV) infection is an important cause of morbidity and mortality in kidney transplant recipients. **Which one of the following statements regarding CMV is CORRECT?**

A. Seronegative recipients when received a kidney from seropositive donor (D+/R−) are at higher risk for severe primary disease during the first 3 months after transplantation
B. CMV disease causes acute and chronic graft dysfunction as well as long-term graft loss
C. Use of mycophenolate mofetil (MMF) >3 g/day increases the risk of CMV viremia
D. Without antiviral prophylaxis, about 60% of recipients develop severe CMV infection within 100 days of transplantation
E. All of the above

The answer is E

All of the above statements are correct (E). CMV infection is the most common opportunistic infection in kidney transplant recipients. One needs to distinguish CMV infection from CMV disease for purpose of treatment. CMV infection refers to its replication irrespective of symptoms, whereas CMV disease is defined by the evidence of infection and the presence of signs and symptoms of viral syndrome (fever, malaise, leukopenia, thrombocytopenia, and tissue diseases such as pneumonia, or chorioretinitis).

Risk factors for CMV include donor seropositivity and recipient seronegativity, exposure to MMF >3 g/day, T-cell-depleting immunosuppressants, simultaneous kidney-pancreas transplantation, and older donors (>60 years of age). CMV disease causes graft dysfunction as well as graft loss. Also, CMV infection within 100 days of transplant is associated with mortality of the recipient, and CMV disease causes cardiovascular mortality beyond 100 days in some recipients.

Because of the association between CMV infection/disease and recipient complications, antiviral prophylaxis has been advocated. Without prophylaxis, 60% of patients do develop severe CMV infection/disease within 100 days of transplantation.

Suggested Reading

Karuthu S, Blumberg EA. Common infections in kidney transplant recipients. Clin J Am Soc Nephrol. 2012;7:2058–70.

Pilmore H, Manley P. Cytomegalovirus. KHA-CARI adaptation of KDIGO clinical practice guideline for the care of kidney transplant recipients. Nephrology. 2012;2012:96–103.

47. **Which one of the following statements regarding prevention of CMV infection and disease is FALSE?**

A. General prophylaxis is found to reduce the incidence of both CMV disease and CMV-associated mortality in high-risk (D+/R−) patients

B. Preemptive therapy in high-risk patients did not have any effect on CMV-associated mortality
C. Preemptive therapy with viral load monitoring with ganciclovir in moderate (D+/R+) and lower (D−/R−) risk patients is effective in CMV infection
D. The Improved Protection Against Cytomegalovirus in Transplant (IMPACT) study showed that daily oral valganciclovir prophylaxis for 200 days provided a significant reduction in the incidence of CMV disease compared with the 100-day prophylaxis in high-risk patients
E. Full doses of ganciclovir or valganciclovir should be administered to have the maximum effect irrespective of kidney function

The answer is E

Studies have shown that the incidence of CMV disease can be reduced by prophylactic antiviral therapy. Two approaches of prophylaxis have been followed to reduce this incidence: universal or general prophylaxis and preemptive therapy. General prophylaxis is defined as the use of antiviral therapy for all kidney recipients regardless of CMV serostatus. Preemptive therapy refers to monitoring viral load and treating viremia prior to development of symptoms.

Studies have shown that general prophylaxis is associated with reduced incidence of CMV disease as well as mortality in high-risk patients (A is correct); however, preemptive therapy did not have any benefit in these high-risk patients (B is correct). Preemptive therapy has been found to be beneficial in moderate to lower risk patients (C is correct).

The IMPACT study evaluated the long-term (up to 2 years) general prophylactic effect of valganciclovir (900 mg once daily) on CMV disease, acute rejection, graft loss, patient survival, and seroconversion in 318 CMV D+/R− kidney transplant recipients. The treatment was either 200 or 100 days. At 2 years, a significant reduction in CMV disease was observed in those treated for 200 days as compared to 100-day therapy. However, there were no significant differences in other outcomes between 200- and 100-day treatment periods (D is correct).

Table 11.10 **shows the recommended approach for CMV prevention.**

Table 11.10 CMV prevention for kidney transplant patients (adapted from Kotton et al.)

Serostatus	Risk level	Recommendation
D−/R−	Low	Monitor clinical symptoms; consider antiviral prophylaxis against other herpes infections
D+/R−	High	6 months of ganciclovir/valganciclovir or preemptive therapy
R+	Intermediate	3 months of valganciclovir or preemptive therapy

Both ganciclovir and valganciclovir are excreted by the kidneys, and dose adjustment is required depending on kidney function to avoid toxicity (leukopenia). Thus, E is false.

Suggested Reading

Humar A, Limaye AP, Blumberg EA, et al. Extended valganciclovir prophylaxis in D+/R− kidney transplant recipients is associated with long-term reduction in cytomegalovirus disease: two-year results of the IMPACT study. Transplantation. 2010;90:1427–30.

Karuthu S, Blumberg EA. Common infections in kidney transplant recipients. Clin J Am Soc Nephrol. 2012;7:2058–70.

Kotton CN, Kumar D, Caliendo AM, et al. on behalf of the Transplantation Society International CMV Consensus Group. The Third International Consensus Guidelines on the management of cytomegalovirus in solid-organ transplantation. Transplantation. 2018;102:900–31.

Pilmore H, Manley P. Cytomegalovirus. KHA-CARI adaptation of KDIGO clinical practice guideline for the care of kidney transplant recipients. Nephrology. 2012;2012:96–103.

48. **Which one of the following immunosuppressive therapies is associated with lower infection rate of cytomegalovirus (CMV) infection?**

A. Mycophenolate mofetil (MMF)
B. mTOR inhibitors
C. Steroids
D. Calcineurin inhibitors
E. Rituximab

The answer is B

Mallat et al. performed a systematic review and meta-analysis on the rate of CMV infection in kidney transplant patients maintained on mTOR inhibitor or calcineurin inhibitor-based therapy. They included 28 randomized, controlled trials with 6211 participants and classified them into comparison 1: mTOR inhibitor versus calcineurin inhibitor and comparison 2: mTOR inhibitor plus reduced dose of calcineurin inhibitor versus regular dose of calcineurin inhibitor. The data showed decreased incidence of CMV infection in mTOR inhibitor-treated group in both comparisons (answer B is correct).

However, mTOR inhibitor-based therapy was associated with more acute rejections in comparison 1 and no difference in comparison 2. There was no difference in graft loss in both comparisons. There were more proteinuria and wound-healing complications in the mTOR inhibitor-based groups. Thus, there is a reduced rate of CMV infection in patients treated with mTOR inhibitors than those treated with calcineurin inhibitors. MMF increases rather than decreases the incidence of CMV infection and disease (A is incorrect). There are no convincing data about other drugs.

Suggested Reading

Mallat SG, Tanios BY, Itan HS, et al. CMV and BKPyV infections in renal transplant recipients receiving an mTOR inhibitor-based regimen versus a CNI-based regimen: a systematic review and meta-analysis of randomized, controlled trials. Clin J Am Soc Nephrol. 2017;12:1321–36.

49. An 18-year-old man on hemodialysis because of vertical transmission of HIV for 3 months. He asks you about kidney transplant from his girlfriend who is HIV negative and willing to donate her kidney. His CD4 count is >200/mm^2 and his viral RNA titers were undetectable. **Which one of the following statements regarding kidney transplantation in HIV/AIDS patients is CORRECT?**

A. He is not a candidate because his viremia deteriorates after immunosuppressive therapy
B. He does not require any strict screening prior to transplantation
C. Both his CD4 count >200/mm^2 and undetectable viral count make him a candidate for kidney transplantation
D. There is no drug interaction between calcineurin inhibitors and protease inhibitors
E. Patient and graft survival are dismal at 3 years

The answer is C

HIV/AIDS is not a contraindication for either kidney or combined kidney and liver transplantation. A number of studies reported good outcomes in HIV patients (A is incorrect). Because of highly active antiretroviral therapy (HAART), the survival of HIV patients has increased. With this increased survival, many patients with ESKD are seeking kidney transplantation. A thorough screening of both the donor and the recipient is required (B is incorrect). The results of the largest prospective study of 150 kidney transplant patients were published in 2010. Entry criteria into this study were CD 4 count >200/mm^2 and undetectable plasma viremia (RNA levels). Our patient has fulfilled the entry criteria. Thus, C is correct. There is a drug interaction between calcineurin inhibitors and protease inhibitors with resultant elevation in trough levels of cyclosporine or tacrolimus. Therefore, close monitoring of trough levels of the calcineurin inhibitors is warranted (D is incorrect). Underdosing of immunosuppressive agents may cause increased rates of rejection. The 2010 study showed that the patient survival rates at 1 and 3 years were 94.6% and 88.2%, respectively. Similarly, the graft survival rates at 1 and 3 years were 90.4% and 73.7%, respectively (E is incorrect). The authors state that these patient and graft survival rates fall somewhere between those for older kidney transplant recipients and those for all kidney transplant recipients. However, a higher rejection rate was observed at 1 (31%) and 3 years (41%). Thus, kidney transplantation is a reality in HIV patients with ESKD.

It is of interest to note that retransplantation (second transplant) in HIV-positive patients experienced a 3.11-fold increased risk of death and a 1.96-fold increased risk of graft loss compared to HIV-negative retransplant recipients.

Suggested Reading

Agarwal DK, Sharma A, Bahl A, et al. Renal transplantation in HIV patients. Apollo Med. 2013;10:50–6.
Pilmore H, Manley P. Human immunodeficiency virus. KHA-CARI adaptation of KDIGO clinical practice guideline for the care of kidney transplantr recipients. Nephrology. 2012:123–6.

Shelton BA, Mehta S, Sawinski D, et al. Increased mortality and graft loss with kidney retransplantation among human immunodeficiency virus (HIV)-infected recipients. Am J Transplant. 2017;17:173–9.

Stock PG, Barin B, Murphy B, et al. Outcomes of kidney transplantation in HIV-infected recipients. N Engl J Med. 2010;363:2004–14.

50. **Which one of the following statements regarding protease inhibitor (PI) therapy in an HIV with kidney transplant recipient is CORRECT?**

A. PIs should be continued to prevent allograft rejection
B. PIs should be continued to prevent allograft recipient death
C. Switching PI to non-PI therapy may reduce the rate of rejection and death
D. Both non-PI and PI-based therapies cause increased rejection and death
E. The combination of PIs with calcineurin inhibitors causes less nephrotoxicity

The answer is C

Although PIs are effective in controlling HIV viremia and disease, their effectiveness in an HIV transplant recipient may not be that effective. The effect of antiretroviral therapy (ART), in particular PI-based and non-PI-based therapy, on allograft rejection and patient death in HIV+ kidney recipients has not been that well studied. With a novel linkage of the Scientific Registry of Transplant Recipients and Intercontinental Marketing Services Pharmacy with pre- and posttransplantation fills, Sawinski et al. were able to assess the association between PI-based regimens and allograft as well as patient survival in 332 HIV+ kidney recipients. Their analysis showed that the PI-based therapy was associated with a 1.8-fold increased risk of allograft loss with the greatest risk observed in the first posttransplantation year and a 1.9-fold increased risk of death as compared to non-PI-based therapy. Thus, the analysis suggests that whenever possible, recipients should be converted to **a non-PI-based therapy prior to kidney transplantation (answer C is correct). Other answers are incorrect.**

Interaction between PIs and calcineurin inhibitors causes nephrotoxicity. Because of this reason, it is possible that restrictive use of calcineurin inhibitors to avoid nephrotoxicity may have contributed to allograft rejection and death. Control of HIV viremia pre- and posttransplantation with non-PI-based therapy seems ideal for HIV+ patients.

Suggested Reading

Sawinski D, Shelton BA, Mehta S, et al. Impact of protease inhibitor-based anti-retroviral therapy on outcomes for HIV+ kidney transplant recipients. Am J Transplant. 2017;17:3114–22.

51. A 40-year-old woman on hemodialysis due to hypertension is found to be positive for hepatitis C (HCV). She has normal liver function tests (LFTs) with normal albumin. She does not drink or use any illicit drugs. She had a blood transfusion several years ago during pregnancy. Physical examination is normal. She wants to know whether or not kidney transplantation with immunosuppression would lead to reactivation of her HCV, resulting in both renal and extrarenal complications. **Which one of the following statements regarding kidney transplantation in HCV seropositive patient is FALSE?**

A. A liver biopsy is indicated despite normal LFTs to assess the extent of occult liver disease
B. Viral genotype should be considered to predict response to treatment
C. Pretransplantation treatment for HCV is required, if the patient has moderate liver fibrosis
D. There is no benefit of kidney transplantation on patient survival compared to maintenance hemodialysis
E. In patients with both liver decompensation and irreversible kidney damage, simultaneous liver and kidney transplantation should be considered

The answer is D

Evaluation of patients with HCV infection or seropositivity is extremely important to determine stage of disease and the need for antiviral therapy. About 7.8% of hemodialysis patients have HCV antibodies, and the titers of viral RNA are variable. Most of the patients have normal LFTs. However, normal LFTs do not rule out occult liver disease. Therefore, a liver biopsy should be considered in the transplant candidate (A is correct). In addition to liver biopsy, viral genotyping is necessary to predict antiviral treatment (B is correct). If the liver biopsy shows moderate fibrosis, antiviral treatment is required prior to transplantation (C is correct). Patients with HCV and kidney transplantation were found to have better patient survival than those patients

on maintenance hemodialysis. Therefore, D is false. Maintenance dialysis patients with decompensated liver disease (abnormal LFTs, ascites, portal hypertension) require both kidney and liver transplantation simultaneously (E is correct).

HCV infection causes the development of new-onset diabetes mellitus, proteinuria, and glomerulopathy in both native and allograft after transplantation. Therefore, HCV patients should be followed with monitoring of viral load for diabetes, renal, and liver disease after transplantation.

Suggested Reading

Karuthu S, Blumberg EA. Common infections in kidney transplant recipients. Clin J Am Soc Nephrol. 2012;7:2058–70.

Kidney Disease: Improving Global Outcomes (KDIGO) Hepatitis C Work Group. KDIGO 2018 clinical practice guideline for the prevention, diagnosis, evaluation, and treatment of hepatitis C in chronic kidney disease. Kidney Int Suppl. 2018;8:91–165.

Pilmore H, Manley P. Hepatitis C virus. KHA-CARI adaptation of KDIGO clinical practice guideline for the care of kidney transplant recipients. Nephrology. 2012;2012:111–5.

Roth D, Bloom RD, Molnar MZ, et al. KDOQI US Commentary on the 2018 KDIGO clinical practice guideline for the prevention, diagnosis, evaluation, and treatment of hepatitis C. Am J Kidney Dis. 2020;75:665–83.

Terrault NA, Adey DB. The kidney transplant recipient with hepatitis C infection: pre- and posttransplantation treatment. Clin J Am Soc Nephrol. 2007;2:563–75.

52. **Which one of the following statements regarding the feasibility of transplantation of donor HCV-positive (HCV+) kidneys to HCV-negative (HCV−) recipients or transplantation of HCV+ kidneys to HCV+ recipients is CORRECT?**

A. A 5-year graft and patient survival rate is much lower when a deceased kidney from HCV+ donor (D+) is transplanted to an HCV− recipient (R−) when compared to that of D−/R−
B. Transplantation of a kidney from D+ into R+ reduces the waiting time for transplantation and also better chances of survival than HCV+ patients on the waiting list
C. Transplantation of a kidney from D+ into R+ patients is associated with a lower risk of death in recipients older than 50 years of age compared to D+/R− patients
D. Direct-acting antiviral treatment of transplant recipients is well tolerated without increasing rates of rejection
E. All of the above

The answer is E

Gupta et al. analyzed the national Organ Procurement and Transplant Network registry from 1994 to 2014 to compare the outcomes of D+/R− to propensity-matched D−/R− kidney transplants. Both 5-year graft survival and patient survival were significantly lower in D+/R− group compared to D−/R− group (A is correct).

It was shown that transplantation of a kidney from D+ into R+ reduces the waiting time for transplantation. One study reported that the waiting time for D+/R+ was 318 ± 458 days compared to 613 ± 819 days for D−/R− patients. D+/R+ patients spent less time on the transplant waitlist, which contributed to improved death-censored graft survival when compared with D−/R− patients (B is correct).

The survival benefit of kidney transplantation from D+ to R+ seems to be related to age of the recipient. It was shown that D+ transplantation into R− was not associated with a survival benefit of the graft; however, when transplantation from D+ into R+ was done in patients >50 years of age, the graft had a lower risk of death. Thus, graft survival was prolonged in the recipient >50 years of age (C is correct).

There are several reports of direct-acting antiviral treatment of patients in the posttransplantation period for HCV infection. The results are positive and encouraging. R+ patients seem to tolerate the treatment with these antivirals well without any increasing rejection rates. Thus, answer D is correct.

Suggested Reading

Gupta G, Kang L, Yu JW, et al. Long-term outcomes and transmission rates in hepatitis C virus positive donor to hepatitis C virus-negative kidney transplant recipients: analysis of United States national data. Clin Transplant. 2017;31.

Kidney Disease: Improving Global Outcomes (KDIGO) Hepatitis C Work Group. KDIGO 2018 clinical practice guideline for the prevention, diagnosis, evaluation, and treatment of hepatitis C in chronic kidney disease. Kidney Int Suppl. 2018;8:91–65.

Myint T, Wright A, Rose C, et al. The benefit of hepatitis C donor kidney transplantation is limited to hepatitis C positive patients over 50 years of age. Am J Transplant. 2015;15:55–72.

Scalea JR, Barth RN, Munivenkatappa R, et al. Shorter waitlist times and improved graft survivals are observed in patients who accept hepatitis C virus+ renal allografts. Transplantation. 2015;99:1192–96.

53. A 45-year-old man on hemodialysis secondary to HIV nephropathy has hepatitis B virus surface antigen (HBsAg) positivity with normal LFTs. He wants to be on kidney transplant list. **Which one of the following statements regarding hepatitis B virus (HBV) infection and kidney transplantation is CORRECT?**

    A. Chronic HBV infection is a contraindication for kidney transplantation
    B. Normal LFTs always indicate normal liver histology in chronic HBV infection
    C. Currently available induction and maintenance immunosuppressive therapies can be used in HBV-infected kidney transplant recipients
    D. Interferon is a better prophylactic agent than tenofovir or entecavir for HBV-infected kidney transplant recipients
    E. Preemptive prophylaxis has been shown to be better than general prophylaxis in reducing HBV e antigenemia (HBeAg)

    The answer is C

    Both kidney donors and recipients are screened for HBV infection. With the introduction of antiviral agents, HBV infection is not any more a contraindication for kidney transplantation (A is incorrect). Patients on hemodialysis or kidney transplant recipients have normal or lower concentration of alanine transferase (ALT) as compared with general population, and therefore, ALT is unreliable as a marker of liver disease (B is incorrect). Therefore, liver biopsy is indicated to assess the extent of fibrosis. Based on stage of liver fibrosis, either kidney transplant or combined kidney-liver transplant can be planned.

    Any of the currently available induction or maintenance immunosuppressive medications can be used in HBV-infected kidney recipients. Thus, C is correct.

    There are at least seven medications for the treatment of HBV infection: interferon-alfa-2b, pegylated alfa-2a, lamivudine, tenofovir, adefovir, telbivudine, and entecavir. Interferon therapy was found to be associated with graft loss, and is not usually recommended. Although no comparative studies between interferon and tenofovir or entecavir are available, the latter drugs are recommended as prophylaxis for kidney recipients (D is incorrect). Also, tenofovir or entecavir is recommended for treatment of lamivudine-resistant HBV infection.

    Preemptive prophylaxis has been found to be inferior to general prophylaxis in patients with HBV infection (E is incorrect). At least 24 months of prophylactic treatment is recommended. During antiviral therapy, HBV DNA and ALT should be measured every 3 months to monitor the efficacy and resistance of drug therapy. Also, patients with cirrhosis should be followed with ultrasound of liver and α-fetoprotein levels every 12 months for the detection of hepatocellular carcinoma.

    Suggested Reading

Manley P, Pilmore H. Hepatitis B virus. KHA-CARI adaptation of KDIGO clinical practice guideline for the care of kidney transplant recipients. Nephrology. 2012;2012:116–22.

Marinaki S, Kolovou K, Sakellariou S, et al. Hepatitis B in renal transplant patients. World J Hepatol. 2017;9:1054–63.

Said A, Safdar N, Lucey MR. Liver disease among renal transplant recipients. In: Knechtle SJ, Marson LP, Morris PJ, editors. Kidney transplantation: principles and practice. 8th ed. Philadelphia: Elsevier; 2020. p. 539–65.

Tsai M-C, Chen Y-T, Chien Y-S, et al. Hepatitis B virus infection and kidney transplantation. World J Gastroenterol. 2010;16:1387–3887.

54. A 52-year-old African American man on hemodialysis for 4 years receives a deceased donor kidney required postoperative hemodialysis because of oliguria, and the diagnosis of delayed graft function (DGF) was made. **Which one of the following contributes to DGF?**

    A. Hemodynamic instability
    B. Postobstructive urological/surgical complications
    C. Acute tubular necrosis (ATN)
    D. Acute rejection
    E. All of the above

    The answer is E

Although several definitions of DGF exist, one of the definitions is the need for dialysis due to acute kidney injury in the first 7 days of posttransplantation. Oliguria may or may not be present. The most recent occurrence rate of DGF in US centers is 31% in deceased donor kidney transplants. There are several risk factors for DGF, which are donor, recipient, transplant-related as well as kidney preservation-related factors (Table 11.11).

Table 11.11 Selected risk factors for DGF (adapted from Nashan et al. and Mannon)

Donor-related	Recipient-related	Transplant-related	Preservation-related
Female gender	Male gender	Sensitization	Increasing cold ischemic time
Old age	African American ethnicity	HLA mismatches	Increasing warm ischemic time
Obesity	Obesity	ABO blood group incompatibility	
High donor serum creatinine	Previous transplant		
Deceased vs. living donation	Diabetes		
Diabetes	Duration of dialysis		
Duration of brain death	Residual diuresis		

The differential diagnosis of DGF includes hypovolemia, urological/surgical complications (lymphocele, ureteral obstruction, urinary leak, catheter obstruction), ATN, and acute rejection. Thus, E is correct. Also, calcineurin inhibitor-induced renal vasoconstriction, thrombosis of the renal artery or vein, thrombotic microangiopathy, and acute interstitial nephritis should also be considered in the differential diagnosis of DGF.

Suggested Reading

Bahl D, Haddadc Z, Datoo A, et al. Delayed graft function in kidney transplantation. Curr Opin Organ Transplant. 2019;24:82–6.

Mannon RB. Delayed graft function: The AKI of kidney transplantation. Nephron. 2018;140:94–8.

Nashan B, Abbud-Filho M, Citterio F. Prediction, prevention, and management of delayed graft function: where are we now? Clin Transplant. 2016;30:1198–208.

Siedlecki DA, Irish W, Brennan DC. Delayed graft function in the kidney transplant. Am J Transplant. 2011;11:2279–96.

55. **Which one of the following therapeutic modalities regarding management of DGF is CORRECT?**

A. Hydration with crystalloids to correct hemodynamic instability
B. Furosemide to improve hypervolemia
C. Induction therapy
D. Allograft biopsy
E. All of the above

The answer is E

Despite several interventional studies in both deceased donors and recipients to prevent ischemic injury, there is not a single definitive study that can either prolong or minimize the course of DGF. Therefore, the management of DGF is mostly supportive. Correction of hemodynamic instability is extremely important, as hypovolemia and hypotension may impair graft function. Crystalloids are preferred to albumin to correct hypovolemia. Many patients may receive fluids perioperatively, causing hypervolemia, which in turn, may precipitate acute kidney injury. Furosemide (100–200 mg) improves urine output in hypervolemic patients. Induction therapy with either antithymocyte globulin or basiliximab or alemtuzumab has been shown to decrease the risk of acute rejection because of the known increased DGF-induced immunogenicity of the allograft. Most centers perform allograft biopsy in 7–10 days to evaluate the histopathological changes of ATN, acute rejection, or other glomerular diseases for appropriate treatment. Thus, E is correct.

In addition, other treatment modalities have been tried in recipients, including dopamine and superoxide dismutase infusions, fenoldopam, anti-ICAM1, and eculizumab without much success. However, two studies have been published with promising results. One is the continuous hypothermic machine perfusion and the other one is inhibition of classical and lectin complement pathway by C1 esterase inhibitor. Both studies showed lower incidence or shorter duration of DGF and maintenance of kidney function at 1 year in the recipient. Further follow-up of C1 esterase inhibitor study for 3.5 years showed lower incidence of graft failure and maintenance of kidney function in the inhibitor-treated compared to the placebo group. Lim and Bloom summarized a few other studies that are underway.

Suggested Reading

Huang E, Vo A, Choi J, et al. Three-year outcomes of a randomized, double-blind, placebo-controlled study assessing safety and efficacy of C1 esterase inhibitor for prevention of delayed graft function in deceased donor kidney transplant recipients. Clin J Am Soc Nephrol. 2020;15:109–16.

Jordan SC, Choi J, Aubert O, et al. A phase I/II, double-blind, placebo-controlled study assessing safety and efficacy of C1 esterase inhibitor for prevention of delayed graft function in deceased donor kidney transplant recipients. Am J Transplant. 2018;18:2955–64.

Lim MA, Bloom RD. Medical therapies to reduce delayed graft function and improve long-term graft survival. Are we making progress? Clin J Am Soc Nephrol. 2020;15:13–15.

Mannon RB. Delayed graft function: The AKI of kidney transplantation. Nephron. 2018;140:94–8.

Schröppel B, Legendre C. Delayed graft function: from mechanism to translation. Kidney Int. 2014;86:251–58.

Siedlecki DA, Irish W, Brennan DC. Delayed graft function in the kidney transplant. Am J Transplant. 2011;11:2279–96.

Tedesco-Silva H, Mello Offerni JC, Ayres Carneiro V, et al. Randomized trial of machine perfusion versus cold storage in recipients of deceased donor kidney transplants with high incidence of delayed graft function. Transplant Direct. 2017;3:e155.

56. **Which one of the following statements regarding outcomes of delayed graft function (DGF) is CORRECT?**

A. DGF shortens the length of stay
B. DGF does not cause any immunogenicity of the allograft due to upregulation of HLAs on the vascular endothelium
C. DGF causes a significant decrease in graft survival
D. DGF has no association with death with graft function (DWGF) in both deceased and living donor kidney transplant recipients
E. No difference in serum creatinine levels between DGF and non-DGF patients

The answer is C

Several studies have shown that DGF is associated with prolonged hospitalization, higher hospital costs, and increased hospital mortality (A is incorrect). Furthermore, DGF causes increased immunogenicity of the allograft due to upregulation of HLAs on the vascular endothelium and release of inflammatory cytokines (B is incorrect). Also, DGF was found associated with death of both deceased and living donor kidney transplant recipients with adequate kidney function (eGFR 30–60 mL/min). The hazard ratio for DWGF was 1.56 (95% CI 1.45–1.63) in patients with DGF compared to those without DGF. Thus, D is incorrect. Studies have shown that serum creatinine was much higher in the DGF group than non-DGF group during a follow-up of 3.5 years (E is incorrect).

A review and meta-analysis of 33 studies showed that DGF was a significant risk factor for graft survival with a relative risk of 1.41 (95% CI 1.27–1.56). Thus, DGF is associated with reduced graft survival (C is correct).

Suggested Reading

Bahl D, Haddadc Z, Datoo A, et al. Delayed graft function in kidney transplantation. Curr Opin Organ Transplant. 2019;24:82–6.

Lee J, Song SH, Lee JY, et al. The recovery status from delayed graft function can predict long-term outcome after deceased donor kidney transplantation. Sci Rep. 2017;7:13725.

Siedlecki DA, Irish W, Brennan DC. Delayed graft function in the kidney transplant. Am J Transplant. 2011;11:2279–96.

Wu W, Famure O, Li Y, et al. Delayed graft function and the risk of acute rejection in the modern era of kidney transplantation. Kidney Int. 2015;88:851–58.

57. **Which one of the following Banff histologic lesions of kidney allograft rejection is FALSE?**

A. Interstitial inflammation (abbreviated as *i* with grading score 0–3)
B. Tubulitis (abbreviated as *t* with grading score 0–3)
C. End arteritis (intimal arteritis; abbreviated as *v* with grading score 0–3)
D. Glomerulitis (abbreviated as *g* with grading score 0–3)
E. Nodular glomerulosclerosis

The answer is E

Initially, the Banff histologic schema was developed by an expert group of renal pathologists, nephrologists, and transplant surgeons who met in Banff, Canada on August 2–4, 1991. The basic concept was to develop a schema for international standardization of nomenclature and criteria for the histologic diagnosis of renal allograft

rejection. Since then, the Banff classification has undergone numerous revisions based on proliferative evidence-based publications. Table 11.12 **shows the most recent standardized Banff lesion scores that renal pathologists need to report for acute/chronic antibody-mediated or acute/chronic T cell-mediated kidney allograft rejection.**

Table 11.12 Banff lesion scores (adapted from Loupy et al.)

Acute Banff scores Grading (0,1, 2, 3)	Chronic Banff scores Grading (0,1, 2, 3)	Acute and chronic Banff scores Grading (0,1, 2, 3)
i	ci	Ti
t	ct	i-IFTA
v	cv	t-IFTA
g	cg	Pvl
ptc	pctml	
C4d		

i inflammation in non-scarred cortex, scored as 0 (absent/minimal, <10% of non-scarred cortex inflamed), 1 (mild, 10–25%), 2 (moderate 26–50%), 3 (severe, >50%). The subcapsular cortex should not be considered
t tubulitis in cortical tubules within non-scarred cortex, scored as 0 (none), 1 (mild, 1–4 mononuclear leukocytes per tubular cross section or 10 tubular epithelial cells in most severely involved tubule), 2 (moderate, 5–10 mononuclear leukocytes), 3 (severe, >10 mononuclear leukocytes)
v endarteritis (intimal arteritis), scored as 0 (none), 1 (mild, 1 or more leukocytes directly beneath the endothelium of 1 or more arteries; endothelial cells typically appear enlarged with associated subendothelial edema; <25% luminal occlusion), 2 (moderate, as grade 1, but with ≥25% luminal occlusion), 3 (severe, with arterial fibrinoid necrosis or transmural inflammation). Note that only arteries (minimum 2 smooth muscle layers) are scored
g glomerulitis, scored as 0 (none), 1 (mild, with ≥1 leukocyte and associated endothelial swelling occluding >50% of 1 of more capillary lumina in at least one but <25% of glomeruli), 2 (moderate, these changes involving 25–75% of glomeruli), 3 (severe, involving >75% of glomeruli). Ischemic, collapsed glomeruli and glomeruli with >50% sclerosis should not be scored
ptc peritubular capillaritis, scored as 0 (minimal, with <3 leukocytes in the most severely involved cortical PTC and/or leukocytes in <10% of cortical PTCs), 1 (mild, with ≥1 leukocyte in ≥10% of cortical PTCs and 3–4 leukocytes in the most severely involved PTC), 2 (moderate, as grade 1 but with 5–10 leukocytes in most severely involved PTC), 3 (severe, as grades 1–2 but with >10 leukocytes in most severely involved cortical PTC). The extent of PTC inflammation should be documented as focal (10–50% of cortical PTCs) or diffuse (>50%). Note that medullary capillaries are NOT scored
C4d linear staining in PTCs or medullary vasa recta by immunofluorescence (IF) on frozen sections of fresh tissue or immunohistochemistry (IHC) on formalin-fixed, paraffin-embedded tissue, scored as 0 (none), 1 (minimal, staining in >0 but <10% of PTCs), 2 (focal, 10–50% of PTCs), 3 (diffuse, >50% of PTCs)

From the above table, only answers A to D are included in the Banff histologic classification of kidney allograft rejection. In addition, peritubular capillaritis and C4d were included in the Banff lesion scores but not nodular glomerulosclerosis (answer E is incorrect).

Suggested Reading

Loupy A, Haas M, Roufosse C, et al. The Banff 2019 kidney meeting report (1): updates on and classification of criteria for T-cell and antibody-mediated rejection. Am J Transplant. 2020;20:2318–31.
Roufosse C, Simmonds N, Clahsen-van Groningen M, et al. A 2018 reference guide to the Banff classification of renal allograft pathology. Transplantation. 2018;102:1795–814.
Solez K, Axelsen RA, Benediktsson H, et al. International standardization of criteria for the histologic diagnosis of renal allograft rejection: the Banff working classification of kidney transplant pathology. Kidney Int. 1993;44:411–22.

58. **Match the following choices (1–9) with the kidney biopsies shown in Fig. 11.2A–I:**

1. Acute T cell-mediated rejection (Banff classification: Grade IB)
2. Acute T cell-mediated rejection (Banff classification: Grade IIA)
3. Acute T cell-mediated rejection (Banff classification: Grade III)
4. Chronic allograft vasculopathy
5. Chronic active antibody-mediated rejection (transplant glomerulopathy, LM and EM)
6. Acute tubular calcineurin inhibitor toxicity (CIN)
7. Chronic vascular/tubulointerstitial CIN toxicity
8. Polyoma/BK virus nephropathy (LM and immunohistochemistry)
9. CMV glomerulitis/glomerulopathy (LM and immunohistochemistry)

Answers: 1 = A; 2 = B; 3 = C; 4 = D; 5 = E; 6 = F; 7 = G; 8 = H; 9 = I (all figures with permission from Springer and Dr. S.V.Seshan)

In Banff grade IB classification of kidney allograft pathology, acute T cell-mediated rejection is characterized by "interstitial inflammation involving >25% of non-sclerotic cortical parenchyma (i2 or i3) with severe tubulitis (t3) involving 1 or more tubules, not including tubules that are severely atrophic." Figure A **shows these changes (1 = A).**

In Banff grade IIA classification, acute T cell-mediated rejection is characterized by "mild to moderate intimal arteritis (v1), with or without interstitial inflammation and/or tubulitis." Figure B **shows these characteristics (2 = B).**

In Banff type III acute T cell-mediated rejection, there is "transmural arteritis and/or arterial fibrinoid necrosis involving medial smooth muscle with accompanying mononuclear cell intimal arteritis (v3), with or without interstitial inflammation and/or tubulitis." Figure C **shows these changes (3 = C).**

Figure D **shows chronic allograft vasculopathy with expansion of intima and deposition of fibrotic tissue in the intima. Duplication of the internal elastica, normal or thickened media, and sparing of arcuate and large arteries characterize hypertensive rather than chronic rejection changes. In chronic rejection, the arterioles are usually spared, as opposed to CIN nephrotoxicity and thrombotic microangiopathy (4 = D).**

Figure E **shows transplant glomerulopathy, which is characterized by duplication of glomerular basement membrane (GBM) in multiple capillaries (arrows on the left). On the right, the EM of a capillary shows duplication of GBM with interposition of cellular components and matrix between the two layers of GBM (arrows) (5 = E).**

Acute tubular CIN causes three pathologic types: acute nephrotoxicity, chronic nephrotoxicity, and thrombotic microangiopathy (TTP/HUS). Acute nephrotoxicity is characterized by isometric vacuolization (defined as cells filled with uniform-sized vacuoles) of the proximal tubule and loss of brush borders. Figure F **shows these characteristics (6 = F).**

Chronic CIN is characterized by interstitial fibrosis, tubular atrophy, and hyaline deposits in the arterioles. However, these changes are nonspecific. Therefore, it has been suggested that newly developed nodular arterial hyalinosis. Findings shown in Fig. G **are suggestive of chronic CIN (7 = G).**

Polyoma/BK virus nephropathy is initially characterized by enlarged tubular epithelial cells, and recognition of viral nuclear bodies (arrow in upper Fig. H**) is the key finding in the diagnosis of this viral infection. During the early changes, the renal medulla is preferentially affected before the infection spreads to the cortex. Interstitial fibrosis and tubular atrophy with mononuclear infiltration are rather common. Polyoma/BK virus nephropathy is confirmed by immunohistochemistry the presence of simian virus (SV) 40 antigen** (Fig. H; **lower figure) in the biopsy specimen. Also, the presence of polyoma/BK viral DNA can be demonstrated in the biopsy specimen (8 = H).**

Although CMV infection is rather uncommon because of universal prophylaxis, it does occur in certain cases with nephritis. The diagnosis is made by demonstrating enlarged tubular epithelial cells with cytopathic changes. In these cells, the large nucleus contains a prominent viral inclusion body (arrow in Fig. I**). In the glomerulus, the endothelial cells are the ones that are affected most frequently with CMV infection (CMV glomerulitis). The interstitium is also affected with mononuclear infiltration, and immunohistochemistry for CMV confirms the presence of viral particles. Thus,** Fig. I **corresponds to CMV nephritis (9 = I).**

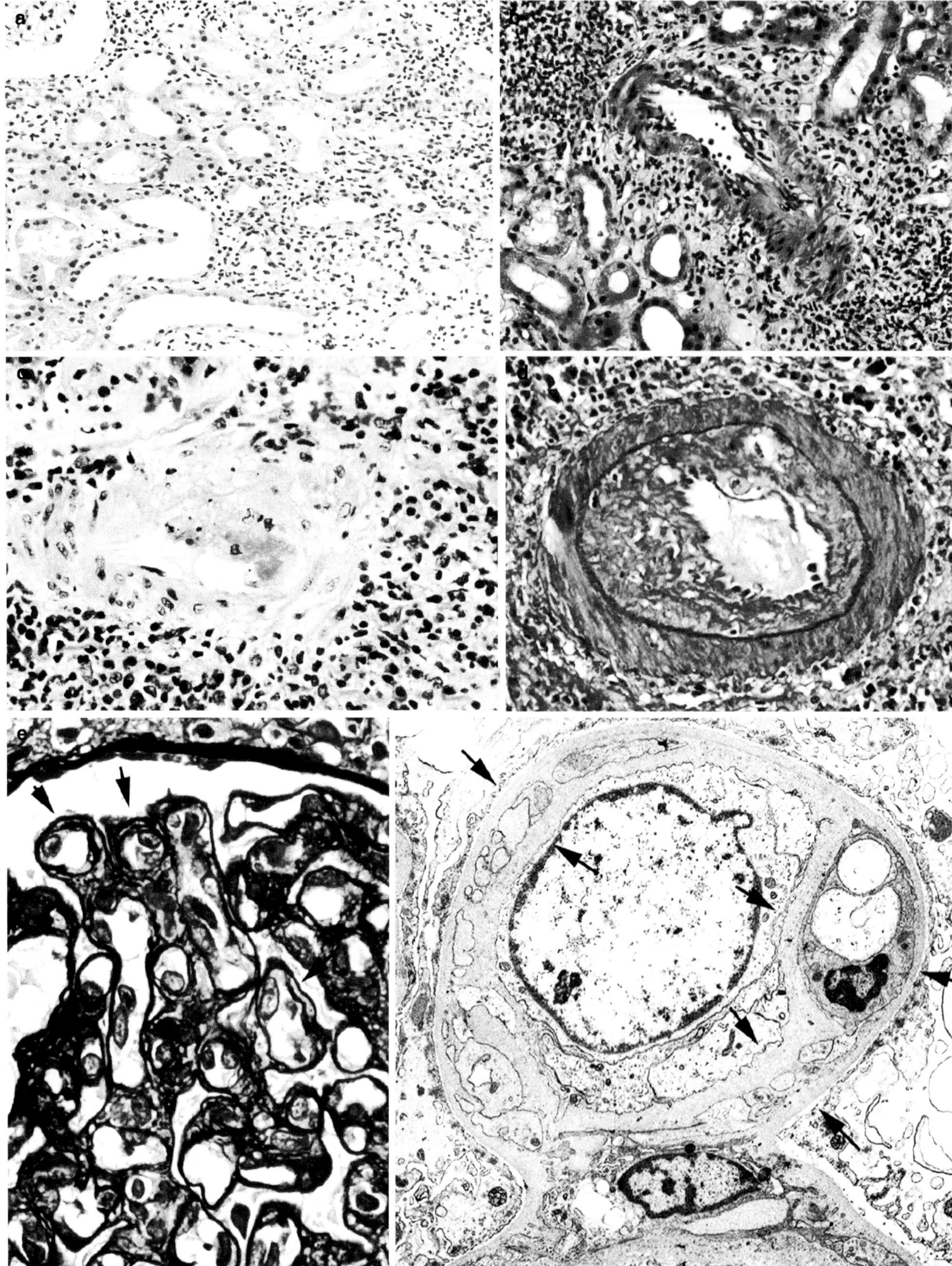

Fig. 11.2 Light, electron, and immunofluorescence pictures of the kidney

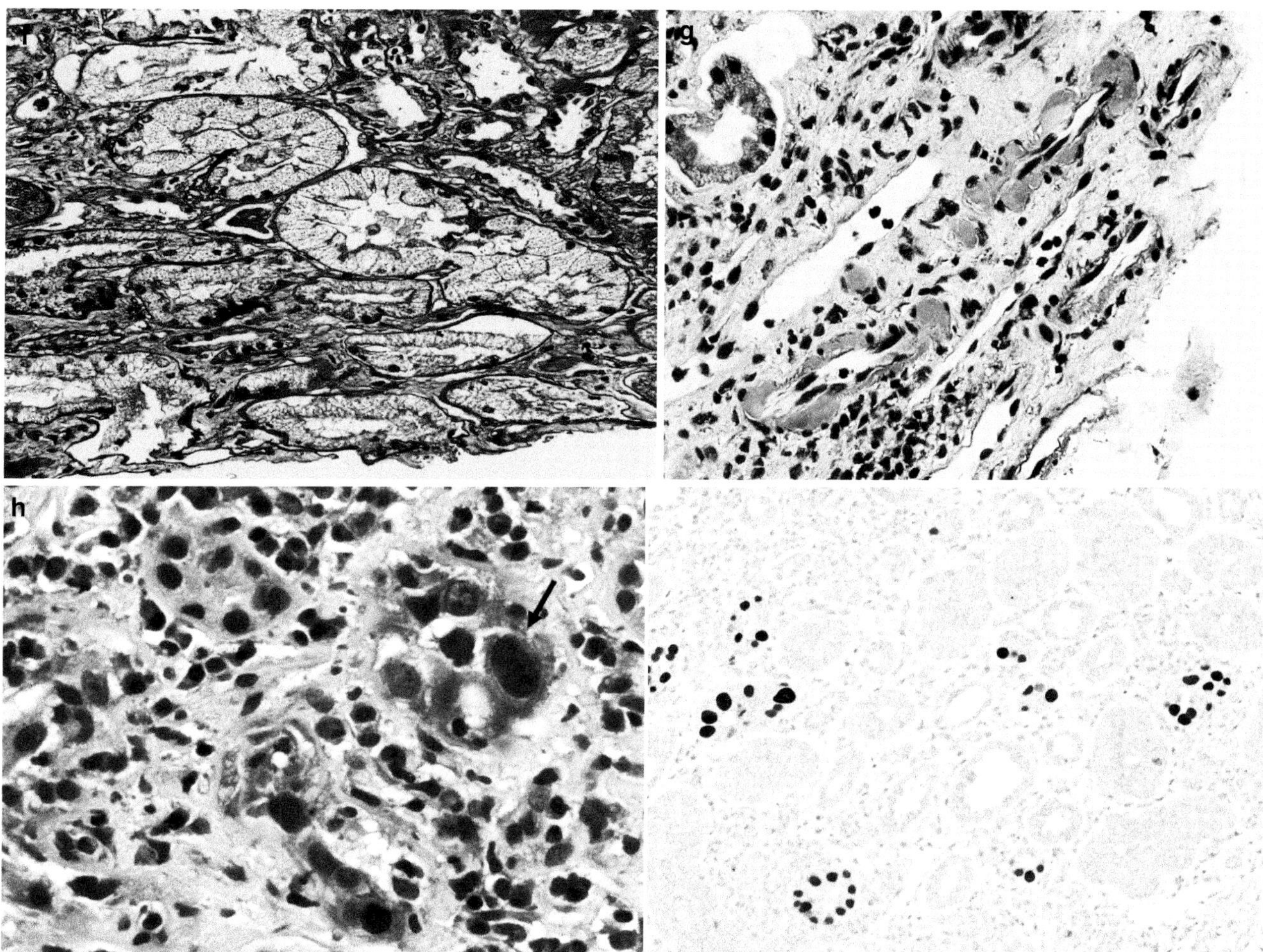

Fig. 11.2 (continued)

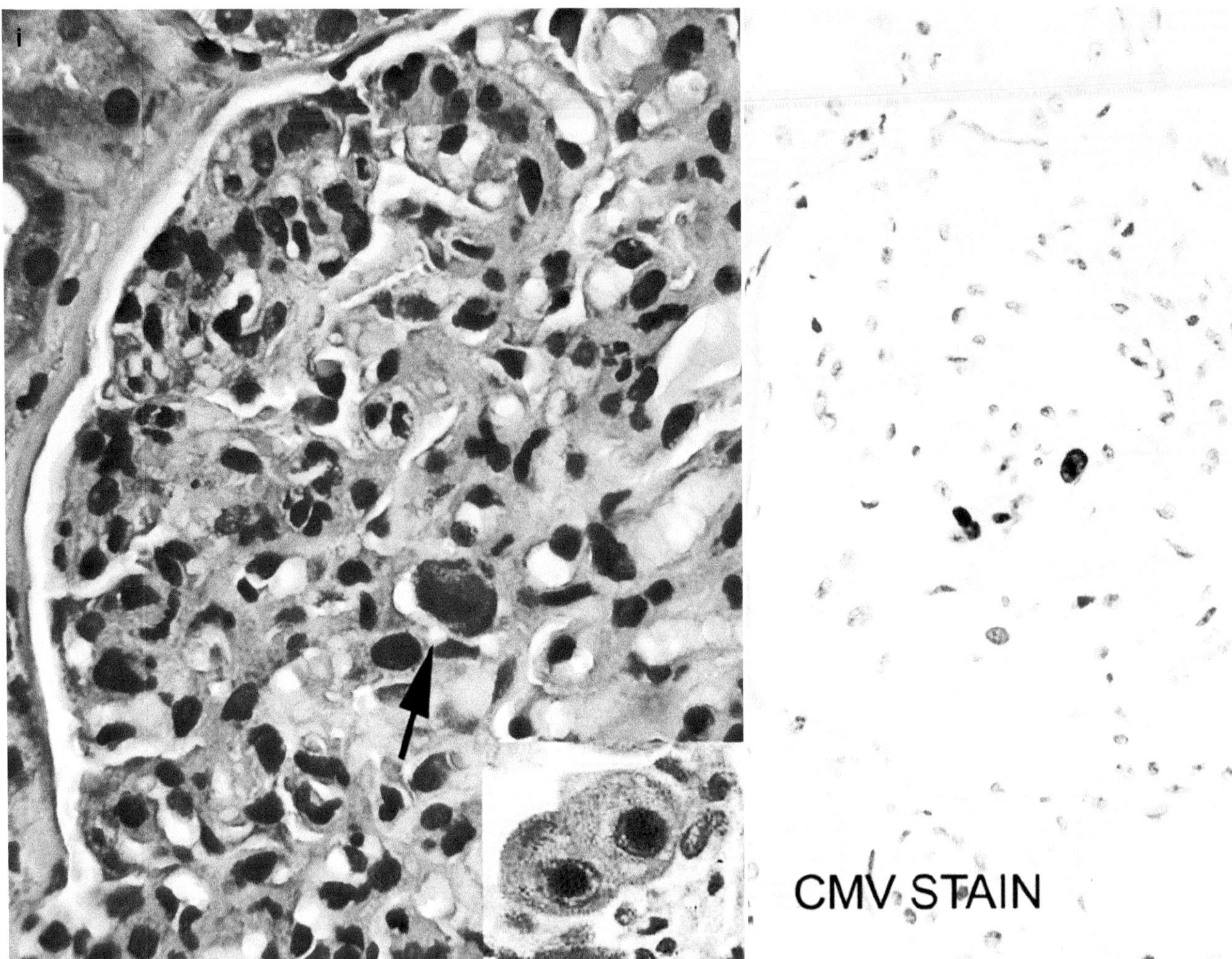

Fig. 11.2 (continued)

Suggested Reading

Drachenberg C, Papadimitriou JC. Practical renal allograft pathology. In Weir MR, Lerma EV (eds). Kidney Transplantation. Practical Guide to Management. New York, Springer, 2014, pp 355–375.

Fogo A. Fundamentals of Renal Pathology. New York, Springer, 2014, pp 1–230.

Loupy A, Haas M, Roufosse C, et al. The Banff 2019 kidney meeting report (I): updates on and classification of criteria for T-cell and antibody-mediated rejection. Am J Transplant. 2020;20:2318–31.

Naesens M, Kuypers DRJ, Sarwal M. Calcineurin inhibitor nephrotoxicity. Clin J Am Soc Nephrol. 2009;4:481–508.

59. A 32-year-old woman with SLE presents to the clinic with weakness and malaise for 2 weeks. She received a deceased donor kidney 5 months ago with 2/6 match. She is on tacrolimus and mycophenolate mofetil, and prednisone 5 mg/day. Tacrolimus levels were undetectable. Her serum creatinine is 1.9 mg/dL, which was 1.1 mg/dL 1 month ago. Urinalysis is benign. Donor-sensitive antibody (DSA) titers are present. Fluid administration did not lower creatinine levels. Biopsy of the allograft shows microvascular infiltrates and intimal arteritis. Linear C4d staining is positive in peritubular capillaries. There is no chronic tissue injury. **Which one of the following is the MOST likely diagnosis in this patient?**

    A. Chronic active antibody-mediated rejection (ABMR)
    B. Active ABMR
    C. Acute T cell rejection (TCR)
    D. Acute tubular necrosis (ATN)
    E. Prerenal AKI

The answer is B

According to the 2019 Banff classification of the histologic evidence for active ABMR includes (simplified partial list):

1. **Mild to moderate microvascular inflammation**
2. **Intimal or transmural arteritis**
3. **Acute thrombotic microangiopathy in the absence of any other cause**
4. **Acute tubular injury in the absence of any other cause**
5. **Linear C4d staining in peritubular capillaries**
6. **Serologic evidence of donor-specific antibodies (DSA to HLA or other antigens)**

Based on kidney biopsy findings (microvascular inflammation, intimal arteritis, C4d staining), the most likely diagnosis in this patient is active ABMR (B is correct). Chronic active ABMR may be considered but biopsy did not show any chronic tissue injury, including new-onset arterial intimal fibrosis or transplant glomerulopathy. Thus, answer A is incorrect. Acute TCR can also be considered but biopsy findings are not that severe to include conclusively this diagnosis (C is incorrect).

ATN should be included in the differential diagnosis, but urinalysis is benign without evidence of kidney tubular cells or renal tubular cast, suggesting that ATN is unlikely (D is incorrect). Prerenal AKI is unlikely, as serum creatinine did not improve after hydration (E is incorrect).

Suggested Reading

Loupy A, Haas M, Roufosse C, et al. The Banff 2019 kidney meeting report (1): updates on and classification of criteria for T-cell and antibody-mediated rejection. Am J Transplant. 2020;20:2318–31.

Schinstock CA, Mannon RB, Budde K, et al. Recommended treatment for antibody-mediated rejection after kidney transplantation: The 2019 Expert Consensus from the Transplantation Society Working Group. Transplantation. 2020;104:911–22.

60. **Which one of the following treatment strategies for antibody-mediated rejection (ABMR) is CORRECT?**

A. Plasmapheresis
B. Intravenous immunoglobulin (IVIG)
C. Rituximab
D. Lymphocyte-depleting antibody
E. All of the above

The answer is E

The rationale for treatment of ABMR is to remove existing antibodies and to inhibit further formation of antibodies. All of the above treatment strategies alone or in combination with or without steroids have been suggested by the KDIGO guideline (E is correct). A review by Roberts et al. identified only five small randomized and eight nonrandomized studies out of 10, 388 citations regarding treatment of acute ABMR. These studies showed benefit from plasmapheresis, rituximab, and bortezomib. Combinations of plasmapheresis and rituximab, or other agents were found to be beneficial in the treatment of ABMR. However, there are no large randomized controlled studies that compared the safety and efficacy of different therapeutic strategies.

Suggested Reading

Cooper JE. Evaluation and treatment of acute rejection in kidney allografts. Clin J Am Soc Nephrol. 2020;15:430–38.

Djamali A, Kaufman DB, Ellis TM, et al. Diagnosis and management of antibody-mediated rejection: current status and novel approaches. Am J Transplant. 2014;14:255–71.

Kasiske BL, Zeier MG, Chapman JR, et al. KDIGI clinical practice guideline for the care of kidney transplant recipients: a summary. Kidney Int. 2010;77:299–311.

Roberts DM, Jiang SH, Chadban SJ. The treatment of acute antibody-mediated rejection in kidney transplant recipients: a systematic review. Transplantation. 2012;94:775–83.

Schinstock CA, Mannon RB, Budde K, et al. Recommended treatment for antibody-mediated rejection after kidney transplantation: the 2019 Expert Consensus from the Transplantation Society Working Group. Transplantation. 2020;104:911–22.

61. A 42-year-old woman received a deceased donor kidney (2/6 match) 3 months ago. Her creatinine 1 week ago was 1.2 mg/dL. She comes to the clinic with a complaint of decreased urine output for 7 days, and creatinine is found to be 2.3 mg/dL. Her creatinine did not improve with hydration, and after excluding other causes of AKI, a kidney biopsy was done. On light microscopy, there was moderate to severe (26–60%) interstitial inflammation involving >25% of non-sclerotic cortical parenchyma with moderate tubulitis (5–10 mononuclear leukocytes) involving 1 or more non-sclerotic tubules. Based on the above histologic findings, acute T cell-mediated rejection (according to Banff 2019 classification-Grade 1A TCMR) was made. **Which one of the following initial treatment strategies is APPROPRIATE for this patient?**

A. Oral prednisone 60 mg per day
B. Methylprednisolone 250–500 mg per day IV for 3 days followed by tapering doses of prednisone
C. Tacrolimus until the trough levels are >20 ng/mL
D. Mycophenolate mofetil 3 g per day
E. Basiliximab

The answer is B

The treatment of choice for acute T cell-mediated rejection is methylprednisolone 250–500 mg per day for 3–5 days (depending on the center) with tapering to a maintenance dose (B is correct). If kidney function does not improve in 5–7 days, steroid dose can be repeated, or T cell-depleting biologic agents such as thymoglobulin or alemtuzumab can be used. The Banff 2019 class grade IA histology, as described above, generally responds to pulse steroids. Other options are incorrect.

Suggested Reading

Cooper JE. Evaluation and treatment of acute rejection in kidney allografts. Clin J Am Soc Nephrol. 2020;15:430–38.
Kanellis J, Mulley W. Treatment of acute rejection. KHA-CARI adaptation of KDIGO clinical practice guideline for the care of kidney transplant recipients. Nephrology. 2012;2012:47–52.
Kidney Disease: Improving Global Outcomes (KDIGO) Transplant Work Group: KDIGO clinical practice guideline for the care of kidney transplant recipients. Am J Transplant. 2009;9 Suppl 3:S1–55.
Loupy A, Haas M, Roufosse C, et al. The Banff 2019 kidney meeting report (1): updates on and classification of criteria for T-cell and antibody-mediated rejection. Am J Transplant. 2020;20:2318–31.
Zhang R. Clinical management of allograft dysfunction. Open J Organ Transplant Surg. 2014;4:7–14.

62. A 61-year-old man with a deceased donor kidney transplant 15 years ago presents to the clinic with slowly progressive decline in kidney function with creatinine of 3.2 mg/dL, malaise, and fatigue. After excluding hemodynamic causes of AKI, a kidney biopsy was done, and the diagnosis of chronic active antibody-mediated rejection (ABMR). **Which one of the following histologic features characterizes the chronic active ABMR?**

A. Positive C4d staining
B. Transplant glomerulopathy
C. New-onset arterial intimal fibrosis
D. Presence of donor-specific antibodies (DSAs)
E. All of the above

The answer is E

The Banff 2019 classification defines chronic active ABMR as follows:

1. Acute tissue injury with one or more of the following:
   (a) Transplant glomerulopathy (cg: chronic glomerulitis >0)
   (b) Severe peritubular capillary basement membrane multilayering
   (c) Arterial intimal fibrosis of new onset
2. Evidence of current/recent antibody interaction with vascular endothelium with one or more of the following:
   (a) Linear peritubular capillary C4d staining
   (b) Moderate microvascular inflammation
   (c) Increased expression of endothelial injury-associated gene transcripts in biopsy tissue

3. Serological evidence of donor-specific antibodies

It is evident that the biopsy findings of the patient include all of the criteria shown in the above classification (answer E is correct). Transplant glomerulopathy is characterized by duplication of the glomerular basement membrane, mesangial expansion with intracapillary presence of mononuclear cells, and lobular appearance of the glomerular tuft, resembling membranoproliferative glomerulonephritis type 1. On EM, the multi-lamination of peritubular capillary basement membrane characterizes the chronic active ABMR.

Arteriolopathy is a cardinal feature of chronic rejection. Arterial intimal fibrosis of new onset characterizes chronic active ABMR. The presence of DSAs should be confirmed in chronic active ABMR.

Suggested Reading

Loupy A, Haas M, Roufosse C, et al. The Banff 2019 kidney meeting report (1): updates on and classification of criteria for T-cell and antibody-mediated rejection. Am J Transplant. 2020;20:2318–31.

Roufosse C, Simmonds N, Clahsen-van Groningen M, et al. A 2018 reference guide to the Banff classification of renal allograft pathology. Transplantation. 2018;102:1795–814.

63. **In the above patient, which one of the following immune and nonimmune treatment modalities is CORRECT?**

A. Control of BP
B. Lifestyle modification
C. Control of glucose and lipids
D. Rituximab alone or rituximab/IVIG
E. All of the above

The answer is E

All of the above choices are correct (E). Chronic ABMR is difficult to treat and reverse chronic pathologic changes in the allograft. However, stabilization of kidney function can be achieved by controlling BP preferably with an ACE-I or ARB, smoking, hyperglycemia, and hyperlipidemia. Since ABMR is mostly a B cell-mediated process, rituximab alone or in combination with IVIG can stabilize kidney function. Several single-center studies have shown beneficial effects of these agents in many patients with chronic active ABMR.

Suggested Reading

Cooper JE. Evaluation and treatment of acute rejection in kidney allografts. Clin J Am Soc Nephrol. 2020;15:430–38.

Djamali A, Kaufman DB, Ellis TM, et al. Diagnosis and management of antibody-mediated rejection: Current status and novel approaches. Am J Transplant. 2014;14:255–71.

Garces JC, Giusti S, Staffeld-Coit C, et al. Antibody-mediated rejection: a review. Ochsner J. 2017;17:46–55.

Sun Q, Yang Y. Late and chronic antibody-mediated rejection: main barrier to long term graft survival. Clin Develop Immunol. 2013;859761:1–7.

64. **Which one of the following conditions is an indication for kidney allograft biopsy?**

A. Persistently unexplained increase in serum creatinine
B. New-onset proteinuria
C. No response in serum creatinine after treatment for acute rejection
D. Failure to achieve expected kidney function in 1–2 months after treatment
E. All of the above

The answer is E

All of the above conditions require allograft biopsies to determine the cause for unexplained elevation in serum creatinine and proteinuria. However, there are no randomized clinical studies that evaluated the indications for allograft biopsies. Kidney biopsies may uncover such disease states as acute or chronic rejection, infection, drug toxicity (calcineurin inhibitor toxicity), malignancies such as posttransplant lymphoproliferative disorders, and recurrent or de novo disease. The clinical utility of these biopsies is to treat the condition appropriately.

Suggested Reading

Han Y, Guo H, Cai M, et al. Renal graft biopsy assists diagnosis and treatment of renal allograft dysfunction after kidney transplantation: a report of 106 cases. Int J Clin Exp Med. 2015;8:4703–07

Kasiske BL, Zeier MG, Chapman JR, et al. KDIGO clinical practice guideline for the care of kidney transplant recipients: a summary. Kidney Int. 2010;77:299–311.

Mulley W, Kanellis J. Kidney allograft biopsy. KHA-CARI adaptation of KDIGO clinical practice guideline for the care of kidney transplant recipients. Nephrology. 2012;2012:62–67.

65. **Which one of the following statements regarding protocol biopsies is CORRECT?**

A. Protocol biopsies are unnecessary risk to the patient, as they do not have any prognostic significance
B. Protocol biopsies can detect subclinical pathology in an otherwise patient with stable kidney function
C. Normal histology on protocol biopsy allows the nephrologist to increase immunosuppression
D. The complication rate of protocol biopsy such as bleeding, hematuria, and graft loss may exceed 10%
E. The cost of protocol biopsies is extremely low

The answer is B

Protocol or surveillance biopsies are elective biopsies performed at predetermined time points after transplantation irrespective of kidney function. They are helpful in detecting subclinical pathologic changes such as acute rejections, calcineurin nephrotoxicity, and posttransplant lymphoproliferative disorders, so that appropriate protocols can be employed (B is correct). Thus, protocol biopsies can improve long-term graft and patient outcomes (A is false).

Normal histology on protocol biopsy with stable kidney function can allow the nephrologist to judiciously reduce immunosuppression (C is false). The safety of protocol biopsies has been well studies. The risk of complications such as bleeding, hematuria, graft loss, ureteral obstruction due to bleeding, and peritonitis is approximately 1% (D is false). One study showed that protocol biopsies cost $114,000 to detect one case of acute rejection (E is false). Therefore, the need for protocol biopsies requires careful evaluation.

Suggested Reading

Fu MS, Lim SJ, Jalalonmuhali M, et al. Clinical significance of renal allograft protocol biopsies: A single tertiary center experience in Malaysia. J Transplant. 2019;20149:9153875.

Mulley W, Kanellis J. Kidney allograft biopsy. KHA-CARI adaptation of KDIGO clinical practice guideline for the care of kidney transplant recipients. Nephrology. 2012;2012:62–7.

Rush D. Protocol biopsies for kidney transplantation. Saudi J Kidney Dis Transplant. 2010;21:1–9.

66. A 30-year-old woman receives a deceased donor kidney transplant. **Which one of the following orders regarding monitoring allograft function is CORRECT?**

A. Measure urine volume every 1–2 h for at least 24 h after transplantation, and then daily until graft function is stable
B. Measure urine protein once in the first month, then every 3 months during the first year, and then annually
C. Measure serum creatinine with eGFR daily for 7 days or until hospital discharge, or 2–3 times per week for 2–4 weeks, weekly for months 2–3, every 2 weeks for months 4–6, monthly for months 7–12, and then every 2–3 months
D. Measure serum lipids month 1 and every few weeks
E. A, B, and C

The answer is E

Graft function is universally practiced to avoid posttransplant complications. The tests mentioned under orders A, B, and C are the minimum recommended tests by the KDIGO and other guidelines. Measurement of lipids, although important, is not warranted that frequently. Thus, D is incorrect.

Suggested Reading

Kasiske BL, Zeier MG, Chapman JR, et al. KDIGO clinical practice guideline for the care of kidney transplant recipients: a summary. Kidney Int. 2010;77:299–311.

Mulley W, Kanellis J. Kidney allograft biopsy. KHA-CARI adaptation of KDIGO clinical practice guideline for the care of kidney transplant recipients. Nephrology. 2012;2012:62–7.

67. A 39-year-old woman receives a deceased donor kidney with no posttransplant complications. Her serum creatinine is stable at 1.0 mg/dL. **Which one of the following maintenance immunosuppressive therapies is APPROPRIATE for this patient?**

A. Cyclosporine, azathioprine, steroids (prednisone or prednisolone)
B. Tacrolimus, mycophenolate mofetil (MMF), sirolimus
C. Basiliximab, MMF, steroids
D. Tacrolimus, MMF, steroids
E. Tacrolimus, MMF, basiliximab

The answer is D

Either cyclosporine or tacrolimus in combination with antiproliferative agents (azathioprine, MMF) and corticosteroids are used to prevent rejection. Cyclosporine is largely replaced by tacrolimus and azathioprine by MMF. The KDIGO and other guidelines suggest continuation of corticosteroids, if they are used beyond the first week after transplantation. Therefore, the common practice in the United States and most Western countries is a combination of tacrolimus, MMF, and prednisone (5 mg daily). MMF can be switched to enteric-coated mycophenolate sodium (MPS). In 2011, about 59% of patients in the United States were discharged from hospital on tacrolimus, MMF/MPS, and prednisone. Thus, D is correct. Patients with low immunological risk and induction therapy may be treated with tacrolimus and MMF after rapid tapering of corticosteroid within the first week. Other combinations are not universally accepted.

Suggested Reading

Kasiske BL, Zeier MG, Chapman JR, et al. KDIGO clinical practice guideline for the care of kidney transplant recipients: a summary. Kidney Int. 2010;77:299–311.
Kidney Disease: Improving Global Outcomes Transplant Work Group. KDIGO clinical practice guideline for the care of kidney transplant recipients. Am J Transplant. 2009;9 Suppl 3:1–155.
Neuwirt H, Rudnicki M, Schratzberger, P et al. Immunosuppression after renal transplantation. Magz Eur Med Oncol (memo). 2019;12:216–21.
Rogers NM, Russ GR, Coates PT. Long-term maintenance immunosuppressive medications. KHA-CARI adaptation of KDIGO clinical practice guideline for the care of kidney transplant recipients. Nephrology. 2012;2012:25–29.

68. **Which one of the following choices about monitoring immunosuppressive medications is FALSE?**

A. Determinations of immunosuppressive drug concentrations by high-performance liquid chromatography (HPLC) provide actual values than those determined by immunoassays
B. Calcineurin inhibitor (CNI) levels should be measured frequently in the immediate posttransplant period until target levels are reached
C. Only 12-h trough or 2-h post-dose cyclosporine levels need to be followed
D. Only trough tacrolimus levels need to be followed
E. Mycophenolate mofetil (MMF) levels should be measured routinely on a fixed dose of the drug

The answer is E

Frequent monitoring of immunosuppressive drugs is required to adjust not only the dose of these drugs but also to prevent their toxicity. HPLC method determines the parent compound, whereas the immunoassays measure the parent compound as well as its metabolites. As a result, the levels obtained by immunoassays are much higher than those determined by the HPLC method (A is correct).

In the immediate posttransplant period, CNI levels should be monitored frequently until therapeutic levels are achieved (B is correct). When cyclosporine is used, either the trough or 2-h post-dose levels should be followed (C is correct). However, only trough levels are recommended for tacrolimus (D is correct).

Routine monitoring of MMF levels is not recommended (E is incorrect). However, the KHA-CARI guidelines recommend monitoring MMF levels in the following conditions:

1. **In high immunological risk patients**
2. **When there is a significant change in clinical parameters, concomitant immunosuppression or medications that may affect drug levels**
3. **When there is concern regarding over- or under-immunosuppression**

4. **Unless a loading dose strategy has been used**

Table 11.13 **shows approximate therapeutic blood levels of CNIs**

Table 11.13 Ideal maintenance levels of CNIs

Drug	0–2 months	2–6 months	>6 months
Cyclosporine (ng/mL)[a]	200–350	100–250	100–200
Tacrolimus (ng/mL)[b]	8–15	5–10	4–8

[a]Chemiluminescence immunoassay (CMIA) or HPLC methods
[b]CMIA

Suggested Reading

Eris J, Wyburn K. Initial maintenance immunosuppressive medication. KHA-CARI adaptation of KDIGO clinical practice guideline for the care of kidney transplant recipients. Nephrology. 2012;2012:17–24.

Rogers NM, Russ GR, Coates PT. Long-term maintenance immunosuppressive medications. KHA-CARI adaptation of KDIGO clinical practice guideline for the care of kidney transplant recipients. Nephrology. 2012;2012:25–9.

69. A 32-year-old type 1 diabetic woman with a deceased donor kidney transplant 1 year ago presents to the clinic with muscle weakness, pain, and fine tremor. Her maintenance immunosuppressive medication includes tacrolimus, MMF, and prednisone (5 mg daily). She refused to take flu shot because of severe reaction last year. Pertinent serum chemistry includes K^+ 6.5 mEq/L, creatinine 1.5 mg/dL (1.1 mg/dL last month), and glucose 102 mg/dL. **Which of the following tests and history are MOST helpful in the management of her kidney function?**

A. Glycated HbA1c
B. Lipid profile
C. Tacrolimus trough levels
D. MMF levels
E. T lymphocytes

The answer is C

Tremor and hyperkalemia are adverse effects of tacrolimus. Therefore, measurement of tacrolimus trough levels is the most appropriate test to guide further management (C is correct). Other laboratory tests are important but not that helpful in her management at the present time.

The tacrolimus levels were 20 ng/mL, and her tremor and hyperkalemia were attributed to tacrolimus toxicity. On further questioning, she took clarithromycin for her flu-like symptoms prescribed by her primary care physician. It should be noted that erythromycin and other macrolides can increase calcineurin inhibitor levels. Her hyperkalemia improved with veltassa (patiromer), and her tremor also improved following withholding of her tacrolimus. Repeated tacrolimus levels were 8 ng/mL, and her original dose of tacrolimus was restarted.

Suggested Reading

Alquadan KF, Worner KL, Casey MJ. Immunosuppressive medications in kidney transplantation. In: Feehally J, Floege J, Tonelli M, et al., editors. Comprehensive clinical nephrology. 6th ed. Philadelphia: Elsevier; 2019. p. 1154–62.

Chang PC-W, Hricik DE. What are immunosuppressive medications? How do they work? What are their side effects? In: McKay DB, Steinberg SM, editors. Kidney transplantation: a guide to the care of kidney transplant recipients. New York: Springer; 2010; p. 119–35.

Sievers TM, Lum EL, Danovitch GM. Immunosuppressive medications and protocols for kidney transplantation. In: Danovitch GM, editor. Handbook of kidney transplantation. 7th ed. Philadelphia: Lippincott Williams & Wilkins; 2017. p. 101–63.

70. A 58-year-old man with a deceased donor kidney transplant 2 years ago is found to have an increase in serum creatinine from 1.1 to 1.5 mg/dL (eGFR >40 mL/min) and proteinuria of 100 mg/g creatinine. A kidney biopsy shows chronic allograft injury. He is on tacrolimus, MMF, and prednisone (5 mg daily). **According to the KDIGO guidelines, which one of the following changes appears MOST acceptable in this patient?**

A. Increase steroid dose
B. Decrease tacrolimus dose

C. Replace tacrolimus with sirolimus
D. Start belatacept
E. Continue the current regimen

The answer is C

The patient seems to have tacrolimus (CNI) nephrotoxicity. Although the CONVERT trial showed no benefit of change from CNI to sirolimus, other studies such as the SPARE the NEPHRON showed that switching MMF/CNI to MMF/sirolimus improved GFR at 12 and 24 months. A benefit in graft function was observed after conversion from CNI-based therapy to mTOR inhibitor-based therapy (CONCEPT trial). It is suggested that patients with CNI nephrotoxicity with eGFR >40 mL/min and proteinuria <500 mg/g creatinine can be switched to sirolimus to prevent further CNI nephrotoxicity. However, this decision should be considered on individual basis with follow-up on kidney function and proteinuria. Thus, C is the most appropriate answer for this patient.

Increasing steroid dose with a decrease in tacrolimus dose is not appropriate. Also, starting belatacept is not appropriate without any evidence of efficacy and safety in patient with chronic allograft injury.

Suggested Reading

Kasiske BL, Zeier MG, Chapman JR, et al. KDIGO clinical practice guideline for the care of kidney transplant recipients: a summary. Kidney Int. 2010;77:299–311.

Schena FP, Pascoe MD, Alberu J et al. Conversion from calcineurin inhibitors to sirolimus maintenance therapy in renal allograft recipients: 24-month efficacy and safety results from the CONVERT trial. Transplantation. 2009;87:233–42.

Wong G, O'Connell P. Treatment of chronic allograft injury. KHA-CARI adaptation of KDIGO clinical practice guideline for the care of kidney transplant recipients. Nephrology. 2012;2012:54–7.

71. Recurrent/de novo glomerular disease is common after kidney transplantation. **Which one of the following statements regarding the prevalence and clinical manifestations of recurrent/de no disease is FALSE?**

A. The Renal Allograft Disease Registry (RADR) reports recurrence/de novo rates of 3.4% after 65 months of follow-up
B. Registry data from Australia and New Zealand report that 8.4% of all allograft loss occurs from recurrent disease 10 years after transplantation
C. Clinical recurrence of disease is manifested by proteinuria, microscopic or macroscopic hematuria, and graft dysfunction
D. Always de novo disease occurs much earlier than recurrent disease
E. The development of calcineurin inhibitors-induced thrombotic microangiopathy (TMA) can occur within the first few months after transplantation

The answer is D

Recurrence is defined as the occurrence of the same native disease in both the native and transplanted kidneys, whereas de novo disease is the occurrence of a new disease other than native kidney disease. The incidence of glomerular disease recurrence in kidney allograft is largely confined to the availability of data from several large registries and single-center reports from the United States, Australia, and New Zealand. The RADR is a consortium of six American transplant centers, which reported the recurrent and de novo glomerular disease at a rate of 3.4% during a mean follow-up of 65 months (A is correct). Briganti et al. reported from the registry data of Australia and New Zealand that 8.4% of all allograft loss occurs from recurrent disease at 10 years after transplantation (B is correct). Expanded evaluation of the above registry data showed that the incidence of disease recurrence after transplantation for the four most common glomerulonephritis (GN) subtypes (IgA nephropathy, membranous GN, focal segmental glomerulosclerosis, and membranoproliferative GN) was approximately 10%. Of those with reported recurrence, 45% lost their allografts within 5 years after the disease recurred (Allen et al.). The common manifestations of recurrent or de novo disease are proteinuria, hematuria, and graft dysfunction (C is correct).

Recurrent kidney disease can occur immediately after posttransplantation (focal segmental glomerulosclerosis) or after a decade of transplantation (IgA nephropathy or diabetic kidney disease). In contrast, de novo disease can take years to occur in the majority of transplant patients except the development of anti-GBM disease in Alport syndrome and calcineurin or mTOR inhibitor-induced TMA which can occur within few months after transplantation. With these exceptions, de novo disease is a late manifestation of transplantation. Thus, D is false.

Suggested Reading

Allen PJ, Chadban SJ, Craig JC, et al. Recurrent glomerulonephritis after kidney transplantation: risk factors and allograft outcomes. Kidney Int. 2017;92:461–9.

Briganti EM, Russ GR, McNeil JJ, et al. Risk of renal allograft loss from recurrent glomerulonephritis. N Engl J Med. 2002;347:103–9.

Cosio FG, Cattran D C. Recent advances in our understanding of recurrent primary glomerulonephritis after kidney transplantation. Kidney Int. 2017;91:304–14.

Hariharan S, Adams MB, Brennan DC, et al. Recurrence and de novo glomerular disease after renal transplantation: a report from Renal Allograft Disease Registry (RADR). Transplantation. 1999;68:635–41.

Lim WH, Shingde M, Wong G. Recurrent and de novo glomerulonephritis after kidney transplantation. Front Immunol. 2019;10:1944. https://doi.org/10.3389/fimmu.2019.01944.

72. **Which one of the following glomerular diseases has the LOWEST recurrence rate in the allograft?**

A. Focal segmental glomerulosclerosis (FSGS)
B. IgA nephropathy
C. Membranoproliferative glomerulonephritis, type 1 (MPGN 1)
D. Membranous nephropathy
E. Fabry's disease

The answer is E

It is well documented from several studies that glomerulonephritis (GN) is one of the leading causes of end-stage kidney disease (ESKD) worldwide, and it is the most common indication for kidney transplantation. It is well known that GN may recur after kidney transplantation, with reported rates from various studies to range from 2.6% to 50%. The recurrence rates for various primary and secondary diseases are shown in Table 11.14. **From this table, it is evident that the least recurrence rate has been reported for Fabry's disease (<5%). Therefore, E is correct.**

Table 11.14 Recurrent rates and risk of graft loss after transplantation

Disease	Recurrence rate (%)	Graft loss after 5–10 years (%)
FSGS	30–50	20–30 (collapsing FSGS >50%)
IgA nephropathy	30–60	10–30
Membranous nephropathy	10–40	30–50
MPGN 1	20–50	10–20
Dense deposit disease	80–100	30–60
Lupus nephritis	2–10	3
Diabetic kidney disease	80 (by histology)	<5%
aHUS	65	65
HSP	25–50	10
ANCA-associated diseases	20–25	5
Anti-GBM disease	5–10	5
Oxalosis	80–100	80
Fibrillary glomerulonephritis	50	30–50
Fabry's disease	<5%	<5%

aHUS atypical hemolytic uremic syndrome, *HSP* Henoch-Schonlein purpura

Of all the above diseases, collapsing FSGS, dense deposit disease, aHUS, and primary oxalosis occur more frequently in the allograft. Although diabetic kidney disease recurs in >80% by histology, the graft loss is usually low. The recurrence rate of Fabry's disease, anti-GBM disease, and congenital nephrosis in the allograft is <5%. Therefore, choice E is correct.

Suggested Reading

Allen PJ, Chadban SJ, Craig JC, et al. Recurrent glomerulonephritis after kidney transplantation: risk factors and allograft outcomes. Kidney Int. 2017;92:461–9.

Cosio FG, Cattran D C. Recent advances in our understanding of recurrent primary glomerulonephritis after kidney transplantation. Kidney Int. 2017;91:304–14.

Ivanyi B. A primer on recurrent and de novo glomerulonephritis in renal allografts. Nat Clin Pract Nephrol. 2008;8:446–57.

Lim WH, Shingde M, Wong G. Recurrent and de novo glomerulonephritis after kidney transplantation. Front Immunol. 2019;10:1944. https://doi.org/10.3389/fimmu.2019.01944.

Morozumi K, Takeda A, Otsuka V, et al. Recurrent glomerular disease after kidney transplantation: An update of selected areas and the impact of protocol biopsy. Nephrology. 2014;19 Suppl 3:6–10.

Ponticelli C, Glassock RJ. Transplant recurrence of primary glomerulonephritis. Clin J Am Soc Nephrol. 2010;5:2263–2372.

Ponticelli C, Moroni G, Glassock RJ. Recurrence of secondary glomerular disease after renal transplantation. Clin J Am Soc Nephrol. 2011;6:1214–21.

73. **Which one of the following diseases does NOT develop de novo in the allograft?**

A. Membranous nephropathy
B. Diabetic kidney disease
C. Primary oxalosis
D. aHUS
E. Anti-GBM disease

The answer is C

Except for primary oxalosis, all other diseases develop de novo in the allograft. Thus, C is correct. It should be noted that all of the above diseases recur in the allograft. De novo membranous nephropathy seems to develop in 0.7–9.3% of allografts. It has been reported that de novo diabetic kidney disease occurred after a mean of 5.9 years after new onset of diabetes. Atypical HUS develops de novo in 0.8–14%, and the risk factors for this disease are younger age, females, and initial use of sirolimus. Anti-GBM disease develops in recipients of Alport syndrome. Plasmapheresis has been shown to be beneficial.

Primary oxalosis develops due to a deficiency of hepatic enzyme, resulting in accumulation of oxalate, kidney stones, and kidney failure. The disease does not develop de novo, but recurs in about 80% of patients with high rate of graft failure.

Suggested Reading

Dube GK, Cohen DJ. Recurrent and de novo disease after renal transplantation. In: Weir MR, Lerma EV, editors. Kidney transplantation. Practical guide to management. New York: Springer; 2014. p. 159–72.

Ivanyi B. A primer on recurrent and de novo glomerulonephritis in renal allografts. Nat Clin Pract Nephrol. 2008;8:446–57.

Lim WH, Shingde M, Wong G. Recurrent and de novo glomerulonephritis after kidney transplantation. Front Immunol. 2019;10:1944. https://doi.org/10.3389/fimmu.2019.01944.

74. **Match the following recurrent and de novo glomerular diseases with their potential therapeutic interventions:**

Disease	Potential intervention (s)
A. FSGS	1. Plasmapheresis, rituximab, galactose, steroids, immunoadsorption with either a protein A or anti-IgG column
B. Membranous nephropathy	2. Rituximab
C. Anti-GBM disease	3. Plasmapheresis, cyclophosphamide, steroids
D. ANCA vasculitis	4. Plasmapheresis, cyclophosphamide, steroids, rituximab
E. IgA nephropathy	5. Steroids, cyclosporine
F. aHUS	6. Eculizumab

Answers: A = 1; B = 2; C = 3; D = 4; E = 5; F = 6

Plasmapheresis, 3 times a week until remission, is usually performed for recurrent idiopathic FSGS. However, some patients may require chronic plasmapheresis to maintain remission. Immunoadsorption with either a protein A or anti-IgG column is beneficial because it removes the circulating permeability factor. Rituximab with plasmapheresis has also been shown to be beneficial. Younger patients and those with normal albumin seem to respond to rituximab treatment. Other treatment options for recurrent FSGS include steroids, cyclosporine, and galactose (A = 1).

Rituximab has been shown to be beneficial in some patients with recurrent membranous nephropathy. Other studies showed the beneficial effects of ACE inhibitors, cyclophosphamide, and high-dose steroids on proteinuria in recurrent disease (B = 2).

For anti-GBM disease, which can develop immediately or after several years after transplantation, plasmapheresis, cyclophosphamide, and steroids have been tried with variable success (C = 3).

Patients with recurrent ANCA vasculitis require the same treatment as nontransplant patients, which includes high-dose steroids, plasmapheresis, and cyclophosphamide. Rituximab alone can be as effective as cyclophosphamide regimen (D = 4).

In one study, the recurrence of IgA nephropathy was 32%. Normal urinalysis was found in 52% of patients with recurrent disease. Cyclosporine was found to stop the recurrence in 79% of patients. In another study, steroid use for 1 year was found to be associated with a reduced recurrence of IgA nephropathy. Also, early withdrawal of steroids was found to elevate the risk for all forms of glomerulonephritis (E = 5).

aHUS is a genetic disease with mutations in complement factors H, I, and membrane cofactor protein. The recurrence rate is 70–90% in patients with factors H and I abnormalities. Eculizumab, an anti-C5 antibody which prevents the formation of the membrane attack complex, has been found to be useful in the treatment of aHUS (F = 6).

Suggested Reading

Clayton P, McDonald S, Chadban S. Steroids and recurrent IgA nephropathy after kidney transplantation. Am J Transplant. 2011;11:1645–49.

Dube GK, Cohen DJ. Recurrent and de novo disease after renal transplantation. In: Weir MR, Lerma EV, editors. Kidney transplantation. Practical guide to management. New York: Springer; 2014. p. 159–72.

Lim WH, Shingde M, Wong G. Recurrent and de novo glomerulonephritis after kidney transplantation. Front Immunol. 2019;10:1944. https://doi.org/10.3389/fimmu.2019.01944.

Ortiz F, Gelpi R, Koskinen P, et al. IgA nephropathy recurs early in the graft when assessed by protocol biopsy. Nephrol Dial Transplant. 2012;27:2553–58.

75. A 36-year-old African American woman on hemodialysis due to FSGS for 4 years and no urine output receives a deceased donor kidney 8 months ago. On a routine visit, she is found to have proteinuria of 1600 mg/day. She is on tacrolimus, MMF, and prednisone. Her creatinine is 1.0 mg/dL. **Which one of the following choices is the cause of her proteinuria?**

A. Acute rejection
B. Tacrolimus (CNI) toxicity
C. Tubulointerstitial fibrosis
D. Recurrent glomerular disease
E. Acute tubulointerstitial disease (aTID)

The answer is D

Shamseddin et al. reported that the incidence of posttransplant proteinuria ranges from 7.5% to 45%. Proteinuria, even 150 mg/day, is a risk factor for graft loss. In general, proteinuria from the native kidney disappears in <4 months. Any proteinuria after this period is assumed to be from the allograft. In this patient, the proteinuria is from her allograft. Several studies have shown that the histologic diagnosis of the kidney is dependent on the degree of proteinuria. Generally, proteinuria >1.5 g/day is associated most frequently with the development of recurrent and transplant glomerulopathy (D is correct). Allograft biopsy showed FSGS and minimal changes of CNI pathology.

In the differential diagnosis, acute and chronic rejection, CNI toxicity, tubulointerstitial fibrosis, as well as recurrent/de novo disease and chronic antibody-mediated transplant glomerulopathy should be considered. Renal biopsy of the allograft in new-onset proteinuria can differentiate one disease from the other.

Suggested Reading

Akbari A, Knoll GA. Post-transplant proteinuria: differential diagnosis and management. In: Weir MR, Lerma EV, editors. Kidney transplantation. Practical guide to management. New York: Springer; 2014. p. 335–40.

Shamseddin MK, Knoll GA. Posttransplantation proteinuria: an approach to diagnosis and proteinuria. Clin J Am Soc Nephrol. 2012;6:1786–93.

Tsampalieros A, Knoll GA. Evaluation and management of proteinuria after kidney transplantation. Transplantation. 2015;99:2049–60.

76. The nephrologist wants to manage her proteinuria by lifestyle modification, and other agents, including switching tacrolimus to another immunosuppressive agent. **Which one of the following agents is contraindicated in this patient?**

   A. Low salt diet
   B. Candesartan
   C. Switch tacrolimus to sirolimus
   D. Low protein diet
   E. Belatacept

   The answer is C

   Lifestyle modification such as low salt diet has been shown to lower proteinuria in transplant and nontransplant CKD patients. Addition of an ACE-I or an ARB is additive in lowering proteinuria. Although low protein diet does improve proteinuria, this approach has to be individualized to avoid malnutrition.

   Treatment of HTN with an ACE-I or an ARB has been advocated by many transplant nephrologists because of their beneficial effects on proteinuria and cardiovascular complications. However, some nephrologists believe that these renin-AII-aldosterone axis inhibitors elevate creatinine and K^+ levels. For this reason, ACE-I or an ARB is not recommended routinely in transplant patients.

   The Study on Evaluation of Candesartan Celexitil after Renal Transplantation (SECRET) showed that candesartan lowered BP and decreased proteinuria, as compared with patients on placebo. Thus, this study showed the safety of an ARB in kidney transplant patients.

   The effect of belatacept on proteinuria in renal transplant patients has not been studied, although the drug is approved for such a study. However, it has been reported that belatacept improves proteinuria in patients with FSGS.

   Sirolimus has been shown to increase proteinuria by decreasing the expression of nephrin on podocytes. Also, sirolimus reduces the glomerular expression of the vascular endothelial growth factor. Thus, option C is correct.

   Suggested Reading

Akbari A, Knoll GA. Post-transplant proteinuria: differential diagnosis and management. In: Weir MR, Lerma EV, editors. Kidney transplantation. Practical guide to management. New York: Springer; 2014. p. 335–40.
Philipp T, Martinez F, Geiger H, et al. Candesartan improves blood pressure control and reduces proteinuria in renal transplant recipients: results from SECRET. Nephrol Dial Transplant. 2010;25:967–76.
Reiser J, Alachkar N. Abate or applaud belatacept in proteinuric kidney disease. Nat Rev Nephrol. 2014;10:128–30.
Shamseddin MK, Knoll GA. Posttransplantation proteinuria: an approach to diagnosis and proteinuria. Clin J Am Soc Nephrol. 2012;6:1786–93.
Tsampalieros A, Knoll GA. Evaluation and management of proteinuria after kidney transplantation. Transplantation. 2015;99:2049–60.
Tsampalieros A, Knoll GA. Evaluation and management of proteinuria after kidney transplantation. Transplantation. 2015;99:2049–60.

77. A 42-year-old woman with liver failure due to hepatitis C and acute kidney injury received a liver transplant 4 years ago. She is maintained on tacrolimus, MMF, and prednisone. On a routine clinic visit, she is found to have a dipstick-positive proteinuria (1+). A 24-h protein excretion was 1.6 g. Her serum creatinine has increased from 1.1 mg/dL to 1.4 mg/dL (eGFR <60 mL/min). **Which one of the following is the possible cause of her declining kidney function and new-onset proteinuria?**

   A. Calcineurin inhibitor toxicity (CNI)-induced thrombotic microangiopathy (TMA)
   B. Acute tubular necrosis (ATN)
   C. Hypertensive nephrosclerosis
   D. Primary glomerular diseases
   E. All of the above

   The answer is E

All of them are correct (E). Schwarz and colleagues performed renal biopsies in patients with nonrenal transplant recipients with declining kidney function and new-onset proteinuria (bone marrow, liver, lung, and heart). In liver transplant patients (*n* = 39 and 41 biopsies), 49% had ATN, 13% had arteriolar hyalinosis, 18% had global glomerular sclerosis, 26% had primary glomerular diseases (IgA nephropathy, minimal change disease, MPGN), 41% had benign nephrosclerosis, and 13% had TMA. Thus, the cause for kidney failure and proteinuria is multifactorial.

Another biopsy study by Kim et al. in liver transplant patients (mostly due to hepatitis C) with reduced kidney function and new-onset proteinuria showed primary glomerular diseases in 42% and only 16% with CNI toxicity. Thus, both studies suggest that reduced kidney function and new-onset proteinuria are most likely related to glomerular diseases rather than CNI toxicity alone.

Suggested Reading

Kim JY, Akalin E, Dikman S, et al. The variable pathology of kidney disease after liver transplantation. Transplantation. 2010;89:215–21.

Schwarz A, Haller H, Schmitt R, et al. Biopsy-diagnosed renal disease in patients after transplantation of other organs and tissues. Am J Tranplant. 2010;10:2017–25.

78. You are asked to see a 52-year-old woman with liver transplant 15 months ago due to hepatitis B for an increase in serum creatinine from 1.1 mg/dL to 1.6 mg/dL. Following adequate hydration, her creatinine remains at 1.6 mg/dL. She is on tacrolimus (trough level 6 ng/mL), MMF, and prednisone 10 mg daily. Her hepatitis B viremia is negligible. **Which one of the following risk factors may account for chronic kidney disease (CKD) in this woman?**

    A. Old age
    B. Calcineurin inhibitor (CNI) nephrotoxicity
    C. High Model for End-Stage Liver Disease (MELD) score prior to liver transplantation
    D. Low pretransplant eGFR
    E. All of the above

The answer is E

All of them are correct (E). A study by Lee et al. analyzed the development of CKD (eGFR <60 mL/min) in 431 Korean liver transplant recipients and found by multivariate analysis that old age recipients (>40 years), CNI toxicity, low pretransplant eGFR, hepatorenal syndrome, severity of posttransplant renal dysfunction, high Child-Pugh and MELD scores, and pretransplant proteinuria. The cumulative incidence of CKD was 32%. About 85% of these patients had hepatitis B-related cirrhosis and hepatocellular carcinoma.

Another study reported a cumulative incidence of CKD in 45% after 5 years of liver transplantation. In this study, pretransplant eGFR was the only independent predictor of CKD. Other studies also reported several other risk factors for CKD in liver transplant patients.

Suggested Reading

Giusto M, Berenguer M, Merkel C, et al. Chronic kidney disease after liver transplantation: pretransplantation risk factors and predictors during follow-up. Transplantation. 2013;15:1148–53.

Kalisvaart M, Schlegel A, Trivedi PJ, et al. Chronic kidney disease after liver transplantation: impact of extended criteria grafts. Liver Transplant. 2019;25:922–33.

Lee JP, Heo NJ, JooKW, et al. The risk factors for consequent kidney impairment and differential impact of liver transplantation on. Nephrol Dial Transplant. 2010;25:2772–85.

79. A 48-year-old man with liver cirrhosis due to alcoholism develops progressive hepatic failure during an 8-month discontinuation of alcohol. His MELD score is 35. **Which one of the following medical eligibility criteria for simultaneous liver and kidney (SLK) transplantation is CORRECT?**

    A. CKD with an eGFR of <60 mL/min for >90 days prior to listing and an eGFR of <35 mL/min at the time of listing
    B. Sustained acute kidney injury (AKI), as defined by a combination of dialysis and an eGFR <25 mL/min for 6 consecutive weeks' duration
    C. Metabolic disease such as hyperoxaluria
    D. All of the above
    E. A and C only

The answer is D

The Organ Procurement and Transplantation Network (OPTN) has revised its policy in 2016 that includes the above mentioned criteria (options from A to C) for SLK. Thus, D is correct. Table 11.15 **provides further details of its recommendations.**

Table 11.15 Medical eligibility criteria for SLK, including "safety net"[a]

Confirmation of diagnosis by transplant nephrologist	Documentation in medical record of the patient by the transplant program
CKD with an eGFR of <60 mL/min for >90 days prior to listing	At least one of the following: Maintenance dialysis Most recent measured or calculated creatinine clearance or GFR ≤35 mL/min at the time of registration on the kidney waiting list
Sustained AKI	At least one of the following: On dialysis for at least for 6 consecutive weeks Measured or calculated creatinine clearance or GFR ≤25 mL/min for at least 6 consecutive weeks, and this needs to be documented in patient's chart every 7 days since the first documentation of the above GFR Document any combination of the above 2 for 6 consecutive weeks
Metabolic disease	An additional diagnosis of at least one of the following: Hyperoxaluria aHUS from mutations in factor H and possibly factor I Familial nonneuropathic systemic amyloid Methylmalonic aciduria

[a]Adapted from https://optn.transplant.hrsa.gov/media/1240/05_slk_allocation.pdf

There is another medical eligibility criterion called "safety net" for liver recipients who continue to be on the kidney waiting list after liver transplant. Simply, this safety net applies to liver transplant alone recipients who do not recover their kidney function and develop dialysis dependency or have an eGFR ≤20 mL/min within 60–365 days of transplant. These liver transplant alone recipients are qualified for increased priority for kidney allocation. The safety net, thus, avoids prolonged maintenance dialysis in liver transplant alone individuals by prioritizing kidney allocation.

Suggested Reading

Formica RN, Aeder M, Boyle G, et al. Simultaneous liver-kidney allocation policy: a proposal to optimize appropriate utilization of scarce resources. Am J Transplant. 2016;16:758–66.

Goyes D, Nsubuga JP, Medina-Morales E, et al. New OPTN simultaneous liver-kidney transplant (SLKT) policy improves racial and ethnic disparities. J Clin Med. 2020;9(12):3901.

Hussain SM, Sureshkumar KK. Refining the role of simultaneous liver kidney transplantation. J Clin Transl Hepatol. 2018;6(3):289–95.

80. A 27-year-old woman develops ESKD due to HTN and is on hemodialysis. She receives a living-related donor kidney and had an unremarkable postoperative course. She is on tacrolimus, MMF, and prednisone. **Which one of the following medico-legal issues needs to be discussed regarding pregnancy with the kidney transplant recipient?**

A. Pregnancy must be delayed for at least 1 year after transplantation with appropriate contraception
B. Although normal birth rate is expected, still the pregnancy is considered high-risk, and she should be informed of the development of preeclampsia, new-onset diabetes, preterm delivery with low birth weight, and miscarriage
C. The adverse effects of immunosuppressive agents on the fetus should be explained during pregnancy and breastfeeding. Referral to genetic counseling should be made, if appropriate
D. The mode of delivery, either vaginal or cesarean section, should be explained
E. All of the above

The answer is E

All of the items listed above are to be discussed with the patient and spouse many weeks prior to conception, and the patient should become pregnant in a planned manner. The American Society of Transplantation (2005) recommends that the recipient could become pregnant in a year provided: (1) the allograft function is stable

(creatinine <1.5 mg/dL and proteinuria <500 mg/day); (2) no acute rejection; and (3) no infection, or no teratogenic drug use such as valganciclovir. Current recommendation for normal kidney function is an eGFR >60 mL/min and proteinuria 300–500 mg/day. In Europe, waiting for 2 years after transplantation is recommended.

The other issues listed above should also be discussed with the patient and the spouse (partner) or family with consent of the patient. The cesarean delivery rate seems to be higher in the transplant recipients compared to the rate in the general population.

The following are the factors that reduce the risk of posttransplant pregnancy complications:

1. **Pregnancy at least after 1 year**
2. **Good kidney function (eGFR >60 mL/min and proteinuria 300–500 mg/day)**
3. **No acute rejection**
4. **Normal allograft ultrasonography**
5. **Maintenance of target BP (<140/90 mm Hg)**
6. **Low-dose immunosuppression with recommended drugs**
7. **Patient compliance with medications and clinic visits**
8. **No recurrent urinary tract infections**
9. **Discontinuation of potentially teratogen drugs for at least 6 weeks**

Suggested Reading

Ahmad M, Pyrsopoulos N. Transplantation and pregnancy. Medscape. 2014.

Cabiddu G, Spotti D, Gernone G, et al. on behalf of the Kidney and Pregnancy Study Group of the Italian Society. A best-practice position statement on pregnancy after kidney transplantation: focusing on the unsolved questions. The Kidney and Pregnancy Study Group of the Italian Society of Nephrology. J Nephrol. 2018;31:665–81.

McKay D, Josephson M. Reproduction and transplantation: report on the AST consensus conference on reproductive issues and transplantation. Am J Transplant. 2005;5:1–8.

Ong SC, Kumar V. Pregnancy in a kidney transplant patient. Clin J Am Soc Nephrol. 2020;15:120–2.

81. The above patient decides to have a baby. **Which one of the following immunosuppressive drugs needs to be discouraged (discontinued) in this patient?**

A. Corticosteroids
B. Tacrolimus
C. Cyclosporine
D. MMF
E. C and D

The answer is D

Almost all of the above drugs can be used during pregnancy except MMF, which is contraindicated because of fetal structural abnormalities. Thus, D is correct. Corticosteroids are used at lower doses, whereas calcineurin inhibitors can be used with close monitoring of their plasma levels.

Sirolimus (mTOR inhibitor) seems to have antifertility effect in men. Therefore, this drug should not be used in men who wish to become fathers.

Table 11.16 **summarizes the main immunosuppressive drugs that are used in transplant patients with FDA rating.**

Table 11.16 Immunosuppressive drugs with FDA rating used in pregnancy

Drug	FDA rating	Comment
Safe to use		
Corticosteroids (prednisone, methylprednisolone, and prednisolone)	C	Risk of premature rupture of membranes has been reported. Other relevant side effects include infectious risk and the increased risk of gestational diabetes
Cyclosporine	C	Small for gestational age babies and preterm delivery have been reported
Tacrolimus	C	Same as cyclosporine
Azathioprine	D	Increased risk of malignancy, predominantly skin cancer and reticulum cell or lymphomatous tumors. Therefore, immunosuppressive drug therapy should be maintained at the lowest effective levels
Drugs to be avoided		
Mycophenolate mofetil (all preparations)	D	Fetal malformations such as cranial as well as cardiovascular malformations were reported. Discontinuation for at least 6 weeks, to stabilize kidney function, is usually indicated after kidney transplantation
mTOR inhibitors	C	KDIGO guidelines suggest discontinuation, but Transplant Pregnancy Registry International (2017 annual report) concludes "To date, sirolimus exposure during pregnancy does not appear to be associated with a pattern of birth defects. Data are limited regarding everolimus exposure during pregnancy"[a]
Rituximab	C, D	Too few studies to allow safe use in pregnancy

FDA rating: Controlled human studies show no risk; B no evidence of risk in studies; C risk cannot be ruled out; D positive evidence of risk; X contraindicated in pregnancy
[a]Transplant Pregnancy Registry International (2017 Annual Report Issued October 16, 2018)

Suggested Reading

Ahmad M, Pyrsopoulos N. Transplantation and pregnancy. Medscape. 2014.
Cabiddu G, Spotti D, Gernone G, et al. on behalf of the Kidney and Pregnancy Study Group of the Italian Society. A best-practice position statement on pregnancy after kidney transplantation: focusing on the unsolved questions. The Kidney and Pregnancy Study Group of the Italian Society of Nephrology. J Nephrol. 2018;31:665–81.
Chittka D, Hutchinson JA. Pregnancy after renal transplantation. Transplantation. 2017;101:675–9.
Ong SC, Kumar V. Pregnancy in a kidney transplant patient. Clin J Am Soc Nephrol. 2020;15:120–2.

82. **Compared to control subjects, kidney transplant recipients are at high risk for which one of the following outcomes during their pregnancy?**

A. Hypertension
B. Preeclampsia
C. Gestational diabetes
D. High rate of cesarean section
E. All of the above

The answer is E

Generally, the majority of pregnancies following kidney transplantation are successful; however, these are considered high risk. Compared to control subjects, kidney recipients have a significantly higher risk of hypertension, preeclampsia, gestational diabetes, cesarean section, preterm delivery, and intrauterine growth restriction (E is correct). Table 11.17 **shows the data of pregnancy outcomes from several sources.**

Table 11.17 Selected pregnancy outcomes in kidney transplant women (adapted from Ong and Kumar)

Outcome (%)	Deshpande et al.	TPR	Shah et al.	US general population*
Hypertension in pregnancy	54.2	48	24.2	N/A
Preeclampsia	27.0	31.0	21.3	3.8
Gestational diabetes	8.0	8.0	5.7	9.2
Cesarean section	56,7	52.0	62.6	31.9
Preterm (<37 week)	45.6	51	43.1	12.5
Acute rejection during pregnancy	4.2	1.0	9.4	N/A
Postpartum rejection	N/A	1.3	N/A	N/A
Graft loss within 2 year (postpregnancy)	8.1	4.6	9.2	N/A
Live births	73.5	75.0	72.9	62.0
Neonatal deaths	N/A	1.4	3,8	0.4
Still births	2.5	2.0	5.1	0.6
Mean birth weight (g)	2420	2571	2470	3389

TPR Transplant Pregnancy Registry International, * data from Deshpande et al. and Shah et al.

Suggested Reading

Deshpande NA, James NT, Kucirka LM, et al. Pregnancy outcomes in kidney transplant recipients: a systematic review and meta-analysis. Am J Transplant. 2011;11:2388–2404.

Moritz MJ, Constantinescu S, Coscia LA, et al. Transplant pregnancy registry international 2017 annual report, gift of life institute, Philadelphia; 2018.

Ong SC, Kumar V. Pregnancy in a kidney transplant patient. Clin J Am Soc Nephrol. 2020;15:120–2.

Shah S, Venkatesan RL, Gupta A, et al. Pregnancy outcomes in women with kidney transplant: meta-analysis and systematic review. BMC Nephrol. 2019;20:24.

83. A 64-year-old nonobese man on hemodialysis due to hypertensive nephrosclerosis for 3 years receives a deceased donor kidney. On a routine clinic visit, he is found to have a fasting glucose level of 130 mg/dL with HbA1c of 7.8%. **Which one of the following risk factors is implicated in the development of posttransplantation diabetes mellitus (PTDM)?**

A. Increasing age
B. Male gender
C. Non-Caucasian race
D. Immunosuppressive medications
E. All of the above

The answer is E

In an international consensus meeting, the members of the committee decided to replace the conventional term "new onset of diabetes after transplantation (NODAT)" with the new term "posttransplantation diabetes mellitus (PTDM)" to represent the development of diabetes after kidney transplantation.

All of the above risk factors are implicated in the development of PTDM (E is correct). The development of PTDM occurs during the first 6 months of immunosuppression. Only fasting glucose or glucose tolerance test is recommended in the first 3 months of transplantation. The HbA1c is not recommended during this 3-month period because new Hb may not have been synthesized and glycated. PTDM develops in about 20% of patients who did not have either fasting hyperglycemia or impaired tolerance to glucose (tested by oral glucose tolerance tests) prior to transplantation.

Several risk factors have been identified, including old age (>60 years), male gender, African American, Hispanic, and other non-Caucasian race, obesity, family history of diabetes, corticosteroids, CNIs (tacrolimus is more diabetogenic than cyclosporine), mTOR inhibitors, polycystic kidney disease, acute rejection, and hepatitis C infection.

Suggested Reading

Dhital SM. Diabetes in kidney transplant recipients. In: Parajuli S, Aziz F, editors. Kidney transplant management. A guide to evaluation and comorbidities. Springer Nature Switzerland AG; 2019. p. 113–31.

Ghisdal L, Van Laecke S, Abramovicz A, et al. New-onset diabetes after renal transplantation. Diabetes Care. 2012;35:181–8.

Sarno G, Muscogiuri G, De Rosa P. New-onset diabetes after kidney transplantation: prevalence, risk factors, and management. Transplantation. 2012;93:1189–95.

Sharif A, Hecking M, de Vries APJ, et al. Proceedings from an international consensus meeting on posttransplantation diabetes mellitus: recommendations and future directions. Am J Transplant. 2014;14:1992–2000.

Yates CJ, Fourlanos S, Hjelmesaeth J, et al. New onset diabetes after kidney transplantation-changes and challenges. Am J Transplant. 2012;12:820–8.

84. **In the above patient, which one of the following immunosuppressive drug combinations poses the highest risk for PTDM?**

   A. MMF and cyclosporine
   B. MMF and sirolimus
   C. Tacrolimus and sirolimus
   D. Azathioprine and belatacept
   E. MMF and belatacept

   The answer is C

   Immunosuppressive drugs that cause hyperglycemia include corticosteroids, CNIs, and mTOR inhibitors. Antiproliferative agents such as MMF, azathioprine, and belatacept were not found to be associated with PTDM.

   Corticosteroids enhance glucose production by the liver and also cause insulin resistance. Between cyclosporine and tacrolimus, the former causes less hyperglycemia than the latter. One large study showed that 26% of cyclosporine-treated patients developed PTDM compared to 33.6% tacrolimus-treated patients. Sirolimus causes direct β-cell toxicity and inhibits insulin-induced suppression of hepatic glucose production and insulin resistance by hypertriglyceridemia caused by the drug itself.

   Although the combination of MMF and cyclosporine may cause PTDM, it is not as severe as that of tacrolimus and sirolimus (A is incorrect). Also, the combination of MMF and sirolimus is not the highest risk for PTDM (B is incorrect). Compared to these both combinations, the combination of tacrolimus and sirolimus causes severe hyperglycemia and poses the highest risk in this patient. Thus, C is correct.

   The other combinations of azathioprine and belatacept and MMF and belatacept are not risk factors for PTDM (D and E are incorrect).

   Suggested Reading

Dhital SM. Diabetes in kidney transplant recipients. In: Parajuli S, Aziz F, editors. Kidney transplant management. A guide to evaluation and comorbidities. Springer Nature Switzerland AG; 2019. p. 113–31.

Ghisdal L, Van Laecke S, Abramovicz A, et al. New-onset diabetes after renal transplantation. Diabetes Care. 2012;35:181–8.

Sarno G, Muscogiuri G, De Rosa P. New-onset diabetes after kidney transplantation: Prevalence, risk factors, and management. Transplantation. 2012;93:1189–95.

Yates CJ, Fourlanos S, Hjelmesaeth J, et al. New onset diabetes after kidney transplantation-changes and challenges. Am J Tranplant. 2012;12:820–8.

85. **The above patient has PTDM. Which one of the following outcomes is expected in this patient?**

   A. Poor survival
   B. Poor graft survival
   C. Increased cardiovascular complications
   D. Increased risk of infections and ophthalmic as well as neurologic complications
   E. All of the above

   The answer is E

   All of the above outcomes have been reported with PTDM (E is correct). Poor survival of the patient as well as the graft has been reported. Also, PTDM increases the risk for cardiovascular mortality by 1.8-fold and overall mortality by 1.5-fold. Also, acute complications of hyperglycemia such as ketoacidosis, hyperglycemic hyperosmolar syndrome, and chronic complications such as retinopathy and neuropathy have been reported. Also, PTDM increases the cost for management of a transplant recipient.

Suggested Reading

Dhital SM. Diabetes in kidney transplant recipients. In: Parajuli S, Aziz F, editors. Kidney transplant management. A guide to evaluation and comorbidities. Springer Nature Switzerland AG; 2019. p. 113–31.

Ghisdal L, Van Laecke S, Abramovicz A, et al. New-onset diabetes after renal transplantation. Diabetes Care. 2012;35:181–8.

Sarno G, Muscogiuri G, De Rosa P. New-onset diabetes after kidney transplantation: prevalence, risk factors, and management. Transplantation. 2012;93:1189–95.

Yates CJ, Fourlanos S, Hjelmesaeth J, et al. New onset diabetes after kidney transplantation-changes and challenges. Am J Transplant. 2012;12:820–8.

86. A 30-year-old woman with type 1 diabetes and creatinine of 4.1 mg/dL (eGFR 18 mL/min) asks you about transplant options. **Which one of the following is considered the BEST option for this patient?**

A. Living-related kidney transplant alone
B. Cadaveric kidney transplant alone
C. Pancreas transplant alone (PTA)
D. Simultaneous pancreas and kidney (SPK) transplant
E. Pancreas after kidney (PAK) transplant

The answer is D

Although all of the above options are available, SPK is the best treatment modality for her because she becomes insulin-independent after transplantation. Also, the patient and graft survival are superior to PAK and PTA. Regression of renal pathologic changes has been observed in SPK patients. Retinopathy either improves or becomes stable after SPK. Thus, D is correct.

It is of interest to note that the number of SPK, PAK, and PTA procedures in type 1 diabetic patients has been decreasing for unexplained reasons despite good outcomes of all the above transplantations. The number of clinical islet transplants has also declined over time.

Despite this decline, a study from the United Kingdom compared the outcomes between LDK and SPK in ESKD patients with type 1 diabetes. There was no significant difference in patient or kidney graft survival between LDK and SPK. However, SPK recipients with a functioning pancreas experienced better kidney graft and patient survival than LDK recipients or those with a failed pancreas graft.

Survival of patients with pancreas transplant alone (PTA) is generally inferior to other pancreas transplantation (SPK, PAK) patients. Also, survival after PTA depends on center variability. For example, pancreas transplant survival is better at high-volume compared with low-volume centers.

Suggested Reading

Al-Qaoud TM, Odorico JS, Redfield RR, III. Pancreas transplantation in type 2 diabetes: expanding the criteria. Curr Opin Organ Transplant. 2018;23:454–60.

Barlow AD, Saeb-Parsy K, Watson CJE. An analysis of the survival outcomes of simultaneous pancreas and kidney transplantation compared to live donor kidney transplantation in patients with type 1 diabetes: a UK Transplant Registry study. Transplant Int. 2017;30:884–92.

Serrano OK, Vock DM, Dunn TB, et al. Maximizing utilization in pancreas transplantation: phenotypic characteristics differentiating aggressive from nonaggressive transplant centers. Transplantation. 2018;102:2108–19.

Wiseman AC, Stites E, Kennealey P. Defining kidney allograft benefit from successful pancreas transplant: separating fact from fiction. Curr Opin Organ Transplant. 2018;23:448–53.

87. Sepsis is the most common adverse event within the first year after among simultaneous pancreas and kidney (SPK) transplant recipients. **Which one of the following is a risk factor for sepsis?**

A. Female gender
B. Low body mass index (BMI)
C. Cytomegalovirus (CMV) seronegativity
D. Acute cellular rejection
E. All of the above

The answer is E

Schachtner et al. studied the incidence of infection in a cohort of 134 patients with SPK and reported 36 of 134 (26.9%) patients developed sepsis. Among these 36 patients, 13 patients (36.1%) experienced severe sepsis/septic shock. A group of SPK without sepsis and another group of deceased donor kidney transplant recipients (KTRs) served as controls. Among KTRs, 11.3% had sepsis. Female sex, low BMI, CMV seronegativity, CMV disease, and acute cellular rejection increased the risk for sepsis (E is correct).

Gram-positive and fungal sepsis were more common among SPK recipients compared to KTRs. Patient and allograft survival rates were not different between patients with sepsis and without sepsis, but sepsis patients had inferior kidney allograft function. Mortality from severe sepsis was 29% among SPK recipients compared to 58% among KTRs. Lower sepsis-related mortality may reflect younger age and more timely diagnosis.

Suggested Reading

Schachtner T, Zaks M, Otto NM, et al. Factors and outcomes in association with sepsis differ between simultaneous pancreas/kidney and single kidney transplant recipients. Transpl Infect Dis. 2018;20(2):e12848.

88. **Which one of the following statements regarding pancreas transplantation in type 2 diabetic patients with eGFR 18 mL/min is FALSE?**

A. The proportion of type 2 diabetic patients who received simultaneous pancreas and kidney (SPK) transplants increased to 11.7% in 2016 from 10.5% in 2015
B. SPK transplants were much higher than pancreas after kidney transplants (PAK) and pancreas transplants alone (PTA) from 1995 to 2015
C. Pancreas allograft survival is similar between type 1 and type 2 diabetic patients
D. Age is not associated with an increased risk of posttransplant major adverse cardiovascular events (MACE)
E. All of the above

The answer is E

Type 2 diabetic patients comprise 90–95% of all the diabetic population. Less than 10% comprises type 1 diabetic patients. Because type 1 diabetics lack insulin, they are considered the prime subjects for pancreas alone or SPK transplantation. However, some type 2 diabetics behave like type 1 diabetic subjects in terms of insulin requirements and hypoglycemic episodes. According to UNOS (United Network for Organ Sharing), the eligibility for pancreas transplantation for type 1 and 2 diabetics includes (1) insulin dependency, and either (2) C-peptide ≤2 ng/mL with no BMI restriction (assumed to be type 1 diabetes) or on insulin and C-peptide >2 ng/mL with a BMI ≤30 kg/m^2 (assumed to be type 2 diabetes). Current UNOS policy lifted the restriction on BMI to accommodate more type 2 diabetic patients for SPK transplants.

Data from OPTN/SRTR 2018 Annual report showed that the proportion of type 2 diabetic patients who received simultaneous pancreas and kidney (SPK) transplants increased to 11.7% in 2016 from 10.5% in 2015 (A is correct).

Gruessner et al. identified 1514 pancreas transplants in type 2 diabetic patients from the International Pancreas and Transplant Registry (IPTR) data from 1995 to 2015. Of these 1514 transplants, 1318 (88%) were SPK, 140 (9%) were PAKs, and 50 (3%) had PTA, and the remaining 33 had pancreas retransplants (B is correct)

Five-year survival for all pancreas transplants in 2011–213 performed in recipients with type 1 diabetes was 91.1% compared with 95.2% in recipients with type 2 diabetes (C is correct).

Several studies have suggested that age is an independent risk factor for major adverse cardiovascular events (MACE) after pancreas transplantation. However, a study by Montagud-Marrahi et al. did not show any difference in MACE among <50-year- and >50-year-old pancreas transplant recipients during a mean follow-up of 9.4 ± 4.9 years (D is correct).

Suggested Reading

Al-Qaoud TM, Odorico JS, Redfield RR, III. Pancreas transplantation in type 2 diabetes: expanding the criteria. Curr Opin Organ Transplant. 2018;23:454–60.

Gruessner AC, Gruessner RW. Pancreas transplantation of US and non-US cases from 2005 to 2014 as reported to the United Network for Organ Sharing (UNOS) and the International Pancreas Transplant Registry (IPTR). Rev Diabet Stud. 2016;13:35–58.

Kandaswamy R, Stock PG, Gustafson SK, et al. OPTN/SRTR 2018 Annual data report: pancreas. Am J Transplant. 2018;18 Suppl 1:114–71.

Kandaswamy R, Stock PG, Gustafson SK, et al. OPTN/SRTR 2018 Annual data report: pancreas. Am J Transplant. 2020;2020:131–92.

Montagud-Marrahi E, Molina-Andújar A, Pané A, et al. Outcomes of pancreas transplantation in older diabetic patients. BMJ Open Diab Res Care. 2020;8:e000916. https://doi.org/10.1136/bmjdrc-2019-000916.

89. A 34-year-old type 1 diabetic woman receives a deceased donor kidney transplant and immunosuppressive regimen. However, her urine output declined. Shown below is her duplex Doppler tracing with resistive index (RI) of 0.61. **Which one of the following is the likely cause of her declined urine output?**

A. Acute rejection
B. Acute tubular necrosis (ATN)
C. Vascular thrombosis
D. Hydronephrosis
E. Hemodynamic abnormality

The answer is E

Ultrasound is the most frequently used imaging technique in kidney transplant patients for evaluation of morphologic characteristics of the transplanted kidney. The addition of color/power and duplex Doppler ultrasound technique allows the evaluation of renal parenchymal blood flow as well the patency of renal arteries. The Doppler-derived renal resistive index (RI) has been used as a marker of normal and abnormal renal blood flow as well as structural abnormalities such as thrombosis, stenosis, or AV fistulas in CKD and kidney transplant patients. The use of RI has been extended to patients with HTN and renal and overall outcomes in critically ill patients.

Normal Doppler arterial waveform is shown in GREEN in the figure (Fig. 11.3)**. The waveform shows a systolic peak (top white circle) and an end diastole (bottom white circle) form. Based on these waveforms, the RI can be calculated as follows:**

$$\text{RI}\left(\text{resistive index}\right) = \text{PSV} - \text{EDV} / \text{PSV}$$

where PSV is peak systolic velocity, and EDV is end-diastolic velocity.

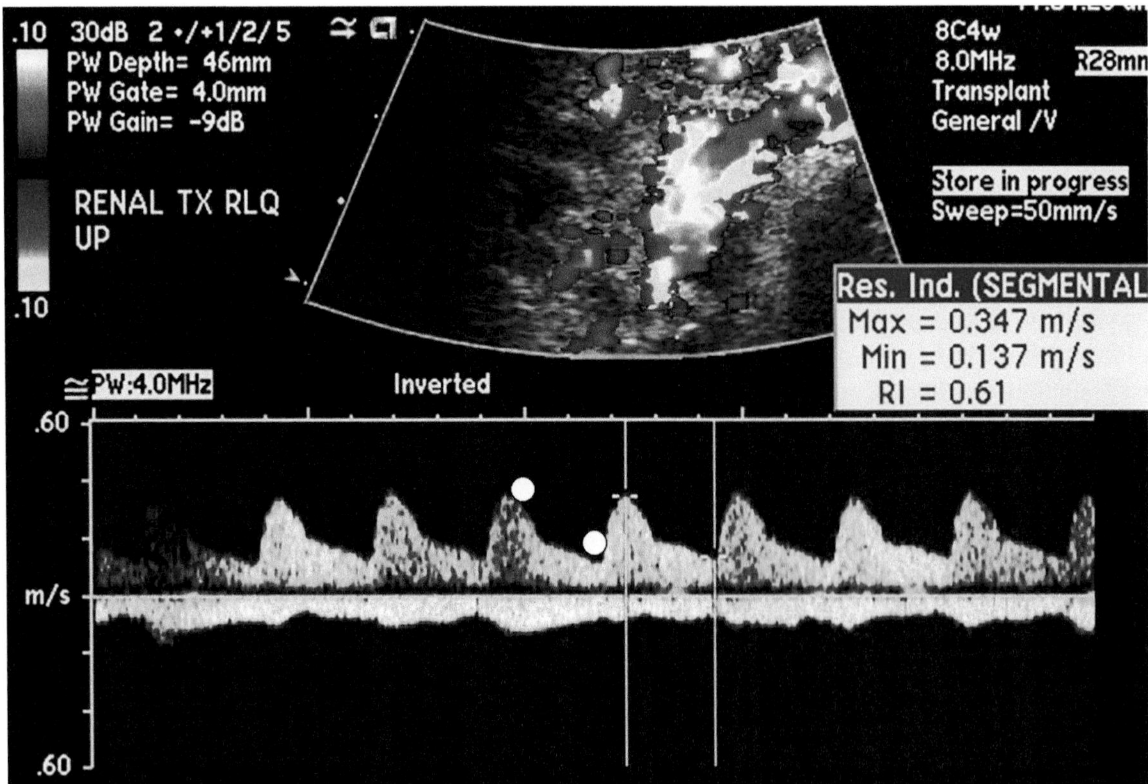

Fig. 11.3 Duplex Doppler ultrasound of the kidney

A normal RI is 0.6, whereas a value >0.7 is high in adults. RI values depend on local vascular status rather than kidney function. Acute rejection, ATN, thrombosis, and hydronephrosis cause high RIs. In this patient, the RI is 0.61. Therefore, the patient has no vascular abnormalities, and the reason for declined urine output is hemodynamic abnormality such as hypovolemia (E is correct).

Suggested Reading

Manning M, Wong-You-Cheong J. Imaging of the renal transplant patient. In: Weir MR, Lerma EV, editors. Kidney transplantation. Practical guide to management. New York: Springer; 2014. p. 377–400.

Viazzi F, Leoncini G, Derchi LE, et al. Ultrasound Doppler renal resistive index: a useful tool for the management of the hypertensive patient. J Hypertens. 2014;32:149–53.

90. A 60-year-old African American man had a deceased donor kidney transplant 12 years ago after 4 years on hemodialysis. His ESKD was due to hypertension, which was complicated by his drinking of moonshine. His medications include tacrolimus, MMF and prednisone (5 mg daily), allopurinol 100 mg twice daily, atorvastatin 20 mg daily, amlodipine 10 mg daily, and losartan 50 mg daily. His creatinine is 1.4 mg/dL, and uric is 8.5 mg/dL. He had symptoms of gout prior to his transplantation and occasionally after transplantation. **Which one of the following therapeutic strategies is INAPPROPRIATE in this patient?**

A. Colchicine 0.6 mg daily
B. Febuxostat
C. Switch tacrolimus to cyclosporine
D. Rasburicase
E. Purine-rich vegetables

The answer is C

Hyperuricemia and gout are rather common after solid organ transplantation. About 10–30% of kidney and cardiac transplant recipients develop gout. Liver transplant recipients have much lower incidence of gout. Asymptomatic hyperuricemia (>6.5 mg/dL) is also much common in kidney transplant recipients.

Risk factors for hyperuricemia and gout in kidney transplant recipients include pretransplant gout, immunosuppressive drugs such as cyclosporine and tacrolimus, alcohol consumption, obesity, and diuretic use.

Cyclosporine has been shown to cause both hyperuricemia and gout in 30–84% and 2–28%, respectively. Tacrolimus causes gout in <3% of patients. Therefore, switching tacrolimus to cyclosporine causes more harm to this patient by precipitating both hyperuricemia and gout. Thus, C is incorrect. The remaining choices are correct and appropriate.

In the management of hyperuricemia, the goal uric acid level is <6.5 mg/dL in order to prevent recurrent gouty attacks. Colchicine 0.6 mg once daily can be used in this patient. This drug causes myopathy and diarrhea. In a patient on statin, careful use of colchicine is needed, and frequent history of myopathy and CK levels need to be monitored.

Febuxostat, similar to allopurinol, is a xanthine oxidase inhibitor. It can be used in those allergic to allopurinol. However, the long-term effect of febuxostat is not fully understood in kidney transplant recipients. Both allopurinol and febuxostat should be used cautiously in patients on azathioprine because xanthine oxidase inhibits the metabolism of azathioprine, thereby increasing its levels and profound myelosuppression.

Rasburicase and pegylated pegloticase are uricases, which convert uric acid into allantoin lower uric acid rapidly. They are usually used when other drugs fail.

Diet that is rich in purines increases not only uric acid levels, but also predisposes to gouty attacks. Purine-rich foods such as meat, seafood, beer, and some alcohols increase the risk for gout; however, purine-rich vegetables (peas, beans, lentils, spinach, mushrooms, oatmeal, and cauliflower) and low-fat dairy products are not associated with an increased risk of gout.

Suggested Reading

Choi HK, Atkinson K, Karlson EW, et al. Purine-rich foods, dairy and protein intake, and the risk of gout in men. N Engl J Med. 2004;35:1093–103.

Stamp LK, Chapman PK. Gout and organ transplantation. Curr Rheumatol Rep. 2012;14:165–72.

91. A 30-year-old Caucasian woman with type 1 diabetes receives a living-related donor kidney transplant 1 year ago. On a routine clinic visit, she complains of mild hip pain for 2 weeks. She is on tacrolimus, MMF, and prednisone (5 mg daily). Her tacrolimus levels are 5 ng/mL. Serum Ca^{2+}, phosphate, alkaline phosphatase, and PTH levels are within normal limits. Her creatinine is 1.3 mg/dL, and HbA1c is 6.8%. 25 vitamin D (25(OH)D_3) levels are low (15 ng/mL; normal >30 ng/mL) with normal calcitriol levels. DXA (dual-energy X ray absorptiometry) scan shows osteoporosis of femoral neck. **Which one of the following therapeutic strategies is APPROPRIATE for this patient?**

A. Bisphosphonates only
B. Ergocalciferol (Calciferol) 50,000 U/3×/week
C. Ergocalciferol, 25,000 U 3×/week, calcitriol (Rocaltrol) 0.25 µg/day, and calcium 1 g/day
D. Recombinant human PTH (teriparatide)
E. Calcitonin

The answer is C

Posttransplantation bone loss is very common in the first 6 months due to corticosteroids and calcineurin inhibitors. Bone loss is 5.5–19.5% in the first 6 months, 2.6–8.2% during 6–12 months, and 0.4–4.5% during subsequent years. Causes of posttransplant bone loss include (1) corticosteroids, (2) CNIs, (3) estrogen or testosterone deficiency, (4) tertiary hyperparathyroidism, (5) inadequate Ca^{2+} intake, and (6) smoking. Diabetes also predisposes to osteoporosis.

Treatment includes all of the abovementioned strategies depending on bone mineral density (BMD) parameters. Bisphosphonates have been shown to increase BMD and reduce fractures of femoral neck rather than vertebral fractures. However, a study showed no superiority of addition of ibandronate to a regimen of calcitriol (0.25 µg/day) and calcium (500 mg twice daily) in increasing BMD compared to calcitriol and calcium. Thus, bisphosphonates alone are not sufficient to improve BMD (A is incorrect).

Ergocalciferol alone may increase 25(OH)D_3 levels, but not sufficient to improve osteoporosis (B is incorrect). Administration of recombinant human PTH (teriparatide) for 6 months did not improve BMD in the lumbar spine or radius compared to placebo. Therefore, routine use of teriparatide cannot be recommended (D is incorrect). Calcitonin effect on BMD in transplant patients has been to be inconsistent; therefore, routine use is not recommended (E is incorrect).

The appropriate management in this patient is to improve 25(OH)D_3 levels initially with calciferol and concomitant use of calcitriol as well as calcium to improve BMD density (C is correct). Regular follow-up is required with evaluation of BMD parameters (Ca^{2+}, phosphate, alkaline phosphate, PTH, and vitamin D levels). HbA1c should be maintained between 6 and 6.5%. Once 25(OH)D_3 levels are normalized, calciferol can be switched to cholecalciferol (1000 U/day).

Suggested Reading

Bouquegneau A, Salam S, Delanaye P, et al. Bone disease after kidney transplantation. Clin J Am Soc Nephrol. 2016;11:1282–96.
Kalantar-Zadeh K, Molnar MZ, Kovesdy CP, et al. Management of mineral and bone disorder after kidney transplantation. Curr Opin Nephrol Hypertens. 2012;21:389–403.
Vangala J, Pan J, Cotton RT, et al. Mineral and bone disorders after kidney transplantation. Front Med (Lausanne). 2018;5:11.
Wiegel JJ, Descourouez JL. Post kidney transplant: bone mineral disease. In: Parajuli S, Aziz F, editors. Kidney transplant management. A guide to evaluation and comorbidities. Springer Nature Switzerland AG; 2019. p. 165–77.

92. A 28-year-old woman on hemodialysis for a year receives a live donor kidney 3 months ago. During her clinic visit, she asks you about some cosmetic issues because of her immunosuppression (tacrolimus, MMF, and prednisone (5 mg daily)). **Which one of the following cosmetic issues needs to be discussed with this young patient?**

A. Gingival hyperplasia
B. Hirsutism
C. Alopecia
D. Moon facies
E. All of the above

The answer is E

The cosmetic issues should be discussed with all transplant patients irrespective of the immunosuppressive drugs used because of switching from one to another drug during the course of management. Gingival hyperplasia is common with cyclosporine use, which is not related to cyclosporine levels. Conversion to tacrolimus results in regression of gum changes within weeks. Surgery is the correct option for gingival hyperplasia. Oral hygiene, discontinuation of calcium channel blockers, and appropriate antibiotic use help gum hyperplasia to regress, in addition to switching cyclosporine to tacrolimus.

Hirsutism occurs in over 20% of cyclosporine-treated patients, which can be aggravated by concomitant use of corticosteroids, or minoxidil for HTN. Conversion to patient to tacrolimus is the best treatment for hirsutism. This patient is on tacrolimus, and she will have rare chances of developing hirsutism.

Alopecia is a complication of tacrolimus rather than cyclosporine. Usually, alopecia induced by tacrolimus resolves spontaneously, but switching to cyclosporine may invite other cosmetic complications, as described above. Lowering tacrolimus dose may reduce the severity of alopecia. Thus, E is correct.

Other problems associated with chronic use of steroids such as moon facies should also be discussed with the patients, in addition to planned pregnancy.

Suggested Reading

Fernando ON, Sweny P, Varghese Z. Elective conversion of patients from cyclosporine to tacrolimus for hypertrichosis. Tansplant Proc. 1998;30:1243–44.

Kohnle M, Lutkes P, Zimmermann U, et al. Conversion from cyclosporine to in renal transplant recipients with gum hyperplasia. Transplant Proc. 1999;31:44S–5S.

Sievers TM, Lum EL, Danovitch GM. Immunosuppressive medications and protocols for kidney transplantation. In: Danovitch GM, editor. Handbook of kidney transplantation. 7th ed. Philadelphia: Lippincott Williams & Wilkins; 2017. p. 101–63.

93. **Which one of the following electrolyte and acid-base disorders in kidney transplant patients is CORRECT?**

A. Hypophosphatemia
B. Hypercalcemia
C. Hyperkalemia
D. Hyperchloremic metabolic acidosis
E. All of the above

The answer is E

Several electrolyte and acid-base abnormalities are rather common after kidney transplantation, including those presented above (E is correct). Hypophosphatemia is a common electrolyte abnormality in kidney transplant recipients. The causes are (1) secondary hyperparathyroidism which may exist for many months (>12 months) or tertiary hyperparathyroidism; (2) excess FGF-23 levels; (3) drugs such as corticosteroids and diuretics; and (4) low levels of 25(OH)D_3 and 1,25$(OH)_2D_3$ levels (A is correct).

Hypercalcemia and hypophosphatemia develop in approximately 50% of kidney transplant recipients, often most pronounced 2–8 weeks after transplantation. It is related to persistent hyperparathyroidism, skeletal resistance to parathyroid hormone, and increasing activity of active vitamin D_3 (1,25$(OH)_2D_3$ or calcitriol). Tertiary hyperparathyroidism exists in some patients. Posttransplant hyperparathyroidism is a risk factor for acute kidney allograft injury, graft loss, fractures, and mortality.

Hyperkalemia is rather common in transplant recipients. There are several causes for hyperkalemia, including diet and sodas that contain high potassium, calcineurin inhibitors (CNIs), uncontrolled glucose, constipation, and urinary tract obstruction. CINs cause hyperkalemia by several mechanisms: (1) hyporeninemic hypoaldosteronism, (2) blocking K^+ channel in the distal nephron, (3) inhibition of Na/K-ATPase, and (4) increased Cl^- shunt in the distal tubule with induction of Gordon-like syndrome with hyperkalemia and hypertension.

Hypomagnesemia is extremely common due to gastrointestinal (GI) and renal losses. GI losses include diarrhea and medications such as proton pump inhibitors and patiromer as well as infections. Renal losses include diuretics, calcineurin inhibitors, and sirolimus. Calcineurin inhibitors downregulate the expression of the magnesium transporter TRPM6 in the distal tubule, which is the main site for active transcellular reabsorption for magnesium. There is evidence that cyclosporine downregulates renal epidermal growth factor production, which in turn leads to inhibition of TRPM6. The net result is loss of magnesium in the urine, causing hypomagnesemia.

The discussion of metabolic acidosis has largely been neglected in kidney transplant patients because of paucity of literature on the subject. Among various types of acid-base disorders, renal tubular acidosis (RTA) is the most frequently encountered disorder in renal transplant recipients. The prevalence of RTA varies from 12% to 58.1% in a review of 12 studies. In most of these studies, the serum HCO_3^- level was <22 mEq/L. Interestingly, metabolic acidosis develops at higher GFR levels in transplant patients compared to those with CKD who develop at lower GFRs.

Proximal RTA (type II) develops in approximately 19% of cases during the first 3 months of transplantation and then resolves spontaneously. This acid-base disorder is due to HCO_3^- wasting caused by ischemic tubular necrosis that is partially attributed to the harvest procedure. If proximal RTA develops after 2 years following transplantation, chronic rejection should be suspected. Distal RTA (type 1) is rather common. It may develop as early as the first 3 months and may last up to 9 years. Causes for its development include chronic rejection and calcineurin inhibitors (cyclosporine or tacrolimus). Tacrolimus seems to be the major reason for RTAs than cyclosporine.

Both proximal and distal RTAs can occur early after transplantation with spontaneous resolution of proximal RTA. Distal RTA can persist for long periods of time (up to 9 years). Alkali therapy is indicated for patients with distal RTA.

Type 4 RTA is seen most frequently with cyclosporine and tacrolimus use as well as other drugs that lower aldosterone levels.

The mechanisms for RTAs in kidney transplant patients are not completely understood, although immunologic mechanisms have been implicated. Also, calcineurin inhibitors seem to impair the activity of transporters involved in acid-base balance in the proximal and distal tubules. Appropriate treatment is recommended to prevent bone disease and other complications of metabolic acidosis.

Suggested Reading

De Waele L, Van Gaal PJ, Abramowicz D: Electrolytes disturbances after kidney transplantation. Acta Clin Belg. 2019;74:48–52.

Messa PG, Alfieri C, Vettoretti S. Metabolic acidosis in renal transplantation: neglected but of potential clinical relevance. Nephrol Dial Transplant. 2016;31:730–6.

Miles CD, Westphal SG. Electrolyte disorders in kidney transplantation. Clin J Am Soc Nephrol. 2020;15:412–4.

Pochineni V, Rondon-Berrios H: Electrolyte and acid-base disorders in the renal transplant recipient. Front Med (Lausanne). 2018;5:261.

Raphael K, Shihab FS. Acidosis and kidney allograft survival. J Am Soc Nephrol. 2017;28:1667–74.

94. Serum phosphorus levels are associated with mortality in patients with ESKD and after transplantation. **Which one of the following statements regarding phosphorus abnormalities and allograft function/mortality is CORRECT?**

A. Each 1 mg/dL serum phosphorus level increase above baseline value (3.1 mg/dL) was associated with a greater risk of transplant failure and total mortality but not cardiovascular disease (CVD) risk
B. Serum phosphorus level 1 year after transplantation exhibits a U-shape association with death-censored graft failure and patient mortality in kidney transplant patients
C. Hyperphosphatemia is associated with CVD but not with graft failure risk
D. Hypophosphatemia has no effect on graft failure
E. A and B only

The answer is E

Serum phosphorus levels have a significant impact on outcomes after kidney transplantation, particularly, allograft failure and total mortality. Folic Acid for Vascular Outcome Reduction in Transplantation (FAVORIT) trial examined the associations between serum phosphorus level and the development of CVD outcomes, transplant failure, or all-cause mortality in 3138 transplant recipients with a median follow-up of 4 years. Mean serum phosphorus level was 3.07 ± 0.68 mg/dL. Proportional hazards modeling revealed that each 1 mg/dL higher serum phosphorus level was associated with a significant increase in transplant failure (72% greater risk) and total mortality (34% greater risk) but not CVD risk (6% greater risk). Thus, answer A is correct.

Jeon et al. examined the role of phosphorus in allograft and patient survival in a retrospective, multicenter cohort study involving 2786 kidney transplant patients. These patients were classified into seven groups according to serum phosphorus levels 1 year after transplantation, with intervals of 0.5 mg/dL (lowest group, 2.5 mg/dL;

highest group, ≥5.0 mg/dL with reference group 3.5–3.99 mg/dL). During a median follow-up of 78.5 months, they observed that both lowest and highest serum phosphorus groups were associated with higher mortality as compared with the reference group. Also, there was a higher death-censored graft loss in the lowest and highest groups. Thus, they observed a U-shape association between serum phosphorus levels and graft loss and patient survival (B is correct). Earlier studies have shown that both hyper- and hypophosphatemia have significant effect on both graft failure and patient survival in kidney transplant recipients (answers C and D are incorrect).

Suggested Reading

Benavente D, Chue CD, Moore J, et al. Serum phosphate measured at 6 and 12 months after successful kidney transplant is independently associated with subsequent graft loss. Exp Clin Transplant. 2012;10:119–24.

Jeon HJ, Kim YC, Park S, et al. Association of serum phosphorus concentration with mortality and graft failure among kidney transplant recipients. Clin J Am Soc Nephrol. 2017;12:653–62.

Merhi B, Shireman T, Carpenter MA, et al. Serum phosphorus and risk of cardiovascular disease, all-cause mortality, or graft failure in kidney transplant recipients: an ancillary study of the FAVORIT trial cohort. Am J Kidney Dis. 2017;70:377–85.

Moore J, Tomson CR, Tessa Savage M, et al. Serum phosphate and calcium concentrations are associated with reduced patient survival following kidney transplantation. Clin Transplant. 2011;25:406–16.

95. Kidney transplant recipients (KTRs) have an increased risk of premature cardiovascular disease (CVD). **Which one of the following statin therapies in KTRs is CORRECT?**

A. Statin therapy is beneficial only in pretransplant patients
B. Statin therapy lowers LDL cholesterol but no effect on major adverse cardiac events (MACE) in KTRs
C. Statin therapy reduces the risk of MACE but not graft or patient survival
D. Statin therapy reduces MACE, graft loss, and patient survival
E. None of the above

The answer is C

The ALERT (Assessment of LEscol in Renal transplantation) study showed that fluvastatin lowered mean LDL cholesterol from 159 mg/dL to 98 mg/dL compared to placebo. Also, there was a reduced risk of MACE and a 29% reduction in cardiac death or definite nonfatal MI. Total mortality and graft loss did not differ significantly between groups. However, there was no difference in either total graft loss or mortality between fluvastatin and placebo groups (C is correct). All other answers are incorrect.

Suggested Reading

Holdaas H, Fellstrom B, Cole E, et al. Assessment of LEscol in Renal Transplantation (ALERT) Study Investigators: long-term cardiac outcomes in renal transplant recipients receiving fluvastatin: the ALERT extension study. Am J Transplant. 2005;5:2929–36.

Palmer SC, Navaneethan SD, Craig JC, et al. HMG CoA reductase inhibitors (statins) for kidney transplant recipients. Cochrane Database Syst Rev. 2014;(1):CD005019.

96. **As per the 2020 KDIGO guideline, which one of the following patients is NOT recommended for preemptive kidney alone transplant evaluation?**

A. Multiple myeloma unless the patient is in remission and stable
B. AL amyloidosis with significant extrarenal involvement
C. Severe irreversible obstructive or restrictive disease
D. Severe uncorrectable and symptomatic cardiac disease
E. All of the above

The answer is E

The 2020 KDIGO clinical practice guideline recommends all patients with CKD 4–5 (G4-G5) who are expected to reach ESKD, except the above patients, should be informed of, educated about, and considered for kidney transplantation regardless of socioeconomic status, sex, gender identity, or race/ethnicity. Thus, answer E is correct.

In addition, patients with light chain deposition disease or heavy chain deposition disease unless they are in remission and progressive central neurodegenerative disease are also not recommended. The physician should document and inform the reasons for not referring them for transplant evaluation. For decompensated cirrhotic patients, simultaneous liver and kidney transplantation should be recommended.

Suggested Reading

Kidney Disease: Improving Global Outcomes (KDIGO) Kidney Transplant Candidate Work Group. KDIGO Clinical practice guideline on the evaluation and management of candidates for kidney transplantation. Transplantation. 2020;104:S1–103.

Correction to: Absolute Nephrology Review

Correction to:
Chapter 6 and Chapter 10 in: A. S. Reddi, *Absolute Nephrology Review*, https://doi.org/10.1007/978-3-030-85958-9

The book was inadvertently published with incorrect questions in chapter 6 and incorrect figure caption in chapter 10. These have been updated in the book.

The updated original versions of the chapters can be found at
https://doi.org/10.1007/978-3-030-85958-9_6
https://doi.org/10.1007/978-3-030-85958-9_10

A. S. Reddi, *Absolute Nephrology Review*, https://doi.org/10.1007/978-3-030-85958-9_12

Index

A. S. Reddi, *Absolute Nephrology Review*, https://doi.org/10.1007/978-3-030-85958-9

B

C

I

J

K